Dispensing of Medication

Editorial Review Board

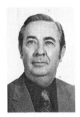
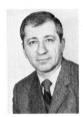
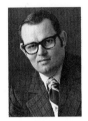
Authors

Kenneth E. Avis, DSc *(Chapter 10)*—Professor and Director, Division of Parenteral Medications, Department of Medicinal Chemistry, College of Pharmacy, The University of Tennessee, Memphis, TN 38163.

Albert A. Belmonte, PhD *(Chapter 1)*—Assistant Professor of Pharmaceutics, School of Pharmacy, Auburn University, Auburn, AL 36830.

Roger E. Booth, PhD *(Chapter 13)*—Manager, Control Records and Services, The Upjohn Co., Kalamazoo, MI 49001.

Donald E. Cadwallader, PhD *(Chapter 9)*—Professor of Pharmacy, School of Pharmacy, University of Georgia, Athens, GA 30602.

Ben F. Cooper, PhD *(Chapter 1)*—Dean, School of Pharmacy, Auburn University, Auburn, AL 36830.

Jack K. Dale, PhD *(Chapter 13)*—Vice President/Quality Control, Carter-Glogau Laboratories—Chromalloy Pharmaceuticals, Glendale, AZ 85301.

Bernard Ecanow, PhD *(Chapters 4, 6, and 8)*—Professor of Pharmacy, College of Pharmacy, University of Illinois at the Medical Center, Chicago, IL 60680.

Werner Lowenthal, PhD *(Chapter 2)*—Professor of Pharmacy and Professor of Educational Planning and Development, School of Pharmacy, Medical College of Virginia, Virginia Commonwealth University, Richmond, VA 23298.

Marvin C. Meyer, PhD *(Chapter 1)*—Associate Professor of Medicinal Chemistry and Biopharmaceutics, College of Pharmacy, The University of Tennessee Center for the Health Sciences, Memphis, TN 38163.

William A. Miller, PharmD, MSc *(Chapter 10)*—Associate Professor and Director, Division of Clinical Pharmacy, Department of Pharmaceutics, College of Pharmacy, The University of Tennessee, Memphis, TN 38163.

Harvey Mintzer, MS *(Chapter 11)*—Vice President, Technical Sales and Services, Armstrong Laboratories Div., Aerosol Techniques, Inc., West Roxbury, MA 02132.

John D. Mullins, PhD *(Chapter 9)*—Director, Dermatology Dept., Science and Technology Div., Alcon Laboratories, Fort Worth, TX 76101.

Henry A. Palmer, PhD *(Chapter 1)*—Associate Clinical Professor of Pharmacy, School of Pharmacy, The University of Connecticut, Storrs, CT 06268.

G. Briggs Phillips, PhD *(Chapter 10)*—Director, Becton, Dickinson & Co. Research Center, Research Triangle Park, NC 27709.

James M. Plaxco, Jr., PhD *(Chapter 7)*—Professor of Pharmacy, School of Pharmacy, University of South Carolina, Columbia, SC 29208.

Edward J. Rowe, PhD *(Chapter 3)*—Professor of Pharmacy, College of Pharmacy, Butler University, Indianapolis, IN 46208.

Farid Sadik, PhD *(Chapters 4 and 5)*—Associate Professor of Pharmaceutics, College of Pharmacy, University of South Carolina, Columbia, SC 29208.

Roger L. Schnaare, PhD *(Chapter 8)*—Associate Professor of Pharmacy, Philadelphia College of Pharmacy and Science, Philadelphia, PA 19104.

Frederick P. Siegel, PhD *(Chapter 6)*—Professor of Pharmacy, College of Pharmacy, University of Illinois at the Medical Center, Chicago, IL 60680.

Harun Takruri, PhD *(Chapter 8)*—Senior Pharmaceutical Chemist, The Lilly Research Laboratories, Indianapolis, IN 46206.

Manuel Tubis, PhD *(Chapter 12)*—Radiopharmacy Program, US Veterans Administration/Wadsworth Hospital Center, Los Angeles, CA 90073.

Walter Wolf, PhD *(Chapter 12)*—Radiopharmacy Program, School of Pharmacy, University of Southern California, Los Angeles, CA 90033.

A practical manual on the
formulation and dispensing of
pharmaceutical products

Dispensing of Medication

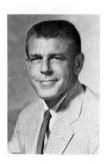

Editor

John E. Hoover, BSc

Managing Editor, *Remington's Pharmaceutical Sciences*
Managing Editor, *American Journal of Pharmacy*
Director of Administration,
Philadelphia College of Pharmacy and Science

Eighth Edition
Mack Publishing Company
1976

Dedication

In loving memory, to my father, Lloyd M. Hoover. . .
A sensitive, generous man and a patient-oriented
clinical pharmacist well ahead of his time.

Preface

*Thy Eternal Providence has appointed me to watch
over the life and health of Thy creatures ... Grant
me strength, time, and opportunity always to correct
what I have acquired, always to extend its domain;
for knowledge is immense ... here am I ready for my
vocation.*

Attributed to Marcus Hertz
German Physician, 18th Century
(Often attributed to Maimonides.)

The spirit of this oath serves as a continuing reminder to all members of the health care team of the ultimate reason for their existence—the patient.

The very heart of pharmacy's important role in patient care is to make every attempt to ensure that the patient receives appropriate medication of the finest quality and both understands and complies with the proper instructions for use.

To serve this important role, this eighth edition was completely redesigned to aid the patient-oriented pharmacist, very often the last health professional to interact with the patient prior to the initiation of therapy. It is a practical text and reference for both pharmacy practitioners and students, as well as for physicians, nurses, and other health professionals involved in prescribing and administering medication.

This eighth edition contains perhaps the most comprehensive compilation of significant compounding and dispensing (patient) information in print for more than 1,400 of the most widely used drug entities and pharmaceutical products, as well as up-to-date dispensing aspects of the prescription itself, bioavailability, product formulation, and the various dosage forms. Each chapter also contains a useful bibliography of the significant citations on the subject for easy access into the literature.

The Editor is indeed indebted to the many persons who made this volume possible through willing and gracious counsel, providing drug and product data, manuscript preparation, proofreading, plus design and production assistance: the authors and editorial reviewers; the staff of Mack Publishing Company and Mack Printing Company—in particular Mr. Walter Kowalick, Miss Mary Brogan, Mr. H. Leslie Varley, Mr. Charles M. Todaro, Mrs. Evelyn M. Sloyer, and Mrs. Evelyn Tarsi; the pharmaceutical manufacturers; the staff of the Philadelphia College of Pharmacy and Science—in particular Dr. Arthur Osol, Dr. Edwin T. Sugita, Dr. Thomas C. Snader, Dr. William S. Bond, and Mrs. Ellen P. Gilligan.

And, finally, my family—for their ongoing support, understanding, and patience.

Swarthmore, Pennsylvania
June, 1976

John E. Hoover
Editor

Contents

1

Medication orders

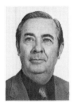

Ben F. Cooper, PhD
Dean, School of Pharmacy
Auburn University
Auburn, AL 36830

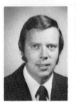

Marvin C. Meyer, PhD
Associate Professor
of Medicinal
Chemistry and
Biopharmaceutics
College of Pharmacy
The University of Tennessee
Center for the Health
Sciences
Memphis, TN 38163

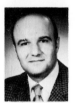

Henry A. Palmer, PhD
Associate Clinical
Professor of Pharmacy
School of Pharmacy
The University of
Connecticut
Storrs, CT 06268

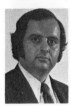

Albert A. Belmonte, PhD
Assistant Professor
of Pharmaceutics
School of Pharmacy
Auburn University
Auburn, AL 36830

Dr. Cooper and **Dr. Belmonte** prepared the sections on *Interpreting and Processing the Order, Compounding Accuracy,* and *Stabilization.* **Dr. Meyer** prepared the section on *Complexation.* **Dr. Palmer** prepared the section on *Packaging and Storage.*

Medications may be *ordered* for a patient by a licensed physician or other authorized prescriber. The order is usually recorded by the prescriber on a *prescription form* (Fig. 1) or a *physician's order form* (Fig. 2). Customarily, the prescription form is utilized for office patients and hospital outpatients, and the physician's order form for hospital inpatients.

Oral transmission of the medication order by the prescriber is permitted, except for certain controlled substances (see page 8). Documentation of an oral medication order should be made on the appropriate form.

Medication orders utilizing the prescription form are usually issued to the

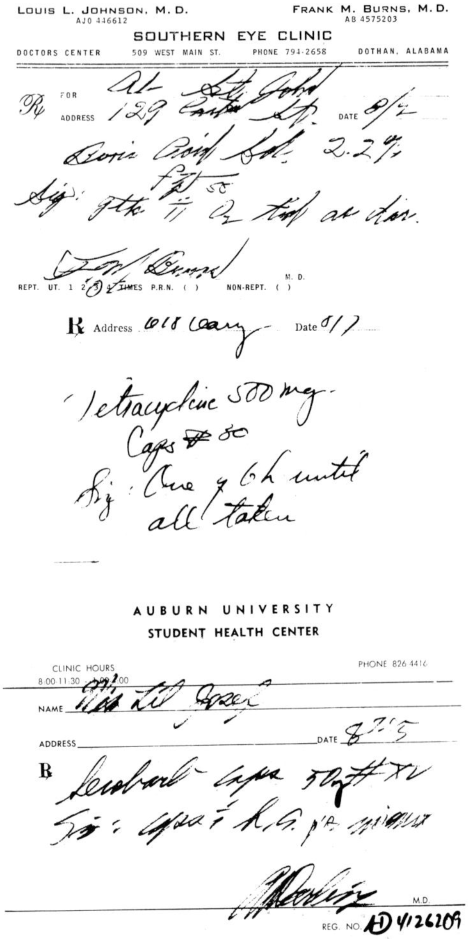

Fig. 1—The prescription.

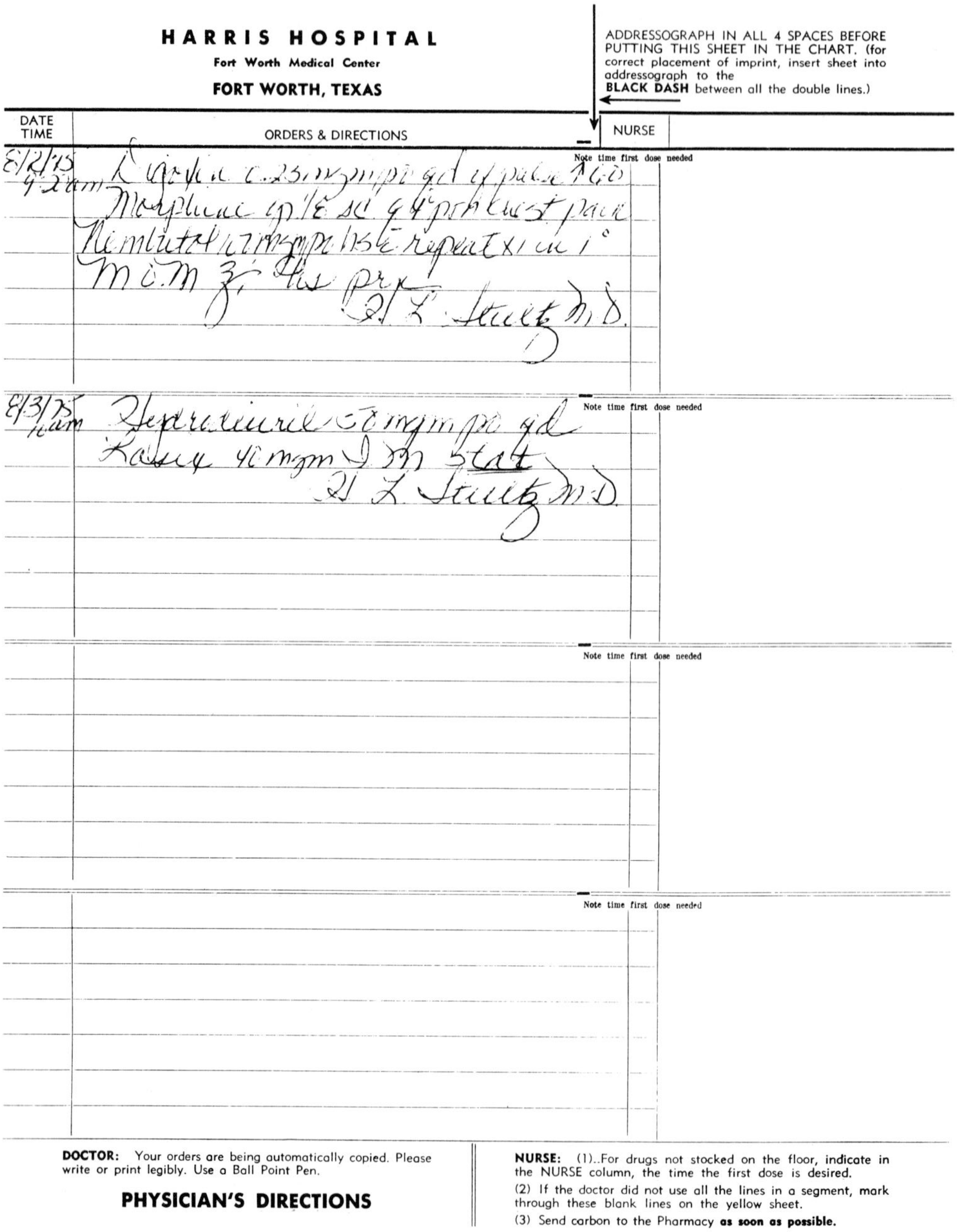

HARRIS HOSPITAL
Fort Worth Medical Center
FORT WORTH, TEXAS

ADDRESSOGRAPH IN ALL 4 SPACES BEFORE
PUTTING THIS SHEET IN THE CHART. (for
correct placement of imprint, insert sheet into
addressograph to the
BLACK DASH between all the double lines.)

DATE TIME	ORDERS & DIRECTIONS	NURSE
8/2/75 9:20 am	*[handwritten medication orders]* Note time first dose needed	
8/3/75 10 am	*[handwritten medication orders]* Note time first dose needed	
	Note time first dose needed	
	Note time first dose needed	

DOCTOR: Your orders are being automatically copied. Please write or print legibly. Use a Ball Point Pen.

PHYSICIAN'S DIRECTIONS

NURSE: (1)..For drugs not stocked on the floor, indicate in the NURSE column, the time the first dose is desired.
(2) If the doctor did not use all the lines in a segment, mark through these blank lines on the yellow sheet.
(3) Send carbon to the Pharmacy **as soon as possible.**

Fig. 2—Physician's order form.

patient and completed by a pharmacist for *dispensing* to the patient. Medication orders utilizing the physician's order form are often issued to a nurse, who obtains the medication from a pharmacist and *administers* it to the patient. A limited number of medications may be supplied by the pharmacist to the nurse (or nursing station) in advance as *floor or ward stock,* from

Table 1—Abbreviations in Medication Orders

Abbreviation	Word	English
a̅a̅	Ana	Of each
ad	Ad	Up to
ad Lib.	Ad libitum	At will
ā	Ante	Before
a.c.	Ante Cibos	Before meals
aq.	Aqua	Water
a.u.	Aures utrae	Each ear
a.d.	Aurio dextra	Right ear
a.l. (s.)	Aurio laeva (sinister)	Left ear
b.i.d.	Bis in die	Twice a day
b.m.	—	Bowel movement
b.p.	—	Blood pressure
caps.	Capsula	Capsule
c̅	cum	With
et	et	And
gtt.	Gutta	Drop
h.	Hora	Hour
ha.	—	Headache
h.s.	Hora sommus	At bedtime
M	Minimum	Minum
n̅o̅c̅.	Nocturnal	In the night
non rep.	Non repetatur	No refills (do not repeat)
O	Octarius	A pint
o.u.	Oculo utro	Each eye
o.d.	Oculus dexter	Right eye
o.l. (s)	Oculus Laevus (Sinister)	Left eye
p.c.	Post Cibos	After meals
p.o.	Per os	By mouth (orally)
p.r.	—	Per rectum (rectally)
p.r.n.	Pro re nata	As needed (for)
pulv.	Pulvis	Powder
p.v.	—	Per vagina (vaginally)
q	Quiaque	Every
q.s.	Quantum sufficiat	As much as sufficient
q.i.d.	Quater in die	Four times a day
rep.	Repetatur	Repeat
s̅s̅	Semis	Half
sig.	Signa	Label to patient
s̅	Sine	Without
stat.	Statim	Immediately
supp.	Suppositorium	Suppository
tab.	Tabella	Tablet
t.i.d.	Ter in die	Three times a day
ung.	Unguentum	Ointment
ut dict. (u.d.)	Ut dictum	As directed
w.a.	—	While awake

which the nurse may obtain the medication pursuant to the physician's order and administer it to the patient.

Interpreting the Order

The physician's original written medication order should be carefully checked by the pharmacist for legibility and accuracy. In the case of oral transmission by the prescriber, the pharmacist should document it in writing immediately and completely. Transmission of a medication order to the pharmacist by a third party by any means other than the original written form should be discouraged due to the increased possibility of error.

Abbreviations

Most medication orders contain abbreviations. However, there is no "official" or standard list of abbreviations. Most of the commonly used abbreviations are derived from Latin words, but some may be symbols and shorthand notations adopted as a matter of custom. A selected list of commonly used abbreviations is given in Table 1.

Legibility

Legibility is a problem requiring alertness and critical judgment on the part of the pharmacist. Careless handwriting and similarity in spelling or pronunciation of names of different drugs add to the difficulty. Some examples of drug names that look alike and/or sound alike are:

Aldactone .... Aldactazide
Aldoril .... Aldomet
Ambenyl .... Ambodryl
Benadryl .... Bentyl
Benadryl .... Benylin
Bicillin .... V-Cillin
Butisol .... Butibel
Delalutin .... Deladumone
Dialose .... Dialose Plus
Digitoxin .... Digoxin
Dimetane .... Dimetapp
Doriden .... Doxidan
Dyrenium .... Dyazide
Elavil .... Aldoril
Feosol .... Fer-In-Sol
Gantrisin .... Gantanol
Hycomine .... Hycodan
Hydropres .... Diupres
Isordil .... Isuprel
Keflex .... Keflin
Marax .... Atarax
Myleran .... Mylicon
Nitroglycerin .... Nitroglyn
Omnipen .... Unipen
Orinase .... Ornade
Otobione .... Otodyne
Otobiotic .... Otobione
Percodan .... Percobarb
Phenaphen .... Phenergan
Phenobarbital .... Pentobarbital
Prednefrin .... Prefin
Prednisone .... Prednisolone
Quinidine .... Quinine
Regroton .... Hygroton
Sterazolidin .... Butazolidin
Tepanil .... Temaril
Thyrar .... Thyrolar
Tuinal .... Tylenol
Tyzine .... Visine

Dosage Regimen

The dose of each ingredient should be evaluated for safety and efficacy. Daily or cumulative, as well as individual, doses should be evaluated because safety and efficacy may depend on frequency of administration as well as size of each dose. The USP and NF have established usual adult doses for official drugs for general guidance, but prescribed doses often deviate therefrom.

Factors Which Affect Dose—The increasing potency and complexity of modern drugs have increased the importance of exact determination of dosage. The optimum dose for a particular patient is highly individualistic, and must be determined after careful analysis of the patient's history, examination, and diagnosis.

The optimum dose depends on:

History and Examination—Age, sex, weight, body surface area, previous illnesses, emotional state, tolerance, and idiosyncrasy.

Diagnosis—Type and severity of disease, presence of other pathological conditions.

Prescribed Regimen—Dosage form, time of administration, frequency of administration, combination with other drugs.

Patient's Environment—Location, facilities, seasonal time, and temperature.

Particular attention should be given to extended, delayed, or repeat action dosage forms. A large number of sustained-release dosage forms, special coatings, and improved dosage forms are commonly prescribed.

Formulation factors may influence the bioavailability, and hence the dose, of a drug. Additives (such as diluents, fillers, and preservatives), particle size, salt form, dissolution rate, pH, viscosity, and other formulation factors have been shown to cause variations in pharmacologic effect of the active ingredient. Different "brands" of the same active ingredient may be formulated in various ways, resulting in possible variations in therapeutic response. A partial list of drugs for which differences in bioavailability of chemically equivalent products has been demonstrated is listed as follows:

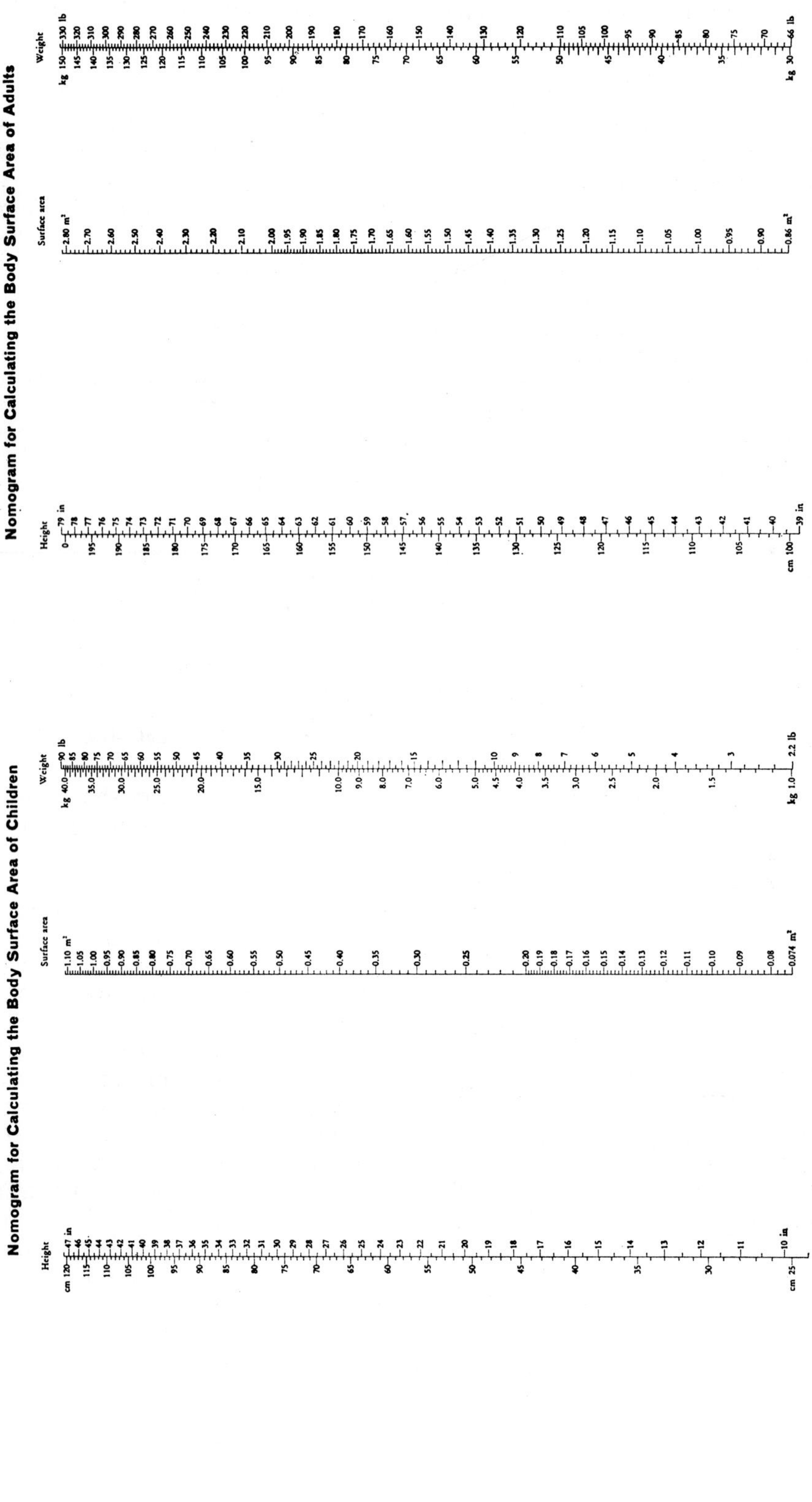

Nomogram for Calculating the Body Surface Area of Children

Nomogram for Calculating the Body Surface Area of Adults

Fig. 3—Nomograms for calculating body surface area.[1]

Table 2—Calculation of Child's Doses

| Age | Weight[a] (kg) | Height[a] (cm) | Body surface area (m²) | Fraction of Adult Dose | | |
				Young's rule	Clark's rule	BSA method[b]
Birth	3.4	50.5	0.21	—	0.05	0.12
3 mos	5.7	59.9	0.29	0.02	0.08	0.17
6 mos	7.5	65.8	0.35	0.04	0.11	0.20
1 yr	9.9	74.7	0.44	0.08	0.15	0.25
2 yrs	12.5	86.9	0.54	0.14	0.18	0.31
3 yrs	14.5	96.0	0.61	0.20	0.21	0.35
4 yrs	16.5	103.4	0.68	0.25	0.24	0.39
5 yrs	19.1	110.5	0.76	0.29	0.28	0.44
6 yrs	21.5	116.8	0.84	0.33	0.32	0.49
7 yrs	24.2	123.2	0.91	0.37	0.35	0.53
8 yrs	26.9	129.0	0.98	0.40	0.39	0.57
9 yrs	29.5	134.1	1.04	0.43	0.43	0.60
10 yrs	32.3	139.4	1.12	0.45	0.47	0.65
11 yrs	35.5	144.5	1.20	0.48	0.52	0.69
12 yrs	39.1	150.9	1.28	0.50	0.57	0.74

[a] Average measurements.
[b] Body Surface Area Method, based on average adult surface area of 1.73 m².

Acetazolamide
Acetylsalicylic acid
Acetaminophen
Aminophylline
Aminosalicylic acid (para-aminosalicylic acid)
Ampicillin trihydrate
Chloramphenicol
Chlordiazepoxide
Chlorothiazide
Digitoxin
Digoxin
Erythromycin
Griseofulvin
Hydrochlorothiazide
Nitrofurantoin
Oxytetracycline
Phenylbutazone
Phenytoin (diphenylhydantoin)
Prednisone
Salicylamide
Sulfadiazine
Tetracycline hydrochloride
Tolbutamide
Warfarin

Pediatric Dosage—Infants and children generally (but not always) require a smaller dose than adults. A child's dose is usually calculated as a fraction of the adult dose by one of several formulas available. Young's Rule (based on age) and Clark's Rule (based on weight) are the most widely used.

Young's Rule:

$$\frac{\text{Age (yr)}}{\text{Age (yr)} + 12} \times \text{Adult dose} = \text{Child's dose}$$

Clark's Rule:

$$\frac{\text{Weight (kg)}}{68.2} \times \text{Adult dose} = \text{Child's dose}$$

These rules are intended as general guides only, and there are exceptions which require caution in their application. For example, digitalis therapy for children requires larger doses than for adults when calculated on a body weight basis. The larger dose required in pediatric therapy may be explained on the basis that digitalis dosage depends on the concentration of the drug on a per-cell basis. Generally, children also require proportionately smaller doses of narcotics and larger doses of belladonna, alcohol, and cathartics. In addition, many manufacturers indicate appropriate dosages, as a function of body weight, in their product literature.

The use of body surface area as a criterion of dosage has gained favor in recent years. It is claimed that body surface area is a more accurate indication of the active metabolism of the body and therefore should be used in preference to age or weight when dosage calculations must be extremely accurate. This view is supported by evidence that many physiological properties—such as plasma volume, oxygen consumption, glomerular filtration, and requirements

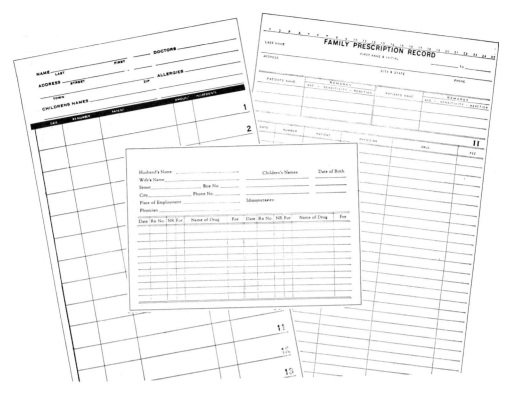

Fig. 4—Patient medication record system.

for fluids, electrolytes, and calories— are proportional to body surface area. This proportionality also holds true for body weight to the $\frac{2}{3}$ power, but not to body weight itself. Nomograms for estimating body surface area of children and adults are shown in Fig. 3. A comparison of Young's Rule, Clark's Rule, and calculations based on body surface area is shown in Table 2.

Patient Medication Records

The proper evaluation of a medication order for safety and efficacy requires some knowledge of the patient's medical history. This knowledge may be obtained by interviewing or consulting with the patient, review of the patient's medical record, and/or review of a specially designed and maintained *medication record system*.

The patient's medical record is usually not available to the pharmacist at the time and point of dispensing medication. Therefore, many pharmacists have

designed and maintain a medication record system, which consists of pertinent information recorded on a form for each patient or family (see Fig. 4). The following types of information are considered important and useful:

Full name and address of patient.
Birth date.
Telephone number.
Place of employment.
Name and address of spouse (if married), guardian, or next of kin.
Names and birth dates of children.
Drug idiosyncrasies and sensitivities.
Name of family physician and other physicians who have been visited.
Serial number of medication order.
Date medication order was dispensed.
Name of drug, including form, strength, and amount dispensed.
Type of medication order (new, refill, controlled).
Medication charge or fee.

A medication record system is useful for (1) protecting the patient against adverse drug reactions, (2) detection of conflicting therapy by different physicians, (3) answering questions or supplying information about the patient's medication history, (4) locating a medication order by patient's name when the serial number is unavailable, and (5) providing patients with a complete medication expenditure record for income tax, insurance, or other necessary reports.

Processing the Order

The medication order must be processed in accordance with applicable state and Federal laws. These laws may be modified at frequent time intervals and may vary from state to state. Therefore, the pharmacist is advised to review and keep current on legal requirements applicable to a locality at a particular point in time.

Legal Controls

The most significant Federal requirements are contained in the Controlled Substances Act of 1970, a Federal law which became fully effective on May 1, 1971, and which is administered by the Drug Enforcement Administration of the Department of Justice. A brief review of selected portions of the regulations is given below. A complete set of the regulations appears in Volume 21, part 300 to end, of the *Code of Federal Regulations*.

The Controlled Substances Act specifies five schedules of controlled drugs with the following designations:

Schedule	Symbol
Schedule I	I or C-I
Schedule II	II or C-II
Schedule III	III or C-III
Schedule IV	IV or C-IV
Schedule V	V or C-V

Schedule I—Drugs in this schedule have a high potential for abuse, no currently accepted medical use in the US, and no accepted safety. Drugs in this schedule include selected narcotic and hallucinogenic substances such as heroin and LSD. Medication orders are illegal for drugs in this schedule.

Schedule II—Drugs in this schedule have accepted medical usefulness and a high potential for abuse which may lead to severe psychological or physical dependence. Examples include selected narcotic, stimulant, and depressant substances such as morphine, amphetamine, and secobarbital. All orders must be in writing (oral orders are permitted under certain emergency conditions). No order may be renewed or refilled. Records of orders must be kept separately from orders for other drugs.

Schedule III—Drugs in this schedule have accepted medical usefulness and a lesser degree (than Schedule II drugs) of abuse potential which may lead to moderate physical or psychological dependence. Examples include selected narcotic, stimulant, and depressant substances such as APC with codeine, phendimetrazine, and butabarbital. Orders may be oral or written and may be renewed up to 5 times within 6 months after the date issued if authorized by the prescriber. Records of orders must be kept separately or be readily retrievable from orders for other drugs.

Schedule IV—Drugs in this schedule have accepted medical usefulness and a lesser degree (than Schedule III drugs) of abuse potential which may lead to moderate physical or psychological dependence. Examples include selected stimulants and depressants such as diethylpropion and phenobarbital. Orders may be oral or written and may be renewed up to 5 times within 6 months after the date issued if authorized by the prescriber. Records of orders must be kept separately or be readily retrievable from orders for other drugs.

Schedule V—Drugs in this schedule have accepted medical usefulness and a lesser degree (than Schedule IV drugs) of abuse potential which may lead to low physical or psychological dependence. Examples include narcotic drugs containing other nonnarcotic active medicinal ingredients such as terpin hydrate with codeine. Orders may be oral or written and may be renewed as authorized by the prescriber. Records of orders must be kept separately or be readily retrievable from orders for other drugs.

Labeling

Medication orders for drugs that are dispensed to the patient for self-administration should be labeled with the following information:

Date of dispensing.
Name and address of pharmacy.
Serial number of the order.
Name of patient.
Name of prescriber.
Directions for use and cautionary statements.

Medication orders for drugs that are dispensed for institutionalized patients when the drug is not in the possession of the patient may be labeled in a different manner, provided the system employed by the pharmacist is adequate to identify the supplier, the product, and the patient.

Pricing

One of the most complex variables in pharmacy practice is the medication price. Medication pricing has been done in one of three ways: (1) an intuitive method not easily quantitated, and often relying on "get what the market will bear"; (2) a simple markup procedure based on the cost of the drug; and (3) a professional fee system.

The price charge for dispensing a medication must be sufficient to cover the cost of ingredients, container, time required for dispensing, professional services, overhead expense, and in addition, yield a profit. Every pharmacy should develop or adopt some pricing policy which combines these factors into a fair, realistic pricing system.

In 1915 there was great diversity and confusion concerning prescription prices. As a result the American Pharmaceutical Association (APhA) appointed a prescription pricing committee with the goal of suggesting a suitable mechanism for prescription pricing which would guarantee a profit for pharmacists. This study resulted in the markup on cost method.

This method is popular because (1) it is easy to use and pricing schedules can be designed to cover various cost prices and (2) it produces an average markup on all prescriptions dispensed. A disadvantage is little consideration for the difference in costs generated by particular items. Additionally, turnover is an ignored factor and little regard is given to demand elasticity.

The professional fee is defined as an amount that covers the cost of providing services and overhead, and a justifiable profit for the pharmacist. The combination of ingredient cost(s) plus a professional fee has gained wide acceptance as a medication pricing formula. The fee system has been endorsed by private and public third party plan payers.

The professional fee philosophy is based on the following principles. A prescribed drug is not an ordinary article of trade, capable of being bought and sold by anyone. It is for the exclusive use of the patient who cannot sell or transfer this item as any other article of trade. Also, neither the cost of dispensing nor the professional or legal responsibility involved is a function of the cost of ingredients used. The pharmacist's ability to do this is inherent to the same extent for each and every prescription dispensed.

One major problem in determining the professional fee is to determine the actual cost to the pharmacy to dispense medication. Several cost-allocation methods have been detailed. However, allocating costs can be difficult since there is a variety of allocations based on changing overhead costs. In the past, gross margin of an average medication order has been the usual and customary fee.

The professional fee is the addition of the cost of dispensing plus profit. The medication price (charge) can be given by

Medication price = Drug cost +
Professional fee

It is conceivable that the professional fee may be varied depending on the practitioner's environment. The fee could be for a community practice, an institution (or a department or service within an institution), inpatients, for outpatients, or some other subdivision in which professional services and/or overhead are incurred.

If i is used for a practice environment, the professional fee for i is the sum of the cost of dispensing in i plus a profit, if one is desired or dictated by administrative policy. Thus,

$$PF_i = COD_i + \text{Profit}$$

where i is the practice environment: community, institution, inpatient service, outpatient service, a department, or some other subdivision, PF is the professional fee, and COD is the cost of dispensing.

The cost of dispensing can be equated to the professional services and overhead encountered in that environment,

Table 3—Professional Fee Based on Operating Expense[a]

$$\frac{A + [B \times C]}{D} + E = \text{Professional fee}$$

A = Proprietor's or manager's salary
B = Percent of prescription sales to total sales
C = Expenses less proprietor's or manager's salary
D = Total number of prescriptions
E = Net profit per prescription (desired or actual)

[a] Courtesy, *American College of Apothecaries.*

or expenses not related to drug cost.

COD_i = (Professional services rendered + Overhead)$_i$

or

$$COD_i = \left(\frac{\text{Total expenses} - \text{Drug costs}}{\text{Number medication orders dispensed}}\right)_i$$

For example, suppose a hospital pharmacy department expended its $500,000 budget: $350,000 was used to purchase drugs. If the department had dispensed 75,000 medication orders and no profit was desired, a professional fee of $2 should have been charged.

$$COD_{\text{hospital}} = \frac{\$500,000 - \$350,000}{75,000} = \$2$$

$$PF_{\text{hospital}} = \$2 + \text{no profit} = \$2$$

In summary, the professional fee system offers several advantages and disadvantages to the practitioner. Advantages include a consistent prescription price which is not difficult to explain, and it allows practitioners to compare their fees with those offered by third-party carriers and rationally decide whether it is profitable to participate as a program vendor. A disadvantage of the professional fee system seems to be little consideration for competition.

Community Practice — Several methods for determining the professional fee in community practice have been published. One method based on *operating expenses* has been reported by the American College of Apothecar-

Table 4—Professional Fee Based on Operating Expense[a]

	Lilly Digest 1974
Total sales	$259,122
R$_X$ sales	$122,615
Percent R$_X$ sales to total (B)	47.3
Proprietor's or manager's salary (A)	$ 21,050
All other expenses (C)	$ 62,697
Total number of prescriptions (D)	27,019
Net profit (percent)	3.8
Average R$_X$ charge	$ 4.54
Net profit per R$_X$ (E)	$ 0.172
Cost of dispensing	$ 1.88
Fee using formula	$ 2.05

[a] Courtesy, *Lilly Digest 1974.*

ies and is shown in Table 3. The formula relates the professional fee computation to five variables: proprietor's or manager's salary, percent of prescription sales to total sales, total expenses less manager's or proprietor's salary, total number of prescriptions, and the net profit per prescription. Table 4 illustrates the professional fee based on data obtained from the *Lilly Digest.* Using this method a professional fee of $2.05/prescription has been calculated.

Another method used to compute the professional fee is based on *average gross margin.* This method, shown in Table 5, employs an eight-step process.

Table 6 illustrates the charge based on 40% margin or a professional fee of $2.05, for a drug which costs $4.25/100. Using a 40% margin the cost of 50 tablets is divided by 0.6 to arrive at a charge to the patient of $3.55. Similarly, using a professional fee of $2.05, the same prescription would cost the patient $4.20. For a prescription of 100, the patient would pay $7.10 on a 40% margin basis, but only $6.30 using the professional fee system. By using the professional fee a number of prescriptions would automatically experience a price rise. However, there would be a corresponding price decrease of a number of prescriptions, particularly those dispensed in larger bulk quantities.

Table 5—Professional Fee Based on Average Gross Margin[a]

Step 1	Record medication costs and selling prices on an adequate sample of prescriptions. *Sample*—Should be drawn from all four calendar quarters using the same number of days in each quarter, *e. g.*, Feb. 10, May 10, Aug. 10 and Nov. 10. *Sample Size*—Total of the four quarters should aggregate at least 600 prescriptions, 1000 or 1200 would be better. Only noncompounded prescriptions should be included. *Recorded Data*—Record the following data. R_X number (for reference purposes), cost of medication, and selling price
Step 2	Total medication costs.
Step 3	Total prescription selling prices.
Step 4	Determine the gross margin by subtracting the total medication costs from the total selling prices.
Step 5	Determine the average gross margin per prescription by dividing the gross margin (*Step 4*) by the total number of prescriptions tabulated.
Step 6	Arrange the samples in ascending order of medication costs (the lowest medication cost first and the highest medication cost last).
Step 7	Inspect the sample to determine approximately where the medication cost + the average gross margin per prescription (*Step 5*) will equal the selling price. This may be referred to as the "break point"—prescriptions with lower medication costs are not carrying their share of overhead and profit; higher prescriptions are carrying more than their share.
Step 8	Consider whether a professional fee should be set which would have the effect of leaving the average gross margin per prescription unchanged. This choice is, of course, made on the assumption that the total number of prescriptions dispensed would continue unchanged.

[a] Courtesy, *Medical Data Services, Inc.*

It has been shown that if the average gross margin/prescription was used as a pharmacy's professional fee, approximately 10% of the lower priced prescriptions would experience a price rise. Therefore the practitioner should assess his position with patrons regarding a change in prescription prices.

Institutional Practice—One difference in most institutional practices is ward or floor stock medication. This medication may be charged to patients in two ways. First, the patient may be charged for specific floor stock medication received; or, the patient may be charged on a daily basis (per diem) for availability of floor stock regardless of use.

Three different areas exist in institutional practice which may call for different prescription pricing policies: (1) dispensing to inpatients; (2) dispensing to patients in ambulatory care centers, extended-care facilities, or other insti-

Table 6—Pricing a Prescription Using Margin and a Professional Fee

R_X drug cost ($4.25/100)	40% margin (divide cost by 0.6)	Professional fee ($2.05)
#50 $2.13	$3.55	$4.20
#100 $4.25	$7.10	$6.30

tutional divisions; and (3) outpatient dispensing. The professional fee concept in the institutional environment is not new and has been recommended by the American Society of Hospital Pharmacists for some time. The professional fee system can be employed equally well in community or institutional practices. However one caution is to determine accurately what constitutes a valid prescription.

Medication orders generated in an institution usually arrive at the pharmacy in one of three forms: (1) the physician writes an original medication order and

Table 7—Exact Equivalents[a]

Apothecaries oz	Apothecaries grains	Avoirdupois lb	Avoirdupois oz	Avoirdupois grains	Metric Equivalents g or ml	Fluid ounces	Fluid minims	Decimal Equivalent
32	72.4	2	3	119.9	1000	33	391.1	33.815
30	204.1	2	1	166.6	946.333	32	....	32
29	80.0	2	..	....	907.185	30	324.6	30.676
16	36.2	1	1	278.7	500	16	435.6	16.907
15	102.1	1	..	302.1	473.167	16	....	16
14	280.0	1	..	....	453.592	15	162.3	15.338
12	....	..	13	72.5	373.242	12	298.1	12.621
8	....	..	8	340.0	248.828	8	198.7	8.414
7	291.0	..	8	151.0	236.583	8	....	8
7	140.0	..	8	....	226.796	7	321.1	7.669
6	206.5	..	7	24.0	200	6	366.2	6.763
4	....	..	4	170.0	124.414	4	99.4	4.207
3	385.5	..	4	75.5	118.292	4	....	4
3	310.0	..	4	....	113.398	3	400.6	3.835
3	103.2	..	3	230.7	100	3	183.1	3.381
2	....	..	2	85.0	62.207	2	49.7	2.104
1	432.8	..	2	37.8	59.146	2	....	2
1	395.0	..	2	....	56.699	1	440.3	1.917
1	291.6	..	1	334.1	50	1	331.5	1.691
1	....	..	1	42.5	31.1035	1	24.9	1.052
..	456.380	..	1	18.88	29.5729	1	....	1
..	437.5	..	1	....	28.350	..	460.15	0.959
..	385.8	..	..	....	25	..	405.78	0.845
..	308.6	..	..	....	20	..	324.62	0.676
..	154.3	..	..	....	10	..	162.31	0.338
..	19.02	..	..	....	1.232	..	20	....
..	15.4324	..	..	....	1	..	16.23	....
..	9.51	..	..	....	0.616	..	10	....
..	5	..	..	....	0.324	..	....	....
..	4.75	..	..	....	0.308	..	5	....
..	1	..	..	....	0.06480	..	1.0517	....

[a] Courtesy, *USP.*

it is sent to the pharmacy, (2) a duplicate copy of the medication order is sent to the pharmacy, or (3) and least desirable, the physician's order is transcribed by nursing personnel onto a pharmacy order blank and this is sent to the pharmacy. Such a medication order can have a professional fee added to it if the quantity dispensed is clearly defined. For example, a physician prescribes aqueous penicillin G, one million units IM every 6 hours. Is the prescription for one dose, one day, or ten days? In many institutions parenteral medication is administered on a 24-hour basis. In this case it would be taken to be four 1-million unit doses and this would constitute the prescription to which a fee would be added. More importantly, however, whatever definitions are set down should be consistent since problems in pricing policy can occur. An initial step in a professional fee system would be to review ordering policy such that rational prescription pricing can be accomplished in the institutional environment.

Filing

Medication orders for institutionalized patients are usually written on the physician's order form and remain in the patient's permanent medical record. For controlled drugs, an additional record of dispensing and administration is kept for purposes of control and accountability.

Medication orders for noninstitutionalized patients are usually written on a prescription order form and filed in numerical order according to the assigned serial number. The filing system of prescription order forms for controlled drugs, however, must conform to provisions of the Controlled Substances Act described below. These provisions are designed to allow easy and reasonable inspection of prescriptions for controlled substances.

Prescriptions for Schedule II controlled drugs must be filed separately from noncontrolled drugs. Prescriptions for drugs in Schedules III, IV, and V may be filed together on a separate file, or on the file containing Schedule II drugs, or on the file containing noncontrolled drugs. When combined with prescriptions for Schedule II or noncontrolled drugs, prescriptions for Schedules III, IV, and V drugs must be stamped with the letter "C" in red, at least 1 in. in height in the lower right-hand corner.

Thus, prescription files may be maintained in one of the following ways:

1. *Two Files*
   a. One file for Schedule II prescriptions.
   b. One file for Schedules III, IV, and V, and noncontrolled prescriptions, provided that prescriptions for controlled drugs are stamped with the letter "C" in red at least one inch in height in the lower right hand corner.
2. *Two Files*
   a. One file for Schedules II, III, IV, and V prescriptions, provided that prescriptions for Schedules III, IV and V are stamped with the letter "C" in red at least one inch in height in the lower right hand corner.
   b. One file for prescriptions for noncontrolled drugs.
3. *Three Files*
   a. One file for Schedule II prescriptions.
   b. One file for Schedules III, IV, and V prescriptions.
   c. One file for noncontrolled prescriptions.

Compounding Accuracy

The problem of improper equivalents when translating from one system of

Table 8—Metric System Abbreviations

Ci = curie
mCi = millicurie
μCi = microcurie
nCi = nanocurie
m = meter
cm = centimeter
mm = millimeter
μm = micrometer[a]
nm = nanometer[b]
kg = kilogram
g = gram
mg = milligram
μg;mcg = microgram
ng = nanogram
l = liter
ml = milliliter
μl = microliter

[a] Formerly, the abbreviation μ (micron) was used.
[b] Formerly, the abbreviation mμ (millimicron) was used.

weights and measures to another has been a source of error in compounding for many years. The official compendia use the metric system; however, for conversion of values not in the metric system, exact equivalents must be used. In all cases exact equivalents should be rounded to three significant figures. Table 7 shows equivalents for weights and measures in the metric, avoirdupois and apothecary systems. The practitioner should always use exact equivalents as approximate equivalents can introduce errors as great as 7–8%.

Table 8 shows the metric system of weights, measures, and abbreviations commonly employed. Several abbreviations require additional comment. The micrometer (micron), microgram, and microliter are similar in nature, depending on length, mass, or volume, respectively. The microgram is abbreviated *mcg* or μg; mcg is more frequently used in practice, while μg is more often used in publications and formal writing. Occasionally the term gamma, shown by γ, is used for microgram quantities in other textbooks. The nanometer (nm) was formerly abbreviated as *millimicron* (mμ) but is no longer used. The milliliter is used as the equivalent of cubic centimeter (cc).

Measuring Devices

Prescription Balances—A prescription balance is an instrument adapted to weighing medicinal and other substances required in pharmaceutical practice. The balance most frequently employed is the Class A prescription balance. Most Class A prescription balances have a maximum capacity of 120 g. Characteristics of the Class A prescription balance include meeting criteria for four basic tests assuring accuracy and precision in compounding.

1. The balance must be sensitive and pass a *sensitivity requirement test.* Simply stated, the test certifies the rest-point will be shifted not less than one scale division on the index plate each time a 6-mg weight is added.
2. The Class A prescription balance must also pass an *arm ratio test* which is designed to check the equality of length of both arms of the balance.
3. The *shift test* assures the arm and lever components of the balance are correct.
4. The *rider and graduated beam test* assures the weight-beam graduation on the balance is correct when compared to two test weights.

In order to avoid errors of 5% or more, not less than 120 mg of any material should be weighed. This value can be obtained using the following equation:

$$LAW = \frac{100}{\% \text{ error}} (SR)$$

where *LAW* is least amount weighted and *SR* is sensitivity requirement. If a smaller amount of material is required an aliquot must be prepared.

Weights—Suitable sets of weights should be maintained for use with the prescription balance. These weights should be kept protected and handled with forceps. The NF recommends the use of Class P (analytical) or Class Q weights for prescription use. Class Q weights have tolerances well within the limits of accuracy of the prescription balance and retain their accuracy for a long time with proper care. If apothecary weights are to be used, they should have the same general construction as metric weights. The coin-type, disk-shaped apothecary weights should not be used. They corrode and undergo weight change easily.

Liquid Measuring Devices—Pharmaceutical devices for measuring volumes of liquids include burets, pipets, cylindrical graduates, conical graduates, and medicine droppers. Cylindrical graduates are preferred to conical graduates since the smaller diameter generally results in a greater degree of accuracy. The practitioner should have at his disposal a variety of graduates in various capacities to complement his prescription work. The capacity of a graduate is designed such that it will contain or deliver, as indicated, at the specified temperature. When liquids are measured, a graduate is selected with a capacity equal to or just exceeding the volume to be measured. Measurements of small volumes in large graduates should be avoided since large volume errors can be introduced.

Several other characteristics of liquids often can lead to sources of error in compounding prescriptions for liquid preparations. The graduate should not be tilted when used. The graduation mark, meniscus of the liquid, and line of sight should be in alignment. This parallax effect can result in considerable error if the graduation mark and the bottom of the meniscus do not align with the eye. If the meniscus cannot be perceived, the background should be altered. Certain liquids because of their meniscus, opaque nature, or physical characteristics, may lead to errors in draining or volume measurements. This must be considered with such dosage forms as suspensions, emulsions, and syrups. In addition, care should be taken in dispensing or compounding preparations containing glycerin, vegetable oils, and mineral oil.

When faced with measuring a small amount of liquid, it may be advantageous to calibrate a dropper. The calibration is done by counting drops of the liquid when added to a graduate until a measurable volume is achieved. The correct number of drops to deliver the required volume then can be calculated.

Measuring the Dose

After the prescription has been accurately compounded, the pharmacist is responsible for seeing that means are available for the patient to self-administer the drug. For liquid preparations, this usually means one of three measuring devices: the teaspoon, the tablespoon, or the dropper. The mechanics by which the patient administers a prescription medication is the responsibility of the pharmacist.

Teaspoon—The average volume contained in a teaspoonful of water has changed remarkably over the years. In the times of Benjamin Franklin, the teaspoon contained approximately 3 ml. The teaspoon gradually grew until by current day standards it contains about 5 ml. The standard American teaspoon has been established by the American National Standards Institute as containing 4.93 ± 0.24 ml. Preparations intended for teaspoon administration should be formulated on the basis of 5-ml units. Other devices used in conjunction with the teaspoon should be calibrated to deliver 5 ml wherever a teaspoon is indicated. The volume error incurred in measuring liquids for an individual dose should not be greater than 10% of the indicated amount.

Although 5 ml has been recognized as the standard teaspoon, household teaspoons may vary from 3–7 ml. The volume contained in a teaspoon for any given liquid is related to the liquid's viscosity and surface tension, among other influencing factors. Thus, when extremely accurate dosing is required, a solid dosage form or liquid concentrate with calibrated dropper should be used.

There are 6 teaspoonfuls in 1 ounce, and this should not be confused with 8 fluid drams to the fluid ounce, formerly used in the apothecary system. Normally practitioners transcribe 1 fluid dram as one teaspoonful. This can be a source of error particularly in compounded prescriptions and for this reason all prescriptions should be written using the metric system of measure. Many physicians have discarded the habit of writing 1 fluid dram when they actually mean a teaspoonful and are writing the word teaspoonful, its abbreviation, or actually 5 ml. This should help alleviate a potential source of dispensing error.

Tablespoon—The household tablespoon contains 15 ml or the equivalent of 3 teaspoonfuls. One tablespoonful is a convenient method of delivering ½ ounce of liquid medication. Stated in other terms, if 1 ounce of medication is desired, it could be labeled as 2 tablespoonfuls.

Tablespoons, like teaspoons, can vary in size from 10 to 30 ml. The patient should be forwarned when tablespoon dosages are indicated. If there is cause for concern the patient may take 3 teaspoonfuls in place of 1 tablespoonful.

Medicine Dropper—Small doses of liquid medication are most accurately delivered by means of the medicine dropper. The medicine dropper is defined as a tube made of glass or other transparent material, fitted with a collapsible bulb, and, while varying in capacity, should deliver 20 drops/ml. Few medicinal liquids have the same surface and flow characteristics as water; therefore, the size of drops varies from one material to another. In addition, it is possible to produce drops of different sizes using the same dropper because of variations in pressure applied to the bulb and the speed in which the drops are formed.

Many concentrated liquid preparations have specially calibrated droppers supplied by the manufacturer. The USP states the volume error incurred in measuring any liquid by means of a calibrated dropper should not exceed 15% under normal conditions.

Other Means—Other means of accurately measuring liquids include the pipet, buret, and syringe. Syringes can be utilized for measuring small amounts of liquid, particularly from 1–10 ml.

Complexation

A drug dosage form may contain several ingredients which can interact, resulting in the formation of complexes. Such complexes may be thought of as distinct entities composed of two or more different species, which may or may not exhibit physical or chemical properties different from the properties of the individual species. Examples of desirable interactions include the use of complexes to improve the stability or the solubility of the drug in the dosage form. On the other hand, the formation of an unanticipated complex may result in decreased product efficacy, as in the case of preservative inactivation, or the formation of an insoluble precipitate. The pharmacist should also be aware of the potential for complexation to occur *in vivo* when dosage form ingredients are exposed to constituents of the gastrointestinal tract, or when the dosage form is administered concomitantly with other pharmaceutical preparations. As discussed later, certain of these interactions may result in decreased drug effectiveness due to reduction of drug available for absorption from the gastrointestinal tract.

The general equilibrium reaction for the formation of a complex may be given as:

$$a(A) + b(B) \overset{K}{\rightleftarrows} (A_aB_b)$$

where a and b are the number of molecules of each component (A and B) present in the complex, and the stability constant, K, is defined in terms of the concentrations of the species:

$$K = \frac{(A_aB_b)}{(A)^a(B)^b}$$

The larger the value of K the more stable the given complex. It is important to recognize that the extent of complex formation is a function of the stability constant and the concentrations of interacting species.

Bonding Forces

In order to understand the phenomenon of complexation and have a basis for anticipation of the formation of a complex between two or more individual species, it is helpful to review briefly the major types of forces which may be operative in such interactions.

van der Waals Forces—Although many molecules may not have a formal positive or negative charge, they may exhibit, naturally or by induction, a partial positive charge in one portion of the molecule and a partial negative charge in another. As a result, the molecule is said to have a polar character. For example, water and ethanol:

$$\overset{\delta+}{H} - \overset{\delta-}{O} \atop | \atop \underset{\delta+}{H} \quad CH_3CH_2 - O^{\delta-} - H^{\delta+}$$

In these examples there is a partial negative charge in the vicinity of the oxygen atom due to the electronegativity of this atom relative to the other atoms present. The hydrogen atom exhibits a partial positive charge due to the depletion of electrons which have been attracted toward the oxygen. As a consequence of the partial charges, there may be an attraction between adjacent neutral molecules. Species which interact as a result of van der Waals forces may involve an attraction between two dipolar molecules, a dipolar molecule and a molecule with an induced dipole, or two molecules with induced dipoles.

Other Types of Bonding Forces—In addition to van der Waals forces, other types of bonding forces may be important in the formation of pharmaceutical complexes. Ion-dipole and ion-induced dipole interactions involve the formation of complexes between ionic species and molecules which have either dipole or induced dipole properties.

Hydrogen bonding is another type of dipole–dipole interaction in which a proton provides the positive center for interaction with an electronegative atom of a dipolar molecule. The hydrogen involved in the bonding is usually covalently bonded to an oxygen, carbon, nitrogen, or fluorine atom. The proton interacts with strongly electronegative atoms such as fluorine, oxygen, or nitrogen.

Chelates (Gk., crab or lobster claw)—This term is descriptive of the complex in that a metal atom is bound to a species known as a *ligand,* through more than one bond, resulting in a ring structure which includes the metal atom. In order to function as a chelating agent a ligand must have at least two functional groups which can donate a pair of electrons to the metal atom. Further, these groups must be positioned on the ligand such that the groups may simultaneously interact with the metal atom.

Miscellaneous Interactions

Sorption, ion-exchange, and surfactant-drug interactions are usually not included in a formal discussion of complexation. However, these phenomena often involve the reversible associations of various species whose interactions may be included within the broad definition of a complex given earlier.

Sorption—This general term describes the interaction between a given species and a solid substance with active sites on and/or within the structure of the solid. Here, only sorption from solution will be considered. Sorption is said to have occurred when the concentration of sorbed species (sorbate) is higher within the vicinity of the solid than in the bulk fluid with which the solid is in contact. When the interaction occurs at the surface of the solid then the term *ad*sorption is employed. In the event the sorbate is able to penetrate within the structure of the solid, *ab*sorption is used to describe the process. We may, to some extent, anticipate the degree of sorption of a sorbate from knowledge of the properties of the solid, sorbate, and solvent present in the system. In general, the greater the solubility of the sorbate in the solvent, the less it will tend to interact with the solid. Thus, the sorption of a polar species, from a polar solvent, onto a nonpolar solid such as charcoal will not be favored. However, the sorption of a nonpolar molecule, from a polar solvent, onto a nonpolar solid will be favored.

Ion-Exchange—Ion-exchange reactions are reversible and involve the re-placement of ions associated with the ion-exchange matrix with ions present in the surrounding solution. An anion-exchange resin is a polymeric, insoluble material which usually contains primary, secondary, or tertiary amino groups or quaternary ammonium groups and has associated with it exchangeable anions. A cation-exchange resin usually contains carboxyl, phosphate, or sulfonate groups which exchange cations. Certain pharmaceutically important materials, such as clay-suspending agents like bentonite and attapulgite, may interact with ions in solution through both ion-exchange and sorption mechanisms.

Surface Activity—A portion of the molecule of a surface-active agent is polar or hydrophilic, the remainder of the molecule being nonpolar or lipophilic. The polar groups may be anionic as in sodium lauryl sulfate; cationic as in benzalkonium chloride; or nonionic as in the Tweens, Spans, and Brijs. Monomers of these compounds would be expected to exhibit limited water solubility because of the hydrophobic character of a portion of the molecule. However, they may be dispersed in water in relatively high concentrations because of orientation of the molecules in such a manner that their hydrophobic regions are in close proximity. Thus, the polar portion of the molecule associates with the water and the nonpolar portion associates with other hydrophobic groups present in adjacent surfactant molecules. The resulting structured arrangement of these surfactant molecules is known as a micelle. The concentration at which the surfactant molecules begin to associate into micelles is known as the *critical micelle concentration* (CMC).

Other species present in solution may interact with the surfactant molecules in a variety of ways. The interaction may be mediated by the types of forces previously considered, such as van der Waals forces or hydrogen bonding. At surfactant concentrations above the CMC, the interactions generally involve

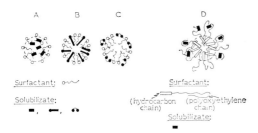

Fig. 5—Mechanisms involved in surfactant-small molecule interactions.[2]

residence of the molecules within or about the micelle. Interactions between nonpolar hydrocarbons and surfactants may be represented as dissolution of the hydrocarbon within the interior, hydrophobic portion of the micelle (see Fig. 5A). Compounds containing both polar and nonpolar groupings, such as long chain alcohols and amines, are thought to orient themselves among the surfactant molecules (see Fig. 5B). Highly polar compounds, such as polyhydroxy alcohols (e.g., glycerin) may be adsorbed onto the surface of the micelle (see Fig. 5C). Finally, with surfactants such as the nonionic polyoxyethylenes, the interacting molecules may become entrapped within the curled polyoxyethylene chain (see Fig. 5D).

While a more detailed discussion of the nature of the various types of bonding forces and resulting interactions is beyond the scope of this chapter, several references are provided in the *Bibliography* which consider this topic in greater detail. Examples of a variety of molecular complexes, involving agents of pharmaceutical importance, are provided in Table 9, as an indication of the variety of drugs which have been observed to be capable of interacting to form a complex.

Complexation and Drug Therapy

Before considering the application of complexation in the preparation of pharmaceutical dosage forms, it is useful to consider briefly several examples of therapeutic agents which are either available in the form of a complex or function as a complexing agent.

A number of hematinics, which are iron-containing products utilized for the treatment of iron-deficiency anemia, are marketed in the form of a complex. For example Ferrolip tablets and syrup (*Flint*) contain an iron–choline citrate complex. Jectofer (*Astra*) and Imferon (*Lakeside*) are parenteral products containing iron–sorbital–citric

Table 9—Examples of Pharmaceutical Complexes

Complexing agent	*Agent which is complexed*
Boric acid	Glycerin
Xanthines (various)	Benzoic acid, sulfonamides, benzocaine, PABA, barbiturates, organic acids
Polyvinylpyrrolidone (PVP), Polypropylene glycol, Polyethylene glycol (PEG)	Phenolic compounds—phenol, salicylic, benzoic, and tannic acids, resorcinol
Polyvinylpyrrolidone	Sulfathiazole, procaine hydrochloride, salicylates, xanthines, antibiotics, cortisone, hexylresorcincl
Polyethylene glycol	Barbiturates, phenolics, organic acids, iodine
Sodium carboxymethyl-cellulose	Cationic drugs—quinine, diphenhydramine, procaine, pyribenzamine
Methylcellulose	Preservatives—benzoic acid and parabens
Saccharin	Xanthines, amides, and phenolics
Riboflavin	Xanthines
Tetracyclines	Aromatic hydroxy acids, saccharin sodium
Aromatic hydroxy acids	Xanthines, steroids, phenacetin, PEG, methylcellulose, PVP, gelatin

acid and iron–dextran complexes, respectively. The rationale proposed for the use of iron complexes, rather than the simple iron salts such as ferrous sulfate, carbonate, etc., is that the complexes are purported to result in increased absorption following oral administration and less gastrointestinal irritation or irritation at the site of injection.

Two topical preparations further illustrate marketed products formulated as complexes. Butesin Picrate (*Abbott*), a topical anesthetic which is a 2:1 complex of butyl *p*-aminobenzoate and picric acid, is shown below:

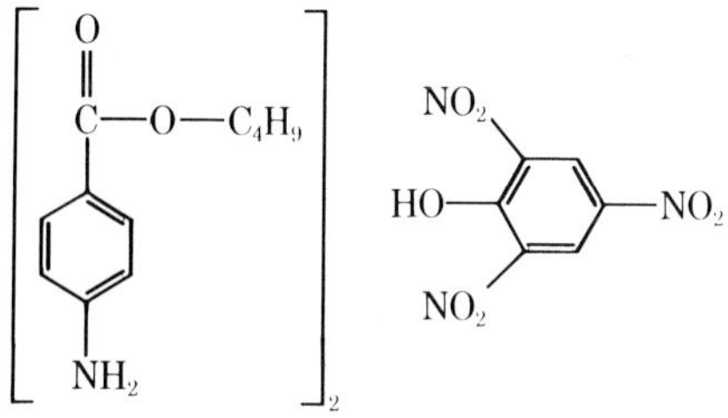

In the product Betadine (*Purdue-Frederick*), iodine is complexed with polyvinylpyrrolidone to enhance the stability and solubility of the iodine. The product is said to slowly release the iodine upon topical application, resulting in a mild antimicrobial effect.

The principles of ion-exchange have also been applied to pharmaceutical products. For example, cholestyramine resin [Cuemid (*MSD*), Questran (Mead Johnson)] is a quaternary ammonium anion-exchange resin. It is used in the relief of pruritus associated with excessive bile absorption from the intestine due to biliary obstruction and also as adjunctive therapy to diet in the management of hypercholesterolemia due to primary Type II hyperlipoproteinemia. The resin functions by exchanging chloride ions for the bile acids present in the intestinal tract. The resin itself is not absorbed and, as a result, the elimination of the bile acids through the feces is increased. Another such product is Kayexalate (*Winthrop*). This is a sodium polystyrene sulfonate cation-exchange resin which exchanges sodium ions for potassium ions present in the intestinal tract, and is used in the treatment of hyperkalemia. Ion-exchange principles have also been applied to the preparation of prolonged-release products, as exemplified by those marketed by Strassenburgh (Biphetamine and Tussionex) and Squibb (Rezipas).

Diagnostics is another area in which complex formation is used. For example, Technetium 99m, a radionuclide, has been prepared in the form of a citrate complex for use in determination of kidney function and glomerular filtration rate. Another diagnostic agent, Diagnex Blue (*Squibb*) is commercially available for the detection of achlorhydria or lack of gastric hydrochloric acid secretion due to conditions such as carcinoma, pernicious anemia, etc. This product is a complex of a dye, azure A, coupled with a carbacrylic cation-exchange resin. The test procedure involves administration of the complex orally and subsequent collection of urine. In the presence of hydrochloric acid in the stomach the blue dye will be displaced from the resin by the hydrogen ions, absorbed systemically, and excreted in the urine. The intensity of the color of the urine is a measure of the extent of acidity present in the stomach.

Other clinical examples of the application of complexation include the oral use of activated charcoal in the treatment of poisonings to adsorb toxic materials, and the use of chelating agents to interact with heavy metal ions. Ethylenediaminetetraacetic acid (EDTA), for example, is commonly employed as an anticoagulant for stored blood, and functions by chelating calcium ions. Penicillamine [Cuprimine (*MSD*)] is a copper chelating agent which is employed in the treatment of Wilson's disease, which results from a deficiency or absence of a specific copper binding plasma protein, ceruloplasmin. The chelation of copper by penicillamine is illustrated in the reaction at the top of page 20.

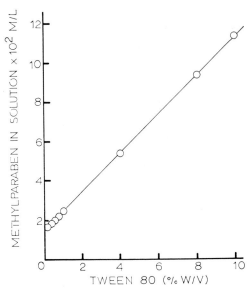

Fig. 6—The apparent solubility of methylparaben in water at 27° as a function of nonionic surfactant concentration.[3]

Application to Compounding

The major areas where complexation is of importance in the preparation of pharmaceuticals are the solubilization and stabilization of active ingredients, and the prevention of incompatibilities.

Solubilization—One problem which often faces the formulator of a pharmaceutical product, whether as a community practitioner or in an industrial setting, is a limited solubility of one or more of the active ingredients of the preparation. Several approaches may be employed in solving this problem. Sometimes a change in the solvent or an adjustment of pH suffice. However, in some instances the principles of complexation are utilized. For example, potassium iodide is commonly employed to facilitate the preparation of aqueous solutions of iodine. The increased solubility of the iodine is believed to be related to the formation of a complex between the ion and the molecule:

$$I_2 + I^- \rightleftarrows I_3^-$$

The principle involved in using complexation to increase the solubility of a drug is to form a soluble complex with some other material; then, as a result, both uncomplexed and complexed drug will be in solution. Thus, if we attempt to dissolve 100 mg of a drug, with an aqueous solubility of 1 mg/ml, in 10 ml of water, only 10 mg of drug will go into solution. If we now add a complexing agent, which interacts with the drug to form a complex with a solubility of 1.5 mg/ml, an additional 15 mg of drug will be solubilized in the 10 ml of water.

Many studies have focused on the complexation between xanthines and a variety of other drugs. Caffeine and sodium benzoate is an example of a commercial injectable product which takes advantage of this interaction. The preparation, which is used as a central nervous system stimulant, is approximately an equal weight mixture of caffeine and sodium benzoate. Caffeine complexation by the benzoate increases the apparent aqueous solubility of the caffeine from about 1 g/46 ml to about 1 g/2.5 ml. Citrated Caffeine NF XIII illustrates a similar use of complexation to increase solubility. It should be noted, however, that the utilization of these types of complexes to enhance drug solubility has not been extensively used. One obvious drawback to this approach is the fact that many agents, such as the xanthines, which could potentially serve as useful complexing agents, possess their own intrinsic pharmacological activity. Thus, in actual practice, the pharmacist is generally not able to solubilize a given drug through the addition of such complexing agents to the prescription formulation.

Of the various agents utilized to solubilize drugs, the most widely employed are the surface-active agents. The pri-

Table 10—Interaction of Preservatives with Other Agents

Preservative	*Complexing agent*
Quaternary ammonium compounds (e.g., cetylpyridinium chloride, benzalkonium chloride)	Tween 80, PVP, methylcellulose
p-Hydroxybenzoic acid esters	Tween 80
Phenylmercuric nitrate, hydroxybenzoate esters, cetyltrimethyl ammonium bromide	Tween 80
Cationic agents (various)	Sodium alginate
Chlorobutanol, benzyl alcohol, phenylethyl alcohol	Tween 80, PVP, methylcellulose
Parabens and phenols	Tween 80
Quaternary ammonium compounds (various)	Hexachlorophene
Parabens (various)	Celluloses, PEG
p-Hydroxybenzoic acid, sorbic acid	Starches
Parabens, phenols, chlorocresol, sorbic acid, dehydroacetic acid	Tween 80, PRG 1000-monocetyl ether

mary mechanism of solubilization involves the incorporation of the solubilized material within the micelles, as discussed earlier. Some interaction between the given drug and the surfactant may also lead to increased solubility even at low surfactant concentrations, in the absence of appreciable micelle formation. Fig. 6 illustrates the increase in solubility of methylparaben in the presence of increasing concentrations of a nonionic surfactant, Tween 80. Typical examples of drugs which may successfully be solubilized with surfactants include phenolic disinfectants such as cresol and coal tar preparations, iodophors, vitamin formulations containing oil-soluble vitamins such as Vitamins A and E, and various steroids such as estradiol and hydrocortisone.

Stabilization—The stabilization of ingredients present in a pharmaceutical preparation against hydrolysis, oxidation, and other forms of degradation is another instance where complex formation has been shown to be useful. The use of complexation to enhance drug stability is discussed on page 25.

Incompatibilities—A complex may have physical or chemical properties which are different than those of the individual species. Thus, it is logical to as-

sume that, in some instances, the end-result of such interactions may be the formation of a complex with poor stability characteristics, or other undesirable properties, which could lead to the formation of precipitates or alteration in the physical appearance of suspensions or emulsions. A typical example is the flocculation of calamine lotion suspension with the addition of phenol, resulting from an interaction between phenol and the polyethylene glycols present in the formulation. An example of an interaction which can occur if two different preparations are employed simultaneously is the formation of an insoluble complex between the polyvinyl alcohol contained in some contact lens wetting solutions and the boric acid found in many ophthalmic irrigating solutions.

Another type of interaction, which is particularly important in ophthalmic solutions and other preparations which contain a preservative to prevent microbial contamination, is the inactivation of the preservative due to complex formation. Considerable effort has been directed toward investigation of interactions between preservatives and other constituents present in a formulation. Various studies have indicated that

Table 11—Extent of Interaction between Methyl and Propylparaben and Various Macromolecules[a]

Macromolecules 2% w/v	% Methyl-paraben free	% Propyl-paraben free
Gelatin	92	89
Methyl-cellulose	91	87
Polyethylene glycol 4000	84	81
Polyvinyl-pyrrolidone	78	64
Myrj 52	55	16
Tween 20	43	14
Tween 80	43	10

[a] Data from the work of Bakley[4] as summarized by Lachman.[5]

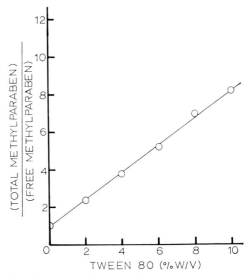

Fig. 7—A plot of the ratio, R, of total methyl p-hydroxybenzoate to free methyl p-hydroxybenzoate, at 30°, in aqueous solutions containing varying concentrations of Tween 80.[3]

many of the commonly employed preservatives strongly interact with materials such as suspending and emulsifying agents, and with various excipients present in a dosage form. The result of such interactions may be to reduce the concentration of unbound preservative to such a level that it is no longer an effective antimicrobial agent. Anionic, cationic, and nonionic preservatives are capable of interacting with ionic and nonionic compounds. Examples of studies of preservative inactivation by various agents are summarized in Table 10. The data in Table 11 summarize the interactions which may occur between some common pharmaceutical materials and two widely employed preservatives.

The potential for such interactions does not necessarily preclude the use of a given preservative in combination with certain ingredients. Knowledge of the extent of the interaction should permit a rational selection of the appropriate quantities of the preservative to use. A scheme has been suggested for the calculation of preservative concentration required, when it is present with some inactivating agent (see Fig. 7). These data illustrate a plot of the ratio (R) of total methylparaben to free methylparaben, present in a system containing a fixed concentration of methylparaben and various concentra-

tions of Tween 80, as determined from complexation studies. At a Tween 80 concentration of 2%, for example, about 58% of the total methylparaben present in the system will be bound by the Tween 80. It has been observed that only the free, unbound preservative has antimicrobial activity. Therefore, if the concentration of preservative necessary to be effective against a certain organism is known and a plot of (R) vs. surfactant concentration is available, the concentration of this preservative required in the presence of surfactant may be calculated. For example, a methylparaben concentration of 0.08% will act as a preservative against the organism *Aerobacter aerogenes*. This preservative in the presence of 2% Tween 80, will require a methylparaben concentration of about 0.19–0.20%, as may be calculated from Fig. 7.

The use of complexation may also enhance the activity of a preservative. An agent such as EDTA (0.1%) can increase the effectiveness of benzalkonium chloride (1/7500) solution against *Pseudomonas aeruginosa*. The EDTA, which does not have any antibacterial activity of its own, may act by chelation of divalent metal ions within the cell membrane and thus alter bacterial cell wall permeability.

Several other types of interactions should be mentioned, which do not actually involve complexation in the strict sense, but do result in a decreased drug concentration in the final dosage form. The first of these concerns drugs which interact with their containers, particularly those packaging materials which are polymeric such as plastics and rubber. Such interactions, discussed elsewhere in this chapter in greater detail, primarily involve sorption of the active drug onto the polymer surface, and possibly penetration of the drug into the polymer matrix. The net result of this process is a reduction in effective drug concentration present in the dosage form. Thus, the pharmacist should be aware that dispensing a drug dosage form usually requires some type of packaging material, and his responsibility to dispense the most efficacious product possible includes the need to properly package the preparation. A somewhat related topic is the potential for interaction between a drug and other materials, such as filtration aids, utilized during the course of preparing the finished dosage form. A fact sometimes overlooked is that filter paper, specialized filters such as Millipore disks, and other filtration aids, may remove significant quantities of active drug from solution. While the ideal way to deal with such a possibility would be to chemically analyze the product before and after filtration, to detect any loss of potency, this is rarely practical. At least a partial solution to this problem is to filter the solution and discard the initial fraction of filtrate. This practice will tend to saturate active binding sites on the filter, depleting drug from the initial portion of the filtrate but will reduce the sorption of significant quantities of drug from the remainder of the solution.

Influence on Drug Absorption

The influence of complexation on drug absorption is considered in some detail in Chapters 2 and 13. Frequently it may not be a simple matter to make *a priori* predictions of specific effects. For example, data to date suggest that surfactants may increase, decrease, or have no effect on drug action, depending on the drug, the surfactant, the concentration of drug and surfactant present, and the physiological system being evaluated.

It should be apparent that the phenomenon of complexation may have a significant effect on both the formulation and the efficacy of a pharmaceutical dosage form. Drugs are currently being marketed in the form of complexes, and some therapeutic agents owe their activity to the formation of a complex. Further, it has been shown that the stability, solubility, and bioavailability of a drug may be enhanced through the use of complexation. However, much research remains to be done before sufficient data becomes available to permit the pharmacist to select specific complexing agents which will perform in a predictable manner and permit significant enhancement of drug product efficacy. The pharmacist should be able to recognize the purpose for certain ingredients in a formulation, which have been included for purposes of complexing with an active constituent. Further, the pharmacist should be alert to those instances where incompatibilities, altered degradation processes, and altered absorption characteristics may be attributed to the process of complex formation.

Stabilization

Stability of a drug product may be defined as the extent to which the product retains the same properties and characteristics that it possessed at the time of its manufacture. Stability is important to the practitioner in making judgments concerning (1) condition of the drug product when compounded or received, (2) proper storage of the drug product after compound or receipt and (3) shelf life of the drug product until used.

The stability of manufactured dosage forms prior to delivery to the practitioner is generally the sole responsibility of the manufacturer. This implies the wholesaler, if involved, has provided proper storage conditions. The manufacturer is required to prove stability of the dosage form and validate the expiration date and storage specifications which accompany the product. Using analytical methods for determining stability and accelerated stability analyses the manufacturer confirms product shelf-life stability. Testing under ambient storage conditions is generally performed for a period of 5 years after a given product is released to the market.

Drug-product stability is generally recognized as being comprised of five types: chemical, physical, microbiological, therapeutic, and toxicological. Chemical stability relates to the chemical integrity of the drug and its labeled potency. Physical stability refers to original physical properties which include appearance, uniformity, dissolution, and palatability. Microbiological stability concerns resistance of the drug product to microbial growth. This is particularly important in liquid and injectable preparations in which antimicrobial agents may be present and their effectiveness judged. Therapeutic stability infers the therapeutic effect of the drug will remain unchanged throughout the shelf-life of the product. Toxicological stability means no significant increase in toxicity will occur.

Factors Influencing Stability

Each ingredient in a drug product is subject to its own particular problems regarding stability. The stability of the drug product is the net effect of the stability of individual ingredients.

Factors which affect stability generally are of three types: (1) external (environmental) factors such as temperature, light, gases, and moisture; (2) internal factors such as pH, complexation, and microbial growth; and (3) boundary (containers) factors such as container composition, porosity, and dosage-form interaction.

Moisture—Water vapor has been shown to be one of the biggest problems in drug-product stability. The sorption of water can have a pronounced effect on both the physical and chemical stability. Chemically, the presence of moisture usually enhances hydrolysis and subsequent alteration in active drug potency. Physically, moisture causes caking of powders, loss of effervescence, and accelerates the loss of physical cohesiveness of solid dosage forms. Moisture can also produce an environment which promotes mold and bacterial growth.

There are instances in which the presence of moisture is desirable, particularly in dermatological ointments and creams. This will be discussed under *Dehydration*, page 28.

Gases—In addition to water vapor, oxygen may pose a stability problem. Oxygen in the air can serve as the cause of oxidative deterioration in some products. Where this is a problem, antioxidants may be formulated in the product, or the space in the container above the product (the head space) may be purged free of air by adding nitrogen immediately before sealing. This latter method, of course, will no longer be effective after the package is initially opened for use.

Carbon dioxide in the air can affect some drugs by forming insoluble carbonates. This can occur with drugs in solution as well as on the surface of solids such as tablets or granules.

Temperature—Stability is influenced by temperature extremes. Chemically, heat can induce oxidation, polymorphic reversions, and decomposition of drug in a drug product. High temperatures may also accelerate physical changes. These changes may be due to sublimation from a solid, solvent loss from a solution, or chemical decomposition of dyes leading to color fading in solid and liquid dosage forms. The changes can also involve phase separation in emulsions, increased sedimentation in suspensions and ointments, increase in disintegration time of tablets, and the development of cracks in sugar-coated tablets.

Conversely, there are certain drugs which should not be exposed to low temperatures or freezing. Low temperatures, while not responsible for increased rates of chemical decomposition, can be responsible for physical changes in dosage forms which may affect therapeutic efficacy and product appearance. Some of these changes include crystal formation in solutions due to lowered solubility, phase separation in emulsions, increased sedimentation in suspensions, and crazing and cracking of sugar-coated tablets.

High temperature when combined with high relative humidity accentuates the potential for degradation. This can be associated with an increase in hydrolysis, tablets which tend to crumble prematurely or swell, and effervescent formulations which lose their capability of reacting in water.

Light—Light rays, especially in the ultraviolet region, can have adverse effects on drug products. These may lead simply to color fading which might affect product acceptance but not necessarily therapeutic efficacy. However, more serious changes can occur due to photodecomposition of susceptible components. Such an effect has been shown with phenothiazines, vitamin B_{12}, epinephrine, and others. For these reasons a number of drug products in the USP and NF are directed to be protected from light.

pH—An important factor to be considered in the formulation and dispensing of liquid drug products is the pH. Decomposition rates of many drugs are highly dependent on pH. Many products precipitate when mixed with other products which have different pH values. For example, the salt of a strong base and a weak acid will exhibit a relatively high pH in solution; if the pH is lowered significantly, the free acid may begin to precipitate. Similarly, the salt of a strong acid and a weak base may exhibit a low pH in solution; if the pH is raised significantly, the free base will begin to precipitate.

Barbiturates are weak acids with limited solubility in water. The salt forms are usually made from strong bases to increase aqueous solubility. Thus, Butisol Elixir (*McNeil*) contains butabarbital sodium and has a pH of 9.7; if it is mixed with another preparation which will significantly lower the pH, free butabarbital will begin to precipitate.

In institutional practice, pentobarbital sodium (basic pH) is sometimes mixed in a syringe with other drugs. With acidic drug products such as Phenergan (*Wyeth*) or Thorazine (*SK&F*), a haze or precipitate will usually develop within 1 hour due to formation of free pentobarbital which is less soluble in water than its sodium salt.

Microorganisms—Microbial growth also poses a stability problem. Bacterial or mold growth is undesirable from an esthetic point of view. Such growth can pose a therapeutic threat for two reasons: toxicity as a result of microbial ingestion and/or degradation of drug resulting in dosage impotency or toxic products. The obvious use of antimicrobial agents in parenteral drug products is well known and documented. However, one area of concern which has recently emerged is the microbial contamination of solid dosage forms such as lozenges. Using proper technique and good manufacturing practices, the appearance of undesirable microorganisms in pharmaceuticals should not pose a significant stability problem.

Complexation—Stabilization of ingredients present in a pharmaceutical preparation against hydrolysis, oxidation, and other forms of degradation may be accomplished by complex formation. Examples of the use of complexation to enhance drug stability are given in Table 12. Many of these examples involve the formation of molecular complexes in which the interaction of a labile functional group of a drug with a complexing agent may shield the drug from attack by other species present in

Table 12—Examples of Complexation To
Enhance Drug Stability

Stabilizer	Compound stabilized
Caffeine	Procaine, benzocaine, riboflavin, tetracaine
1-Ethytheo-bromine	Benzocaine
EDTA	Papaverine, morphine, procaine, phenylephrine, sulfacetamide sodium, ascorbic acid, antibiotics, epinephrine, prednisolone
Boric Acid	Epinephrine
Schardinger dextrin	Benzocaine
Polyvinyl-pyrrolidone	Hexylresorcinol
α,β-Dextrins	Vitamin A palmitate
Surfactants	Chlorobutanol, benzocaine, aspirin

solution, e.g., hydroxyl ions. In addition, the interaction may alter the usual electronic properties of the drug and result in either increased or decreased stability. Among the drugs which have been most extensively studied in this respect are the local anesthetic esters. These drugs have been stabilized against hydrolysis by complexation with caffeine and various macromolecules. For example, the half-life for procaine in solution has been observed to increase from 26 hours in the absence of caffeine to about 46 hours in the presence of 2% caffeine, and to about 71 hours in the presence of 5% caffeine. Similarily, the use of a boric acid–borax buffer has been shown to enhance both the stability and solubility of chloramphenicol in ophthalmic solutions, likely as a result of the formation of a 1:2 borax–chloramphenicol complex. Unfortunately, as previously discussed in use of complexation to enhance solubility, the dispensing pharmacist may have difficulty in applying these principles to the stabilization of extemporaneously prepared formulations since many of the stabilizing agents have intrinsic pharmacological activity. However, an understanding of these principles should enable the pharmacist to better evaluate stability claims made for commercially available preparations.

In addition to stabilization of labile drugs through interaction with other molecules, the use of chelating agents and surface-active agents have been studied with respect to their stabilizing properties. Metal ions are known to be involved in the oxidative degradation of a variety of drugs including epinephrine, phenothiazine, steroids, and vitamins, as well as certain colors, flavors, and other pharmaceutical additives. Since many degradation reactions are catalyzed by the presence of these heavy metals, it is not surprising the chelating agents such as EDTA may improve the stability of formulations containing these drugs. Surface-active agents can also protect certain labile drugs against degradation. The effectiveness of the particular surfactant will, however, be a function of the charge and the concentration of the surfactant, the type of degradation occurring, and the type of drug and its degree of ionization; thus, it is difficult to predict, *a priori,* the activity of an individual surfactant in a given system. For example, studies of the interaction of the hydroxyl–ion–mediated hydrolysis of chlorobutanol indicated enhanced stability of the labile trichloromethyl groups in the presence of certain nonionic surfactants, but not in the presence of polyethylene glycol 4000, even though both macromolecules interacted to some extent with the chlorobutanol. In a stability study of the ester benzocaine, it was observed that nonionic surfactants did decrease the hydrolytic degradation rate, but not nearly to the extent observed with the cationic and anionic surfactants. The ester was apparently incorporated into the palisade layers of the nonionic polyoxyethylene surfactant micelles. Due to the lack of charge and the degree of hydration of the surfactant, hydroxyl ions were still able to attack the ester, although with somewhat reduced ease. In contrast, the incorporation of the ester into micelles formed from cationic and anionic surfactants precluded attack by hydroxyl ion and the degradation rate was significantly reduced. At low concentrations the cationic surfactant slightly increased the degradation rate of the ester. This was due to the rather loose orientation of the micelle at low surfactant concentration, which permitted entry of the hydroxyl ion, and to the attractive force which the cationic portion of the surfactant had for the hydroxyl ion. Somewhat similar studies, involving the stabilization of aspirin by various surfactants, demonstrated that nonionized aspirin was stabilized against hydrolysis by anionic, cationic, and nonionic surfactants. However, ionized aspirin was observed to interact only with the cationic surfactants.

Solid State—Stability of drugs in the solid state has only been studied by a few investigators, and the basic mechanisms which contribute to degradation are not clearly understood. Vitamins have been shown to degrade in the solid state and both oil-soluble and water-soluble vitamins have been studied. Water-soluble drugs, in general, may undergo solid-state degradation in the presence of moisture. One proposed mechanism involves solution of drug dissolved in small amounts of moisture, which are sorbed layers and degradation is confined to this area. Aspirin has been shown to pose a stability problem in this regard. The presence of an acetic acid odor in aspirin or aspirin containing preparations indicates hydrolysis, probably the result of moisture being present. Salicylic acid can also form thin needlelike crystals in the container.

Another problem in solid-state stability deals with surface phenomena and photolysis of surface molecules. Color decay has been shown to be the results of photolysis of surface molecules in these drug products. Still another concern in solid-state stability deals with solid–solid interaction. Studies have been published which show that tablet excipients (so-called inert ingredients) are not inert. Excipients and other tablet ingredients are eligible to interact with active ingredients of dosage forms and may significantly alter their characteristics. Although these considerations exist primarily at the manufacturing level, the practicing pharmacist should be aware of any abnormal changes which occur in drug products.

Routes of Degradation

There are at least five important routes of drug degradation which influence dosage forms, their manufacture, and the practice of pharmacy. The practitioner should be aware of the major routes of drug degradation since they are important in looking at possible toxic reactions from degradation, can be a means for minimizing drug degradation and maximizing stability, and can explain basic mechanisms by which drugs degrade and provide insight in reviewing pertinent literature.

Oxidation—One of the most common pathways of drug degradation is oxidation. Epinephrine is a classic example and when oxidized

Epinephrine

Adrenochrome

turns a reddish-brown color. The institutional practitioner should be aware of this color change particularly in checking old drug cabinets or emergency carts which may not be often used. Oxidation has also been shown with vitamins including vitamin A, the tocopherols, and ascorbic acid. Terbutaline and amitriptyline have also been shown to undergo oxidative degradation under stress conditions in aqueous solution. Substances which contain unsaturated bonding (e.g., fats, essential oils, perfumes, and flavoring agents) can be extremely sensitive to oxidation. Many

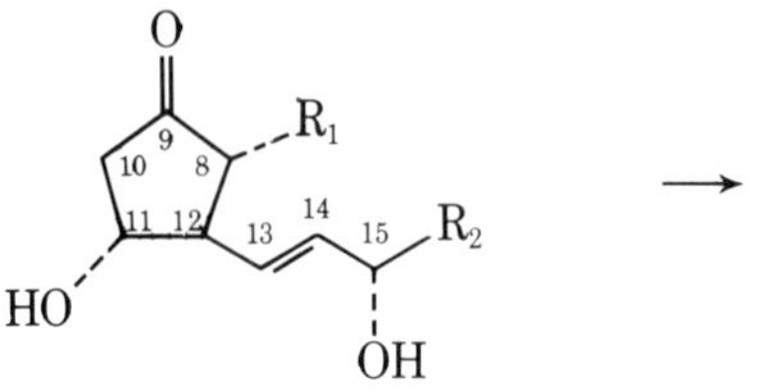

PGE

PGE$_1$: R$_1$ = (CH$_2$)$_6$COOH

      R$_2$ = (CH$_2$)$_4$CH$_3$

PGE$_2$: R$_1$ = CH$_2$CH=CH(CH$_2$)$_3$COOH

      R$_2$ = (CH$_2$)$_4$CH$_3$

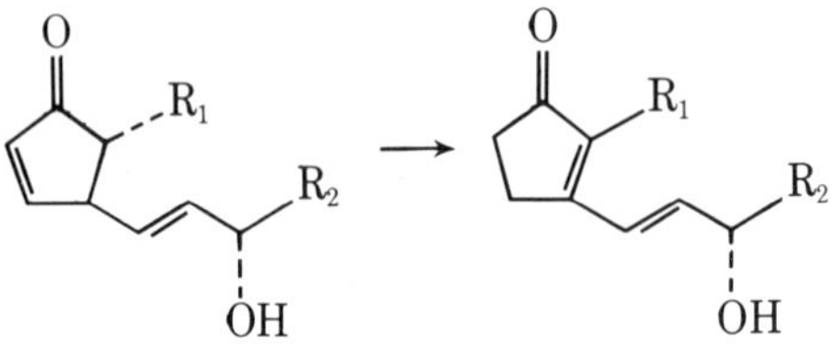

PGA   PGB

Fig. 8—Dehydration and isomerization of prostaglandins E$_1$ and E$_2$ (courtesy, *J Pharm Sci*).

times the oxidative product is extremely unsuitable and gives a characteristic rancid odor or unpleasant taste. This type of reaction is undesirable and materials suspected of having undergone these changes should be discarded.

Hydrolysis—Many drugs contain functional groups which readily undergo hydrolysis. A good example is the decomposition of aspirin in the presence of moisture:

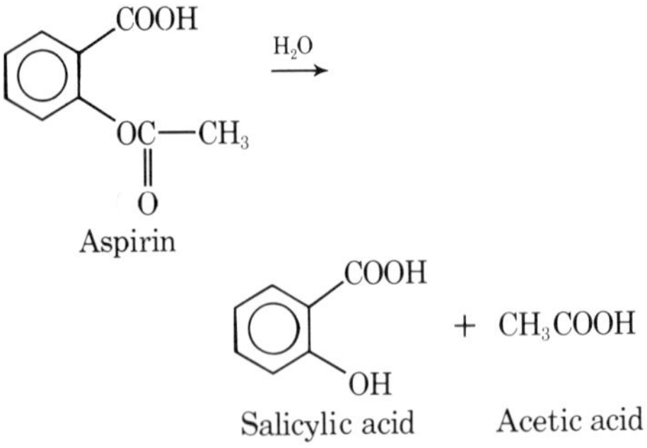

Aspirin

+ CH$_3$COOH

Salicylic acid   Acetic acid

Hydrolysis of aspirin to acetic acid and salicylic acid has been well documented. Therefore, simple aqueous solutions of aspirin are extremely unstable. Hydrolysis of other drugs such as cocaine, atro-

pine, meclofenoxate, barbiturates, erythromycin ethylsuccinate, sulfacetamide, rolitetracycline, benzocaine, corticosteroids, and metronidazole has also been shown.

Generally, kinetic rates of degradation via hydrolysis are changed directly and depend on pH. Thus, hydrolysis is usually catalyzed by either acid or base, depending on the structure and drug.

Dehydration—As has been pointed out previously, moisture is a source of many problems in stability. However, the removal of water from a drug molecule or a drug product can be detrimental and may be considered a route of drug degradation. This can occur in two basic ways: dehydration by desolvation (loss of bound moisture) and dehydration by removal of a proton and hydroxyl group. The former is particularly true with dermatological preparations in which a certain degree of moisture should be present. Ointments and creams may undergo irreversible damage if water is removed from their formulation. The cracking and crumbling of ointments and the caking and formation of suspension gels both adversely affect the stability of the product and are the direct results of dehydration. Dehydration is usually a result of exposure to extremes in environmental temperatures or low humidity, or simply aging and poor formulation. In dispensing suspensions and ointments which may have been previously opened it is important to confirm the consistency and assure that significant dehydration has not occurred.

Drugs which contain water of crystallization also may suffer detrimental effects from desolvation. Drugs which have been shown to degrade by this mechanism include theophylline monohydrate and ampicillin trihydrate.

Dehydration by loss of a proton and hydroxyl group has been shown with tetracyline and more recently with a new chemical class of drugs, the prostaglandins. Fig. 8 shows the dehydration and isomerization of prostaglandins E$_1$ and E$_2$. As these drugs take on greater clinical significance their degradative pathways will take on added importance.

Polymorphic Reversions—A polymorph is a solid crystalline phase of a drug resulting from the possibility of at least two different arrangements of molecules of that compound in the solid state. Some drugs have been shown to exist in more than one crystalline form and these are said to be polymorphic. Polymorphs usually belong to different crystalline systems and when one polymorphic form can change to another reversibly, it is said to be *enantiotropic;* if the transition takes place in only one direction, the change is said to be *monotropic.* Carbon and sulfur may exist in more than one crystalline form and nearly all long-chain organic compounds, especially fatty acids and glycerides, exhibit polymorphism. For a drug to be classified as polymorphic it must exist in different crystalline structures in the solid state but be identical in the liquid and vapor states; thus, polymorphism is the ability of any element or compound to crystallize as more than one distinct crystal species.

Various polymorphs of a given compound are often different in certain properties. Polymorphs of the same compound can exhibit different solubility rates, melting points, hardness, crystal shape, optical or electrical properties, and other physical characteristics. Polymorphism has special significance in the case of slightly soluble drugs where the dissolution rate can be drastically affected. One polymorph may be much more therapeutically active than another if the dissolution rates are different. This has been substantiated by much laboratory and clinical investigation.

Polymorphic reversions are common in cocoa butter (theobroma oil) suppositories. Theobroma oil is capable of existing in four polymorphic forms each having a different melting point. Cocoa butter suppositories prepared by fusion will sometimes liquefy and crystallize into a metastable form which melts at about 23°C. A polymorph of theobroma oil thus formed melts at room temperature, making the suppository impossible to insert.

In preparing physically stable drug products, polymorphism plays an important part in crystal growth and caking of suspensions, creams, and ointments. Due to an improper drug polymorph, phase conversion from the metastable to stable polymorph can occur. This may produce crystal growth resulting in undesirable dosage forms and problems in availability, including caking suspensions which cannot be resuspended easily by shaking. Examples of drugs which exhibit polymorphism are novobiocin, chloramphenicol, ampicillin, methylprednisolone, hydrocortisone, fluprednisolone, various sulfonamides, and barbiturates.

Racemization and Epimerization—The conversion of an optically active compound (one that rotates the plane of polarized light) into its optically inactive form is known as *racemization.* The resultant mixture of equal quantities of dextro- and levorotatory isomers is without effect on plane-polarized light due to external compensation. Racemization can occur from instability and is often the result of resonance, enolization, substitution, or elimination of groups, in which the asymmetry needed to maintain optical activity is destroyed. Thus, a racemic mixture is one which is optically inactive and results from the equal mixing of optical enantiomorphs.

If the enantiomorphs possess different degrees of physiological action, which can be the case, a change in therapeutic response can be expected. A classic example is the biological activity of *l*-epinephrine compared to *d*-epinephrine. The enantiomer, *l*-epinephrine, has been shown to be approximately 15–20 times more active physiologically than *d*-epinephrine. Therefore, racemic mixtures containing equal parts of *l*- and *d*-epinephrine have a reduced pharmacological activity compared to the pure *l*-form. More recently, several anesthetics such as mepivacaine and

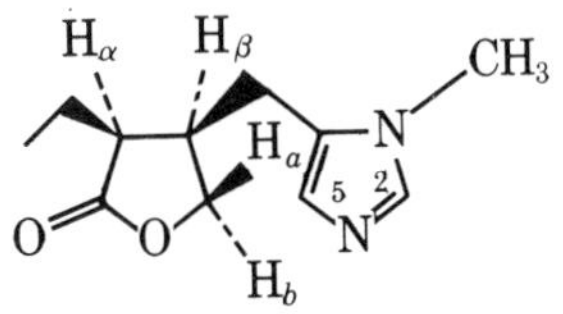

Fig. 9—Pilocarpine (I) epimerization forming isopilocarpine (II) (courtesy, *J Pharm Sci*).

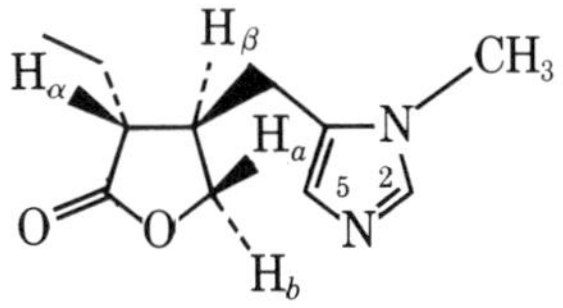

bupivacaine have been shown to undergo racemization.

Epimers are compounds having the same configuration on all but one carbon atom. They are isomers which differ only in the relative positions of an attached H or OH. Tetracycline epimerizes in solution to epitetracycline which has little or no antibacterial activity. Fig. 9 shows the structure of pilocarpine (I) which can epimerize to isopilocarpine (II). This epimerization also results in loss of pharmacological activity.

Reactions such as these are pH-dependent and catalyzed by acids and bases. Optimum conditions for formulation and storage can be predicted from stability studies.

Summary

It is the pharmacist's responsibility to help insure that drugs under his supervision meet acceptable levels of stability. There are some simple techniques which the pharmacist should master to meet his responsibilities regarding the stability of drugs and drug dosage forms. Some of these responsibilities have been discussed in scientific context; however, practical recommendations should be mentioned. Stability plays an important role in the delivery of quality pharmaceutical services to the patient. The USP includes a section on stability in dispensing.[6]

The pharmacist should rotate his stock and be constantly aware of expiration dates to prevent the dispensing of products that have expired. The pharmacist can usually assure this does not happen by dispensing older stock first and continually monitoring expiration dates on drug products, particularly parenterals and biologicals.

The pharmacist must identify products which are designed to be stored under various environmental conditions. The word *refrigerate* should signal a red flag that stability may be a problem with this product and it must be kept under the recommended storage conditions until the expiration date.

If the product is light-sensitive, it must be protected from light, for example, in drawers or cabinets that do not have windows. Generally, excesses in any environmental conditions such as heat, cold, or light (including fluorescent lighting) should be avoided.

The pharmacist has a continuing responsibility to observe products carefully for evidence of degradation, recalling the most common chemical changes occur from hydrolysis, oxidation, and photolysis. Physical changes leave telltale evidence, often more exaggerated than chemical changes. Alterations in color or odor, and the formation of precipitates or cloudiness in solutions should be carefully scrutinized by the practitioner as he dispenses medication. Most changes in physical characteristics are signs of instability and such dosage forms should not be dispensed.

When repackaging or mixing one drug product with another, it is a good policy to mimic the manufacturer as much as possible. If a tightly closed, amber glass bottle was used originally, any repackaging should be done in a similar manner and dispensed in a similar bottle. Special attention should be given to mixtures of parenteral products as in the case of intravenous solutions and IV-admixture programs (see Chapter 10).

Lastly, the pharmacist has a continuing responsibility to educate the public as to the stability of the drugs he dispenses. The pharmacist should tell the patient if a prescription is intended to be stored in a cool place not to store it in the bathroom. Bathrooms traditionally suffer from high temperature and high humidity and are usually a bad place to store medication. The pharmacist should be extremely cognizant of expiration dates as they apply to dispensed medication and point these out to the patient. Auxiliary labeling should highlight expiration dates so that no drug will be used after the manufacturer has declared it unsuitable. Patients should be encouraged to discard older medication, including nonprescription drugs.

Many patients ask practitioners, "Is this medication still all right to use?" Patients should be counseled to an awareness that prescriptions dispensed by the pharmacist are not good forever. In addition, the concept behind the prescription (i.e., a particular medication for a particular patient for a particular condition at this particular time) should be kept in mind.

Packaging and Storage

A drug product may become a useless and even hazardous therapeutic agent if it reacts with packaging materials or decomposes because of improper storage. This may happen regardless of how well it is formulated, manufactured, and tested or how sophisticated the technology applied by the pharmaceutical manufacturer may be.

Drug products are subjected to extremes in storage conditions as they move in commerce from manufacturer to consumer. Therefore, since manufacturers are highly concerned about maintaining the integrity of their products, they are cognizant of the need to package them properly and to store them in the proper environment. The consumer, however, is not always aware of these needs. Accordingly, the pharmacist who is the key professional in the distribution chain has the duty to inform the patient concerning proper storage, ex-

pected shelf-life, expiration date, and common external signs of product deterioration. He also has the responsibility to select containers for repackaging that will not hasten deterioration or interact with the drug product.

Storage

The effect of storage environment on stability is well known and has been discussed previously. Extremes of environment have been used to accelerate aging of drug products in order to predict stability at normal temperatures as well as to determine actual long-term stability at the extremes. The experimental environmental conditions usually include exposure to extremes of temperature, relative humidity, light, and various gases.

High temperatures are, of course, known to accelerate the rate of chemical reactions and, consequently, temperature control within specified limits is a means of controlling the stability of the active chemical principles in drug products. Containers will not generally serve as a protective barrier from the ravages of temperature extremes. However, the increased volatility and subsequent loss of product components that can occur at high temperatures can be reduced by proper choice of container.

High relative humidity increases the potential for hydrolysis of susceptible drugs and often induces physical changes in solid dosage forms, as has been mentioned previously. These deleterious effects can be diminished by proper container choice and with desiccants such as silica gel.

In the normal storage history of a drug product, few gases, other than water vapor, present a problem relative to stability. Oxygen in the air can serve as the cause of oxidative deterioration in some products. Where this is possible, antioxidants are frequently formulated in the product and are sometimes incorporated within the package liner. Other gases can be encountered in drug shipping or warehousing. Noxious vapors such as chlorine, ammonia, and

Table 13—Compendial Storage Temperature Definitions

Cold—Any temperature not exceeding 8° (46°F). A refrigerator is a cold place in which the temperature is maintained thermostatically between 2° and 8° (36° and 46°F). A freezer is a cold place in which the temperature is maintained thermostatically between −20° and −10° (−4° and 14°F).

Cool—Any temperature between 8° and 15° (46° and 59°F). An article for which storage in a cool place is directed may, alternatively, be stored in a refrigerator, unless otherwise specified in the individual monograph.

Room Temperature—The temperature prevailing in a working area. Controlled room temperature is a temperature maintained thermostatically between 15° and 30° (59° and 86°F).

Warm—Any temperature between 30° and 40° (86° and 104°F).

Excessive Heat—Any temperature above 40° (104°F).

Protection from Freezing—Where, in addition to the risk of breakage of the container, freezing subjects a product to loss of strength or potency, or to destructive alteration of the dosage form, the container label bears an appropriate instruction to protect the product from freezing.

---

gasoline engine exhaust fumes can have a deleterious effect on the flavor and aroma of a drug product and hence affect its patient acceptance.

Storage and Packaging Requirements—The detrimental effects of improper packaging and storage are recognized by the manufacturer, the pharmacist, and the official compendia. This recognition has led to the establishment of official restrictions for storage and definitions of storage environments and containers. The compendial restrictions regarding storage and their definitions appear in Table 13. These are taken from the USP and NF and differ somewhat from those formerly official.

Although the term "cool place" has a specific compendial definition (which for all practical purposes in a pharmacy means a refrigerator), it is used by many manufacturers who do not define it by compendial standards. This leads to confusion as to the appropriateness of storage conditions for the products of these manufacturers. Pharmacists should seek clarification of these terms when they are improperly used and request that these manufacturers make changes in their labeling.

In addition to these general terms used to restrict storage environments, the compendia state specific restrictions in certain individual drug monographs applicable to particular drug products.

While there are no compendial statements directly affecting the protection of a substance from vapor attack or loss, such protection is affected by the application of the officially defined limitations for containers. See *Compendial Definitions for Containers.*

Containers for drug products can be selected to assure protection of the drug product from only certain of the environmental factors mentioned such as light and vapors, but not from heat. Insofar as factors which can be controlled are concerned, the container provides an immediate local environment for the drug product which can markedly differ from the environment surrounding the container. Additionally, the choice of container is governed by the potential for loss of a drug-product component by passage outward through the container. Volatile components such as flavors, perfumes, solvents, preservatives, and some active ingredients can migrate from the drug product and thus alter its character.

The choice of container is obviously a major factor affecting drug stability since the container must (1) protect against adverse effects of the environment and (2) prevent loss of drug product components.

Packaging

The increasing concern for proper drug storage and packaging that has evolved through the years can be followed by examining past editions of the official compendia. Following adoption of standards for containers and storage, there has been a steady increase in the stringency of these standards.

Compendial Definitions for Containers—The container is the device that holds the drug and that is or may be in direct contact with the drug. The immediate container is that which is in direct contact with the drug at all times. The closure is a part of the container.

Prior to its being filled, the container should be clean and, except in the case of containers for liquids, dry. Special precautions and cleaning procedures may be necessary to ensure that extraneous particulate matter is not introduced into the drug.

The container does not interact physically or chemically with the article placed in it so as to alter the strength, quality, or purity of the drug beyond the official requirements.

The USP requirements for the use of specified containers apply also to articles as packaged by the pharmacist, unless otherwise indicated in the individual monograph.

Light-Resistant Container—Protects the contents from the effects of light by virtue of the specific properties of the material of which it is composed, including any coating applied to it. Alternatively, a clear and colorless or a translucent container may be made light-resistant by means of an opaque covering, in which case the label of the container bears a statement that the opaque covering is needed until the contents have been used. An example of this stipulation is seen in the case of Aldomet tablets (*MSD*). Where it is directed to "protect from light" in an individual monograph, storage in a light-resistant container is intended.

Well-Closed Container—Protects the contents from extraneous solids and from loss of the drug under the ordinary or customary conditions of handling, shipment, storage, and distribution.

Tight Container—Protects the contents from contamination by extraneous liquids, solids, or vapors, from loss of the drug, and from efflorescence, deliquescence, or evaporation under the ordinary or customary conditions of handling, shipment, storage, and distribution, and is capable of tight re-closure. Where a tight container is specified, it may be replaced by a hermetic container for a single dose of a drug.

A gas cylinder is a metallic tight container designed to hold gas under pressure. As a safety measure, for carbon dioxide, cyclopropane, ethylene, helium, nitrous oxide, and oxygen, the Pin-index Safety System of matched fittings is recommended for cylinders of Size E or smaller.

Hermetic Container—Impervious to air or any other gas under the ordinary or customary conditions of handling, shipment, storage, and distribution.

Single-Unit Container—Designed to hold a quantity of drug intended for administration as a single dose promptly after the container is opened. Preferably, the immediate container and/or the outer container or protective packaging shall be so designed as to show evidence of any tampering with the contents.

Single-Dose Container—A single-unit container for articles intended for parenteral administration only. A single-dose container is labeled as such. Examples are disposable syringes, prefilled syringes, cartridges, fusion-sealed containers, and closure-sealed containers when so labeled.

Unit-Dose Container—A single-unit container for articles intended for administration by other than the parenteral route as a single dose, direct from the container. Each unit-dose container shall be labeled to indicate the identity, quantity and/or strength, name of the manufacturer, and lot number of the article.

Multiple-Unit Container—Permits withdrawal of successive portions of the contents without changing the strength, quality, or purity of the remaining portion.

Multiple-Dose Container—A multiple-unit container for articles intended for parenteral administration only.

While the rather simple definitions given above for "tight" or "well-closed" containers have long appeared in the compendia, it is only in the current USP and NF that the standards of a quantitative nature have been established. These standards are based on a determination of moisture permeation into *multiple-unit* containers. The methods for determining compliance to standards are such that they may be performed in any pharmacy. It is the intent of the compendia to establish similar standards for unit-dose containers and packaging materials.

Packaging Materials

Through the years, many different materials have been used to fabricate containers for drug products. Today, most drug containers are composed of the following materials, singly or sometimes in combination: paper, metal, glass, and plastic.

Paper—Paper is used in fabricating drug containers ranging from the envelopes used by a dispensing physician to hold a few tablets to the fiber drums used by a manufacturer to hold thousands. Envelopes and boxes have, of course, long been used by pharmacists for prescription packaging as well as for nonprescription drugs. However, few, if any, of the paper containers sold to pharmacists or used by physicians offer suitable protection against moisture or oxygen.

It is possible to modify paper by coating it with plastic, foil, waxes, or other material to improve its barrier properties. In such cases, however, the coating material rather than the paper provides the protection. Such specialized types of paper and paperboard containers may be used by the pharmaceutical industry but are generally not available to community pharmacists.

This does not infer that paper may not be used for packaging drugs dispensed on prescription but its use should be based on a knowledge of the stability of the drug involved and an appreciation for the storage conditions likely to be experienced.

Metal—Metal containers have had greatest use in pharmaceutical packaging in the form of collapsible tubes for ointments and shaker cans for dusting powders. Pressurized packages of metal are also employed for aerosol products.

Collapsible metal tubes provide good product protection from atmospheric conditions and at the same time provide convenience and economy for the consumer. They are also a more sanitary package for ointments since only the extruded product is exposed to contamination rather than the entire contents, i.e., with wide-mouth ointment jars.

Full tubes can be labeled easily and adequately and they present an appealing appearance. However, they may be easily punctured unless carefully overwrapped. Also, during use, as they collapse, their labeling usually can become less legible and their appearance suffers as does their ease of storage.

Metal tube manufacturers generally use three metals: aluminum, tin, and lead. Aluminum in the form of an alloy of about 99% purity is the material most commonly used today. It produces light, strong tubes which may be conveniently labeled by a direct printing process.

Tin tubes are also light, stronger than aluminum, and less reactive, characteristics that make them desirable for ointments where aluminum incompatibility is a problem.

Lead and lead alloys are not used for pharmaceuticals because of the hazards of lead poisoning. Tin-coated lead or lined tubes of lead alloys may be used for some ointments but their use is dwindling.

Glass—Containers made of glass are the ones most commonly used in the pharmaceutical industry. It is the only packaging material in use for all dosage forms from bulk powders to parenteral solutions. There are many reasons for the widespread use of glass containers, including the four following ones.

Inertness—Although the alkalinity of glass can sometimes present problems with pharmaceutical solutions, glass in comparison with other packaging materials may be considered inert and free from incompatibilities. The choice of glass type can obviate the problem of alkalinity for a given application. The USP recognizes four types of glass and describes tests and limits for the chemical resistance of each. The four types are: Type I, a highly resistant, borosilicate glass; Type II, a treated soda-lime glass; Type III, a soda-lime glass; and Type NP, a general purpose soda-lime glass. Types I, II, and III are intended for packaging parenteral products while Type NP is intended for nonparenteral products, i.e., those intended for oral or topical use.

Visibility—The clarity of glass allows for product recognition and eye appeal. This advantage may diminish somewhat when light protection for a product dictates the use of a colored glass which blocks the passage of light rays.

Stability—Glass itself does not deteriorate under extremes of environment and it protects drugs from some of the environmental factors which may hasten their decomposition.

FDA Acceptance—Glass containers are permitted for use in packaging all pharmaceuticals. Indeed any other packaging material proposed by a manufacturer is tested in comparison with glass as the standard before it can be used for drug packaging.

There are some disadvantages to glass containers, the most obvious of which is their fragility. This necessitates care and added expense when

Table 14—Properties of Plastic Container Materials[7]

Material	Acrylic multipolymer	Polyethylene — Low density	Polyethylene — High density	Propylene-modified polyvinyl chloride	Polystyrene and compounds	Polyvinyl chloride
Resin density	1.09–1.14	0.92	0.95–0.96	1.35–1.42	1.0–1.1	1.2–1.4
Permeability to:						
Water vapor	High	Low	Very low	Low	High	Moderate to low
Alcohol	High	Low	Low	Low	Moderate	Low
Oxygen	Low	High	Moderate	Low	High	Low
Mineral oil	Low	High	Moderate	Very low	Moderate	Very low
Petroleum distillates	Low to high	High	High	Low	High	Very low
Resistance to impact	Poor to good	Excellent	Good	Poor to excellent	Poor to good	Poor to excellent
Chemical attack resistance[a]	Fair	Good	Good	Good	Poor	Good
Clarity of natural material	Clear to opaque	Milky transparent	Milky translucent	Clear to opaque	Clear to opaque	Clear to opaque
FDA grades available	Yes	Yes	Yes	Yes	Yes	Yes

[a] Depends on various factors such as product, temperature, and use.

packing and shipping whether they are empty or filled with medication. Glass weighs more than plastic and other materials, a characteristic which also contributes to increased shipping expense. Thicker walls are required for glass bottles than for plastic containers; this increases the volume (or cube) of the package, which is another disadvantage with regards to shipping and storage.

Plastic—The use of plastics for packaging drug products began to increase dramatically during the period following 1965. This increase was largely due to the variety of plastics available and their adaptability to many package forms such as bottles, boxes, pouches, syringes, and tubes. Other advantages of plastics include reduced weight, cube, and fragility of containers, as well as consumer appeal.

Acceptance of plastics by the pharmaceutical industry and the FDA did not come easily because of the many potential and actual problems when drugs are in contact with these materials. These problems have been divided into five broad categories: (1) *permeation*, (2) *leaching*, (3) *sorption*, (4) *chemical reaction*, and (5) *alteration or stability of the material*. In some cases the problems can be predictably avoided by a knowledge of the physical properties of the plastic and the chemical stability of the drug product. Table 14 compares some of the properties of plastics commonly used in bottle manufacturing.

The USP describes test procedures for plastic containers. These are both biological and physiochemical in nature. The biological test procedures are designed to test the suitability of plastic materials used to package or administer parenteral products. Physiochemical tests are used to determine extractable material in the plastic.

Both types of tests are supplemented by actual product compatibility tests under extremes of environments to assure both the chemical and physical stability of the drug product. Such testing procedures have been carried out extensively in the pharmaceutical industry.

Closures

Container closures are usually fabricated of metal or plastic with liners of various other materials usually combined in a laminate. The closure or cap does not generally contact the product in the container. However, the closure lining does and some attention must be given to its composition to assure that, like the container, it does not react with the contents. Vinyl-coated paper pulp is the type of liner used most often in drug packages, especially in prescription containers used by pharmacists.

In some instances a waxed-paper inner liner may be used by a manufacturer to serve as a tamperproof seal which may afford some extra measure of product protection. Extra protection against water vapor has also been shown to occur with the use of laminated paper-foil-polyethylene inner seals with both polyethylene and glass bottles.

Specialized closures (dispensing closures) have been designed to increase the convenience of product removal and use. Examples are the dropper-tip closure on ophthalmic solution bottles, the glide-on and roll-on closures used for antiperspirants and some liniments, the sifter tops used for dusting powders, and the push-pull closure used for viscous lotions packaged in squeeze bottles.

Attention has also been given to the design of closures which deter easy removal of product. These are the "safety closures" or "child-proof" caps intended to reduce the incidence of accidental poisoning of children with drugs and other toxic products. A number of types of these closures have been designed, evaluated, and marketed over the years for use on prescription containers.

Few of these closures found widespread voluntary usage and acceptance by pharmacists or consumers. It required an act of Congress in 1970 to give acceptance to safety closures. This legislation began with requirements for aspirin-containing products, extended to controlled drugs, and finally in 1974 was extended to all oral prescription drug products, with few exceptions.

The law requires the use of child-proof closures for oral dosage forms unless the prescriber or patient makes a request to the contrary. There has been some controversy as to the appropriateness of the pharmacist making this option known to the patient. Clearly, when the use of these closures presents an inconvenience to an infirmed patient and when there are no children in the household, the option should be mentioned. The alternative solutions used by these patients (i.e., leaving the cap off or transferring drugs to inappropriate containers) are probably more hazardous and more detrimental to the drug product.

The use of these containers, even if universal, should not obviate the need for storage of drugs and all toxic substances in locked locations out of the reach of children. No closure or container can be as effective in preventing poisoning as inaccessibility of the poison.

Unit-Dose Packaging

A unit-dose package contains an ordered amount of a drug in a dosage form ready for administration to a particular patient by the prescribed route at the prescribed time. A single-unit package is one which contains one discrete pharmaceutical dosage form, e.g., one tablet, one capsule, or a 5-ml quantity of an oral liquid. A single-unit package becomes a unit-dose package when the physician happens to order that amount of drug for a patient.

Unit-dose packages are unique and of interest not simply because of their departure from conventional drug packaging but because they allow the implementation of an improved drug-distribution system. Thus far the unit-dose system has found primary applications in hospitals; however, some community pharmacists who provide pharmaceutical services to extended-care facilities find it applicable in their practice also.

The system essentially is a method for distribution, administration, and charging of medication which is at all times properly labeled, packaged, and "patient-ready" up to the point of administration.

Advantages of the system are that the medication is always identifiable, medication errors are decreased, contamination due to handling is eliminated, "pouring" time of nurses is eliminated, and drug inventories may be more closely controlled.

Disadvantages are related to problems of space, standardization, availability, and cost. The storage of drugs packaged as unit doses requires more space since the packaging material increases the bulk of the dosage form. Unit-dose packages commercially available are quite variable in size, shape, labeling format, and packaging material. This further complicates space and storage problems. Some manufacturers are reluctant to supply their products in unit-dose packages until the unit-dose distribution system is more widely accepted. The lack of commercially available unit-dose packages has not deterred some hospitals who package their own medications in patient-ready forms within the hospital. Equipment to carry out this type of packaging for oral solids, liquids, and injectables is readily available and relatively easy to use. The last disadvantage, that of cost, is real even if consideration is only given to the additional cost of packaging. The cost factor is reduced to a more favorable level, however, if the reduction in nursing time is calculated and also, if the incalculable worth of increased patient safety due to decreased medication errors is considered.

An additional safety consideration may be given this type of packaging if it is used for drugs with high accidental poisoning potential such as children's aspirin and barbiturates. A unit-dose package is a difficult one for children to open and when opened makes available only one tablet for ingestion.

While unit-dose packaging is seldom used in the normal course of community practice, a related type of packaging is seen consisting of packages containing a dosage regimen of a drug which is supplied as such by the manufacturer and which does not require repackaging by the pharmacist. The most notable examples of drugs so packaged are the oral contraceptives. They come packaged in amounts required for a month's use (or multiple thereof) in containers designed to remind the patient of the proper dosage scheduling.

The use of such mnemonic dispenser packaging is slowly extending to other drug products and has been shown in at least one study to improve patient compliance with a medication regimen. Examples commercially available include antibiotics, hypoglycemics, diuretics, synthetic thyroid products, and corticosteroids.

Container Selection

When dispensing medications, the pharmacist is responsible for selecting a proper container. His selection should be made based on his knowledge of the stability of the drug product, properties of the container, patient safety and convenience, and legal requirements.

Both official and manufacturer's requirements can be obtained easily from the official compendia and labeling, respectively. Patient safety and convenience are also parameters which are easily appreciated by the pharmacist.

Another example of legal requirements, in addition to that cited in reference to child-resistant containers, is that attached to the dispensing of nitroglycerin tablets.

The extremely volatile nature of this product and studies on its stability in various containers has led to rather stringent requirements for its packaging and dispensing.

These requirements limit the dispensing container to the original, unopened container supplied by the manufacturer. The container must be glass and have a metal screw-cap. Further, the number of tablets/container may not exceed 100. It should be noted that these requirements apply to the so-called stabilized nitroglycerin formulations as well as those with no indication of enhanced stability.

It is unfortunate that pharmacists do not make more use of collapsible tubes in packaging ointments. Tubes make the use of ointments much more convenient and sanitary for the patient; however, they are inconvenient for the pharmacist to fill. Their lack of ready availability, when compared to ointment jars, also probably contributes to their infrequent use by pharmacists.

Frugality should be abandoned relative to container selection for medication dispensing. Many pharmacists, perhaps remembering leaner times, find it difficult to discard old bottles. A great deal of time is frequently spent attempting to render old bottles fit for reuse. However, there is seldom any guarantee that residue of the previous contents is not still present to contaminate the future contents of these bottles. It is not too farfetched to imagine an allergic reaction of a patient to some unknown residue. Because of the very real likelihood of such an occurrence, the reuse of old bottles is a habit to be condemned.

For the same reason the reuse in prescription packages of cotton headspace filler from bulk containers of tablets or capsules, should likewise be condemned.

The outward appearance of the prescription drug package is the only tangible basis for the patient's judgment of a pharmacist's care and skill. It should, accordingly, be a point of pride with pharmacists to dispense prescriptions whose appearance bespeaks this care and skill.

References

1. Reproduced from Documenta Geigy Scientific Tables by permission of J. R. Geigy S. A., Basle, Switzerland; from the formula of DuBois and DuBois, *Arch Intern Med 17:*863, 1916.
2. Shinoda K, Nakagawa T, Tamamushi B, Isemura T: *Colloidal Surfactants,* Academic, New York, 135–142, 1963.
3. Patel NK, Kostenbauder HB: *JAPhA Sci Ed 47:*289, 1958.
4. Bakley EL: *Am Perf Aromat 73:*33, 1959.
5. Lachman L. *Bull Parent Drug Assoc 22:*127, 1968.
6. Stability considerations in dispensing practice. *USP XIX,* Mack Publ. Co., Easton, PA, 707, 1975.
7. *Modern Packaging Encyclopedia,* McGraw-Hill, New York, 268, 1970.

Bibliography

Review Manual of Patient Record Systems, APhA, Washington, DC, 1975.
Office of Technology Assessment Report on Bioavailability, USGPO, Washington, DC, 1974.
Rodowskas CA Jr: *JAPhA NS 13:*8, 1973.
Martin AN, Swarbrick J, Cammarata A: *Physical Pharmacy,* 2nd ed, Lea & Febiger, Philadelphia, 1969.
Remington's Pharmaceutical Sciences, 15th ed, Mack Publ. Co., Easton, PA, 1975.
Carstensen JT, Osadca M, Rubin SH: *J Pharm Sci 58:*549, 1969.
Cooper J, Rees JE: *Ibid 61:*1511, 1972.
Ho NFH, Goeman JA: *Drug Intel 4:*69, 1970.
Carstensen JT: *J Pharm Sci 63:*1, 1974.
Haleblian J, McCrone W: *Ibid 58:*911, 1969.
Chafetz L: *Ibid 60:*335, 1971.
Smart R, Spooner DF: *J Soc Cos Chem 23:*721, 1972.
Haleblian JK, Goodhart FW: *J Pharm Sci 64:*1085, 1975.
Parrett EL: *JAPhA NS 6:*73, 1966.
Autian J: *Drug Cos Ind 102:*47, 1968.
*Ibid:*54, 1968.
*Ibid:*79, 1968.
Palmer H, Di Cenzo R: *Mod Packaging 42:*111, 1969.
Chmielewski DH: *JAPhA NS 11:*16, 1971.
Linkewich JA, *et al: Drug Intel Clin Pharm 8:*10, 1974.
Edelman BA, *et al: JAPhA NS 1:*30, 1971.

2

Bioavailability

Werner Lowenthal, PhD
Professor of Pharmacy and
Professor of Educational
Planning and Development
School of Pharmacy
Medical College of Virginia
Virginia Commonwealth
University
Richmond, VA 23298

Bioavailability (biological availability, physiological availability) is a relatively new concept in drug therapy. In 1945, Oser, *et al,* recognized the need to determine the bioavailability of water-soluble vitamins in pharmaceutical products. The work was continued in 1954 by Campbell and his co-workers at the Food and Drug Directorate in Canada who published a series of articles on bioavailability of various drugs from different dosage forms. They considered an efficacious product as one where at least 70% of the drug is physiologically available. This can be considered the beginning of interest by pharmacists in the problems of bioavailability. The application of kinetic theory to drug studies dates back to Widmark in 1919, with more direct applications made by Teorell in 1937 and Dominguez in 1950. The current intense interest in the application of kinetics to bioavailability problems can be considered to have been initiated by Swintosky and co-workers in 1956 who showed the applicability of kinetics to drug delivery systems.

In this chapter, physiology, physical chemistry, and pharmaceutical technology will often be blended together. For example, the particle size of a drug (a physical characteristic) affects dissolution rate (a physicochemical characteristic), which may affect bioavailability (a pharmaceutical dosage form characteristic) and absorption (a physiological characteristic), which affects the final pharmacodynamic action of the drug. Even though this chapter is divided into sections, overlapping occurs because no fact should be taken alone, but all facts should be put into the context of a drug delivery system.

This chapter helps link together many of the chapters in this text. An understanding of bioavailability is particularly pertinent to the preparation of efficacious dosage forms, how they are compounded and dispensed, and the problems that may occur in these processes. In order to deliver safe and efficacious medication to the patient the pharmacist must be familiar with the full significance of the need to have medications become biologically available after they are administered. This chapter, therefore, discusses various dosage forms, interactions of ingredients within dosage forms, and interactions of the dosage forms within the body. To a limited extent biological (physiological) incompatibilities are mentioned as they affect bioavailability. Interactions among different drugs are covered in Chapter 13.

The biopharmaceutic characteristics of dosage forms are more important elements of the drug delivery system than taste, color, odor, and elegance because they determine its bioavailability and if the drug is delivered to the patient's blood stream.

Various terms used in discussing the biological availability of medications may be defined as follows:

1. **Biopharmaceutics**—The study of the factors influencing the extent and rate of absorption and release of a drug from its various dosage forms.

2. **Pharmacokinetics**—The study concerned with the kinetics of absorption, distribution, metabolism, and excretion of drugs. Pharmacokinetics can be considered a tool to quantify biopharmaceutics.

3. **Physiological Availability**—The per cent of drug absorbed into the blood stream from a given dosage form. It usually refers to a solid oral dosage form such as a capsule or tablet, and may be roughly expressed, according to one of its many definitions, as:

$$\frac{\text{Amount excreted in urine}}{\text{Amount administered}} = \text{fraction biologically available}$$

$$\frac{\text{Amount excreted in urine}}{\text{Amount excreted in urine from a standard preparation}} \times 100 = \text{relative availability}$$

The amount excreted in the urine includes unchanged drug plus that in the form of metabolites.

4. **Generic Name** (Nonproprietary Name)—The established or official name given to a drug and its dosage forms.

5. **Brand Name**—The registered trademarked name given to a drug and its dosage forms.

6. **Chemical Equivalents**—Those multiple-source drug products which contain the same amounts of the identical active ingredients, in identical dosage forms.

7. **Biological Equivalents**—Those chemical equivalents which, when administered in the same amounts, will provide essentially the same bioavailability.

8. **Clinical Equivalents** (Therapeutic Equivalents)—Those chemical equivalents which, when administered in the same amounts, will provide essentially the same therapeutic effect.

Physiological Factors

Physiological mechanisms concerned with bioavailability include drug absorption, distribution, storage, biotransformation, and excretion. The structures most intimately involved with these mechanisms are the epithelial cell and the various biological membranes.

The Epithelial Cell—The epithelial cells lining the serous cavities, whose linings secrete serum, and the inner surfaces of the blood and lymph vessels are flat and elastic and are held together by a cement-like substance. The skin consists of several layers of epithelial cells superimposed upon each other. It covers the outer surfaces of the body including the ear canal. The top layer or layers are mainly flat and scaly and are called stratified squamous epithelium. The epithelial covering in the mouth is similar to the skin but does not have as many layers. Similar stratified squamous epithelium lines the anus, intravaginal portion of the cervix, uterus, vagina, and vulva, anterior third of the nasal cavity, laryngeal parts of the pharynx and respiratory passages, alveoli, conjunctiva, and cornea. The internal surface of the stomach and intestine are lined by simple columnar epithelium (tall, column-like cells). Sometimes there are special cells which are ciliated, e.g., nose and respiratory passages, or which contain mucus and serous glands as in the nose, mouth, and gastrointestinal tract.

Biological Membranes—The three fundamental properties of biological membranes are:

1. The existence of low surface tension at their surface.

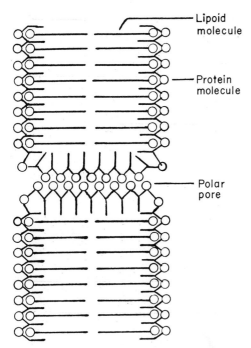

Fig. 1—Davson-Danielli model of membrane structure.[1]

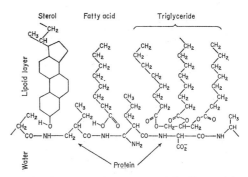

Fig. 2—A suggested arrangement for the protein and lipids in the Davson-Danielli model.[2]

2. Preferential permeability to lipid-soluble substances.

3. High electrical resistance.

These properties suggest that a biological membrane consists of lipids with a protein layer on the surface. The membrane covering the individual cell was shown to be composed of cholesterol, phospholipids, and protein. A membrane structure has been postulated which appears to fit most of the data, such as the lipoprotein barrier (bimolecular lipid leaflet) illustrated in Fig. 1. Fig. 2 shows a more detailed view. The polar groups of the protein are in roughly the same plane as those of the fatty molecules, and the hydrocarbon parts of the protein extend into the fatty layers. The upper limit of thickness of the lipid layer is 100 Å. Lipid solubility, molecular volume, specific chemical groupings, and position of the groups on the molecule affect penetration of the membrane. As can be seen in Fig. 1, the lipid molecules form a bimolecular layer with the hydrocarbon chains toward the center and perpendicular to the protein

molecules. Fig. 1 also shows an aqueous pore through which small, lipid-insoluble substances may pass. This model is too simple to explain the varied activities of the membrane and will be modified as our knowledge increases.

The membrane should also be considered as dynamic rather than inert. The protein covering may contain polysaccharides and proteins which are active sites and agents for constant modification. The amount and configuration of protein and lipid may vary depending on the required functions. In addition, calcium ions act as an adhesive in sticking cells together, increase rigidity of cytoplasmic surfaces, decrease ionization at the membrane, and reduce permeability.

Gastrointestinal Absorption and Transport across Membranes

Since the membrane through which all substances to be absorbed must pass consists of lipoproteins, a drug to be absorbed must be lipid-soluble and preferably nonionized.

Drugs may pass through oral and gastrointestinal membranes by one or more of the processes discussed under *Passive Transport* and *Active Transport*.

Passive Transport or Simple Diffusion—The characteristics of this process are:

1. The membrane acts as a lipoprotein barrier with charged and uncharged water-filled pores.

2. There is little or no energy expended by the body.

3. The rate of transport is proportional to the concentration gradient across the membrane.

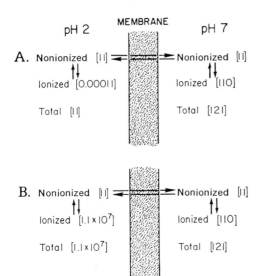

Fig. 3—*A*: Nonionized and ionized concentrations of a weak acidic drug with a pK_a of 6 in fluids with pH of 2 and pH of 7 separated by a membrane; *B*: nonionized and ionized concentrations of a weak basic drug with a pK_a of 8 under the same conditions as in *A*.

Aqueous soluble molecules may pass through the pores if the molecule size is smaller than that of the pores. If the pore is charged it attracts the molecules of the opposite charge and repels those of the same charge. Hydrostatic or osmotic pressure differences may exist to cause the flow of water through the membrane, e.g., glomerular filtration in the kidney. This causes water-soluble molecules of sufficiently small size to be "dragged" with the water.

pH   Partition   Theory—Ionizable drugs may distribute unequally because of pH differences or because of Donnan type of distribution. Donnan distribution occurs when a solution on one side of the membrane contains some ions (such as proteins) which cannot cross the membrane. This may cause transport of ions that can cross the membrane in order to equalize charge difference.

Simple diffusion through a membrane is probably the most common process by which drugs are absorbed in the body, regardless of the location of the membrane. Diffusion through the membrane depends on lipid solubility, as evidenced by lipid-water partition coefficients, and the degree of ionization of the drug. This latter property is affected by the pH of the fluids on both sides of the membrane and the pK_a of the drug. The nonionized molecule is more lipid soluble than the ionized form. The pH-partition theory was developed to explain the existing data on the absorption of drugs under varied conditions of pH and lipid solubility. This is important because most drugs are either weak acids or weak bases.

First, consider the pH effect alone. When the pH is different for the fluids on opposite sides of the membrane, e.g., the gastrointestinal tract fluid and the blood, the degree of ionization of either a weak acid or weak base differ in the fluids, resulting in different concentrations. The respective concentrations of the drug are functions of the pH's of the dissolving fluids and the pK_a of the drug, the significance of which is illustrated in Fig. 3.

A weakly acidic drug is thus transferred from an acid medium (pH 2) to a more alkaline one (pH 7) because of the greater concentration of the nonionized form in the acid medium. The weakly basic drug is highly ionized in the acid fluid so that relatively little is transferred. If the pH 2 fluid is gastric fluid and the pH 7 fluid the blood, weakly acidic drugs are well absorbed from the stomach and weakly basic drugs are poorly absorbed. In the intestinal tract the reverse will become true because the increasing pH in the intestine causes weak acids to be more highly ionized and weak bases more completely nonionized.

The reverse transfer from blood to gastric fluid can also occur depending on the pK_a of the weak acids and bases. This means weak bases which are not absorbed from the stomach, e.g., mecamylamine, are more readily transferred from plasma to gastric fluid than weak acids. Weak acids would tend to concentrate in alkaline fluids.

In the late 1950's a series of articles

nonionized to be absorbed

appeared to establish the pH-partition theory. It was found that in using rat stomach, containing 0.1 M HCl, acids with $pK_a > 2.3$ were well absorbed but strong acids were not absorbed. Bases with $pK_a > 2.5$ were poorly absorbed but bases with $pK_a < 2.5$ were moderately absorbed.

If the stomach contained 0.15 M NaHCO$_3$(pH 8), the absorption of acids decreased as pK_a decreased while the absorption of bases increased as the strength of the base decreased. In addition, absorption increased as the chloroform-water partition coefficient increased, as shown in Table 1. It was concluded that the gastric mucosa is selectively permeable to the undissociated drug form in animals and man.

In studies involving the rat intestine, absorption of weak acids was found to decrease as pH of the solution in the intestinal lumen increased. Absorption of weak bases from the intestinal lumen increased as the pH was increased. Highly lipid-insoluble drugs are generally poorly absorbed. Again, the intestinal mucosa is preferentially permeable to nonionized drugs. Acids with pK_a greater than 2.9 and bases with pK_a less than 8 were relatively rapidly absorbed from the rat intestine.

Other evidence showed that absorption from the stomach and intestine was by simple diffusion; i.e., the process was noncompetitive and nonsaturable.

The intestinal absorption of steroids decreased as polarity of the compound increased and as lipid solubility decreased.

In addition, tetracycline absorption, which occurs mainly in the intestine, is incomplete because of the formation of zwitter ions which are poorly lipid-soluble.

It was reported that weak acids with pK_a above 4.3 and weak bases with pK_a below 8.5 were generally absorbed rapidly from the colon. As the pH was decreased in the colonic lumen, absorption of acids which became more nonionized, increased; e.g., 12% salicylic acid was absorbed at pH 7 and 42% at

Table 1—Effect of Chloroform-Water Partition Coefficient on Gastric Absorption of Barbiturates[3]

	pK_a	% absorbed from 0.1 M HCl	K_{CHCl_3/H_2O}
Barbital	7.8	4	0.7
Secobarbital	7.9	30	23.3
Thiopental	7.6	46	100

pH 4. Absorption of basic drugs was also dependent on their degree of ionization, e.g., 20% quinine was absorbed at pH 7 and only 9% at pH 4. Comparing nine barbiturates with pK_a values of 7.4 to 8.1, it has been found, in general, that the greater the chloroform-water partition coefficient, the greater the absorption. The rapid absorption of some drugs from the colon explains the effectiveness of rectal administration.

A high oil-water partition coefficient also resulted in increased absorption from the oral mucosa. There may be an optimum coefficient because if the lipid solubility is too high the drug will not dissolve sufficiently in the aqueous salivary fluids.

It may be inferred from the previous discussion that the ratio of nonionized to ionized molecules is important in predicting sites of absorption in the gastrointestinal tract. In fact, a critical proportion of 1:200 for nonionized to ionized forms has been proposed for maximum absorption. The Henderson-Hasselbalch equation can be used to calculate the ratio of nonionized to ionized forms of acids and bases when pK_a of the drug and the pH of the fluid are known.

For acids:

$$pH = pK_a + \log \frac{[\text{Ionized acid}]}{[\text{Nonionized acid}]} \quad (1)$$

For bases:

$$pH = pK_a + \log \frac{[\text{Nonionized base}]}{[\text{Ionized base}]} \quad (2)$$

Fick's First Law of Diffusion—This law describes passive diffusion through an inert membrane. Since biological membranes are not inert, but dynamic systems, Fick's law is only an approximation. However, it helps to visualize some of the factors affecting transport of substance across a membrane. Fick's law indicates that the rate of diffusion is directly proportional to membrane surface area and the concentration gradient, and inversely proportional to the membrane thickness.

Active Transport—The characteristics of an active transport process are:

1. Involvement of membrane components.
2. Specificity for chemical structure.
3. Transport against a concentration gradient or electrochemical potential.
4. Prevention by metabolic poisons (interfere with cell metabolism).
5. Upper rate limit (saturable).
6. Expenditure of metabolic energy.
7. Functioning of a carrier mechanism.

Several foreign sugars, 5-fluorouracil, and 5-bromouracil are absorbed by active transport. Riboflavin may also be absorbed by this mechanism because the process appears to be saturable and site specific.

Facilitated diffusion has the above characteristics except that transport against concentration gradients does not occur and metabolic energy is not required.

Pinocytosis and Phagocytosis— These processes are characterized by engulfment of the substances by membrane movement and subsequent release. This involves the formation of invaginations and vesicles by the membrane. Trace amounts of protein, macromolecules, and fat droplets may be transported in this manner.

Summary of Absorption Theory— Absorption of drugs from the mouth, stomach, small intestine, and colon are strongly influenced by the following principles:

1. The canal from the oral cavity to the anus may be considered to consist of segments that are bounded by a continuous lipoidal barrier, with small aqueous pores and specialized transport systems in certain sites.
2. The rate of absorption is proportional to drug concentration and the drug lipid-water partition coefficient.

3. The rate of absorption is affected by the pH of the canal at the site of absorption and the pK_a of the drug. These control the degree of ionization of the drug and hence its lipid solubility. The nonionized species are more lipid soluble and appear preferentially absorbed. It should be remembered that ionic forms of the drug may be absorbed, possibly through the pores. Both ionic and nonionic forms of salicylate and pentobarbital have been reported to diffuse across the isolated mesenteric membrane. Although quaternary ammonium compounds are completely ionized at every physiological pH, they seem to be absorbed.

4. Weakly acidic drugs are nonionized in an acid pH. Therefore they are preferably absorbed from the stomach, and as the pH rises their rate of absorption decreases.

5. Weakly basic drugs are nonionized in a neutral or alkaline pH, hence are preferably absorbed from the intestinal tract. They are poorly absorbed from acidic fluids.

6. Most drugs are absorbed by passive diffusion because the process is not saturable.

Gastrointestinal Tract Physiology

Anatomy (Fig. 4)—The term membrane was used earlier in this chapter to indicate the outer covering of the cell, a thin coating structure 75–150 Å thick. Here, membrane, in the histological sense, includes the epithelium and underlying connective tissue. It varies in thickness (measured in mm) and toughness. For example, mucous membranes consist of surface epithelium, a basement membrane, and connective tissue.

The epithelial cells from the cardia of the stomach to the anus are similar except for specialized cells. In the intestine there are a series of folds which run across the lumen. The epithelial cells form villi and microvilli which increase the surface area in the intestine many thousands of times over what it would be if the lining were smooth. The microvilli are also the sites of hydrolytic digestion of carbohydrates and proteins and for active transport. In contrast, the surfaces of the gastric rugae and of the colon are smooth.

The position of the person modifies the size and shape of the stomach. It holds 1 to 1.5 liters of gastric juice containing 0.4–0.5% HCl (pH about 1.2), pepsin, mucus, and various inorganic monovalent and divalent anions and cations. The pH of gastric juice may be higher in the resting stomach and also increases with the age of an individual.

The intestine is divided into the duodenum (about 1 foot long), the jejunum (about 9 feet long), and the ileum (about 13 feet long). The surface area of the intestine is about 300 m². Enzymes like maltase, nuclease, and lipase are secreted by intestinal glands. Intestinal secretions have a pH of about 8.3. Pancreatic juice, which enters into the duodenum, contains amylase, lipase, trypsinogen, bicarbonate ions, and other enzymes and inorganic anions and cations. It has a pH of about 8. Bile also enters into the duodenum and contains cholesterol, lecithin, and sodium and potassium salts of bile acids (e.g., cholic acid, desoxycholic acid, chenodesoxycholic acid, and lithocholic acid) conjugated to glycine or taurine to form the corresponding bile salts (glycochenodesoxycholates, glycocholates, glycodesoxycholates, taurocholates, etc.). Bile acids are reabsorbed in the terminal portion of the ileum. In the liver the pH of the bile is 8–8.6, whereas in the gallbladder it is about 7 or perhaps slightly alkaline.

The colon is about 5 feet long, absorbs water, and secretes mucus. The rectum is structurally similar to the colon and the feces maintain a pH of about 7–7.5.

The first part of the meal and unabsorbed drug taken at meal time reach the cecum in about 4 hours and the entire meal enters the colon in 8–9 hours.

The ratio of ionized to nonionized species for a basic drug and the ratio of nonionized to ionized species for acidic drugs are given in Table 2. Aspirin with a pK_a of 3.5 and barbital with a pK_a of 7.6 are weak acids and antipyrine with a pK_a of 1.4 is a weak base.

Physiological factors other than pH can affect drug absorption. Bile or bile salts may increase the permeability of the intestine to drugs, increase the solubility or rate of solution of drugs, or help decrease agglomeration of powders. The mucus normally present in

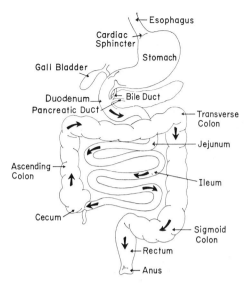

Fig. 4—The gastrointestinal tract.

the intestine may inhibit the absorption of drugs.

Another effect of physiological pH is the precipitation of an insoluble acidic drug in the stomach from an aqueous solution of its soluble salt. It has also been shown that the salt form of the drug generally results in higher blood levels than the administration of the acid form. This may be a particle size effect where the precipitated acid species has very small particle size that will redissolve rapidly as the nonionized form is absorbed. For example, potassium and calcium salts of penicillin V are more rapidly absorbed and give higher peak levels than penicillin V acid. Similar results could occur with soluble salts of other weak organic acids, e.g., barbiturates.

Table 2—Effect of pH on Ionization

pH of fluid	Aspirin[a]	Barbital[a]	Antipyrine[b]
1.2	200	2.5×10^6	1.59
3.6	0.794	10^4	0.00631
5.6	0.00794	100	6.31×10^{-5}
7.0	3.16×10^{-4}	3.98	2.5×10^{-6}
7.5	10^{-4}	1.26	7.94×10^{-7}

[a] Nonionized/ionized.
[b] Ionized/nonionized.

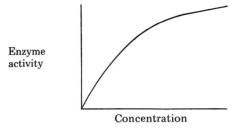

Fig. 5—Effect of substrate concentration on enzyme activity.

Enzymes and Drug Biotransformation

Enzymes and drug biotransformation (metabolism) are important components of bioavailability because:

1. Some drugs are biotransformed by enzymes in the gastrointestinal tract in a manner that affects absorption; e.g., hydrolysis of esters.
2. Enzymes detoxify drugs and modify their distribution in the body.
3. "Prodrugs" are biotransformed to pharmacologically active drugs; e.g., carbenicillin indanyl sodium is biotransformed to carbenicillin.
4. Bacteria develop resistance to anti-infectives, because the bacteria develop alternate metabolic pathways, so that the drugs are no longer effective.
5. Microorganisms can develop enzymes to detoxify drugs, e.g., penicillinase biotransforms penicillin.
6. One drug may enhance or inhibit the biotransformation of another drug. This is covered in Chapter 13.

Enzymes consist of protein only (pepsin, trypsin, etc.), protein plus a cation (carbonic anhydrase, alkaline phosphatase, etc.), or protein plus a nonprotein, low molecular weight organic compound called a coenzyme or prosthetic group (catalase, pyruvate oxidase, etc.). They are catalysts causing specific biochemical reactions to proceed faster and with less input of energy. The type and amount of enzyme required varies with the animal species, individual, sex, age, nutrition, and other factors. An enzyme may not develop until a few weeks after birth, reach a maximum during early adulthood, and decline with aging.

The following are examples of some of the types of biotransformation catalyzed by enzymes.

Hydrolysis:
De-esterification: Aspirin →
                      acetic acid + salicylic acid
Reduction:
(a) Chloral hydrate—$CCl_3CH(OH)_2$ →
                      $CCl_3CH_2OH + H_2O$
(b) Prontosil → sulfanilamide
Conjugation:
(a) *Glucuronide formation:* Salicylic acid + glucuronic acid → salicyl glucuronides
(b) *Glycinate formation:* Salicylic acid + glycine → salicyluric acid
Hydroxylation:
Salicylic acid → gentisic acid + 2,3-dihydroxybenzoic acid + 2,3,5-trihydroxybenzoic acid
Oxidation:
(a) *Aliphatic side chain:* Pentobarbital → 3-hydroxypentobarbital
(b) *Deamination:* Amphetamine → phenylacetone
(c) *Sulfoxidation:* Chlorpromazine → chlorpromazine sulfoxide

Enzyme Kinetics—The kinetic order of a reaction (see *Applied Pharmacokinetics*) may change as the concentrations change and products accumulate. A reaction involving an enzyme may initially be zero order when the substrate concentration is high (see the following) and then may become first order when the substrate concentration is low.

The following are factors affecting the rate of enzymatic reaction:

1. *Concentration of Substrate*—Above a certain concentration, the rate does not increase because all the enzyme is being used and reused at its maximum rate (e.g., see Fig. 5).
2. *Concentration of Enzyme*—The rate is proportional to enzyme concentration.
3. *Concentration of Reaction Products*—Reaction products may inhibit the rate of reaction because they form a more stable complex with the enzyme (see the following).
4. *Effect of pH*—Each enzyme has an optimum pH.
5. *Temperature*—The rate increases with temperature. For practical purposes, the temperature is constant because body temperature will be constant.
6. *Enzyme Poisons*—These are substances which will inactivate or inhibit enzymes; e.g., heavy metals, fluoride ion, iodine, and oxidizing agents. Drugs often inhibit an enzyme; e.g., atropine inhibits choline esterase, sulfanilamide inhibits carbonic anhydrase, and tranylcypromine inhibits monoamine oxidase (MAO).

Most enzyme kinetics are based on the work of Michaelis and Menton. The reaction used to describe enzyme activity is:

Enzyme + Substrate ⇌
    Enzyme-Substrate Complex →
        Enzyme + Products

or

$$E + S \underset{k_2}{\overset{k_1}{\rightleftharpoons}} ES \overset{k_3}{\rightarrow} E + P$$

where k_1, k_2, k_3 are the reaction rate constants.

The Michaelis–Menton equation is concerned with the effect of substrate concentration on reaction rate.

Enzyme systems are needed to biotransform drugs and this process may be competitive for similar drugs. For example, Levy and co-workers showed that the co-administration of salicylamide and sodium salicylate in humans results in decrease of the formation of the total glucuronides of the drugs. This may result in enhanced action.

Another aspect of enzyme activity can be seen with aspirin. As the dose of aspirin is increased from 250 mg to 2 g, the per cent drug excreted as salicyluric acid decreases and the per cents of salicylic acid and salicyl glucuronides increase. When the aspirin dose is small and the process is first order, the biological half-life ($t_{1/2}$) of salicylate is 2.9 hours. When the dose is so large that the formation of salicyluric acid is negligible, $t_{1/2}$ may be as high as 22 hours. Man has a limited capacity to form the salicyluric acid conjugate.

The rate of absorption can also affect the amount of drug biotransformed. Slow absorption may increase the amount biotransformed because the drug (substrate) does not saturate the enzyme system, e.g., salicylamide.

Renal Elimination

The kidneys are the major organ for drug elimination from the body. Its unit, composed of a glomerulus and tubules, is called a nephron (see Fig. 6). There are about 2 million nephrons in the two human kidneys with about 40 miles of tubules. In each nephron, plas-

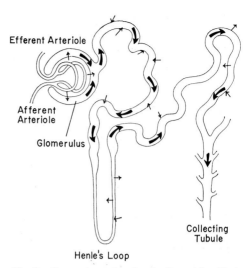

Fig. 6—The nephron showing the flow of the filtrate (dark arrows) and secretions into the tubule and reabsorption from the tubule (small arrows).

ma enters through arterioles into a network of fine blood vessels, the glomerulus. The epithelium separating the glomerulus and the fluid in the surrounding Bowman's capsule is very thin. As the fluid passes through the vessels, it filters from them into the capsule to form urine which passes into the tubules (100 liters/day). Its composition is changed due to tubular reabsorption of the water (almost 99%) and other components, and secretion. Drugs may be both filtered in the glomeruli, secreted by the tubules, and reabsorbed by the tubules.

Renal Clearance—The adult kidney filters about 1.2–1.3 liters of plasma/min and forms about 1 ml of urine/min. The filtered fluid passes through the proximal convoluted tubule into the loop of Henle, into the distal convoluted tubule, and out through the collecting ducts. The tubules are supplied with blood vessels for secretion and reabsorption.

The rate of flow of renal plasma can be measured by a substance such as *p*-aminohippuric (PAH) acid. It is filtered and secreted by the tubular cells and is 90% extracted by a single circulation through the kidney. This can therefore serve as a measure of renal plasma flow and is calculated from:

$$\frac{\text{(PAH concentration in urine)} \times \text{(volume of urine)}}{\text{PAH concentration is plasma}} \quad (3)$$

This is also called the *clearance* of PAH and the average value is about 650 ml/min in man. In this manner, kidney function can be measured by determining values different from the normal. They can also be used to determine the rate of drug extraction and clearance by the kidneys and monitor any changes.

Glomerular Filtration—The glomerular filtration rate (GFR) can be determined by measuring the excretion and plasma levels of a substance; e.g., inulin, which is freely filtered through the glomeruli. The substance used to measure GFR should not be secreted or reabsorbed by the tubules, nor be metabolized, stored, or protein bound, and it should not affect the filtration rate. GFR can be calculated by the following equation:

$$GFR = \frac{\text{(Concentration in urine)} \times \text{(Urine flow/unit time)}}{\text{Concentration in artery}} \quad (4)$$

This shows that approximately 180 liters/day in man are filtered but since the urine volume is about 1.5 liters/day, 90–99% of the water is reabsorbed. If the clearance value exceeds the GFR, the substance is secreted by the tubules, and if it is less, the substance is reabsorbed. Unbound drugs are excreted by glomerular filtration.

Materials may be reabsorbed by an active transport mechanism which can become saturated. Uric acid reabsorption can be inhibited by probenecid, phenylbutazone, and certain other drugs. Hence, these drugs may be used in gout. Probenecid inhibits the secretion of penicillin by competing for sites on the enzyme involved, thus prolonging penicillin levels in the body and potentiating the drug. Ionized drugs may be excreted in the proximal tubules by active transport.

Effect of Urine pH on Drug Excretion—Just as the pH in the gastrointestinal tract affects ionization of the drug and influences absorption, so does the pH of the urine affect the excretion of the drug. In the gastrointestinal tract the nonionized form is desired to achieve maximum absorption. A nonionized drug in the urine may be reabsorbed by the tubules. A pH of the urine that causes ionization of the drug increases its excretion rate. Increasing urine pH (e.g., administration of bicarbonate ion) increases the rate of excretion of acidic drugs such as salicylic acid, phenobarbital, sulfadiazine, and nalidixic acid. Acidifying urine pH (e.g., administration of ammonium chloride) will hasten the excretion of basic drugs such as amphetamines, chloroquine, imipramine, procaine, and quinine. Normally, urine pH may vary from 4.5 to 8.

To summarize, excretion of weak acids and weak bases depends on urine pH. Clearance of bases is higher in acid urine and clearance of acids is higher in alkaline urine. The effect of urine pH on the rate of drug excretion was demonstrated by investigators who reported that $t_{1/2}$ of sulfaethidole at pH 5 was 11.5 hours, whereas at pH 8 the $t_{1/2}$ was 4.2 hours.

Urine Flow Rate—Urine flow rate can also affect the rate of excretion. For example, under constant urine pH the rate of excretion of chlorpheniramine in man appeared to be directly related to changes in urine flow rate, e.g., high flow rate resulted in high excretion. The use of water to insure adequate quantities of urine in drug evaluations may change urine pH and affect excretion. Whether the patient is upright or recumbent could also affect urine flow.

Other Factors

In addition to renal elimination, the following elimination and storage factors also play a role in bioavailability of medications.

Salivary Glands—Nonionized, lipid-soluble molecules can be excreted in the saliva. Drugs excreted in saliva can be swallowed and reabsorbed, and thus enter an enterosalivary cycle. The appearance of drugs in saliva seems to depend upon three main characteristics: (1) molecular size, (2) lipid solubility, and (3) degree of ionization.

Sweat Glands—Excretion appears to be by the nonionized form across a lipid membrane.

Lungs—Volatile chemicals, including acetone and gaseous anesthetics, are excreted mainly by the lungs.

Mammary Glands—Transport into the mammary glands seems to follow the same principles as absorption from the gastrointestinal tract into the blood or from the blood into the urine.

Liver—A variety of drugs and their metabolites occur in the bile; e.g., steroids, penicillin, streptomycin, and tetracyclines. Drugs excreted in the bile may be reabsorbed and thus enter into an enterohepatic cycle which results in prolonged blood levels. Drug biotransformation by the liver also is a factor. After an oral dose, the first pass through the liver may cause a decrease in effect when compared to an intravenous dose of, e.g., levodopa.

Tissue Storage—Certain drugs with high lipid solubility (e.g., thiopental and DDT) may be stored temporarily in body fat, giving rise to the possibility of subsequent release which produces a longer duration of action. Tetracyclines are stored in bones and teeth. Quinacrine, an antimalarial, is stored in large quantities in the liver.

Protein Binding—Binding of a drug to protein in the blood, membrane, or tissue may cause a loss of action because the bound drug cannot readily cross membranes or become attached to receptor sites. The rate of biotransformation and rate of excretion may also be decreased. If a drug (e.g., an antibiotic) is extensively bound, it may have to be given in a larger dose to achieve proper blood levels for the free drug. Binding is reversible and bound drug exists in equilibrium with unbound (free) drug. Binding may be competitive where one drug displaces another drug or substance, e.g., aspirin displacing penicillin. Phenylbutazone displaces warfarin sodium and other oral anticoagulants from proteins, resulting in an increase in prothrombin time (a drug interaction). Suramin, a trypanocide, is effective several months after intravenous injection due to binding and subsequent slow release.

Binding in the blood is usually mainly to albumin. Albumin has terminal amino acids and mercapto groups which may react to bind drugs. Binding appears to be pH-dependent; the pH has an effect on ionization of both the protein and drug.

Blood-Brain Barrier—The blood-brain barrier is complex. The brain receives a higher percentage of blood and more rapid blood flow than the rest of the body. This barrier appears between the plasma and extracellular fluid of the central nervous system, and that transport between the brain and cerebrospinal fluid (CSF) may encounter a similar barrier. Barbital and thiobarbital eventually achieve the same concentrations in the brain, but the latter drug enters at a much faster rate. Some drugs achieve the same concentration in the brain as in the plasma, while others do not. The rate of transport across the blood-brain barrier is roughly proportional to the lipid-water partition coefficient. The degree of ionization in the plasma is important, because the greater the concentration of nonionized drug, the greater the potential for ready transport across membranes.

Drugs may pass out of the CSF rapidly after injection into the CSF, if they do not normally appear in this fluid, e.g., sucrose, dextran. Such compounds appear to leave by other routes that are not affected by molecular size or lipid solubility. Normally, compounds leave at a rate related to lipid solubility.

Placenta—The placenta appears to function as a lipoid barrier. Drugs that penetrate into the CSF, e.g., barbiturates, salicylates, meperidine, tetracyclines, reserpine, and thyroxin, also cross the placenta. Placental transfer of most drugs seems to occur by simple diffusion. Vascularity and blood flow affect this transfer.

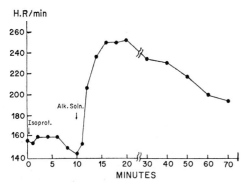

Fig. 7—The effect of alkaline solution on the gastric absorption of isoproterenol in the anesthetized dog with the pyloric sphincter ligated. A dose of 15 mg of isoproterenol was given at the beginning followed by 10 ml of 5% Na_2CO_3 at the tenth minute as indicated by the arrows. The initial gastric pH was 3–3.5 compared with pH of 10–10.5 on termination.[4] (H.R = heart rate.)

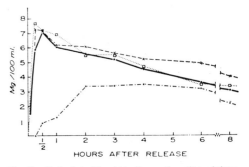

Fig. 8—Salicylate blood level as a function of time, following release at several sites in the GI tract of a 16 kg dog. Dose was 275 mg - - X - - X, sodium salicylate released in stomach; - - □ - - □, drug release 12–15 in. past pylorus; – · – · –, released 26 in. past pylorus; ☉ — · — · ☉, released in cecum.[5]

Other Physiological Factors

In addition to the factors influencing gastrointestinal absorption, distribution, biotransformation, and excretion of drugs that were discussed above, a number of other characteristics of the patient, medication, and environment may have a profound influence on bioavailability. They are considered in that order below.

Patient Factors

Absorption Sites—A drug may only be absorbed at specific sites so that unless it reaches a given site or once it has passed this site, it will not be absorbed to any significant extent. There are now several examples of site specificity for drugs. This may be related to degree of ionization of the drug or active transport. Isoproterenol is poorly absorbed from the stomach at pH 3–3.5. Absorption increases when $NaHCO_3$ is added to raise the pH and decrease ionization (see Fig. 7). On the other hand, sodium salicylate is well absorbed from various areas of the gastrointestinal tract in dogs (see Fig. 8).

Age—Generally there is a decrease in body activity and function with age so that body systems involved with absorption, distribution, biotransforma-

tion, and excretion show declining activity. In the older person, absorption may be slower and more erratic. Metabolism may also be slower and less complete, necessitating a lower dose than that for a young adult. Young children may not absorb some drugs readily and they may not have certain systems completely developed, e.g., metabolizing enzymes, so that they also require smaller doses. Thus, for the same dose, drug blood levels may vary with the age of the patient.

Ambulatory vs Recumbent Patients—Activity and posture of patients influence drug absorption and metabolism. Ambulatory subjects have a lower amount of free benzylpenicillin excreted, and a higher rate constant for the metabolism of the drug than the same subjects during bed rest. It has been suggested that changes in plasma volumes or blood flow rate may cause these changes. Therefore, there may be a difference in pharmacokinetics between the patient in the hospital and the same patient when he comes into a pharmacy.

Biological Variability—People differ in more ways than just fingerprints, e.g., slow and fast absorbers, slow and fast excretors, and slow and fast metabolizers.

Rapid inactivators of isoniazid (INH), an antitubercular drug, had a $t_{1/2}$ of 45–80 min while slow inactivators

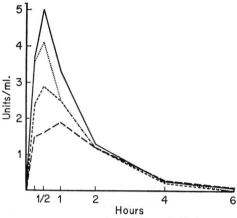

Fig. 9—The average levels of penicillin after a dose of 400,000 units in the plasma of 10 fasting subjects. — penicillin V potassium; . . . penicillin V calcium; - - - penicillin V acid, and – – – penicillin V sodium.[6]

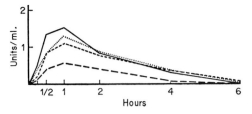

Fig. 10—The average levels of penicillin after a dose of 400,000 units in the plasma of 10 nonfasting subjects. The curves have the same meaning as in Fig. 9.[6]

had a $t_{1/2}$ of 140–200 min, for the acetylation biotransformation.

Body Weight—The volume of body fluid affects the volume of distribution of a drug. Patients with smaller volumes of fluids and of lighter weight usually have higher blood drug levels. However, whether the body weight is lean body mass or fat mass significantly affects drug distribution and dose. Both males and females may differ in the amount of each. Blood levels may decrease with the weight of the patient, e.g., acetaminophen. Pregnancy affects body volume.

Children's doses calculated from adult dose based on weight differences are only an estimate. The square meter surface area rule is considered a more accurate estimate for calculating doses. See page 6.

Gastric Emptying Time—Gastric emptying is affected by the presence of food and the type of food; e.g., carbohydrates are emptied most rapidly, followed by proteins, and fats last. Drug retention in the stomach may enhance absorption of acidic drugs, delay absorption of those mainly absorbed in the intestine, or may cause increased decomposition by gastric fluids.

Intestinal Surface Area and Blood Supply—The rate and extent of drug absorption increase with an increase of surface area and blood supply of the intestinal membranes.

Heredity—It was found that the $t_{1/2}$ of phenylbutazone ranged from 1.2 to 7.3 days in a group of individuals. Identical twins exhibited similar $t_{1/2}$'s, while fraternal twins had different $t_{1/2}$'s. Some persons lack cholinesterase in the plasma so that they fail to hydrolyze succinylcholine normally. This can become life-threatening during surgery.

Because of the effect of heredity on drug action, a new area of study called *pharmacogenetics* has arisen. Among Eskimos 95.4% were rapid inactivators of INH while 44.9% of US and Canadian whites and 47.5% of US Negroes were rapid inactivators. Slow inactivators tended to have higher blood levels and more side effects.

Sex—Weight distribution, hormone systems, and other sex characteristics and functions differ; all may affect bioavailability in yet unknown ways. For example, female dogs reportedly showed higher blood levels of dicloxacillin than males.

Normal vs Sick Individuals—Temperature, diarrhea, achlorhydria, liver or kidney disfunctions, blood flow changes, diseases of the gastrointestinal tract, and many other conditions of the patient may affect drug absorption, distribution, biotransformation, and excretion.

Pregnancy—The physiology of the woman is changed during pregnancy. In addition to drug effects on the fetus, the woman may react differently to a drug.

In a normal pregnancy, the total body water increases 6–8 liters which could affect drug distribution.

Food—Absorption of drugs may be enhanced in the presence of food due to a decrease in intestinal transit rate, e.g., vitamin B_2. Tablets may disintegrate more rapidly when ingested with water. Figs. 9 and 10 show the difference in penicillin levels between fasting and nonfasting subjects. This is why a patient is often directed to take oral medication before meals or with fluids. The absorption of many drugs has been shown to be enhanced or decreased by the presence of food.

Food may coat the drug to decrease absorption. The increase in viscosity of the fluid in the gastrointestinal tract due to food may also decrease diffusion of the drug to the membranes. Conversely, a high-fat diet may affect the absorption of griseofulvin.

Medication Factors

Dose—The dosage of some drugs affects its biological half-life; e.g., the $t_{1/2}$ increases as the amount and frequency of the dose of dicumarol or bishydroxycoumarin increases. Half-lives that change with dose and time may undergo zero-order kinetics.

Drug Interactions—Drug interactions in the gastrointestinal tract affect absorption. Thus, tetracyclines react with antacids and constituents of milk to form unabsorbable complexes. Antacids also interfere with the absorption of quinidine and warfarin. Anticholinergics can increase or decrease the bioavailability of a poorly absorbed drug. Kaolin may adsorb pseudoephedrine. This subject is covered in greater detail in Chapter 13.

Alteration of Absorption, Excretion, and Distribution through Molecular Modification

Drug latentiation may be defined as the chemical modification of a drug to form a new compound, which *in vivo* will liberate the parent compound. La-

tentiation can affect absorption, distribution, and enzymatic biotransformation. Examples are phenacetin yielding acetaminophen, or iron-dextran complex which is a suitable transport form of iron to overcome problems of absorption, toxicity, and stability.

Drugs may be produced that have prolonged action due to an increase in lipid solubility, resulting in fat storage, different biotransformation rate, increased absorption, or increased excretion rate. A compound may have a delayed onset of action because it must first be converted to active drug. Due to a change in solubility, higher concentration could occur in target tissues, e.g., increased concentration in the brain.

It was postulated that disodium edetate increases permeability of membrane by increasing pore size or widening spaces between cells through removal of calcium ions. This could increase the rate of absorption of drugs. Surfactants may also alter membrane permeability or delay gastric emptying.

Ion pairs reportedly increase drug absorption in the rat; e.g., benzomethamine with acetate or propionic and butyric acids. Certain amides may enhance absorption of prednisone and prednisolone.

"Protoammonium" compounds cyclize to form quaternary compounds. If cyclization can be delayed, absorption may be increased because the "protoammonium" compounds are more nonionized. After absorption the compounds may then cyclize to form pharmacologically active drugs in the body.

Carbonate and carboxylic esters reported as "prodrugs" of acetaminophen have higher oil/water partition coefficients than the parent drug. Hetacillin is an ampicillin precursor with better aqueous solubility. This could lead to better absorption.

Absorption can also be modified by the drug itself by:

1. Irritating and damaging the absorbing membrane, e.g., salicylate.
2. Changing the pH of the intestines, e.g., antacids.

3. Modifying drug diffusion in the gastrointestinal tract fluid.
4. Blocking enzyme or transport mechanisms.
5. Drug metabolism in the intestinal membrane.

6. Upsetting the intestinal flora, e.g., antibiotics.

See Chapter 1 for further discussion.

Physicochemical Factors

Pertinent physical and chemical aspects of bioavailability include the pharmacokinetics of drug absorption, distribution and elimination, the derivation of mathematical models to simulate the kinetics of these functions, and the analysis of biopharmaceutic factors that influence them. Fundamental to all of these considerations is recognition of the part played by drug solubility.

Drug Solubility

A drug, to be absorbed through a membrane, must be in solution. Therefore, all drugs absorbed through the gastrointestinal tract must possess a certain amount of solubility. Poorly soluble drugs are absorbed with difficulty. The effect of pH on drug solubility and on the oil/water partition coefficient has already been discussed. The rate of solution has also been found to be a critical factor. Before the importance of the rate of drug solution was recognized, bioavailability was correlated to tablet disintegration, e.g., vitamins. This is illustrated in Table 3, where rate of solution of riboflavin from various products is related to the disintegration time and bioavailability. Unfortunately, such correlations are not always seen.

All the conditions that occur in the gastrointestinal tract cannot be simulated for disintegration or dissolution studies so that the results can at best only give a guide. A drug that takes a long time to dissolve in an *in vitro* test may not be available for absorption. *In vitro* tests only have significance if they can be related to *in vivo* results. Once such a relationship has been established, the *in vitro* test can be used as a quality control test. The effect of food, enzymes, pH, and mucin on bioavailability has already been discussed.

Theoretical Aspects of Drug Solubility—The rate at which solids dissolve is directly proportional to the surface area of the solid (S) and to the difference between the concentration of a saturated solution (C_s) and the concentration of the solid at a given time (C_t).

$$\frac{dw}{dt} = K_2 S(C_s - C_t) \qquad (5)$$

where dw/dt is the rate of dissolution and K_2 is a constant. This means as the particle size decreases and surface area increases, the rate of solution will increase. Factors that affect C_s such as more soluble salts and polymorphic forms will also directly affect the rate of

Table 3—Relationship between Disintegration Time and Dissolution Rate on Physiological Availability of Riboflavin in Sugar-Coated Tablets[7]

Tablets	In vitro		Physiological availability (%)
	Disintegration time (min)	Dissolution rate $T_{1/2}$ (min)	
Multivitamin and minerals	151	114	58 ± 10[a]
Multivitamin and minerals	45	25	87 ± 4
Multivitamin	101	83	36 ± 10
Multivitamin and minerals	45	38	88 ± 11
Multivitamin	20	11	94 ± 7
Multivitamin and minerals	98	124	12 ± 5
Multivitamin	20	11	98 ± 5

[a] Standard error of the mean.

solution. Griseofulvin plasma levels are directly related to its rate of solution.

The following factors affect the rate of solution of a drug and therefore its bioavailability.

Viscosity—Viscosity can affect the rate of solution by decreasing the ability of molecules to diffuse away from the particle surfaces. This becomes important for poorly soluble drugs as the viscosity of gastrointestinal fluids may inhibit diffusion of drug to the intestinal membrane.

Crystallizing Solvate—*Tert*-Butyl acetate esters of prednisolone and hydrocortisone might be better absorbed as monoethanol solvates than the anhydrous esters.

Salt Form—The aluminum salt of aspirin dissolves slower in either acid or alkaline fluids than aspirin. After the first 2 hours about $2\frac{1}{2}$ times more salicylate from aspirin than from aluminum aspirin was excreted. After 15 hours, salicylate excreted with the aluminum salt is only 80% of that excreted with aspirin.

Various salts of tolbutamide give better absorption and greater lowering of blood sugar levels than the acid form in human subjects due to more rapid dissolution of the salts. The rate-limiting step in absorption for many drugs seems to be the dissolution rate of the drug.

Particle Size—Some of the physical effects of particle size have been known for many years, but only recently have its effects been appreciated in pharmacodynamics. Absorption of such drugs as sulfadiazine, griseofulvin, phenothiazine, diphenylhydantoin, chloramphenicol, tolbutamide, dicumarol, medroxyprogesterone acetate, and spironolactone are all affected by particle size. Particle size becomes increasingly important as the solubility of the drug decreases. Small particles can be obtained by micropulverization of the drug before manufacture. Small particles may also be obtained *in vivo*. For example, the acid form of water-soluble salts are precipitated in a very finely subdivided form in the acid pH of the stomach.

A fine particle size may not always be desirable. It was found in dogs that a 80–200 mesh particle size range of nitrofurantoin gives optimum absorption with minimal emesis. Small particles increase the incidence of emesis and larger size crystals decrease absorption.

Decreasing the particle size of a drug may decrease its stability in the gastrointestinal tract. For example, penicillin and erythromycin are unstable in gastric fluids, so that rapid dissolution in the stomach may increase decomposition. More insoluble forms, although more slowly dissolved result in higher blood levels.

Dissolution tests are included in the official compendia for Indomethacin Capsules and for the following tablets: Acetohexamide; Digitoxin; Ergotamine Tartrate and Caffeine; Hydrochlorothiazide; Methandrostenolone; Methylprednisolone; Nitrofurantoin; Prednisolone; Prednisone; Sulfamethoxazole; Sulfisoxazole; Theophylline, Ephedrine Hydrochloride, and Phenobarbital; and Tolbutamide.

Crystal Form—The crystalline form of chloramphenicol is not absorbed but the amorphous form is. The anhydrous form of ampicillin is more soluble than the trihydrate. This difference in solubility appears to result in better absorption of the ampicillin. A difference in rate of solution exists between two anhydrous forms and a hydrous form of prednisolone. Only amorphous novobiocin is pharmacologically active.

Surfactant—There appears to be no general agreement on the effect of surfactants on bioavailability and absorption of drugs. The effect is apparently highly selective. Surfactants may increase the wettability of powders and aid in the removal of air from the surfaces, especially hydrophobic powders, and in this manner increase their rate of solution. Surfactants can solubilize certain drugs by complex or micelle formation (see Chapter 1), which may retard absorption because the new structures are too large to be absorbed.

Surfactants may enhance absorption by emulsifying oils. This is a form of particle-size reduction. Polysorbate surfactants may enhance vitamin A absorption yet they do not increase absorption of various antibiotics. Polysorbate 80 may increase the action of certain drugs administered as ophthalmic drops by acting as a wetting or spreading agent. The type of emulsion form, e.g., O/W or W/O, may affect bioavailability.

Eutectic Mixtures and Solid Solutions—The use of eutectic mixtures and solid solutions as a method of increasing the rate of solution of poorly soluble drugs has been recommended. When a water-soluble, "physiologically inert" material and a drug were used to form a eutectic or solid solution (e.g., sulfathiazole-urea) it was suggested that the particle size of the drug was reduced in the process and that this resulted in an increase in solution rate.

A coprecipitate of sulfathiazole and polyvinylpyrollidone (PVP) was found to increase the dissolution rate of the sulfathiazole from compressed tablets. Reserpine–PVP and reserpine–cholanic acid coprecipitates also have been reported.

Applied Pharmacokinetics

The application of chemical kinetic concepts to drug absorption, distribution and elimination is not new, but most of the work in this area has occurred since about 1955. The availability of small digital and analog computers has greatly aided in performing the required calculations.

The first concept that must be kept in mind is that the dose of drug equals, at any given time, the amount that has

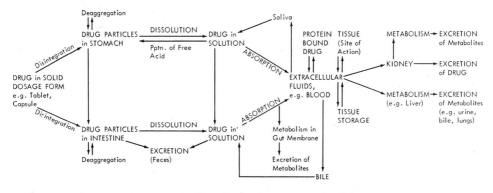

Fig. 11—Potential routes a drug may take from dosage form to excretion. Each arrow indicates a rate is involved.

been excreted by all routes plus the amount remaining at the absorption sites plus the amount distributed in the body plus the amount already metabolized. That this is a very complicated situation is seen from examination of Fig. 11.

Derivation of Mathematical Models—An interesting concept that has evolved is that of deriving models to simulate physiological systems. Theoretical models that have been derived are quite detailed. In practice, the models have been simple because data collection has been limited by time, amount of data available, and the number of organs or tissues that could be sampled. In human subjects only blood and urine samples can be collected. For example, drug absorption may involve several steps. See Fig. 11. Distributions into various tissues may be at different rates and reversible and the drug may be biotransformed into several products which may vary with the mode of administration. The proper model can be useful because it pictorially describes the data and shows the mathematics that are required. The following questions should be answered before accepting a pharmacokinetic model:

1. Are the assumptions stated?
2. What are the physiological or biochemical inferences and are they valid?
3. Are there other models that explain the data equally well?

4. How close is the fit between observed and calculated data?
5. Are there trends in areas of poor fit?
6. Will the model provide accurate predictions if the system is modified?

Only the simplest concept will be discussed here.

The rate of elimination from the blood (dc/dt) or the change in concentration with time, of a drug has been found to be proportional to the concentration (C) of the drug in the blood. This can be written as:

$$\frac{dc}{dt} = kC \qquad (6)$$

The proportionality constant, k, is called the rate constant. In most cases C is the first power. The one major exception is when a saturable enzyme system becomes involved. Since C is to the first power, we have a *first order* rate of elimination. If the equation is rewritten and integrated we get:

$$\ln \frac{C_o}{C} = kt \qquad (7)$$

where C_o is the blood concentration at zero time. Again rewriting the equation to get in a form of $y = mx + b$, we have:

$$\ln C = -kt + \ln C_o$$

and converting natural logs to logs base 10,

$$\log C = \frac{-kt}{2.303} + \log C_o$$

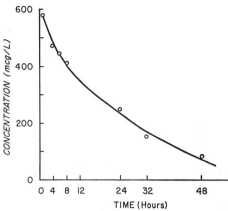

Fig. 12—Plasma concentration of 2-sulfanilamido-5-methylpyrimidine at various times after IV administration of 2 g of the sodium salt to a 75-kg, 45-year-old male.[8]

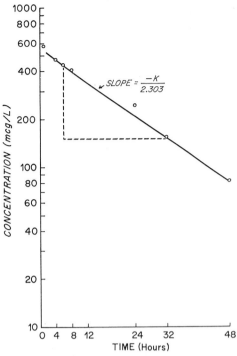

Fig. 13—Semi-log plot of data in Fig. 12.

If C is plotted against t, the curve seen in Fig. 12 is obtained. But if log C is plotted against t the curve seen in Fig. 13 results. The plot also indicates rapid tissue distribution. The y intercept is log C_o and the slope is equal to $-k/2.303$, so that we can solve for the rate constant,

$$(2.303)(\text{Slope}) = -k$$

Going back to Eq. 7 and converting to $\log_{10}$, we get:

$$\log \frac{C_o}{C} = \frac{kt}{2.303}$$

If C is equal to ½ of C_o, the equation becomes:

$$\log \frac{C_o}{\frac{1}{2}C_o} = \frac{kt_{1/2}}{2.303}$$

cancelling C_o, cross multiplying and solving the equation we finally obtain:

$$t_{1/2} = \frac{0.693}{k}$$

$T_{1/2}$ is called the biological half-life, the time it takes the peak concentration of a drug to decrease ½ after the absorption has ceased. The proportionality constant, k, is called the rate constant and is a measure of how fast the reaction proceeds.

Using previously published data[8] for plasma concentration of 2-sulfanilamido-5-methylpyrimidine after intravenous administration of 2 g of the sodi-

um salt in a 75-kg 45-year-old male, the following calculations were made:

Time after administration (hours)	Drug blood level (μg/l)
1	579.8
4	473.4
6	445.0
8	412.0
24	245.4
32	153.2
48	82.0

The data are plotted in Fig. 12. Using the semi-log plot in Fig. 13, we can obtain the elimination rate constant (k) for the drug in the following manner:

1. 33-hour concentration is
    150 μg/l, the log being   2.1761
   6-hour concentration is
    445 μg/l, the log being 2.6484
   27-hour time lapse   −0.4723
2. Slope = (−0.4723/27 hr) = −0.01749 hour⁻¹
   (the slope is negative)
3. Slope = $-k/2.303$, therefore $-k$ = (slope) (2.303)
   $-k$ = 2.303 × −0.01749 hr⁻¹ = 0.04028 hour⁻¹
   k = 0.04028 hour⁻¹ (the unit of a first order rate constant is reciprocal of the time, usually hour⁻¹)

The biological half-life of the drug can be found by the following two methods:

1. $t_{1/2} = (0.693/k) = (0.693/0.04028 \text{ hour}^{-1}) = 17.21$ hours
2. At 8 hours the concentration is 412 μg/l
   At 25 hours the concentration is 206 μg/l (half of first concentration)

   25 hours
   −8 hours
   _____
   17 hours the time it took for the concentration to decrease by 0.5

To determine the slope or $t_{1/2}$ graphically we can use any portion of the straight line portion of the graph. In the above example, it was shown that the elimination of the sulfa drug from the blood appeared to be first-order kinetics.

Types of Models—The equation for the above apparent first-order drug disappearance from the blood may be written as:

$$A \xrightarrow{k_d} B$$

where A is the body compartment and B the urine. Compartment-wise it is represented as:

$$\xrightarrow{\text{IV dose}} \boxed{A} \xrightarrow{k_d}$$

This is a single-compartment open system. This model can also be used to simulate the transfer of a drug across a membrane (gastrointestinal tract, skin, cornea, and other sites).

Most drugs appear to be absorbed and eliminated from the body by first-order kinetics. This means that the rate of absorption by passive diffusion is dependent on drug concentration at the absorption sites. The elimination of a drug from the body and its distribution into various tissues are dependent on the blood concentration of the free drug. The rate of reentry of a drug into the blood is assumed to be dependent of the drug tissue concentration, therefore, apparent first-order rate also.

If the process of absorption and elimination are combined we can write:

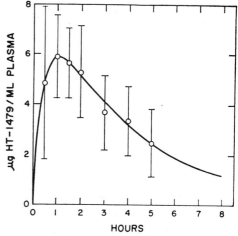

Fig. 13-1—Mean plasma concentration of HT-1479, an experimental drug, in six dogs after administration of an oral solution of the drug. The vertical lines are the standard deviations.[8a]

$$A \xrightarrow{k_a} B \xrightarrow{k_d} C$$

where k_a is the apparent first-order absorption rate constant and k_d is the apparent first-order elimination rate constant. To use the above "two consecutive reactions" as a model to determine apparent absorption and elimination rate constants from blood level data, several assumptions are made:

(1) The processes are first order.
(2) The drug dissolution process is rapid compared to the absorption process.
(3) There is no significant lag time before absorption occurs.
(4) The distribution and metabolism processes can be ignored.

Using these assumptions, the equation that describes two consecutive first-order processes is:

$$C = \frac{a_o k_a}{V_d(k_a - k_d)}(e^{-k_d t} - e^{-k_a t}) \qquad (8)$$

where C is the drug concentration in the blood in mg/ml, a_o is the dose in mg/kg body weight, t is time, V_d is the apparent volume of drug distribution in l/kg, and k_a and k_d are the apparent first-order absorption and elimination rate constants. Fig. 13-1 shows that the calculated curve using Eq. 8 describes the experimental data points. This equation may also be used to determine k_a, k_d, and V_d. Since there are three un-

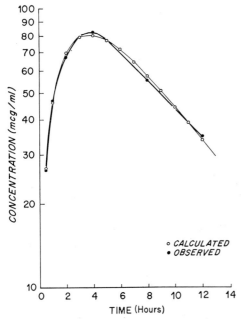

Fig. 13-2—Average salicylate plasma levels for four individuals as a function of time. Amount of aspirin given was 20 gr. Concentrations represented by open circles (O) were calculated by computer using Eq. 8. Concentrations represented by dark circles (●) were the observed data.[8b]

known parameters, and only the blood concentration at various times and the dose are known, the calculations are very tedious when carried out manually. But the three unknown parameters can be readily calculated using a digital computer.

Another set of data that was solved by the above biexponential equation was that of Wood and Syarto.[8b] The observed (black circles) and calculated (open circles) blood concentrations are shown in Fig. 13-2 which is a semi-log

compartments outside the blood are ignored. The next step in model simulation is the addition of a tissue compartment to give a two compartment open model, as follows:

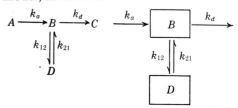

"D" is the tissue compartment and k_{12} and k_{21} the apparent first-order rate constants for leaving the blood and leaving the tissues, respectively. "B" is called the central compartment. Riegelman and co-workers[8c] derived equations and gave examples for this model. The equation for this model is:

$$C_p = Ae^{-\alpha t} + Be^{-\beta t}$$

where C_p is the concentration of drug in plasma, and α and β are hybrid rate constants which are dependent on all four specific rate constants. $C_p{}^0$, the plasma concentration at zero time, equals $A + B$. V_p is the volume of the central compartment and equals Dose/$C_p{}^0$.

A model to explain the distribution of LSD by correlating the action of LSD as determined by a performance test with the LSD blood concentration after intravenous administration of 2 μg/kg body weight to five human subjects was developed. It was found that a tri-exponential equation best explained the results. The equation,

$$C_p = Ae^{-k\alpha t} + Be^{-k\beta t} + Ce^{-k\gamma t}$$

represents the model shown below:

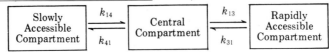

plot of concentration vs time after administration. The calculated constants are:

$k_a = 0.435$ hr^{-1}, $k_d = 0.154$ hr^{-1} and
$$V_d = 9.11 \text{ l/kg}$$

The above model simulates a simple system where drug distribution into

The slowly accessible compartment represents the tissue where LSD exerts its action affecting performance.

Several attempts have been made to derive equations for multidosing with drugs. The most detailed studies were done by Krüger-Thiemer and co-workers. This extension is necessary because the patient rarely takes only one tablet or capsule to cure or prevent a disease, so that knowledge of the initial dose, maintenance dose, and dosing time interval become important. The following assumptions were stated as necessary for dose regimen calculations:

(1) Activity is due to free drug in plasma water.

(2) Quasi equilibrium exists between plasma and tissue.

(3) Binding to protein is described by law of mass action.

(4) Absorption and elimination rates are by first-order kinetics.

(5) $C_p{}^0$ is proportional to dose/body weight.

Using experimental data from various sulfonamide drugs, it was found that to maintain the free drug level in the blood above the minimum inhibitory concentration, the ratio of initial dose to maintenance dose equals two and the dose interval equals $t_{1/2}$. This prevents levels from falling or rising cumulatively. To calculate the ratio of initial dose to maintenance dose requires knowledge of k_a and k_d. In addition, to calculate the maintenance dose requires knowledge of volume of distribution, maximum binding capacity of the plasma proteins, drug concentration in plasma water at half saturation binding, minimum inhibitory concentration, a proportionality constant between the minimum inhibitory concentration and the minimum concentration for a 95% therapeutic effect, protein and water content of plasma, molecular weight of the drug, and the patient's weight. The investigators found that a smaller dose administered more frequently gave more constant levels and resulted in a lower total dose per day.

A more detailed study of the use of models to access bioavailability may be found in the article by Barr (see *Bibliography*).

Kinetics of Absorption and Elimination of Parenteral Products

The kinetics of subcutaneous and intramuscular absorption are similar to those of oral absorption. The main difference is location of the depot—the gastrointestinal tract, under the skin, or in the muscle.

The kinetics of intravenous injection may be viewed as a simplification of intramuscular or subcutaneous kinetics where there is instantaneous absorption. Rapid intravenous injection is a good method of determining the rate of elimination of the drug from the blood, because absorption of the drug does not complicate the calculation. But there may be a slight delay caused by the mixing of the drug with the blood and the establishing of equilibrium between the blood and tissues.

Teorell[8d] postulated that after rapid intravenous injection, if tissue distribution and inactivation can be neglected when considering kidney elimination, the equation for the amount of drug in the blood (y) at time (t) is:

$$y = N_o e^{-kt}$$

where N_o is the dose and k the apparent first-order elimination constant. The time of appearance of maximum tissue drug concentration is independent of dose, but the height of peak concentration is directly proportional to dose. The slower the drug distribution into tissue, the lower the maximum concentration and the later its appearance.

For drugs administered by intravenous infusion, Teorell stated that after sufficient time there is a constant rate of elimination and biotransformation. After sufficient time, drug concentration in the blood and tissue is identical, directly proportional to the rate of infusion, and inversely proportional to elimination. Again, if tissue distribution can be neglected then,

$$Y = \frac{r}{k} (1 - e^{-kt})$$

where Y, t, and k have the same meaning as above and r is the rate of infusion. $r = N_o/v$, where N_o is the dose and v the duration of infusion. When the rate of infusion is constant, the maximum drug blood concentration will be proportional to the dose and after a sufficiently large dose, a constant limiting concentration occurs. Depending upon the rate of infusion, identical doses can produce different blood concentrations and hence different pharmacological effects. Increasing the rate of infusion beyond a certain limit does not produce any appreciable increase in blood drug concentration.

Volume of Distribution of a Drug

Volumes of distribution of drugs in the body have been calculated, but defined differently and hence interpretation varies and physiological significance becomes obscure. The volume of distribution depends upon the pharmacokinetic model. It may be concluded that it is not necessary to introduce a fictitious volume constant to describe a fictitious concentration. The meaning of this constant becomes more confusing because it does not account for the usual drug binding to proteins. This volume for a drug is usually calculated by determining the drug concentration in plasma or serum (central compartmen) at various time intervals. Riggs (see *Bibliography*) defines the volume

of distribution as: $V_{dist} = Q_{tot}/C_{ref\ eq}$, where Q_{tot} is the total quantity of drug in the body and $C_{ref\ eq}$ is the equilibrium concentration in the reference fluid, blood. Another way of calculating the volume in the central compartment (V_p) is:

$$V_p = \frac{\text{Dose of drug}}{C_p^0} \qquad (9)$$

where C_p^0 is the theoretical drug concentration at zero time. The assumption is that all the drug is absorbed and the concentration of the central compartment (blood) is the same as all other tissue and fluids.

Some workers say that these calculations actually estimate the volume of two compartments, the central and the peripheral. The volume may also be determined from:

$$V_d = \frac{\text{Dose of drug}}{(\text{Area under curve})\ (k_d)} \qquad (10)$$

where the area "under the curve" refers to the blood concentration *vs* time plot and k_d is the elimination rate constant for that drug.

Pharmaceutical Factors

The effect of adjuncts on the bioavailability of a drug are sometimes significant. The effect of surfactants on rate of solution was previously discussed. The effect of various additives and adjuncts has caused many controversies.

Effect of Additives

Several reports in 1957–58 showed that tetracycline phosphate complex, tetracycline sodium metaphosphate mixture, tetracycline hydrochloride plus citric acid or tetracycline plus glucosamine give higher drug blood levels than tetracycline hydrochloride, tetracycline base, or chlortetracycline alone. At that time dicalcium phosphate was used as an "inert" filler for the capsule formulations. It was then discovered that calcium and magnesium ions de-

press the absorption of tetracycline. When the dicalcium phosphate was removed from the formulas, the additives no longer had an enhancing effect.

In the studies of aspirin-containing products, calcium acetylsalicylate carbamide complex tablets and aspirin buffered with aluminum glycinate and magnesium carbonate had $t_{1/2}$ <5 min whereas six different plain aspirin tablets had $t_{1/2}$ values ranging from 8.5 to 13.75 min. Degree of local irritation and absorption rate were thought to be a function of aspirin dissolution rate. Other researchers found the following sequence of rates of absorption of aspirin from different dosage forms: solution of sodium acetylsalicylate > effervescent aspirin (Alka-Seltzer) > aspirin in hot water > buffered aspirin tablets > plain aspirin tablets.

Table 4—Effect of Additives on Aspirin[9]

Product	Amount in solution at 10 min	Disintegration with disks (sec)	Amount excreted (mg)
1. Calcium acetylsalicylate	242.2	256	24.3
2. Buffered drug with Al glycinate and $MgCO_3$	205.0	35	18.5
3. Plain drug	165.1	<10	18.1
4. Plain drug	157.6	13	13.6
5. Plain drug	126.8	10	12.1

A comparison of various aspirin products showing disintegration time, dissolution rate, and cumulative apparent amount excreted in 1 hour in human subjects after administration of two 0.3 g tablets is shown in Table 4. The tablet disintegration test cannot distinguish between rapid and slowly dissolving small granules or primary particles. Also, it cannot reflect changes due to particle size or crystalline structure.

A study comparing different types of aspirin products and placebo involved the effect on electrical energy levels and variability of left occipital electroencephalograms (EEG) in normal subjects. The threshold dose for significant EEG effects was found to be two tablets. "Brand" aspirin, "brand" buffered aspirin, and effervescent aspirin gave an onset of action within 1 to 2 hours. "Brand" buffered aspirin gave the longest effect.

Magnesium hydroxide mixed with Pemoline in a 1:1 ratio was about eight times more potent than the drug alone in rate of acquisition and retention of a conditional avoidance response in rats. It has been suggested that absorption may be enhanced by a complexing agent which keeps the drug in solution in the gastrointestinal tract; e.g., ergotamine tartrate and caffeine, sugar amines and coumermycin A, surfactants and vitamin A, sulfisoxazole, dienestrol, and griseofulvin.

Another effect of complex formation is shown when drug absorption across a rat intestinal segment is inhibited. Phenobarbital forms an apparent complex with polyethylene glycol 4000 which reduces solubility. Yet, pentobarbital, barbital acid, or barbituric acid did not show the same tendency. This type of complex formation is difficult to predict and may go undetected.

Adsorption of drugs by other drugs, fillers, or adjuvants is always a potential problem. The adsorbed drug may not be available for absorption or absorption may be delayed. For example, various drugs such as the phenothiazines are adsorbed on silicates such as talc and kaolin. The extent to which this occurs depends on the pH and ionic strength of the medium. Activated charcoal may adsorb aspirin and reduce absorption.

Effect of Formulation

The ingredients of a formulation and the processing procedures strongly affect bioavailability. In discussing the total dosage form, however, it becomes very difficult to differentiate the various factors that affect the bioavailability of a given drug. Tablet disintegration is affected by compression pressure, binder type and concentration, aging, lubricant, fillers (water-soluble or insoluble), and disintegrant. Drug particle size, granule size, amount of fluid, pH of fluid, crystalline form of drug, enzymes, mucin, food, and bile salts also affect tablet disintegration and rate solution of a drug. Many variables may interact among themselves to yield optimum conditions for bioavailability of a given drug from the formulation. It becomes difficult to generalize that the addition or omission of an ingredient in a formula has an effect on bioavailability. In the following discussion, the effect of physical and chemical factors are presented as single variables or multiple variables affecting one parameter. This brings us into the area of the "generic equivalen-

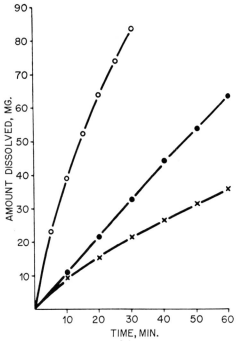

Fig. 14—Effect of lubricants on the dissolution rate of salicylic acid from tablets. Tablets contained 300 mg drug, 60 mg starch and 9 mg lubricant. Key: X, 3% magnesium stearate; ●, no lubricant; O, 3% sodium lauryl sulfate. Each data point is an average of 10 tablets.[10]

Table 5—Effect of Filler[11]

Time (min)	Lactose[a]	Terra Alba[a]
5	81	—
10	92	50
20	99	67
30	100	80

[a] Drug:filler ratio of 1:3.

Table 6—Effect of Binder[11]

Time (min)	Terra Alba[a] PVP	Terra Alba[a] Gelatin	Lactose[a] PVP	Lactose[a] Gelatin
5	58	25	16	5
10	70	40	35	33
20	82	55	69	65
30	90	67	89	86

[a] Drug:filler ratio of 1:3.

Table 7—Effect of Surfactant[11,a]

Time (min)	Sodium Lauryl Sulfate	Polysorbate 20
5	36	51
10	63	81
20	87	94
30	93	96

[a] Drug 100 mg, lactose 300 mg, gelatin 15 mg.

cy" and "therapeutic equivalency" controversy, and whether chemical equivalent dosage forms made by different manufacturers have the same therapeutic efficacy. Potential nonequivalencies may be due to formulation variables illustrated below.

Effect of Vehicle—Ethinylestradiol or its 3-cyclopentyl ether were reported to be absorbed more slowly from sesame oil solution than from aqueous suspensions in rats. Bile and pancreatic secretions aided absorption of the ether derivative from the oil solution.

Formulation Ingredients and Processing Variables—An explanation given for a recent increase in untoward effects in patients taking 100 mg diphenylhydantoin tablets (Dilantin) was that the excipient was changed from calcium sulfate (insoluble) to lactose (soluble). Binders may decrease dissolution rate, but a hydrophilic binder may aid solubility of a hydrophobic drug. It was suggested that hydrophobic tablet lubricants (e.g., magnesium or aluminum stearate, stearic acid, or talc) cause the solvent to be repelled and retard dissolution, while water-soluble lubricants such as sodium oleate or sodium lauryl sulfate do not do this and may actually enhance the dissolution rate. Because these two water-soluble lubricants are also surfactants, they may cause better penetration into the tablet. This can be seen in Fig. 14. The data given in Tables 5–9 illustrate the effect of various formula ingredients on the % of triamterene dissolved at the specified time intervals.

Rapid disintegration of the tablet or capsule and use of a water-soluble filler aids bioavailability.

Table 8—Effect of Starch Disintegrant[11]

Time (min)	Gelatin[a]	Gelatin and starch
10	6	52
20	29	82
30	50	90

[a] Binder.

Table 9—Effect of Magnesium Stearate Lubricant[11]

Time (min)	Terra Alba[a]	Lactose[a]
10	42	85
20	62	93
30	73	97

[a] Drug:filler ratio of 1:2.

The content of some hard gelatin capsules may dissolve slowly because it forms a powder pack. Magnesium stearate could further reduce water penetration into the pack.

Product Comparisons

In the following section, blood levels and efficaciousness of various dosage forms of the same drug are compared; the studies reviewed were usually conducted in human subjects. Occasionally not only are the dosage forms compared, but also other variables. It is not usually possible to separate the effects of the different variables because the dosage form is a complex mixture and its efficacy is affected not only by the formula but also by manufacturing techniques and physicochemical properties. As a general rule, the rate of absorption from various dosage forms is, in order of decreasing rate: solutions > suspensions > capsules > tablets > coated tablets.

To achieve a reasonable rate of solution for drug absorption the drug particles must first be released from the tablet or capsule, then the drug may have to be deaggregated from granules or a powder pack.

Several studies involving tolbutamide, an oral hypoglycemic agent available from many different sources, have been reported. Two reports noted that diabetic patients who had been adequately controlled with tolbutamide went out of control after taking the product made by a different manufacturer. When the reported clinically ineffective brand was compared with a clin-

Table 10—Disintegration Times and Dissolution Rates of Tolbutamide Tablets[12]

Products	Disintegration time (min)	Dissolution times (min) gastric fluid pH 1.5 (40%)	Intestinal fluid pH 7.5 (90%)
A	8	16	19
B	10	92	43
C	3	44	7
D	35	120	69
E	1	72	9

ically effective one, it was found that the time for 50% of the ineffective drug to dissolve was 43 versus 22 min for the effective one. Another study compared dissolution rates of 18 commercially available brands of the same drug product. The amount of drug dissolved after 60 min varied from 30 to 76% and the $t_{1/2}$ ranged from 16 min to greater than 44 min. A double-blind clinical study on three purported poor products and two brand-named preparations in 22 stable diabetics was reported. The daily dose of 1 to 2 g was kept constant for each patient. Statistical analyses showed no significant differences between the five products, except the fasting blood sugar which was slightly better controlled by one brand, D. Clinical observations revealed no differences between these preparations. The disintegration time and dissolution rates are shown in Table 10. Due to the possible superiority of Product D in the clinical study, a slow dissolution rate may be desirable. Further study on 26 lots of tolbutamide from 21 manufacturers showed that two lots had disintegration times greater than 60 min. Lot-to-lot variation from

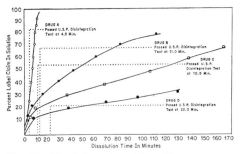

Fig. 15—Dissolution rates of four different tetracycline capsules. Drug A is Achromycin.[13]

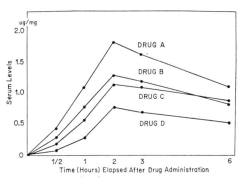

Fig. 16—Average tetracycline serum levels in 12 volunteers.[13]

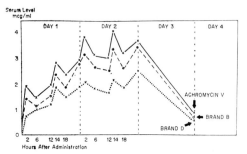

Fig. 17—Average serum tetracycline levels for three products given to a group of nine males. The dosage schedule was 250 mg drug every 6 hours for 48 hours.[13]

one source showed disintegration times of 17, 35, and 3 min.

Orinase (tolbutamide) was compared with another tolbutamide product that was deliberately made to illustrate the effect of formulation. The second product contained only ½ of the disintegration agent, Veegum (colloidal magnesium aluminum silicate). The disintegration time for the tablet and dissolution time for the drug was 2 and 7.6 min and 3.8 min and 103 min, respectively. Orinase gave continuously higher levels. Serum glucose levels at 5 and 8 hours were the same for both products, but Orinase produced lower glucose levels at 1.5 and 3 hours.

Sulfisoxazole (Gantrisin) tablets were absorbed slightly faster and showed a higher peak at 1 hour than two generic products. After 2 hours the blood levels of the three products were similar and amounts excreted in the urine after 24 hours did not differ significantly. A dissolution rate study showed the brand-name product dissolved more rapidly.

Crushed tablets in capsules narrowed the difference between the brand-name and a generic product. Another study of three different makes of sulfisoxazole tablets indicated that the most rapidly dissolving product gave higher blood levels at 0.5 and 1 hour. At 2, 3, 4, 6, 8, and 24 hours there was no significant difference in blood levels, nor was there a significant difference clinically.

In comparing brand-name diphenylhydantoin capsules against two generic brands, it was found that one generic product gave significantly greater absorption than the other products. Although both the rate and degree of absorption of the brand-name preparation appeared greater than the second generic product the difference was not statistically significant. Dissolution rates showed that both generic brands were absorbed faster initially.

Several reports have been made on the bioavailability of the antibiotic tetracycline. The peak blood values of 250-mg capsules of tetracycline hydrochloride from nine different sources, ranged from 0.9 to greater than 2 $\mu g/ml$. Some tablets of this drug failed to show measurable levels, while others showed delayed absorption with peak values below 0.4 $\mu g/ml$. Later a study related dissolution rates and serum levels of Achromycin V (product A) and three generic preparations. Figs. 15 and 16 illustrate this. Urine recoveries of the drug up to 8 hours showed similar re-

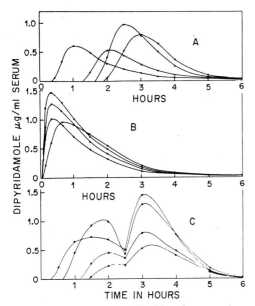

Fig. 18—Average serum dipyridamole concentrations in three groups of four volunteers each. Curves A resulted after taking 25-mg intact tablets. Curves B resulted after taking the drug as crushed tablets. Curves C resulted after intact tablets were taken 2 hours before lunch.[14]

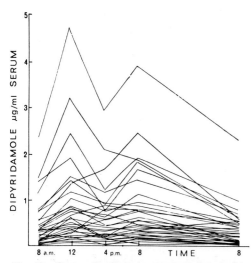

Fig. 19—Serum dipyridamole concentrations in 31 cardiac patients who had been under treatment with the drug for more than 1 month.[14]

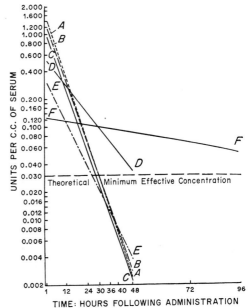

Fig. 20—Average penicillin blood concentrates produced by single IM injections of 300,000 units each. A: penicillin G sodium in peanut oil with 4.8% w/v beeswax; B: penicillin G sodium in peanut oil with 2% aluminum monostearate; C: penicillin G procaine in oil; D: penicillin G procaine in peanut oil with 2% w/v aluminum monostearate (large particle); E: penicillin aluminum in peanut oil with 2% w/v aluminum monostearate; F: penicillin G procaine in peanut oil with 2% w/v aluminum monostearate (small particle).[15]

lets and capsules, and also that an encapsulated product is not always better than a tablet. Triamterene is soluble to the extent of 45 mg/ml. The 24-hour urinary recovery data given below shows this:

24-Hour urinary recovery (mg)[13a]

Capsule	24.7
Initial tablet	13.3
Rapid dissolving tablet	32.4
Micropulverized drug tablet	22.1
Capsule with 16 mesh "slugged" granules	11.2

Fig. 18 taken from a study of Persantin (dipyridamole), a drug used in coronary insufficiencies, illustrates the effect of whole tablet, crushed tablet and food eaten 2 hours after drug intake. The individual variation among patients taking 25 mg of the drug three times a day for more than a month can be seen in Fig. 19.

sults for all products. Apparent differences in serum levels for three 250-mg products given every 6 hours for 48 hours is shown in Fig. 17.

Another study on triamterene illustrates relative bioavailability from tab-

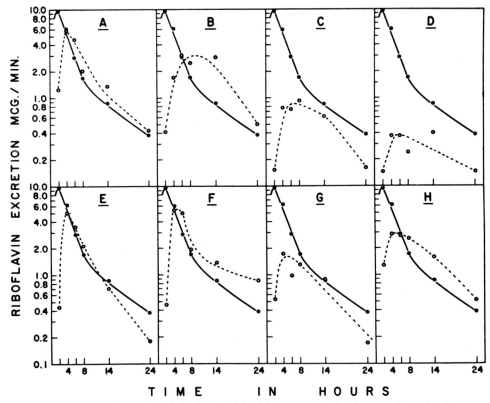

Fig. 21—Urinary excretion curves of riboflavin obtained from sugar coated tablets taken after breakfast. O - - - - O: products under study; ●——●: rapidly disintegrating standard tablet.[16]

Procaine penicillin G in peanut oil gave 24 hours duration of action in human subjects. With larger drug size particles (75–150 μm) in peanut oil gelled with 2% aluminum monostearate, about 48 hours duration of action was obtained. With <5-μm particles, 96 hours duration was obtained. Fig. 20 illustrates the effect of the vehicle of six different repository penicillin preparations as reflected in serum concentration in humans.

An investigation of eight sugar-coated multivitamin tablets showed that disintegration times for products A through H were: 69, 75, 75, 120, 78, 69, 69, and 62 min, respectively. Fig. 21 compares riboflavin excretion from these products.

Among the many studies involving salicylates, the following illustrate the effect of salt form and formulation on absorption or excretion of salicylate.

Similar results can be expected from *p*-aminosalicylic acid.

Using urinary salicylate excretion as the criterion, 12 subjects were given 0.65 g aspirin or equivalent in six different preparations. The preparations tested consisted of two brands of nationally distributed plain aspirin tablets, aspirin plus aluminum glycinate and magnesium carbonate, an aqueous solution of the buffered aspirin, an aqueous solution of sodium salicylate, and a commercial solution of choline salicylate. The amounts of salicylate excreted during the first hour after ingestion were:[16a]

Choline salicylate solution	26.5 mg
Sodium salicylate solution	25.0 mg
Aspirin solution and buffers	22.3 mg
Buffered aspirin	17.2 mg
Aspirin tablet A	12.5 mg
Aspirin tablet B	14.6 mg

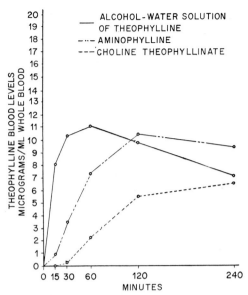

Fig. 22—Average blood theophylline levels in 15 patients after oral administration of equal doses of three different theophylline products. [17]

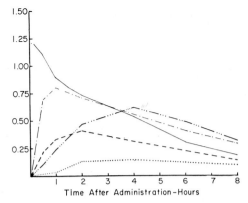

Fig. 23—Average blood theophylline levels in mg/ 100 ml adjusted to standard body weight of 70 kg, after administration of aminophylline in the amounts and by the routes indicated. ——: intravenous, 500 mg; — · —: retention enema, 500 mg; — · · · —: oral tablets—pl., 500 mg; – – – – –: oral tablets— pl., 300 mg; ·········: rectal suppository, 500 mg. [18]

A study with 640 mg of aspirin in various dosage forms indicated that salicylate level reached a peak in approximately 2 hours after tablets taken orally and disappeared from the blood uniformly. During the first 3 hours salicylate levels were significantly higher for tablets than for suppositories. In addition, salicylate levels from the suppository dosage form were erratic. Absorption after rectal administration of crushed tablets was even slower and more erratic. No salicylate could be detected in the blood after rectal administration of finely powdered tablets suspended in a 0.25% tragacanth solution. Total urinary salicylate recovery indicated that bioavailability from tablets taken orally and from suppositories given rectally was similar. Both these dosage forms gave significantly larger amounts in the urine than the crushed tablets administered rectally or the suspension given rectally. The calculated $t_{1/2}$ were for suppositories 3.0 hours, tablets orally 3.7 hours, crushed tablets rectally 6.6 hours, and rectal suspension 10.7 hours. The proportions of metabolites formed were similar regardless of

dosage form and route of administration.

Diazepam in tablets gave earlier peak blood levels and the levels decreased more rapidly than those from a syrupy suspension. The tablets gave a relatively constant blood level for 3 hours, whereas the suspension gave a relatively constant level for 6 hours. Diazepam tablets gave an average blood level twice as high as the suppositories. Some ingredient in the suspension seems to have caused a delay in dissolution of the drug or interferes with drug absorption.

Theophylline derivatives and dosage forms have been studied over the years because this drug is an important vasodilator in coronary disease, and the mistaken belief that tablets caused gastric irritation. Serum theophylline values in human subjects were compared after administration of aminophylline in various dosage forms. After administration of drug equal to 212.5 mg theophylline, the peak value was 4.25 μg/ml serum in 2 hours for capsules, 3.20 μg in 1 hour for rectal suppositories, and 5.68 μg in 2 hours for a hydroalcoholic solution of theophylline.

Similar results were obtained when approximately the equivalent of 400 mg theophylline was administered to human subjects. A hydroalcoholic solution of theophylline, 200-mg coated tablets of choline theophylline, and 100-mg uncoated tablets of aminophylline were compared. See Fig. 22. The solution yielded peak blood levels most rapidly, followed by uncoated tablets, with the coated tablets a poor third. The hydroalcoholic solution gave good levels for at least 4 hours with no gastrointestinal complaints and had a high level in 15 min. Also, absorption from the hydroalcoholic solution was equal to or greater than absorption from an intramuscular injection in human subjects. Another study in patients with normal cardiac and renal function compared aminophylline and theophylline-sodium glycinate. As seen in Fig. 23, the intravenous injection and retention enema were similar after 1 hour. Suppository absorption was slow and overall poor.

Various studies evaluating different dosage forms may not always be consistent. The original articles must be consulted to see if the vehicle, solvent or base could enhance or delay absorption. Particle size of drug, effect of food, and other factors must be checked to determine whether the data from different studies are comparable.

Thioridazine (Mellaril) appears rapidly in the blood and the peak level appears in about 2 hours from a liquid concentrate. Crushed tablets of the drug produce lower blood levels and a later peak. Appearance of blood levels from intact tablets and the sustained-release form (Spacetab) are delayed for more than 1 hour with a corresponding delay in peak levels. The levels from the sustained-release form are more uniform than either the "twice a day" or "three times a day" dosage regimen. However, a 150-mg dose of thioridazine in the regular product is also reported to be equal to the 150-mg sustained-release product when judged by blood levels and duration of levels.

An intravenous dose of 2.5 μg of isoproterenol in dogs increases the heart rate by about 100 beats/min and has a $t_{1/2}$ of 1.2 min. A 1.7-mg oral dose is needed to increase the heart beat to the same degree. The maximum heart rate is obtained in 5 min, and then slowly decreases to normal in 120 min. A rectal retention enema with 2 mg of drug in solution gives a rapid peak level, and the heart beat rate decreases to normal in 2 hours. Rectal administration is more efficient than the oral route. The apparent oral absorption rate constant is 0.735 hour^{-1} and for rectal administration it is 0.40 hour^{-1}, with similar threshold doses. Orally administered isoproterenol is less efficient than intravenous injection due to inactivation of a large portion of the drug by biotransformation to a sulfuric acid ester either before or during absorption from the small intestine. The remaining free drug is then subject to deactivation by the liver, thus only a small portion of the original amount reaches the sites of action.

The effect of the vehicle and dosage form on the drug indoxole, a nonsteroid anti-inflammatory agent is illustrated below. The drug is soluble only to the extent of 0.1 μg/ml. The dosage forms studied were:

(1) An emulsion which consisted of indoxole dissolved in the internal oil phase of Lipomul-Oral;

(2) A soft elastic capsule which contained the drug dissolved in polysorbate 80;

(3) Indoxole suspended in an aqueous vehicle of 0.1% nonionic surfactant Pluronic F-68 (polyoxyethylene-polyoxypropylene block polymer molecular weight 8350), 50% sucrose, preservatives, and a flavoring agent; and

(4) A hard gelatin product which consisted of the drug mixed with small amounts of dioctyl sodium sulfosuccinate, sodium benzoate, and magnesium stearate.

Fig. 24 shows that the emulsion and soft elastic capsule dosage forms give similar serum levels after the first and sixth dose of the drug. The aqueous suspension is a poor third and the hard gelatin capsules give the lowest levels. Table 11 shows the average peak concentrations and the time the peak levels occur. Analyses of the areas under the serum concentration curves and drug dose show that the emulsion and the soft elastic capsules are equipotent

Table 11—Peak Serum Concentrations of Indoxole and Time of Occurrence
of Peak Serum Concentrations in an 8-Hour Dosage Interval Following Oral
Administration of Indoxole in Four Dosage Forms to Eight Subjects[19]

Dose of indoxole (mg)	Dosage interval	Peak serum concentration of indoxole (μg/ml)		Time of peak serum concentration of indoxole (hours)	
		Average	*Range*	*Average*	*Range*
Emulsion					
366	First	1.99	1.16–3.52	3.1	3–4
366	Sixth	3.09	0.94–5.62	2.3	2–3
Soft elastic capsules					
408	First	1.89	1.14–2.67	2.6	2–4
408	Sixth	3.03	2.18–4.18	2.1	2–3
Aqueous suspensions					
361	First	0.64	0.21–1.35	3.3	3–4
361	Sixth	0.90	0.21–3.44	2.8	0–8
Hard capsule					
389	First	0.24	0–0.56	4.0	3–8
389	Sixth	0.41	0–0.94	1.8	0–6

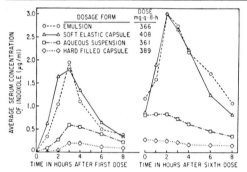

Fig. 24—Average serum concentrations of indoxole in 17 adult subjects following first and sixth doses of four different dosage forms.[19]

after the first dose. The aqueous suspension is 47% and the hard gelatin capsules are only 16% as potent. After the sixth dose the potencies of the soft capsules and aqueous suspension decrease, relative to the emulsion, and the hard gelatin capsule remain the same. Because indoxole is excreted in the bile, it may be reabsorbed, and the rate of absorption could be enhanced by an emulsion or oily vehicle.

The efficaciousness of nafcillin sodium was tested in three different dosage forms, 250-mg tablets, 500-mg sterile powder for intramuscular administration, and 250-mg capsules. The capsule dosage form was further modified so

that one formula consisted of 250 mg of nafcillin sodium, a second one was the sodium salt buffered with calcium carbonate, and a third formula contained 250 mg of the nafcillin acid. The tests showed that in human subjects after intramuscular injection a peak level is obtained between ½ and 1 hour. Administration of oral probenecid cause peak levels about twice as high in 1 hour and cause levels at 8 hours which are comparable to 6-hour levels when probenecid is not given. The intramuscular product at 500 mg dose level gives higher blood levels at all times than those of 1 g drug given orally before or after breakfast. In the capsule dosage form, the drug with the calcium carbonate gives the highest levels at ½ and 1 hour after which the acid form gives the highest levels and also the most sustained level. Nafcillin sodium capsules give the lowest levels.

Enteric-Coated Tablets

A coating that prevents a tablet from disintegrating in the stomach but allows the tablet to disintegrate in the intestine and release the drug at some location beyond the pyloric sphincter, is called an enteric coating. Enteric coatings have been used either to protect

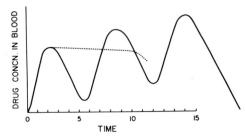

Fig. 25—Curve (——): three consecutive doses; curve (. . . . .): idealized prolonged-action product.

the drug against decomposition in the stomach or to protect the stomach from the irritant action of the drug. Over the years many different enteric-coating materials have been used. They were supposedly insoluble in an acid pH and soluble in a slightly alkaline pH. This specification was based on the erroneous assumption that the stomach fluid is always acidic and the intestinal fluid is always alkaline.

The problems that must be overcome to achieve an efficacious enteric-coated product are many. The random nature of gastric emptying can lead to overdosing. Thus, if one tablet takes 4 hours to leave the stomach, and the next tablet, taken 4 hours after the first one, leaves the stomach in 30 min, then two doses of the drug reach the intestine ½ hour apart. Food and other factors may cause this situation by affecting disintegration and gastric emptying time. When disintegration is delayed, absorption is delayed. Slow absorption of a drug may result in increased biotransformation of the drug, compared with a rapidly absorbed drug. The time of occurrence of the peak blood level and its magnitude for enteric-coated tablets is different, generally delayed and lower than that for regular tablets. Generally, bioavailability is more erratic. Variability within and between patients is also a critical factor that influences the disintegration of enteric-coated drug products, and may result in low or no drug levels in the blood.

A solution of aspirin made with calcium carbonate, sodium bicarbonate, and citric acid gives a peak level in 1 hour

while enteric-coated aspirin tablets (Ecotrin) gives only ½ the peak level in 4 hours. Reproducibility of plasma salicylate levels with the enteric-coated product was poor, possibly due to variation in gastric emptying time. Yet there is no difference between the solution and enteric-coated tablet in urinary recovery to total salicylates.

Prolonged-Action Medications

Products that release a drug over a period of time are known as prolonged-action, sustained-release, sustained-action, continuous-action, timed-disintegration, or timed-release medication.

These products are formulated to provide an initial amount of drug sufficient to cause a rapid onset of action and an additional amount of drug that maintains the response at the desired level for a number of hours beyond the activity resulting from a single dose. The desired therapeutic response is maintained because the drug is released at the rate of drug elimination from the body.

Advantages—The most important reason for formulating sustained-release products is to maintain the therapeutic effect for a longer period than can be obtained after the administration of a single dose. Other reasons are to:

1. Reduce the number and frequency of doses, e.g., nighttime dose.
2. Eliminate peaks and valleys in drug blood levels (Fig. 25) and thus maintain an even level of drug concentration in the body.
3. Lessen the possibility of the patients forgetting to take their medication.
4. Reduce the incidence and intensity of undesirable side effects caused by high peak blood levels of drug.

Contraindications and Disadvantages—Certain drugs should not be administered in a prolonged-acting dosage form, for example

1. Drugs whose precision of dosage is important; e.g., anticoagulants, digoxin, and digitoxin.
2. Drugs whose absorption from the gastrointestinal tract is impaired or erratic.
3. Drugs that are known to have narrow margins of safety between their therapeutic and toxic ranges.

4. Drugs which require an immediate onset of action; e.g., nitroglycerin.

5. Drugs having an inherently long biologic half-life; e.g., long-acting sulfonamides and digoxin.

Disadvantages of prolonged-release products include

1. They are more costly.

2. They do not permit prompt termination of therapy when this is required.

3. They are limited usually to a single available dose.

4. They are designed on the basis of an average elimination rate to provide the desired therapeutic effect.

Since the rates of drug elimination vary, there is the possibility of either *drug accumulation* because of too slow an elimination or *underdosage* because of too rapid an elimination.

Methods of Prolonging Absorption—The relative elimination rate of salicylate decreases with increasing dose above about 600 mg and high doses administered in rapidly absorbed form have a prolonged-action effect. Nevertheless, it is usually dangerous to produce a prolonged blood level by giving large doses. Other methods involving physiological factors for prolonging drug action are: slowing inactivation, slowing excretion (or elimination), and slowing absorption.

Slowing Inactivation and Excretion—Inactivation of a drug may be slowed by inhibiting the enzymes that metabolize the drug in the liver. The activity of acetylcholine is inhibited by cholinesterase; therefore, by using an anticholinesterase like neostigmine that combines with cholinesterase, the hydrolysis of acetylcholine is slowed and its activity is prolonged.

Renal elimination depends on glomerular filtration, secretion by the tubules, and tubular reabsorption. Drugs which are reabsorbed by tubular cells may have a prolonged stay in the body; e.g., sulfamerazine. A method used to slow drug urinary excretion consists of the reversible inhibition of renal excretion. Probenecid (Benemid) has been used to prolong and maintain the therapeutic effect of penicillin by slowing renal tubular excretion of penicillin. Probenecid also interferes with the renal tubular excretion of *p*-aminosalicylic acid, as well as *p*-aminobenzoic acid, by inhibiting their conjugation with glycine, thus prolonging their high blood levels. However, the practical problem of conveniently maintaining an effective concentration of the interfering drug has restricted this method of slowing excretion of a drug.

Slowing Absorption—The rate and the extent of absorption are very important factors in influencing blood and tissue levels and, therefore, in affecting the intensity and duration of pharmacological action.

The principle common to the factors providing prolonged action by slowing absorption is to decrease the rate of solution of the drug in the circulating body fluids. Among the many formulation factors, physiochemical and physiological properties of the drug involved in a slowing of the rate of absorption are: vasoconstriction (blood flow), vehicle miscibility with body fluids, drug dissolution rate, drug solubility, drug ionization (pH of vehicle), drug particle size and surface area, surface tension of the dissolution media, viscosity of the vehicle, esterification of the drug, adsorption of drugs, rate of hydrolysis of drug ion-exchange resin compound, rate of drug hydrolysis from drug complex with large molecules, and rate of drug release from the dosage form.

Injectable Products—Drugs in a pellet may be implanted under the skin to be slowly absorbed. Such pellets are small rod or ovoid-shaped, sterile tablets consisting of drug without excipients. These are intended for subcutaneous implantation in body tissue to serve as a depot for providing slow release of drug over a period of weeks or months. Six 75-mg testosterone pellets implanted into both thighs give 4–6 months of drug action. A 25-mg estradiol pellet provides the drug for 3–4 months.

Oils are immiscible with tissue fluids and this immiscibility provides a slower release and greater duration of action by decreasing the rate of drug dissolution. Injectable products, to be given subcutaneously or intramuscularly, containing vegetable oils with or without fatty substances (such as aluminum stearate), release the suspended drug over a longer period of time; e.g., various hormones in vegetable oils. The amount of solvent also may effect the release of the drug.

Solubility usually affects dissolution rate, and dissolution rate usually affects absorption rate, so that relatively insoluble drugs may be considered to have a slow rate of absorption. When suspensions are injected either intramuscularly or subcutaneously, the suspended material, deposited in the tissues, causes prolonged release of medication. A suspension having a high solid/liquid ratio may be more effective in further slowing drug absorption. An even longer duration of action may occur with oleaginous vehicles, e.g., sterile epinephrine suspension in an oil.

The simplest formulation of prolonged-acting suspension is the combination of a water-soluble substance in a nonaqueous vehicle. The first successful method for prolonging penicillin blood levels was the development of the Romansky formula. This contained penicillin G sodium in a vehicle of vegetable oil and beeswax.

Because of the rapid excretion of aqueous solutions of water-soluble penicillin G potassium, intramuscular injections must be given repeatedly to maintain therapeutic blood levels. However, using an intramuscular aqueous suspension of penicillin G procaine with aluminum stearate in oil, detectable concentrations of penicillin may be found in the blood for longer periods of time. At the same dose, prolonged blood levels are usually obtained at the expense of concentration; that is, lower blood levels are obtained over a longer period of time. With an even less water-soluble derivative such as penicillin G benzathine, penicillin remains in the blood at significantly lower levels for even longer periods of time.

Particle size and particle-size distribution are important factors in the absorption of drugs since solution rate is directly related to surface exposed to the solvent. When the particle size is greater than about 10 μm, the rate of dissolution is directly proportional to the surface area. However, when particles below 10 μm are considered, the particle size, and not the surface area, may be more important. Finely divided particles dissolve at a faster rate and may have higher solubilities than large particles of the same drug.

Generally, drugs in large particles are more slowly absorbed than drugs in small particles. The size of estrone (Theelin) crystals in an aqueous suspension is important in determining the duration of estrogenic effect; greater duration of action was obtained when most of the crystals were large.

The viscosity of the vehicle may prolong drug action regardless of whether the drug is in solution or suspension. A vehicle consisting of a gelatin solution is used for such drugs as adrenocorticotropic hormone (ACTH) to provide more prolonged effects than when administered in aqueous solution. Polyvinylpyrrolidone and dextrans have also been used as thickening agents to prolong the action of intramuscular injections.

Slow absorption may be obtained by the use of esters that provide a therapeutic effect only after hydrolysis releases the active drug. Estrogens esterified as benzoates (e.g., estradiol benzoate) have a prolonged action due to prolonged metabolism in the body in addition to delaying absorption at the site of injection. The carbamate of the spasmolytic drug mephenesin has a longer action than the unesterified drug.

Adsorption is the concentration of a substance upon the surface of a liquid or solid. The mechanism of adsorption is obscure; however, it has suggested that the adsorbent enters into a loose chemical combination with the material absorbed. When a colloid, or other adsorptive substance absorbs a drug, the absorption of the drug may be slowed. Use has been made of this action of protein to prolong the effect of insulin. Corticotropin zinc hydroxide suspension contains corticotropin adsorbed on zinc hydroxide, and injection of the product results in a prolonged therapeutic effect.

Oral Products—Many factors are theoretically involved in controlling the absorption of orally administered products. Some of these include disintegration time, particle aggregation, formulation components, tablet-compression force, pH of intestinal fluids, the presence of interfering factors such as gastric mucus, food, and factors mentioned under *Injectable Products*.

Ideally, with orally administered prolonged-action medication, the purpose is to produce a dosage form which permits smooth and sustained release of the drug over 8 to 12 hours. However, the ideal has been difficult to attain because of the nature and variability in the gastrointestinal tract (i.e., the time required for stomach emptying, presence of food, vascularity of the gastrointestinal tract).

The rate at which the maintenance portion must be absorbed for a predetermined number of hours may be computed from a knowledge of biological half-life. For example, if 0.333 g of drug provides a peak response and the elimination rate is 15%/hour, then 15% of the drug must be provided in the maintenance portion/hour; that is, 0.333 g $\times$ 0.15 = 0.05 g/hour. If the dosage unit is to act h hours, the total drug in the dosage unit may be determined from the relationship:

$$W_t = W_0 + W_0 kh \qquad (11)$$

where W_t is the total weight of drug in the dosage unit, W_0 is the weight of the quick-release portion, k is the elimination constant, h is the time in hours during which sustained action may be

required, and $W_0 kh$ is the weight of the maintenance portion. Thus, if $W_0 = 0.333$ g, $k = 15\%$/hour, and $h = 10$, $W_t = 0.333$ g + (0.333 g $\times$ 0.15 $\times$ 10), and $W_t = 0.833$ g.

The following methods of obtaining prolonged action in oral products will be discussed briefly: ion-exchange resins, complexation, plasma protein binding, and slowing dissolution of drug from the formulation.

Ion-Exchange Resins—Ion exchange refers to the ability of certain insoluble resins to extract one species of charged ion out of solution and exchange it for another. Ion-exchange resins used to replace anions with other anions are anion-exchange resins, and ion-exchange resins used to replace cations with other cations are cation-exchange resins.

The following illustrates the formation and *in vivo* release of drugs from ion-exchange resins:

Cation-exchange resin + basic drug → drug resinate
Anion-exchange resin + acidic drug → resin salt

In the stomach

Drug resinate + hydrochloric acid → cation-exchange resin + drug HCl
Resin salt + hydrochloric acid → anion-resin exchange + acidic drug

In the intestine

Drug resinate + NaCl → cation-exchange resin + drug HCl
Resin salt + NaCl → anion-exchange + sodium salt of the drug.

The most common cation-exchange resins contain either carboxylic or sulfonic acid groups. Carboxylic acid resin with higher binding capacities releases drugs more rapidly in acid solution than the sulfonic acid resins. Polyamines are used for anion-exchange resins.

Pennwalt has been marketing a number of preparations based upon drugs forming complexes with ion-exchange resins. If the proper ion-exchange resin is chosen, the rate of dissociation with the gastrointestinal fluids can be controlled to produce a uniform rate of release of the drug over a period of time which depends on the concentration of available ions; e.g., Biphetamine (dextroamphetamine and amphetamine as cation-exchange resin complexes).

Complexation—Complex compounds are primarily those molecules in which most of the bonding structure is ionic or covalent, or one or more of the bonds are somewhat anomalous and, therefore, complex. Accordingly, the process of preparing such compounds is referred to as complexation. A drug contained in a complex is usually pharmacologically inactive and must dissociate in the body before it can exert its usual pharmacological action.

Organic amines are converted to tannates by tannic acid which, in the presence of aqueous solutions, provides a gradual release. of the therapeutic amine. Since gastric fluid could cause too-rapid a release of amine from its tannate, polygalacturonic acid is used to protect the tannate from too-rapid hydrolysis in the stomach. The release of medication from such tablets and liquids is independent of the emptying time of the stomach, the motility of the intestinal tract, and the varying pH of the stomach and intestinal tract.

Many hydrocolloids are polyanionic (e.g., carboxymethylcellulose and alginic acid) and can enter into interactions with cationic drugs such as antihistamines to form highly insoluble complexes with prolongation of therapeutic activity. Likewise, in injectables, either zinc- or tannic acid-insoluble complexes (e.g., pitressin tannate) have been used to provide various degrees of increased duration of release. With vitamin B_{12}, neither zinc nor tannic acid alone has any marked influence on the retardation of the absorption of the vitamin. However, the reaction product of vitamin B_{12}, tannic acid, and zinc provides a complex derivative with prolonged absorption when injected.

Plasma Protein Binding and Tissue Storage—Drugs are bound to varying extent to plasma proteins and exist in the blood in part as free drug and in part as a drug-protein complex. Since only the free drug can diffuse into other tissues, the greater the degree of protein binding, the smaller the amount of free drug which is available to extravascular sites. The bound drug could provide a reservoir which is converted into the active free form to maintain a constant blood level over extended periods of time; e.g., suramin strongly binds with plasma and tissue proteins, and the complex acts as a reservoir to release the drug slowly and permit it to exert its antitrypanosomal activity over a period of months following a single dose.

Certain drugs, e.g., chlorotrianisene (TACE) are lipid-soluble and are deposited in the adipose tissue after administration, acting as a depot from which the drug is gradually released to provide a prolonged effect.

Slowing Drug Dissolution—Suspending the drug in an emulsion is another method of obtaining prolonged action. For example, a suspension of sulfisoxazole acetyl (Lipo Gantrisin) in a digestible vegetable oil-in-water emulsion provides high blood levels over a longer period of time. This form of the drug is administered in approximately double the concentration but only ½ as frequently as the aqueous forms.

Xerogel entrapment using polymer emulsions may be used to disperse drugs for controlled release.

Silicone rubber has been used for implants and intrauterine-implantable devices. Medroxyprogesterone acetate, desoxycorticosterone acetate, melengesterol acetate, and atropine have been tested. Reportedly the amount released depends on the molecular structure of the steroid, solubility of the steroid in the polymer, and the use of filters such as siliceous earth.

Methods of prolonging release of drugs from capsules and tablets include wax-fatty substance-coated pellets and granules either encapsulated or compressed into tablets; wax-fatty substance matrix for tablets forming an insoluble plastic matrix which allows the drug to be leached out; and hydrophilic matrices which slowly erode allowing the drug to dissolve over a period of time. Hydroxypropyl methylcellulose/ethylcellulose films and hydroxypropyl cellulose/polyvinyl acetate films also have been used to prolong drug release from tablets. These methods are discussed in greater detail in Chapters 3 and 5.

Ophthalmic Products—Ophthalmic products require special manufacturing and handling; e.g., they must be sterile, nonirritating, and ointments must be free from particles. A viscosity-increasing agent (e.g., methylcellulose or PVP) is added to increase drug action by decreasing drainage of the solution. Surfactants such as polysorbate 80 increase action by allowing better contact with the eye. Drugs can bind with the proteins in the lacrimal fluid thus decreasing drug action. The rate of drainage of solutions increases with the volume instilled, and blinking will squeeze the solution out of the eye. Application of additional solutions will only increase the loss of the solution instilled earlier.

Ocusert employs a polylaminated structure from which the drug slowly diffuses out. The drug-containing core is covered with a polymer membrane (made of ethylene and vinyl acetate) on both sides to control drug release; e.g., pilocarpine (Pilo 20) delivers 20 μg of pilocarpine (±20%)/hour over a 7-day period.

Studies—In the past, studies showed that three types of urine level patterns occurred:

(1) Essentially the same curve as a solution of the drug, indicating no sustained excretion.
(2) Lower and later peak level compared to a solution preparation but a slightly longer excretion time.
(3) Prolonged excretion with a more or less constant urine level.

A pelleted capsule preparation containing 15 mg dextroamphetamine-^{14}C gives similar levels to 5 mg of the drug given every 4 hours for three doses. A single 15-mg dose of a conventional product gives higher levels for the first 12 hours. All three dosage regimens give

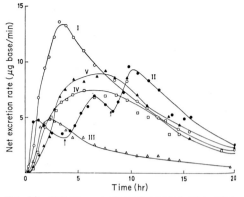

Fig. 26—Urinary excretion of amphetamine after oral administration of dextroamphetamine sulfate. *I*: 15-mg "Free Capsule"; *II*: 5-mg "Free Capsule" given three times at 4-hour intervals indicated by arrow (↑), first dose given as unencapsulated pellets; *III*: 5-mg "Free Capsule"; *IV*: Preparation A; *V*: Preparation B.[20]

equivalent average cumulative urinary excretion at 24 and 48 hours.

Another study of sustained-release dextroamphetamines also compared various products and dosage regimens. The urinary excretion levels of the drug in human subjects whose urine was maintained acidic were used to judge the sustained effect. The pH of urine was kept constant because urinary pH can affect the rate of amphetamine excretion. The products tested were:

1. Encapsulated sugar pellets coated with dextroamphetamine sulfate (Free Capsule).
2. Drug pellets not encapsulated.
3. Product A containing 20% uncoated drug pellets, 30% of drug pellets coated with a thin lipid film, 10% of drug pellets coated with a thicker lipid film, and the remainder of coated drug pellets with intermediate thickness.
4. A commercial capsule of pellets coated with a dialyzing membrane (Preparation B).

As seen in Fig. 26, the 5 mg given at 4.0 and 8 hours shows a characteristic staircase effect. The high peak level of the single 15-mg dose of encapsulated uncoated pellets and the proportionally lower levels of a 5-mg dose are illustrated. The sustained levels of the two sustained-release products can be seen. These levels are not as high as the 15-mg dose, nor are the length of time of the levels greater than the 15-mg dose, but the levels are more uniform than the three times a day regimen. The rise is faster in the initial level of the three times a day regimen than that of the single 5-mg dose because the initial 5-mg dose of the former was not encapsulated.

An informative study compared 400-mg tablets of meprobamate (Equanil), encapsulated coated meprobamate granules (Meprospan), a similar sustained-release product made by Wyeth, and a placebo. Human subjects were given an 800-mg dose of the drug. The study indicated that there is no significant difference at 4 hours between the products, the two sustained-release capsules give significantly higher levels at 8 and 12 hours, but only the Wyeth sustained-release capsule gives significantly higher levels at 24 hours at the 800-mg dose level. The sustained release products give higher 24-hour total drug excretion than the tablets but this is not statistically significant. In the normal subjects used, clinical efficaciousness could not be related to blood levels or products.

Twelve human subjects were tested with 200-mg doses of pentobarbital sodium as conventional capsules or as a sustained-release preparation (Gradumet). Over a 24-hour period average serum levels were greater for the capsules than sustained-release products. There was some evidence of delayed and more uniform absorption from the Gradumet. Eleven subjects rated the capsules as more intense and ten subjects as having longer duration. On the Clyde mood scale, the capsules at 2 and 4 hours were rated more efficacious and at 8 hours the sustained-release product more efficacious. Attempts to correlate serum levels to mood scale scores were unsuccessful.

Dermatological Preparations

The skin protects the body and prevents dehydration. The epidermis consists of a layer of keratinized cells, a thin layer of flat cells, another layer of flat cells which act as a barrier, and a layer of reproducing cells which replace the dead cells. The dermis consists of the blood vessels, nerves, hair follicles, and sweat glands. Most of the research on dermatological preparations has been conducted with ointments and creams. These preparations have been commonly tested *in vitro,* or in mice or rabbits. Animals have different skin characteristics than humans because animals lack sweat glands, have more hair and hair follicles, and their skin is thinner. The use of animals to test dermatological preparations only gives a qualitative rank ordering of the efficaciousness. But then the lack of knowledge of drug transport through the skin is no greater than our ignorance of drug transport across the gastrointestinal tract membranes.

Further complications in the investigation of efficaciousness of dermatological products result from variations in the characteristics of human skin. It varies, from region to region, in thickness, number of hair follicles, size and rate of growth, and the diverse distribution of sweat glands. The variable characteristics of drugs such as particle size, solubility, partition coefficient, and vehicle composition cause complications also.

The so-called penetrating power of the dermatological vehicle is often measured by the amount of drug absorbed through the skin. This assumes that the penetration of the vehicle is related to drug transport. The drug may diffuse through the vehicle and skin without any movement of the vehicle into the skin. This is also true for suppository vehicles. The terms absorption and penetration of the drug into the skin are used synonymously.

Surfactants in dermatological bases may help or hinder drug transport through the base and skin in a similar manner to their action in the gastrointestinal tract. They may increase water loss from the skin. In creams or emulsion vehicles surfactants are already present, therefore care in the selection of these vehicles must be taken so that they do not adversely affect bioavailability of the drug.

In general, dermatological products are applied to achieve local pharmacological action. Therefore, for this purpose a fast rate of drug absorption is not desirable for it removes the drug from the desired site before it has a chance to exert its local action. Also, indiscriminate use of drugs such as appreciably absorbed corticosteroids may give rise to unwanted side effects. Action *on* or *in* the skin may be desired. The vehicle can determine whether the drug stays on the skin or penetrates into the deeper layers of the skin, but at the same time it is difficult to control the amount of drug that penetrates.

Percutaneous (through unbroken skin) absorption may occur by the following routes:

1. *Transepidermal,* through or between the cells of the stratum corneum (outer layer of the skin).
2. *Transfollicular,* through the walls of the hair follicles.
3. Through the walls of the sebaceous or sweat glands.

Hydration of the skin increases absorption. Thus, the use of certain bases or occlusive dressings that minimize loss of water (perspiration) from the skin promote hydration and absorption. Some substances, such as salicylic acid, may promote absorption by irritation.

The effect of solvents on percutaneous absorption has been reported many times, with conflicting results. It has been claimed that washing with organic solvents dissolves the skin fats and thereby permits far better penetration. The same has been claimed for washing with detergents before applying the preparation. Solvents for the drug such as vegetable oils, alcohol, propylene glycol, tetrahydrofurfuryl alcohol, dimethylsulfoxide (DMSO), and water have all been reported to aid drug absorption from the skin.

Factors that affect absorption of a drug from the skin are: skin thickness, drug particle size, drug partition coefficient, pH of the vehicle, patient's age, size of area applied, area of body applied, time left on the skin, and inunction.

Studies of absorption of several drugs in various bases indicate that hydration may increase skin permeability. Degree of hydration depends on rate of sweat secretion, rate of sweat evaporation and amount of water in vehicle, and also appears to increase as the product becomes more occlusive. The rate at which a drug diffuses from the dermatologic preparation to the skin depends on its solubility in the base or external phase of an emulsion base. Diffusion is more rapid if the drug is in its molecular state, and appears directly proportional to drug concentration. Penetration by the drug appears to be proportional to time of application and as long as a concentration gradient exists.

Although hydrous bases or ones containing water generally may be better for drug absorption from skin, an occlusive base may occasionally be better. The former causes hydration initially, but the water will slowly evaporate because there is nothing to keep it at the skin surface. An occlusive base allows perspiration to collect and minimizes its evaporation; e.g., reportedly, fluocinolone acetonide is more efficacious in white petrolatum than a water-washable cream.

Radioactive dexamethasone-^{14}C is absorbed by stripped skin much more rapidly from a gelled base (50% gelled isopropyl myristate, 27% Wax B white square, 22% lanolin alcohols, and 1% inorganic buffers) than from petrolatum, during the first 5 hours. Within 24 hours the rates from the two bases become equal and considerably slower possibly due to regeneration of the skin barrier. Very often dermatological preparations are applied to abraded or inflamed skin, so that studies on intact, healthy skin may not give an accurate picture of the clinical situation.

Parenteral Products

When a drug is delivered directly into the blood stream, e.g., intravenous injection, the patient may not receive instant relief. If an ester derivative is used to solubilize the drug, the molecule may first have to be hydrolyzed to yield the pharmacologically active part, before relief is obtained. Thus, hydrolysis is necessary with erythromycin esters. The toxicity of the drug and of all the formula ingredients becomes more acute when a product is administered intravenously. A substance may be "nontoxic" when administered orally because it is decomposed in the gastrointestinal tract or is not absorbed, but it may become toxic when placed directly into the blood stream. Extra care in the selection of antioxidants, antimicrobial preservatives, chelating agents, solubilizing agents, and solvents must be used because of potential detrimental effects, e.g., hemolysis of red blood cells. Intramuscular injection of a drug does not insure efficacy, e.g., chloramphenicol sodium succinate is ineffective when given intramuscularly.

Subcutaneous tissue is supplied with both blood capillaries and lymphatic vessels. Muscular tissue is supplied with capillaries and only a limited number of lymphatic vessels. Activity increases the flow of both blood and lymph in these areas, and thus may increase the rate of absorption. This rate may vary with the site, e.g., arm or thigh. Massage of the injection site increases absorption from the depot site because the injected fluid is dispersed, and a larger surface area is exposed to the capillaries. Absorption from intramuscular or subcutaneous sites may be by simple diffusion as explained by Fick's Law, or by pinocytosis and phagocytosis. Absorption may occur in the venous part of the capillaries when the osmotic pressure of the extracellular fluid surrounding the vessels exceeds the hydrostatic pressure of the fluid in the vessels. Solvent drag may become an important mechanism. When the flow from the capillaries equals the flow into the capillaries, diffusion may predominate. The area covered by the fluid given intramuscularly or subcutaneously varies with the vehi-

cle; an aqueous vehicle or one miscible with the intercellular fluids spreads more readily than a nonaqueous or immiscible one. The pH of the vehicle affects the ionization of the drug which in turn affects the rate of absorption. Precipitation of the drug due to a pH change at the injection site limits spreading and decreases the absorption rate.

Smaller molecules with larger diffusion coefficients are absorbed more rapidly. Large molecules such as polymers are absorbed more slowly. The lymphatic system may be the preferred route for absorption of macromolecules.

Since the kinetics of absorption from subcutaneous or intramuscular depots is similar to that of oral absorption, if absorption from an intramuscular site is slowed, prolonged-release is obtained. Intravenous infusion is another method of delivering a drug over a prolonged period of time and thereby provides continuous drug blood levels.

Insulin products provide examples of what can be done to modify the time of onset and rate of absorption of a drug. Insulin Injection USP is a solution which gives rapid onset and 5–7 hours duration of action. Protamine Zinc Insulin Suspension USP is slowly absorbed (onset 4–6 hours) and lasts about 36 hours. Isophane Insulin Suspension USP, which is a mixture of regular insulin and protamine zinc insulin in a 2:1 ratio, has a fairly rapid onset due to the plain insulin and has a 24–28 hour duration due to the protamine zinc insulin. In Extended Insulin Zinc Suspension USP a crystal size of 10–40 μm causes slow dissolution and gives slow onset and 36 hour duration of action. Prompt Insulin Zinc Suspension USP consists of 2 μm amorphous particles for more rapid dissolution and absorption. This product has a 12–16 hour duration of action. Finally, Insulin Zinc Suspension USP is a mixture of 30% amorphous form and 70% Extended Insulin Zinc crystals to give a product with a 24–28 hour duration similar to Isophane Insulin Suspension. Thus by varying particle size or molecular derivative, products with a different onset and duration of action can be obtained. There is no significant difference in rate of absorption of lente insulin from intramuscular and subcutaneous injection sites, but there may be a delay when the thigh is used as the site instead of the arm.

The rate of absorption from subcutaneous sites may be decreased by histamine, estrogenic hormones, or epinephrine; e.g., the action of local anesthetics such as procaine hydrochloride is prolonged with epinephrine, a vasoconstrictor. The rate of absorption may be increased by the coadministration of hyaluronidase. Hyaluronidase hydrolyzes hyaluronic acid, a component of tissue ground substance, and thereby allows more spreading to occur. Certain adrenal glucocorticoids such as cortisone may also increase absorption from subcutaneous sites.

Physicochemical factors that affect the rate of absorption and general efficaciousness of parenteral products are:

1. Particle-size distribution.
2. Recrystallization of suspended particles.
3. Sterility.
4. Resuspendibility.
5. Drainage from the container walls.
6. Viscosity and rheological characteristics of the preparation.
7. Polymorphic forms.

Another problem that may arise during manufacture of parenteral products concerns the safety of the products due to the presence of microorganisms and foreign particulate matter. Foreign particles separated, especially during autoclaving, from the container and rubber closures as well as particles from the metal equipment may enter the product. In addition, coring of the rubber closure and skin deposits foreign material into the body. These foreign particles may increase tissue inflammation or cause arterial or pulmonary granulomas.

One group of investigators concluded that basically only surface area, diluents, and solubility of the implants in body fluids affect absorption rates.

However, site of implantation and body movement also have an effect. Factors that appear not to affect absorption rate are pellet density, crystal size used in implant preparation, phagocytosis, physiological need or sex of the animal, encapsulation, "ghost" formation, and age of the animal (if it is not young). Crumbling of the pellets may result in increased absorption and overdosage.

Rectal Products

Suppositories and retention enemas are the most common rectal dosage forms. Suppositories resemble both dermatological products, because they are often used to relieve local irritation and inflammation, and oral dosage forms because the drug in a suppository or enema may be absorbed by the lower part of the gastrointestinal tract. Suppositories are discussed in greater detail in Chapter 7. This section deals with absorption of drugs from suppository vehicles in the specific instance where systemic action is desired. A few examples compare absorption from the rectum with absorption from other dosage forms.

Factors such as particle size, drug solubility, rate of diffusion of the drug to the absorbing membrane, and partition coefficient, that affect absorption from the upper gastrointestinal tract, also affect absorption from the rectum. The chemical composition of the base and its melting point may also affect the absorption and therefore the bioavailability of the drug, e.g., aspirin reportedly is rapidly absorbed from a polyethylene glycol or cocoa butter base and sodium salicylate is rapidly absorbed from a cocoa butter base. The surfactant effect is variable, aiding absorption in some instances and in other cases having no apparent effect. Acetaminophen absorption has been related to the dielectric constant of the base; i.e., absorption increases with an increase in dielectric constant. In studies with human subjects involving a long-acting sulfonamide, sulfadimethoxine (Madribon), lower doses of the drug were more com-

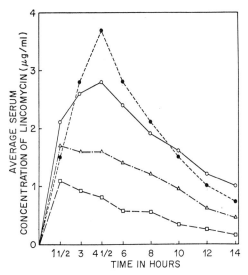

Fig. 27—Average serum concentrations of lincomycin in 10 adult subjects. ● - - - ●: capsule, oral, fasting; O—O: solution rectal, preceded by enemas, fasting; △ – · – △: solution, rectal, without enema, nonfasting; □ - - - □, suppository, rectal, without enema, fasting.[21]

pletely absorbed rectally than higher doses. Therapeutically effective concentrations reportedly were readily maintained with this drug given rectally. The two-compartment model of Teorell did not fit the blood level data. This latter observation is not surprising because of the long biological half-life of the drug and the latent period before measurable blood levels appear. In later studies, with various suppository bases containing sodium salicylate or salicylic acid, the drug blood-level curves in dogs appear to follow the kinetics of a single compartment open model of Teorell.

Recently, lincomycin hydrochloride absorption was determined with a rectal preparation and compared with that of other dosage forms. In human subjects given 500 mg of the drug (see Fig. 27) oral capsules apparently give the highest peak, a rectal solution preceded by an enema in fasting subjects gives the second best levels; a rectal solution without the enema in nonfasting subjects is poorer than the above two, and a rectal suppository made with a polyethylene glycol base given without

an enema but to fasting subjects gives the lowest levels. The rectal solution given after an enema to fasting subjects yields levels similar to those from the capsules but the curve has a different shape. The rectal solution without enema in nonfasting patients gives levels only about ½ of those from the capsule. In children, after multiple dosing with lincomycin hydrochloride, an oral syrup and rectal solution give similar serum concentrations. However, in the study yielding these findings the rectal dose was 30 mg/kg while the oral dose was only ½ as much, 15 mg/kg.

Drug Interactions

In addition to the effects of formulation and processing on bioavailability, drug interactions are also very important. They include physical and chemical incompatibilities as well as therapeutic incompatibilities. For example, such interactions occur when drugs interfere with the gastric emptying time, change gastrointestinal tract pH, or adsorb or bind or otherwise alter the action of other drugs. Other interactions take place when drugs alter urine pH, change amount of protein binding, or stimulate or inhibit biotransformation of a second medicament. The intensity and length of drug action may be changed by urine pH or urine flow and inhibition or stimulation of kidney secretion. This subject is further discussed in Chapters 1 and 13.

Generic, Chemical, and Therapeutic Equivalency

Originally, controversy over this subject led to direct comparison of brand name drug products with generic drugs. This was an oversimplification because all individual drugs have generic names and anyone can obtain a brand name for his drug product. It was also illogical because the generic drug is only one ingredient of a brand-name product. Comparing a generic drug with a brand-name product is as senseless as trying to compare flour with a loaf of bread containing softeners, preservatives, and the many other ingredients. The problem does not lie with the pure drug material but with the formulation of the pure drug into efficacious dosage forms. The products may be generic and chemical equivalents as determined by tests and assays, but the products still may not be therapeutically equivalent. Nonequivalency has been found in products from large and small manufacturers, and among both generic and brand name products. It is due to tablet-hardness variation, tablet lubricants, fillers and other formula adjuvants, tablet coatings, all the other factors previously mentioned, and probably some as yet unknown. The length of time a product has been used and the frequency of its use, however, does not necessarily correlate with efficaciousness; it may only indicate lack of information on what to look for or force of habit. It is interesting to note that of the 200 most frequently prescribed products in 1974, 15 were generic drugs and the rest could only be obtained from a single manufacturer.

To minimize nonequivalencies due to manufacturing procedures, the 1962 amendments to the Food, Drug and Cosmetic Act specified that products should be made by current good manufacturing practices. Regulations have been issued by the FDA detailing what these practices should be. The Defense Personnel Support Center, Directorate of Medical Material, which buys pharmaceuticals for the US government also has specifications for the drug products it purchases, some may be more stringent than those of the USP or NF.

Sometimes the tablet-disintegration times have been correlated to bioavailability. Dissolution tests have been recommended as a more sensitive indicator of both bioavailability and equivalency. Some NF and USP monographs include a dissolution test. Currently, bioavailability is best judged by blood levels, although in some instances amounts excreted in the urine can be used. This assumes that products made by different manufacturers or by different formulas,

giving the same blood levels are therapeutically equivalent.

The following criteria may be useful in judging product equivalence:

1. Peak drug blood concentration.
2. Time of peak drug blood concentration.
3. Superimposable curves of test product and a standard.
4. Area under the concentration–time curve.
5. Cumulative amounts excreted in the urine and the rate of excretion.

Since the early 1970's several studies have been reported comparing digoxin tablets from various manufacturers to determine the extent of bioequivalence. This drug is a potent cardiotonic that has a small range between ineffective, effective, and toxic doses. This drug is also poorly absorbed, i.e., about 80% from a solution and only about 60% from tablets. Due to difficulty in making efficacious digoxin tablets, batch certification of all marketed products has been instituted. Lanoxin (*Burroughs-Wellcome*) has become the standard. In this case, dissolution tests reflect bioavailability.

Because of the difficulty the individual pharmacist has in gaining useful data to help him determine bioequivalence, the American Pharmaceutical Association instituted the Bioavailability Pilot Project. The initial report (Dittert LW, DiSanto AR: *JAPhA NS13:* 421, 1973) published data on ampicillin, digoxin, diphenylhydantoin, nitrofurantoin, oxytetracycline, and prednisone. In 1975 they published an update on digoxin (Colaizzi JW, Wagner JG: *JAPhA NS15:* 43, 1975). Additional articles will be published in the near future. These are important readings for all pharmacists because the reviews describe all available data submitted by independent manufacturers and data published by individual investigators.

The Academy of Pharmacy Practice and Academy of Pharmaceutical Sciences also have published information (*JAPhA NS13:* 278, 1973; *NS14:* 556, 1974) helpful to pharmacists in product selection. The latter Academy divided drugs into three groups.

The first group listed those drugs which have the least likelihood of exhibiting significant bioavailability differences: acetaminophen, butabarbital sodium, codeine sulfate, chlorpheniramine maleate, chlorpromazine hydrochloride, diphenhydramine hydrochloride, isoniazid, meperidine hydrochloride, nicotinic acid, papaverine hydrochloride, pentobarbital sodium, phenobarbital, phenazopyridine hydrochloride, propantheline bromide, propoxyphene hydrochloride, reserpine, secobarbital sodium, sulfisoxazole, tripelennamine hydrochloride.

The second group is those solid dosage forms which exhibit the most serious bioavailability and/or quality assurance problems: chloral hydrate, conjugated estrogens, dexamethasone, digoxin, diphenylhydantoin sodium, erythromycin and its derivatives, nitroglycerin, prednisone, quinidine sulfate and other salts, thyroid, triamcinolone, warfarin sodium, and bishydroxycoumarin.

The third group is those solid dosage forms where there is insufficient information available at present to state categorically there is or isn't a potential for bioequivalence and/or quality assurance problems: ampicillin, chloramphenicol, nystatin, oxytetracycline, penicillin G potassium, penicillin V potassium, tetracycline, aspirin compound with codeine, ferrous sulfate, griseofulvin, hydrochlorothiazide.

For the present, drugs and products that are

1. Poorly soluble, e.g., less than 1%.
2. Polymorphic structures, e.g., steroids.
3. Antibiotics, e.g., penicillins and tetracyclines.
4. Enteric-coated tablets, e.g., aspirin, methenamine mandelate.
5. Sustained-release dosage forms.
6. Poorly absorbed.
7. Slow disintegrating tablets or capsules.
8. Unstable and require special storage conditions.

have a potential for therapeutic nonequivalency. In addition, when a small difference in dose may cause a marked change in effect and when rate of absorption may affect the effectiveness of a drug, bioinequivalence may result. For additional thoughts on this problem consult the recent literature.

Experimental Design

The proper design or layout of an experiment is necessary if the experiment is to have meaning. This is especially important in biological systems. Experimental design is a complex subject covered by a vast array of publications.

Variables have been discussed that affect the design of pharmacological and bioavailability experiments. The following paragraphs are meant only to explain some of the terms previously used.

A *single-blind study* refers to the fact that the subjects do not know whether they are taking a drug or a placebo but the physician knows whether the subjects are taking an active ingredient or a placebo. The products being studied look and taste alike.

In a *double-blind study*, the products being tested look and taste alike and even the investigators do not know the identity of the products. Only after all the data have been collected and are being analyzed are the investigators made aware of the identity of the products, e.g., which is the placebo and which is the active drug product.

To study therapeutic equivalency a *cross-over* experimental design is often used. The test subjects are divided into two equal groups. One group is given Treatment A (reference product) and the other group is given Treatment B (test product). At a later time the first group is given Treatment B and the second group, Treatment A. The difference in results due to the time interval should be small. The physiological conditions affecting bioavailability should be kept constant. Blood (serum, plasma) levels of either drug or metabolites or both and amounts in urine and feces may be determined. The treatments may be compared by means of levels in the blood, amounts excreted, or areas under various curves. The data can also be statistically analyzed by the use of tools such as analysis of variance. Enough data should be collected to draw meaningful curves, at least seven points covering two to three half-lives.

In conclusion, let the pharmacist remember that research is conducted by human beings on other human beings, so that errors in interpretation can be made, especially if complete information is not available or there is no previous experience in knowing what to look for. See the discussion on tetracycline and calcium phosphate filler (see index). There is need to know blood levels, not just total amounts excreted, because levels may never rise above the minimum effective concentration yet the drug may be completely absorbed. The smallest particle size range may not necessarily be the best. See the discussion on nitrofurantoin (see index). Averaging data may give a false sense of security because the individual data could range from no drug to near toxic amounts being absorbed but the average of the resulting extreme blood levels represents an apparently satisfactory level. The pharmacist must therefore constantly read the literature with a questioning mind.

References

1. Danielli JF: Recent developments in cell physiology. In Kitching JA, ed: *Proceedings of the 7th Symposium of the Colston Research Society,* 1954.

2. Davson H, Danielli JF: *The Permeability of Natural Membranes,* Cambridge Univ. Press, New York, 60, 1943.

3. Schanker LS, Shore PA, Brodie BB, Hogben CAM: *J Pharmacol Exp Ther 120:*528, 1957.

4. Minatoya H, Lands AM, Portman GA: *J Pharm Sci 54:*968, 1965.

5. Eriksen SP, Swintosky JV, Seross EJ, Lin TH, Abrams J, Sturtevant FM: *J Pharm Sci 50:* 151, 1961.

6. Juncher H, Raaschou F: *Antibiot Med Clin Ther 4:*497, 1957.

7. Middleton EJ, Davis JM, Morrison AB: *J Pharm Sci 53:*1378, 1964.

8. Kruger-Thiemer E, Eriksen SP: *J Pharm Sci 55:*1249, 1966.

8a. Weigand RG, Sanders PG: *J Pharmacol Exp Ther 146:*271, 1964.

8b. Wood JH, Syarto, J: *J Pharm Sci 53:*877, 1964.

8c. Riegelman S, Loo J, Rowland M: *J Pharm Sci 57:*117, 1968.

8d. Teorell T: *Arch Int Pharmacodyn 57:*205, 226, 1937.

9. Levy G: *J Pharm Sci 50:*388, 1961.

10. Levy G, Gumtow RH: *J Pharm Sci 52:*1139, 1963.

11. Yen JKC: *Can Pharm J 97:*493, 1964.

12. Lu FC, Rice WB, Mainville CW: *Can Med Ass J 92:*1166, 1965.

13. MacDonald H, Pisano F, Burger J, Dornbush A, Pelcak E: *Drug Inform Bull 3:*76, 1969.

13a. Rosen E, Tannenbaum PJ, Crosley AP Jr, Flanagan T: In Goldstein SW: *Safer and More Effective Drugs,* APhA, Washington, DC, 111–120, 1968.

14. Mellinger TJ, Bohorfoush JB: *Arch Int Pharmacodyn 163:*471, 1966.

15. Buckwalter FH, Dickison HL: *JAPhA Sci Ed 47:*661, 1958.

16. Morrison AB, Chapman DG, Campbell JA: *JAPhA Sci Ed 48:*634, 1959.

16a. Levy G, Gumtow RH, Rutowski JB: *Can Med Assoc J 85:*414, 1961.

17. Schluger J, McGinn JT, Hennessy DJ: *Am J Med Sci 233:*296, 1957.

18. Truitt EB, Jr McKusick VA, Krantz JC, Jr: *J Pharmacol Exp Ther 100:*309, 1950.

19. Wagner JG, Gerard ES, Kaiser DG: *Clin Pharmacol Ther 7:*610, 1966.

20. Beckett AH, Tucker GT: *J Pharm Pharmacol (Suppl) 18:*72S, 1966.

21. Wagner JG, Carter CH, Martens IJ: *J Clin Pharm J New Drugs 8:*154, 1968.

Bibliography

Cressman WA, Sugita ET: Bioavailability and bioequivalency testing. In *Remington's Pharmaceutical Sciences,* 15th ed, Mack Publ. Co., Easton, PA, 1368, 1975.

Wagner JG: *J Pharm Sci 50:*359, 1961.

Brown F, Danielli JF, Bourne GH: *Cytology and Cell Physiology,* Academic, New York, 241, 1964.

Rothfield L, Finkelstein A: *Ann Rev Biochem 37:*464, 1968.

Branton D: *Ann Rev Plant Physiol 20:*209, 1969.

Stoeckenius W, Engelman DM: *J Cell Biol 42:* 613, 1969.

Schanker LS: In Harper NJ, Simmonds AB, eds: *Advances in Drug Research,* Academic, New York, 71, 1964.

Gibaldi M, Kanig JL: *J Oral Ther Pharmacol 1:*440, 1965.

Parke DW: *The Biochemistry of Foreign Compounds,* Pergamon, New York, 1968.

Brodie BB, Erdos EG, eds: *Metabolic Factors Controlling Duration of Drug Action* (1st Inter Pharmacol Mtg, vol 6), Pergamon, London, 1962.

Patton AR: *Biochemical Energetics and Kinetics,* Saunders, Philadelphia, 81–95, 1965.

LaDu BN, Mandel HG, Way EL, eds: *Fundamentals of Drug Metabolism and Drug Disposition,* Williams & Wilkins, Baltimore, 1971.

Meyer MC, Guttman DE: *J Pharm Sci 57:*895, 1968.

Kalow W: Pharmacogenetics: *Heredity and the Response to Drugs,* Saunders, Philadelphia, 93, 1962.

Harper NJ: *J Med Chem 1:*467, 1959.

Sinkula AA, Yalkowsky SH: *J Pharm Sci 64:* 181, 1975.

Wurster DE, Taylor PW: *Ibid 54:*169, 1965.

Levy G: *Am J Pharm 135:*78, 1963.

Fincher JH: *J Pharm Sci 57:*1825, 1968.

Gibaldi M, Feldman S: *J Pharm Sci 59:*579, 1970.

Wagner JG: *Ann Rev Pharmacol 8:*67, 1968.

Wagner JG, ed: *Biopharmaceutics and Relevant Pharmacokinetics,* Drug Intel Publ, Hamilton, IL, 1971.

Barr WH: *Pharmacol 8:*55, 1972.

Riggs DS: *The Mathematical Approach to Physiological Problems—A Critical Primer,* Williams & Wilkins, Baltimore, 193–220, 1963.

Levy G, ed: *Clinical PharmacoKinetics,* APhA, Washington, DC, 1974.

Wood JH: *Pharm Acta Helv 42:*129, 1967.

Symposium on formulation factors affecting therapeutic performance of drug products. *Drug Inform Bull (Jan/June),* 1969.

Rosen E, Tannenbaum PJ, Crosley AP Jr,

Flanagan T: In Goldstein SW, ed: *Safer and More Effective Drugs,* APhA, Washington, DC, 111, 1968.

Barr WH: *Drug Inform Bull 3:*27, 1969.

Ballard BE, Nelson E: Prolonged-action pharmaceuticals. In *Remington's Pharmaceutical Sciences,* 15th ed, Mack Publ. Co., Easton, PA, 1618, 1975.

Montagna W: *The Structure and Function of Skin,* 2nd ed, Academic, New York, 1962.

Hadgraft JW: *J Mond Pharm 10:*309, 1967.

Wurster DE: *Am Perfum 80:*21, 1965.

Ballard BE: *J Pharm Sci 57:*357, 1968.

Schou J: *Pharmacol Rev 13:*441, 1961.

Ballard BE, Nelson E: *J Pharm Sci 51:*915, 1962.

Diller W, Burger P: *Arzneim-Forsch 15:*1445, 1965.

Guidelines for Biopharmaceutical Studies in Man, APhA, Washington, DC, 1972.

3

Capsules

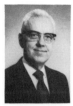

Edward J. Rowe, PhD
Professor of Pharmacy
College of Pharmacy
Butler University
Indianapolis, IN 46208

Gelatin capsules were first prepared in France by Mothes and Dublanc and patented by them in 1834. The two-piece telescoping hard gelatin capsule was invented by James Murdock of London in 1848. In the USP capsules are defined as "solid dosage forms in which the drug is enclosed in either a hard or a soft, soluble container or 'shell' of a suitable form of gelatin."

The administration of drugs, both liquid and solid, enclosed in hard or soft gelatin capsules is very popular. Of all prescription medications dispensed, about one out of five is in a capsule dosage form. The advantage of this form of medication is that drugs having an unpleasant odor or taste are completely enclosed in the practically tasteless shell. Since the pharmacist can prepare capsules quickly and conveniently, the physician is able to vary the dosage and combination of drugs to suit each individual case.

Capsules are unsuitable for the administration of very-soluble compounds such as potassium or calcium chloride, potassium bromide, or ammonium chloride. In such cases, when the partly dissolved capsule comes in contact with the stomach wall, the concentrated solution may cause localized irritation and gastric distress.

Capsules have been reported to produce both better and poorer absorption rates than tablets of a particular drug. Phenoxymethyl penicillin, e.g., has been shown to be more rapidly absorbed from hard gelatin capsules than from tablets, and aspirin less rapidly absorbed from capsules than from tablets. However, the availability of a drug for absorption from a well-formulated capsule generally will be better than, or equal to, that available from a tablet. The gelatin shell dissolves in about 10 to 20 min after ingestion, although a range of as low as 2½–6 min has been reported in an *in vivo* disintegration study for capsules filled with sodium bicarbonate. When the gelatin shell dissolves, its contents may also dissolve or remain as an aggregate for some time.

Much depends on the formulation. Factors that may influence the rate of absorption of a drug from a capsule include particle size, crystalline form, and choice of fillers, lubricants, and deaggregants, as well as interactions of these with the drug.

Administration

For oral administration, the capsule is placed near the tip of the tongue and swallowed with a drink of water. The capsule may be dipped in water just before placing on the tongue if desired.

Occasionally, the patient is directed to dissolve the contents of the capsule in water or a medicated liquid and use the resulting preparation as illustrated in R 1, written by a dentist:

1

R   Aureomycin 250 mg   #28
    Sig: Dissolve contents of one cap. in ¼ glass
    distilled water and rinse mouth 4xd for 7 days.

Although capsules are seldom administered rectally, this method may be directed by the physician in some cases, as in R 2:

2

R   Nembutal Caps. 50 mg.   #xii
    Sig: Caps iii–iv in rectum every 2–3 hrs. as
    needed.

For rectal administration, the capsule should be dipped in water just before use to facilitate insertion. To hasten the action, as in administering capsules of barbiturates rectally to infants, each end of the capsule may be perforated.

Sometimes capsules are also administered vaginally.

Various proprietary items are marketed in capsules. A number of manufacturers give special names to their particular capsule dosage form as shown in R's 3–7.

3

R   Benadryl   50 mg.
    D.T.D. Kapseals No. xv.
    Sig: One capsule B.I.D. with water.
    (*Note:* Kapseals (*Parke-Davis*) are hard capsules which are sealed by a band of gelatin.)

4

R   Spansule Dexedrine DTD #30   10 mg.
    Sig: one daily in a.m.
    Refill 4 x   LABEL
    (*Note:* Spansule (*SK&F*) are sustained-release pellet-containing capsules.) See page 95.

5

R   Prenatal
        Dri-Caps   #100
    Sig: Label by name. i t.i.d.
    (*Note:* Dri-Caps (*Lederle*) are dry-filled sealed capsules.)

6

R   Co-Pyronil Pulvule
        Disp. 100
    Sig: 1 or 2 daily prn nasal drip
    (*Note:* Pulvules (*Lilly*) are filled hard capsules.)

7

R   Medrol Medules   4 mg.
                                         #30
    Sig: i q. 4 h. 1st 48 h. around the clock, then i
    q. 5 h. 2nd 48 h. around the clock, then 1 q. 6 h.
    3rd 48 h. around the clock.
    (*Note:* Medules (*Upjohn*) are capsules containing sustained-action pellets.)

Just as in the case of powders, the physician sometimes writes the total amount of each of the ingredients and directs that they be mixed and the mixture divided into a certain number of doses in capsules. Prescriptions of this type are seen in R's 8 and 9.

8

R   Phenacetin   gr xxiv
    ASA   gr xxxvi
    Codeine Sulfate   gr iii
    M. & ft. in caps.   #xii
    Sig: 1 prn pain.

9

R   Ephedrine Sulfate   gr. xiiss
    Amytal   gr. xxv
    Aspirin   gr. cl
    M.   50 capsules
    Sig: One t.i.d.

It may not always be clear on the prescription whether the total amount of each of the ingredients is to be divided. In such a case it is important to consider the use, dose, and the frequency of the dose of the medication.

In many instances the prescription will be written for a single dose of medicine in a capsule, with directions that a certain number of such doses be dispensed. R's 10 and 11 are of this type.

The individual quantities for each capsule are multiplied by the number of capsules to be dispensed. Note that quantities of ingredients in a prescription may sometimes be given in a mixture of both apothecary and metric systems in a single prescription.

10

R　Atropine　　　　　　　　$\frac{1}{150}$ gr.
　　Phenobarb.　　　　　　　$\frac{1}{2}$ gr.
　　Demerol　　　　　　　　100 mg.
　　M. caps. D. T. D. #15
　　S.—i stat; i in 2 hrs.; then i q. 4–6 h.

11

R　Phenobarbital　　　　　　gr. ss
　　Belladonna　　　　　　　gr. $\frac{1}{10}$
　　Dexedrine　　　　　　　　3 mg.
　　Mft caps 40 such.
　　Sig:　1—2xd

Filling

When dry powders are prescribed in capsules, mixing of the powder is carried on according to the same general principles as those applied when dealing with powders to be dispensed in powder papers. Capsules are generally filled by punching, i.e., by placing the compounded powder on paper and arranging it in a uniform pile of a depth of about ⅓ the length of the capsule, and

then repeatedly pressing the open end of the body of the capsule downward into the powder firmly and uniformly with a rotary motion until it is filled. A sense of touch should indicate the fullness of packing of the powder. The cap is then applied to close the capsule. To insure accuracy of dosage, each filled capsule should be weighed using an empty capsule of the same size as a tare. The capsule should have a completely filled appearance. To accomplish this the filled capsule may be rotated gently between the thumb and finger or the cap end tapped gently on a hard surface. Some powders do not pack readily and tend to drop out of the body of the capsule during filling. A procedure for handling this problem is to push the powder into the capsule with a spatula.

In compounding capsule prescriptions for less than 25 capsules, many pharmacists calculate 5 to 10% more capsules than the number to be dispensed. In any case the calculation is for whole units of capsules. This procedure insures greater accuracy by compensating for the loss of ingredients through adherence to the mortar, the pestle, and any surface with which the powder mixture comes in contact; ample material is thus available for filling the last few capsules.

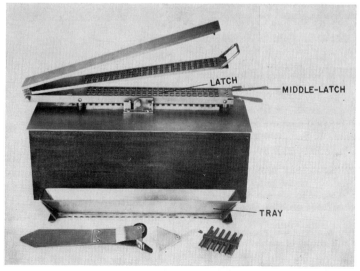

Fig. 1—Universal Model hand-operated capsule-filling machine (courtesy, *ChemiPharm*).

Before compounding capsule prescriptions, it is a good idea to count the actual number of empty capsules to be used. This avoids returning capsules, possibly contaminated with a drug or other substance, to stock containers.

Very efficient capsule-filling machines are used for filling hundreds of thousands of hard capsules daily. A significant development in the capsule field has been the construction of a single machine which automatically and in a continuous process performs the entire operation of making the hard gelatin capsules and filling them. References containing a description of hard capsule-filling machines used commercially are included in the *Bibliography.*

Capsule fillers for use at the prescription counter are available and in use in some pharmacies. One such machine is the Universal capsule-filling machine (Fig. 1). With it, up to 24 capsules of one size can be filled at a time. The capsules are placed in the machine by hand and the caps removed mechanically. The capsules are then filled with the aid of a tray and tamper, after which the caps are replaced mechanically. The machine will accommodate capsule size numbers 3, 2, 1, and 0. Larger models are available which allow filling of up to 144 capsules at a time, depending upon the size of the capsule.

Sanitary Handling

Since hard gelatin capsules are untouched by human hands during mass manufacture, special precautions are taken by the pharmacist during extemporaneous filling so that the capsule surfaces are not soiled and marred with fingerprints. Considering that capsules are taken orally, the pharmacist should at least carefully wash and dry his hands just before filling capsules in order to remove perspiration, dirt, and bacteria. If he is interrupted and leaves his task to make a sale and handle money, he should rewash and redry his hands before resuming the filling of the capsules.

To insure sanitary capsule filling and

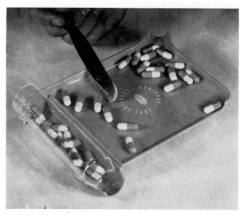

Fig. 2—Sanitary capsule counting tray (courtesy, *Abbott*).

avoid finger imprints, some pharmacists use clean or sterile thin latex gloves, disposable plastic gloves, or finger cots, a procedure highly recommended. The use of gloves is also advantageous in encapsulating drugs which may elicit a topical allergic response.

Prescriptions for prefabricated capsule medication comprise the major share by far of the capsule prescriptions that a pharmacist fills. To insure sanitary handling of such filled capsules during pouring from the bottle and counting, a simple yet very effective device is a specially designed counting tray. See Fig. 2. With this device and a spatula the pharmacist can rapidly count and transfer capsules to a vial or other container as well as return excess capsules of the count to the stock bottle without so much as touching them.

The tray should be cleaned after each counting of capsules or tablets to avoid contamination of one medicament with another. This is especially important to persons sensitive to certain drugs such as penicillin. Some pharmacists go so far as to reserve a counting tray only for capsules or tablets of such drugs. In addition, the counting tray should be kept in a location removed from the normal work area to minimize possible drug dust contamination. In cleaning the counting tray a dampened cleansing tissue may be employed but care must be taken to thoroughly dry the tray before use.

Cleaning

Since one of the primary reasons for enclosing drugs in capsules is to avoid the odor and taste of the drug, it is obvious that this purpose is defeated if some of the drug gets on the outside of the capsule. In the more commonly used methods of capsule filling, such as pressing the open end of the capsule into a pile of the powder, the outside of the capsule necessarily comes into contact with the drug. For capsules containing hygroscopic substances the presence of powder adhering to the outside of the capsule may hasten deterioration. These circumstances necessitate cleaning the filled capsules.

One way to remove powder from the outside of capsules is to wipe each capsule with clean surgical gauze or cleansing tissue. Some pharmacists wet the gauze with alcohol if the powders are soluble in alcohol (or with diluted alcohol if the powders are water-soluble) and then wipe with a dry cloth.

Another method of cleaning capsules is to place them between folds of surgical gauze, a towel, or cleansing tissue and lightly roll them back and forth.

Capsules may be polished by rolling them in a towel which has been lightly sprayed with mineral oil (liquid petrolatum) by means of an atomizer. However, if the capsule surface is deeply etched with soil and/or fingerprints, cleaning and polishing measures will prove futile.

Identification

It is not unusual for the pharmacist to be asked the identity of an unknown capsule, particularly when the question of poisoning arises or when a physician wants to know what medication a patient had been receiving or another physician has prescribed. As an aid, some manufacturers include in their price lists or product information booklets identification charts showing the exact size, strength, color, and markings of the capsules they market.

A section on product identification, which consists of color plates showing in

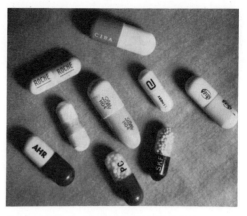

Fig. 3—Capsule branding and identification.

actual size and markings many capsules and tablets of several manufacturers, has been included in the *Physician's Desk Reference* since 1961. The need for such a guide has been recognized by physicians, toxicologists, and pharmacists, as well as by personnel in hospital emergency receiving rooms, poison-control centers, law-enforcement agencies, and the pharmaceutical industry.

The imprinting or "branding" of capsules by manufacturers with their name, initial, code number, or symbol is now required, as with all dosage forms, and greatly facilitates identification (see Fig. 3). Other features such as the colored band on Kapseals (*Parke-Davis*), the tapered body of Pulvules (*Lilly*), or the "taper-end" cap and body of SK&F products are also helpful in identification.

Colored Capsules—Most proprietary capsules are distinctively colored (by using suitable dyes) as a product identity aid. Only transparent, colorless, or pink capsules are made available to the community pharmacist. Colorless capsules may be given a distinctive color by mixing the contents with charcoal or other suitable color additives approved for drug use by the Food and Drug Administration. In choosing color additives, care should be taken to make certain that the additive does not interact with the capsule contents or contribute a physiological effect of its own. For example, commercial pink capsules colored with erythrosine (FD&C red

#3 dye, tetraiodofluorescein) have been reported to elevate protein-bound iodine in PBI tests.

The colorless capsule is used for practically all extemporaneous capsule prescriptions. The physician generally specifies the color, should he prefer other than a colorless capsule. Only in special cases should a colored capsule be used as, e.g., when prescriptions for different capsules, similar in appearance, are dispensed for one person or family. Whenever a colored capsule is dispensed, this should be noted on the filed prescription for future guidance. Indiscriminate use of colored capsules for extemporaneous compounding is not advisable.

Special Problems

The following are some of the problems which may be encountered in prescription work with discussions that describe methods of solving them.

Deliquescent Powders—Capsules containing deliquescent or hygroscopic drugs should always be dispensed in moisture-tight containers, such as screw-top glass capsule vials. In a study of water-vapor sorption and diffusion through hard gelatin capsules, it was shown that gelatin capsules exposed to high relative humidities offer little protection to contents which are hygroscopic, and may even give up moisture to such content. A gelatin capsule normally contains 9–12% moisture. Capsules filled with potassium acetate, e.g., become brittle and crack.

While capsules dispensed in moisture-tight vials require no addition of an absorbent, in the hands of the patient where the vial is opened and closed with some frequency the addition of an absorbent such as starch may prolong the stability of the capsule.

Eutectic Mixtures—In filling prescriptions for powder mixtures to be dispensed in capsules, pharmacists sometimes encounter difficulties due to liquefaction or formation of a pasty mass caused by a mixture having a eutectic point below room temperature.

One method of handling the difficulty is to keep the ingredients separated from one another by use of a diluent to prevent the mixture from liquefying. Effective diluents for this purpose are substances such as magnesium carbonate, light magnesium oxide, and kaolin. Heavy magnesium oxide and starch are comparatively less effective. In some instances the use of light or heavy magnesium oxide causes the contents of capsules to change into a hard, cement-like mass. Since insoluble masses of this kind would probably pass through the alimentary tract without disintegrating, it is important that the pharmacist take precautions to prevent their formation. Usually cement-like masses do not form when magnesium carbonate is used as the diluent.

It is often better first to mix one potent eutectic ingredient with the diluent or to mix each potent eutectic ingredient with a separate portion of the diluent. Generally a weight of diluent equal to that of the substances being protected is adequate. Heavy trituration hastens liquefaction. Likewise, the use of too small a capsule hastens liquefaction due to the tightness of packing.

Exposure of capsules to air or moisture usually has little or no effect on the liquefaction of a eutectic mixture.

Another method suggested for handling eutectic mixtures in capsules is to liquefy the eutectic intentionally and absorb it on magnesium carbonate. This method gives an acceptable capsule. While it is difficult to predict how much absorbent will be required to prevent liquefaction, this method avoids the possibility of subsequent liquefaction or softening because of too little diluent being used. However, more absorbent is likely to be needed to absorb a eutectic than to prevent it.

Capsules should be stable for at least the length of time that would normally elapse before all the capsules are used. Perhaps too much attention in the past has been given to the appearance of the capsules at the time they are dispensed, and too little consideration to the changes which may occur before all the capsules are used. Both considerations are important.

Obviously, the use of an inert powder increases the size of the capsule to a certain extent, depending on the relative quantity of powder used and its bulkiness. This factor must always be kept in mind since many patients find it difficult to swallow the larger capsules. In exceptional cases it may be necessary to divide the material into twice the number of capsules designated and to double the dose as to number of capsules. The ratio of the potential eutectic ingredients may have a bearing on the quantity of absorbent necessary.

Addition of Inert Powders—In some cases it is necessary to add inert powders to the ingredients prescribed before filling into capsules. This is done to increase the quantity of material/capsule to achieve greater accuracy in weighing small amounts of potent ingredients and to provide sufficient bulk so that a convenient size capsule is used for both the pharmacist and the patient.

12

℞	Vit C	25 mg.
	Thiamin B_1	2 mg.
	Nicotinic Acid	25 mg.

Make 25 such caps.
Sig: i cap. twice a day.

The pharmacist added 5.6 g of lactose to make the proper bulk.

Use of Tablets or Capsules—As the source of an active ingredient, many pharmacists are accustomed to using tablets or capsule contents (1) to avoid the necessity of weighing extremely small quantities of potent drugs, (2) because the prefabricated form is the only source of the ingredient, or (3) because the compounding is more convenient. See ℞ 17.

13

℞	Demerol Hydrochloride	50 mg.
	Atropine Sulfate	600 µg.

DtD caps. #24.
Sig: 1 q. 6–8h. for pain

In compounding this prescription the pharma-

cist triturated 24 tablets of demerol hydrochloride (50 mg each) with 24 hypodermic tablets of atropine sulfate (600 µg each), weighed the mixture, and filled 24 capsules with it.

Sometimes a physician directs ingredients to be incorporated with the contents of a prefilled capsule. The following prescriptions were filled by opening the prefilled capsule and inserting the prescribed ingredient in the form of a tablet:

14

℞	Phenaphen caps.	
	Morphine Sulfate	8 mg

D. t. d. #6
Sig: One at bt. (bedtime)

15

℞	Blank HT	#12
	Atropine Sulf. 300 µg	#12
	Pentobarb. Sod. 50 mg	#12

Sig: ut dict.

The pharmacist dispensed 12 capsules of pentobarbital sodium into each of which was inserted a tablet of the placebo and of atropine sulfate.

In other instances it may be expedient to triturate tablets and encapsulate the resulting powder when the dosage quantity of the tablet prescribed is not manufactured, as in ℞ 16:

16

℞	Cytoxan	85 mg.

D.T.D. #14
Sig: i q.d.

Cytoxan is available as tablets containing 50 mg of the active ingredient, cyclophosphamide. The average weight of a tablet was found to be 580 mg. The pharmacist dispensed 28 capsules (#0), each containing 500 mg of the powdered tablets. The directions were changed to read: "Take two (2) capsules daily."

Some pharmacists find it advantageous to use compressed tablets as a source of ingredients to fill capsule prescriptions, as seen in ℞ 17:

17

℞	Aminophylline	100 mg.
	Ephedrine sulf.	25 mg.
	Chlor-Trimeton	4 mg.
	Phenobarbital	30 mg.

DTD #36
Sig: 1 q 6–8 h prn SOB

To compound, the pharmacist triturated 36 of each of the following commercially available tablets and encapsulated the powder mixture: Combined aminophylline (100 mg) − phenobarbital (30 mg), Chlor-Trimeton (*Schering*) (4 mg), and ephedrine sulfate (25 mg).

An extension of the idea of tablets in capsules is seen in the use commercially of a tablet in a capsule to avoid an incompatibility. The case in point is Epragen Pulvules (*Lilly*) in which ephedrine hydrochloride in the form of a specially coated tablet (Sphercote) is embedded in a mixture of aspirin, phenacetin, amobarbital, and diluent.

Use of Two Capsules—Similar to using a tablet in a capsule to overcome an incompatibility, as mentioned, is the use of a capsule within a capsule. Pharmacists have long recognized that sometimes the problem of two mutually incompatible ingredients in a prescription can be handled by placing one of the ingredients in a small capsule and then enclosing it in a larger capsule containing the remaining ingredient.

Liquids—Oils and other liquids which will not dissolve gelatin may be dispensed in hard capsules, as shown in R 18 and 19.

The oil may be dropped into the body of the capsule, using a medicine dropper, measuring pipet, or a buret. The inside rim of the cap portion is moistened with hot water which may be applied with a glass rod or cotton-tipped applicator and the cap is then put in place with a rotary motion.

18

R   Trichloroethylene   0.6 ml./cap. #36
   Sig: Pierce and inhale prn.

Another method for sealing liquids in hard capsules is to allow the cap of the capsule to stand on a piece of wetted filter paper during the time that it takes to fill the body of the capsule with the given liquid. This is usually enough time for the rim of the cap to become sufficiently moist to effect a satisfactory seal. Capsules which show signs of leaking due to imperfect sealing should be rejected.

19

R   Castor Oil   7.5 ml
   Dispense 12 capsules
   Sig: 2 caps. at night

(The pharmacist used #11 veterinary capsules.)

Storing

It is best to store capsules in a cool place of moderate humidity, as they tend to lose water and become brittle if kept too long in a warm, dry place. Excess moisture tends to soften gelatin so that the separation of the cap from the body of the capsule presents a problem. Many pharmacists transfer their stock of empty capsules to screw-cap wide-mouth bottles for protection from variations in humidity.

Dispensing

Capsules should be dispensed in glass or plastic containers (see Figs. 5 and 6). The advantages such containers offer in convenience of handling and portability and in protecting the capsules from moisture and dust make them more desirable than cardboard boxes. Unit dose packaging may also be advantageous.

If capsules containing deliquescent or hygroscopic substances are dispensed, the pharmacist should advise the pa-

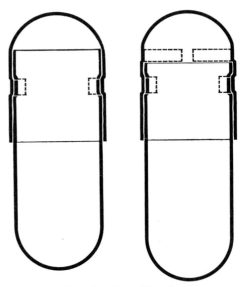

Fig. 4—Lok-Caps (courtesy, *Elanco*).

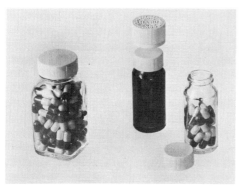

Fig. 5—Glass containers for capsules with slip-on overcaps to make child-resistant closure (courtesy, *Brockway Glass Co., Inc.*).

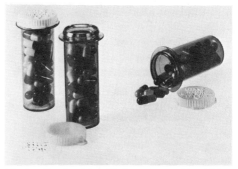

Fig. 6—Plastic vials with interchangeable child-resistant and regular snap-cap closures (courtesy, *Brockway Glass Co., Inc.*).

tient to keep the vial well-closed after removal of the prescribed dose.

Not to be overlooked is the requirement to dispense certain capsule medications in light-resistant containers. Information of this nature is usually included in the labeling for the market product. However, if the pharmacist has doubts, he can take a cue from the container used for the market package, and select amber or flint vials accordingly.

To prevent capsules from rattling, a tuft of cotton may be placed over or under the capsules in the vial.

When dispensing capsules, it is advisable to inform the patient on how best to take the capsule orally. Patients have been known to return the empty capsules from their prescription medication for refilling.

In some pharmacies, to facilitate prompt dispensing, the more commonly prescribed hand-filled capsule prescriptions of various physicians are made up in advance and kept in stock.

Closures—Several manufacturers have devised special means for keeping filled hard-shell capsules from coming apart during shipment and handling. Kapseals (*Parke-Davis*) have a gelatin band around the middle of the capsule which serves as a seal. Spansules (*SK&F*) are sealed by pinpoint fusion of the cap to the surface of the capsule body. Lok-Caps (*Elanco*) (Fig. 4) contain a slightly raised segmented collar around the inside shoulder. The collar

provides a locking action. In addition to keeping the capsule from coming apart, these techniques tend to render the capsules tamper-proof.

In extemporaneous compounding no particular problem is encountered with filled capsules coming apart provided the capsule is properly closed and not overfilled by tamping excessive quantities of the contents into the cap.

Quality Control

Quality control is an essential part of hard and soft capsule production. Numerous tests and inspections are involved before the capsule reaches the consumer. In the production of empty hard-shell capsules, the tolerances are controlled so that the capsules will join properly when they are filled. Physical dimensions—wall thickness, length, and overall joined length are checked. Capsules leaving the automated machines are visually inspected; those with air bubbles, dents, cracks, loose caps, and other faults are sorted out. On filled capsules, both the hard and soft, the controls include tests for drug content, moisture content, fill-weight, disintegration, dissolution, stability, and, in the case of capsules containing liquids, for leaking and other defects. Since the control of the quality of prefabricated capsules rests largely with the manufacturer, the pharmacist must rely on the reputation of the manufacturer. The pharmacist should make every effort to acquaint himself with the quality-con-

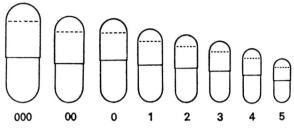

| 000 | 00 | 0 | 1 | 2 | 3 | 4 | 5 |

Fig. 7—Actual relative sizes of hard gelatin capsules.

trol capability and quality consciousness of the manufacturer.

In the extemporaneous preparation of capsule medication, the pharmacist also exercises a personal degree of quality control by making certain that the drug substances used are obtained from highly reputable sources and that the procedure and technique used in compounding will result in a capsule medication that is within accepted accuracy and uniformity of content and is free of controllable environmental contaminants.

Control tests included in the USP and the NF are for weight variation of the contents of both hard and soft capsules, content uniformity, and dissolution.

Types

Hard Capsules

Hard-shell gelatin capsules are made from a mixture of gelatin, sugar, and water, with or without suitable coloring agents. Sulfur dioxide is used as a preservative. Capsules are made opaque with titanium dioxide.

Sizes—Hard capsules are available in a variety of sizes and are designated by numbers from 000 to 5. Capsule sizes are shown in Fig. 7. Manufacturers also make available numbers 10, 11, and 12 for veterinary use. The latter have relative capacities of 1, ½, and ¼ oz, respectively. Usually the pharmacist selects the proper size by actual trial. However, for general guidance he may refer to tables printed on the box of empty capsules which gives the approximate capacity of capsules in the apothecary and metric systems for several drugs of

Table 1—Capacity of Empty Capsules

Capsule number	Quinine sulfate (gr)	Acetylsalicylic acid (gr)	Sodium bicarbonate (gr)	Bismuth subnitrate (gr)
000	10	16	22	28
00	6	10	15	20
0	5	8	11	14
1	3½	5	8	10
2	3	4	6	8
3	2	3	5	6
4	1½	2½	4	4
5	1	1½	2	2

varying densities. See Table 1. The capacity, of course, varies with the degree of pressure used in filling.

It is important for the dispensing pharmacist to write the size of the capsule on the prescription in the event that the prescription is refilled. Fluffy powders may be triturated in a mortar to reduce the bulk, thus allowing a smaller capsule to be used for a given weight of powder.

Prescriptions—The following prescription illustrates the dispensing of a single drug in powdered form in hard capsules. Such substances should be in the form of fine powders; this makes it easier to place the material in capsules and makes the drug more soluble or diffusible when liberated in the stomach.

20

R̸   Magnesium oxide (Hvy)   150 mg. #90
     Mft capsules
     Sig: 1—3 x d

Occasionally, a physician may prescribe a colored prefilled capsule to be dispensed as a placebo, the capsule not being available *per se.* In R̸ 21 the pharmacist emptied the prefilled capsules specified and refilled them with lactose.

21

℞ Pulvule Amytal   65
    Placebo #30
    Sig: 1 q 6 h prn nervousness NMT 3 x d

To open the pulvule for refilling with lactose, the cap should be first rotated slightly and then gently pulled.

The ℞ 22 and 23 are typical powder mixtures prescribed in capsules.

22

℞ Codeine Phosph.   0.6 g
    Phenobarbital   1 g
    Acidi Acetylsalicyl.   8 g
    M. ft. cap. No. XL.
    Sig: One cap. q. 4 hrs.

23

℞ Cod. sulf.   15 mg
    Papav.   100 mg
    Ft. cap #1   disp. 15
    Sig: 1 q. 3–4 h p.r.n. pain

See also *Miscellaneous Prescriptions* at the end of the chapter.

Soft Capsules

Soft capsules, also called "soft shell," or "soluble elastic" capsules are made from gelatin to which glycerin or some other polyol, such as sorbitol or propylene glycol, has been added as a plasticizer. The distinctive feature of this dosage form is its one-piece construction with the fill material literally wrapped inside of a sealed, gelatin matrix. Hard gelatin capsule manufacture, on the other hand, is generally a two-step process in which the shells are made on one type of machinery and the filling operation is performed on another. There is a large variety of shapes and sizes in which soft capsules are prepared. Cosmetics, flavors, food concentrates, detergents, and other items are enclosed in soft capsules, as well as pharmaceuticals. Spherical or ovoid capsules are sometimes called pearls or globules. Soft capsules are formed and filled in one continuous operation on complicated semiautomatic and automatic machines. Developments in this area include a machine that is specially designed for filling dry powders and granular materials into a soft gelatin capsule. Studies of dissolution rates have shown that dry-fill materials are assimilated much more readily than an oleaginous liquid or paste. References containing a description of commercial soft-capsule filling machines are included in the *Bibliography*.

Long-Acting Capsules

Included among a variety of prolonged-action medications are some which involve capsules. Several of these capsular dosage forms and the mechanisms by which they provide prolonged action are briefly described here.

The Spansule (*SK&F*), introduced in 1952, consists of a hard gelatin capsule containing a mixture of tiny medicated beads, some of which are coated with different thicknesses of ingestible lipid materials, such as beeswax or glyceryl monostearate, and some of which are uncoated. The uncoated beads provide the initial release of medication, while the coated beads slowly disintegrate in the gastrointestinal tract and release the medicament over an extended period of time. By appropriate blending of uncoated and coated beads a desired prolonged-action pattern is obtained. Medicament release from the Spansule is independent of pH; the release is primarily controlled by moisture vapor permeability of the lipid coat which in turn is a function of the composition and thickness of the coat. The Dexamyl Spansule is an example of this type of prolonged-action dosage form.

The Medule (*Upjohn*) capsular dosage form also consists of coated and uncoated medicated beads. Here the sustained-release portion of the beads is coated with different thicknesses of a styrene-maleic anhydride copolymer which is pH-sensitive, thereby preventing dissolution of the coated beads in the stomach. Medrol Medules is an example of this type of prolonged-action dosage form.

Another variation of the encapsulated sustained-release bead-type product involves microdialysis. Beads containing the drug are coated with different thicknesses of an inert, flexible, insoluble, semipermeable polymer. Cells in the semipermeable membranous coat absorb water, and the water dissolves the drug. The drug then dialyzes through the coat into the gastrointestinal fluids. The rate of dialysis depends primarily on the thickness of the coat. An example of this capsular dosage form is Nitrospan Capsules (*USV*).

Encapsulation of tiny beads of drug resinates offers still another means of prolonging drug action. Antihistamines, sympathomimetics, or narcotics may be released from a sulfonic acid cation resinate by an exchange with cations present in the gastrointestinal fluids. Drug release depends on the pH and the total concentration of cations of the gastrointestinal fluids. An example of this type of capsular dosage form is Tussionex Capsules (*Pennwalt*).

Patients taking prolonged-action dosage forms should be advised of the nature of formulation from the standpoint of administration intervals so as to avoid overdosage. In the following prescription the pharmacist in consultation with the prescriber changed the directions to the patient to read "Take one capsule every 12 hours as needed."

24

℞ Pyma Timed Capsules #30
    Sig: 1 cap prn.

Occasionally a prescription may call for a portion of a dose of a prolonged-release capsule, as in the following:

25

age 4 yrs.

℞ Ornade Spansule DTD #10
    Sig: ½ cap q. 12 h.

(Instructions to the parent were to empty half of the "beads," close the capsule, and give it.)

The composition of the prolonged-release capsule determines the feasibility of dispensing only a portion of a dose. In this case it is not advisable to administer a partially filled capsule.

There is no assurance of a uniform dose since the capsule contains a mixture of uncoated and coated beads, with the coated beads having different thicknesses of coats as well.

Enteric-Coated Capsules

See Chapter 5.

Miscellaneous Prescriptions

26

℞ Butazolidin Alka caps
    #20
    Sig: 1 QID c̄ 2 ASA
    Label
    Refill 1x

The pharmacist noted the additive effects of Butazolidin with aspirin. The physician then directed that the doses be alternated every 2 hours.

27

℞ Placidyl   100 mg
    Mft caps #32
    Sig: 1 cap ea. a.m. & p.m.

28

℞ Nembutal   gr. iss
    #12 NaHCO₃ blank
    Sig: One at bedtime prn sleep

29

℞ Cap Vistaril   50 mg.
    Disp. #30
    Sig: Label by name. One h.s. daily
    Refill prn.

30

℞ Ku-Zyme
    Disp. 12 caps.
    Sig: Sprinkle opened capsule on high protein vegetables

The pharmacist took time to show the patient how to open the capsule.

31

℞ Pyrroxate Capsules
      Codeine gr. s̄s̄
    Mft. caps #12
    Sig: 1 q. 4 h. p.r.n. pain.

32

Age 5 years

℞ Ekko Jr.
    #100
    Sig: 1 bid. Empty cap in tsp. and give.

33

℞ Caps. Fiorinal
    Dispense 40

Sig: i q 4 h. prn pain or muscle and joint soreness.
Refill prn

34

R̞ Acogesic caps #12
Darvo-tran #12
Sig: 1 of ea q. 4 h.

35

R̞ Noctec 0.5 g
DTD #50
Sig: 500 mg. p. o. h. s.
Label

36

R̞ Cap. Vitamin A (50,000 units) No. L.
Sig: i capsule daily.

37

R̞ Bism. Subgall. caps.
#50
(Fill a #0 cap till full)
Sig: 1–2 prn
LABEL
Refill—ut dict

38

R̞ Atropine sulfate gr. $\frac{1}{32}$
Ephedrine sulfate gr. ii
Salicylamide gr. xxv
Pentobarbital gr. iv
M ft cap. no. xii
Sig: 1 cap ut dict

39

R̞ Talwin 50 mg.
(Patient has difficulty swallowing tabs.)
Mft caps #36
Sig: 1 q. 3–4 h.

40

R̞ Ferro-Sequels #30
Sig: 2 capsules daily

Note: This is a dry-filled soft gelatin capsule. Sequels (Lederle) are sustained-release capsules.

Bibliography

Hostetler VB, Bellard JQ: Hard capsules. In Lachman L, Lieberman HA, Kanig JL (eds): *Theory and Practice of Industrial Pharmacy,* Lea & Febiger, Philadelphia, 359, 1970.

Jones BE: Hard gelatin capsules. *Mfg. Chem Aerosol News Feb:* 25, 1969.

Strickland WA Jr, Moss M: Water vapor sorption and diffusion through hard gelatin capsules. *J Pharm Sci 51:* 1002, 1962.

Newton JM, Rowley G: On the release of drug from hard gelatin capsules. *J Pharm Pharmacol 22 Suppl:* 163S, 1970.

Newton JM, Rowley G, Tornblom JVF: The effect of additives on the release of drug from hard gelatin capsules. *J Pharm Pharmacol 23:* 452, 1971.

Samyn JC, Yin Jung W: In vitro dissolution from several experimental capsule formulations. *J Pharm Sci 59:* 169, 1970.

Stempel E: Patents for prolonged action dosage forms. *Drug Cos Ind 98(1):* 44, 118, 1966.

Stanley JJ: Soft gelatin capsules. In Lachman L, Lieberman HA, Kanig JL (eds): *Theory and Practice of Industrial Pharmacy,* Lea & Febiger, Philadelphia, 359, 1970.

Lazor T: Soft gelatin capsules for pharmaceuticals. *Drug Cos Ind 114 (Jan–Jun):* 42, 109, 1974.

King RE: Tablets, Capsules, and Pills. In *Remington's Pharmaceutical Sciences,* 15th ed, Mack Publ. Co., Easton, PA, 1576, 1975.

4

Powders

Bernard Ecanow, PhD
Professor of Pharmacy
College of Pharmacy
University of Illinois at the
Medical Center
Chicago, IL 60680

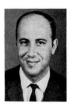

Farid Sadik, PhD
Associate Professor of
Pharmaceutics
College of Pharmacy
University of South Carolina
Columbia, SC 29208

Dr. Sadik prepared the section on *Comminution.*

There is no official pharmaceutical definition for the term powder. In general, however, a powder may be described as the fine particles which result from the comminution of any dry substance. Comminution is a broadly used term referring to many types of processes such as triturating, levigating, grinding, and pulverizing. Finely divided powders may also be prepared by carefully controlled chemical and physical reactions such as precipitation and crystal growth, followed by appropriate treatment and drying of the finely divided particles. See *Comminution,* page 100.

Powders consist of particles ranging from about 10,000 micrometers (μm) (1 μm = 0.001 mm)–0.1 μm. The most useful range for pharmaceutical powders as dosage forms is in the paracolloidal and colloidal region (10–0.1 μm). Despite the fact that powdered dosage forms have a continuous history of use since antiquity, the lack of any restrictive definition reflects the art of their formulation rather than the science of powder technology. The fineness of particles, in pharmaceutical terminology, is defined by the USP in descriptive terms: *very coarse, coarse, moderately coarse, fine,* and *very fine.* Such designations generally correspond to groups of standard mesh sieves which are identified by sieve numbers.

The nominal dimensions and descriptive terminology of powdered chemicals of various degrees of fineness are given in Table 1. Since the classification scheme refers to the number of wire strands in its construction, it should be noted that sieves with the higher sieve numbers retain finer particles than those with the lower numbers.

The physicochemical properties of powders are largely a function of the size and surface area of the particles. Fine particles approaching the colloidal range diffuse in a manner similar to a gas. The rate of settling of very small particles (up to 200 mesh) depends on the viscosity of the fluid suspension medium. Larger size particles settle at a

Table 1—Fineness of Powdered Chemicals

Sieve[a] number	Sieve opening mm	Sieve opening µm	Descriptive standard	Particle size (range of)
2	9.52	9520	Very coarse	Granulated effervescent salts and powders for compressed tablets
8	2.38	2380		
10	2.00	2000		
20	0.84	840	Coarse	
30	0.59	590		
40	0.42	420	Moderately coarse	
50	0.297	297		Powdered effervescent salts and divided powders
60	0.250	250	Fine	
80	0.177	177	Very fine	
120	0.125	125		
200	0.074	74		
325	0.044	44		
	Theoretical			
625	0.020	20		Divided powders for dusting; adsorbents; inhalants; and micronized sulfonamides, cortisone, penicillin, etc.
1250	0.010	10		
2500	0.005	5	Micronized (not USP terminology)	
5000	0.0025	2.5		
12500	0.001	1		

[a] Sieves which meet USP and National Bureau of Standards specifications are made of wire cloth woven from brass, bronze, or other suitable wire, and are not coated or plated.

rate which depends primarily on the difference between the density of the particle and that of the dispersion medium (Stokes' law). High concentrations of particles or aggregates of large particles do not follow Stokes' law, however, and in such cases the settling characteristics are related to the type of aggregate which the particles form, structure density of the aggregates, and particle geometry. Dosage forms consisting of powdered materials, either in the dry or suspended state, reflect the characteristics which result from the surface interactions of the particles. Particle size and surface activity influence such physical characteristics as ease of mixing, dispersibility, and pharmaceutical elegance. Attempts to deal with particle size diameters as a function of surface/unit volume have provided important information concerning adsorption, dissolution, and particle-particle interactions. These same physicochemical parameters may profoundly influence such important biopharmaceutic characteristics as degree of solubility, bioavailability, pharmacological onset, and duration of drug action.

Knowledge of interfacial conditions and aggregation phenomena in dry powders represent significant considerations for the pharmacist. As with other dosage forms, powders are subject to the general processes of aggregation. Most aggregations in powders result directly from the interaction of adsorbed films such as water or gases present on the particulate surface. The absence of such surface impurities generally reduces the tendency for the particles to aggregate under the normal gravitational conditions and similarly increases the rate of solution in most solvents. Although the absolute solubility in any solvent remains relatively unaffected by traces of adsorbed impurities in surface films, the dissolution rates may be markedly altered. Crystals of boric acid are usually recommended for the preparation of extemporaneous solutions such as eye washes. Yet, if the crystals are first powdered before being dissolved, the rate of solution is considerably greater than that observed for the commercially powdered boric acid, which, with time, has acquired a film of adsorbed gases. Since freshly powdered boric acid has not been in prolonged contact with the atmosphere, it possesses very little adsorbed contaminants. The relatively greater surface area permits the powder to dissolve more rapidly than the crystalline material. In general, absolute solubility does not depend on particle size except for particles in the subcolloidal range. Very small particles (below 1 μm) possess unusually high surface free energy which results in increased absolute solubility. Such considerations may be important in the industrial manufacture of powdered dosage forms and may have biopharmaceutical significance, but they rarely influence the extemporaneous compounding of prescription powders. The beneficial use of wetting agents to increase the dispersibility of powders which are extemporaneously compounded with liquid vehicles should be kept in mind. Often, levigation of the dry powder with a small amount of glycerin, alcohol, propylene glycol, or other suitable liquid improves the efficacy and pharmaceutic elegance of the finished powder-liquid dispersion, regardless of whether the system is a suspension, emulsion, ointment, or aerosol. The use of wetting agents increases contact between the particle surface and the dispersion medium.

Comminution

Comminution refers to the process of reducing the particle size of a solid substance to a finer state of subdivision. The USP and the NF express the fineness of a powder in descriptive terms and relate it to the number assigned to a standard sieve.

In the past, the reduction of particle size and the uniformity of fineness of medicinal substances were primarily considered for their effect on the formulation of powders and other dosage forms. However, for the last two decades particle size reduction has gained added importance because of its influence on drug availability in biological systems. The main objectives of comminution are to (1) increase the surface area of a drug thereby increasing its dissolution and absorption rates and (2) aid in the formulation of pharmaceutically acceptable dosage forms including powders.

Methods of Comminution

Operations such as contusion, grating, cutting, slicing, and chopping are less important today than they were in the past. The cutting process is employed mainly on crude vegetable drugs such as leaves and roots. Grating is applied to a few drugs such as cocoa butter preparatory to making suppositories. Present methods employed by drug manufacturers involve the use of numerous and diversified types of machines that reduce drugs to powders of varying degree of fineness.

The type of equipment employed for particle size reduction depends largely on the physical properties of the drug. Different drugs vary in their ease of grinding. Factors such as hardness, structure, water of crystallization, hygroscopicity, moisture content, and sensitiveness to change in temperature may affect the grindability of a drug. Hard, crystalline materials may be reduced effectively by the attrition and impact action of the hammer mills. Fibrous crude drugs such as roots, leaves, and barks can be sufficiently subdivided by a cutting action. Drugs such as sodium sulfate give off water of crystallization at comparatively low temperature, causing clogging of the mill. Likewise, moisture absorbed by hygroscopic drugs as well as moisture content give to drugs elasticity which makes it difficult to pulverize. Certain materials tend to soften, burn, or degrade with the increase in temperature resulting from the milling process.

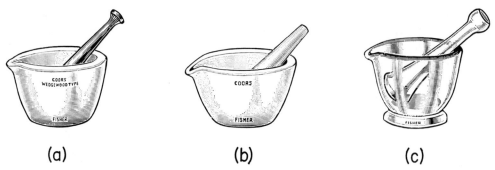

Fig. 1—Mortars and pestles: (a) Wedgwood type, (b) porcelain, and (c) glass (courtesy, *Fisher Sci. Co.*).

Manual Comminution

The operations used manually by pharmacists for particle size reduction are trituration and pulverization by intervention.

Trituration (L. *triturare*, rub to pieces) is the grinding of a solid substance to a fine powder by continued rubbing of the particles in a mortar with a pestle—this term is also employed to designate the process by which two or more powders are mixed together. Trituration is best accomplished by rotating the firmly held pestle in a circular movement with a downward pressure starting at the center of the mortar and gradually moving in successive circles until the side of the mortar is touched and then back again toward the center. In order to ensure uniform mixing and better grinding, powder that adheres to the sides of mortar and pestle should be scraped off with a spatula. The trituration process should be continued until a uniformly mixed fine powder is obtained. The subdivision of the powder is accomplished by grinding the particles entrapped between the pestle and the roughened sides and bottom of the mortar.

In general, trituration is performed in a mortar and pestle made of Wedgwood ware, porcelain, or glass (Fig. 1). Wedgwood ware mortars are durable but stain easily and after continued usage become smooth. Porcelain mortars are either glazed or unglazed and are useful for preparing emulsions and solutions. Pestles made of porcelain are easily broken and should not be used when trituration is combined with contusion. Glass mortars and pestles are objectionable because of their smooth surfaces. However, because they are nonporous they are preferred for making solutions which stain Wedgwood or porcelain mortars. They have an additional usefulness for triturating small quantities of potent drugs. The shape of mortars best suited for trituration are those having flat bottoms.

For other considerations regarding the use of mortar and pestle see *Trituration*, page 108.

Pulverization by Intervention is the process of reducing a substance to a fine powder by means of utilizing a solvent which can be removed easily. The best known example is camphor which, when triturated in a mortar to reduce it to a powder, becomes a pliable mass. However, when camphor is triturated with a few drops of alcohol, ether, or chloroform, it can be pulverized without difficulty. The solvent added evaporates rather quickly leaving behind the finely subdivided camphor.

Mechanical Comminution

Large-scale mechanical comminution is carried out mostly by different kinds of mills that have the capability of producing powders having a wide range of particle size.

Ball or Pebble Mills—These mills, which are also called jar mills, consist of cylindrical containers or jars made of porcelain or steel either unlined or lined with buhrstone, porcelain, rubber, or high-density alumina. The jar contains different-sized balls or pebbles made of steel, porcelain, or flint which act as the grinding media. Pulverization is accomplished by placing the material to be ground in the jar along with the balls or pebbles. The cover is sealed tightly and the jar is fitted with shafts and rotated about its longitudinal axis at a predetermined speed until pulverization is achieved. Another method of rotating the jar is by placing it on motor-driven friction rolls mounted on a steel frame.

Particle size reduction is affected by the rolling, sliding, and tumbling of balls or pebbles on the material being pulverized as well as by size and speed of the balls.

Ball or pebble mills are economical, simple to operate, versatile, and easy to clean. They can be used for pulverizing and/or mixing wet or dry mixtures.

Wiley Mill—The structure of the Wiley mill involves four knives on a rotor with a shearing action against six stationary knives on the frame. The material to be comminuted is introduced into the loading hopper. As the rotor revolves, the material is carried to the grinding chamber where it is ground after which it passes through a screen to a receiving compartment. The size of the particle is controlled by the screen aperture.

The Wiley mill operates by successive shear action of the knives and this makes it useful for comminuting fibrous materials that cannot be reduced by grinding or crushing.

Hammer Mills—A hammer mill is composed of a high-speed horizontal or vertical rotor shaft carrying hammers or beaters which may be T-shaped, stirrups, bars, or rings. The rotor revolves with its hammers in a grinding chamber containing grinding liners. A screen encloses the rotor and serves as an internal size classifier by keeping coarse particles in the grinding chamber until they are fine enough to pass through the screen.

The fineness of the product is affected by the type of hammers, rotor speed, and size of the screen opening.

Hammer mills are available in many types which include the Mikro-Pulverizer and Mikro-Atomizer.

Fluid-Energy Mills—These mills, which are also known as jet mills, basically have no moving parts. Jet pulverization is achieved by subjecting the material to be micronized to a stream of fluid energy (compressed air, steam, or inert gas) which causes the particles to accelerate to great speeds inside the grinding chamber. The particles are impacted against each other or against the mill wall and as a result they are reduced in size.

Materials that break readily under high-speed impact are suitable for use in such mills. Fibrous, elastic, or sticky materials cannot be pulverized effectively. Depending on the material being pulverized these mills can produce particles as small as 0.5 μm. In general, the particle size of the finished powder is controlled through variation of the feed flow rate and the fluid energy flow rate. Fine particles are obtained with slow feed and high fluid energy rate.

Spray Drying—A spray dryer consists of a cone-shaped drying chamber through which hot air is circulated, an atomizer, and a powder-collecting device. A solution or suspension of the material to be pulverized is sprayed by an atomizer into the top of the drying chamber producing small droplets which are almost instantly dried by the hot dry air circulating in the chamber. In this way an extremely fine powder is formed which falls to the bottom of the chamber and is collected by a collector.

Lyophilization—This procedure, which is also known as freeze-drying, is the process of drying substances at very low pressure by direct vaporization (sublimation) of water from the frozen state to vapor without intermediate passage through the liquid state. The temperature of the frozen material should be between −10° to −40° C.

The basic elements of a freeze-drier consist of a vacuum chamber, source of heat, condenser, and vacuum pump capable of reducing the pressure in the vacuum chamber to between 0.01 and 0.05 mm of mercury. An aqueous solution or dispersion of the material to be lyophilized is frozen by placing it in a container which is then immersed in a freezing bath consisting of a mixture of solid carbon dioxide (Dry Ice) and solvents having low freezing points such as alcohol and acetone. In large-scale operations, freezing the liquid can be accomplished by an internal cooling source inside the vacuum chamber. In any case, it is advisable to have the thickness of the frozen material in the container not greater than $7/8$ in. in order to facilitate the diffusion of water vapor through the ice. The container is then quickly transferred from the freezing bath to the vacuum chamber which is then sealed promptly and immediately subjected to vacuum in order to prevent thawing of the frozen material. When the absolute pressure reaches 3 mm or lower, frozen water sublimes and is collected in the condenser. As frozen water vaporizes heat is removed from the frozen material and consequently the temperature of the material steadily drops. In order to facilitate the drying process, external heat such as infrared heating is employed. When the water content of the frozen material is reduced to 1% or less the temperature of the material rises until it approaches that of the heating medium. The temperature elevation indicates the completion of the drying process. Lyophilization is utilized mainly for drying heat-sensitive materials such as biological products, antibiotics, enzymes, and hormones.

Particle Size Specifications

Because standardization of particle size is essential in controlling the quality of medications, specific methods of classifying and measuring particles have been developed.

Particle Size Classification

In order to produce a powder of a uniform particle size it is important to subject the powdered material to a process of size classification in which the material is separated into two or more fractions. Particle size classification is accomplished either after the material has been pulverized or during milling where pulverization and classification processes are performed inside the mill. Size classifiers or separators may be divided into gravity, centrifugal or air types.

Gravity Separation—Gravity classification of particle size involves the use of one or more sieves. The process is referred to as sieving (sifting, screening) and is accomplished by separating a powdered sample composed of various particle sizes into two or more fractions with a sieve. The types of screen surfaces most frequently used include (1) punched plates made of sheet steel, (2) woven wire screen made of brass, copper, bronze, iron, or steel, (3) silk bolting cloth, and (4) micromesh sieves made by electroforming nickel. Sieves for pharmacopeial testing are of wire cloth woven, not twilled, except the cloth for Nos. 230, 270, 325, 400, from brass, bronze, stainless steel, or other suitable wire, and are not coated or plated.

Sieves are numbered according to two standard designations: the Tyler Standard Sieve series and the US Standard Sieve series. The difference is that the Tyler Standard Sieves are identified by a number which designates the number of openings/linear inch, whereas the US Standard Sieves are identified by millimeters or micrometers. Table 1 correlates the official classification of powders with the particle size of each class that passes through standard sieves. Table 2 gives the nominal dimensions of standard sieves.

Sieving may be performed either manually or mechanically. In manual sieving the material is placed on top of the sieve which is shaken by a circular motion until sieving is practically complete. Powder that passes through the sieve is accepted while that retained on the sieve is rejected for further grind-

Table 2—Openings of Standard Sieves

	Sieve opening	
Number	*mm*	*μm*
2	9.52	9520
3.5	5.66	5660
4	4.76	4760
8	2.38	2380
10	2.00	2000
20	0.84	840
30	0.59	595
40	0.42	420
50	0.297	297
60	0.250	250
70	0.210	210
80	0.177	177
100	0.149	149
120	0.125	125
200	0.074	74
230	0.063	63
270	0.053	53
325	0.044	44
400	0.037	37

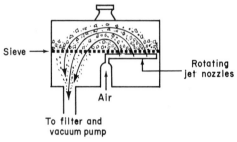

Fig. 3—Alpine Laboratory Air Jet Sieve.

ing. Mechanical sieving is accomplished by means of a variety of devices. An example is the Ro-Tap Sieve Shaker (Fig. 2). The various sieves are arranged in a stack, including a bottom pan, with the coarsest sieve at the top. The sample to be sieved is placed on the top sieve and the whole nest of sieves is shaken. The shaker, which produces a uniform circular and tapping motion, causes the undersize to pass downward through the nest of sieves until they rest on a sieve with openings smaller than the parti-

cles. As a result the sample is separated into fractions according to particle size range.

Centrifugal Separation—Centrifugal classifiers operate at high rotor speeds (13,000–15,000 rpm). The powder is introduced into the classifier where it falls on a rotating distributor which deflects the powder into the classification zone. Centrifugal force causes the coarse particles to be removed through the coarse discharge outlet while fine ones are carried inward and are discharged into the collector.

Air Separation—Air classification is affected with the aid of a stream of air. An example is the Alpine Laboratory Air Jet Sieve illustrated in Fig. 3. Air is sucked through the machine by means of a vacuum pump. The entering air is distributed through the base of the sieve by rotating jet nozzles located below the sieve. When the material to be sifted is placed on the surface of the sieve the air jet keeps the sieve openings clear and the return flow of air carries the undersize with it. The undersize is collected by a filter while the oversize is retained on the sieve.

Particle Size Measurement

A powdered material is normally composed of particles of various size ranges. The result of particle size measurement of a sample can be graphically depicted by a size-frequency distribution curve which is obtained by plotting frequency (the percentage weight of each fraction of the sample or the number of particles occurring in a definite size range) against the mean particle

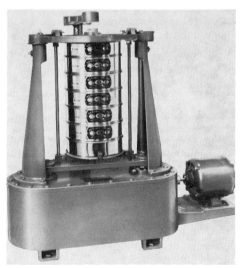

Fig. 2—Ro-Tap Sieve Shaker (courtesy, *W. S. Tyler Co.*).

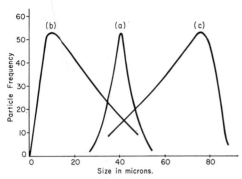

Fig. 4—Particle size distribution curves of various powders: (a) symmetrical, (b) negatively skewed, and (c) positively skewed.

size of each range. The shape of the size-frequency distribution curve differs from one powder to another. Some powders may have a particle size distribution that results in a symmetric or normal curve (Fig. 4a). Other powders may produce asymmetric or skewed curves. A powder which contains a greater number of coarser particles than finer ones produces a positively skewed curve (Fig. 4c) while a powder which contains a greater number of finer particles produces a negatively skewed curve (Fig. 4b). An S-shaped cumulative frequency curve may result when the number of particles in each size range are added consecutively to those in the previous range and the cumulative percentage is plotted against the particle size.

Measurement of particle size may be made by a wide variety of instruments and techniques which include sieving, microscopy, sedimentation, elutriation, particle volume measurement, light scattering, air permeability, or gas adsorption.

Sieving is the simplest method of determining the particle size distribution of powdered solids, particularly vegetable drugs and coarser particles. The various sieves are arranged in a stack with the coarsest sieve at the top. A sample of known weight is placed on the top sieve and the whole stack is shaken either manually or mechanically for a predetermined period of time by an oscillating motion. The powder retained

on each sieve is weighed and the percentage weight of each fraction is obtained.

Sieving is simple, economical, and allows the use of a large quantity of powder, thus minimizing sample error. It is employed in particle size analyses over a size range from 50 to 1000 μm.

Microscopy has the advantage of giving direct observation on shape, structure, and surface characteristics of particles. However, the method is tedious and time-consuming because a large number of particles, approximately 1000, should be measured to ensure a representative count. A specimen weighing approximately 1 mg (depending somewhat on fineness of the powder) is placed on a microscopic slide. One or two drops of dispersant, in which the powder is insoluble, are added and the mixture is incorporated with a spatula until a smooth dispersion is obtained. The particle size is estimated by comparing its image with a series of circles on a graticule placed on the microscope field of view. To facilitate microscopic particle size measurement, the field either can be projected onto a screen or photographed for subsequent projection. Direct counting and measuring of particles from a photomicrograph can be performed automatically by means of electronic particle sizers such as the Zeiss Particle Size Analyzer.

A white-light microscope can be used to measure particles having a size range of from 0.2 to 100 μm. The ultramicroscope can detect particles as small as 0.01 μm, while the electron microscope is useful in revealing particles in the Ångstrom (Å = 1 $\times$ 10^{-8} cm) range.

Sedimentation methods are all based on the relationship between the particle size and the settling rate derived from Stokes equation which shows that larger particles settle more quickly than smaller. The majority of the sedimentation methods utilize liquid dispersion of the powder to be analyzed but gas can be used as sedimentation medium. The particle size distribution of the powder is obtained by studying the concentration changes occurring within a settling suspension.

Elutriation is the process of separating powders into two or more fractions of different sizes by suspending the particles in a fluid, such as water or air.

Air elutriation is based on the fact that an air stream moving upward at a specific velocity is capable of carrying particles smaller than a given size while larger particles settle to the bottom. Thus, the powder is separated into two fractions of different sizes. Several fractions can be obtained by changing the velocity of the air stream. Size analysis is obtained by weighing the powder in each fraction.

In liquid elutriation the powder is mixed with a liquid in which it is insoluble. The mixture is agitated and allowed to stand. Coarser particles, being heavier, settle to the bottom of the elutriater while finer particles remain suspended temporarily. The liquid holding the fine particles is decanted and evaporated to dryness.

Particle Volume Measurement— An instrument which is based on this method is the Coulter Counter. It consists of an electronic cabinet and a sample stand. The sample stand consists of an aperture tube with electrodes located on either side of the aperture, a beaker that contains the suspended particles to be analyzed and a mercury manometer connected to the aperture tube by means of a stopcock.

The particles to be analyzed are suspended in an electrically conductive liquid. The concentration of the suspension is such that particles pass through the aperture one at a time. When the stopcock is opened, the suspension in the beaker is drawn through the aperture by means of an external vacuum system. This flow unbalances the mercury manometer. The stopcock is closed and the flow of suspension is continued by the siphoning action of the mercury column. When a suspended particle passes through the aperture, it replaces its own volume of electrolyte and this momentarily increases the resistance

between the two electrodes. The change in resistance produces a short duration voltage pulse, the magnitude of which is proportional to the particle volume. The pulses are electronically amplified, scaled, and counted. In order to select the pulse size to be counted, the pulses are also fed to a threshold circuit. A particle size distribution can be obtained by taking a series of counts on a constant sample volume at selected threshold levels. Thousands of particles can be counted within a few seconds enabling one to obtain a complete particle size distribution in a relatively short period of time.

The Coulter Counter is capable of measuring particle size in the 0.5–400 μm range. This range can be accommodated by utilizing a set of aperture tubes each of which has a specific particle size range. The main advantages of the Coulter Counter are its accuracy, versatility, and speed.

Light Scattering—Particle size analysis using light scattering techniques is based on the fact that the amount of light scattered by particles in a fluid stream is in accordance with their size. The sample liquid is passed through an intense beam of light. The particles present in the liquid scatter bursts of light as they pass through this beam. Each scattered burst is collected by a photodetector and converted to an electrical pulse. The amount of light scattered is a function of the size of the passing particle.

Air permeability techniques are based on the fact that a current of air flows more easily through a bed of coarse powder than through a bed of fine powder that is equal in apparent volume, bed shape, and percentage of voids. The particles in the path of regulated air flow will resist that air flow in relationship to their sizes; i.e., the greater the surface area/gram of powder, the greater the resistance to air flow.

Gas Adsorption Methods—Solid surfaces, particularly those having large specific surface areas, tend to adsorb gas that comes in contact with them.

The volume of the gas adsorbed depends on the nature of the gas, nature and surface area of the solid material, pressure, and temperature. By measuring the quantity of gas required to cover a powdered solid with a complete monomolecular layer of gas molecules, the surface area of the powder can be calculated, using the cross-sectional area of the gas molecules. The gas adsorption data can be represented by the so-called gas adsorption isotherms which plot the volume of gas adsorbed, usually expressed in milliliters of gas/gram of powdered solid, against the equilibrium pressure at a constant temperature.

Powders as a Dosage Form

Advantages of Powders

The availability of drugs in powdered form allows the physician to prescribe the precise amount of medication the individual patient requires in each dose. Powders are usually more stable than liquid dosage forms because chemical reactions between drugs in the dosage form and between drugs and the atmospheric conditions generally occur more slowly for powders than liquids. The smaller particle size of powders promotes more rapid dissolution in the body fluids than is obtained from compressed solid dosage forms such as tablets. Rapid dissolution produces higher blood levels in a shorter time and lessens the chance for irritation of the gastrointestinal tract which may result from unusually high local concentrations of the drug.

In addition, powders are usually easy to swallow even in large bulk, especially when mixed with food or drink. Hospitalized patients who are fed through tubes terminating in the stomach itself may have powders administered directly with the feeding. Tablets, on the other hand, must be crushed prior to administration and capsules should be emptied before use wherever possible, with the contents dosed as a powder which is mixed with the regular feeding through stomach tubes.

Disadvantages

Drugs which deteriorate upon exposure to atmospheric conditions should be dispensed in a dosage form protected against these conditions. Bitter, nauseating, or corrosive drugs usually cannot have these characteristics conveniently masked when dispensed in a powder form.

Most compounded prescriptions are more time-consuming in their preparation than prefabricated dosage forms. Because powders are usually compounded extemporaneously by the pharmacist, their preparation is more time-consuming, and therefore, usually more costly than the corresponding tablets or capsules prepared by a pharmaceutical manufacturer.

Characteristics of Good Powders

In the great majority of cases a properly prepared powder has the finest state of subdivision that is practical to obtain. A very small particle size permits the preparation of a more homogeneous powder. A perfectly homogeneous preparation of two or more materials has each particle of one material as nearly adjacent as possible to a particle of each of the other materials. This may be achievable in mixing miscible fluids of low viscosity but is not obtainable with powders. However, for most practical purposes, the mixing of finely subdivided particles gives a sufficiently homogeneous preparation.

Small particle size and large specific surface give insoluble powders a highly adsorptive capacity which is important in antacid, antidiarrheal, and other types of medicaments intended for local treatment of the skin and gastrointestinal tract. Certain types of dosage forms such as capsules, suspensions, aerosols, or tablets are merely powders in differing types of vehicles, enclosures, or states of compaction. They are most effective when the primary powder particles are released as individual entities rather than agglomerates at the time the dosage form is administered.

Categories

Physician's prescriptions or individual patient requests for powdered dosage forms fall into two general categories: *divided powders* and *bulk powders*. Divided powders (*chartulae*) refer to single doses of the powdered drug mixture individually enclosed in paper, cellophane, or metallic foil wrappers or packets. Bulk powders are intended to be administered in dosage quantities which are safe for the patient himself to measure. Bulk powders are frequently used as dusting powders, aerosols, dentifrices, antacids, laxatives, and dietary nutrient supplements, or in the preparation of douches.

Preparation

A mixing process is used primarily to prepare a homogeneous powdered dosage form. However, the mixing process affects the physical state, i.e., particle size, compactness, etc., of the powder and thereby such physical properties as solubility, dispersibility, and dissolution rate. Chemical reactions may be promoted or hindered depending on the mixing process that is chosen. Mixing or tapping of powders consisting of a large range of particle size can result in stratification. Coarse particles rise to the top as the fine particles slip through the voids and go to the bottom. When possible, powdered ingredients should be reduced to uniform particle size before mixing.

Stratification may also occur when powders containing particles of greatly different densities are mixed. Heavier particles sink to the bottom and lighter particles layer out at the top. The use of a mixing tumbler is one effective approach to this problem.

The nature of the finished product controls the choice of a mixing process. A product in which the particles do not aggregate, but are light and readily diffusible, requires a different mixing procedure than does the preparation of a compact, less bulky powder. In some cases it is advantageous to use a volatile solvent to obtain particle size reduction and uniform distribution of an ingredient. In solution, the ingredient is in the molecular or colloidal size range. The solution is then mixed with the insoluble powders and upon evaporation of the volatile solvent the ingredient remains as small particles dispersed throughout the preparation. This procedure is known as *pulverization by intervention.*

In the following prescription, e.g., the iodine may be distributed in the boric acid with the aid of a small amount of alcohol.

1

℞ Iodine   2%
    Powdered boric acid   qs   30 g
    Mft. pulv.
    Sig: Dust on toes q A.M.

Hand Mixing Methods

Most chemicals are available in powdered or granular form; larger crystals should be reduced to a powder before weighing. Usually it is best to have each ingredient in finely powdered form before mixing. The mixing methods most commonly used are spatulation, trituration, sifting, and tumbling.

Spatulation—Small   amounts   of powders, having the same range of particle sizes and densities, may be conveniently mixed on a sheet of paper or on a tile with a spatula. Little particle size reduction or compacting of the powder results from spatulation. The finished powder is light and readily dispersible in liquids.

Trituration—Powders   may   be mixed in a mortar by gentle trituration with a pestle when it is desired that the finished products have the properties of lightness and diffusibility in liquids.

Heavy and prolonged trituration results in a finer and denser powder. Heavy trituration is employed when it is desired to reduce granular salts to a finer powder or to change fluffy, bulky powders to a more compact form. In the case of resinous vegetable powders, heavy trituration should be avoided because it may cause the powder to cake.

A homogeneous product is particularly important when a small amount of a potent drug is to be mixed with a large amount of diluent. The general procedure known as *geometric dilution* may be useful in preparing such a distribution. First the entire quantity of potent drug is reduced to a fine powder and triturated with an *equal volume* of diluent of the same particle size and density as the drug. Then twice the volume of diluent is added and the trituration continued. This process is repeated, each time adding a volume of diluent equal to the volume of the material in the mortar, until all the diluent is used. An equal volume of a contrasting colored powder may be added to the potent drug to evaluate the progress of the mixing. Geometric dilution may also be used in mixing powders consisting of several contrasting ingredients. As the mixing process continues, the appearance of a uniformly-colored powder mixture indicates homogeneity. Any suitable certified coal-tar color permitted for drugs by the FDA can be used. White powders, in general, require incorporation of less than 0.1% of dye to impart a pastel color. Carmine serves as the coloring agent in R 2.

2

R Chloramine   0.6 g
   Carmine   *colouring agent*   0.1 g
   Saccharin sodium   0.3 g
   Cinnamon Oil   *flavor*   0.5 g
   Sodium Chloride   qs   100.0 g
   Mft. Powder.
   Sig: ¼ teaspoonful to a cup of water as a mouth wash.

The dye may be dry-blended into the powder by trituration in a mortar or added in the form of a solution. A volatile solvent should be used to prepare the dye solution. The solution is added in portions, with efficient mixing, and the solvent is allowed to evaporate from the powder. This procedure must be used with caution, however, since studies have shown that small amounts of dyes may significantly reduce the dissolution rates of certain powdered drugs.

Wedgewood or porcelain mortars and pestles are best for general trituration in prescription compounding because the surfaces of these materials are relatively rough. Wedgewood or porcelain surfaces which have become smooth with routine use may be suitably roughened by occasionally triturating a small amount of sand or emery powder in the mortar. The pharmacist must remember, however, that as mortars become smooth, the surface is being worn away, and with certain types of mortars the resulting contamination of the material being triturated is appreciable.

In certain prescription compounding situations the use of relatively porous mortar materials such as wedgewood and porcelain may be undesirable. Drugs such as iodine, potassium permanganate, and dyes which tend to stain composition mortars should be triturated in glass mortars. The smooth, less-porous surface of a glass mortar allows less particle size reduction, and therefore, less chance for packing effects to occur. While glass mortars are more fragile than other types, they are very easily cleaned. Furthermore, it is a simple matter to observe the homogeneity of a colored mixture in a transparent glass mortar. Visual inspection of the material against the mortar walls will quickly reveal any areas of nonuniform color.

Sifting—Where free-flowing, light powders are desired the ingredients may be brushed through a sieve. Ordinary household sifters may be used in sifting pharmaceutical powders. Standardized prescription sieves, however, give much better control of the particle size. Routine sifting of powder prescriptions is recommended to insure the removal of larger sized foreign materials and the dispersal of particles which have agglomerated. Agglomeration in powder mixtures is primarily due to interaction of hydration films surrounding each particle.

Tumbling—When simple mixing of powders is desired, without reduction in particle size and compaction which normally accompanies trituration, wide-mouthed closed containers may be used for tumbling. The powders should not occupy more than $\frac{1}{3}$ to $\frac{1}{2}$ the volume of the container. The tumbling should be of such a nature that the powders do not slide down the sides of the container; rather, the particles should float freely downward in the air after the tumbling. The mouth of the container should be sufficiently large so that upon emptying no orifice effect, such as packing or stratification, occurs. Tumbling is recommended for mixing powders with considerable density differences.

Tumbling may also be accomplished by placing the powders on a sheet of paper and lifting alternate corners of the paper. When properly done, the powders are randomly tumbled over each other, not slid down the sides. Under these conditions, mixing occurs with a minimum of pressure exerted upon the powders.

Dividing Powder Mixtures

When powders are prescribed in divided doses, the total quantity of powders to be dispensed is prepared and then divided into the proper number of doses. Several methods of dividing powders are commonly used.

Weighing Each Powder—The most accurate and professional method of dividing powders is to weigh each dose separately. During the mixing of powders there is some unavoidable loss of material. Consequently, when the individual powders are accurately weighed, there will not be enough material available to provide full weight for the last powder. Usually this difficulty is avoided by weighing a sufficient amount in the compounded mixture for one more powder than the number to be dis-

pensed, and discarding the fraction of one powder which remains at the end. In the case of narcotics this cannot be done since the Federal Narcotic Regulations do not recognize such dispensing losses. A ±5% error is a reasonably achievable standard of accuracy in dispensing powders. Within these limits the prescribed amount of powdered narcotic can be prepared and the prescribed number of dosages dispensed.

Blocking and Dividing—The compounded powder mixture is placed on a pill tile or glazed paper and blocked into an even rectangular pile which is then divided into the desired number of parts. The parts should be made as nearly equal as possible by the eye; division is accomplished by placing the edge of a clean spatula into the powder surface. The parts are then separated slightly with the spatula and transferred to individual powder papers. Because this method does not insure accuracy, the weight of the powder blocks should be checked with a sufficient number of weighings to be sure that reasonable accuracy has been attained. Many powders flow so readily that much time and accuracy are wasted in trying to block and divide the mixture on a tile. In these instances the weighing procedure previously described offers the advantage of increased accuracy and may actually represent a time-saving over the method of blocking and dividing.

Powder Measures—Various sized scoops, spoons, and mechanical powder dividers have been introduced periodically. Specially designed cups used to measure Seidlitz powder and dietary nutrient supplements are examples of powder measures. A disadvantage of such devices is their inaccuracy. Powder measures are useful only when the powder contains no potent ingredients and when the inherent dose variation which results from the use of the measure does not affect the intended therapeutic response.

Choice of Method—The method to be selected for dividing powder mixtures is largely a matter of professional judgment. However, with an emphasis on accuracy in dispensing, weighing of each powder should be recognized as the only proper method. The other methods offer a marginal time-saving at the expense of accuracy. A skilled pharmacist can carry out the weighing process quickly and efficiently.

Enclosing Powders

Various powder enclosures are available. Extemporaneously prepared divided prescription powders are usually packaged in papers or packets containing individual doses.

Powder Papers—A powder paper should fold readily, hold the finished fold without springing back, remain clean with handling, be impermeable to atmospheric conditions, be water-repellent, and present a pharmaceutically elegant appearance when packed in a box. Parchment and thin white light-weight bond are frequently used for powder papers. Parchment is somewhat water-repellent and impermeable; bond paper has neither of these desirable features. However, both readily retain their folded forms and present an elegant appearance. Both a glazed material known as glassine paper and waxed paper are relatively water-repellent and impermeable to atmospheric conditions. For hygroscopic substances double wrapping is commonly employed: the inner paper being parchment or glassine and the outer being ordinary bond powder paper.

Powder papers are available in different sizes which are usually designated by numbers. However, there is no standardized numbering system.

Methods of Folding—Folding powder papers is an art best learned by actual demonstration and practice. Care should be taken to obtain uniformity in each of the following steps.

1. The long edge of each paper is folded over from ¼ to ½ in. From three to six papers may be folded at one time. If too many papers are folded at once, the folds vary in size between papers and are not straight.

2. The separated papers are conveniently arranged on the counter with the folded margins up and away from the pharmacist.
3. The proper quantity of powder for a single dose is placed in the center of each paper.
4. The lower edge of the paper is brought under the top fold and into the crease. The top fold is brought forward, toward the pharmacist, and gently creased.
5. Additional folds are now made from the top so that the height of the folded paper is slightly greater than the depth of the powder box.
6. The folded paper is placed lengthwise on an open powder box, and the ends of the paper are folded down while the sides of the box are pressed slightly inward. A box of the same size as that in which the powders will be placed is used as a guide for folding the powders. When the procedure is accurately followed, each folded powder paper will be of a uniform length and height to permit easy removal from the box in which it is dispensed.

The powders are placed in the powder box one at a time, generally with the folds up and facing away from the pharmacist. Occasionally powders are placed alternately with the fold upward then downward. This procedure lessens the tendency of all the powders springing from the box when one powder is removed.

Envelopes—Newer materials and methods for enclosing powders are continuously becoming available. The alert practitioner adopts those techniques which offer ease in enclosing the powder, increased stability for ingredients, and pharmaceutical elegance for the prescription product. Among the newer developments is the use of cellophane and plastic envelopes and bags. After the individual dose is placed in the envelope, the open end is folded over and closed. Air-tight closures may be achieved with special zipper-like tracks which run the length of the plastic bag or by means of heat sealing the ends of the packaging material. Heat-sealed packets are tamper-proof and may be prepared in any desired shape and size. Aluminum foil and pliofilm-bonded white paper have many of the desirable characteristics of a powder paper. They are readily available in various-sized rolls.

Powder Boxes—The most useful powder box is the shouldered type with a hinged cover. The permanent attachment of the lid prevents its loss or acci-

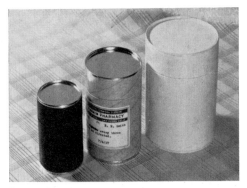

Fig. 5—Containers for bulk powders or capsules.

Table 3—Hygroscopic and Deliquescent Powders

Ammonium bromide	Phenobarbital
Ammonium chloride	sodium
Ammonium iodide	Physostigmine
Calcium bromide	hydrobromide
Calcium chloride	Physostigmine
Ephedrine sulfate	hydrochloride
Hydrastine	Physostigmine
hydrochloride	sulfate
Hydrastine sulfate	Pilocarpine
Hyoscyamine	alkaloid
hydrobromide	Potassium acetate
Hyoscyamine sulfate	Potassium citrate
Iron and ammonium	Sodium bromide
citrate	Sodium iodide
Lithium bromide	Sodium nitrate
Pepsin	Zinc chloride

dental interchange with the lid from another box. The label with directions for the patient is glued on the lid. Powder boxes with completely removable lids are also available. Frequently when only two or three powders are required, they may be dispensed in a small envelope which contains an appropriately prepared label.

Bulk powders are dispensed in containers like those shown in Fig. 5.

Special Problems

Many of the special problems which arise in compounding powder dosages occur when mixtures of powders either liquefy or become pasty. The general approach to these problems is to obtain proper-sized powder particles, to incorporate an inert, finely powdered absorbent such as light magnesium oxide or magnesium carbonate, and to double wrap the powder. Each ingredient should be triturated separately with some absorbent, and the ingredients mixed by a process which applies little or no pressure upon the powders.

Hygroscopic and Deliquescent Powders—Substances which absorb moisture from the air are termed *hygroscopic*. A few examples are given in Table 3. Hygroscopic substances which absorb moisture from the air to the extent that they liquefy by partially or wholly forming a solution are termed *deliquescent*. Hygroscopic and deliquescent substances are not well-suited for dispensing in powder papers. When

they are prescribed as powders, several precautions should be observed. Hygroscopic substances are usually supplied in a granular form in order to expose less surface to the air. The pharmacist should not powder the hygroscopic substance more finely than is necessary. Such powders should, of course, be doubled wrapped. The following prescriptions contain hygroscopic materials.

3

R Phenobarbital sodium		0.05
Sodium bromide		
Sodium bicarbonate	aa	0.3
D.T.D. #12		

Sig: Pulv. j1/2° before retiring.

4

R Aspirin	1.5
Sodium phenobarbital	0.5
Potassium citrate	5.0
Mft. pulv. #5	

Sig: One in H_2O b.i.d.

In very humid weather or when compounding extremely deliquescent ingredients, it is advisable to use aluminum foil or plastic film packets. The addition of light magnesium oxide to the powder mixture often reduces its tendency to become damp. The pharmacist should keep in mind the adsorbing capacity of light magnesium oxide and its antacid and/or laxative effect if taken in quantity. No ingredients should be indiscriminantly added to a prescription which will alter the therapeutic response to the drug mixture. Additionally, it

Table 4—Efflorescent Powders

Alums	Quinine bisulfate
Atropine sulfate	Quinine hydrobromide
Caffeine	Quinine hydrochloride
Calcium lactate	Scopolamine
Citric acid	hydrobromide
Cocaine	Sodium acetate
Codeine	Sodium carbonate
Codeine phosphate	(decahydrate) 10 H₂O
Codeine sulfate	Sodium phosphate
Ferrous sulfate	Strychnine sulfate
Morphine acetate	Terpin hydrate

Table 5—Substances Which Liquefy When Mixed

Acetanilid	Camphor
Acetophenetidin	Chloral hydrate
Acetylsalicylic acid	Menthol
Aminopyrine	Phenol
Antipyrine	Salol
Betanaphthol	Thymol

should be remembered that the absorption of moisture from the air depends on the relative humidity. A powder which is dry and free-flowing in the low humidity of an air-conditioned pharmacy may become damp rapidly in the moist atmosphere of a medicine cabinet in the patient's home.

Efflorescent Powders—Crystalline substances which become powdery and liberate their water of crystallization are said to be *efflorescent*. Some examples are given in Table 4. The liberation of water may be due to a change in relative humidity or it may occur during the trituration process itself. The water liberated by efflorescence can cause a powder to become pasty or to liquefy. This difficulty may sometimes be overcome by using the corresponding anhydrous salt. The anhydrous salt usually tends to attract moisture from the air and should be handled in the manner suggested for hygroscopic powders. (When using an anhydrous salt in place of one with water of crystallization, the dose must be carefully adjusted to allow for the weight of active material.)

Eutectic Mixtures—A eutectic mixture is defined as that proportion of components which will give the lowest melting point. Frequently the melting points of many eutectics encountered in pharmacy are below room temperature. In the practical sense, a eutectic mixture may be recognized by the liquefaction of two or more substances upon their admixture. One method of avoiding the formation of a eutectic mixture is to separate its component ingredients by dispensing them as separate sets of

powders with directions that one powder of each kind shall be taken as a dose.

The general technique of adding an absorbent powder such as those previously mentioned, or starch, talc, lactose, calcium phosphate, etc., may help solve the problem. When substances which liquefy are present in small proportion along with other ingredients, the liquefiable substance should first be triturated together, forming the eutectic. All other liquid components are added, and the other substances in the form of fine powders are gradually incorporated. This procedure insures that the powders absorb the maximum amount of liquid which may appear in the prescription. It also allows the pharmacist to add exactly the amount of absorbent needed to assure the preparation of a dry powder mixture.

A number of substances which form eutectic mixtures are listed in Table 5. Two or more of the chemicals may produce a eutectic mixture. Occasionally two chemicals will remain as a dry mixture, and the addition of a third results in the formation of the eutectic. The extent of liquefaction is affected by the proportions of each substance as well as the amount of trituration and the pressure exerted in mixing. The following prescriptions contain eutectic mixtures.

5

R	Menthol	0.1
	Camphor	0.2
	Zinc stearate	0.8
	Zinc oxide	8.0
	Talc	31.0

Mix.
Sig: Dust on prickly heat.

6

R̶ Aminopyrine   1.0
   Aspirin   2.0
   Belladonna extract   0.065
   Mft. charts #6
   Sig: One u.d.

Incorporation of Liquids—When a relatively small proportion of liquid is to be incorporated into a powder, the liquid may be triturated with an equal weight of the powder, and the remainder of the powder added in several portions with trituration. An absorbent is incorporated, if necessary, to produce a dry powder.

7

R̶ Tragacanth   100   g
   Sassafrass oil   1.5 ml
   Mix.
   Sig: Use as a denture adhesive.

When larger portions of tinctures or fluidextracts are prescribed as components of powders, the liquid volume should be reduced by evaporation on a water bath to a syrupy consistency. Lactose or some other inert diluent may then be added and the evaporation continued to dryness. The diluent acts as a carrier for the residue, thereby avoiding the formation of sticky gum when evaporation is completed. Wherever possible, powdered extracts should be used to replace a tincture or fluidextract prescribed in a powder mixture.

Incorporation of Extracts—Some extracts are available in both pilular and powdered forms; the latter are selected for use in powders whenever possible. The powdered extract is handled in the same way as any other powder. When necessary, the pilular extract may be mixed with a quantity of lactose and reduced to a dry powder by evapo-

Table 6—Oxidizing and Reducing Agents

Oxidizing agents	Reducing agents
Potassium chlorate	Charcoal
Potassium dichromate	Hypophosphites
Potassium nitrate	Sulfur
Potassium	Sulfides
permanganate	Tannic acid
Sodium peroxide	Volatile oils
Silver nitrate	Organic substances
Silver oxide	in general

ration before incorporation with other ingredients. Care must be exercised in heating all natural products, since the potency may be reduced by the action of the heat.

Explosive Mixtures and Incompatible Salts—When an oxidizing agent such as potassium chlorate is triturated in a mortar with a reducing agent such as tannic acid, a violent explosion may result. Examples of potentially explosive materials are given in Table 6.

The following mixture is an example of a potentially explosive combination of prescription ingredients.

8

R̶ Potassium chlorate   0.6 g
   Tannic acid
   Sucrose   aa   0.3 g
   D.T.D. #20
   Sig: Chart j in glass of water as gargle.

Other chemically incompatible salts, when triturated together, may produce powders which show discoloration, chemical deterioration, or loss in potency. The compounding of these types of prescription powders should be accomplished with a minimum of pressure. Tumbling the powders in a jar or on a sheet of paper is a convenient method for mixing potentially reactive compounds. Each substance should be powdered separately in a clean mortar and then combined with all other ingredients and gently mixed. An alternative method is to powder each substance separately and dispense them in separate powder papers with appropriate directions to the patient.

Potent Drug Triturations—The limitations in the accuracy of a Class A prescription balance require special procedures for weighing small quantities of potent drugs. Suitable diluents, such as lactose, are mixed in a definite proportion (by weight) with the potent drug which has been powdered. A homogeneous dispersion is prepared; such a powder mixture is known as a *trituration*. Official triturations commonly contain 10% of the potent drug by weight. Very fine powders must be used in the preparation of titurations. The mixing procedure should employ the method of geometric dilution as previously described. An example of a prescription utilizing a potent drug trituration is:

9

℞ Vitamin B_{12} 2.0 mg
   Desiccated liver extract   2.0 g
   Mft. Charts #20.
   Sig: Chart j t.i.d. a.c.

Special Powders

A number of special types of powders require particular methods of preparation and packaging.

Effervescent Salts

Granules or powders consisting of sodium bicarbonate, a suitable organic or inorganic acid, and medicinal ingredients are known as *effervescent salts*. In the presence of water, the acid and the base react to liberate carbon dioxide, thereby producing an effervescence. The resulting pleasantly carbonated solution masks the saline taste of certain salts and the bitter taste of many objectionable medications. A prescription for effervescent powders may require the preparation of either a bulk powder mixture or divided individual doses. Effervescent powders are much simpler to prepare than the granules. The main difficulty in preparing effervescent medications is keeping the ingredients perfectly dry during compounding in the pharmacy and during storage by the patient in order to prevent premature reaction. The acidic and basic components are sometimes packaged in separate powder papers of contrasting colors to prevent the reaction from occurring until shortly before the mixture is administered to the patient. At the time of dosing, he is directed to mix the contents of one of each of the colored papers in a quantity of water. The liquid is consumed just after the reaction begins to subside.

The binding of powder particles into larger size effervescent granules may be accomplished by (1) the addition of a liquid binding agent or (2) heating

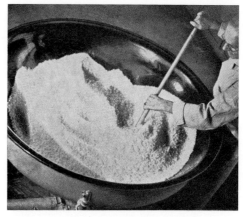

Fig. 6—Fusing granular effervescent salts.

uneffloresced powders to liberate the water of crystallization which then acts as the binding agent. Sodium bicarbonate is used in a dry powdered form. Most commonly the acids are either tartaric or citric. Sodium acid phosphate is frequently used as a commercial alternative for the more costly organic acids, (see Fig. 6).

Uneffloresced citric acid contains one molecule of water of crystallization/molecule of acid. It is kept in the crystalline form and is not powdered until just before use to prevent loss of the water of crystallization. During the process of efflorescence the water liberated from the powdered citric acid acts as the binding agent in the dry method of granulation.

Alcohol USP is frequently used as the binding agent in the wet method of granulation. The powders are mixed without pressure in a suitable container. Alcohol is added in portions, with stirring, until a doughlike mass is formed. The material is then passed through a #6 sieve and the granules are dried at a temperature not exceeding 50°C. The granules are again passed through the sieve and then packaged in airtight containers.

Granules prepared by the dry method are compounded in the following manner. All ingredients except the citric acid are dried and passed through a #60 sieve; the powders are thoroughly mixed and the freshly-powdered citric acid is added last. The mixture is spread in a shallow dish or on a sheet of paper and placed in an oven (95–105°C) without stirring, until the powders become moist and form a doughy mass. The mass is then granulated by passage through a #6 sieve and dried as before.

A generally more convenient method for the pharmacist requires the use of a water bath surrounding a beaker in which the powders are stirred to prevent local overheating. A pasty mass is soon formed. Granulation, drying, and regranulation are then carried out. The proportions of citric acid and tartaric acid used in the formulations may be varied provided that the total acidity is kept equivalent to the acidity in the official monograph. *NF VII* was the last official compendium to give general directions for preparing granular effervescent salts.

Dusting Powders

Powders for external use must possess the characteristics of all properly compounded powders plus those which are unique for their particular use. Therefore, dusting powders must be homogeneous and free from the potential of causing local irritation. The powder should flow easily, spread uniformly, and cling to the skin on application. Additionally, dusting powders should possess good covering capability, adsorptive and absorptive capacity, and be capable of protecting the skin against chafing and irritation caused by friction, moisture, or chemical irritants. Medicated dusting powders may be applied either to the intact skin or to open wounds and mucous membranes. The powder particles present a large surface area which promotes the evaporation of surface fluids and radiation of heat.

Highly sorptive powders should not be used on areas exuding large quantities of fluids because a hard crust is usually formed. Water-repellent powders, on the other hand, prevent evaporation and do not cake on oozing surfaces. The proper selection and blending of different substances with special

properties produce a dusting powder with the precise characteristics desired. Starch has the general qualities of a dusting powder, but unfortunately it is an organic substance which can support bacterial growth. Talc is chemically inert, but it is readily contaminated and may represent a potential source for infection; therefore, talc must be sterilized before it is used in compounding medicated dusting powders.

A powder-base vehicle may not always be required for dusting powders; a medicament may be applied as a pure drug in powdered form. Dusting powders are generally dispensed in sifter-topped cans. They may be applied with a powder puff, a soft brush, or a sterile gauze pad. Care must be taken to avoid mechanical irritation of damaged skin surfaces. Light, fluffy powders may be inhaled by patients if proper care is not taken. It is recommended that dusting powders for infant care be dispensed in self-closing sifter-topped containers which bear the warning "Keep Out of the Reach of Infants."

Dentifrices

Powders used to clean the teeth are called *dentifrices*. The preparation of dentifrices should utilize the same general principles already discussed for the incorporation and mixing of powders. It is important to obtain the cleansing action chiefly by the detergent properties of the powder rather than through the use of harmful abrasives. A very mild degree of abrasion is desirable and may be obtained by the incorporation of finely precipitated calcium carbonate or hydrous dibasic calcium phosphate. Excessive abrasiveness has been shown to damage tooth structure. Dentifrices used by the dentist are far too abrasive to be used daily. Finely powdered pumice imparts the abrasive action to these professional formulations.

Insufflations

Finely divided powders intended for application to body cavities such as tooth sockets, ears, nose, vagina, and throat are known as *insufflations*. The apparatus used to deliver a stream of finely divided powder particles to the site of application is called an *insufflator*. A typical insufflator consists of a bulb, chamber, and delivery nozzle. The powder is placed into the chamber and, when the bulb is compressed, the resulting current of air distributes the fine powder particles in the stream of gas and delivers them through the nozzle to the point of application. Advances in aerosol technology have resulted in the production of pressurized powdered insufflations in self-contained units with accurately reproducible metering dosage valves.

Intranasal insufflation has the advantage of not only producing local effects, but also systemic effects with those drugs whose therapeutic activity is reduced or lost if taken orally. Disadvantages of the older insufflators include the difficulty of obtaining accurate metering to give a uniform amount of drug and the tendency to generate electrostatic charges which cause the powder particles to stick to each other and to the walls of the insufflator. The newer powder aerosols have largely eliminated these problems.

Powder Aerosols

Many of the objections to the use of powders may be overcome by dispensing them as aerosols in pressurized, "push-button" containers. Many different formulations have been tested for their suitability as powder aerosols. Recently, aerosolized powder formulations have gained popularity as antiperspirants and deodorants, feminine hygiene sprays, body sprays, insufflations, and dry lubricants.

Aerosol packaging is usually done by the manufacturer, but the pharmacist should be familiar with the general advantages of the aerosols which he dispenses. The environment is controlled so that the powder is not attacked by chemicals, moisture, light, or other atmospheric conditions. Powders dispensed under pressure deliver a homo-

geneous dose. And finally, the maintenance of sterility in an aerosol container is no problem.

Typical Prescriptions

The following prescriptions illustrate various points discussed in the text and represent powders which require compounding. They are to be dispensed as directed.

10

R Belladonna extract	15 mg
Charcoal, activated	100 mg
Dried aluminum hydroxide gel	300 mg

Mft charts D.T.D. #24
Sig: ½° p.c.

11

R KMnO$_4$	31
Powdered alum	60
Sodium perborate	100
Oil of peppermint	0.1

Mft Charts #50
Sig: Chart j in qt. warm water as douche 3x weekly.

12

R Heavy magnesium oxide		
Sodium bicarbonate	aa	1
Codeine Sulfate		.15
Cinnamon oil		.1

D.T.D. pulv. #10
Sig: One q.i.d. prn abdominal pain.

13

R Hexachlorophene	2%
Sterilized talc	10%
Fragrance	qs
Freon 11: Freon 12; 2:1	qs

Mft. aerosol
Sig: Use as deodorant daily.

14

R Aspirin	0.3
Calcium phosphate	0.2
Citric acid	1.1
Sodium bicarbonate	2.0

D.T.D. charts #5
Sig: One q 3h in water prn headache and fever.

15

R Aluminum hydroxide		
Magnesium hydroxide	aa	2 g
Peppermint oil		1 ml
Aerosol OT		0.5 g

D.T.D. charts #10
Sig: One p.c.

16

℞ Salicylamide *analgesic*   0.200
potentiating Methapyriline HCl *anti H*   0.025
     Scopolamine HBr   0.0002
Mft. D.T.D. charts #XXV
Sig: Charts j or ij h.s.

17

60 mg/mg dose
120 mg
℞ Phenolphthalein   0.1
turn urine red Methylcellulose   qs   4.0
Chart D.T.D. #10
Sig: j h.s. with 8 oz water.

18

℞ Zinc sulfate   0.25%
   Magnesium sulfate   20.0 %
   Boric acid   3.00%
   Oil of lemon   0.2 %
   Lactose   qs
Mft. pulv.
Sig: ʒj (dram) pint warm water as douche.

19

℞ Methylbenzethonium Cl   1:1200
   Starch
   Magnesium carbonate   aa   qs
Sig: Dust on diaper rash.

20

℞ ZrO₂ *remove*   1.0
   Calamine   2.0
   ZnO   10.0
   Starch
   Talc   aa   20.0

Benzocaine *shake well*   10.0
Phenol   0.5
Mft. powder
Sig: Dust on poison ivy t.i.d.

21

℞ Salicylic acid powder   5%
   Benzoic acid   6%
   Camphor   1%
   Menthol   0.2%
   Phenol   0.1%
   Starch   qs
Mft. pulv.
Sig: Sprinkle between toes AM and PM.

Bibliography

Dare JG: *Australian J Pharm 45:* S-58, 1964.
Higuchi T: *JAPhA Sci Ed 47:* 657, 1958.
Neumann BS: In Hermans JJ: *Flow Properties of Disperse Systems,* Interscience, New York, Chap. 10, 1953.
Harwood CF, Pilpel N: *Chem Process Eng (Jul.):* 1968.
Train D: *JAPhA 49:* 265, 1960.
Miles JEP: *J Soc Cos Chem 21:* 53, 1970.
Williams JC, Rahman MA: *Ibid:* 3, 1970.
Ecanow B, Balagot RC, Bandelin V: *Am Rev Resp Dis 99:* 106, 1969.
Martin AN, Swarbrick J, Cammarata A: *Physical Pharmacy,* 2nd ed, Lea & Febiger, Philadelphia, Chap. 17, 1969.
Hogg R, Mempel G, Fuerstenau D: *Powd Techn 2:* 223, 1969.
Fowler H: *Mfg Chem Aerosol News 40:* 29, 1969.

5

Tablets and pills

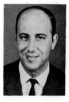

Farid Sadik, PhD
Associate Professor of
Pharmaceutics
College of Pharmacy
University of South Carolina
Columbia, SC 29208

Tablets

The USP and NF describe tablets as "solid dosage forms containing medicinal substances with or without suitable diluents." Different tablets vary in shape and differ greatly in size and weight, depending on the amount of the medicinal substance and the intended mode of administration.

Tablets are an efficient, versatile, and practical form of medication. The vast popularity and the extremely wide usage of tablets as medicinal agents clearly demonstrate that they represent an efficient, a highly practical, and, in fact, an ideal form for the administration of orally active therapeutic agents. Generally speaking, tablets are the most widely accepted form of adult medication because of the following advantages:

1. Bitter, nauseating, or unpleasant drugs can be rendered acceptable and even palatable by covering the entire tablet or the tablet granule with a suitable protective coating. This coating need only be designed to protect during the normally short time of exposure while the tablet is in contact with the taste buds.

2. A marked advantage of tablets is the ease of administering an accurate dose. If desired, the dose can be uniformly distributed throughout the tablet to facilitate accurate, fractional dosage when the tablet is cleaved, or one or more of the therapeutic agents can be segregated into specific areas as a layer, a pellet, or a granule for improved therapeutic results.

3. Tablets exhibit the absence of alcohol. Alcohol is frequently necessary to promote the solubility or stability of other forms of medication. The absence of alcohol in tablets normally decreases manufacturing costs and increases the scope and range of patients to which the medication can be prudently administered.

4. Tablets are readily adaptable to the manufacturing of various dosages of medicinal agents. Therefore, the proper concentration of medicinal agent is easily, conveniently, and economically available to the prescriber, the patient, and the pharmacist. Thiamine chloride tablets represent an unusually broad example of varying sizes that are commercially available; e.g., 0.1, 0.15, 0.25, 0.33, 0.50, 1.0, 3.3, 5.0, 10, 12, 15, 20, 25, 50, and 100 mg tablets.

5. The very nature of a tablet—inherent in such striking qualities as ease of portability, compact form, rugged stability, impressive economy compared with other dosage forms, broad flexibility, ready availability, ease of administration, etc.—

insures the proper psychological impression for almost universal patient acceptance.

6. The convenience associated with the use of tablets clearly establishes that they are an extremely practical and efficient form of medication. Tablets are convenient to the pharmacist because of the ease of packaging and dispensing and the favorable professional connotation inherent in their use. Tablets also embody convenience to the manufacturer in ease of production, storage, transporting economy, applicability to mass production, etc.

When tablets are designed, manufactured, distributed, and stored with a full realization of the limitations demanded by the chemical, physical, and therapeutic properties of the ingredients, they have very few disadvantages. The most significant disadvantage is that some individuals experience psychological difficulty in administering or swallowing a tablet. A lesser disadvantage is the general impracticality of preparing tablets extemporaneously.

Types—Classification of tablets is usually based on the method of manufacture and on the intended usage.

Compressed Tablets

Tablets Delivered into the Gastrointestinal Tract
1. Conventionally Compressed Tablets (CT)
2. Multiple Compressed Tablets (MCT)
3. Enteric-Coated Tablets (ECT)
4. Sugar-Coated Tablets (SCT)
5. Film-Coated Tablets (FCT)
6. Chocolate-Coated Tablets
7. Effervescent Tablets
8. Chewable Tablets
9. Sustained-Action Tablets

Tablets Used in the Oral Cavity
1. Buccal and Sublingual Tablets
2. Lozenges or Troches
3. Dental Cones

Tablets for Miscellaneous Use
1. Vaginal Tablets
2. Implantation Tablets
3. Diagnostic Tablets

Molded Tablets
1. Tablet Triturates (TT)
2. Hypodermic Tablets (HT)
3. Dispensing Tablets (DT)

Tablets Delivered into Gastrointestinal Tract

Oral tablets intended for use in the gastrointestinal tract are administered either for systemic effect (aspirin, phenobarbital) or for local action in the stomach and intestine (aluminum hydrogel, kanamycin). These tablets may be swallowed intact usually with a drink of water, chewed before swallowing, or dissolved in water before administration.

Conventionally Compressed Tablets are prepared by single compression cycle and usually are composed of the active ingredient(s), alone or in combination with a diluent such as lactose, a binder such as sucrose solution or starch paste to give adhesiveness, and a disintegrator such as starch to cause disintegration of the tablet when it contacts the gastrointestinal fluid.

Multiple Compressed Tablets are conventionally compressed tablets prepared by subjection to more than a single compression cycle. Thus, a finished multiple compressed tablet is composed of two or more layers or cores.

Enteric-Coated Tablets are conventionally compressed tablets covered with a coating which resists dissolution in the stomach but dissolves in the intestinal tract. The coating may be composed of a material which is pH-dependent, i.e., insoluble in the acid medium of the stomach but dissolves in the less acidic or mildly alkaline environment of the intestinal tract, is susceptible to chemical or enzymatic action within the intestinal tract, or may erode due to the time in contact with moisture as the tablet passes through the intestinal tract. The reasons for the use of enteric coated tablets are:

1. To prevent excessive irritation of the gastric mucosa caused by irritating (potassium chloride) or nauseating (emetine, diethylstilbesterol) drugs.
2. To prevent inactivation of drugs by the gastric juice.
3. To delay release of the drug.
4. To deliver the active ingredients in optimum concentration for local action in the intestinal tract as in the case of intestinal antiseptics and anthelmintics.

Sugar-Coated Tablets are conventionally compressed tablets which are coated with several successive thin layers of colored or uncolored sucrose solution. Such coating is useful because it protects the medicinal agents by acting as a barrier to moisture and air, conceals medications having objectionable odor or taste, and improves the appearance of the tablet.

Film-Coated Tablets are conventionally compressed tablets coated with a colored or uncolored thin film of a water-soluble material which disintegrates readily in the gastrointestinal tract. The film coating serves the same function as sugar coating with the added advantage of being less bulky, as well as less time-consuming for the coating operation.

Chocolate-Colored Tablets are conventionally compressed tablets coated with chocolate which serves as a coloring material. Today, iron oxides have largely replaced chocolate as a colorant.

Effervescent Tablets are conventionally compressed tablets which effervesce (liberate carbon dioxide) when in contact with water; the tablet should be allowed to dissolve in water before administration. Release of carbon dioxide occurs as a result of an acid-base reaction between citric acid and/or tartaric acid and sodium bicarbonate which are usually included in the tablet. These additives provide fast disintegration or dissolution of the tablet and help in masking unpleasant tastes of some of the medicinal agents present. Effervescent saccharin tablets represent the use of an effervescent disintegrator to promote rapid disintegration and solution of the saccharin tablets without external stirring. Effervescent tablets are made by granulating the alkali (sodium bicarbonate) and acid (citric and/or tartaric acid) separately; other ingredients may be mixed with acid or with the alkali or with both. The granules are then pressed into tablets. Another method used in preparing these tablets is by granulating the acid, alkali and the rest of the medicinal agents by using a binder such as alcohol; the mixture should be dried quickly and thoroughly before pressing it into tablets. Irrespective of the method used, mixing and granulating the powders should be performed rapidly and in an environment of low humidity. Keeping the mixture and granules dry is an important factor in the success of manufacturing effervescent tablets.

Chewable Tablets are compressed tablets designed to be sucked or chewed before swallowing. In addition to the active ingredients, chewable tablets contain mannitol, which has been pleasantly flavored, as their base. Mannitol is a chemically inert, nonhygroscopic, thermally-stable powder rather ideally suited as a tablet base for sensitive medicinal chemicals (e.g., the water-soluble vitamins). Many chewable multivitamin tablets, antacid tablets, and some other ethical and proprietary tablets use a specially flavored and/or colored mannitol (25+ %) as a basic excipient. These chewable tablets can be taken without water. The disintegration is smooth, rapid, and produces a pleasantly cool, sweet taste. Thus, mannitol-base tablets are relatively free of the objectionable chalkiness or grittiness frequently associated with the dissolution of tablets in the mouth. These tablets are especially favored by parents for administration of multivitamins to children and by adults who dislike swallowing or chewing non-mannitol-based tablets.

Sustained-Action Tablets are those which provide an initial sufficient amount of drug to cause a rapid onset of desired therapeutic response, and an additional amount of drug that maintains the response at the initial level for a desired number of hours beyond the activity resulting from a conventional dose; the initial desired therapeutic response is maintained because the rate of release of the desired therapeutic concentration is equal to the rate at which the drug is eliminated or inactivated.

Advantages of sustained-action tablets are to:

1. Maintain the therapeutic effect for a longer

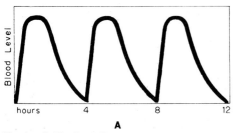
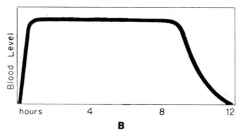

Fig. 1—*A:* The "peak" and "valley" effects which are inevitable with divided doses; *B: the effect of orally-administered prolonged-action medication.*

period than can be obtained after the administration of conventional single-dose medication.

2. Reduce the number and frequency of doses administered.

3. Eliminate decreases in drug concentration which are inevitable with divided doses and thus maintain an even level of drug concentration in the body (see Fig. 1).

4. Eliminate the inconvenience of night-time administration of drugs.

5. Lessen the possibility of the patient's defaulting from treatment by forgetting to take this medication.

6. Reduce or prevent the irritation of the gastrointestinal tract caused by some orally-administered drugs released in high concentration.

Sustained-action tablets are available in various types. Sustained-action tablets with slow-release cores consist of a layer containing an immediate-release dosage to achieve the therapeutic level and another layer containing a sustained-release dosage to maintain a therapeutic level of the medication over an extended period of time. These tablets may be prepared by intimately mixing the drug(s) with a molten mass of a slowly dissolving substance or a mixture of substances such as carnauba wax, beeswax, stearyl alcohol, and glyceryl monostearate to produce a pasty mass. The mass is stirred until congealed and then reduced to granules. The aforementioned granulation is introduced into a tablet die cavity and compressed to form a single solid layer, then the immediate-release medicated granulation is introduced on top of the previously compressed layer and compressed to form a second solid layer that adheres firmly to the first.

Repeat-action tablets consist of two cores and may be prepared by compressing the outer core which contains the initial dose of the drug around a core that contains a second dose which is released at a later interval. The two cores are separated by a barrier coating. A conventional method for making these tablets consists of preparing a core containing active ingredient(s) and then coating the core with a substance which will not be affected by stomach juices but will be dissolved by intestinal fluids; to this coated core another layer of active ingredient is applied, by means of pan-coating. The outer core releases the first dose and after the protective coat has had time to disintegrate, the active material in the inner core is released and the patient receives the second or subsequent dose of medication. With such tablets, the patient receives an initial dose that may be followed by a short period of no drug release. Thus, this type is not a true sustained-action type according to the definition used earlier. The blood levels obtained with repeat-action tablets is similar to those obtained with two individual doses of drugs. Repetabs (*Schering*) consist of an outer layer of medication available for immediate release and rapid action, a laminated time barrier that is not enteric-coated (yet defers release of the inner core ingredients for 4 to 6 hours regardless of exposure to acid or alkaline secretions), and an inner core containing another full therapeutic dose.

Tableted mixed-release granules are made of two or more groups of granules. One group which carries the initial dose of the drug is prepared by the conventional method (i.e., active ingredient(s), excipients, and binders). The other group(s) which carries the sustained-release dosage contains the active ingredient(s) coated with slowly digestible or poorly soluble material. The two groups of granules, which usually have two different colors, are mixed, lubricated, and compressed into tablets. The resultant tablets are usually speckled.

Gradumet (*Abbott*), connoting gradual-release medicament, has been applied to a tablet consisting of a physiologically inert plastic pellet containing thousands of interstitial passages filled with a "channeling agent" and the active ingredient(s). The main function of the channeling agent is to attract gastrointestinal fluids into the passages where the active ingredient(s) will leach out at a continuous even rate during 8 to 12 hours; the inert plastic pellet is excreted unchanged, in the feces.

Sustained-action tablets can be achieved by employing ion-exchange resins. The most common cationic exchangers contain either carboxylic or sulfonic acid groups distributed throughout the resin particles. A drug-resinate complex is formed by passing a solution of a cationic drug through a column containing an ion-exchange resin. The reaction is

vide systemic action by placing them in the buccal pouch between the cheek and the gums (buccal tablets) or beneath the tongue (sublingual tablets) and allowed to dissolve there. Absorption of drugs used in these tablets occurs directly through the oral mucosa. The drug enters general circulation from the oral venous drainage system to the right heart, bypassing the stomach and liver; thus, first-pass destruction of the drug by gastric juice and metabolism by enzymes of the liver are avoided.

Lozenges or Troches are disk-shaped, solid dosage form made of medicinal substance and flavoring agent intended for slow dissolution in the mouth for continuous local application of the drug to the mucous membrane of the oral cavity. On a large scale, lozenges are made by a compression process as in the manufacture of compressed tablets. The process differs slightly from tablet-making because lozenges are intended to dissolve slowly in the mouth, while tablets are intended to disintegrate rapidly in the stomach. Accordingly, in the manufacture of lozenges by compression, more gum is used

$$n[(\text{Drug})^+\text{X}^-] + \left[\begin{array}{c} \text{SO}_2\text{—O}^-\text{Na}^+ \\ \\ \text{CH—CH}_2\text{—} \end{array}\right]_n \rightleftharpoons n[\text{Na}^+\text{X}^-] + \left[\begin{array}{c} \text{SO}_2\text{—O}^- \, (\text{Drug})^+ \\ \\ \text{CH—CH}_2\text{—} \end{array}\right]_n$$

The resultant drug-resinate is then washed and may be formulated into tablets. Sustained-action from the tableted drug-resinate results from the slow rate of the displacement reaction that takes place between the ions in the digestive juices of the gastrointestinal tract and the drug-resinate; liberation of the drug from the complex occurs over an extended period of time.

Tablets Used in Oral Cavity

Buccal and Sublingual Tablets are compressed tablets which are usually flat, oval in shape, and intended to pro-

in order to secure a harder, more cohesive product, and no disintegrating substance is used. Otherwise, the material is granulated as for compressed tablets and is compressed in the usual tablet machine, using punches and dies of the desired shape and setting the punches to give a somewhat higher compression than for tablets. Lozenges can be prepared manually in a manner similar to that for pills. The drug is mixed with a diluent such as acacia and an excipient, usually water. The mass is rolled into a cylinder and cut into disks of the desired size, after which the disks are allowed to dry. Slightly medicated candies such as cough drops are manufactured in a manner similar to that of the manufacture of confectionery. The process is usually one of molding a hot mass which solidifies on cooling.

Dental Cones are used to prevent multiplication of pathogenic microorganisms in the empty socket following tooth extraction. In addition to the active ingredients, dental cones contain additives such as sodium bicarbonate, sodium chloride, or lactose. Such additives are usually formulated so that the dental cone disintegrates in 20–40 min after it is placed in the socket.

Tablets for Miscellaneous Use

Vaginal Tablets are ovoid or pear-shaped conventionally compressed tablets intended for insertion into the vagina where dissolution and release of the medication takes place. Vaginal tablets usually contain antiseptics, astringents, or steroids and may be buffered to produce the desired pH. The most common bases for these tablets are lactose and sodium bicarbonate. Vaginal tablets are usually inserted by means of a plastic-tube inserter in order to ensure that the tablet is inserted into the upper part of the vagina; the tablet disintegrates in the vaginal fluid.

Diagnostic Tablets are intended for the diagnosis of certain diseases. The tests are usually carried out either by the patient or in the clinic.

Implantation Tablets also known as pellets, are prepared under aseptic technique and intended for subcutaneous implantation of drug. Implantation tablets are about 3.2 × 8 mm in size and slowly release the medication over a prolonged period of time ranging from 3 to 6 months or longer.

Molded Tablets are small tablets made by molding a soft mass which usually consists of potent medicament diluted with lactose and moistened with alcohol.

Tablet Triturates are administered sublingually or by placing them on the tongue and swallowing them with a drink of water. In the community pharmacy, these tablets are prepared by molding but produced industrially by compression with a tablet machine.

Hypodermic Tablets are tablet triturates for use by the physician to prepare extemporaneous injection by dissolving the tablet in sterile water for injection and the resulting solution is injected hypodermically. Hypodermic tablets were once popular because the physician could carry them along with a suitable vehicle in his medicine bag. However, these tablets are little used today because it is difficult to achieve sterility and safe, sterile, and stable drugs are available in the injectable form. Hypodermic tablets are prepared either by molding or compression and the base used should be water-soluble.

Dispensing Tablets are for use by the pharmacist in compounding solid or liquid dosage forms. The diluent of these tablets is usually water-soluble to produce a clear solution. Most dispensing tablets contain toxic or potent drugs.

Compressed Tablets

Components

Compressed medicinal tablets may be considered as being composed of two basic groups of ingredients: (1) the medicaments, which are always present, and (2) the excipients, which may or may not be present. The term "excipient" is of Latin origin and refers to all materials in a compressed tablet except the medicament. Therefore, an excipient is an inert substance used to give a preparation a suitable form of consistency. The excipients used in the manufacture of compressed tablets may be conveniently assigned a function in the general process and, hence, classified on this basis; i.e., excipients may function as a diluent, binder, disintegrator, lubricant, coloring agent, or flavoring agent. Frequently, one excipient may serve two or more functions; e.g., sucrose may serve as both diluent and binder. The fabrication of most tablets does not require the presence of all of these functioning components; e.g., many tablets are neither colored nor flavored. The terms used to designate the functions of the excipients are descriptive and self-explanatory.

Diluents are added to tablet formulations to increase the bulk of the individual tablet to a practical and convenient, workable size. This is especially true when the dose of drug in each tablet is very small, e.g., 10 mg methyltestosterone tablets. Diluents must be compatible with the drug, physically stable, physiologically inert, and nonreactive with the ingredients. The following powdered materials are examples of diluents: lactose, sucrose, sodium chloride, mannitol, selected milk solids, starch, kaolin and other purified clays, calcium carbonate, calcium sulfate, and dicalcium phosphate. Equal parts of lactose and dicalcium phosphate granulated with starch paste are frequently used as a granular diluent. Obviously, all components, including the diluent of a tablet intended for the preparation of solutions, must be soluble.

Binders are adhesive materials used to hold powders together as granules and to assist in ultimately holding the compressed tablet together. The following materials are examples of binders: water, alcohol, acetone, starch paste (10–17%), sucrose syrup (50–85%), gelatin solutions (10–20%), acacia mucilage (10–20%), glucose solutions (25–50%), alcohol–glucose solutions (50% alcohol, 25% glucose, and 25% water), starch-paste (5% starch and 2% acacia in water), methyl cellulose—400 cps (4%), ethyl cellulose (5%) in alcohol, confectionery (arsenic-free) shellac (25% in alcohol), sodium carboxymethylcellulose, polyethylene glycol 4000 or 6000, and polyvinylpyrrolidone in aqueous, alcoholic, and hydroalcoholic solutions. Water, alcohol, and acetone, or mixtures thereof, are not binders in their own right. They act by means of their solvent effect upon ingredients; e.g., sucrose in a tablet formula.

Disintegrators are substances which are added to tablet formulations, when required, to induce the tablet to disintegrate after administration. The factors which influence the rate of solution or the rate of disintegration are the (1) physical and chemical properties of the materials in the tablet formulation, (2) tablet hardness, and, to a far less extent, (3) surface area (of certain special tablets). Dried corn or potato starch and cellulose derivatives [e.g., Solka-Floc (*Brown*) Avicel (*Am. Viscose*)] are the most popular disintegrating agents.

Lubricants are added to tablet granulations, when needed, to

1. Improve the flow properties of granules.
2. Eliminate adhesion to the surfaces of the punch and die.
3. Reduce die-wall friction and thus facilitate the ejection of the finished tablet.
4. Reduce excessive punch and die wear.

Many finely powdered substances (80–200 mesh) are used as lubricants. The proper selection of a lubricant is related to the purposes of lubricants mentioned above. Examples of "glidants," which improve the flow properties of granules: calcium stearate, magnesium stearate, starch, sodium chloride, and talc. The elimination of adhesion to the surfaces of the punches and dies is best accomplished by soft materials such as cocoa butter and other natural fats, hydrogenated vegetable oils or fats, liquid and solid petrolatum, sodium stearate and other soaps, paraffin wax, stearic acid, and waxes or waxlike materials. Lubricants added to reduce excessive punch and die wear and to reduce the die wall friction are calcium stearate, magnesium stearate, and talc.

Coloring Agents—When a colored tablet is desired, a certified FD&C color is normally added by:

1. Dissolving the dye in the binding solution.
2. Spraying the granules with a special solution of the dye.
3. Distributing the dye through the dry mix and then employing wet granulation.
4. Adding a triturate of the dye to starch or calcium sulfate (suitable for pastel shades only).

Such dye triturates are commercially

Table 1—Optimum Mesh Size
of Granulations

Diameter of tablet	Granulation
3/16 in.	20 mesh
7/32-5/16 in.	16 mesh
11/32-13/32 in.	14 mesh
7/16 in. and over	12 mesh

available. A No. 40 mesh granulation, or finer, is necessary to avoid mottled tablets.

Flavoring Agents—If a flavored tablet is desired, it is usually accomplished by spraying an alcoholic or ethereal solution of volatile oil or other flavoring agent onto the dry granules before the compression of the finished tablets. After spraying, the granules are tumbled and sometimes stored in sealed containers to allow greater permeation of the flavor. Frequently, fruit flavorings are also incorporated into the original powder mix before granulation.

Manufacture

The satisfactory compression of tablets requires the material to (1) be free-flowing, (2) possess suitable binding properties, and (3) freely separate from the punches and dies without any sticking. Since few materials satisfactorily meet these requirements, the general process of fabricating compressed tablets consists in correcting these defects by suitably altering the material so that these requirements are fulfilled.

The modern tablet machine may not function properly unless the material to be compressed is largely in the form of granules equivalent to approximately a No. 12 to a No. 20 mesh. Larger granules may not feed into the dies as evenly or compress as well as particles of the proper size. Fine powders likewise may not flow into the dies evenly. It is not necessary that all of the material be in No. 12 to No. 20 granules; usually, a small proportion of finer material does no harm, and may even do some good by producing a smoother tablet. Normally, the presence of as much as 12 or 15% of fine powder is not objectionable.

No general statement can be made safely regarding the acceptable limits of "fineness." In all probability it varies with each specific granulation. If the granulation has satisfactory free-flowing and binding properties, the practical upper limits to the acceptable amount of fineness may approach 100% and perhaps even finer than a No. 100 mesh. The optimum mesh size of granulation varies with the diameter of the tablets to be made (see Table 1).

It should be clearly understood that this is but a convenient guide, best used to represent the maximum diameter of the granules and not the minimum. Properly formulated granulations, which are much finer than suggested above, can be easily compressed, and at extremely high speeds.

The pharmaceutical industry uses three distinct methods for the production of compressed tablets: direct compression, wet granulation, and dry granulation.

Direct Compression—The term direct compression is applied to the general process of manufacturing compressed tablets when little or no preliminary treatment (e.g., granulation) is necessary before feeding the material into the tablet machine. Some few materials have the necessary free-flowing and binding characteristics. Generally, such suitable materials are granular, have marked ionic properties, possess crystalline structures with good planes of slippage, and are comparatively soft materials (i.e., low in the scale of hardness). Obviously, materials suitable for direct compression must be reasonably stable under the working conditions and must possess, or be capable of reduction to the proper physical size. Examples of materials which can be compressed directly are ammonium chloride, sodium chloride, sodium bromide, sodium bicarbonate (lubricant required), sodium phenolsulfonate, sodium salicylate (free-flowing crystals plus lubricant), potassium chloride, potassium bromide, potassium iodide, potassium nitrate, potassium chloride, potassium permanganate, methenamine (lubricant advisable), chloral hydrate, camphor, aspirin crystals, and naphthalene (slightly moistened with water). Most of these materials are also self-lubricating.

The introduction of the induced die feed frame on modern rotary tablet machines has extended the range of direct compression. Many materials, which formerly required some type of granulation, can now be directly compressed into finished tablets.

Wet Granulation—Fine powders require special treatment for conversion into the granular form. This process is known as wet granulation. The steps involved in this method are:

1. Weighing and mixing the ingredients.
2. Sieving and wet massing.
3. Wet granulation.
4. Drying.
5. Dry granulation.
6. Lubrication.
7. Tableting by compression.

The first step in the wet granulation process consists of weighing and uniformly mixing the powdered medicinal agents with the diluent and, perhaps, a portion of the disintegrator. The mixture thus obtained is passed one or more times through a suitable screen (usually a No. 30–60-mesh) and subjected to additional blending. This is followed by careful moistening with the proper binding solution until the mixture has the consistency of a crumbly mass. The uniform distribution of the binding solution is imperative. The quantity of the proper binder is also relatively critical. Insufficient binder leads to poor adhesion, soft tablets, and "capping" (chipping). Excessive binder yields a tablet with longer disintegration time and greater hardness. In addition, the wet screening operation may be infinitely more difficult if excessive binder is present. The wet mass is then screened. The screen size may vary from a No. 6–20-mesh. Small quantities are conveniently hand-screened through a No. 14–20-mesh screen. If larger quantities of materials are to be hand-screened, it is common to use a

No. 6- or a No. 8-mesh screen. Industrially, this screening is done mechanically with a suitable granulating or comminuting machine. The wet granules are then air-dried at room temperature or in forced-air drying ovens at about 50°C. They may be vacuum-dried in heated tumbling chambers. After drying, the granules are broken up and passed through the proper screen to obtain the desired granule size.

A method of granulation used by many pharmaceutical manufacturers is as follows. The moistened material is forced through a No. 4- or a 6-mesh screen so as to break it up into large particles. The granules are then dried either on trays in forced hot-air cabinets or in special vacuum rotating driers or in air-suspended fluidized bed-driers. After the material has dried, the coarse granulation is reduced to a No. 12–20-mesh granulation by running it through a granulator. The advantage of the oscillating granulator is that as soon as a particle is reduced to the proper mesh size, it falls through the screen away from the grinding action and is not reduced further in size. A disadvantage of grinding tablet granulations in an ordinary grinder is that an exceptionally large amount of fine powder is formed.

In some mixers the moistening liquid is added slowly as a fine spray. When treated in this manner, some materials form granules with a minimum of liquid (e.g., alcoholic PVP solutions), thus making it unnecessary to run the wet material through a granulator.

To the granules prepared by either of these methods outlined above, a lubricant is next added to insure uniform feeding into the dies and to prevent the material from adhering to the punches and dies after compression. Common lubricants, previously discussed, usually constitute ½–3% of the total tablet weight. Powdered lubricants are screened or bolted on a thin layer of the granules, followed by gentle agitation in order that the lubricant may be distributed as evenly as possible. On a large scale the granules are mixed with lubricant in a tumbling mixer, twin-shell blender, ribbon blender, etc. More lubricating powder must be used in granulations in which there is considerable fine powder since the fine powder has a greater tendency to stick to the face of the punch.

Another lubrication method is to spray an ethereal solution of liquid petrolatum (mineral oil) or petrolatum on the granules and allow the ether to evaporate. The proportion of these lubricants should not exceed 1 or 2% of the weight of the granules since excessive amounts of hydrocarbons tend to render the tablets impervious to water, thus interfering with proper disintegration.

In the case of tablets of insoluble chemicals, it is common to add 10–20% of starch dried at 100°C to the dry granules before compression. When the tablet reaches the stomach, the particles of starch attract water and the tablet disintegrates, thus exposing a greater surface of the medicament. Some of the starch may be mixed with the medicaments prior to granulation in order to break apart the individual granules on subsequent contact with water.

When appreciable proportions of liquid medicaments are to be included in tablets, it is usually necessary to use some rather inert material such as an absorbent. Starch is an efficient absorbent; lactose is a good absorbent for extracts; magnesium carbonate is excellent for oily substances; aqueous or alcoholic liquids such as tinctures, fluidextracts, etc., may be mixed with the moistening liquid, or they may be evaporated to dryness and mixed with the powders prior to granulation.

Incompatibility of two ingredients may be successfully handled in some cases by granulating the troublesome ingredients separately and then mixing the granulations.

Dry Granulation—This method is also known as "slugging" or "precompression." The process of wet granulation is obviously unsuitable for substances which are sensitive to heat or moisture and for mixtures which are incompatible in the presence of moisture. In such cases dry granulation is applicable. The steps involved in this method include weighing and mixing the ingredients, slugging, dry granulation of the slug, lubrication, and tableting by compression. For example, following weighing and mixing the ingredients, granulations of aspirin may be made by compressing a mixture of finely divided acetylsalicylic acid and dried starch into large, flat-faced tablets called slugs, which are subsequently reduced to a granular form. Formerly, considerable difficulty was encountered with this method because the tablet machines available were not suitable for the compression of powders. The precompression of a fine powder into slugs is best carried out in a special, heavy-duty rotary tablet machine frequently fitted with a special feed-frame. The die-cavities are usually $3/4$–$1 3/8$ in. in diameter. Since considerable dust results from the liberation of air entrapped in the powder, it is advisable to have the working parts well-housed and to use some form of dust-collecting device at the point of compression. Some powder mixtures do not have sufficient binding qualities; in such cases the binding qualities may be improved by adding suitable dry excipients. The slugs are reduced to proper granule size with a granulator, or other suitable device. The resulting granulation is lubricated and then compressed into the finished tablets in the usual way. In some cases the lubricant is added at the time the ingredients are mixed.

In tablets made by the dry granulation method, any possible reactions or deterioration due to heat and moisture are avoided. The resulting tablets are more uniform in content of active ingredients than tablets made by the process of mixing two or more separate granulations; in the latter method the different granulations may tend to separate in the feeding device. Tablets made by dry granulation disintegrate more rapidly than tablets made by other methods because the starch used as a disintegrating agent is more intimately mixed with the other substances, and its disintegrating action has not been impaired by absorption of some of the binder. These advantages, together with the lower costs for equipment, labor, and handling account for the growing popularity of dry granulation. This is a very important and widely used procedure in the pharmaceutical industry.

Tablet Machines—A tablet machine suitable for making lots of a few thousand tablets is the hand single-punch tablet machine (Fig. 2). The granulated material is placed in a hopper and from there it feeds into a die, where it is compressed by the action of two punches: the one operating from above the die is the upper punch, and the one working from below is the lower punch. The lower punch is adjusted so that at its highest point it is exactly flush with the top of the die, and so that at its lowest point it leaves a space in the die exactly sufficient to hold the quantity of granulated material necessary for one tablet. The pressure which is brought to play on the granulated material is regulated by the position of the upper punch. The compression should be great enough to prevent breaking or crumbling the tablets during handling, but should not be so great that solution or disintegration will be impeded. A practical rule for judging proper compression is that the tablet should be readily broken when pressed between the thumb and fingers but should not break when dropped on the floor. A higher degree of compression is desirable for tablets intended to be dissolved slowly in the mouth. Great care should be taken to prevent punches and dies from becoming scratched or rusted. After use, they should be carefully cleaned and kept under oil or coated with petrolatum.

The simplest tablet machine is the single-punch machine which makes one tablet at each revolution (e.g., the hand tablet machine). Power-driven single-punch machines have an output of 40,000–50,000 tablets/working day. By

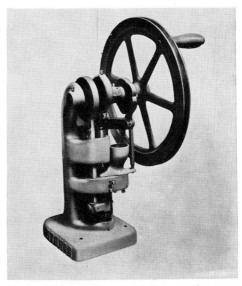

Fig. 2—Eureka single-punch tablet press (courtesy, *F. J. Stokes Corp.*).

using different sets of punches and dies a variety of sizes and shapes can be made on such a machine. Because of their comparative simplicity and low cost, power-driven single-punch machines are well-suited for tablet production on a moderate scale.

In the multiple-punch machine, 2–12 punches operate simultaneously in corresponding holes in a single die, thus producing a number of tablets/revolution. Such machines speed up production, but there is a greater tendency to a lack of uniformity in the tablets due to irregular filling of the holes in the die.

Most tablets manufactured today are compressed on high-speed "rotary tablet machines," which have the dual advantage of low processing costs and a large production capacity of uniform tablets. When single-punch machines are operated at speeds in excess of 100 tablets/min, the weight variations of the finished tablet may fluctuate excessively because of the short die-filling and compression times. Rotary machines have a comparatively long die-filling time. The unique arrangement of feeding the granules and the special positioning of the lower punches combine to produce a uniform filling of the dies.

This is very effective in controlling variations in tablet weight. Rotary tablet machines may produce tablets with less internal stress because of the gradually increasing pressure and the comparatively long compression time. These factors may lower the compression rebound and the elastic recovery of the tablet.

Correction of Difficulties—To prevent undue wear and insure proper operation, all moving parts of a tablet machine must be sufficiently lubricated, avoiding an excess of lubricant which might contaminate the tablets. Since many drugs have a corrosive action on metal, the machine should be thoroughly cleaned after each run. If a machine is used continuously, it should be cleaned at intervals to prevent dust accumulation around the moving parts.

The dust which arises in tablet making is usually carried away by a suction system terminating in openings at the compression points, as well as a suction system for each individual machine's cubicle. If this is not done, the dust from each machine will contaminate other products and also cause discomfort to people in the room.

Improper feeding may result from operation at an excessive speed which does not allow sufficient time to uniformly fill the dies. Induced die feed-frames on rotary machines largely eliminate this problem and greatly increase the machines' productivity. The same difficulty is encountered if the granulation is too damp, too fine, or too coarse, or if it contains an excess of powder. It is necessary to check the weight and hardness of the tablets from time to time during a run so that any loosening of adjustments on the machine may be corrected.

Tablet makers use the term *capping* to designate splitting off of the upper surface of the tablet. When this is encountered it is usually due to poor adhesion, compression rebound, or a large elastic recovery. In such cases it may be necessary to regranulate the material, alter the pressure adjustment, or reduce the speed of the tablet machine. Capping may also be due to worn punches.

Capping and splitting of tablets is sometimes caused by having too soft a granulation; regranulation, which results in a hardening of the granules, usually eliminates this difficulty. A hard granulation permits a higher percentage of fine powder than a soft granulation. Capping may also occur if there is not enough fine powder in the granulation, particularly in the compression of crystalline substances such as methenamine or sodium bromide. For example, difficulty encountered with crystals of No. 16 mesh may be corrected by forcing the material through a No. 20-mesh screen to provide some fine powder. The addition of stearic acid ($\frac{1}{2}$–1%) sometimes remedies capping and splitting, especially with granulations containing powdered sugar.

Sometimes the punch picks out a small area of the surface of the tablet; this difficulty is known as *picking*. The trouble occurs more frequently with the upper punch and is due to adherence of the material to the face of the punch. One cause of picking is a scratched punch; if the scratch is only slight it may be smoothed with fine emery cloth and a trace of oil, but if this does not suffice, it is necessary to regrind the punch. Picking also may result from compressing a granulation which is not quite dry. Sometimes picking is corrected by adding fats of waxlike materials with the lubricant.

In some cases the tablet material may stick to the die and cause binding of the lower punch. This may be due to slight dampness of the granulation, an excess of powder, or worn punches and dies. Binding of the lower punch may occur with substances such as calcium lactate. When the granulation tends to take up moisture from the air, it is helpful to minimize exposure by transferring the warm granulation directly from the dryer into the hopper of the tablet machine. However, some granulations cannot be compressed in humid weather unless air-conditioning facilities are provided. Frequent repolishing and cleaning of the punches and dies helps to prevent binding.

Difficulties encountered in compression may be prevented by studying each substance or mixture individually to determine the best moistening and lubricating agents. For instance, sodium salicylate gives difficulty with aqueous granulating liquids, but favorable results can be obtained using powdered sucrose and 7% alcohol in making the granulation and using 3–4% magnesium stearate as a lubricant.

Sometimes it will be observed that the tablets have a peripheral ridge which may break off in sifting (leaving a ragged edge) or after packing in bottles (making dust in the container). This is caused by using excessively worn punches and dies, which allow a slight amount of material to squeeze between the die and the punch, thus forming a rim on the tablet. Naturally, there is a constant wear on punches and dies. The only solution is to install a new set of punches and dies. The use of unduly worn tablet machines is generally unsatisfactory as the weight of the tablets may vary.

Lettered Tablets—Tablets bearing letters or designs may be made by using suitable punches. Some ingredients are well adapted to raised letters while others give better results when the lettering is indented. For lettered tablets, a No. 30 or 40 granulation is used since coarser particles do not fill as evenly into the engraving on the punches. There is a tendency to compress lettered tablets harder than usual in order to make the letters stand out.

Solubility and Ease of Disintegration—Compressed tablets composed of insoluble medicament should disintegrate within a few minutes when dropped into water. In lozenges, where a continued local effect is sought, disintegration should be very slow; in hypodermic tablets, very rapid solution is necessary. Obviously, a tablet which is swallowed must dissolve or disintegrate within a reasonable time if it is to have any medicinal effect. A tablet that will pass through the alimentary tract without disintegrating is not only useless, but is worse than useless, for it not only fails to have the desired effect, but through the confidence wrongly placed in it, stands in the way of other treatment which might prove beneficial.

The solubility of a tablet depends, to a certain extent, on the solubility of its ingredients. Tablets composed entirely or almost entirely of soluble materials offer no difficulties in this respect. In the case of insoluble substances, the treatment will differ according to whether or not the substance possesses a cellular structure. Vegetable powders, such as ground roots, barks, etc., swell in water; this property assures disintegration of a tablet largely composed of material of this nature. For tablets of insoluble chemicals, something must be done to cause the tablet to disintegrate after it is swallowed. A very common method is to incorporate 10–20% dry starch in the tablet; when the tablet comes in contact with water the wicking effect of the starch causes the tablet to break up. Starch to be used in tablets should be dried at 100°C before use, and tablets containing starch should be kept in air-tight containers. Commercial cornstarch, potato flour, and rice flour may contain 9–14% moisture; this moisture content should be reduced to 1.5% or less to secure maximum disintegrating effect and to prevent deterioration of easily hydrolyzed drugs such as aspirin. In the wet granulation process the dried starch must be added to the dry granules just before compression, thus avoiding contact with the moistening liquid. In the slugging method some starch can be added just before compression into tablets. Subsequently, in contact with water, this starch will aid in breaking up the tablet into granules; some starch may also be used in the original powder mixture in order to separate the granules into smaller particles. Another method is to incorporate a small amount of sodium bicarbonate and citric (or tartaric) acid in each tablet. When such a tablet is dropped into water, there is an effervescence and the tablet falls apart. Sodium bicarbonate may also be used without acids since the acid of the gastric juice will be sufficient to cause effervescence and disintegration. Excessive hardness of a tablet, the use of too much gum or gelatin, and the excessive use of oil as a lubricant are factors which tend to hinder disintegration.

Essential Qualities of a Good Tablet

The essential qualities of a good tablet are the evident criteria which are used by everyone wishing to determine the general or precise nature of the character excellence (in fact, the quality itself) of tablets from a given lot. These are the criteria used alike by the pharmacist, scientist, physician, patient, and layman. The significant difference between these individuals in determining the quality of a tablet is the variation in the degree of perception and in the depth of investigation. The necessary purity of ingredients and dosage accuracy, e.g., may not be readily available to the patient, but it is well-known, or can be determined, by the scientists of the pharmaceutical industry and the US Food and Drug Administration. There is, however, a clear-cut, implied warranty on the part of the manufacturer and the dispensing pharmacist to the ultimate purchasing consumer that such qualities do, in fact, exist in the dispensed tablet. Therefore, it is prudent, on the part of the pharmacist, to use reasonable care in determining the qualities of the tablets he elects to dispense.

Accurate and Uniform Weight—Legal, regulating, and licensing agencies of the various world governments (e.g., the US Food and Drug Administration, a division of the Department of Health, Education and Welfare) precisely demand that tablets contain the specifically designated medication in either the therapeutically required or the stated quantities. This is tantamount to concisely stating that any sampling within a specific batch of tablets would reveal the tablets to be both uniform and accurate with respect to weight and content. The limits of deviation (alternately termed tolerance, variability limits, potency, etc.) for the thousands of different tablets commercially available are, thus, directly specified or indirectly implied by the responsible, legal controlling agencies.

The acceptable limits of deviation depend on the special problems associated with the production of the particular tablet. The official compendia normally specify that a certain number of tablets (frequently 20) be weighed, finely powdered, analytically sampled, and assayed. Some tablets, which exhibit relatively large unit dosages of medicinal agents (e.g., aspirin 0.3 g; or sodium chloride, 0.3–1.0 g), are fabricated with comparative ease. Note that these chemicals have been widely studied and rigidly standardized to exacting specifications and are of known purity and established stability. Under such circumstances the allowable deviation would be expected to be reasonably small, e.g., ±5%. Official compendia such as the USP normally express the limits of deviation in such cases as "not less than 95% and not more than 105% of the labeled amount."

Conversely, some medicinal tablets require greater tolerances. The necessity for a small tablet or a relatively small therapeutic dose/tablet adversely effects accuracy and drastically magnifies slight deviations in weight when expressed as a percentage [e.g., atropine sulfate tablets—dosage (400 μg), tolerance (90–110%)]. Hence, greater deviations are allowed. Since some medicinal agents are subject to gradual decomposition during processing, greater tolerances are then permitted [e.g., nitroglycerin tablets—dosage (0.2–0.6 mg), tolerance (80–112%) and ascorbic acid tablets—dosage (25 mg–1 g), tolerance (95–115%)]. Medicinal agents that are difficult to purify or standardize are also permitted wider tolerances [e.g., polymixin B sulfate tablets—dosage (50 mg), tolerance (not less than 85%); thyroid tablets—dosage (30–180 mg), tolerance "contains an amount of iodine in thyroid combination equivalent to 0.17–0.23% of the labeled amount of thyroid"]. A larger tolerance is also acceptable with some materials which are normally obtained and employed as a mixture of two or more components [e.g., tablets or lozenges of tyrothricin, a crystallizable polypeptide which occurs as a mixture of approximately 80% tyrocidine and 20% gramicidin—dosage (varies), tolerance (90–120% of the labeled potency)].

The official compendia throughout the world prescribe the limits of "weight variation" of individual tablets. For example, the USP broadly denotes that the average weight of uncoated tablets conforms to the tolerances given in Table 2 unless otherwise provided in the individual monograph. The USP directs that 20 unbroken tablets are first weighed individually and then the average weight/tablet is calculated. The USP exacts that the weight of not more than *two* (i.e., 10%) of the tablets differ from the average weight by more than the percentages listed in Table 2 and that no *one* (i.e., 5%) tablet differs by more than *double* that percentage. Thus, the essential quality of accurate and uniform weight in a tablet, which in effect implies controlled and correct dosage, is explicitly dictated.

Content Uniformity—To assure uniform potency for tablets, a content uniformity test is applied in which a sample of 30 tablets are selected and 10 are individually assayed. The requirements are met if the content of each of not less than 9 of the tablets is within the limits of 85–115% of labeled potency and if the content of none of the tablets falls outside the limits of 75–125% of labeled potency. If the content of not more than 2 tablets falls outside the limits of 85–115%, the remaining 20 tablets should be individually assayed. The requirements are met if the content of each tablet falls within the limits of 85–115%.

Table 2—Limits of Deviation in Tablets

Average weight/tablet	Maximum percentage difference	
	Two tablets	One tablet
13 mg or less	15	30
More than 13 mg and including 130 mg	10	20
More than 130 mg and including 324 mg	7½	15
More than 324 mg	5	10

Homogeneity—This essential quality of a good tablet is closely linked with the accurate and uniform weight requirement discussed previously. Both single and multiple compressed tablets must exhibit a reasonably accurate distribution of the active ingredient or ingredients (i.e., homogeneity) to insure:

1. Compliance with the regulations affecting the industry.
2. Acceptance by the dispensing pharmacist.
3. Physicians' confidence.
4. A pleasing and psychologically acceptable appearance to the patient.

Since appearance is a key factor in visually recognizing a lack of homogeneity, tablet manufacturers strive to excel in this quality to insure a satisfactory and homogeneous appearance.

Multiple compressed tablets are frequently laminated into two or more distinct layers or contain a separate core tablet, i.e., a tablet within a tablet. The reasons for this procedure are highly diverse. They vary from the necessity of avoiding physical and chemical incompatibilities to enhancing the tablet's acceptability for increased sales appeal. It should be noted, however, that a high degree of homogeneity must exist within each separate layer comprising the laminated tablet or within each phase of the tablet within a tablet type. Tablet manufacturers frequently accentuate the layering effect by impressively coloring each layer with attractive complementary dyes.

A further necessity for the uniform distribution of the active ingredients in a tablet (single and multiple com-

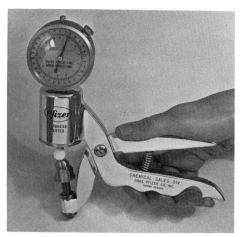

Fig. 3—Pfizer Tablet Hardness Tester.

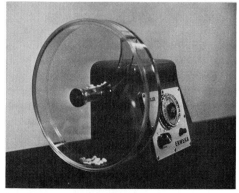

Fig. 4—The Roche Friabilator.

pressed) is to present a tablet that can be divided with reasonable assurance of administering that divided portion of the total tablet dosage. Many tablets are scored to facilitate convenient division into halves or even quarters. Obviously, such a scored tablet carries an implied warranty that the active ingredients are uniformly distributed throughout the entire volume of the tablet.

Absence of Incompatibilities— Tablets must be essentially free of incompatibilities in order to assure the labeled potency for the maximum shelf life and to assure the desired therapeutic effect. The absence of incompatibilities from a pharmaceutical and medicinal standpoint means chemical constancy and freedom from undesirable physiological effects. Naturally, this is of paramount importance to everyone concerned: the patient, pharmacist, physician, and pharmaceutical manufacturer.

Tablets with mild incompatibilities frequently exhibit these defects by visible or odoriferous changes on aging. The usual methods of accelerating the rates of chemical reactions increase the ease of observing chemical incompatibilities.

Stability and Hardness—Tablets must be stable to assure that the intended therapeutic quantity of the drug is received by the patient. Stability,

from a pharmaceutical or medical standpoint, normally means physical constancy. Hence maximum tablet stability requires that tablets be fabricated to withstand the physical factors to which they can be expected to be subjected. Tablets must be properly formulated and compressed to attain a satisfactory hardness. Hardness determination is usually made during production in order to make the necessary pressure adjustments of the tablet machine. The degree of hardness varies with different manufacturers and with different tablets (lozenges and buccal tablets which are intended to dissolve slowly are deliberately manufactured hard), but tablets must be sufficiently hard to maintain their shape during the expected life of the tablet. Hardness can be determined by using a Pfizer Hardness Tester (Fig. 3) or similar device. Exceptionally soft tablets may powder or crumble, while excessively hard tablets may chip or fracture. The Roche Friabilator (Fig. 4) represents a convenient device to determine the "wearing qualities" of tablets. The tablets to be tested are weighed and then allowed to tumble in the rotating Friabilator. After a certain number of rotations, the tablets are weighed again and the loss in weight is determined. Stable tablets show no appreciable loss or damage during the test.

Tablets are subject to varying conditions that can adversely affect their stability. Some tablets must be protected from climatic extremes such as temperature, relative humidity, and actinic irradiation. Excessive heat is very damaging to many tablets.

Excellent tablet stability requires the anticipation of the effect of all probably antagonistic physical factors and the correct counteraction to neutralize them efficiently.

Disintegration—Tablets must disintegrate in the stomach or intestinal tract so that the medication can exert its therapeutic effects. Some medicinal agents possess this desired property. Most medicinal tablets, however, require that suitable materials, termed disintegrating agents, be incorporated in the formula to produce the desired collapse of the tablet after oral administration.

USP and NF tablets must pass the official Tablet Disintegration Test. The apparatus used (Fig. 5) consists of a basket-rack assembly containing 6 open-ended glass tubes held in a vertical position. A No. 10-mesh stainless steel wire screen is attached to the bottom of the assembly. Through a mechanical device the basket rack is raised and lowered through a distance of 5–6 cm at a frequency of 28–32 cycles/min. During testing, one tablet is placed in each tube and the basket rack is allowed to move up and down a 1-liter beaker of water, simulated gastric fluid, or simulated intestinal fluid at 37° ± 2°. Not all tablets are designed to disintegrate at the same rate. In fact, the time required for disintegration varies with different tablets and different uses. For uncoated tablets, buccal tablets, and sublingual tablets water maintained at 37° ± 2° is used as immersion fluid unless another fluid is specified in the monograph. Uncoated tablets and sublingual tablets must disintegrate at the end of the time limit specified and buccal tablets must disintegrate within 4 hours. The disintegration test for plain coated tablets consists of removing the external coating by immersing the tablets in water at room temperature for 5 min. Then the tablets are

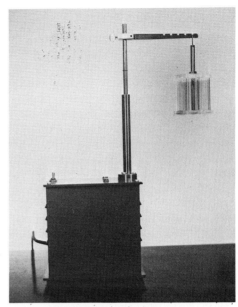

Fig. 5—Tablet disintegration tester.

placed in the basket rack. The apparatus is operated using simulated gastric fluid at 37° ± 2° as the immersion fluid. If the tablets have not disintegrated completely within 30 min, simulated intestinal fluid maintained at 37° ± 2° should be used as the immersion fluid, and the test is continued for a period of time equal to the time limit specified in the individual monograph. For enteric-coated tablets, the test consists of immersing the tablets in water at room temperature for 5 min to wash off any soluble external coating after which the tablets are subjected to the test using simulated gastric fluid maintained at 37° ± 2°; 1 hour later, the tablets should show no distinct evidence of dissolution or disintegration. The tablets are then immersed in simulated intestinal fluid maintained at 37° ± 2° for specified time during which the tablet should have disintegrated. In all aforementioned tests, if one or two tablets fail to disintegrate completely, the test should be repeated on 12 additional tablets, not less than 16 of the total of 18 tablets tested should disintegrate completely.

Size and Shape for Administra-

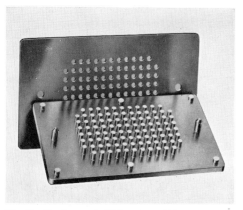

Fig. 6—Hand-operated triturate mold (courtesy, *Arthur Colton Co.*).

tion—Tablets are designed and fabricated into many different sizes and shapes to serve a wide variety of purposes. The intended method and/or route of administration of the medicament in the tablet form dictates that both its shape and the size must be of reasonable dimensions. Tablets intended for oral administration by the usual method of swallowing accompanied by a large volume of an aqueous fluid such as water normally vary from $\frac{1}{8}$ to $\frac{1}{2}$ in. in diameter. The thickness of these tablets is usually held to less than 50% of the tablet diameter. Tablet thickness depends largely on die-fill and compressive load. Thus, in order to produce uniform thickness, the same volume of fill and the same pressure must be employed. During production, the thickness of each tablet may be measured with a micrometer to ensure a consistent thickness.

Molded Tablets

Preparation

Very fine powders are used in the preparation of tablet triturates (TT's). The methods of mixing are the same as those described in Chapter 4, with emphasis on uniform distribution of the medicament in the diluent.

Diluents—Lactose, dextrose, sucrose, and mannitol are the most generally used diluents. Lactose (preferably beta-lactose which dissolves faster than alpha-lactose) gives a triturate which is a little too friable for ordinary handling, while sucrose yields a tablet which is a little too hard. For this reason mixtures of lactose and finely powdered sucrose (5–25%) are frequently used. For tablet triturates of substances such as potassium permanganate and silver nitrate, which would be reduced by carbohydrates, kaolin or precipitated chalk may be used as diluents. Sodium bicarbonate is a traditional diluent for TT's of calomel. Both soluble and nonsoluble diluents are used for orally administered molded tablets, but only soluble diluents (e.g., beta-lactose) are suitable for hypodermic tablets.

Molds—The molds are made of hard rubber or metal and consist of an upper plate perforated with holes and a lower plate with pegs which fit into the holes when the upper plate is placed on the lower one (Fig. 6). Molds for hypodermic tablets have smaller holes than those for ordinary tablet triturates.

Developing a Formula—The amount of moistened diluent necessary to fill a certain number of holes in the mold should be determined. This is done by molding a certain number of tablets using the moistened diluent and then drying and weighing the resulting tablets. A determination of this kind should be made for each new mold and kept on record for future use. From the figure thus obtained the weight of diluent needed for the required number of triturates is calculated. The weight of medicament to be used is subtracted from the weight of diluent, leaving the amount of diluent to be used. A trial batch may be made to determine whether the calculated quantities exactly fill the holes; if necessary, a slightly greater or smaller quantity of diluent is used to adjust for variations in the specific volume of the diluent and the drug.

Process of Molding—The well-triturated powder is moistened with alcohol or a mixture of alcohol and water. The use of 50% alcohol gives favorable results; higher percentages yield tablet triturates which tend to powder during normal handling. The use of water alone is necessary when the triturates contain strong oxidizing agents which would react with alcohol. The proportion of moistening liquid should be kept low since excess liquid may cause discoloration and yield tablets which are harder and more slowly soluble. For 4 g of lactose, the use of 0.8 ml of 50% alcohol is suitable. The mass must be moist enough to adhere, but not so wet that the resulting triturates are too hard. The upper plate of the mold is set on a glass plate and the mass is forced into the holes with a spatula. After a few moments, the upper plate is placed over the lower plate and gently pressed down, the triturates thus being forced upward out of the hole. The triturates are allowed to remain in position on the pegs until they dry.

Tablet machines may be used for making tablet triturates by using punches and dies of the proper shape and setting the machines for light compression.

Dispensing

Tablets are dispensed in many different types of containers and in various manners uniquely applicable to special situations. Many hospital pharmacists are deeply interested in dispensing each individual dose of tablet medication in a special foil or laminated polyethylene film pack. Some hospital pharmacies are using this system. Tablets are generally dispensed in glass or plastic vials or in specially fabricated pasteboard boxes. Glass bottles are also widely used.

Tablets should receive a minimum of direct handling during the dispensing operation. This increases cleanliness, minimizes moisture absorption, and conveys a professional appearance. Several pharmaceutical manufacturers supply convenient and sanitary counting trays which completely eliminate the necessity for touching a tablet with the hands. Tablets should not be handled with the fingers or poured into the hand

for counting. This is particularly important for coated tablets, because the warmth and moisture of the hand tend to dull the coating, and the tablets remaining in the hand after counting the desired number may contaminate other tablets when returned to their container.

If a counting tray is not available, considerable skill in counting tablets without touching them directly can be easily acquired with a little practice. A few tablets are poured into the closure cap of the stock bottle or onto an arched paper and then transferred to the dispensing package.

Typical Prescriptions

1

℞ Quinidine   gr. iii
    30 tablets
Sig: One daily

2

℞ Tab. Feosol   #100
Sig: 2 tablets t.i.d.p.c.

3

℞ Mysoline Tablets   250 mg.   #30
Sig: 1 tablet t.i.d.

4

℞ Belladenal Spacetabs   #20
Sig: i tablet b.i.d.

5

℞ Empirin Compound Tablets   #30
Sig: 1 tablet p.r.n. for headache

6

℞ Fero-Grad 500   #30
Sig: 1 tablet daily

7

℞ Ilosone Chewable   125 mg.
    Tabs #20
Sig: 1 tab. q. 6 hrs.

8

℞ Ilotycin (Enteric-Coated)   250 mg.
    Tabs #30
Sig: 1 tab. t.i.d.a.c.

9

℞ Strychnine Sulf   gr $\frac{1}{60}$

    Tab. No. XX
Sig: i t.i.d.

10

℞   Nilstat Vaginal Tabs   100,000 U
        No. 30
    Sig: Insert i tab. daily

11

2   Tempra Tablets   #30
    Sig: i tab. q. 4 h p.r.n. for pain

12

℞   Dimetane Extentabs   8 mg.
        Tabs #20
    Sig: i b.i.d.

13

℞   Libritabs   5 mg.
        Tabs #30
    Sig: i t.i.d. and at h.s.

14

℞   Tabs of Potassium Permanganate   5 gr.
        #XX
    Sig: Dissolve i tab in a quart of water. Bathe
    feet 10 min at night

15

℞   Nitroglycerin   0.4 g.
        Tabs #50
    Sig: As directed

16

℞   Thantis Lozenges
        No. 24
    Sig: Dissolve 1 lozenge in the mouth q. 4 hrs.

17

℞   Alka-Seltzer
        Tabs #25
    Sig: Dissolve 1 tab in ½ glass of water p.r.n. for
    headache

18

℞   Phenergan   25 mg.
        Tabs #20
    Sig: i tab b.i.d. during attack

19

℞   Luminal Tabs   gr 1½
        #30
    Sig: i h.s.

20

℞   Meprobamate   400 mg.
        Tabs #20
    Sig: As directed

Pills

Pills are small, round or egg-shaped, solid bodies for internal use. Most pills weigh 65–300 mg, exclusive of coating. Very small pills are sometimes known as *parvules* or *granules;* a very large pill, usually for veterinary use, is known as a *bolus*. A pill is administered by placing on the tongue and swallowing with water.

Because of their smallness of bulk, pills offer ease of administration and concealment of taste. Certain formulas are not suitable for incorporation into tablets or capsules; pills are still the best dosage form for them. Pills containing resinous drugs dissolve slowly, which is an advantage where slow continuous action is desired such as with cathartics.

Pills are unsuitable when rapid action is required since a pill possessing the characteristic firmness usually disintegrates slowly as it passes through the intestinal tract. In fact, there have been cases where pills passed through the intestinal tract almost unchanged and were eliminated in the feces. They are not suitable for the administration of bulky powders or for liquids, except in small doses. Drugs which may be irritating in concentrated form should not be made into pills.

Despite the fact that the community pharmacist very rarely is called upon to make them, pills are a form of medication and a pharmacist should be able to prepare satisfactory pills.

Ingredients of Pills

Diluents and Excipients—Frequently, the amount of medicinal agent prescribed has insufficient bulk to make pills. In such cases the pharmacist should add a solid known as a *diluent* to supply sufficient bulk. It should be chemically and physiologically inert, and it should not alter appreciably the color of the pill mass. The most commonly used diluents are powdered glycyrrhiza or licorice, glycyrrhiza extract, starch, althea, tragacanth, or mixtures of these. The amount to be added should be sufficient to allow the pharmacist to work efficiently (as in filling capsules) but not enough to make the pill too large. The usual custom is to make the finished pill weigh about 120 mg.

Ordinarily, the ingredients prescribed will not of themselves yield a mass having the desired properties, and it is necessary to add a liquid, a solid, or both to obtain a suitable mass. The material added for this purpose is the *excipient*. The choice of excipient is usually left to the pharmacist and is of great importance since the bulk and nature of the excipient determine the size, solubility, and stability of the pill. It must be chemically and physiologically inactive and preferably should have a stabilizing action on the medicinal substance.

Excipients may be classified in various ways. They may be divided into *adhesive* (liquid glucose, syrup, honey, and tragacanth and acacia mucilages), *liquid* (water, alcohol and glycerin), *dry* or *absorbent* (powdered glycyrrhiza, acacia, tragacanth, and calcium phosphate), and *oleaginous* or *fatty* excipients (waxes and hydrogenated oils).

Conspergents (dusting powders) are used to prevent the pill mass from sticking to the hands or machine and to prevent the pills from adhering to each other in the container. All excess powder should be removed, and no powder should be visible on the finished pills. Conspergents should not be used on pills to be coated.

The choice of conspergent depends chiefly on the color of the pill, the object being to make the dusting powder as inconspicuous as possible. The most commonly used conspergents are lycopodium, powdered licorice root or extract, magnesium carbonate, powdered althea, flour, and starch.

Manufacturing

Pills are made by hand or by machines. The hand method consists of the following steps: making the mass, dividing the mass, and shaping and finishing.

Hand Method

Making the Mass—In a pill formula containing several dry ingredients uniform distribution can be accomplished readily by means of geometric dilution. If there is only one potent dry substance it should be reduced to a fine powder and diluted with several times its weight of powdered diluent before incorporation with any other ingredients. If potent dry substances are to be mixed with liquid or semiliquid material, the potent drug should be diluted with a dry diluent to ensure even, uniform distribution.

If a liquid excipient is required, this is added little by little, and the material is kneaded with the pestle. The liquid excipient must be added very gradually unless the exact amount required is known. The beginner usually adds too much and the mass becomes too soft. It is better—particularly if the excipient is a thick, viscid substance such as glucose—to transfer the excipient to the head (not the side) of the pestle to facilitate handling.

Much more effort and pressure are required to form a pill mass than to triturate dry powders. The necessary pressure may be exerted with a minimum of effort by using the pestle as a lever and the side of the mortar as a fulcrum. By holding the pestle so that the end rests on the fleshy part of the hand near the wrist, and by exerting a twisting motion, the mass can be worked easily and rapidly. It is necessary to scrape the material from the side and bottom of the mortar from time to time, using a heavy pill spatula. As the massing progresses, as shown by the tendency of the mass to peel from the sides of the mortar, some pharmacists prefer to complete the process by kneading the mass with the fingers and hands.

Dividing the Mass—The mass is removed from the mortar as completely as possible and rolled in the hands into the form of a rough cylinder. The warmth of the hands and the heat generated by massing and rolling aids in forming the mass and keeping it in proper condition.

Using a broad spatula or a flat board fitted with a handle, the short cylinder is rolled into a long, thin cylinder (usually called a *pipe*). The cylinder is rolled until it has a uniform diameter, approximately that of the finished pill, or until its length corresponds to the number of divisions of the scale on the pill tile.

Care must be exercised constantly so that the diameter is uniform and the pipe does not become hollow. The pipe is placed on the division lines of the pill tile, dusted lightly with conspergent, scored, and cut into the desired number of segments. The tip of a thin spatula may be used for this purpose, but a sharp cutting edge such as a single-edge razor blade is preferred. The blade must be held at right angles to the pipe and each segment cut the same size.

Shaping and Finishing—The segments cut from the pipe are rolled with the fingers into approximately globular form, care being taken that the edges formed during cutting are pressed into the pills. Shaping is especially important when alcohol is used as an excipient since alcohol evaporates rapidly and the pills become brittle and less plastic.

The pills may be rolled individually in the palm of one hand with the fingers of the other hand. The rounding of the pills is completed under a pill finisher (a boxwood having a round shape), using light pressure at the beginning, increasing the pressure, and finally finishing with light pressure. If a pill finisher is not at hand, the top of a large pill or powder box may be used, or the pills may be finished by rolling between the palms of the hands. The pills should remain exposed to the air for a few minutes to aid in hardening the surface, to prevent sticking, and to aid in retaining their shape. They may be dusted, with all excess powder removed, unless they are to be coated.

Pill Machines

Although many machines and devices have been used to make pills extemporaneously, only one is in use today. It is used for lots of a few dozen to a few thousand pills, after the pill mass has been made by machine or hand. It consists of two parts, an upper and lower plate with grooves and knife edges which correspond exactly when superimposed. The pill pipe is placed on the lower plate, dusted lightly with dusting powder, and the upper cutter placed lightly upon it. The upper cutter is moved backward and forward several times with increasing pressure, cutting the pipe into pills and rolling the segments into globular form within the tubes formed by the matching grooves. The main disadvantage is its inflexibility; a machine will make only one size pill and it is necessary to have several machines on hand to meet all contingencies. If the volume of the pill is less than that made by the pill machine, its volume may be increased by the addition of a suitable diluent.

For the commercial manufacture of pills, elaborate machines have been devised. The mass is prepared in a machine such as the double worm mixer which requires about 1 hour to prepare a suitable mass. This mass must have the property of remaining plastic for several days as it may take this time to complete the rolling of the pills. The prepared mass is placed in the hopper of one section of the pill machine which forms the mass into cylinders by pressing it through a round orifice by means of a worm drive.

As the cylinder is ejected, it is cut into short pieces by a mechanical knife, sprinkled with dusting powder, rolled into a ball by passing between two revolving and oscillating belts, and transferred by a conveyer to the second section of the machine. The balls are formed into pipes by passing between belts moving in opposite directions, and the pipes are cut into roughly shaped pills by passing between two rollers which have grooves and knife edges. The pills are rounded by passing between revolving and oscillating belts and are passed through perforated troughs which reject the oversized and undersized pills.

Dispensing

Pills prepared extemporaneously should be dispensed in pill or powder boxes to allow them to dry thoroughly. All excess dusting powder should be removed before the pills are placed in the box. If the surface of the pills is dry and firm, cotton may be placed in the bottom of the container to prevent rattling.

As with tablets, manufactured pills should not be counted in the hand. To prevent contamination and the loss of the gloss coating they should be poured onto a tablet counting tray or a piece of paper. They should be dispensed in glass or plastic capsule vials. Cotton may be placed in the bottom of the vial or on top of the pills to prevent rattling and breaking of the coating.

Typical Prescriptions

21

R	Ferrous Sulfate, exsiccated	60.0 mg.
	Aloe extract	60.0 mg.

	Apiol	0.06 ml.
	Oil of Savin	0.06 ml.

M ft. pil D.T.D. # 24.
Sig: One t.i.d.

22

R	Pulv. digitalis	gr x
	Pulv. colchicum sem.	gr xx
	Sod. bicarb.	gr xxx

M ft. pil # 20
Sig: One b.i.d.

23

R	Ferr. reducti	gr ii
	Quin. bisulf	gr iss
	Strych. sulf	gr 1/100

M and Ft. Pil D.T.D. No. 100
Sig: One b.i.d.

24

R	Aloin	0.013 g
	Strychnine	0.0005 g
	Belladonna ext.	0.008 g
	Cas. Sag. ext.	0.0325 g

M ft. pil D.T.D. # 24
Sig: Ut dict.

25

R	Aloe	0.13 g
	Myrrh	0.065 g

M ft. pil D.T.D. # 30
Sig: One b.i.d.

Coating

There are four types of tablet and pill coating: sugar coating, film coating, compression coating, and air suspension.

Sugar Coating

Probably the most commonly used coating for tablets on a commercial scale is a sugar coating in which successive thin layers of the coating material are applied to the tablets as they rotate and tumble in the coating pan. Coating pans (Fig. 7) are available in various sizes and shapes but are essentially spherical vessels, usually made of copper or stainless steel and are mounted on the end of a shaft so that they may be made to rotate. Polishing pans frequently are coating pans that have been lined with canvas, or they may be canvas drums. Since the sugar coating of tablets is accomplished by adding the coating material in solution or suspension form, coating pans are equipped with air blowers to force hot or cold air through the pans to facilitate drying. Exhaust ducts are used to remove moisture and dust from the pans. Although this pocess is in common use, it possesses a number of disadvantages: it is time-consuming, plus the coating may promote the growth of microorganisms, cracks readily on exposure to temperature, and may absorb atmospheric moisture (causing an increase in the tablet weight).

Tablets which are to be coated are

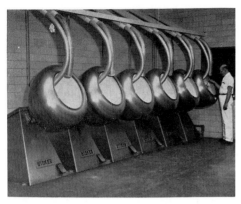

Fig. 7—Stokes' tablet coating pans (courtesy, *Ciba*).

made with convex surfaces approaching a spherical shape since flat tablets are difficult to coat. Dust and broken tablets should be removed before tablets are placed in the coating pan.

The usual stages of coating consist of

1. Waterproofing to prevent penetration of moisture into the tablet.
2. Subcoating to fill out and build up the tablets.
3. Smooth coating to produce a hard smooth surface.
4. Coloring and finishing to obtain the desired color.
5. Polishing to give the finished product a high gloss.

Dusting and Waterproofing—Excessive dust should be removed before sealing. This is achieved by placing the tablets in a rotating coating pan under a directed current of air. Since the vehicle for sugar coating is water, most tablets require an initial sealing coat to prevent moisture from penetrating the tablet and destroying its ingredients. This is accomplished by applying one or two coats of arsenic-free shellac, cellulose derivatives such as ethylcellulose, or silicones. Waterproofing materials must be applied sparingly since excess material may retard disintegration time of the coating and even result in an unwanted enteric coating.

Subcoating—As the tablets rotate in the coating pan, a heavy syrup usually containing acacia and sugar in water is added. The tablets should tumble freely in the pan until they become sticky. A dusting powder consisting of starch and powdered sugar is then applied and rotation of the pan is continued until the tablets have dried. Precipitated chalk, powdered acacia, or talc may also be added to the subcoating powder. The process of adding the solution and powder is repeated until the edges of the tablets are sufficiently covered and rounded.

Smoothing—Following subcoating, a heavy sugar syrup is added to the rotating tablets. The smoothing syrup is added slowly to moisten the tablets and warm air is used to hasten drying. A dusting powder may or may not be used in conjunction with the syrup. A sufficient number of coats are applied to give a smooth surface and to build the tablets to a specific size.

Coloring—To avoid a mottled appearance, color is built up gradually with diluted colored syrups; these are made by dissolving certified water-soluble dyes in syrup and then several different dilutions of color are made by adding plain syrup to the colored syrup. Several coats of the lightest colored syrups are applied, followed by several coats of the next dilution. The other dilutions are added in order, with the undiluted colored syrups being applied last. Drying is necessary between each coat and it is customary to dry the last coat very slowly by manually turning the pan every few minutes to prevent the tablets from sticking together and to promote slow drying.

Polishing—After the coloring coats have been applied, the coated tablets are polished by rotating them in the polishing pan with the addition of a solution of the wax in a volatile solvent. Beeswax, carnauba wax, or chlorinated waxes are among the most commonly used waxes.

Since in the standard sugar-coating procedure much time is spent in sealing, rounding, and smoothing the tablet and overcoming the white background during the coloring phase, a revised procedure has been advanced. An undercoating adhesive suspension consisting essentially of acacia, gelatin, sucrose, and water is mixed with a stock coating formulation of dioctyl sodium sulfosuccinate, insoluble coloring material, titanium dioxide, and syrup. This undercoating suspension is applied to the rotating tablets and followed by dusting the tablets with powdered acacia. The procedure is repeated once. The tablets are then sealed with one coat of a material such as shellac and are finished by applying approximately 25 coats of the stock coating formulation diluted with coating syrup. The tablets are then polished in the usual fashion. With this procedure, colored coatings can be applied to the subcoating and the application of smoothing coats is eliminated.

Film Coating

A more recent coating method employs a soluble polymeric film to coat tablets. Thin coats, or films, are sufficient and since subcoating and smooth coatings are unnecessary, coating time is quite rapid. Coating materials may be applied to the tablets as a solution in volatile, anhydrous vehicles and waterproofing prior to coating is unnecessary. Tablets retain their original shape and essentially their original size. The films may be colored with soluble dyes or rendered opaque with pigments or materials such as titanium dioxide.

The materials used for film coating are cellulosic high polymers such as sodium carboxymethylcellulose, Carbowax 6000, and a combination of carboxymethylcellulose and Carbowax 6000. Film coating employs coating pans, such as those used for sugar coating, and the tablets are tumbled in the pan and the solution of the coating material is added to the tablets. The solution may be poured or sprayed onto the tumbling tablets.

Compression Coating

Compression coating is also referred to as "dry coating" since the coating (in the form of a fine granulation) is compressed around the tablet by punches. This method may be utilized when

water, as in the sugar-coating operation, causes decomposition or degradation of the tablet ingredients. Incompatible materials may also be combined by placing one material compressed on the core and second coat containing the other incompatible material may be compressed on the core and first coat. Repeat-action or sustained-action tablets may be produced by coating the core tablet with an appropriate material.

Compression coating may be applied by feeding previously compressed core tablets into the dies of a specially designed tablet press used as a coating machine. Each die has previously received a measured amount of the coating material, the core tablet is fed onto this and another measured amount of coating material is fed into the die. The tablet is then compressed between the punches of the press. Compression coating may also be produced by coupling two or three tablet presses together so that the first press produces the core tablet and transfers it to the second press which presses the coating material on the tablet. The coated tablet may then be transferred to a third press for the application of the second coating.

Air Suspension

A rapid method of coating drug particles of various sizes and shapes has been developed. The process consists of supporting particles or tablets in a vertical column with an upwardly moving airstream during which time the coating solution is sprayed onto the suspended particles. The coating chamber consists of a vertical column constricted at the bottom and expanded at the top. Air velocity in the constricted area is sufficiently strong so that tablets entering this area are propelled upwards. In the upper, or expanded area, the air velocity is greatly decreased so that the velocity will not support the tablets and they fall to the bottom of the chamber.

This process may be used to apply various types of coating materials such as suspensions of insoluble materials in coating solutions as well as film-type coating materials dissolved in volatile solvents. It is not readily adaptable to the typical sugar coating. Coating time with air suspension is very rapid and batch uniformity is readily achieved.

Enteric Coating

Dosage forms such as tablets that are to be enteric-coated are processed in a manner depending on the material to be used. The general process for tablets includes waterproofing the tablet by coating with shellac in a coating pan and then adding the enteric-coating material to the rotating tablets to build up the coat. A sugar coating may be applied over the enteric coating. Some coating materials may be applied by other methods such as spraying the coating material on the tablets or by air suspension.

Among the materials used in enteric coating are shellac, cellulose acetate phthalate, lipids, and synthetic resins.

Shellac—This resinous material is soluble in aqueous solutions which are alkaline but not in those which are neutral or acid. An alcoholic solution of arsenic-free shellac may be sprayed on tablets or capsules in a coating pan and the solvent evaporated by means of a current of air. Ammoniated shellac, as well as combinations of shellac with other coating substances, gives effective coatings. Shellac is also used to waterproof tablets prior to sugar-coating to prevent moisture in the syrups from reacting with the tablet and when used for this purpose, care must be exercised to avoid forming an enteric coating on the tablets.

Cellulose Acetate Phthalate—This coating material has been found to have considerable merit as an enteric coating and is used commercially for this purpose. It disintegrates due to the hydrolytic effect of intestinal esterases, even when the intestinal contents are acid. It has been found to withstand the action of artificial gastric juice for a long period of time but will readily disintegrate in intestinal juice.

Cellulose acetate phthalate is applied to tablets as a solution in volatile organic solvents such as ethyl acetate-3A denatured alcohol solution. Tablets that have been coated with this material may be sealed with a coating of wax to improve water impermeability. Cellulose acetate phthalate when combined with polyethylene glycol has also been used as a water-soluble film coating. The use of starch and amylose acetate phthalate as an enteric-coating material has also been reported.

Lipids—These have been combined with other ingredients to give favorable enteric coatings. One such combination is a mixture of myristic acid, hydrogenated castor oil, castor oil, cholesterol, and sodium taurocholate. The mixture is dissolved in ethylene dichloride, benzene, and absolute ethyl alcohol for application. Coating mixtures containing lipids such as waxes or hydrogenated oils in combination with fillers may be granulated and applied to core tablets by compression coating.

Synthetic Resins—Resins have been applied as enteric coatings on a commercial basis and in general are applied as a solution in volatile solvents. Among the resins that have been proposed as ingredients in various coating formulations are polyvinyl acetate phthalate, phenolic anhydride, styrene-maleic acid copolymers, and poly (methylvinyl ether)/maleic anhydride.

Extemporaneous Methods—While the coating of dosage forms such as tablets is a process best performed by manufacturing companies, it is possible for the pharmacist to coat these dosage forms extemporaneously if the proper materials and methods are used.

Some traditional methods, such as the use of phenyl salicylate (salol) or the dipping of capsules into formaldehyde solution for the extemporaneous enteric-coating of capsules, have fallen into disfavor because of the unreliability of the coatings.

For a convenient and satisfactory extemporaneous enteric coating for tablets, capsules, or pills, the following process may be used. A mixture composed of *n*-butyl stearate (45 parts), carnauba wax (30 parts), and stearic acid (25 parts), is heated on a water bath to 75°C. The tablet, pill, or capsule is held at one end with tweezers and dipped into the liquid. As the object is withdrawn, the coating solidifies rapidly. After the coating of each of the capsules, or other dosage form, in this manner, the uncoated end is dipped in the melted mixture to a depth that will give an overlap of the coating material over the previously coated end. Two coats are sufficient.

Another extemporaneous method for enteric-coating of capsules utilizes polyvinyl acetate polymers. The recommended formula is:

Vinac ASB-10 or	
Gelva C-3	10–12%
Castor oil	10% *v*/*v*
Acetone	80–78% *v*/*v*

Approximately 2 ml of the coating solution/25 capsules is added to the capsules in a 400–600 ml beaker which is then swirled until the capsules are coated and become tacky. A second 2-ml portion of the coating solution is added and swirling of the beaker is repeated. The procedure is repeated until 8–10 coats have been applied. The capsules are then tossed onto gauze or a towel and allowed to air dry for 8–12 hours or overnight. This technique produced capsules which withstand immersion in simulated gastric fluid TS for 3 hours and dissolve in simulated intestinal fluid TS in less than 1 hour.

Testing and Evaluation

Coated dosage forms may be tested by *in vitro* and *in vivo* methods for both disintegration and dissolution rates. With the present emphasis on the physiological availability of drugs from dosage forms, it is necessary to determine the effect of a coating on the release of a drug by both *in vitro* and *in vivo* methods.

Particularly with enteric and timed-release coatings, there is some disagreement among various investigators as to the relative value of different types of coating materials. Much of the disagreement is due to variations in the coating materials, the methods of application, and to the dissimilarity of techniques used to determine the efficiency of the coatings. Physiological factors such as stomach emptying time and absorptive sites of the gastrointestinal tract also contribute to disagreements in the evaluation of enteric coatings.

To insure batch uniformity in control procedures, *in vitro* methods may be used to determine disintegration and dissolution rates and automated methods for prolonged determination of dissolution rates have been devised which may be adapted for this purpose.

Determination of the efficiency of coatings by *in vitro* tests involves the use of simulated digestive fluids. An official test for plain-coated and enteric-coated tablets has been discussed earlier in this chapter.

The USP also provides a procedure for the determination of dissolution rates for tablets and capsules. Various methods, similar in nature to the USP method, have been devised to measure dissolution of drugs from coated tablets and capsules which in turn permit the evaluation of the specific coating materials. In general, the various methods have modifications in the dissolution medium and in the extent and type of agitation.

Since barium sulfate is opaque to x-rays, it may be used in experimental enteric-coated products so that the behavior of the product in the gastrointestinal tract may be determined by roentgenoscopy or roentgenography. At various time intervals the position and condition of the enteric-coated product may be determined with disintegration being indicated by a scattering of the barium sulfate. This procedure is quite suitable for comparative testing of different enteric coating materials.

In vitro disintegration tests are suitable for comparative evaluation of coating materials but further *in vivo* tests must be conducted to determine the influence of the coating on the absorption or physiological availability of the drug. This testing includes such methods as the measurement of the concentration of a drug in the blood at periodic time intervals or the measurement of urinary excretion of a drug.

Bibliography

Banker GS: In Dittert LW, ed: *Sprowls' American Pharmacy,* 7th ed, Lippincott, Philadelphia, 345, 1975.

King RE: In *Remington's Pharmaceutical Sciences,* 15th ed, Mack Publ. Co., Easton, PA, 1576, 1975.

The United States Pharmacopeia, 19th rev., Mack Publ. Co., Easton, PA, 704, 1975.

The National Formulary, 14th ed, Mack Publ. Co., Easton, PA, 937, 939, 1975.

Becker BA, Swift JG: *Toxicol Appl Pharmacol 1 (1):* 42, 1959.

Wurster DE: *JAPhA Sci Ed 48:* 451, 1959.

Cook CH, Webber MF: *Am J Hosp Pharm 22:* 95, 1965.

Gross HM, Endicott CJ: *Drug Cos Ind 86:* 170, 1960.

Swintosky JV: *Ibid 87:* 464, 1960.

Morrison AB, Campbell JA: *J Pharm Sci 54:* 1, 1965.

Lazarus J, Cooper J: *Ibid 50:* 715, 1961.

Seidler WMK, Rowe EJ: *Ibid 57:* 1007, 1968.

6

Dermatologicals

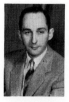

Frederick P. Siegel, PhD
Professor of Pharmacy
College of Pharmacy
University of Illinois at the
Medical Center
Chicago, IL 60680

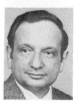

Bernard Ecanow, PhD
Professor of Pharmacy
College of Pharmacy
University of Illinois at the
Medical Center
Chicago, IL 60680

Dermatologicals are dosage forms that are applied to the skin for therapeutic or protective functions. In addition, they may be designed to provide a cosmetic function, e.g., to mask the unsightliness of various skin afflictions.

Classification According to Physicochemical Characteristics

Dermatologicals may be classified as liquid, solid, semisolid, or aerosol preparations.

Liquid Dermatologicals

From a physicochemical standpoint, liquid dermatologicals are identical with any other liquid dosage form, in that they may exist as solutions, suspensions, colloidal dispersions, etc. of therapeutic and supplementary ingredients in aqueous, hydroalcoholic, or nonaqueous (usually oily) vehicles. The fact that these liquids are applied externally, however, permits a somewhat larger selection of vehicles. For example, vehicles such as propylene glycol, polyethylene glycols, butylene glycol, isopropyl alcohol, anhydrous ethanol, acetone, ethyl ether, isopropyl myristate, and isopropyl palmitate have been employed in dermatological products.

The classical definition of a lotion focuses on aqueous preparations containing insoluble materials which are applied to the skin without friction. Calamine lotion and White lotion illustrate this definition. However, many of these classical products represented the technology of their era, and accordingly, in the light of modern advancements, they often represent something less than acceptable formulations from both therapeutic and esthetic standpoints.

The innovation of newer additives and suspending agents that produce more nearly ideal viscosities has yielded lotions in the form of suspensions that are more permanent, more stable, easier to manufacture, and more cosmetic in appearance than the older ones. Replacement of the natural gums (Acacia USP and Tragacanth USP) and the natural clay (Bentonite USP) with su-

147

perior viscosity additives, plus the use of emulsions to provide the body of the lotion, has yielded more ideal products. These viscosity additives include Methylcellulose USP and its derivatives Carboxymethylcellulose USP and Hydroxypropyl Methylcellulose USP; the Carbopols represented by Carbomer NF, Alginic Acid NF, and Sodium Alginate NF; Xanthan Gum NF represented by Keltrol, Microcrystalline Cellulose NF, and the combination product Microcrystalline Cellulose and Sodium Carboxymethylcellulose NF; fumed silica official as Colloidal Silicon Dioxide NF; and the series of Veegums. See Chapter 8.

The term lotion has been expanded in meaning, as is evident upon inspection of a number of proprietary lotions. Today, from a commercial sense, "lotion" includes any liquid dermatological. Products are referred to as lotions whether they are classical suspensions, emulsions, combination emulsion-suspensions, or aqueous or nonaqueous solutions. A clear hydroalcoholic system may be used as a cleansing lotion

Table 1—Official Lotions

	Type
Benzoyl Peroxide Lotion USP	Suspension or suspension in O/W emulsion
Benzyl Benzoate Lotion NF	Emulsion
Betamethasone Valerate Lotion NF	Suspension
Calamine Lotion USP and Phenolated Calamine Lotion USP	Suspension
Dimethisoquin Hydrochloride Lotion NF	Solution in O/W emulsion
Gamma Benzene Hexachloride Lotion USP	Suspension in O/W emulsion
Hexachlorophene Detergent Lotion USP	Micellar solubilized in O/W emulsion
Hydrocortisone Lotion USP	Suspension in O/W emulsion
Monobenzone Lotion NF	Suspension in O/W lotion
Selenium Sulfide Lotion USP	Suspension
White Lotion NF	Suspension

(Bonne Bell cleansing lotion) or a clear hydroalcoholic system or creamy lotion as a sunscreen (Sundare Lotions). Pre-Sun lotion is a hydroalcoholic solution of the sunscreen, PABA. Baker's P & S Liquid is an unusual lotion in that it consists of two separate phases—a mineral oil and an aqueous phase. Medicated shampoos such as zinc omadine liquid shampoos, selenium sulfide liquid shampoos, and medicated skin cleansers such as pHisoHex may be regarded as lotions although their resident time on the skin and scalp is transient.

Nonaqueous Systems

Most liquid dermatologicals are aqueous or hydroalcoholic systems with just sufficient ethyl alcohol to permit solubilization of the component(s) and/ or to hasten the evaporation of the solvent from the skin surface. Where solubility or stability preclude the use of aqueous or low alcohol containing aqueous systems or, on occasion, where more rapid permeation of the epidermis is required, then the pharmacist may have to resort to higher alcohol containing aqueous systems or totally nonaqueous systems. Some of the more common vehicles in this latter category are absolute alcohol and isopropyl alcohol, the glycols—glycerin, propylene glycol, and the liquid polyethylene glycols. PEG 400 is the most widely used liquid polyethylene glycol, however, PEG 300 and 600 are sometimes used. They are all three official products. Admixtures of alcohols or glycols or combinations of alcohols plus glycols are finding greater use currently. Oils such as light liquid petrolatum, isopropyl myristate, diethyl sebacate, and other synthetic esters are used. Acetone has been used to hasten evaporation of tinctures (Merthiolate, Zephiran) and on rare occasion chloroform is used as a solvent (anthralin, chrysarobin). In some cases the active ingredients, without solvents, have been used as nonaqueous dermatologicals. The counterirritants such as methyl salicylate lotions (liniments) best illustrate this.

Table 2—Some Currently Prescribed
Nonaqueous Dermatologicals

R product	Vehicle
Cantharidin collodion	Ether-ethanol
Salicylic acid collodion	Ether-ethanol
Glycerite of peroxide	Glycerin
Auralgan	Glycerin
Thimerosal glycerite	Glycerin
Tannic acid glycerite	Glycerin
Methoxsalen solution	Propylene glycol
Fluocinolone acetonide topical solution	Propylene glycol
Fluorouracil 1% solution	Propylene glycol
Tretinoin	PEG 400-ethanol
Tolnaftate 1% solution	PEG 400
Cuprex	Tetrahydronaph- thalene, acetone, mineral oil
Chrysarobin 5%	Chloroform
Podophyllum resin 25%	liquid petrolatum
Haloprogin topical solution	Diethyl sebacate- ethanol

Collodions are uniquely different nonaqueous dermatologicals. They are usually solutions of drugs (rarely a suspension) in flexible collodion. On application to the skin, in a thin layer, it leaves a transparent, tenacious, plasticized film of pyroxylin. Collodions are usually employed to provide a sustained source of a keratolytic agent such as salicylic acid (Salicylic Acid Collodion USP) as in the treatment of corns and warts. Cantharone is a cantharidin collodion intended for the removal of benign epithelial growths.

Table 2 lists some examples of current items used in prescription practice.

Solid Dermatologicals

Solid dosage forms used as dermatological agents include tablets and powders intended for the preparation of solutions, as illustrated by Domeboro tablets and powder packets. Solutions prepared from these dosage forms are employed as wet dressings and soaks. Potassium permanganate tablets and mercuric chloride tablets may be employed similarly. Dusting powders are usually employed to couple the therapeutic ef-

fect of the active ingredient, e.g., zinc undecylenate in Desenex powder, with the moisture absorbing effect of the powdered vehicle designed to keep the skin surface dry. Adsorbent powders such as kaolin, talc, zinc oxide, and zinc stearate have been used.

Powders are contraindicated in weeping dermatoses where the possibility of encrustation may lead to a secondary infection.

Semisolid Dermatologicals

Semisolid dosage forms, unlike liquid and solid forms, are nearly all dermatologicals. These dosage forms include the classical ointments, pastes, creams, and other preparations seldom prescribed such as cerates and poultices.

As with many dosage forms which have been developed largely as an art, these semisolid dermatologicals have never been rigorously defined. Hence it is quite difficult to distinguish between even the classical dosage forms. What distinguishes an ointment from a cream? The classical ointment base, rose water ointment, is commonly referred to as a cream (cold cream).

Important considerations in the formulation of a dermatological preparation are degree of stiffness, ease of flow, and adhesiveness upon application to the skin. Since flow properties significantly differentiate between the various dermatological dosage forms, their rheology can supply the basis for meaningful definitions.

A *lotion*, therefore, in rheological terminology, is a fluid preparation showing essentially Newtonian flow characteristics. When applied to the skin, it offers no resistance (yield value) and it flows under the force of gravity.

A *cream* is a semisolid preparation showing essentially pseudoplastic flow properties. When applied, creams have very little yield value but will not flow under the influence of gravity. However, a small additional amount of force will readily produce flow. As the cream is rubbed onto the skin, the ease of flow increases and it can approach the flow of a lotion. As rubbing ceases so does the flow.

An *ointment* is a semisolid preparation which shows plastic flow characteristics. When the ointment is applied, there is a definite yield value and the resistance to flow drops as the application to the skin is continued.

A *paste* is a semisolid dermatological which shows essentially dilatant flow. When applied, the paste possesses a definite yield value and resistance to the flow increases with increased force of application. Pastes are usually prepared by adding significant amounts of insoluble powders (usually 20% or higher) to conventional ointment bases so as to alter the plastic flow of the ointment to yield a dilatant flow.

Cerates are semisolid preparations containing a relatively high wax content, whose yield point is too great to permit it to be applied directly to the skin. It is usually spread on material with a cloth backing before use.

Plasters are solid preparations which cannot be spread at room temperature. They are prepared by melting the mass and spreading the melt upon a material backing.

Cataplasms or *poultices* are defined as wet masses of solid matter applied to the skin in order to reduce inflammation and in some cases to act as a counterirritant. Historically the poultices have been composed of either clays such as kaolin or flaxseed.

Thus the desired properties of structure and flow are indicated by choice of the dosage form—lotion, cream, ointment, etc. The specific effect desired upon the skin can be obtained by selection of the appropriate physicochemical structure of the dosage form. Hence, an ointment with a gel, an emulsion or a suspension structure may be selected. This discussion permits a more systematic classification of the wide variety of dosage forms whose physical properties are similar even though their physicochemical structures are completely different. Classification of the finished product on the basis of flow properties

is readily accomplished by the normal procedures of application and does not require analysis, as does classification by means of the physicochemical system (emulsions, suspensions, solutions, etc.) or the chemical structure (aliphatic alcohols, glycerides, waxes, etc.).

The importance of these considerations to proper practice is indicated by a typical complaint made that a desired prescription was obtained as a lotion instead of a higher viscosity cream.

Dermatological Aerosols

With the advent of aerosol packaging, dermatological products are becoming more popular in this form. The nature of the basic dosage form is similar to all of the dermatological dosage variations considered in this chapter. Aerosol packaging, however, provides a more novel and a more nearly ideal method of providing a single dose of medication at the desired site of application.

Several fundamental delivery systems may be utilized in an aerosol. The first is a spray of either a solution or suspension of medicament. The second is a foamed product, either a quick-breaking foam or a foam of the shaving cream type. The third is a semisolid dermatological which is delivered from an accordion bag liner inside an aerosol can where the propellant and dermatological are isolated and not in intimate contact as in the first two systems. The advent of a twin valve system using a bag within a bag permits isolation of the ingredients until just prior to activating the button. This holds potential for incompatible systems, which theoretically could be mixed just before administration of a single dose. A review of aerosol systems (see Chapter 11) recalls their limits in terms of the stability of active ingredients in the presence of the usual solvents and propellants and interactions between the dosage form and its container. The major point to stress is that the dosage forms that go into the aerosol container are the dermatological dosage forms that are discussed throughout this chapter.

Medicated Tapes

Recently there has been introduced a surgical tape in which the active ingredient is distributed in the adhesive components of the tape. The intent is to provide a convenient dosage form where the therapeutic activity is enhanced by the water impervious tape which in turn increases skin hydration and medicament absorption. Cordran (*Dista*) is illustrative of this category. Their expense and inapplicability to moist lesions and intertriginous areas, coupled with the fact that all advantages of the product can be built into a dermatologic base, limits their utility.

Classification According to Aqueous Content of the Base

The classical method for classifying dermatological bases emphasizes the degree of supposed skin penetrating ability. *Epidermatic* bases possess no skin penetrating properties. *Endodermatic* bases have the power to penetrate into the layers of the epidermis. *Diadermatic* bases have the greatest skin penetrating ability. They ultimately reach the dermis, and apparently facilitate absorption of therapeutic ingredients into the circulatory system. Unfortunately, very little literature linking bases to the extent of penetration is available and much confusion in regard to the properties of bases and their relationship to the active ingredient exists.

A more current, practical classification is based on the relationship of water to the composition of the dermatological base. This leads to the following classification:

Oleaginous Bases—These are insoluble in water and hence not water washable nor can they absorb or contain water.

Absorption Bases—These are insoluble in water and not water washable. Although they are essentially anhydrous systems these bases can absorb water.

Emulsion Bases—These are subdivided on the basis of emulsion type. W/O emulsion bases are insoluble in water but contain water in the internal phase and they may absorb water. They are not water washable. O/W emulsion bases are insoluble in water but contain water in the external phase. They absorb water and are water washable.

Water-Soluble Bases—These are water soluble and water washable. They may be essentially anhydrous or they may contain water. In either case they absorb water to the point of solubility.

Oleaginous Bases

These bases consist of water-insoluble, hydrophobic oils and fats. The most important group comprises the hydrocarbons—the mineral oils, the petrolatums, and the paraffins. Combinations of these materials can produce a wide range of melting points and viscosities. Mineral oil can be gelled with colloidal silica to form transparent gels. Plastibase utilizes polyethylene as the gelling agent for mineral oil. Animal and vegetable lipids are used to some extent and they include almond oil, castor oil, cottonseed oil, olive oil, peanut oil, persic oil, soybean oil, and wool fat (lanolin). Some exotic oils such as mink oil, turtle oil, and avocado oil have also been used in cosmetic products. All of these oils contain glycerides which are subject to rancidification through double bond oxidation of the unsaturated fatty acid moiety. In addition, these natural glycerides and wool fat (a mixture of esters and polyesters of aliphatic, steroid, and triterpenoid alcohols) may possess undesirable, difficult-to-mask odors.

A number of synthetic esters have been employed as oleaginous constituents. They include glyceryl monostearate, isopropyl myristate, isopropyl palmitate, isopropyl lanolate (esters of the mixed lanolin derived fatty acids), butyl stearate, and butyl palmitate. Many vegetable oils can be gelled with aluminum stearate or the Bentones. A number of longer chain alcohols such as cetyl alcohol, stearyl alcohol, and the polyalkylene glycols (Ucons) may be used as part of the hydrophobic system.

Several lanolin derivatives have found their way into common usage in dermatologicals and cosmetics, e.g., an oily dewaxed fraction of lanolin referred to as lanolin oil (Lantrol) and a hydrogenated lanolin. Lanolin oil has been used as an emollient in antipruritic bath oils (Alpha-Keri).

A number of the oily silicones have also been used as hydrophobic oils particularly in barrier protective products. These hydrophobic materials are essentially epidermatic and are sometimes used singly but usually in combination when it is desired to place an occlusive film on the skin. These occlusive dressings hydrate the epidermis by preventing water loss from the exposed epidermal surface and thus permit the dermal water to penetrate the tough, nonviable keratin layer from beneath. Normal hydrated epidermis is supple and resilient. Emolliency is based on this mechanism of epidermal hydration. Oleaginous bases, unfortunately, because of their oiliness and occlusiveness may lack cosmetic appeal.

White petrolatum is the most commonly prescribed oleaginous base. It should be remembered that most drugs are extremely insoluble in petrolatum.

Absorption or Emulsifiable Bases

These bases are essentially anhydrous systems composed of the hydrophobic ingredients discussed under oleaginous bases. These water-insoluble components are rendered somewhat hydrophilic through the addition of W/O emulsifiers. Hence, the addition of water results in the uptake or "absorption of water" by the base through the mechanism of W/O emulsion formation. The base maintains its semisolidity after the addition of water since the water participates as the internal phase of the emulsion system. As the water content of the internal phase increases the viscosity of the base increases.

The incorporation of water, directly, at room temperature, into an absorption base is rather difficult, messy, and less than quantitative. Prior melting of the base and admixture with hot water at a temperature somewhat above the melting point of the base, followed by vigorous agitation (with a blender) and cooling, permits combination with greater ease. Hydration of the base also can be accomplished by softening the base in a warm mortar and incorporating the aqueous phase, in increments.

Hydrophilic Petrolatum USP is white petrolatum combined with 8% white beeswax, 3% stearyl alcohol, and 3% cholesterol which are added as the W/O emulsifiers. Aquaphor (*Duke*) employs wool wax alcohols to render white petrolatum emulsifiable and Polysorb (*Fougera*) utilizes sorbitan sesquioleate, an Arlacel (Arlacel 83) as the W/O emulsifier. A form of hydrophilic petrolatum was introduced in 1975 as Kessolin (*Armak Co.*) and appears to be superior to the USP base and Aquaphor in its ability to absorb larger quantities of water. It possesses a water number in excess of 800. Anhydrous Lanolin USP is a naturally derived absorption base which tends to be quite sticky, unctuous, somewhat odorous, and color unstable.

The water absorption bases permit the inclusion of water-soluble medicaments through prior solution and uptake of the solution as the internal phase. Since the emulsifiers are nonionic in nature, the bases generally are stable over a broad range of electrolyte concentrations and of pH values. See R's 1 and 2.

1

R	Burows Solution		10 ml
	Aquaphor	q.s. ad	30 g

2

R	Solution of Formaldehyde 2%		30 ml
	Hydrophilic Petrolatum	q.s.	90 g

The use of absorption bases such as hydrophilic petrolatum in their anhydrous form seems to provide no advantage over oleaginous bases such as petrolatum.

pHisoHex, a commercial skin cleanser and surgical scrub containing entsufon and hexachlorophene, represents an unusual use of absorption base. A hydrophilic petrolatum is emulsified in water by surfactants to produce an O/W emulsion. The resulting system provides a creamy emulsion appearance to the product and, presumably, modifies any irritant tendency of the ingredients.

Emulsion Bases

Emulsion bases are classified according to the nature of the emulsion, W/O or O/W. As already indicated, absorption bases upon addition of water yield W/O emulsions. These hydrated absorption bases can therefore be classified as emulsion bases. All W/O bases are not water-washable since the oil is in the external phase.

The classical illustration of the W/O base is cold cream. Cold creams are generally beeswax-borax, W/O systems. They usually contain about 75% of oil phase, of which 20–25% is the oil-soluble, primary emulsifier—beeswax or a combination of beeswax and spermaceti. The borax, on aqueous hydrolysis, affords hydroxyl ions, essential for neutralizing small amounts of free fatty acid present in the wax to yield a sodium soap. While beeswax produces a W/O emulsion, it is unstable *per se*. The presence of a small quantity of sodium soap (an O/W emulsifier) stabilizes the beeswax system. The use of small amounts of O/W emulsifiers to stabilize the less stable emulsion type is common practice. Presently, there are two official cold creams. The only significant difference is that Rose Water Ointment NF uses expressed almond oil while Cold Cream USP (nonscented) employs an equivalent amount of mineral oil. Both cold creams contain 19% water in the internal phase. Cold creams, unlike the absorption bases, are susceptible to emulsion splitting with medicaments that are incompatible with sodium soaps. Acids and insolubilizing cations, for example, cause this emulsion splitting. Under the general information section of the USP and NF, both texts refer to cold cream as a water-absorption base. This is misleading because this W/O system will not tolerate very much water above and beyond its original composition without emulsion breakdown.

Hydrous wool fat (lanolin) is a W/O emulsion containing about 25% water. Its disadvantages are mentioned under wool fat. Unlike cold cream which is incapable of any appreciable further hydration, lanolin is a partially hydrated anhydrous lanolin and is capable of further hydration (water number of about 100–200) and hence can still be considered an absorption base.

W/O emulsion bases, generally, are easier to spread on the skin and are more cosmetically elegant than the oleaginous or absorption bases. They act effectively as occlusive dressings that prevent water loss from the epidermis. Keep in mind that for a given drug there may be significant differences in bioavailability from W/O emulsion bases as contrasted to oleaginous systems.

The second category of emulsion bases comprise the O/W dermatological bases. These are the ones which are most easily spread across the skin surfaces. They tend to vanish into the skin, on continued rubbing, as the result of the relatively higher water content and comparatively lower oil content than those of the oleaginous, absorption, or W/O emulsion bases. These products are generally the most cosmetically elegant of all the different types of dermatological bases because of their creamy appearance and their water washability. They are frequently referred to as creams.

Hydrophilic Ointment USP is a classical example of an O/W base, particularly one with a high concentration of oil phase (50%). Petrolatum and stearyl alcohol represent the oil phase in this product. While hydrophilic ointment only contains 37% water it easily incorporates larger amounts in the external phase and retains its semisolidity (soft cream). Further additions of water can produce lower viscosities and yield O/W lotions.

This principle has been applied in dermatological practice with products such as Cordran cream, a topical steroid cream in an O/W emulsion base consisting of stearic acid, cetyl alcohol, mineral oil, glycerin, water, and polyoxyl 40 stearate as the emulsifier. Dermatologists have prescribed an equal mixture of Cordran cream and water which results in a soft cream practically indistinguishable in viscosity and texture from the original cream. On other occasions, dermatologists have requested the preparation of lotions from the same cream through the addition of several multiples of water.

Interestingly, the emulsifier polyoxyl 40 stearate (Myrj 52) is a polyoxyethylene surfactant. These ethylene oxide type adjuncts should be checked for possible interaction with the medicament. Hydrophilic ointment utilizes sodium lauryl sulfate, one of the most efficient O/W emulsifiers. However, this surfactant has been known to be a skin irritant. The Tweens, Myrjs, and Brijs tend to require larger concentrations of nonionic surfactant for emulsification but they also tend to be nonirritating to the skin.

The formulation given in ℞ 3 represents an elegant, soft, water washable base evolved from triethanolamine stearate, which serves as emulsifier and viscosity additive.

3

℞	Stearic Acid		7
	Cetyl Alcohol		2
	Glycerin		10
	Light Mineral Oil		20
	TEA		2
	D. Water	q.s.	100

The product shown in ℞ 3, when prepared with 50% of these ingredients, provides an elegant, viscid lotion. See ℞ 4.

4

℞	Stearic Acid		3.5
	Cetyl Alcohol		1
	Glycerin		5
	Mineral Oil		10
	TEA		1
	D. Water	q.s.	100

The inclusion of significant amounts of free stearic acid in O/W emulsions results in products referred to as "vanishing creams." In these products, a portion of the stearic acid is converted to a soap emulsifier through the inclusion of a source of hydroxyl ions such as sodium or potassium hydroxide or carbonate, or a neutralizing amine such as triethanolamine. Part of the stearic acid remains unneutralized and is emulsified as part of the internal oil phase by the stearate emulsifier. The product, shortly after manufacture, takes on a metallic or pearlescent luster which has been attributed to the free stearic acid aggregates. Noxzema skin cream illustrates a typical vanishing cream base. The formulation given in ℞ 5 is typical of a vanishing cream base.

5

℞	Stearic Acid		18
	Mineral Oil, Light		2
	Lanolin		0.5
	Arlacel 83		2
	Pot. Hydroxide		0.7
	Sorbitol Soln 70%		3.7
	D. Water	q.s.	100

Humectants are essential for the preparation of vanishing creams and are usually incorporated in most O/W dermatological bases to retard the surface evaporation of the high water containing product. Glycerin, propylene glycol, and 70% sorbitol solution have been used as humectants, usually in concentrations of 2–5%. Excessive amounts of humectant have been used in such products as clay poultices where the pack should remain moist. Excessive use of a humectant in any dermatological base may prevent rapid drying and may withdraw moisture from the skin area, not unlike the role of glycerin in glycerin suppositories.

Self-Emulsifying Waxes—There are several commercial products available which are waxlike in appearance and anhydrous, and which contain a combination of lipid material plus emulsifier in an ideal ratio for the preparation of O/W systems, when blended with other oils and water. Cera Emulsificans BP contains stearyl alcohol, cetyl alcohol, and the sulfated derivatives of these fatty alcohols as the anionic emulsifiers.

Glyceryl monostearate may be purchased as the pure material or in combination with an emulsifier. Several self emulsifying glyceryl monostearates are available as combinations with anionic surfactants such as sodium lauryl sulfate or with nonionic surfactants such as Arlacel 165 and Kessco 636. The nonionic combinations have the advantage of improved compatibility with electrolytes and acids. Thus a Burow's cream prepared from Burow's solution is stable in a system using the nonionic combination. Polawax (*Croda*) is a nonionic ethoxylated stearyl alcohol which performs very well as a general O/W emulsifier for creams and lotions. ℞ 6 illustrates the use of self-emulsifying waxes.

6

℞	Glyceryl Monostearate, S.E.		12
	Stearyl Alcohol		1
	Cetyl Alcohol		1
	Mineral Oil, Light		5
	Glycerin		5
	D. Water	q.s. ad	100

Water-Soluble Bases

This category represents both anhydrous and hydrous dermatological nonemulsion bases which are water-soluble and contain no oil phase.

Polyethylene Glycol Ointment USP represents a blend of water-soluble polymeric glycols (polyethylene glycol 400 and polyethylene glycol 4000) that yield a semisolid base capable of solubilizing water-soluble medicaments and solubilizing (dispersing) certain water-insoluble medicaments. Anhydrous polyethylene glycol bases have been used in preparing enzyme-containing dermatologicals. Biozyme ointment combines proteolytic enzymes in an anhydrous base consisting of PEG 400 and 4000 plus stearyl alcohol.

Tinactin is available as an anhydrous solution of the antifungal ingredient tolnaftate in a liquid polyethylene glycol such as PEG 400. Tinactin cream is an anhydrous system composed of tolnaftate in PEG 400 gelled with a Carbopol, using monoamylamine as the neutralizing agent. Again, as was pointed out in a previous discussion, the formulator must be certain that any ethylene oxide polymer does not interfere by attenuating the activity of the medicament through interaction.

Propylene glycol and propylene glycol–ethanol systems are becoming increasingly popular as dermatological vehicles. Hydroalcoholic systems and propylene glycol–alcohol systems can form clear gels with about 2% of hydroxypropyl methylcellulose.

Hydrous systems may be best described as aqueous systems to which sufficient viscosity additives have been added to provide the base consistency (semisolidity) desired. A lubricating jelly employing tragacanth or one of the synthetic gums such as carboxymethylcellulose illustrates such a simple base.

A colloidal magnesium aluminum silicate known commercially as Veegum is an excellent thickener and suspending agent. Concentrations of about 5% produce fine thixotropic lotions and concentrations of about 10% produce excellent semisolid dermatological bases. Generally, the use of humectant is advisable in these systems.

Combinations of microcrystalline cellulose and carboxymethylcellulose sodium provide useful dermatological bases. Methylcelluloses and their derivatives yield high viscosity aqueous gel-like systems. Unfortunately, where a large amount of the methylcellulose must be employed (as in the low viscosity methylcelluloses) the final base may have the undesirable feature of roll-off when the product is rubbed onto the skin. That is, solid balls of methylcellulose roll off the skin on rubbing, thus giving the appearance of removing dead skin.

The Carbopols, particularly Carbopol 934 and Carbopol 940, are excellent gelling agents for aqueous systems. They provide, weight for weight, the greatest viscosity attributes. The powdered carboxyvinyl polymer is first dispersed in water using high speed agitation. After dissolving or dispersing the other ingredients, hydroxyl ion is added to promote hydration of the polymer. The synthetic polymer is more stable and less susceptible to microbiological influences than most of the other gums. Carbopol 934 can provide transparent aqueous gels while Carbopol 940 produces more transparent hydroalcoholic systems. The tolerance of the Carbopol system to appreciable concentrations of other ingredients can be increased by employing certain organic amines as neutralizers in lieu of inorganic alkalis. These gels tend to liquefy readily on application to the skin.

Water-soluble or "greaseless ointment bases" are nongreasy but afford no protective or emollient characteristics. Their ease in washability make them readily removable by perspiration. Water-soluble bases may in some instances be irritating to inflamed or denuded areas of the skin.

Practical Aspects of Dermatologicals

Perspective concerning the functions of dermatological prescriptions must be gained before they can be skillfully prepared.

Functions

Dermatologicals have three main functions. The first function is to protect injured areas from the environment and thus permit rejuvenation of an injured or diseased area. The second function is to provide skin hydration or emollient effects. This is important in the treatment of dry or chapped skin. The third function is to provide a means of conveying a medicament to the skin for the purpose of inducing a specific topical activity. This function may include provision for absorption through the epidermal barrier (percutaneous absorption). Obviously a dermatological product may be called upon to perform any combination of these functions of acting as a protective, emollient, or dosage form.

In regards to the third function, wherein the base acts as a drug delivery system, both pharmacist and physician ideally should have some qualitative picture of the mission or objective of the dermatological. This assists them in spelling out the properties of a base that will fulfill these objectives.

In regards to the various classes of dermatological bases spanning the extremes of hydrophobic, oleaginous to total aqueous systems, it should be kept in mind that the functionality of a base as defined above can alter with the change in the original base composition once applied to the skin. In particular, as the volatile phase of a base evaporates, such as water, the base characteristics may change. If a simple aqueous solution is applied to the skin, ultimately microcrystals of solute may be the only surface residue. O/W emulsions when spread on the skin will lose their external phase and produce a reversion to a W/O system and finally a film of oil. The drug may be "microencapsulated" by the oil film. It is the ultimate nature of these residual films which will affect function, particularly, drug absorption.

Dermatologicals are quite different in one major respect from most of the other dosage forms. Drug activity of the usual dosage forms may be related quantitatively to a specific dose of drug when all other variables are held constant. In dermatologicals, on the other hand, concentrations of drug in a base must be related to the amount of dose delivered topically or percutaneously. The first consideration is the availability of the drug from its base to the skin. In general, the rate for a drug release process dq/dt, at any given time, as a first approximation, can be expressed as a driving force (ΔF) divided by a resistance (R).

Thus

$$\frac{dq}{dt} = \frac{\Delta F}{R}$$

This equation must be in the form of a differential because as the operation proceeds, the driving force changes and hence the rate changes.

The driving force may be considered to be the difference in concentration between the base containing the drug and the skin, initially containing no drug. But a more useful way to describe this driving force mathematically is to compare the difference in chemical potential of the drug in the base with the chemical potential of the drug on the epidermis. The chemical potential of any molecule is a measure of its tendency to escape from its surrounding environment (phase).

A drug incorporated into a base in which it is difficultly soluble has a strong tendency to come out of solution and therefore it has a high chemical potential in that base. If the drug then diffuses into the skin where it is more soluble, the drug tends to accumulate in that tissue. Hence, the drug has a low chemical potential in the skin.

The resistance to drug diffusion varies with such factors as the viscosity of the base and the nature of the interfacial barriers as the molecule passes from one phase into another. The condition of the skin at the interface between vehicle and skin is of particular importance. The amount of drug that penetrates into the skin is considered to be a function of the pressure and vigor of rubbing, surface area covered, and condition of the skin. The number of pores and sweat glands which empty onto the surface of the skin tend to facilitate passage of drugs to some extent through the epidermal barrier. Drug penetration appears to involve both passive diffusion through the epidermis and conveyance via the skin openings (sweat glands, hair follicles).

In general, drug penetration through normal skin epidermis will depend on the state of hydration of the stratum corneum. The state of hydration includes the quantity of water and the degree of structuring of that water. See Chapter 8.

Normal stratum corneum usually contains approximately 20% water and values of approximately 10% and less results in the characteristic symptoms of "dry skin." Normal stratum corneum maintains an equilibrium between structured, bound water and the more mobile bulk water (Fig. 1). Bulk water is the form of water through which more polar drug species will readily migrate, while the water more firmly structured

will enhance the diffusion of less polar drug species. Agents which break the structured water are called water structure breakers. If these materials are presented to the stratum corneum, they will shift the equilibrium between the water phases to produce more mobile water which is free to diffuse throughout the stratum corneum and ultimately diffuse to the skin surface where it would be subject to evaporation. Incidentally, the moisturizing properties attributed to urea (usually employed at a 10–20% level in O/W bases) could be explained by it's water structure breaking activity. Urea is soluble in both the bulk water and the less-polar, coacervate-structured water. The application of a urea-containing dermatological favors the conversion of structured to bulk water which temporarily hydrates the milieu of the stratum corneum. If the formulation, in addition, provides some barrier properties then the free-to-evaporate bulk water would be held in the stratum corneum and at its surface. This hydration phenomenon has implications not only in the physical moisturizing of skin but in drug absorption from the interface.

Dehydrating solvents such as the alcohols and glycols serve as water-structure breakers as well as solvents for the lipid barrier coat on the epidermal surface. Both phenomena favor loss of water from the stratum corneum and result in skin drying. As bulk water evaporates from the skin surface the phospholipid, and other lipids associated with the epidermis (such as ethyl linoleate), become more concentrated and bind the remaining water into a coacervate structure. The vapor pressure of the bound water becomes less as more structuring occurs and, hence, the drying process is, to some extent, self-limiting. Conversely, as the skin becomes more highly hydrated (as via occlusive barrier bases) the bulk-water phase increases and polar drugs can diffuse through this increased bulk volume. A higher degree of bulk water via skin hydration will generate more of the

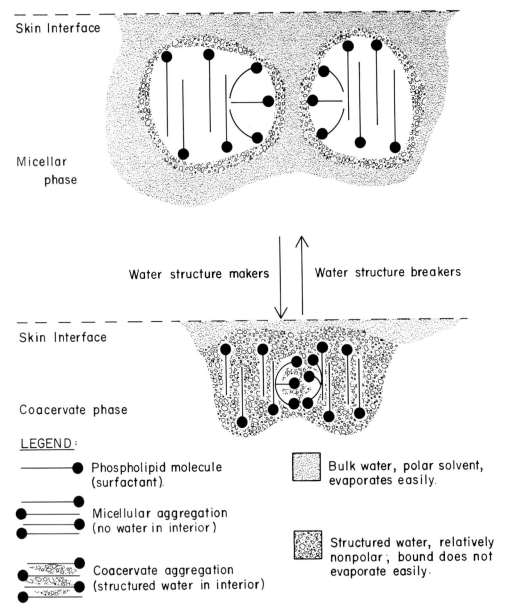

Skin Interface

Micellar
phase

Water structure makers | Water structure breakers

Skin Interface

Coacervate phase

LEGEND:

●————● Phospholipid molecule
(surfactant).

Micellular aggregation
(no water in interior)

Coacervate aggregation
(structured water in interior)

Bulk water, polar solvent,
evaporates easily.

Structured water, relatively
nonpolar; bound does not
evaporate easily.

Fig. 1—Skin tissue in equilibrium between micellar and coacervate phases as conceptualized by Ecanow and Siegel.

phase containing the phospholipid micelles dispersed in bulk water, which will permit nonpolar drug species to be transported readily by solubilization in the micelles and then diffusing through the remaining structured, nonpolar water of the epidermis. Thus a high degree of epidermal hydration has a seemingly paradoxical effect in that it increases the absorption of both water-soluble and insoluble drugs.

Preparation of Dermatological Prescriptions

The preparation of liquid dermatologicals entails the same basic knowledge of solution, emulsification, and suspension technology as any other liquid dosage form. All solids to be suspended should be previously triturated to fine powders. The powders should then be levigated in a mortar with an appropriate liquid to ensure the production of a sufficiently small particle size, prior to incorporation of the insoluble solids to the main bulk of the liquid composition. Increased surface area of the suspended solids provides for a better suspension, a more uniform and adhering protective coat to the epidermal surface and it also provides a more optimum dissolution of the insoluble drugs to insure a bioavailability that will provide therapeutic levels to the affected epidermal and dermal sites. Some solids such as precipitated sulfur and salicylic acid require more vigorous trituration plus levigation or else the microcrystalline aggregates will produce an undesirable gritty product. A small amount of the levigated phase can be gently rubbed on the skin to ascertain whether grit-free comminution has been attained.

Hydrophobic solids such as sulfur may be best levigated with a small amount of surface-tension-reducing aids such as ethyl alcohol, glycerin, or surfactants and then incorporated into the suspending medium.

Occasionally, prescriptions may be received calling for an active ingredient which is not commercially available as the bulk chemical.

The pharmacist may resort to other sources of pure drug such as the sterile powder for intravenous injection. Also, the compounder might select an injectable solution or suspension as the source of drug, assuming the solvent or vehicle (usually water) can be tolerated by the dermatological base. If this is the only source of raw material the dermatological vehicle may have to be altered to accommodate the injectable solution or suspension. Hydrophilic Petrolatum could replace petrolatum, for example, to accommodate an aqueous system. If the pharmacist changes the dermatological base called for on the prescription, he should do so only after weighing all

the implications such as specific use, area of application, and biopharmaceutics. This decision may require communicating with the physician depending on the nature and extent of the change. Other dermatological dosage forms may serve as the source of drug. Thus, 5% ammoniated mercury ointment could serve as the starting point for a 3% ointment. Steroid creams could serve as a source of the steroid for creams and lotions requiring lesser concentrations of the steroid.

Tablets may have to be used as the only source of drug or the physician may, on occasion, call for the use of a commercial tablet as a component of a dermatologic · prescription. Unfortunately, while inert tablet ingredients are not disclosed to the pharmacist, they could provide a compounding problem. Tablets should be crushed and triturated to a fine powder, then levigated (as with any insoluble solid) prior to incorporation. If the tablet bears a coating, it may be carefully removed with a pledget of solvent moistened cotton (water, water-alcohol). The tablet can be dried with absorbent paper and then reduced to a powder.

7

| R̸ Erythromycin Stearate | 500 mg |
| Propylene Glycol q.s. | 60 ml |

R̸ 7, intended for topical application in acne therapy, could be prepared from one 500-mg or two 250-mg erythromycin stearate tablets. The tablet(s) should have their coating removed and be powdered and levigated with the propylene glycol or with a few ml of alcohol. The use of the lactobionate or other water-soluble forms of erythromycin, as found in the powders for IV injection should be discouraged since there is a distinct difference in the biopharmaceutics of the water-soluble forms vs the stearate or free base.

Any liquid dermatological containing either suspended solids or an emulsion should be packaged in a prescription bottle bearing a "Shake Well Before Using" label.

Similarly, understanding the preparation of powders for internal use provides the background needed for preparation of dermatological powders. Dusting powders should be sieved (100-mesh sieve) to assure a grit-free product. These powders should be dispensed in a sifter-top container to facilitate the dusting onto the skin surface. See Chapters 4 and 8.

Since semisolid dosage forms are the types principally used in dermatology, we will emphasize the preparation of prescriptions in semisolid dermatological bases. There are two primary methods for preparing dermatological prescriptions that require extemporaneous compounding.

Incorporation—The first method for the extemporaneous preparation of dermatologicals utilizes incorporation or admixture of the ingredients by levigation on an ointment slab or pad or by trituration in a mortar. This is the most widely employed and generally the most facile method, since most dermatological compounding entails the admixture of several proprietary dermatologicals or the admixture of solids or liquids into a dermatological base.

Stainless steel spatulas with long broad blades that have sufficient flexibility should be used for levigating. In the event that a potential exists for interaction of the metal blade with the materials involved, for example, with elemental iodine and mercuric salts, a hard rubber spatula is available.

The mortar and pestle is preferred when relatively large volumes of liquid must be incorporated. Insoluble substances which are not already in the form of an impalpable powder should be powdered very finely in a mortar. The powder may then be worked in a mortar with a pestle or on a slab or pad with an equal quantity of base until a smooth, grit free concentrate is obtained. The remainder of the base is then added in increments. In order to facilitate levigation of powders into the base, a small portion of melted base may be used to decrease the viscosity of the concentrate or a small amount of a levigating aid such as mineral oil, water, glycerin, etc. may be used to produce a grit free concentrate. The choice of levigating aid must be compatible with the specific nature of the base. Light mineral oil serves well with oleaginous, absorption, or W/O bases, while water or glycerin functions well in O/W and other water-miscible bases.

Water-soluble solids such as salts may be incorporated into the least possible amount of water and the concentrated solution incorporated into the base directly, if compatible, or indirectly by employing sufficient absorption base to take up the water and maintain the solidity of the product.

It is usually inadvisable to use solvents such as ether, alcohol, or chloroform for dissolving crystalline organic medicaments because the drug may tend to crystallize out as the solvent evaporates. The use of solvents as levigating aids is permissible if the solution is permitted to evaporate while the solid is being rubbed into a fine powder (i.e., camphor) prior to incorporation into the base (pulverization by intervention).

In compounding a collodion, the active material may be solubilized by stirring directly into the flexible collodion, as with salicylic acid. If the quantity of salicylic acid approaches 25% or higher, the solution process may be more easily handled by first dispersing the solid in a few ml of a solution of 25% ethyl alcohol in ether and then stirring in the flexible collodion, to the final volume. Cantharidin is not as soluble in the collodion, so it can be dispersed in a few ml of acetone and then adding a sufficient quantity of the flexible collodion.

Collodions are dispensed in containers with a soft brush (similar to those found in nail polishes) or in the more prevalent glass-rod applicator bottles.

Remember if nonaqueous dermatologicals are dispensed in regular prescription containers, their solvency may affect the cap liner. Precoating the protective liner with a layer of petrolatum

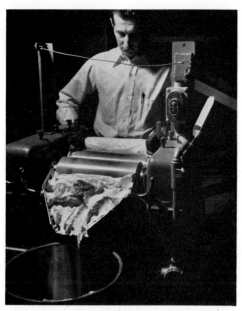

Fig. 2—Operator supervising the preparation of an ointment with an ointment mill (courtesy, *Abbott*).

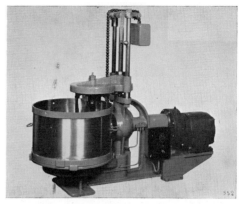

Fig. 3—Motor driven paste mixer (courtesy, *Arthur Colton Co.*).

or paraffin or using aluminum foil as an additional inner liner may be useful.

Fusion—The second method for preparing dermatological prescriptions involves fusion and incorporation of ingredients. This method pertains to prescriptions which specify the components of the dermatological base (base prepared *in situ*), particularly higher melting point solids such as waxes, cetyl alcohol, glyceryl monostearate, etc. This method is also particularly suitable for solid medicaments which are readily soluble in the melted base. Another ideal use of the fusion method was discussed under absorption bases, that is, for the incorporation of significant amounts of water into absorption bases.

In preparing a dermatological by fusion, the oil phase should be melted separately starting with the highest melting point materials. Other oil phase ingredients are then added in order of decreasing melting points. In this way the whole base is not heated up to the highest temperature, and the cooling process is hastened considerably. The water phase ingredients are combined and heated separately (assuming there is such a phase). The water phase is

heated several degrees above the temperature of the melted oil phase and the two phases are then combined. If a W/O system is to be formed, the hot-water phase is added to the hot-oil phase, in increments, with agitation. If an O/W system is to be prepared, the order of addition is reversed. Volatile substances such as perfumes, menthol, camphor, iodine, alcohol, etc., should be added after the base has cooled to about 40°C. If the medicament is a solid which is insoluble in the base, it is triturated to a fine powder and then levigated with a portion of the melted base; the remainder of the base is allowed to cool, slowly, with frequent stirring, before combining with the levigated concentrate.

The above principles underlying the preparation of dermatologicals are usually applied in large-scale manufacturing with the aid of specialized equipment such as the ointment mill shown in Fig. 2 and the paste mixer shown in Fig. 3.

Containers

The two containers most commonly used for packaging dermatological semisolid prescriptions are ointment jars and tubes. Ointment jars are available in glass or plastic. The glass jars are either transparent green, amber, or opaque white.

Ointments are usually packaged in jars by spatulating them into the container while taking care to avoid air

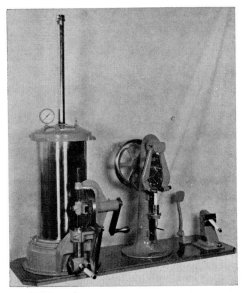

Fig. 4—Paste filler, tube closer, and crimper (courtesy, *Arthur Colton Co.*).

id preparation into a cylinder of parchment paper of such a diameter that it will fit when inserted into the tube. The paper is then removed by carefully pressing together the open end of the tube by means of a small spatula blade and withdrawing the paper while firmly holding the end of the tube together. It is usually necessary to remove the cap of the tube during the filling operation to eliminate air pockets at the top of the tube.

In Fig. 4 are shown a paste filler, tube closer, and crimper which may be used for small scale production of frequently prescribed specialty formulations, not available on the market, which are prepared for local physicians.

Labeling

Ointment jars may be labeled with an available assortment of labels that are self adhesive in nature or which must be premoistened to activate the adhesive. As an added precaution, a wide strip of Scotch tape may be wrapped around the label and jar to protect the label and prevent the directions from being obscured. Self-adhesive strip labels are recommended for tubes since the conventional gummed label usually fails to adhere appropriately to the tube surface. Ointment tubes may be protected by placing them in a cardboard box or plastic tube container. The box or tube is usually labeled in addition to the ointment tube as an additional precaution.

pockets. The surface of the ointment is usually rendered smooth by manipulating the spatula tip across the ointment surface or it is formed into a glossy surface by briefly exposing the surface to heat.

Tin and aluminum tubes are available for packaging ointments which are not too stiff and easily extrudable (products with either a very high or a very low viscosity are not ideal for this packaging). Tubes are available in various sizes complete with cap and may be purchased with special fittings such as a rectal tip. They may be filled at the prescription counter by rolling the semisol-

7

Suppositories

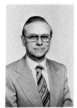

James M. Plaxco, Jr., PhD
Professor of Pharmacy
School of Pharmacy
University of South Carolina
Columbia, SC 29208

Suppositories are solid medications of various sizes and shapes suitable for insertion into a cavity of the body, usually the rectum, vagina, or urethra. They either melt at body temperature or dissolve or disintegrate in the aqueous secretion of the cavity into which they are inserted. Tablets designed for insertion into the vagina are loosely termed vaginal suppositories.

The use of suppositories as a form of medication dates back at least as far as the time of Hippocrates. Early forms of suppositories were carved pieces of wood or bone dipped or soaked in the medicinal agent. Many other agents such as pieces of leaves, rags, etc. were used as bases, but it was not until the discovery of cocoa butter in the 18th century and especially its recommendation as a suppository base in 1852 by A. B. Taylor that they received much recognition. Suppositories account for only 1% of the prescriptions in the US but the use of OTC suppositories is widespread. Their use in Europe is much more widespread than in the US. The great majority of published reports are in European literature.

Suppositories are frequently employed for local action such as relief of hemorrhoids or infection in the rectum, vagina, or urethra. Glycerin suppositories have long been used to evacuate the lower bowel. Because drugs are absorbed from the rectum, suppositories have been used for systemic medication when oral administration was not suitable, such as in infants, debilitated persons, comatose patients, or patients with nausea, vomiting, and gastrointestinal disturbances. There is a plethora of conflicting reports in the literature as to the efficacy of medicating by suppositories. Studies have shown that some drugs are absorbed as readily from rectal administration as from oral administration.

Drug Absorption

A lengthy discussion of the kinetics of absorption and elimination of drugs administered by suppositories is not with-

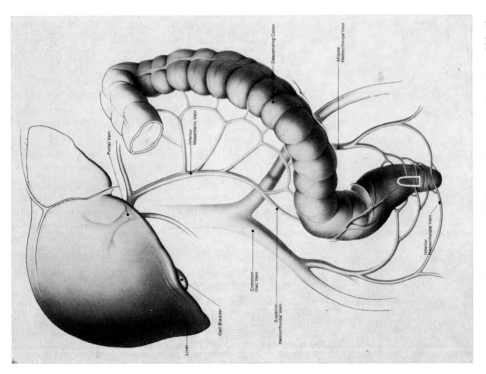

Fig. 1—The vascular supply and drainage of the rectum (courtesy, *Abbott*).

in the scope of this chapter. For convenience of discussion, it is helpful to categorize some of the factors influencing absorption from the rectum into two broad categories, namely, the physiological factors and the physicochemical factors.

Physiological Factors—The rectum, the terminal end of the intestine, begins at the rectosigmoid junction and ends at the anus. It has a length in the adult of about 15 cm. Normally it is empty except for a small amount of mucus which averages about 2 ml and has a pH of about 7.4. See Fig. 1.

The rectum has no primary absorptive functions as evidenced by the absence of villi. However, diffusion takes place readily and once through the mucosa the abundant supply of lymph and blood vessels rapidly distributes the drug throughout the body. It has been generally accepted that lymphatic flow, which is very slow compared to venous flow, does not contribute materially to transportation of drugs from the rectum. However, it has been found that in dogs, slightly more sulfanilamide was transported by the lymph system than the venous system.

The venous circulation of the rectum consists of three veins:

The *inferior hemorrhoidal vein* near the anal sphincter.
The *middle hemorrhoidal vein,* which receives blood from the capillaries of the middle region of the rectum.
The *superior hemorrhoidal vein,* which drains the upper end of the rectum.

The inferior and middle hemorrhoidal veins drain into the vena cava, thus bypassing the portal system.

The superior hemorrhoidal vein drains into the mesenteric vein which empties into the portal vein. This venous structure has given rise to the assumption that drugs administered rectally go directly to the vena cava, bypassing the liver where the biotransformation of most drugs occurs. Even if the assumption that $\frac{2}{3}$ of absorbed drugs bypass the liver during their first circulation is true, the short time (15 to 30 sec) it takes the blood to circulate makes this immaterial.

It has been shown by x-ray studies using radiopaque substances in suppositories that once inserted, regardless of depth of insertion, a suppository comes to rest 4–6 cm above the anal sphincter. As it melts or dissolves, it spreads over essentially the entire area of the rectum. For most drugs it is immaterial into which hemorrhoidal vein the drug is carried.

Although the importance of pH in affecting the absorption rates of drugs has been described in Chapter 2, it is useful to reiterate certain factors that are peculiar to the rectal environment. Rectal fluids are reported to have very little buffer capacity; therefore, medication that is dissolved in these fluids may largely determine the pH of this environment. If adjustment of pH is critical for efficient absorption of a therapeutic agent, suitable buffering agents may be required in the formulation to create a favorable pH.

Physicochemical Factors—In selecting the type of suppository base to be used for any particular therapeutic agent, the factor of lipid-water solubility must be considered because of its relationship to rate of release and intensity of action. Generally, if an oil-soluble drug is incorporated into an oily base, the rate of absorption is somewhat less than that achieved with a water-soluble base. The oil-soluble drug tends to remain dissolved in the oily pool produced by the melting of the suppository and to have a minimal tendency to escape into the aqueous medium of the mucous secretions from which it is ultimately absorbed. On the other hand, a water-soluble drug tends to pass more rapidly from the oily phase to the aqueous phase. Therefore, if rapid onset of action is sought, the water-soluble form of the drug and an oily base should be selected. However, if a more gradual release of the drug is desired, the lipid-soluble form of the drug provides a longer duration of action.

The importance of proper selection of

base material has been verified since it has been found that when a water-soluble barbiturate salt was administered rectally in cocoa butter base, the onset of action was faster than when it was administered in a water-soluble polyethylene glycol base. However, with the latter base the duration of action was longer. When the plasma levels achieved after rectal absorption of aspirin from bases of cocoa butter, polyethylene glycol, and glycerinated gelatin were compared with plasma levels observed after oral administration, it was found that the levels were about 93% from polyethylene glycol, 66% from cocoa butter, and 53% from glycerinated gelatin. Administration of aspirin in glycerinated gelatin caused a high incidence of irritation.

In recommending a base for procaine hydrochloride, it has been suggested that, if a quick effect is sought, the drug should be incorporated as a suspension in a base in which the salt is not soluble, i.e., a fatty base.

It was also found that drugs which were suspended in the suppository were released only at the melting point. Below the melting point but above the softening point only about 15% as much drug was released.

In studies comparing the release of salicylates from fatty bases use was made of both *in vitro* and *in vivo* techniques. While the *in vitro* model showed marked differences in the release of relatively water-insoluble aspirin (acetylsalicylic acid) and freely-soluble calcium acetylsalicylate and sodium salicylate, in human test subjects data obtained for the absorption of aspirin and calcium acetylsalicylate were identical. Even though both calcium acetylsalicylate and sodium salicylate are freely soluble, the sodium salt was taken up more readily by the body.

The inclusion of surface-active agents occasionally has a profound influence on the therapeutic effect of active ingredients administered via rectal suppository. These surface-active agents may alter the surface tension of the mucous blanket which lines the rectal ampulla, and in so doing may create an environment more favorable to the absorption of the drug. In addition, these agents may act as solubilizing agents for the active ingredient and the solubilized forms may be absorbed more readily. However, the opposite effect may also be seen if the surface-active agent forms complexes with the active ingredient and these complexes represent drug bound so firmly that absorption is minimized. The specific surfactant and its concentration in the base mixture ultimately affect the rates of absorption of medicaments from suppositories, as well as other types of dosage forms.

In studying the effect of the inclusion of surface-active agents in suppositories, it has also been found that with ephedrine hydrochloride, aminophenazone, and butabarbital in Witepsol and cocoa butter bases containing emulsifiers, optimum release was observed above HLB 10. These findings are in general agreement with the results determined by studying the effect of a large number of surfactants on the release of aminophylline, ephedrine, and ephedrine hydrochloride from cocoa butter. A later study utilizing rabbits revealed no difference in the rate of absorption from the effect of surfactants. From a study of barbiturate suppositories containing surfactants, it was concluded that salts of pentobarbital are absorbed more readily (by rabbits) if the base contains surfactants. However, it was also determined that although the inclusion of 3% sodium lauryl sulfate increased the absorption rate of sodium aprobarbital from a fatty base in rabbits, this effect was not seen in human subjects. Sodium lauryl sulfate and polysorbates having HLB's of about 10 were incorporated into a polyethylene glycol base for a study on the release of chloramphenicol. Although it was found that the release of the antibiotic was increased by the surfactants, only sodium lauryl sulfate increased the antibiotic activity of the drug over that seen with the base alone.

In an investigation of the effect of nonionic surfactants on the absorption of sulfonamides, it was found that the nonionic surfactants used decreased absorption of the sulfonamide because of entrapment of the drug in micelles which were too large to be absorbed through the rectal mucosa.

It has also been noted that absorption rates of certain sulfonamides were reduced when these agents were incorporated into a number of water-soluble bases. This effect has been associated with the dielectric constants of the bases, and it has been concluded that bases having larger dielectric constants reduce rectal absorption to a lesser degree.

In spite of the contributions of many studies, the relationship of surfactants to drug release and absorption remains obscure and reliable predictions cannot be made for all drugs.

Reliable evaluation of suppository medication in man cannot be based on animal experiments, much less on *in vitro* studies.

Types

Rectal Suppositories

These are usually cylindrical and taper to a point, thus assuming a shape similar to that of a rifle bullet. An improved form has its greatest diameter about ¼ the distance from the tip to the base and gradually decreases in diameter toward the base; this has the advantage that, after it has been inserted, any contractions of the rectum cause the suppository to move inward rather than to be expelled. Rectal suppositories vary in size for infants and adults; those for adults weigh approximately 2 g, while those for infants and children are proportionately smaller. Some commercial rectal suppositories are shown in Fig. 2.

Local Action—Local medication of the anal region is employed most often in the treatment of hemorrhoids; how-

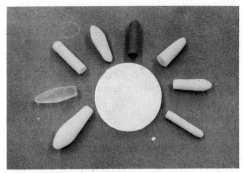

Fig. 2—Commercial rectal suppositories.

ever, suppositories are used for other conditions such as pruritis ani, bacterial infections, and chronic inflammation. Common constituents of rectal suppositories intended for local action include local anesthetics, astringents, antiseptics, and various antibacterial agents.

Suppositories of soap are used as rectal evacuants, particularly for children. The effect is partly mechanical and partly due to a slight irritant action of the soap. The advantages are that prompt results are obtained and the use of laxatives is avoided. In the past it was common practice to cut a rectal suppository from a cake of castile or other mild soap. At present it is more common to use Glycerin Suppositories, USP, in which the soap is sodium stearate. As these suppositories are hygroscopic, they should be kept in tightly closed containers in a cool place.

Systemic Action—The rectum is a convenient route for systemic administration of drugs. The abundant supply of blood vessels and rapid diffusion of drugs through the rectal mucosa permit rapid absorption of many drugs. Many classes of medicaments appear to be well absorbed, e.g., antinauseants, tranquilizers, vasodilators, vasoconstrictors, bronchodilators, sedatives, analgesics, and alkaloids such as those of belladonna and ergot.

At present, systemic medicating is limited to the rectum, although absorption of drugs from the vagina is under investigation.

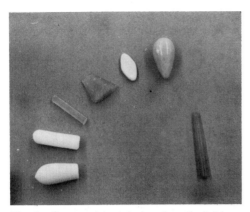

Fig. 3—Commercial vaginal and urethral (lower right) suppositories.

Vaginal Suppositories

Vaginal suppositories are oval in shape and are generally considered to weigh about 5 g but commercial products vary widely in size and shape (see Fig. 3). Drugs are administered to the vagina for a local effect only but it must be kept in mind that systemic absorption can occur. It is common practice to use various antiseptic agents as vaginal douches, although the same concentration of drug in a vaginal suppository may produce a toxic effect. The douche remains in contact with the vaginal lining for only a short time, but the suppository remains long enough for toxic amounts to be absorbed.

Common constituents of vaginal suppositories are antiseptics, contraceptive agents, and various drugs used to treat trichomonal, monilial, or bacterial infections.

In addition to the conventional bases of cocoa butter (theobroma oil), polyethylene glycols, glycerinated gelatin, and various emulsifying agents, vaginal suppositories are also made by tableting processes that utilize bases composed largely of lactose. These tablets may be inserted manually or by use of a special plastic inserter. Dipping the tablet momentarily into water facilitates insertion. Occasionally dry powders such as boric acid are dispensed in large capsules for insertion into the vagina.

Urethral Suppositories

The third route of administering drugs by suppository is via the urethra. This route is limited to local action, usually with anti-infectives. These suppositories are long and tapered, having a length of about 60 mm and a diameter of 4–5 mm (see Fig. 3). The only urethral suppository in common use in the US is the Furacin Urethral Insert which has a base composed of glyceryl monolaurate and polyethylene glycol (4) sorbitan monostearate. Package labeling directs that the suppository be stored at room temperature but to place the suppository in the refrigerator for a short time prior to use to ensure a firm enough suppository for insertion; it should also be moistened.

Suppository Bases

The vehicle in which a drug is distributed exerts a great influence on its action in the body. The drug must be released from the vehicle, dissolve in the fluid of the cavity, diffuse to the mucous membrane, and pass through the membrane, by passive diffusion from the rectum to the bloodstream and hence be transported throughout the body.

A satisfactory base must meet several criteria:

It must remain a firm enough solid for insertion at room temperature, even in warm climates. Preferably it should not soften below 30° C to avoid premature melting during storage.

It should have a narrow or sharp melting range. Preferably there should be not more than 3° between the temperature at which the base begins to soften and the clear or complete melting point.

It should yield a "clear melt" just below body temperature or it should dissolve or disintegrate readily in the cavity fluid. Studies have shown that up to the clear melting point drug release is very slow.

It should be inert and compatible with a wide variety of drugs, especially the ones in the particular formula.

It should be nonirritating and nonsensitizing.

It should be stable, and not exhibit "bloom," i.e., the formation of a white powder-like substance on the outside of the suppository.

From a production viewpoint, there are other considerations:

The fused mass should solidify rapidly to prevent suspended solids from settling. It should give good mold-release, i.e., it should contract and not stick to the mold.

The suppository should not become brittle. This may be avoided by cooling the fused mass slowly or temper the suppositories to prevent crystal formation, or by incorporating 2% monoglycerides into the mass.

Neither USP nor NF specifies suppository vehicles in the monographs. The USP mentions several vehicles: cocoa butter, glycerinated gelatin, hydrogenated vegetable oils, mixtures of polyethylene glycols of various molecular weights, and fatty acid esters of polyethylene glycol. Minor deviations in composition are allowed to maintain suitable consistency of the base under different climatic conditions.

Many suppository bases have been used. A survey of 40 suppositories in a community pharmacy, both those available on prescription only and OTC reveals that approximately ⅓ use cocoa butter or synthetic substitutes, ⅓ use polyethylene glycol polymers, and the remaining ⅓ use a wide variety of components. The following discussion will be limited to those bases readily available in the US.

Bases That Melt

Cocoa Butter USP (Theobroma Oil, Cacao Butter)—Most fats and waxes soften long before they reach melting temperature. An exception is cocoa butter, which has been one of the most widely used suppository bases since its introduction as a base in 1852. It is a firm solid to a temperature of 32° C at which temperature it begins to soften. At 34–35° it melts to produce a thin, bland, oily liquid. It is a good base for rectal suppositories, but is less than ideal for vaginal or urethral suppositories because of its tendency to leak from the cavities and the lack of miscibility with the aqueous secretions.

Cocoa butter is a mixture of triglycerides. Oleic acid contributes approximately ⅓ of the acid constituents. Like many triglycerides, cocoa butter exhibits polymorphism. It may crystallize in any of four crystal forms depending on the fusion temperature and rate of cooling. The stable *beta* crystals exist up to the melting point of 34–35°. Their solidification point is 28°. The presence of these crystals is essential to produce solidification at room temperature within a reasonable period of time. If the base is heated to a "clear melt," the beta crystals are destroyed and no seed crystals remain. The least-stable form, *gamma* crystals, melts at 18°. If allowed to stand undisturbed, there is a transition to the *alpha* form with a melting point of 22°. A second transition yields *beta prime* crystals with a melting point of 27°. A final transition results in the formation of the stable beta crystals, melting just above 34°. Several days are usually required for these transformations, during which time the suppositories should be stored in a cool place, preferably below 20°.

One of the principal drawbacks of cocoa butter is its inability to absorb aqueous solutions. This can be overcome to some extent by the addition of nonionic surfactants to the base; but the resulting suppositories exhibit poor storage stability and become rancid rapidly. Also, the addition of surfactants, with or without water, has been reported to alter the action of drugs in cocoa butter. As noted previously, both increase and decrease in the rate of release and absorption of drugs has been reported. If aqueous solutions are to be incorporated into suppositories, another base should be used, i.e., PEG.

Another shortcoming of theobroma oil is the lowering of the melting point by the addition of certain drugs, i.e., chloral hydrate. The addition of high melting point waxes and fats has been tried but has not been satisfactory, especially with chloral hydrate. It appears that each drug is an individual problem and no generalizations can be made as to amount of wax to add.

Because of the shortcomings of cocoa butter as a suppository base, many combinations of fats and waxes have been suggested as substitutes. Most of

Table 1—Bases That Melt[1]

Vehicle	Composition	Melting range (°C)	Congealing range (°C)
Cocoa butter	Mixed triglycerides of oleic, palmitic, stearic acids	34–35	28 or less[a]
Cotmar	Partially hydrogenated cottonseed oil	35–75	
Dehydag[d]	Hydrogenated fatty alcohols	33–36	32–33
Base I	and esters	37–39	36–37
Base II			
Base III	Glycerides of saturated fatty acids C_{12}–C_{18}	9 ranges	
Wecobee R[b,d]	Triglycerides derived from	33–35	31–32
Wecobee SS[b,d]	coconut oil	40–43	33–35
Witepsol[c,d]			
H-12	Triglycerides of saturated		
H-15	fatty acids C_{12}–C_{18} with	32–33	29–31
H-85	varied portions of the corresponding partial glycerides	33–35	32–34
		42–44	36–38

[a] Depends on melting temperature.
[b] Of the seven Wecobee bases, a high- and a low-melting product were selected.
[c] Of the 12 Witepsol bases the most widely used and the highest- and lowest-melting bases were selected.
[d] The Dehydag, Wecobee, and Witepsol bases all contain a small amount of some emulsifier.

the currently used bases were developed in Europe during World War II, largely as a result of the shortage of cocoa butter. A partial list of suppository bases used in the US is given in Table 1.

Witepsol Bases—Other than cocoa butter, the largest number of published studies concerning melting suppository bases deal with the Witepsol bases. All 12 members of this series of bases are nearly white and almost odorless. Witepsol H 15 melts at almost the same rate and releases drugs at the same rate as cocoa butter. Unlike cocoa butter, the Witepsols do not exhibit polymorphism when melted and cooled. They are composed of natural saturated fats of acid chains between C_{12} and C_{18} with lauric acid being present in greatest concentration. They have a small interval between softening and melting temperature and their solidification point is only a few degrees below their melting point. They solidify rapidly in the mold and contract, making lubrication of the mold unnecessary. High-melting Witepsols can be mixed with low-melting Witepsols to produce combinations covering a wide range of melting points, i.e., 34–44° C. Chloral hydrate produces

a much less pronounced lowering of the melting point than in cocoa butter and it is relatively simple to determine the percentage of various types of Witepsols, i.e., Witepsol H 15 and Witepsol E 85, to produce the required melting point. The Witepsols also contain emulsifiers and will absorb limited amounts of water.

Wecobee Suppository Bases—These bases are derived from coconut oil. The incorporation of glyceryl monostearate and propylene glycol monostearate makes them emulsifiable. The seven members of Wecobee bases, which are available in a range of melting points, appear similar in action to the Witepsol bases but reports of *in vitro* tests have not been found in the literature.

Water-Soluble Bases—These bases are of comparatively recent origin. The principal bases used are based on polymers of ethylene oxide and water. The polyethylene glycol polymers (PEG), best known as Carbowaxes, are available for suppository use in a molecular weight range of 400 to 6000 (see Table 2). At room temperature, PEG 400 is a liquid, PEG 1000 is a soft semisolid,

Table 2—Polyethylene Glycol Polymers

Average mol wt	400	600	1000	1500	1540	4000	6000
Melting range (°C)	4–8	20–25	37–40	38–41	40–46	50–56	60–63
Solubility in water (%)	100	100	70	73	70	62	50

PEG 1500 and PEG 1540 are fairly firm semisolids (and generally can be used interchangeably), and PEG 4000 and PEG 6000 are firm wax-like solids. They are water-soluble, but dissolve slowly, even in an excess of water. In the rectum or vagina, which have little fluid, they are very slow to dissolve but soften and spread. When suppositories of this type are inserted into the rectum, the patient must repress the defecation reflex to avoid expelling the suppository. There is some evidence that several drugs complex with PEG which results in slow rates of release and absorption. Contradictory reports of drug absorption from PEG bases abound in the literature. Evidence supports the view that those bases containing the higher melting point polymers, especially PEG 6000, have slower release and solution rates than those bases composed of lower-melting polymers.

In spite of these many apparent shortcomings, and possibly because of their greater stability at room temperature, these bases are widely used. In the US, approximately ⅓ of the suppositories use the PEG polymers with satisfactory results.

The many polymers can be mixed in varying proportions to give bases with different properties. Many formulas have been tested. The following mixtures of PEG shown in Table 3 have been found to give satisfactory bases, stable at room temperature, and dissolving or softening and spreading within 30–45 min.

Glycerin Suppositories USP consist of 91% glycerin gelled with 9% sodium stearate. They are available as adult and infant suppositories to evacuate the lower bowel.

Hard-gelatin capsules provide a convenient means for the extemporaneous

Table 3—Polyethylene Glycol (PEG) Bases

Base I		
PEG	6000	50%
PEG	1540	30%
PEG	400	20%

A good general-purpose water-soluble suppository base.

Base 2		
PEG	4000	60%
PEG	1000	30%
PEG	400	10%

A good general-purpose base which is slightly softer and dissolves more readily.

Base 3		
PEG	6000	30%
PEG	1540	70%

This base has a higher melting point which is usually sufficient to compensate for the melting-point lowering of drugs such as chloral hydrate and camphor.

preparation of suppositories. The capsule can be filled with drug and inserted as a suppository. Prior to insertion, it is advisable to make a small hole in each end of the capsule with a pin or other similar object to speed solution and rupture of the capsule. Dipping the capsule into water facilitates insertion.

Various substances have been investigated to increase the water-holding power of suppository bases. The author has found that the addition of 5% cetyl alcohol to any of these PEG bases enables the suppository to hold at least 10% water with no evidence of instability. When water-soluble drugs, especially solutions, are to be incorporated into suppositories, these bases, with 5% cetyl alcohol added, are recommended.

Certain synthetic surface-active agents have been suggested for use as hydrophilic suppository bases that may frequently be used without the addition of other materials for the preparation of some formulations. Polyoxyl 40 stearate (Myrj 52) and polyoxyethylene sorbitan monostearate (Tween 61) are two such agents which have been suggested for

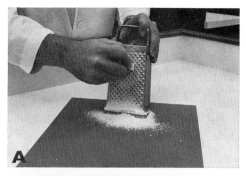

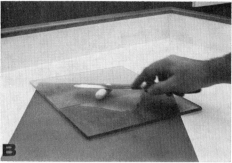

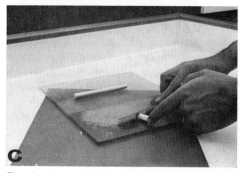

Fig. 4—Hand rolling suppositories: (a) shredding cocoa butter, (b) rolling the cylinder, and (c) tapering.

use in producing hydrophilic suppository bases. The author has found them to dissolve too slowly and to lack sufficient firmness to be used by themselves.

An emulsifying base containing 0.5 to 1% sodium or ethanolamine stearate in combination with propylene glycol monostearate has been suggested. This mixture forms an emulsion in the body fluids and slowly releases incorporated medicaments. An improvement on this formulation utilizes polyethylene glycol 400 monostearate, 20 to 40%, in combination with the propylene glycol monostearate. This mixture softens more

readily at body temperatures. It has been found that a mixture of dioctyl sodium sulfosuccinate, polyoxyethylene 30 stearate, white wax, and water produces a satisfactory base.

Suppository bases utilizing many other ingredients have been studied. Few, if any, detailed reports of rates of drug release and absorption have been found in the literature.

Glycerinated Gelatin Suppositories USP consist of 10% water, 70% glycerin, and 20% gelatin. It is important to select the type of gelatin most suitable for the drug to be incorporated. While either Type A or Type B gelatin is satisfactory for many drugs, in many instances one type is required. The suppositories must be stored in tight containers preferably at a temperature below 35°C. The base is too soft for easy insertion and is seldom used in the US today.

It must be remembered that the inclusion of emulsifying agents may affect the onset, duration, and intensity of the action of the medicament, and that bases should be tested thoroughly before using them for any therapeutic agent. This, of course, holds true whenever the vehicle is changed in any formulation.

Preparation

A willingness and ability to prepare various dosage forms on an individual basis distinguishes the professional pharmacist from the technician. Contrary to many opinions, suppositories are one of the easiest, though time consuming, dosage forms to prepare extemporaneously. They may be made by the cold method, either hand-shaping or compression, or by the fusion method. Attention to a few basic guidelines results in quite satisfactory products.

Cold Hand Shaping—This is the time-honored method for the extemporaneous preparation of cocoa butter suppositories (Fig. 4). It is simple, no elaborate equipment or source of heat is required, and it is not necessary to determine the amount of base displaced by the drug.

The author has found most problems are the result of two common mistakes: (1) Getting and keeping the cocoa butter too cold which results in lack of plasticity and the suppositories are brittle and crack, and (2) using too much starch or other conspergent on the pill tile which also leads to cracking and loss of cohesiveness. The following procedure is suggested.

1. Reduce the drug to an impalpable powder.
2. Grate or otherwise reduce the cocoa butter to small particles.
3. Mix the powdered drug with a small portion of the grated base in a mortar.
4. Add 1 drop of fixed vegetable oil/12 suppositories to give additional plasticity to the mass.
5. Add the remainder of the cocoa butter by geometric dilution, i.e., add the same amount of base as is already in the mortar. Triturate with much pressure until well mixed. The heat generated by the trituration results in a plastic, pliable mass which is cohesive and ready to roll.
6. Quickly wash and dry the hands before the mass has an opportunity to cool and lose its plasticity.
7. Remove the suppository mass from the mortar by scraping with a spatula and quickly roll into an elongated, football-shaped mass in the hands.
8. Place the shaped mass on a pill tile lightly dusted with starch and, using a spatula with a broad blade, roll the mass into a pipe or cylinder having a diameter approximately the diameter of the finished suppository. As the mass lengthens, keep the ends square by shaping with the fingers and spatula blade. Too much starch results in loss of cohesiveness and cracking. Too little starch results in the mass adhering to the spatula blade and pill tile.
9. Score the pipe into the desired number of equal size segments, and cut with a razor blade or other sharp instrument.
10. Use firm pressure with the fingers of one hand and shape one end of segment of mass into a point, forming the suppository. Finish by rolling each suppository lightly with a broad blade spatula to remove finger prints and other imperfections.

Cold Compression—For those pharmacists who are willing and have occasion to prepare suppositories for their patients, the purchase of a compression mold (e.g., a Whitehall-Tatum or Armstrong type) is justified (Fig. 5). There are molds for making 1-g rectal,

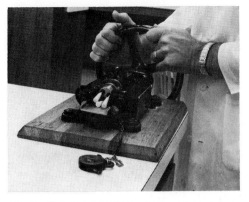

Fig. 5—Rectal suppositories being released from the compression mold.

2-g rectal, and 5-g vaginal suppositories. Compression is applicable only to cocoa butter and a few other bases. When using these devices, the pharmacist must determine the capacity of the individual dies which prepare these suppositories simultaneously. The capacity is easily determined by compressing a sufficient amount of blank cocoa butter into the dies and weighing the finished suppositories. Again, as in the case of the hand-rolled suppositories, the powdered active ingredients are triturated with grated cocoa butter and transferred into a chilled cylinder. The mixture is extruded into the die until firm resistance of the piston is felt. The wheel is backed off just enough to loosen the gate, which is then removed, and with a sharp motion the wheel is advanced forward to expel the suppositories from the die. The gate is replaced and the procedure repeated until the prescription is finished. Because there is some loss of mixture in the equipment, it is advisable to prepare enough formula for one extra suppository.

The volume of active ingredients may have some effect on the amount of cocoa butter required for an individual formula. Some tables of cocoa butter density factors have been published which equate the weights of active ingredients to the amount of cocoa butter which they replace. Table 4 lists cocoa butter density factors for some of the common drugs. However, in many

Table 4—Density Factors of Suppositories

Medication	Cocoa butter
Aloin	1.3
Aminophylline	1.1
Aminopyrine	1.3
Aspirin	1.1
Barbital sodium	1.2
Belladonna Extract	1.3
Bismuth subgallate	2.7
Chloral hydrate	1.3
Cocaine hydrochloride	1.3
Codeine phosphate	1.1
Digitalis leaf	1.6
Dimenhydrinate	1.3
Diphenhydramine hydrochloride	1.3
Gallic acid	2.0
Morphine hydrochloride	1.6
Opium	1.4
Pentobarbital	1.2
Phenobarbital sodium	1.2
Salicylic acid	1.3
Secobarbital sodium	1.2
Tannic acid	1.6

cases, especially with potent drugs, the volume occupied by the active ingredient is so very slight as to be negligible. Still, with other active ingredients which may be present in relatively large volumes, allowance should be made to determine the amount of cocoa butter which should be omitted from the full formula. This determination may be made by calculating the total amount of active ingredient to be used, dividing this figure by the cocoa butter density factor and, finally, subtracting the resulting quantity from the total amount of cocoa butter which would be needed for the required number of dosage forms, if no active ingredient were used.

For example, if 12 suppositories, each containing 300 mg of aspirin, are to be made in a mold which has a capacity of 2 g of cocoa butter, 3.9 g of aspirin is required. (Use enough of all ingredients to make 1 additional suppository.) Dividing 3.9 by 1.1, it is found that this amount of aspirin replaces 3.55 g of cocoa butter. Therefore, instead of using 13 × 2 or 26 g of cocoa butter for the formula, 26 − 3.55, or 22.45 g, of cocoa butter is needed.

Commercially, many suppositories are prepared with the aid of powerful hydraulic compression equipment. Compression molding is suitable only for oleaginous bases such as cocoa butter and special formulations of polyethylene glycol polymer mixtures.

Fusion—This is the principal method of making suppositories commercially. The fusion process can be used with almost all suppository bases and it must be used with the majority of bases. Molds come in sizes to make from 6 to 500 suppositories. They are made of aluminum, brass, or nickel-copper alloys. The inner surface must be smooth to prevent the suppositories from sticking to the mold. When purchasing new molds it is recommended that polytetrafluoroethylene (Teflon)-coated molds be purchased.

As with compression molding, the first step is to determine the capacity of the molds. Sufficient base is melted over a steam bath and poured into the mold (at least 6 holes) and allowed to congeal. The excess is removed by trimming with a sharp blade, and the blanks are turned out of the mold and weighed. After determining the proper amount of base mixture to be used, the components are melted on a steam bath and the active ingredients added. The mixtures should neither be subjected to excessive heat nor poured at temperatures very far above the melting points, so as to avoid decomposition of active ingredients and excessive contraction of the mixture when it cools. See suppositories being cast in Fig. 6.

Special precautions are required when making cocoa butter suppositories by the fusion method. As stated previously, if the cocoa butter melts completely, the beta crystals are destroyed.

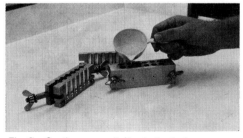

Fig. 6—Casting suppositories in the fusion process.

The cocoa butter is transformed into a metastable form which congeals below 20° C and storage for several days is required for a return to the stable form which melts at 34° C. The following procedure has been found to yield stable suppositories providing careful attention is paid to the temperature.

1. Reduce the drug to an impalpable powder.
2. Carefully "melt" a small portion of the grated cocoa butter in a suitable container suspended in a water bath at 34–35° C.
3. Mix the powdered drug with the "creamy melted" base by stirring.
4. Add the remainder of the grated cocoa butter, stir, and mix.
5. Maintain the temperature at 34–35° C with stirring until the drug is uniformly mixed and the base is "creamy melted." If a "clear melt" results, the beta crystals are destroyed and the congealing and melting point is lowered below 20° C.
6. Pour the "creamy melted" mass into a suppository mold at room temperature which has been very lightly lubricated with mineral oil. Pour each mold continuously to avoid "layering" of the suppository, which leads to breaking.
7. Allow to congeal, then place in the refrigerator for 30 min to harden.
8. Remove from the refrigerator, trim off the top, and press from the mold.

If time permits, it is advisable to allow the suppositories to remain in the mold in the refrigerator for several days to ensure formation of stable beta crystals.

In the case of cocoa butter, density factors may be used, as described previously. However, density factors for other suppository base materials are not generally available. If the volume of the active ingredients is appreciable, a double casting procedure can be used. This technique involves mixing the total active ingredients required for the full number of suppositories with an amount of the base mixture which is inadequate to fill the required number of cavities. This mixture, containing the active ingredients, is poured into the mold and the remaining cavities are filled with the blank base mixture. After congealing, the suppositories are turned out of the mold, remelted, mixed thoroughly, and again cast so as to distribute the active ingredient uniformly throughout the total number of suppositories. By weighing the finished suppositories at this point and subtracting the amount of active ingredients incorporated, the pharmacist can determine the amount of base mixture used. This information should be recorded on the back of the prescription. This precludes the necessity of repeating this double-casting procedure when the prescription is refilled.

Lubrication of fusion molds is frequently advisable. New molds are well made, have highly polished surfaces, and may release the finished suppositories readily; however, after some usage they may become scratched and may not release the suppositories as readily. The lubricant used depends on the type of base mixture to be cast. The best lubricant is one which is immiscible with the base. For cocoa butter suppositories, a thin film of glycerin or mineral oil applied to a well-washed mold usually suffices. At one time green soap tincture was a popular lubricant for this purpose. For suppositories made of polyethylene glycol mixtures, a thin film of mineral oil applied to the mold ensures ready release. Another technique which facilitates removal of the suppositories from the mold is chilling for a short time in the freezer compartment of the refrigerator after the suppositories have congealed at room temperature. The additional contraction may free them from the metal surfaces.

Special Problems

The incorporation of vegetable extracts, especially into cocoa butter, can be facilitated if the extract is moistened with a few drops of alcohol and levigated with a small portion of melted cocoa butter on an ointment slab before final incorporation. This procedure aids in the distribution of the drug throughout the base matrix. When hard crystalline materials—e.g., merbromin, iodine, silver protein, or dyes—are to be incorporated into suppositories, it is most helpful to dissolve these in a minimum of suitable solvent, such as water or glyc-

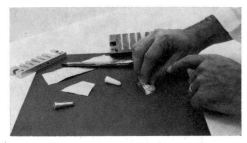

Fig. 7—Wrapping finished suppositories in aluminum foil.

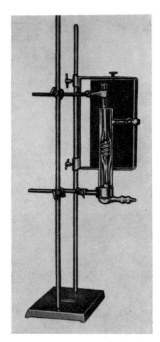

Fig. 9—Suppository melting tester (courtesy, *ChemiPharm*).

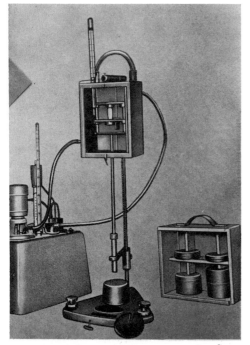

Fig. 8—Fracture point testing apparatus (courtesy, *ChemiPharm*).

erin, prior to incorporation into the base. These solutions then may be picked up with a small amount of anhydrous lanolin (wool fat) and incorporated into cocoa butter, or preferably use one of the PEG bases discussed previously.

Packaging and Dispensing

Suppositories are best dispensed in sectioned suppository boxes, ointment jars, or appropriate-sized capsule vials. The sectioned boxes help keep the individual units from touching and possibly sticking. In some cases it is advisable to wrap the suppositories before final packaging. Wrapping is a simple matter with small pieces of aluminum foil cut in a trapezoidal pattern. See Fig. 7. Chloral hydrate suppositories should always be wrapped to avoid evaporation of the chloral hydrate and dispensed in tightly closed containers, preferably glass. Upon dispensing the prescription, the pharmacist should make certain that the patient understands the proper use of this dosage form. The label should read "Unwrap and insert (via route) . . . ." There are numerous cases where suppositories have been administered by the wrong route or without being unwrapped, and it is the pharmacist's responsibility to clarify the procedure tactfully with the patient. It is also advisable to instruct patients to keep their suppository prescriptions in a refrigerator to avoid melting in overly warm rooms.

Testing Procedures

The development of testing procedures which might give results that can be correlated closely with actual clinical usage has been fraught with the usual problems encountered in the extrapolation of *in vitro* data to the *in vivo* situation. The USP contains but little guidance on the standards and testing procedures by which suppositories may be evaluated.

In addition to the usual instruments available for testing hardness of waxes, e.g., the penetrometer, several instruments are marketed commercially for testing suppositories. These include accessories for the tablet-disintegration apparatus in which the suppositories are placed in small plastic bags with a small amount of water. As the apparatus rises and falls, a set of bars lightly squeezes the bag. Dissolution or melting is observed directly. A fracture-point testing apparatus and suppository melting tester are also available. See Figs. 8 and 9. These two instruments are manufactured in Europe and are distributed in this country by the Chemical and Pharmaceutical Industry Co., Inc., 260 W. Broadway, New York, NY 10013.

Setnikar and Fantelli (see *Bibliography*) devised an excellent apparatus to test the liquefaction time of rectal suppositories. Their apparatus consists of a length of cellulose dialyzer tubing fitted with a glass water jacket which permits circulation of temperature-controlled water. The suppository is held inside the tubing so that the water which passes to the inside aids in effecting liquefaction. This apparatus closely resembles the rectal environment by providing both warmth and moisture. These same investigators proposed weight-uniformity specifications for rectal suppositories which may be useful in establishing official standards.

References

1. Anschel, J, Lieberman HA: *Drug Cos Ind* 97:341, 1965; *Ibid:* 507.

Bibliography

Schwartz TW, in Dittert LW, ed: *Sprowl's American Pharmacy,* 7th ed, Lippincott, Philadelphia, 279, 1974.

Blaug SM, in *Remington's Pharmaceutical Sciences,* 15th ed, Mack Publ. Co., Easton, PA, 1546, 1975.

Guillot BR, Lombard AP: *The Suppository,* Gattefosse Est., Paris, 1973.

Ward WC: *JAPhA Sci Ed 39:*265, 1950.

Whitworth CW, LaRocca JP: *Ibid 48:*353, 1959.

Setnikar I, Fantelli S: *J. Pharm Sci 51:*556, 1962.

8

Liquid medications

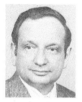

Bernard Ecanow, PhD
Professor of Pharmacy
College of Pharmacy
University of Illinois
at the Medical Center
Chicago, IL 60612

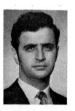

Harun Takruri, PhD
Senior Pharmaceutical
Chemist
The Lilly Research
Laboratories
Indianapolis, IN 46206

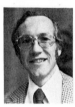

Roger L. Schnaare, PhD
Associate Professor of
Pharmacy
Philadelphia College of
Pharmacy and Science
Philadelphia, PA 19104

Dr. Ecanow prepared the *Introduction* and the section on *Liquid Dosage Forms*. **Dr. Takruri** prepared the section on *Solution Technology*. **Dr. Schnaare** prepared the sections on *Emulsion Technology* and *Suspension Technology*.

Liquid medications will be considered under the general topics of solution technology, emulsion technology, suspension technology, and liquid dosage forms.

In solutions, the medications are dispersed in the liquid vehicle in essentially molecular-sized particles and form a homogeneous mixture. As higher concentrations of the medicaments in the liquid vehicle are desired, the saturation point is exceeded and the drugs exist as aggregates of molecules in the liquid. The aggregates are of different particle size but all tend to separate from the vehicle; i.e., the preparations are heterogeneous, thermodynamically unstable systems. But common to all heterogeneous systems is the fact that the aggregates can exist as dispersed, independent particles (dispersed state), close-packed particles which act as a unit (coagulated state), or aggregated in an open network structure (flocculated state).

Precise definitions are still lacking in the vocabulary dealing with heterogeneous systems, and the student is cautioned to clearly have in mind what is meant by the various terms as they are used by different authors (see *Bibliography*). Each of the different aggregation states have a different set of properties which in turn produce different pharmaceutical and biological effects (see *Bibliography*).

The pharmaceutical knowledge required to properly deal with these liquid systems is discussed in the following sections.

Solution Technology

Solutions are thermodynamically stable, homogeneous systems of two or more components. The components can be gases, liquids, or solids. Gas systems and some alloys are considered to be solutions, but the pharmacist is primarily interested in liquid solutions which result from the dissolution of a gas, liquid, or solid in a liquid. This discussion is limited to this category, referred to simply as *solution*. Most solution dosage forms fall in this category.

Classification

An understanding of the physicochemical forces operating in solution systems requires an understanding of the liquid state which is the most complex and least understood form of matter. As an aid in the study of solutions, they can be classified into three broad classes: micromolecular, micellar, and macromolecular.

Micromolecular Solutions—These are solutions consisting entirely of microunits which can be either molecules or ions, e.g., water, alcohol, sodium ions, chloride ions, sucrose, and glycerin. This class also includes solutions in which components dimerize, trimerize, or form ion pairs. The main criterion that differentiates micromolecular solutions from other classes is the size of the units of solute and solvent. In general the size should be of the order of 1–10 Å.

Micellar Solutions—The solute units in these systems consist of aggregates (micelles) of the solute molecules or ions. The visual properties of these solutions, such as clarity and viscosity, resemble those of micromolecular solutions but the values of measured physical properties such as vapor pressure, osmotic pressure, conductance, and others show marked deviations from the values for micromolecular solutions. The *micelles* in these systems are defined as polymolecular or polyionic aggregates which can reach the colloidal range of particle size. Thus micellar solutions are referred to as solutions of association colloids. The importance of micelles in pharmacy lies in their solubilizing power and in their close resemblance to various biological systems.

Macromolecular Solutions—These are systems where the solute is molecularly dispersed just as in micromolecular solutions. But they differ from these solutions in one important aspect. The molecular weight and size of the macromolecules are of such large magnitude that the system acquires unique properties. Solutions of acacia, carboxymethylcellulose, albumin, DNA, and polyvinylpyrrolidone are examples of this class. These solutions are recognized now as true monophasic, thermodynamically stable systems and the old concept of considering them as heterogeneous dispersions (e.g., colloidal gold) is believed to be inaccurate.

The categorization of solutions into these three broad classes is arbitrary. It does not mean that the physicochemical laws of solutions are not applicable to micellar or macromolecular solutions. It only serves to present a physical picture and a realization of the size and origin of the solute. Thus, a 1% solution of albumin is as true a solution as 1% sodium chloride.

Some of the terms and concepts encountered in any discussion of solutions need clarification. The assignment of the terms solvent or solute to a component is arbitrary. Usually the liquid component is considered to be the solvent and the solid or gaseous component to be the solute, although in systems of amorphous polymers the organic liquids are presumed to "dissolve" in the polymer. If both components are liquids it is advisable to use the term miscibility rather than solubility in describing the mutual affinity of the components. Thus, sorbitol is soluble in water, glycerin is miscible, and chloroform is slightly miscible with water.

Consider a solution of a compound A in water at room temperature, the following types of solution can be obtained:

Dilute solution: very small amount of A in solution.

Concentrated solution: large fraction of the solution consists of A.

Saturated solution: contains the maximum amount of A that can be incorporated in water at a given temperature and pressure.

Supersaturated solution: amount of A is more than its solubility limit in water at room temperature. This solution is unstable and disturbances cause it to revert to the stable saturated solution.

The relationships among these types are interesting. Thus, official aromatic waters are both dilute solutions (approximately 0.2%) and (by definition) saturated. Also, a solution can be concentrated but far from saturated; 50% solutions of potassium iodide or sucrose in water are concentrated but not saturated. This pharmaceutical classification leaves some questions unanswered, such as what type of solution is 10% sucrose, or 30% alcohol, or phenobarbital elixir? These questions emphasize that when dealing with pharmaceutical solutions one must be careful in using the terms of physical chemistry. The physical chemist usually deals with solutions which are less complicated than solution dosage forms and his concept of dilute and concentrated solutions is related to the degree of deviation from ideal behavior. If this concept were applied to pharmaceutical solutions, most of them would be considered to be concentrated solutions, e.g., normal saline solution.

Solvent-Solute Interactions

Dissolution results from interactions between solvent and solute molecules or ions. Despite the complexity of these interactions due to the wide range of solvents and solutes, it is possible to study their net effect in terms of the changes in few thermodynamic functions such as free energy, enthalpy, and entropy. On the other hand, these molecular interactions can be visualized readily by studying the effect of various physical-chemical parameters on solubility behavior. Knowledge of the physical-chemical characteristics of the solvent and solute makes it possible to predict the type of interactions and consequently the extent of solubility.

Physicochemical Factors

Polarity—The well-known rule "like dissolves like" is based on the observation that molecules of similar charge distribution are mutually soluble. Molecules which have asymmetric charge distribution, i.e., polar molecules, are soluble in similar media, while nonpolar molecules can easily be placed in nonpolar media.

The dielectric constant D is a measure of the polarizability of a molecule. Compounds are often classified according to their dielectric constants as either polar, semipolar, or nonpolar:

Dielectric Constant and Polarity

Nonpolar	1–20
Semipolar	20–50
Polar	>50

Table 1 shows the dielectric constants of several compounds at 20°C, in

Table 1—Dielectric Constants at 20°C

Compound	D
N-methylformamide	190
Water	80.4
Glycerin	46.0
Ethylene glycol	41
Methanol	33.7
Ethyl alcohol	26
Acetone	21
Methyl salicylate	9.0
Ammonium chloride	7.0
Chloroform	5.0
Hydrochloric acid	4.6
Castor oil	4.6
Ethyl ether	4.3
Sucrose	3.3
Olive oil	3.1
Dioxane	2.26
Carbon tetrachloride	2.2
Liquid petrolatum	2.5

descending order. Table 2 shows the dielectric constant of water as a function of temperature, and Table 3 shows the dielectric constant of mixtures of solvents. These tables show that the dielectric constant is not necessarily an accurate and sufficient predictive tool for solubility. D for sucrose is 3.3, yet it is very soluble in water. Castor oil and olive oil have close values, yet castor oil is miscible and olive oil is only slightly miscible with alcohol. The dielectric constants of dioxane and mineral oil are essentially similar, yet dioxane is completely miscible with water. The dielectric constant of water decreases with an increase in temperature, yet the solubility of most compounds increases with an increase in temperature, a fact which cannot be predicted from consideration of the dielectric constant alone. The dielectric constant of a two-component

Table 2—Dielectric Constant of Water as a Function of Temperature[1]

T	D
0	88.15
5	86.12
15	82.23
20	80.36
25	78.54
40	73.35
50	70.10
80	61.22
100	55.90

Table 3—Dielectric Constants at 25°C of
Mixtures of Solvents and Water[1]

Water (Wt%)	Eth- anol D	Glyc- erin D	Su- crose D	Di- oxane D
90	72.8	75.5	76.3	69.69
80	67.0	72.9	73.6	60.79
70	61.1	70.0	70.9	51.90
60	55.0	67.1	67.9	42.98
50	49.0	64.0	64.2	34.26
40	43.4	60.0	59.9	25.85
30	38.0	55.6	54.2	17.69
20	32.8	50.6	...	10.71
10	28.1	45.5	...	5.605
0	24.3	40.1	...	2.101

solvent lies between the values for the individual components. The solvent properties of solvent blends having the same dielectric constant are not similar. From Table 3 it can be seen that D for 40% w/w ethanol is very close to that of 70% w/w sucrose, yet these two solvents have different solvent properties.

The dielectric constant of a solvent, therefore, gives only a rough qualitative prediction of the solvent properties and the degree of solubility of polar and nonpolar compounds. Deviations from "expected" solubility patterns should not be surprising.

Cosolvency—Solvent blending to dissolve certain compounds is widely used in the preparation of solution dosage forms. Because of the limited number of solvents that can be used in a dosage form, most solvent mixtures consist of water, alcohol, glycerin, propylene glycol, and syrups. This range of solvents is somewhat expanded with dosage forms intended for external use.

Cosolvency may be considered as either a modification of the polarity of the solvent system to approach that of the solute or the formation of a completely new solvent whose interactions cannot be easily predicted from the interactions of the individual components of the solvent mixture. It is much easier to predict solubilities of nonpolar or semipolar compounds in 20% ethanol in water than to predict solubilities of the same compounds in a water-ethanol-glycerin-sorbitol solvent system. Cosolvency should be differentiated from the closely related phenomenon of solubilization.

Temperature—Most compounds of pharmaceutical value become more soluble as the temperature increases.

Salting-Out—The addition of large amounts of highly soluble salts to aqueous solutions of organic compounds often leads to precipitation or separation of organic solutes. This phenomenon is attributed to competition between the salts and the organic compounds for solvent molecules, i.e., water. The salting-out power of a salt depends on the size and valence of its ions. In general, macromolecules and association colloids are easier to salt-out than other organic compounds.

Salting-In—This is the increase in solubility of an organic compound upon the addition of a salt. The mechanism of this effect is unknown and the phenomenon is rarely encountered or recognized in the formulation of solution dosage forms. The increase in the solubility of nonpolar organic compounds by the addition of micelle-forming electrolytes should not be considered as a salting-in effect but rather a solubilizing effect. An example of salting-in is the solubility behavior of the class of proteins known as globulins. These compounds are insoluble in water and soluble in dilute salt solutions.

Complex Formation—Insoluble compounds often interact with a soluble ingredient to form a soluble complex. The formation of the soluble triiodide complex (I_3^-) from (I_2) and (I^-) is well known. Xanthines are slightly soluble in water, but they form soluble hydrogen-bonded complexes with salicylates, benzoates, and other compounds. Caffeine is soluble to the extent of about 1 g/50 ml of water, while Caffeine and Sodium Benzoate USP is soluble to the extent of 1 g/1.2 ml water. In utilizing this approach for increasing the solubility of a compound, one has to make sure that the complex is reversible, dissociates easily, and releases the active ingredient, otherwise the active ingredient becomes therapeutically ineffective.

Common-Ion Effect—Drugs which are unstable in solution are often formulated as suspensions with the solid particles in equilibrium with their saturated solution. To reduce the amount of drug ions in solution, and thereby increase the stability of the dosage form, a salt of the counter ion of the drug is included in the formulation. Penicillin is very unstable in solutions. A suspension of procaine penicillin is in equilibrium with its saturated solution which contains procaine cations and penicillin anions in amounts governed by the solubility product Ksp of the compound.

$$Ksp = [\text{Procaine}][\text{Penicillin}]$$

If procaine hydrochloride, a soluble ionic compound, is added to the suspension, the concentration term for procaine cations in the above equation is greatly increased. Since the solubility product is constant at constant temperature, it follows that the concentration of penicillin ions in solution decreases drastically. This effectively removes the unstable species from solution and thereby increases the shelf-life of the preparation.

Particle Size—The effect of particle size of the solute on its solubility is manifested only when the particles are submicron in size; an increase of about 10% in solubility is then observed. This increase is due to the large surface free energy associated with small particles. This increase in solubility is important in colloidal systems which are not intended for systemic absorption, such as barium sulfate magma, where a slight increase in solubility might cause harmful effects.

Molecular Size and Shape—The solvent properties of water are due in part to the small size of its molecules. Liquids which are similar to water in polarity, dielectric constant, and hydrogen-bonding may be poor solvents for ionic compounds, because of the larger size of their molecules; it is difficult for them to penetrate and dissolve the crystals.

The shape of the solute molecule is also a factor to be considered in the study of solubility. The high solubility of ammonia in water is attributed in part to the shape of the ammonia molecule which fits without difficulty in the structure of water. The effect of the shape of the solute molecule on its solubility in a given solvent is predominantly an entropy effect.

Macromolecular Solutions

Macromolecules are compounds with molecular weights ranging from 10,000 to millions. Examples of pharmaceutical macromolecules are plasma proteins, enzymes, natural polysaccharides, synthetic cellulose derivatives, and synthetic polymers such as polyvinyl pyrrolidone and carbopol. Solubility behavior of macromolecules depends on molecular weight, ionic character, shape, pH, temperature, and added salts. Aqueous solutions are generally highly viscous and many form gels at low concentrations. These properties are the basis for the extensive use of macromolecules as thickening and suspending agents in dosage forms.

Incompatibilities of macromolecular solutions include binding, and often inactivation, of small molecules and ions. Interaction with other macromolecules results in precipitation or phase separation; and ionic macromolecules exhibit the usual acid-base incompatibilities. In addition, macromolecules are susceptible to microbial attack which results in degradation evidenced by loss of viscosity.

The broad range of molecular weight of macromolecules makes it necessary to express the concentration of their solutions on a percentage rather than on a molar or molal basis. A 5% w/v solution of a polymer whose molecular weight is 100,000 is $0.0005M$. Such low values are inconvenient to deal with routinely.

Association Colloids

The salt sodium formate,

$$\text{H}-\overset{\displaystyle O}{\underset{\displaystyle }{C}}-\text{O}^- \text{Na}^+$$

is soluble in water and the gas ethane, CH_3CH_3 is insoluble. If these two entities are parts of a single molecule as in sodium propionate,

$$CH_3CH_2 - C \overset{O}{\diagup} O^- \ Na^+$$

the molecule consists of hydrophobic and hydrophilic segments. This double property of the molecule leads to two opposing tendencies, one is to dissolve in water and the other to remain insoluble. The net effect of these two tendencies or forces determines the extent of solubility. In the case of sodium propionate, the hydrophilic property predominates and the salt is soluble in water. On the other hand hydrophobic properties predominate in the molecule of sodium hexacosanoate (cerotate),

$$CH_3(CH_2)_{24}C \overset{O}{\diagup} O^- \ Na^+$$

and the salt is insoluble in water.

Compounds which have a molecular weight intermediate between the preceding two examples will exhibit a compromise behavior in aqueous solution. Thus, instead of being dissolved as individual ions or being completely insoluble, the ions aggregate in aqueous media in such a way as to minimize the contact of the nonpolar chains with water. The aggregates, called micelles, fall in the colloidal range, hence the name association colloids. If sodium laurate,

$$CH_3(CH_2)_{10} - C \overset{O}{\diagup} O^- \ Na^+$$

is added in increasing amounts to water, the first few molecules are individually dispersed. The carboxylate group is hydrated while the hydrocarbon chain is somewhat rigidly held in a cage of "iceberg" water. As the concentration increases the ionized molecules aggregate into spherical micelles with the ionic groups oriented toward the water and the hydrocarbon chains buried inside the micelles where they create a nonpolar region. The sodium ions bind to the surface of the highly charged micelle

and the degree of ionization of these micelles is generally low. The driving force for micellization is generally considered to be the entropy increase accompanying the process. This is derived from the entropy increase of water (iceberg → normal) and the entropy increase of the hydrocarbon chain as it goes from an aqueous to a nonpolar environment inside the micelle. The concentration of surface active agents at which micelles form is called the critical micelle concentration (cmc), above which any further increase in the concentration increases the number of micelles in solution. At very high concentrations of very soluble surfactants, the shape and structure of micelles changes from spherical to lamellar or liquid crystalline. At any concentration above the cmc, the micelles are in equilibrium with molecularly dispersed species and this equilibrium can be shifted to increase or decrease the number of micelles in a system.

The practical aspect of micellization is the ability to put into solution compounds which are otherwise insoluble in aqueous solutions. Compounds which are insoluble or slightly soluble in water due to their nonpolar structure, e.g., vitamins A and D, steroids, and volatile oils can be solubilized by being incorporated in the nonpolar interior of the micelles. The resulting solubilized solutions are clear and thermodynamically stable.

Micellization and solubilization are very sensitive to the variables of the system. The cmc, number of molecules of solubilizer/micelle, degree of ionization of micelles, and number of molecules of solubilizate (compounds that are solubilized)/micelle are functions of the concentrations of solubilizer and solubilizate, temperature, electrolytes, and other components such as ethanol, glycerin, urea, fatty acids, and long-chain alcohols. In general, factors which tend to increase the solubility of the surfactant increase the cmc. Soaps do not form micelles in ethanol but exist as molecular dispersions since there is no reason for the alkyl chain of the soap to be removed from the bulk of the solvent. The cmc's of ionic surfactants increase and those of nonionics decrease with an increase in temperature. Of particular interest is the effect of electrolytes on cmc. Electrolytes in low concentrations cause a marked decrease in cmc. The cmc of sodium lauryl sulfate is 0.234% with an average number n of 62 molecules/micelle. In 0.20 *M* sodium chloride the cmc is 0.026% and n is 101.

Association colloids can be either anionic, e.g., sodium lauryl sulfate; cationic, e.g., benzalkonium chloride; or nonionic, e.g., polysorbate 80. Amphoteric compounds such as lecithin are also micelle formers but their use in pharmacy is limited. Most association colloids form micelles in water as well as in nonpolar organic solvents. The shape and structure of micelles in nonpolar solvents is different from those in water. Nonaqueous solubilized systems are rarely encountered in pharmaceutical practice. Nonionic solubilizers are the most widely used group because they are less toxic and more compatible with ionic drugs and formulations than ionic solubilizers.

The effects of solubilization on the solubilizate are complex and depend among other factors on the nature of the components. The chemical stability may be altered in a favorable or unfavorable way. The hydrolysis of an ester for example might be enhanced or retarded upon solubilization. Complex formation or strong binding between solubilizer and solubilizate is also a possibility that affects the release and biological availability of the solubilized active ingredients.

Pharmaceutical Aspects

During the preparation of any pharmaceutically acceptable solution, due consideration must be given to acid-base properties, buffers, isotonicity, viscosity, dissolution rate, toxicity, stability, percentage strength, and its advantages and disadvantages as a form of medication.

Acid-Base Properties—Many drugs are weak acids or weak bases and the preparation, solubility, and incompatibilities of these drugs depend on their acid-base properties. The Brønsted-Lowry theory of acids and bases defines an acid as a proton donor and a base as a proton acceptor. A strong acid releases its protons readily while a weak acid dissociates only slightly. A strong base has a very high affinity for protons while a weak base has a low affinity. The ionization or dissociation constant of a chemical species is a measure of its affinity for protons.

Buffers—A buffer solution is a system that resists changes in pH. Solutions of a weak acid and its salts, a weak base and its salts, or a protein, act as buffers. If a base is added to a solution containing equimolar concentrations of a weak acid and its salt, the base is neutralized by the weak acid forming more of the salt and the resulting increase in pH is slight. Likewise if an acid is added to solutions of weak bases and their salts, only a small decrease in pH is observed. Typical buffer systems used in pharmaceutical preparations include acetate-acetic acid, bicarbonate-carbonate, borate-boric acid, and Na_2HPO_4—NaH_2PO_4.

The properties of buffers are illustrated in the following example: The pH of a solution of sodium acetate-acetic acid is given by the Henderson-Hasselbalch equation

$$pH = pKa + \log \frac{[Acetate]}{[Acetic\ acid]}, pKa = 4.76$$

The addition of a strong base, e.g., NaOH increases the concentration of acetate and decreases by an equal amount the concentration of the acid

$$pH = 4.76 + \log \frac{[acetate + base]}{[acetic\ acid - base]}$$

The efficiency of buffers is measured by the function known as *buffer capacity*. Buffer capacity is defined as the amount, in gram-equivalents per liter, of strong acid or strong base, required to change the pH of a solution by one unit. In the above acetate buffer, the buffer capacity is: moles of NaOH added/change of pH. Analysis of the preceding equation shows that the buffer capacity depends on the absolute concentrations of the salt and acid and on their ratio. It is obvious that a 0.5 M acetate buffer at pH 4.76 has a higher buffer capacity than a 0.05 M buffer. For a fixed total acetate-acetic acid concentration the buffer capacity is maximum at a ratio of 1/1, i.e., when pH = pKa, and decreases steadily as this ratio changes. In choosing a buffer system therefore the pKa of the acid should be close to the desired pH of the final system.

Most weak acids and bases of pharmaceutical value are insoluble or slightly soluble in water while their salts are soluble. Many exceptions of course exist, such as ammonia, acetic acid, citric acid, and triethanolamine, but the previous generalization is necessary since it alerts the formulator to the possible pH-dependent incompatibilities. Such incompatibilities are encountered when salts of weak acids and strong bases are mixed with acidic vehicles. Barbiturate salts for example cannot be prepared in vehicles such as orange syrup or wild cherry syrup, otherwise the insoluble weak acids will precipitate. Likewise, salts of weak bases and strong acids are incompatible with basic vehicles. The specific incompatibilities of acidic and basic drugs and their salts are discussed in Chapter 13.

During the formulation of solutions of acidic and basic drugs, three factors must be considered: (1) the solubility of ionized and unionized forms of the drug, (2) the chemical stability of the drug as functions of the pH and the buffer components, and (3) the therapeutic or pharmaceutical efficacy of the drug. The buffer pH and buffer type are selected to maintain a proper balance between these three variables.

Isotonicity—Biological systems are compatible with solutions which have similar osmotic pressures, i.e., equivalent number of dissolved species. If tissues, cells, or membranes come in contact with aqueous solutions which have osmotic pressures that are not close to that of the biological systems, damage or injury, manifested as cell lysis or irritation and pain, results. The adjustment of solute concentration in a dosage form to make it isotonic with body fluids is therefore necessary to avoid these undesirable effects.

If body membranes are assumed to act as perfect semipermeable membranes, that is, membranes which are permeable only to water and impermeable to all other solute species, the principles of colligative properties can be applied to calculate or measure the concentration of a given drug that is isotonic with blood and other tissue fluids. They can be used to determine the contribution of a given drug concentration to the osmotic pressure of a solution, and thus make it possible to adjust the osmotic pressure or tonicity by the addition of sodium chloride, dextrose, or other inert ingredients. Both blood plasma and 0.9% sodium chloride have the same freezing point of −0.52°C. Thus, red blood cells, blood plasma, and 0.9% sodium chloride solution contain the same number of solute particles and they are iso-osmotic and isotonic. Any drug solution which has a freezing point of −0.52°C is, therefore, iso-osmotic with blood. The therapeutic concentration of many drugs yields hypotonic solutions because of the low concentration of the active ingredient and it is necessary to make these solutions isotonic by the addition of sodium chloride.

The sodium chloride equivalent method is frequently used in the calculation of the amount of sodium chloride necessary to prepare isotonic drug solutions. The sodium chloride equivalent is defined as the amount of sodium chloride that is osmotically equivalent to 1 g of the drug. The sodium chloride equivalent of amphetamine sulfate is 0.22. This means that a 1% solution of amphetamine sulfate is osmotically equivalent to a 0.22% solution of sodium chloride and that it is hypotonic. Addition of 0.9–0.22 = 0.68 g of sodium chloride/100 ml of the 1% solution of amphetamine sulfate results in an isotonic solution. Another method of preparing the 1% solution is to prepare an isotonic solution of amphetamine sulfate by dissolving 1 g in 24 ml of water (0.22 g sodium chloride in 24 ml water is isotonic) and adding 76 ml of 0.9% sodium chloride (actually, 75.5 ml contains 0.68 g). The sodium chloride equivalent varies with the concentration of the drug. For example, the equivalent for morphine sulfate has a value of 0.16 at 0.5% and 0.09 at 5% concentrations.

This discussion is based on the assumption that biological membranes behave as ideal semipermeable membranes. In fact, biological membranes are completely or partially permeable to a number of drugs and in these cases the use of colligative properties data in preparing iso-osmotic solutions with blood is incorrect since the solutions will always be hypotonic. A solution of urea that has the same osmotic pressure and freezing point as 0.9% sodium chloride is not isotonic but rather hypotonic to red blood cells simply because urea molecules pass freely in and out of the red blood cell membrane. Other compounds that exhibit this property are ethanol, glycerin, boric acid, monovalent ammonium compounds, ascorbic acid, lactic acid, etc.

In preparing isotonic solutions for injection or ophthalmic solutions, an approximate adjustment of isotonicity is often satisfactory, particularly if the osmotic or permeability properties of the drug are not known exactly. It should be emphasized that the consequences of the administration of hypotonic solutions are usually more serious than those of hypertonic solutions. The effects also depend on the volume of solution and the site of administration, as for example, subcutaneous injections vs intravenous fluids. It is obvious that the isotonicity of intravenous fluids should be controlled more rigorously than the isotonicity of small volume subcutaneous injections.

Viscosity—Viscosity is a measure of resistance to flow and can be regarded as an indication of friction, on the molecular level, between planes of liquid moving past each other. The degree of interactions and structuring as well as the shape of the components determine the flow characteristics of a solution. The addition of any compound to water changes its viscosity and the change is related to the effects of the compound on the structure of water. Ions which are structure makers increase the viscosity and structure-breaking ions produce the opposite effect.

This effect, especially in dilute solutions, is of little practical value in the preparation of solution dosage forms, however. More important are the viscosity effects observed in solutions of macromolecules, association colloids, and concentrated solutions of micromolecules such as syrups or glycerin-water systems. The high viscosity of these solutions retards all diffusional processes in the system and markedly decreases the dissolution rate. This reduction might be erroneously interpreted as a lack of solubility of the drug. The viscosity of the solution also affects the formation of insoluble compounds, caused by incompatibilities in the system. The addition of a small volume of a solution of sodium phenobarbital to wild cherry syrup should result in the precipitation of phenobarbital but because of the high viscosity of the syrup, precipitation is observed only after an extended period of time. High viscosity of solutions, in some cases, enhances the therapeutic efficacy of a drug. The inclusion of methylcellulose in ophthalmic solutions increases the absorption of active ingredients by increasing the contact time between the solution and the surface of the eye. In this case, increasing the viscosity of the solution increases its resistance to removal by the lacrimal fluid. Finally, the viscosity of a solution affects any diffusion-dependent process, whether it be in the preparation, storage, or application of the solution. It is a general rule that pharmacists never dissolve a solid drug directly in a viscous vehicle but dissolve it in a minimum quantity of water or other solvent of low viscosity and add the resulting solution to the viscous vehicle.

Dissolution Rate—The dissolution rate of a drug in a solvent is distinct from its solubility. Solubility is the amount of drug that can be molecularly dispersed in a given amount of a solvent. The dissolution rate is the rate at which the solute changes from a crystal, powder, liquid, or other state into a molecular dispersion in the solvent. The dissolution rate and the factors that influence it are becoming increasingly more important in determining the biological availability of drugs, particularly those in solid or suspension dosage forms.

The pharmacist may be faced with the problem of dissolving a drug in the shortest possible time. The dissolution rate depends on many factors, such as:

1. Particle size of the solute. Smaller particles have a higher specific surface area and therefore more contact with the solvent which results in higher rates of dissolution.
2. Conditions on the surface of the particle. The adsorption of gases on the surface of fine particles can prevent wetting and decrease the dissolution rate, particularly in aqueous media. Solutions of highly soluble compounds can be prepared by directly adding the crystals to the solvent, while those of slightly soluble compounds can be prepared by adding the freshly powdered drug to the solvent.
3. Viscosity of the solvent. If the solvent has a high viscosity, the diffusion rate of molecules dissolving from the surface of the particle to the bulk of the medium is reduced accordingly and the dissolution rate is thereby affected.
4. Temperature increases the kinetic energy of solvent and solute molecules, decreases the viscosity, and accelerates diffusional processes, thus causing an increase in the dissolution rate. Heat, therefore, is usually employed in accelerating the dissolution of thermostable compounds.
5. Mechanical agitation increases the dissolution rate but complications might arise in preparing solutions of surface active agents, film forming macromolecules, and sensitive biological products such as enzymes. Surfactants, by producing a large volume of foam which may require a long time to collapse, make it difficult to make up to volume. Macromolecules also form very stable and viscous foams and enzymes might be denatured when exposed continuously to the air-water interface. Vigorous agitation is not recommended in these cases.

Difficulties are often encountered in preparing solutions of water-soluble macromolecules such as proteins, polysaccharides, cellulose derivatives, and synthetic polymers. When these solids are added to water, they invariably form large aggregates (clumps) whose dissolution rate is very low. This is attributed to the fact that when water comes into contact with a number of small particles it hydrates the surface and forms a very viscous film that envelopes the particles inside, thus preventing or delaying any further contact with water. These compounds can be put in solution in a short period of time by wetting them with a nonsolvent such as alcohol or glycerin and then adding water. In cases where the use of wetting agents is not feasible, the powders should be added in small increments each of which should be dissolved completely before the next is added.

Toxicity—The primary consideration in the selection of a solvent or a vehicle is its toxicity. An excellent solvent cannot be used as a pharmaceutical solvent if it has any harmful biological effects. It is obvious then that the number of solvents that can be used in preparing dosage forms is very limited.

Water, by far, is the most commonly used solvent and in cases where the drug is insoluble in water alone, its solvent properties can be modified by the addition of alcohol, glycerin, propylene glycol, or nonionic solubilizing agents. Vegetable oils and mineral oil are often used as solvents for nonpolar drugs. Many common solvents such as acetone, chloroform, carbon tetrachloride, and ether *cannot* be used in solution dosage forms because of their toxicity. Other solvents used in dosage forms include polyethylene glycols, propylene carbonate, hexanetriol, benzyl benzoate, and *N,N*-dimethylacetamide.

Stability—It is not sufficient to formulate a solution dosage form that has the desired concentrations of the active ingredients, pH, color, flavor, and ionic strength. The shelf-life or physicochemical stability of the dosage form should also be a major consideration in the formulation. The *chemical* stability of the active ingredients is of primary importance and the formulation should be designed to minimize hydrolysis, oxidation, reduction, polymerization, or any other chemical alteration of the active ingredients. It should be emphasized, however, that stability of a dosage form is not synonymous with chemical stability of the active ingredients. Instability, also includes color fading, flavor loss, cloudiness or precipitation, microbial growth, viscosity decrease, and binding to the container or rubber closures (e.g., multiple-dose vials). It also includes instability of the physicochemical system comprising the dosage form, e.g., caking of suspensions or cracking of emulsions. It is not uncommon therefore to find in relatively simple formulations such additives as buffers, antimicrobials, antioxidants, and polymerization inhibitors. Because of the complexity of preparing solutions with an extended shelf-life, many drugs are prepared as "powders for solution" to be reconstituted immediately before use.

Percentage Solutions—The amount of a drug in a formulation is often expressed as a per cent strength. The USP states that:

Percentage concentrations of solutions are expressed as follows:

Percent weight in weight—(w/w) expresses the number of g of a constituent in 100 g of solution.

Percent weight in volume—(w/v) expresses the number of g of a constituent in 100 ml of solution, and is used regardless of whether water or another liquid is the solvent.

Percent volume in volume—(v/v) expresses the number of ml of a constituent in 100 ml of solution.

The term *percent* used without qualification means, for mixtures of solids, percent weight in weight; for solutions or suspensions of solids in liquids, percent weight in volume; and for solutions of gases in liquids, percent weight in volume. For example a 1% solution is prepared by dissolving 1 g of a solid or 1 ml of a liquid in sufficient quantities of the solvent to make 100 ml of the solution.

In the dispensing of prescription medications, slight changes in volume owing to variations in room temperature may be disregarded.

The strength of a solution can also be expressed as parts of solute per million parts of solution (ppm) or as the number of parts of solution that contain 1 part of the solute (ratio strength). A solution of 1:10,000 of benzalkonium chloride in water contains 1 g of benzalkonium chloride in 10,000 ml of solution. The per cent strength of this solution is 0.01% *w/v*.

In preparing saturated solutions of highly soluble drugs, the volume occupied by the solute should be taken into account. Saturated potassium iodide solution contains 100 g of KI in 100 ml of solution. This does not mean that 100 g are dissolved in 100 ml of water, but rather that enough water is added to dissolve the 100 g to produce a saturated solution. In this case about 87.0 ml of water are required.

Prescriptions

1

| ℞ Sodium iodide | 15 g |
| Aqua q.s. | 180 ml |

Sig: 5 ml diluted p.c.

2

℞ Aluminum chloride	15%
Formaldehyde	2%
Sig: Use as directed	120 ml

3

| ℞ Merthiolate 1-1000 | 120 ml |

Sig: Dilute 1 to 8 parts of water.

4

| ℞ Adrenaline chloride 1:1000 sol. | 30 ml |
| (Parke Davis) | |

Sig: Used as directed.

5

| ℞ Sol. Atropine sulfat. 1:3000 | 15 ml |

Sig: Gtts. ii before nursing.

6

| ℞ Sat. Boric Acid Sol. | 473 ml |

Sig: For wet dressings to leg.

7

℞ Cocaine hydrochloride	130 mg
Sol. epinephrine 1:1000	4 ml
Vehicle, buffered and	
isotonic q.s.	30 ml

Sig: Use in eye as directed.

8

℞ Pilocarpine HCl   50 mg
   Phosphate buffer soln.
        q.s. ad   10 ml
   Sig: Instil 1 drop in each eye as often as neces-
   sary to maintain miosis.

9

℞ Codeine sulfate   130 mg
   Ammonium chloride   4 g

   Elix. terpin hydrate
        q.s. ad   90 ml
   Sig: 5 ml q 3–4 h.

10

℞ Phenobarbital   400 mg
   Tinct. Belladonna   10 ml
   Elix. Lactated Pepsin   q.s.   90 ml
   M. Sig: 5 ml t.i.d. p.c.

Emulsion Technology

A particularly simple and useful definition of an emulsion is:

An emulsion is a heterogeneous system, consisting of at least one immiscible liquid intimately dispersed in another in the form of droplets, whose diameters, in general, exceed 0.1 μm. (Ref. 2.)

This type of system is inherently unstable since if there is no interference the droplets of the dispersed liquid will coalesce (i.e., unite) to form larger droplets. This process will naturally continue until all of the dispersed droplets have coalesced. A third component, an emulsifying agent, is required to prepare a usable emulsion. Its purpose is to prevent coalescence and maintain the integrity of the individual droplets of dispersed liquid.

Emulsion Type and Terminology

Emulsions are generally considered as two-phase systems. The liquid or phase in the form of droplets is called the dispersed phase, the internal phase, or the discontinuous phase; the remaining liquid is termed the dispersion medium, the external phase, or the continuous phase.

Any two immiscible liquids can theoretically form an emulsion; however, in pharmaceutical applications one of the phases is usually water or an aqueous solution. It follows that the remaining phase is nonaqueous, most importantly lipid or oily in nature. Such lipids can range from vegetable or hydrocarbon oils to semisolid hydrocarbons and waxes.

It is customary to describe emulsions in terms of water and oil. Oil is used here as a generic term to refer to the lipid or nonaqueous phase regardless of its composition. If water is the internal phase, the emulsion is classified as a water-in-oil (W/O) type. The converse is true; if water is the external phase, the emulsion is classified as an oil-in-water (O/W) type.

The type of emulsion is influenced primarily by two factors; the ratio of the phases (i.e., the relative phase volume) and the emulsifying agent. The maximum concentration of internal phase for an ideal emulsion composed of uniform perfectly spherical droplets is 74%. This maximum is based on a consideration of packing arrangements of geometric figures in a closed space. Thus, theoretically one could prepare an O/W emulsion containing up to but not greater than 74% oil. This ideal case is usually found to hold true in practice; however, this maximum can be exceeded under certain circumstances.

The more important factor of the two is the nature or properties of the emulsifying agent. Most of them preferentially will form one type of emulsion or the other if the phase volume permits. Acacia, for example, nearly always will form O/W type of emulsions.

Most common O/W emulsions are creamy white in appearance regardless of the oil used. In fact, the color is an indication of the relative droplet size. Fairly coarse emulsions are yellowish in color. The color becomes whiter and develops a bluish tinge as the droplet size becomes smaller. In the extreme, at generally 0.05 μm or smaller the droplets are no longer detected by the human eye and the emulsion appears transparent. These are special preparations termed microemulsions and are usually classified as colloidal dispersions rather than emulsions.

The appearance of W/O emulsions is more glassy and translucent rather than creamy and depends more on the nature of the oil.

Several methods are available to determine the type of emulsion. Some of the more common methods follow.

Drop Dilution Test—This method is based on the principle that an emulsion is miscible with its external phase. Consequently, if water is added to an O/W emulsion, it will readily disperse in the emulsion. If an oil is added, it does not disperse without vigorous agitation. The reverse is true with W/O emulsions.

Dye Solubility Test—This test is based on the principle that a dye disperses uniformly throughout an emulsion, if the dye is soluble in the external phase. Amaranth, a water-soluble dye readily tints an O/W emulsion but not a W/O emulsion. An oil-soluble dye readily tints a W/O emulsion but not an O/W type.

Direction of Creaming Test—Creaming is the process of sedimentation of the dispersed droplets (either upward or downward) due to the difference in densities of the internal and external phases. If the relative densities of the two phases are known, the direction of creaming of the dispersed phase indicates the type of emulsion present. In most pharmaceutical systems the density of the oil or lipid phase is less than that of the aqueous phase; thus, if the emulsion creams upward, the emulsion is the O/W type. Conversely, if the emulsion creams downward, it is of the W/O type.

Electrical Conductivity Test—This test is based on the principle that water or aqueous solutions conduct an electric current while oils do not. If electrodes, placed in an emulsion, conduct an electric current, an O/W emulsion is indicated. If the system does not conduct an electric current, the emulsion is of the W/O type.

Fluorescence Test—Many oils fluoresce when exposed to ultraviolet light. If a drop of an emulsion is examined in fluorescent light under a microscope and the entire field fluoresces, a W/O emulsion is indicated. However, if the emulsion is of the O/W type the fluorescence is spotty.

Pharmaceutical Applications

The first pharmaceutical emulsion dates back to the 2nd century. Galen, born in 130 A.D., was the originator of a formula for a cream that is very similar to Rose Water Ointment NF. In fact, most creams and lotions intended for topical use are emulsions. Oleaginous materials intended for topical application have greater acceptance and appeal if they are in the emulsified state.

By incorporating active ingredients into an emulsion, objectionable-tasting medicinal agents may be rendered more palatable and administered more conveniently. The characteristic unpleasant taste of cod liver oil, e.g., can be masked by incorporating it into the internal phase of an O/W emulsion. The external phase may be suitably flavored to enhance the masking effect. Mineral Oil Emulsion NF is an example of such an application.

The action of certain active ingredients is prolonged by incorporation into a specialized emulsion vehicle. Oil-soluble drugs dissolved in oil and injected as an O/W emulsion into a muscle mass can serve as a depot providing a sustained blood level for hours or even days. Another application of this prolonged-action principle is the preparation of sterile emulsions of allergenic principles where an oil is the external phase. Intravenous emulsions have been formulated to contain fats, oils, carbohydrates, vitamins, and other nutrients to be administered as replacement therapy for debilitated patients. Oil- and water-soluble vitamins are formulated as clear, transparent emulsions.

In the formulation of foam aerosols, the propellant is emulsified with water or some other solvent system that contains the active ingredient. To maintain the emulsion characteristics, this system usually requires agitation prior to dispensing. Such pressurized emulsions present features that are not usually or easily attained with conventional emulsions.

Theory of Emulsions

In general, to understand emulsion systems and the theory associated with the technology of emulsification and stabilization, certain fundamentals of surface chemistry should be reviewed. It is the surface, or more correctly the interface between the two liquids which plays the dominant role in sustaining a dispersed system. The addition of an emulsifying agent or agents affects the interface in such a way that stable emulsions may be achieved. An emulsifying agent or other agents included in an emulsion formula determine, for the most part, the bulk properties of the final product.

Surface Tension of Pure Liquids— In a pure liquid, the molecules in the bulk of the liquid are attracted equally on all sides by the surrounding molecules, whereas at the surface the liquid molecules are pulled inward toward the liquid because of the unbalanced attractive forces. This view is depicted in an idealized manner in Fig. 1. As the surface molecules are pulled toward the bulk liquid, a stress or tension is produced called the surface tension. From an energy point of view, surface tension may be regarded as being due to the tendency of a liquid to reduce its surface to a point of minimum potential energy, a condition requisite for stable surface equilibrium. Since a sphere has the smallest area for a given volume, the tendency of a liquid particle is to draw itself into a sphere is due to the action of surface tension.

To expand the surface of a liquid, energy in the form of work must be exerted to overcome the tendency of the surface molecules to move into the bulk liquid. This statement may be quantitized in the expression

$$\gamma = W/\Delta A \qquad (1)$$

where γ is the surface tension, W is the work required to expand a surface, and ΔA is the increase in the surface area. If W is expressed in ergs and ΔA is given in cm^2, the surface tension would be expressed as $ergs/cm^2$. Surface tension thus may be defined as the work in ergs necessary to generate 1 cm^2 of surface.

Even though the surface tension as $ergs/cm^2$ is quite acceptable, the more conventional unit used in the literature is dynes/cm. Since an erg is equal to a dyne-cm, it can be seen that the numer-

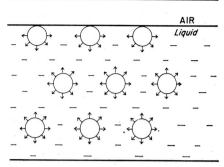

Fig. 1—Forces acting on molecules on the surface and in the interior of a liquid.

ical values for surface tension will be identical no matter which units are used.

It is customary to refer to the tension existing between a liquid and air as surface tension and between two immiscible liquids as interfacial tension. Table 4 includes the interfacial tension of a number of liquids against water. It should be noted that the more closely a liquid resembles water, or the greater the possible interaction across the interface between a liquid and water, the lower will be the interfacial tension. Thus, n-octyl alcohol resembles water more so than does n-octane because of the hydroxyl group and has a lower interfacial tension, 8.52 dynes/cm vs 50.8 dynes/cm.

Surface Tension of Solutions—If an electrolyte such as sodium chloride is added to water, it dissociates into a positive and a negative ion. Each ion is strongly hydrated and prefers energeti-

Table 4—Interfacial Tension of Liquids Against Water at 20°C[3]

Liquid	Interfacial tension (dynes/cm)
n-Hexane	51.0
n-Octane	50.8
Toluene	36.1
Benzene	35.0
Chloroform	32.8
Olive oil	22.9
Oleic acid	15.6
Ethyl ether	10.7
n-Octyl alcohol	8.52
Methyl propyl ketone	6.28

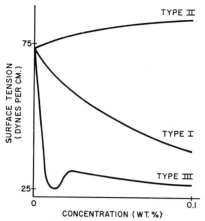

Fig. 2—The principal types of surface-tension concentration curves.[4]

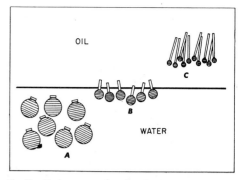

Fig. 3—Three types of molecules having both polar and nonpolar properties: *A*, strong polar group; *B*, polar and nonpolar groups of equal strength, and *C*, strong nonpolar group.

cally to remain in the bulk of the solution rather than to reside at the surface. Consequently, the water molecules at the surface will be attracted more strongly to the bulk of the solution creating a greater tension at the surface. The result is an increase in surface tension as electrolytes or ions are added to water or a solution. Such behavior is indicated by the Type II curve in Fig. 2.

Non-electrolytes such as ethanol or sucrose, on the other hand, are not so strongly hydrated in solution and can be found at the surface as well as in the bulk of a solution. When such molecules reside at the surface they interfere or weaken the water–water interactions and cause a small decrease in the surface tension as indicated by the Type I curve in Fig. 2.

Combining the properties of an ion or electrolyte with a non-electrolyte, or better yet a lipid into a single molecule, results in a compound having a tremendous influence on the surface tension of solutions as shown by the Type III curve in Fig. 2. Such molecules are called surface-active agents.

Surface Orientation—A surface-active agent or surfactant contains a polar group and a nonpolar group and is strongly oriented at the interface of an oil and water mixture. It orients itself in such a way that the polar (hydrophilic) group faces the water, while the nonpo-

lar (lipophilic) group faces the oil. Fig. 3 represents three possible situations. The rectangle and circle are employed to depict the nonpolar and polar groups, respectively.

Consider a molecule having a much larger polar group than nonpolar group. This type of molecule is more soluble in the water and it moves away from the oil and enters the main portion of the water. The molecule with a large nonpolar group migrates into the main portion of the oil phase. A surfactant molecule having equal hydrophilic and lipophilic character would be oriented exactly at the interface.

This picture is extremely idealized and does not truly represent a real system. In a real system, there is always a distribution of molecules so that some are situated in the body of the liquid and some at the interface, whether the molecules possess large polar or large nonpolar groups.

Emulsification Process—The first objective to be attained in emulsification is to reduce the internal phase (oil or water) into small droplets. This can be accomplished only if an external source of energy in the form of work is applied. It is possible to calculate this amount of work required from a rearrangement of Eq. 1:

$$W = \gamma \Delta A \qquad (2)$$

For example, if 1 ml of mineral oil is

dispersed into droplets of 1.0 μm (10^{-4} cm) diameter in 1 ml of water, the surface area of the oil droplets is 6×10^6 cm^2. Using this as an approximation of ΔA and a value of 57 ergs/cm^2 for the interfacial tension between mineral oil and water, the work of emulsification may be calculated from Eq. 2 as

$$W = (57 \text{ ergs/cm}^2) \times (6 \times 10^6 \text{ cm}^2)$$
$$= 34 \times 10^7 \text{ ergs or 8 calories}$$

If a surfactant is added which lowers the interfacial tension to 1 dyne/cm, the work required would be reduced to about 0.14 cal. Thus, the addition of a surface-active agent greatly reduces the amount of energy needed to produce an emulsion.

This energy or work can also be interpreted as surface free energy or excess potential energy which makes an emulsion unstable. No disperse system is truly stable from an energy standpoint unless W approaches zero. There will always be a degree of instability in an emulsion since it is not possible to reduce the interfacial tension to zero.

The surface free energy, however small, will promote coalescence and destruction of the emulsion. Fortunately, emulsifying agents also present some sort of mechanical barrier to coalescence which counterbalances the surface free energy. Three possible mechanisms are

Interfacial Film—Some emulsifying agents (e.g., acacia) do not markedly reduce the interfacial tension but are thought to function primarily by forming a strong pliable film around the dispersed droplet.

Charge Repulsion—Oil droplets in an aqueous phase usually possess an electrical charge developed either from the nature of the emulsifying agent or by adsorbing ions from solution. Such a charge, if great enough, can cause the droplets to repel each other and act as a mechanical barrier to coalescence.

Steric Repulsion—Water droplets in an oily phase are prevented from contacting each other by the long hydrocarbon chain of the surfactant or emulsifying agent molecule.

Experience has shown that an emulsifying agent that is more hydrophilic than hydrophobic usually produces an O/W emulsion, while one that is more hydrophobic usually forms a W/O emulsion. This tendency was noted a number of years ago and it was concluded that the phase in which the emulsifying agent was more soluble would be the continuous or external phase.

The most complete and theoretically sound discussion of the emulsification process has been presented by Davies[8] who demonstrated experimentally and mathematically that an emulsion type can be predicted in model systems. In general it has been postulated that when an emulsion is prepared, an O/W and W/O emulsion form simultaneously. From the original mixture of the two types of emulsion, one type emerges at the expense of the other and directly depends on the rate of coalescence of the dispersed particles in both types of emulsion. In other words, a W/O emulsion finally forms if the rate of coalescence of oil droplets is greater than the rate of coalescence of water droplets.

Emulsifying Agents

Any compound that can lower interfacial tension, form a film at an interface, or orient at an interface can potentially function as an emulsifying agent. The discussion here will be limited to those compounds or agents that are readily available to the practitioner, have been traditionally available to the practitioner, or have some unique property or quality that make them unusually valuable to the practitioner. A short usable list is deemed more valuable than an exhaustive survey.

Hydrophilic Colloids

These are collectively macromolecular materials that do not exhibit a marked reduction of interfacial tension but are thought to function as emulsifying agents primarily by forming strong interfacial films. They are usually anionic, are sensitive to relatively high concentrations of electrolytes and alcohol, and greatly increase the viscosity of the external phase. They also support the growth of microorganisms and require the addition of a preservative.

Acacia is a mixture of salts of arabic acid, precipitates at 30% alcohol or higher, is effective over a wide range of pH, and forms O/W emulsions only. Acacia should be considered the most convenient emulsifying agent for emulsions intended for internal use.

Tragacanth is similar to acacia but is effective at 1/10 the concentration and over a much smaller pH range (about 4–6).

Methylcellulose and **Sodium Carboxymethylcellulose** are used primarily to increase the viscosity of emulsions (see also *Suspending Agents,* page 203).

Wool Fat contains cholesterol as the principal emulsifying agent, forms W/O emulsions only, and is used for external preparations, primarily semisolids (see also *Dermatologicals,* page 147).

Inorganic Solids

Theoretically any solid material can function as an emulsifying agent if the particle size is small enough. At particle sizes approaching colloidal range the particles tend not to be wetted very well by liquids in general. As a result, they tend to orient at interfaces and function in a manner similar to surface-active agents.

The only solids of consequence relative to emulsification are the magmas, primarily magnesia magma and bentonite magma. Preparation involves simply shaking or blending the magma with an equal volume or less of oil. The emulsion is nearly always O/W. A commercial example is Haley's MO which contains 75% magnesia magma and 25% mineral oil.

Synthetic Emulsifying Agents

There are conservatively thousands of compounds classified as synthetic surfactants that could be utilized as emulsifying agents. Needless to say, a complete discussion is beyond the scope of this text.

There is, however, a representative handful of synthetic emulsifying agents that should fill most needs of the practitioner. Many of these are official.

They all contain a relatively large hydrocarbon chain as the lipophilic portion of the molecule; the most common are the stearyl (18 carbon atoms), oleyl (18 carbon atoms) and lauryl or dodecyl (12 carbon atoms) groups.

The hydrophilic group can be anionic, cationic, or nonionic. The common anionic agents contain either a carboxyl, a sulfate, or a sulfonate group as the hydrophilic portion of the molecule. Common cationic groups are the quaternary nitrogen and pyridinium nitrogen. As a class, the cationics are seldom used as emulsifying agents but rather as antimicrobial agents.

By far the largest group of synthetics are the nonionics. The more lipophilic of these contain a polyhydroxyl group such as glycerin or sorbitan as the hydrophilic group. The more hydrophilic agents contain a polyoxyethylene chain as the hydrophilic group.

Soft Soaps—These are salts obtained by reacting a fatty acid with an alkali such as sodium or potassium hydroxide or with an organic amine such as triethanolamine; consequently, they are anionic. They are generally soluble or dispersible in water and form O/W emulsions. The pH of emulsions formed with soft soaps is around 8–10. Such emulsions are incompatible with high concentrations of electrolytes, with acidic compounds and with divalent cations such as zinc, calcium, and magnesium. They also precipitate with cationic compounds of relatively high molecular weight. The emulsifying agent is usually formed *in situ.*

Hard Soaps are salts of fatty acids and di- or trivalent cations. Calcium oleate is the prime example formed by reacting oleic acid with limewater (calcium hydroxide solution). The soap is insoluble in water and forms W/O emulsions. They are also incompatible with acids or acidic drugs.

Sodium Lauryl Sulfate USP is an alkyl sulfate and as such is a strong electrolyte compared to the soaps and is very soluble in water. Since it is very hydrophilic it forms O/W emulsions. It is stable in the presence of acids and much more stable to electrolytes than are the soaps.

Polyoxyl 40 Stearate USP is an ester of polyoxyethylene glycol and stearic acid. It is predominantly hydrophilic and forms O/W emulsions.

Sorbitan Monooleate (Span 80) is an ester of sorbitan and oleic acid and is predominantly lipophilic, forming W/O emulsions.

Polysorbate 80 USP (Tween 80) is sorbitan monooleate copolymerized with ethylene oxide to increase its hydrophilic character; consequently, it forms O/W emulsions.

Glycerol Monostearate NF is quite lipophilic and is not usually suitable as an emulsifying agent by itself. It is used in conjunction with other emulsifying agents and should be considered only as an auxiliary emulsifying agent.

The last four compounds are all nonionic agents. They have the advantage of being stable in the presence of acids and relatively high concentrations of electrolytes and are compatible with divalent cations like calcium. They are also compatible with cationic surfactants.

The one disadvantage of nonionic emulsifiers containing a polyoxyethylene chain is that they are precipitated with phenol. Other phenolic compounds such as salicylic acid may also form inactive complexes with nonionic surfactants.

Preparation

In the pharmacy, several manual methods and various manually or electrically operated equipment can be used in the preparation of emulsions. For extemporaneous compounding at the prescription level, a mortar and pestle may frequently serve as the most efficient apparatus, the best of which is a wedgewood mortar and pestle that is rough on the inner surface so as to provide maximum shearing of the dispersed droplets to produce a fine particle size. Other authors recommend a glass mortar and pestle to prevent oil from being trapped

in the pores of the wedgwood and becoming rancid. The mortar and pestle are especially suitable for preparing emulsions with natural gums as the emulsifying agent.

Electric mixers—such as the malt mixer, blender, or electric egg beater—may also be satisfactory, but these frequently have a tendency to incorporate excessive amounts of air in the finished product, creating problems of stability and packaging.

Hand homogenizers are available at modest cost and produce very satisfactory emulsions. The coarse emulsion is formed in a mortar, or other apparatus, and transferred to the hand homogenizer, wherein it is pumped through a small orifice against a spring-loaded plate. This reduces the size of the droplets as they are forced between the plate and the homogenizer proper. Because some volumes of the preparation are invariably lost in the equipment, it is advisable to use the liquid which serves as the external phase to rinse the mortar and the homogenizer and collect it in the graduated container which receives the finished product.

Dry Gum Method

The dry gum method (Continental Method, 4:2:1 Method) is exclusively used for emulsions prepared from dry gum emulsifiers, especially acacia. A primary emulsion is formed by using the entire quantity of the oil called for in the preparation, ½ that volume of water, and ¼ that amount of emulsifier. Thus the ratio is 4 parts of oil, 2 of water, and 1 of emulsifier. Because the concentrations are not extremely critical, one may use fluid or dry measure interchangeably in determining the appropriate amount of emulsifier; e.g., if the prescription requires 2 fl oz of oil, ½ oz by weight of acacia may be used.

The dry gum is first dispersed in the oil. When the gum is just dispersed, the water is added all at once with rapid trituration. The trituration is continued at high speed, using a spiral motion of the pestle, until a thick primary emulsion is formed. A snapping sound is heard when a good stable primary emulsion has been prepared. It is during this process that the droplet size is reduced to its minimum dimensions and therefore, the time spent in this operation yields dividends in stability of final product. Finally, the remainder of the aqueous phase is added slowly with trituration.

Wet Gum Method

This technique of emulsion formation (also known as the English Method) is suitable for preparing emulsions with mucilages or dissolved gums as the emulsifying agents and uses the 4:2:1 ratio as in the dry gum method. It is necessary to use this method, although it is slower and not as reliable as the dry gum method, if the emulsifying agent is available only in solution or if it must be dissolved before being used, as with perhaps methylcellulose. In this method, a viscous mucilage of the one part of gum is made with the two parts of water and the oil is added in small amounts, with thorough, rapid trituration. When all of the oil has been added, the mixture is brought to volume with water.

Bottle Method

In the preparation of emulsions of volatile and other nonviscous oils, the bottle method frequently provides the most efficient procedure. This method is merely a variation of the dry gum or wet gum method, except that a large bottle or flask is used as the mixing device. The primary emulsion is formed by a vigorous shaking and is then diluted with the external phase.

In these methods it may seem to have been inferred that the emulsifier is always used in a quantity equal to $\frac{1}{4}$ that of the oil. There are, however, exceptions to this, based on the composition of the oil and the particular emulsifier used. It should be remembered that tragacanth is 10 times as effective as acacia and appropriate adjustment must be made in the amount of tragacanth used. Volatile oils, liquid petrolatum, or min-

Table 5—Ratios of Components for Preparation of Primary Emulsions

Oil	Acacia	Tragacanth
Fixed oils	4:2:1	40:20:1
Mineral oil	3:2:1	30:20:1
Linseed oil	2:2:1	20:20:1
Volatile oils	2:2:1	20:20:1

eral oil and linseed oil require greater amounts of emulsifiers than most of the fixed oils. The generally recommended proportions of these exceptions are outlined in Table 5.

In Situ Soap Method

Calcium Soaps—W/O emulsions containing certain vegetable oils and limewater are prepared simply by mixing equal volumes of the oil and limewater and shaking vigorously. The emulsifying agent, primarily calcium oleate, is formed *in situ* provided that the vegetable oil naturally contains free fatty acids. Suitable oils are olive, almond, and linseed. Other vegetable oils such as cottonseed, corn, and peanut and hydrocarbon oils that do not naturally contain free fatty acids can be emulsified by adding oleic acid. A few drops of oleic acid/fluidounce of oil is usually sufficient. A typical example is calamine liniment:

Calamine	80 g
Zinc oxide	80 g
Olive oil	500 ml
Calcium hydroxide solution qs	1000 ml

In order to generate a sufficient quantity of emulsifying agent in this type of preparation, it is necessary to use almost equal parts of the oil and lime water.

Soft Soaps—In this method the base is dissolved in the aqueous phase and the fatty acid in the oil phase. If it is necessary to melt any of the ingredients, the components of the two phases are put into separate beakers in a water bath and heated to the melting point of the highest melting component. When the two phases have reached approximately the same temperature, the external phase is added to the internal phase with stirring. It is important that the emulsion is stirred during the entire period of cooling. Otherwise, the oily layer may rise to the top of the mixture and solidify as a cake on the surface, making it impossible to disperse the oil uniformly throughout the finished preparation.

An example would be the following simple O/W lotion:

(Oil phase)	
Mineral oil	8 g
Stearic acid	15 g
(Aqueous phase)	
Triethanolamine	1.5 g
Water qs	100 g

Usually, insufficient base is added to completely neutralize the acid. This excess acid protects against the irritating effects of excess alkali. The lotion or base is said to be "superfatted."

Synthetic Emulsifiers

In general, the method is similar to the *in situ* soap method using soft soaps with the difference that the emulsifier is added to the phase in which it is more soluble. A reasonable concentration for most emulsifiers is about 2–5%. Emulsification does not occur as readily as with the soaps. Some type of mechanical equipment such as a hand homogenizer is usually necessary.

There are numerous examples in the literature in which the external phase is added to the internal phase. This order of mixing involves emulsion formation by phase inversion; i.e., the opposite type of emulsion forms first, followed by the desired type as more external phase is added. Emulsions formed in this manner may be somewhat more stable than those in which the internal phase is added to the external. However, in the absence of previous experience with a given formulation, it is acceptable to add the internal phase to the external phase, as the emulsifier is usually in the external phase and, therefore, present at maximum concentration during the addition of the internal phase.

In some instances it may not be nec-essary to warm the phases if all of the materials are liquid and soluble at room temperature. The addition of alcohol and some volatile components might be reserved until the emulsion is at least partially cooled, so as to avoid breaking the emulsion and losing the volatile ingredients.

Incorporation of Medicinal Agents

During Emulsion Formation

As a general rule, it is most desirable to incorporate a drug into a vehicle in molecular form; hence, soluble drugs should be dissolved in the appropriate phase. In the following example of a sunscreen lotion, the phenyl salicylate should be dissolved in the oil prior to emulsification.

11

℞ Phenyl salicylate	1.0 g
Almond oil	50 ml
Acacia qs	
Water qs ad	100 ml
M. ft. Emulsion	

Drugs soluble in the external phase of the emulsion should be added as a solution to the primary emulsion.

Preformed Emulsions

The addition of medicinal agents to preformed emulsions may present certain problems which may be overcome easily if one keeps in mind the type of emulsion and the nature of the emulsifier.

O/W Emulsions—It is very difficult to add oleaginous materials to an O/W emulsion once it is formed. Occasionally, small amounts of oily materials may be added, if some excess emulsifier was used in the original formulation. A small quantity of an oil-soluble drug such as menthol may sometimes be added if it is dissolved in a very small quantity of olive oil in a mortar and the preformed emulsion added by the technique of geometric dilution.

The addition of aqueous materials and soluble solids to this type of emulsion usually presents no problem when the added materials do not react with the emulsifying agent. Potential interactions should be expected with cationic compounds and salts of weak bases, i.e., neomycin sulfate, with anionic emulsifying agents. Soaps are particularly incompatible with acidic drugs. Water-soluble drugs can be dissolved in a small amount of water and added to the base with simple trituration or levigation.

Large amounts of very soluble solids such as urea may require so much water for hydration that when added to a lotion vehicle produce a semisolid preparation. The only solution to this problem, if a fluid preparation is desired, is to reduce the concentration of solids.

Insoluble powders such as sulfur, hydrocortisone, and iodochlorhydroxyquin can be incorporated into these emulsions easily, if levigated first with a small quantity of glycerin, propylene glycol, or the emulsion itself to form a smooth paste.

Small quantities of alcoholic solutions can be incorporated directly, provided the solute is compatible or dispersible in the aqueous external phase of the emulsion. With acacia or other gums as the emulsifying agent, the alcoholic solution should be diluted with water before addition. The addition of alcoholic solutions can be accomplished with minimum hazard if they are added to the bulk of the base so that the concentration of alcohol is at a minimal level at all times. Adding alcoholic solutions by geometric dilution techniques frequently breaks the emulsion because of the high concentration of alcohol present in the initial mixture. Should the quantity of alcohol be too great, as in the case of large proportions of coal tar solution, all or some of the alcohol should be evaporated to avoid the possibility of breaking the emulsion.

The following prescriptions illustrate the techniques most suitable for compounding with preformed O/W emulsions.

12

℞	Phenol	0.5%
	Sulfur	6%
	Neutracolor	2%
	Lubriderm qs	120 ml

In a glass mortar levigate the sulfur and Neutracolor with a small amount of glycerin containing the dissolved phenol, then bring to volume with the vehicle, using geometric dilution.

13

℞	Hydrocortisone	0.25%
	Coal tar solution	5%
	Lubriderm qs ad	120 ml

In a glass mortar, levigate the hydrocortisone powder with a few drops of glycerin or propylene glycol. While triturating, add the Lubriderm by geometric dilution until nearly to final volume. Add the coal tar solution, with stirring, and bring to the prescribed volume with the Lubriderm.

Table 6—Some Commercial Emulsion Bases

Product	Type	Emulsifier	Remarks[a]
Allercreme Skin Lotion (*Texas*)	O/W	Triethanolamine stearate	S A Q P
Almay Emulsion Base (*Almay*)	O/W	Fatty acid glycol esters	Nonionic
Cetaphil (*Texas*)	O/W	Sodium lauryl sulfate	S Q
Dermovan (*Texas*)	O/W	Fatty acid amides	Nonionic
Eucerin (*Duke*)	W/O	Wool wax alcohols	Nonionic
HEB Base (*Barnes-Hind*)	O/W	Sodium lauryl sulfate	S Q
Keri Lotion (*Westwood*)	O/W	Nonionic emulsifiers	Nonionic
Lubriderm (*Texas*)	O/W	Triethanolamine stearate	S A Q P
Neobase (*B-W*)	O/W	Polyhydric alcohol esters	Nonionic
Neutrogena Lotion (*Neutrogena*)	O/W	Triethanolamine lactate	S A Q P
Nivea Cream (*Duke*)	W/O	Wool wax alcohols	Nonionic
pHorsix (*Texas*)	O/W	Polyoxyethylene emulsifiers	Nonionic
Polysorb Hydrate (*Fougera*)	W/O	Sorbitan sesquioleate	Nonionic
Velvachol (*Texas*)	O/W	Sodium lauryl sulfate	S Q

[a] Incompatibilities: *S*: salts of weak bases; *A*: salts of weak acids; *Q*: quaternary ammonium compounds; *P*: polyvalent cations.

Some commercial emulsion bases and their general composition are included in Table 6.

W/O Emulsions—The addition of oleaginous materials to bases of this type presents no problem because of the miscibility of the additive with the external phase. Crystalline drugs are incorporated most easily if they can be dissolved in a small portion of oil before addition to the vehicle. It is extremely difficult, if not impossible, to incorporate much water into the W/O emulsion base, unless sufficient quantities of emulsifiers have been provided at the time of the manufacture of the vehicle.

A few emulsion bases are designed to absorb water for the ultimate formation of W/O emulsions. Typical products of this type are the absorption ointment bases (see Chapter 6).

HLB system applies primarily to the synthetic emulsifying agents.

To produce a stable emulsion the emulsifier should have an HLB that agrees with the lipid nature of the oil to be emulsified. Every oil or lipid material has a required HLB value, i.e., the HLB that an emulsifier should have to produce a stable emulsion with that oil. A list of required HLB values for some common oils and lipids is given in Table 7.

Determination of the correct HLB value for the emulsifier system within an emulsion depends on the components of the oily phase. The method of calculating the required HLB for a mixture of oils in an emulsion is based on the percentage of each lipid in the oil phase and is illustrated in the following example:

		a *(% of oil phase)*	*b* *(Req'd HLB)*	*a × b*
Petrolatum	25 g	56	8	4.5
Cetyl alcohol	20 g	44	15	6.7
Emulsifier	2 g			
Preservative	0.2 g			
Purif water qs ad	100 g	Approximate HLB for emulsifier		11.2

The HLB System

Because of the great number of emulsifying agents available for preparation of pharmaceutical products, it has become necessary to devise a method of narrowing the number of agents which might be most useful for any given emulsion system. The HLB system was devised for this purpose. In this system, emulsifiers are given numerical designations between 1 and 20, depending upon the relative strength of the hydrophilic and hydrophobic segments of the molecule. An emulsifier with a low HLB is hydrophobic in nature, whereas one with a high HLB is hydrophilic. Emulsifiers with HLB's below 9 generally produce W/O emulsions, while those having values between 9 and 11 are intermediate and most susceptible to the other factors which influence the type of emulsion ultimately formed. The

Table 7—Required HLB Values of Common Oily Materials for O/W Emulsions

Material	*Required HLB*
Acid, lauric	15–16
Acid, oleic	17
Alcohol, cetyl	15
Alcohol, lauryl	14
Beeswax	9
Carbon tetrachloride	16
Carnauba wax	12
Castor oil	14
Cottonseed oil	6
Kerosene	14
Lanolin, anhydrous	12
Methyl silicone	11
Mineral oil	11
Paraffin wax	10
Petrolatum	7–8

When the optimum HLB for the emulsifier is determined, it is neither necessary nor even always desirable to seek a single emulsifier which has that particular HLB. Usually, the desired HLB can be obtained by using a blend

Table 8—Approximate HLB Values
for a Number of Surfactants

Generic or chemical name	Trademark	HLB
Glycerol monostearate	Tegin 515	3.8
Sorbitan monooleate	Span 80	4.3
Acacia	—	8.0
Tragacanth	—	13.2
Polyoxyethylene sorbitan monooleate (Polysorbate 80 USP)	Tween 80	15.0
Polyoxyethylene monostearate (Polyoxyl 40 Stearate USP)	Myrj 52	16.9
Sodium lauryl sulfate	—	40.0

of two emulsifiers, one more hydrophilic and the other more hydrophobic. The HLB values for a small group of emulsifying agents are given in Table 8.

Any HLB value between 4.3 and 15.0 can be obtained by using the appropriate mixture of Span 80 and Tween 80. As with the calculation of the required HLB for a mixture of oils, the HLB for a mixture of surfactants is based on the percentage of each surfactant in the mixture. For a mixture of two surfactants the percentage of each can be calculated by

$$\%(A) = 100(X-HLB_B)/(HLB_A-HLB_B) \tag{3}$$

$$\%(B) = 100 - \%(A) \tag{4}$$

where X is the required HLB.

Applying these formulas to the preparation above, it is possible to determine the proportions in which Span 80 and Tween 80 should be mixed to prepare the emulsifier for that product. Let A represent the Tween and B the Span, then

$$\%(Tween\ 80) = 100(11.2–4.3)/(15.0–4.3) = 64\%$$
$$\%(Span\ 80) = 100 - 64 = 36\%$$

The determination of a numerical value for the HLB does not absolutely guarantee that every emulsifier having that HLB will work for a particular system; therefore, other factors need to be considered in the ultimate selection of the agents used. It is necessary to consider the chemical makeup of the oils to be emulsified and to try to match it with the general chemical nature of the emulsifier. For example, an emulsion of coconut oil might be prepared best using emulsifiers which are laurate derivatives, while highly unsaturated oils might be emulsified best using oleate derivatives.

Suspension Technology

By simple definition a suspension is a two-phase system composed of a solid material dispersed in a liquid. The particle size of the dispersed solid is usually taken to be greater than 0.5 μm, considerably greater than colloidal dimensions. The liquid can be oily or aqueous; most of the suspensions of pharmaceutical interest are aqueous.

A point should be made to differentiate emulsions (a dispersion of a liquid in a second liquid) and suspensions. Although the two classes of preparations have many properties in common, they should be considered separately. At times, differentiation becomes difficult. A wax, for example, dispersed in an aqueous system above its melting point is technically an emulsion but on cooling below its melting point becomes a suspension. Both are referred to as emulsions in practice. However, dispersions of crystalline solids in aqueous systems are obviously suspensions.

Other dosage forms use the term suspension to refer to a dispersion of a solid in a medium other than a fluid. A suspension-type ointment or a suspension-type suppository refers to a crystalline solid dispersed in a semisolid. Here, the discussion will be limited to fluid suspensions.

Several official classes of preparations fall within the definition of suspensions, specifically lotions (some are emulsions), magmas, and mixtures. These are for the most part preparations that have been official for a long time. Usually a complete formula and a specific method of preparation is given, i.e., Calamine Lotion USP and Kaolin Mixture with Pectin NF.

Other official suspensions indicate only the concentration of the active ingredient(s), allowing the manufacturer a considerable degree of freedom in developing a formula for a given suspension. Flavors and preservatives can be included in Alumina and Magnesia Oral Suspension USP while a "suitable aqueous vehicle" is required for Primidone Oral Suspension USP.

A closely related type of preparation is solids for oral suspension. Certain drugs, notably antibiotics, are not stable in solution or in aqueous dispersions. To circumvent this problem and at the same time provide an oral liquid dosage form, they are packaged in dry form. Water is added at the time of dispensing to complete the suspension. All additives required are present in the dry powder mixture. Allowances for Erythromycin Ethyl Carbonate for Oral Suspension USP include color, flavor, buffer, suspending agent, dispersant, and preservative.

Extemporaneous suspensions at the prescription level are often prescribed indicating only the drug in the type of vehicle:

14

R̸ Magnesium carbonate   15%
   Cinnamon water   qs   120 ml

Other prescriptions include existing commercial suspensions:

15

R̸ Phenobarbital sodium   gr iv
   Kolantyl Gel   qs   f ℥vi

It falls within the realm of professional discretion for the pharmacist to modify such a prescription if necessary to prepare a pharmaceutically elegant and clinically useful product. Justification can also be found in USP policy.

Applications

In general, suspensions afford a dosage form for administering an insoluble drug. Suspensions intended for oral administration are usually aqueous and are usually flavored in order to mask the unpleasant taste of many drugs. The taste of drugs formulated in suspensions is minimal since the intensity of taste is proportional to solubility or the concentration of the drug in solution.

Suspensions of drugs intended for external application are formulated in either aqueous or oily vehicles depending on the intent of the preparation. A small particle size is critical in preventing a gritty feeling on application and in providing a large surface area for maximum contact between the drug and the surface of the skin.

Intramuscular injections are also formulated as suspensions. The absorption from the injection site is normally slower than from a solution. The use of an oily vehicle further slows absorption and can provide a sustained or prolonged action.

Ideal Properties vs Real Behavior

An ideal suspension can be described as one having the following properties:

1. A uniform particle size so that each particle acts like every other particle producing a consistent behavior for the suspension as a whole.

2. No particle–particle interactions. Each particle remains discrete; i.e., there is no aggregation or clumping of particles. Such a suspension is called a monodisperse suspension.

3. No sedimentation. The drug particles are either stationary or move randomly throughout the dispersion medium so that there is always a uniform distribution of drug.

These ideal properties are not usually realized in actual practice. It is, however, possible to approximate them by controlling some fundamental parameters of the suspension: particle size, concentration of solids, particle-particle interactions, and particle movement.

Particle Size—It is desirable both from a pharmaceutical and pharmacological standpoint to have the smallest particle size possible. For particles in the colloidal range, Brownian movement is sufficient to keep the particles moving randomly, thus preventing sedimentation. In suspensions the particle size is too large for thermal energy to keep them suspended and there will al-

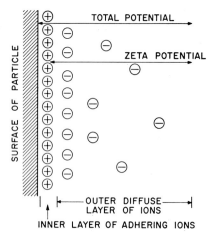

Fig. 4—Diffuse double layer.

ways be some sedimentation.

Stokes' law (Eq. 5) shows a direct relationship between

$$\text{Sedimentation rate} = \frac{d^2(\rho - \rho_0)g}{18\eta} \quad (5)$$

sedimentation rate and the particle diameter. In Eq. 5, d is the particle diameter, ρ the density of the solid, ρ_0 the density of the dispersion medium, g the acceleration due to gravity, and η the viscosity of the dispersion medium. Although Stokes' law is not rigorously valid for real suspensions, it indicates that a small particle size favors a slower rate of sedimentation.

The reduction of particle size for small quantities of crystalline materials is accomplished most conveniently with a Wedgwood mortar and pestle. The lower limit is about 200 μm. It is very difficult to obtain a very uniform particle size with trituration; a rather wide particle size distribution is the usual case, particularly with very hard crystalline materials. Small powder mills are available that are fairly inexpensive and efficient. Many drugs, i.e. zinc oxide and sulfur, are available commercially as fairly fine powders and are usually suitable as such for the preparation of suspensions.

A distinction should be made between actual particle size reduction and the breaking up of aggregates. The latter is necessary in preparing a monodis-perse suspension but is nearly impossible to accomplish by triturating a dry powder. Levigation is the correct technique. The levigating agent coats each individual particle preventing reaggregation.

Concentration of Solids—A high concentration of solids increases the possibility of particle–particle collisions and can be expected to promote particle–particle interactions. Unfortunately, the concentration of solid is usually fixed by the formula or prescription and beyond the control of the practitioner.

Particle–Particle Interactions— From an ideal standpoint, particle–particle interactions are to be avoided. If aggregation of individual particles occurs, the resulting clumps of particles will behave like larger particles and will settle at an increased rate.

Aggregation can be prevented if the particles have a similar electrical charge, i.e., like charges repel. It so happens that solids dispersed in an aqueous system will have some type of charge. There are various ways this charge can develop: (1) ionization of chemical groups on the solid surface, (2) adsorption of surfactant molecules on the solid surface, and (3) adsorption of electrolyte from solution. The latter two mechanisms are most common.

The sign of the charge can usually be predicted if the charge results from adsorption of an ionic surfactant. For example, if sodium lauryl sulfate is used to disperse a solid in water, the solid will most likely carry a negative charge. The sign of the charge by adsorption of electrolytes depends on which ion is adsorbed and is almost impossible to predict. Adsorption will be affected by the properties of the solid surface, concentration of electrolyte, and method of preparation.

The magnitude of the charge is defined as the difference in electrical potential between the charged solid surface and the bulk of the solution. There are several potentials that can be defined as indicated in Fig. 4; the important one in considering suspensions is the Zeta potential calculated from the fixed layer of ions on the particle surface. This layer of ions is tightly bound and moves with the particle. For all practical purposes this fixed layer is considered a part of the particle.

In order to maintain a monodisperse system, the Zeta potential must be great enough for the particles to repel each other. This minimum value is called the critical Zeta potential and is specific for a given suspension.

Particle Movement—Referring to Stokes' law (Eq. 5) it can be seen that if the densities of the solid and the dispersion medium are equal the sedimentation rate would be zero, i.e., ideal conditions would be satisfied. Unfortunately, this is not a practical solution to sedimentation. It is difficult to prepare aqueous solutions with a density great enough to match that of solids commonly used in suspensions. The density of solutions also changes with temperature; therefore, "density matching" is useful only under carefully controlled temperatures.

Stokes' law also indicates that the sedimentation rate is inversely proportional to the viscosity of the dispersion medium. It is important to realize that increasing the viscosity will only decrease the sedimentation rate, not stop it completely. The only way for this to happen would be for the viscosity to approach infinity; however, the suspension would no longer be fluid.

It was pointed out earlier that Stokes' law was not strictly valid for suspensions. One factor that makes this so is the definition of viscosity. For a single particle falling through a liquid, the appropriate viscosity in Stokes' law is obviously the viscosity of that liquid. For a real suspension the viscosity is not so clearly defined and perhaps should refer to the viscosity of the suspension as a whole rather than that of the dispersion medium.

In this context, properties of the solid can affect the viscosity. A smaller particle size results in a larger surface area, a larger degree of interaction with the dispersion fluid, and an increased viscosity. The concentration of solids also directly affects the overall viscosity.

The usual and by far the most practical way to increase the viscosity of the dispersion medium or the suspension is to add a thickening agent or a suspending agent.

Suspending Agents

The materials commonly used as suspending agents are hydrophilic colloids (specifically gums and celluloses), clays, and a few miscellaneous agents. Several of these are the same materials considered previously as emulsifying agents.

Hydrophilic Colloids

Hydrophilic colloids increase the viscosity of water by binding water molecules, thereby limiting their mobility or fluidity. As a class, hydrophilic colloids are strongly hydrated and are considered to be soluble; however, dispersible is perhaps a better term because of their large molecular size. Viscosity is proportional to the concentration of the colloid; many form a semisolid gel at high concentration.

Most hydrophilic colloids are not soluble in alcoholic solutions; about 30% alcohol is the upper limit. The addition of glycols and glycerin also decreases the solubility of the colloid but, instead of precipitation, a gel structure can form. For example, tragacanth mucilage is a 6% dispersion and is a viscous fluid. Ephedrine Sulfate Jelly NF XII (below), on the other hand, is a semisolid containing only 1% tragacanth in an aqueous-glycerin solvent.

Ephedrine sulfate	1%
Tragacanth	1%
Glycerin	15%
Purified water qs	

These suspending agents also support the growth of microorganisms and, therefore, require a preservative. With the exception of methylcellulose, their charge in solution is anionic. Therefore, an incompatibility with quaternary antibacterial agents and other positively charged drugs should be expected.

Acacia (see *Emulsifying Agents,* page 193) is usually used as the official mucilage which is a 35% dispersion in water. The viscosity is greatest between pH 5 and 9.

Tragacanth (see *Emulsifying Agents,* page 193)—The official mucilage is 6%. The viscosity depends greatly on the quality and form of the starting material and is somewhat unpredictable. In general, it is more difficult to use than acacia.

Methylcellulose. is soluble in cold water but not in hot water. Dispersions are prepared by adding the material to boiling water, then cooling to dissolve. Methylcellulose is available in several viscosity grades indicated by a number ranging from 10 to 15,000. The number indicates the viscosity in centipoise (cps) of a 2% solution. Dispersions should be preserved and the polymer is nonionic.

Carboxymethylcellulose (CMC) is available as the sodium salt and is therefore anionic. It is soluble in water and available in three viscosity grades: low, medium and high.

Clays

There are two clays useful as suspending agents: bentonite and Veegum. Chemically, they are both silicates and are anionic in aqueous dispersion. They are strongly hydrated and exhibit thixotropy, the property of forming a gel-like structure on standing and becoming fluid on agitation. This is their outstanding characteristic as suspending agents. Bentonite is official as a 5% magma; Veegum is hydrated to a greater degree and is more viscous than bentonite at the same concentration.

Soaps and Emulsions

Cetyl Alcohol Emulsion is a dispersion of cetyl alcohol in water with sodium lauryl sulfate as the dispersing agent. The emulsion is used as a suspending agent for suspensions intended for topical use.

Cetyl alcohol	3.6%
Sodium lauryl sulfate	0.4%
Purified water qs	

Soap Emulsion—Lime water-vegetable oil emulsions have served as suspending agents for preparing oily suspensions for topical use. An example is calamine liniment:

Calamine	80 g
Zinc Oxide	80 g
Olive Oil	500 ml
Calcium Hydroxide Solution qs	1000 ml

Aluminum Stearate is an insoluble soap used specifically to thicken dispersions in oil such as in Sterile Procaine Penicillin G Suspension with Aluminum Stearate USP. The solid soap is utilized by melting it with the oil to effect dispersion, then stirring until cooled. The viscosity of such oily dispersions is very sensitive to the method of dispersion and the cooling rate.

Viscosity Behavior

It is not really sufficient to just add a suspending agent to a suspension. It is necessary to know something about their viscosity behavior to understand and evaluate their function and to compare different agents.

Newtonian vs Non-Newtonian Flow—Pure liquids and dilute solutions are characterized by a single viscosity value and are classified as being Newtonian in behavior. Glycerin, for example, has a viscosity of about 500 cps at room temperature and is independent of the method of measurement.

Other fluids, particularly dispersions of suspending agents, exhibit a variable viscosity behavior depending on a parameter called the shear rate. For our purposes the shear rate can be described as the degree of agitation or stirring. Shear can be introduced by shaking a container of the fluid or by measuring the viscosity in a viscometer. This variable behavior is called non-Newtonian.

If the viscosity is measured with a viscometer that can vary the shear rate, the behavior pictured in Fig. 5 is observed. The significance of non-Newtonian behavior is that at a very low shear rate the viscosity is very large, i.e., the fluid is very thick. A small particle

Table 9—Shear Rates of Some Pharmaceutical Operations

Operation	Approximate shear rate (sec⁻¹)
Particle settling	less than 0.1
Pouring	100
Rubbing	200
Spraying	1000
Syringing	10,000

Table 10—Comparative Viscosities of Selected Suspending Agents[5]

Suspending agent	% concentration to give 800 cps
Acacia	35%[a]
Tragacanth	2.8
Methylcellulose 100	3.5
Methylcellulose 400	2.4
Methylcellulose 1500	1.7
Carboxymethylcellulose	
Low viscosity	4.1
Medium viscosity	1.9
High viscosity	0.7
Bentonite	6.3
Veegum	6.0

[a] 600 cps.

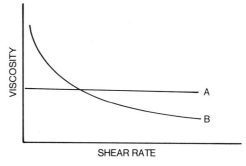

Fig. 5—Viscosity as a function of shear rate: *A*, Newtonian; *B*, non-Newtonian.

would be expected to settle very slowly in such a fluid. At high shear rates, the viscosity decreases, i.e., the fluid becomes thinner. Particles may settle faster but, more importantly, the fluid is easy to pour or apply, as the case may be.

Shear can be developed by any procedure that disturbs the system. Some representative values are given in Table 9.

Suspending Agents of Choice— Table 10 lists the concentration of various suspending agents to produce an aqueous dispersion having a viscosity of 800 cps. This particular viscosity was chosen as an arbitrary standard but is also a reasonable viscosity to consider for actual use. The data can serve as a guide in comparing different agents and for selecting initial concentrations.

Most agents in Table 10 suffer from some serious drawback: acacia has poor viscosity, tragacanth has poor reproducibility, bentonite and Veegum have an unattractive appearance, and CMC plus the above are anionic. They all have po-

tential incompatibilities with quaternary nitrogen compounds, weak acids, and salts of weak bases.

Since methylcellulose is nonionic, it avoids the above incompatibilities and is recommended for use with oral suspensions. Particularly useful is the following suspending vehicle formulated by the Pharmacy Service at the Hospital of the University of Pennsylvania (HUP):*

HUP Suspending Vehicle

Sucrose	250 g
Sorbitol solution 70%	100 ml
Glycerin	25 ml
Saccharin sodium	0.5 g
Methylparaben	1.0 g
Methylcellulose 1500	10–30 g
FD&C Yellow No. 5	0.15 g
Lemon lime flavor	3 ml
Purified water qs	1000 ml

The vehicle is easily formulated, stable, relatively effective as a suspending agent, and accepted well by patients.

For external use cetyl alcohol emulsion is recommended. Its appearance is very pleasing and acceptable cosmetically (compared to bentonite, for example), is effective, and can be prepared as a stock dispersion. The emulsion is usually used in concentration of 15–50% of the suspension volume.

Extemporaneous Preparation

An "ideal" suspension should be a monodisperse system with a zero or at

* The author wishes to acknowledge HUP Pharmacy Service for permission to use their formulation.

least a very slow sedimentation rate. To prepare such a suspension the following steps are generally required when starting with a fine powder.

Wetting the Solid—The purpose is to separate each individual particle and coat it with a layer of dispersion medium. Levigation is the most convenient technique using a glass mortar and pestle with a suitable levigating agent. Occasionally, the levigating agent is specified in the formula particularly if the preparation is official. Otherwise the choice of levigating agent is left to the discretion of the pharmacist.

Surfactants are also effective in wetting solids. The powder can be tumbled gently with a surfactant solution; however, this procedure takes considerable time and is usually not practical on a small scale. Surfactants may also aid the wetting process during levigation.

Addition of Suspending Agent—The suspending agent may be added as a dry powder with the active ingredients prior to wetting, but this is not the best procedure since some of the natural plant materials such as acacia have a tendency to "gum up" into a rubbery mass and are difficult to work with. Other agents, particularly tragacanth, take a long time (e.g., days) to hydrate and develop maximum viscosity.

The recommended procedure is to add the suspending agent in the form of an aqueous dispersion (i.e., acacia mucilage, HUP Suspending Vehicle, or cetyl alcohol emulsion). The dispersion is added to the solid or the levigation of the solid via geometric dilution to insure proper dispersion. The dispersion of the suspending agent can also serve as the levigating agent.

Bringing the Preparation To Volume—This is accomplished with the appropriate vehicle with stirring. If a suspending agent such as HUP Suspendng Vehicle is used, it serves as the complete dispersion medium.

Controlled Flocculation

Problems with Monodisperse Suspensions—The "ideal" monodisperse suspension suffers several disadvantages. The suspension will eventually settle and form a sediment in the bottom of the container. Although this is not very elegant, it is acceptable if the sediment can be redispersed easily on shaking.

A serious problem arises when the sediment compacts to form a dense cake that is not redispersible. While it is true that the particles in a monodisperse system are charged and repel each other, this charge is not great enough to counteract the force of gravity in compacting a sediment. All monodisperse suspensions have the potential for forming a compacted, caked sediment.

The Flocculation Process—Caking can be overcome by using a process called controlled flocculation to prepare suspensions. Practitioners will find it difficult to utilize the method on an extemporaneous basis but should be aware of the concepts to understand the behavior of modern suspensions.

The basic process involves promoting a degree of interaction between suspension particles and several mechanisms are possible; e.g.,

Bridging is the addition of an ion that will interact with more than one particle; e.g., the addition of aluminum ions to a dispersion of negatively charged particles.

Charge Reduction is the addition of an electrolyte to reduce the charge on the particles allowing interaction between particles to occur. The addition of sodium chloride, e.g., will promote interaction with either a positively or negatively charged particle. Higher valence ions are more effective in neutralizing charged particles.

The result of either mechanism is flocculation (the development of a network of loosely bound particles). One consequence is that the effective particle size is larger; i.e., the particles act in clumps rather than as individual particles. Sedimentation will be more rapid and the supernatant fluid will be clear. As before, a suspending agent can be added to slow the sedimentation rate. Flocculation also increases the viscosity of the suspension.

The most important consequence is that the network developed is loose and fluffy and very easy to redisperse. Caking is completely eliminated. The flocculated network should occupy as large a volume as possible. If it occupies the entire suspension volume, there will in effect be no sedimentation.

Thus, a pharmaceutically ideal suspension should be a flocculated system having a sediment volume equal to the volume of the suspension.

Behavior of Flocculated Systems—The flocculation process is a reversible one. If electrolyte is added to a monodisperse suspension, ions will be selectively adsorbed, the Zeta potential will be decreased to below the critical value, and flocculation will occur. If additional electrolyte is added, ions will continue to be adsorbed. It is possible to again develop a charge on individual particles only now the charge will have the opposite sign as the original. If this new charge exceeds the critical Zeta potential, the suspension will again become monodisperse. The suspension is said to be deflocculated, the consequence of which is that electrolytes or ionic drugs can affect a suspension causing flocculation or deflocculation depending on the starting condition of the suspension.

A similar action is observed by the addition of a less-polar solvent such as ethanol. The predominant effect is the reduction of solvent polarity and a corresponding decrease in the efficiency of charge–charge repulsion. If, for example, alcohol is added to a monodisperse suspension, the repulsion between particles is reduced and flocculation is possible. In a flocculated suspension, alcohol will produce a greater attraction between particles producing a more dense network; if it is dense enough, the process is called coagulation and the result is a dense precipitate.

As with electrolytes, the process is reversible. If electrolyte is added to a coagulated suspension resulting from the addition of alcohol, it is possible for the particles to again develop a charge and become deflocculated.

Preparation—Preparation is essentially similar to that for a monodisperse suspension with the exception that somewhere during the process a definite quantity of electrolyte is added to produce the desired degree of flocculation. The amount of electrolyte needed must be determined by experimentation, hence the impracticability for the community practitioner. The procedure might be described as

1. Wet the solid
2. Add electrolyte to flocculate
3. Add suspending agent
4. Dilute to volume.

A commercial suspension can become

quite complex. Even in compounding extemporaneously, some degree of flocculation may occur serendipitously. Some understanding of the flocculation process is necessary to appreciate the potential problems in dealing with suspension.

Dispensing

A slowly settling, nearly monodisperse suspension is about the best the practitioner can hope for. If some flocculation occurs, it is fortunate. At any rate, a degree of sedimentation will occur. Suspensions, therefore, should be dispensed with a "shake-well" label and the patient informed of their proper use.

When sedimentation occurs, in the absence of flocculation, the larger particles naturally settle faster than the smaller ones. The supernatant fluid will remain cloudy, yielding a not particularly elegant preparation. The only remedy is to start with as fine a powder as possible and, more importantly, with as uniform a particle size as possible.

A valid concern in compounding is the chemical stability of a drug in suspension form. With extremely insoluble materials such as sulfur there is probably no need for concern. For other drugs, particularly newer ones, there is no effective way to establish stability at the practitioner level. Some type of expiration dating has been advocated, but this approach has no practical solution. It is fortunate that prescriptions are used only for a relatively short period of time. Recommendation to the patient to store the preparation in a cool place is also beneficial.

Many prescriptions for suspensions are written for active ingredients not readily available in powder form. The pharmacist is forced to utilize other sources of the drug such as capsules or tablets. Reducing a tablet to a fine particle size with a mortar and pestle can be difficult, particularly if the tablet is coated. Since most coatings are soluble, they present difficulties only in trituration to reduce the particle size.

Other components in capsule and tablet formulations such as diluents are for the most part dispersible in water and present no particular problem. Lubricants such as talc or magnesium stearate are usually present in insignificant amounts.

It is possible to use a parenteral preparation as the source of a drug for preparing oral solutions or suspensions, but its solvent system must be carefully considered. Diazepam injection, for example, is prepared in a buffered solvent containing 40% propylene glycol and 10% alcohol. Diluting this solution in an aqueous suspension would most assuredly cause precipitation. No control is possible over particle size, crystal growth, or stability; furthermore, injections often utilize different salts and esters of the parent drug than those used in oral dosage forms. There is much evidence that these variations can profoundly affect the biological activity of a drug.

The only conclusion that can be reached from the above considerations is that it is probably best to utilize dosage forms designed for oral use as the source of a drug in preparing suspensions and try to overcome as many problems as possible with appropriate compounding methodology.

Prescriptions

16

R̸   Zinc sulfate   4
     Sulfurated potash   4
     Purified water   qs   100

This formula for white lotion should be made according to official directions. Traditionally, it has been prepared and dispensed without a suspending agent and as such it is not a pharmaceutically elegant product. About 20% cetyl alcohol emulsion might be used as a suspending agent.

17

R̸   Kaolin mixture with pectin
     Paregoric   aa   f ℥ ii

This mixture gels because the alcohol in paregoric produces a flocculation effect on the kaolin mixture. The addition of electrolyte has been shown to defflocculate the gel. Commercial products like Kaopectate do not exhibit the gelling effect, presumably because of a higher salt content than the official mixture.

18

R̸   Calamine   8
     Zinc oxide   8
     Purified water   qs   100

Bentonite magma can be used as a suspending agent, essentially preparing official calamine lotion. Alternately, cetyl alcohol emulsion would produce a more cosmetically appealing suspension.

19

R̸   Prepared chalk   6%
     Cinnamon water   qs   pint

Since this prescription is intended for oral use, a flavored vehicle such as HUP Suspending Vehicle (page 205) should be considered.

Liquid Dosage Forms

Liquid medications may be subdivided into two major categories: (1) liquid medications for internal use and (2) liquid medications for external application. Oral liquids are usually compounded in the form of aqueous solutions, elixirs, or syrups, but liquid preparations for external use are much more varied. They include aqueous liquids (aerosols, sprays, baths, dental liquids, douches, enemas, gargles and mouth washes, jellies, lotions ophthalmic solutions, and wet dressings including compresses) and nonaqueous liquids (collodions, dental liquids, glycerites, and liniments).

This section reviews the advantages and disadvantages of oral liquid medications, as well as the flavors and vehicles that are used to prepare organoleptically acceptable products. It also reviews the important factors that must be considered in the preparation of external liquid formulations with appropriate characteristics, including order of mixing, pH, and critical dispensing factors.

Internal Liquids

Liquid medications for internal use take on a variety of forms depending on the solvent, vehicle, viscosity, adjuvants, flavor, color, and therapeutic intention. This portion of the chapter is confined to liquid pharmaceutical dosage forms intended for oral administration. These are further considered to include prescription-only medications and the self-medication forms widely known as over-the-counter (OTC) drugs. Formulations associated with the categories named, represent solutions of liquids or solids dissolved in the diluent or vehicle in such a way as to insure drug stability, formulation integrity, and acceptable taste and color. Such liquid pharmaceuticals are available as prefabricated formulations or as extemporaneously compounded mixtures prepared according to prescription order. Mixtures of prefabricated liquid formulations are common and on occasion need to be evaluated as to physical, chemical, or therapeutic incompatibility.

Oral liquid medications are further identified according to the physical characteristics of the formulations based on types of solvents or vehicles used. The major pharmaceutical vehicles are simple aqueous or alcoholic solutions, aromatic waters, spirits, tinctures, syrups, elixirs, and special formulations. These may be flavored or unflavored and artificially colored.

The popularity of this form of medication continues to be based on patient convenience and acceptability, flexibility of dosage levels that may be prescribed, and the variety of drug combinations that may be made available. Prefabricated formulations may be administered individually or as combinations, and compounded prescriptions often involve admixture with additional solid or liquid therapeutic agents.

Advantages of Oral Liquids

A solution as a form of medication has several advantages over other forms. Since solutions are homogeneous mixtures, the medication is uniformly distributed throughout the preparation. The dosage can easily be varied with the preparation. Some drugs are irritating to the gastric mucosa when given in a concentrated tablet or capsule form. This irritation may be reduced when the drug is given in solution because of the dilution factor. Prompt action of the drug occurs because the drug is absorbed faster when administered in solution. Another advantage of solutions is they can easily be flavored, sweetened, or colored. This is particularly advantageous for administration of medication to children or patients who cannot readily swallow tablets or capsules. Drugs intended for external use can be easily and uniformly applied if dispensed in solution. There are also certain drugs which are best prepared in solution because of their natural physical characteristics.

Some medications are available generally in a liquid formulation because of therapeutic advantages (trend toward administration of potassium chloride in solution (as in Ŗ 20 and 21). The bulk of a particular ingredient or the therapeutic intention may dictate a liquid form [Basaljel (*Wyeth*)]. Infants, geriatric and mental patients often require oral liquid medication (Ŗ 22). In general, liquid oral pharmaceuticals offer diversity in the form of medication given to the patient.

20

Ŗ   KCl, 10% soln.   4 oz.
     Sig: 15 cc. t.i.d. with orange juice

The pharmacist may use wild cherry syrup, syrup of cherry, raspberry, lemon-lime; when the KCl is dissolved in 10 ml of purified water, previous to addition to the vehicle, a clearer solution results.

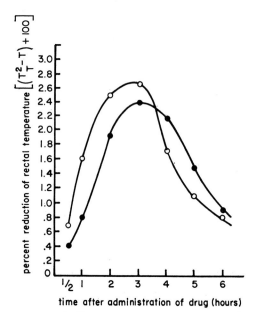

Fig. 6—Comparative effects of aspirin (●) and acetaminophen (O) in reducing fever. This graph shows the time response curve for the mean per cent reduction of original temperature in 50 febrile patients receiving a single dose (based on age) of three agents. (Calculated from data in Ref 44 using the formula $(T^0 - T/T^0) \times 100$, where T^0 is the rectal temperature before medication and T the temperature at a given time after drug-administration.)[6]

21

℞ Kaon Elixir   oz. viii
    Sig: Take 1 tablespoon daily

The pharmacist should be prepared to give mEq wts of K for each tablespoonful.

22

℞ Gevrabon   16 oz.
    Sig: Take 1 teaspoonful A.C.

℞ Poly-Vi-Flor   50 ml
    Sig: Give 1.0 ml daily

One interpretation of Fig. 6 indicates that acetaminophen results in a more rapid onset of action, but a shorter duration of antipyretic effect than aspirin. The acetaminophen was administered in a hydroalcoholic solution and the aspirin was given as crushed tablets. However, the data were collected in order to compare the antipyretic effect of these two therapeutic agents. Tablet forms were not measured with liquid formulations of the same agent in equal concen-

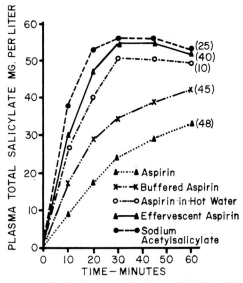

Fig. 7—Plasma total salicylate concentrations following the oral ingestion of various preparations of aspirin in all cases. Figures in parentheses represent the number of human subjects studies in each group.[7]

trations. There are a limited number of studies available in which the therapeutic effect of the liquid and solid forms of the medications are compared, and the data are usually presented as incidental to the main purpose. Many biopharmaceutists take the position that all comparisons of therapeutic activity should be made with a standardized solution of the drug as a reference.

An aminophylline study is another example to illustrate the comparison of drug availability from liquid dosage forms with that from solid dosage forms. A blood level peak of 4.25 mg/ml at 2 hours was obtained for a capsule dosage form, while a blood level peak of 5.68 mg/ml in 2 hours was found for the hydrochloride solution of aminophylline.

Further evidence of the enhanced effect of drugs when administered in solution rather than in a solid dosage form is observed in Fig. 7. The equivalent of 640 mg of aspirin was administered following overnight fast. The sodium acetylsalicylate and effervescent aspirin were given in solution in 120 ml water.

The aspirin and "buffered" aspirin were taken as tablets followed by 2–4 oz of water. The data show that the most rapid absorption and the earliest peak blood levels are obtained in completely dissolved preparations.

Disadvantages of Oral Liquids

There are some disadvantages associated with liquid oral formulations. Patients not having access to accurate measuring devices and a uniform volume from one dose to another are the exception rather than the rule. Teaspoonful sizes vary considerably and measurement of a teaspoonful (5 ml) results in a significant volume difference. A dropper may possibly deliver as little as 45% of the intended dose or 100% in excess.

Bacterial contamination has been found in 8.2% of the liquid medications examined. Organisms considered pathogenic occurred in 17% of those formulations. Potential pathogens were found in 40% of the commercial syrups tested. The establishment of standards in this area is strongly recommended. A count of less than 5 organisms/5 ml of product is well within the capabilities of a good pharmaceutical manufacturing procedure and any organisms present obviously should be nonpathogenic.

Chapter 13 deals with incompatibilities which may result from chemical, physical, or therapeutic drug interactions. The pharmacist on occasion may be in a position to suggest ways in which these incompatibilities can be avoided and stability can be improved. There are occasions when improved palatability may be suggested to the prescriber in order to gain greater patient acceptance. Patient acceptability is related to taste, color, and odor now more than it was a few years ago.

Taste-panel techniques of the pharmaceutical manufacturers have resulted in advancement in the art and science of masking and flavoring unpleasant tasting medications; however, the pleasant taste of liquid formulations may result in overdosage. This is especially hazardous with children.

The community pharmacist is infrequently called upon to compound a liquid prescription formulation. However, the extent of compounding varies from pharmacy to pharmacy and the geographical location. When a mixture of two or more ingredients is required, as in ℞ 23, the pharmaceutical technique is usually quite elementary and is based upon appropriate knowledge gained in various pharmacy technology courses, commonly referred to as fundamental principles and processes.

23

℞ Codeine Phosph.   0.3 g
    Robitussin AC, q.s. ad.   90 ml
    Sig: One teaspoonful q3h prn for cough

There may be a preferred order of mixing to dissolve or to distribute one ingredient in another. The codeine phosphate in ℞ 23 should be dissolved in the least amount of purified water possible and then the vehicle added to volume. The patient's dose of codeine should be noted and proper records made before filing the prescription order.

The chemical and physical properties of drugs and chemicals may require special handling. Physical and chemical compatibility or particle size may require adjustments. The pH may alter the stability or therapeutic activity of medications, as illustrated in ℞ 24.

24

℞ K-Cillin 125 mg/5 ml
    Anamine Syr., q.s.   150 ml
    Sig: One teaspoonful q.i.d.

The stability of potassium penicillin in an acid pH is questionable.

Bulk and fluidity of solutions are two of the main disadvantages. Capsules or tablets occupy less space and are more convenient to carry. Some medications, because of their obnoxious taste and odor, are very difficult to prepare suitably in solution; others are not stable in the presence of water.

Flavoring

Flavor refers to a mixed sensation of

Table 11—Selected Flavor Applications

Drug category	Preferred flavors
Antibiotics	Cherry, maple, pineapple, orange, raspberry, banana-pineapple, banana-vanilla, butterscotch-maple, coconut-custard, strawberry, vanilla, lemon-custard, cherry-custard, fruit-cinnamon
Antihistamines	Apricot, black currant, cherry, cinnamon, custard, grape, honey, lime, loganberry, peach-orange, peach-rum, raspberry, root beer, wild cherry
Barbiturates	Banana-pineapple, banana-vanilla, black currant, cinnamon-peppermint, grenadine-strawberry, lime, orange, peach-orange, root beer
Decongestants and expectorants	Anise, apricot, black-currant, butterscotch, cherry, coconut-custard, custard-mint-strawberry, grenadine-peach, strawberry, lemon, gooseberry, loganberry, maple, orange, orange-lemon, coriander, orange-peach, pineapple, raspberry, strawberry, tangerine
Electrolyte solutions	Cherry, grape, lemon-lime, raspberry, wild cherry syrup
Geriatrics	Black currant, grenadine-strawberry, lime, port wine, sherry wine, root beer, wild strawberry

taste, touch, smell, sight and sound, all of which involve a combination of physicochemical and psychological actions that influence the perception of substances. Today, more than ever before, pharmaceutical formulations must be organoleptically acceptable. Desirable or undesirable therapeutic results may be caused by patient reaction to the taste, odor, and color of medications taken internally. With the expansion of technology in the flavor industry, many artificial or imitation flavors have been created. Manufacturing pharmacy has responded to the public demand for acceptable taste. As a result, many new flavors have been introduced. However, the variety of flavor entities has decreased since 1957, while the use of blends to create distinctive new tastes has increased. Table 11 lists a number of new flavors introduced in recent years.

Flavor selections were gathered from *Physicians' Desk Reference,* correspondence with pharmaceutical manufacturers, and the pharmaceutical literature.

A meaningful discussion of flavor technology is outside the scope of this text and the dispensing pharmacist now has little need for such information. References cited are quite exhaustive and can be referred to for handling a specific flavor problem. The modern flavorist has upset the ancient flavor patterns. Cough syrups, laxatives, sedatives, antihistamines, antibiotics, vitamins, and pediatric and geriatric formulations now are available in a variety of flavors which successfully mask unpleasant tastes without affecting physical and chemical stability. While a large number of flavor blends are represented, it must be realized that these flavors have been selected through the results of elaborate taste-panel studies. Formulators have found that unpleasant taste masking problems can best be resolved by use of blends of distinctive flavors.

The Monte-Bovi peppermint water concentrate should be mentioned.[8] It has the following formula.

Peppermint Oil USP	7.5
Tween 20	42.5
Purified Water qs ad	100

One ml of this concentrate in sufficient purified water to make 100 ml makes a peppermint water equivalent to an aromatic water made by the USP process.

With the expansion of technology in the flavor industry, new artificial flavoring agents have been made available to the formulator and the pharmacist. The flavoring industry will supply literature, samples, and assistance if special taste masking problems arise.

Specific therapeutic agents and associated flavors with unique names individualize certain formulations. An orange-mint flavor is especially effective in disguising diphenhydramine in an expectorant formulation. The use of a spice-vanilla flavor for phenylephrine

Table 12—Flavor Selection Guide

Taste	Masking flavor
Salt	Butterscotch, maple
Bitter	Wild cherry, walnut, chocolate-mint, licorice
Sweet	Fruit, berry, vanilla
Acid	Citrus

and chlorpheniramine maleate preparation has been proposed. Strawberry is well suited to tranquilizer formulations. Maple combined with butterscotch is well suited to improve the taste of adsorbents such as kaolin and pectin. This same flavor combination is recommended for aminophylline and theophylline. Mint is a favorite taste for use in antacid preparations. In some hospitals the pharmacists use a mint flavor effectively to flavor Basaljel.

Table 12 on flavor selection is useful as a general guide.

Vehicles

Compounded prescriptions requiring the selection of a vehicle are practically obsolete as far as dispensing is concerned. Therefore, only brief mention will be made of the vehicles used for internal liquids, namely purified water, aromatic waters, official elixirs, medicinal elixirs, and syrups.

Purified Water—Purified Water USP should be used to dissolve soluble solids for all oral liquid prescription orders calling for water. ℞ 25 and 26 illustrate the use of purified water in a prescription. However, water alone is rarely used as the vehicle.

25

℞ Potassium Iodide Solution 1 oz.
  Sig: gtts. x in juice t.i.d. for lungs

Saturated solution of potassium iodide (SSKI) is intended here.

26

℞ V-Cillin K 125 mg./5 ml 80 ml
  Sig: dr. i orally t.i.d. until bottle empty

Purified Water USP, 52 ml, should be used as directed on the package.

Aromatic Waters—The occasional prescription in which an aromatic water is called for is illustrated in ℞ 27.

27

℞ Phenobarbital Na 2
  Tinct. Belladonna 20
  Peppermint Water, q.s. 240

Order of mixing does not seem to be of special concern. There is a moderate clouding, but no precipitate as may be surmised or as may be described in certain texts. Should a sedimentation (plant extractive matter, which may consist of some active ingredient) appear likely, a "shake well" label should be used. Do not filter.

Official Elixirs—There are two categories of elixirs available as vehicles for medicinal agents: official elixirs and medicinal elixirs.

28

℞ Sod. Bromide 4.5
  Sod. Citrate 3
  Tr. Hyoscyamus 6
  Tr. Belladonna 9
  Aromatic Elixir, q.s. 120
  Sig: One teaspoonful q6h

The sodium citrate should be dissolved in 10 ml of purified water, followed by the sodium bromide. The tinctures are then added to about ½ ℞ volume with Aromatic Elixir USP, to which is added the water mixture. Aromatic Elixir USP is then used to bring the volume to 120 ml.

29

℞ Sod. Bromide 4
  Chloral Hydrate 4
  Elixir Alurate, q.s. 240
  Sig: One teaspoonful in water, 9 a.m., 4 p.m. and at bedtime if necessary

Chloral alcoholate does not form in ℞ 29. The concentrations of alcohol, chloral hydrate and sodium bromide are not sufficient to cause a reaction or salting out. However, chloral alcoholate is known to occur at higher concentrations of sodium bromide and chloral hydrate than that in ℞ 29.

30

℞ Codeine SO$_4$ 0.3
  Elixir Terpin Hydrate
    and Codeine, q.s. ad. 120
  Sig: One teaspoonful q2–3 h, prn cough

Codeine phosphate is 12 times more soluble than the sulfate. The prescriber should permit the change or write another prescription. The phosphate can then be dissolved in 1 ml of purified water, and the dispenser should make a note on the prescription order.

Medicinal Elixirs—This type of vehicle combines the advantages of sweetness, pleasant flavor and alcoholic content. The alcoholic content may vary from as low as 3–5% to as high as 20–25%. Adjustments may be made in the form of the drugs used or in the alcoholic concentration or both to accommodate the solubility characteristics of the ingredients included in a formulation. ℞ 31 illustrates this point.

31

℞ Tinct. Belladonna   4
   Phenobarbital Na   0.4
   Elixir Betalin Comp.
   Aqua, aa, q.s. ad   120
   Sig: One teaspoonful 15 min. ac and q. hs

Phenobarbital should be used in place of the sodium salt and sufficient alcohol to dissolve the base added in place of a portion of the elixir. Prefabricated medicinal elixirs are popularly employed in modern prescription orders. As a rule, few pharmaceutical formulations in this category exhibit incompatibility.

32

℞ Elixir Donnatal   oz. 2
   Amphojel, q.s.   oz. 4
   Sig: Two teaspoonfuls in water for indigestion

Syrups—The use of syrups as vehicles has the advantage of satisfactory masking of unpleasant tastes. Syrups are available in a variety of flavors and flavor blends. Reference to Table 12 will show the selection of certain general flavors that are used to mask the several taste modalities (sweet, sour, salty, bitter). Here again, there are certain official syrups available along with the many commercial liquid medicinal syrups often used as vehicles.

Some drugs are weak acids (e.g., coumarins, nalidixic acid, nitrofurantoin, phenobarbital, salicylic acid, and sulfonamides) and others are weak bases (e.g., amphetamine, antipyrine, chloroquine, mecamylamine, meperidine, procaine, quinidine, theophylline, and some tranquilizers). Accordingly, the pH of the surrounding media affects the rate and extent of absorption and excretion. The therapeutic activity may be destroyed (℞ 24). Phenylbutazone, for example, is not absorbed well in the presence of antacids. Investigators found that 28 tradenamed products consisting of elixirs, syrups and special liquid formulations have a pH range from about 2.75–5.5, with the majority at 2.8–3.5. Nafcillin cannot be added to a solution of diphenhydramine for one is a sodium salt and the other a hydrochloride. Tetracyclines are not absorbed when administered along with antacids (this is largely because of complexation with aluminum, magnesium, and calcium). Aspirin and phenobarbital are more readily absorbed in the stomach having lower pH, where the nonionized form prevails.

Absorption of drugs can be delayed or inhibited depending upon the form of the drug or the improper pH. The pH of liquid formulations used as vehicles or along with other medications may alter the availability of some drugs. Some medications may be partially or wholly inactivated or precipitation may take place.

Therapeutic Information

In this era of rigid control over drug products, the responsibility of the pharmacist in regard to pharmacological and therapeutic knowledge of drug action has expanded. Both the physician and the patient now look to the pharmacist for specialized information. The highly potent and specific medications now available require that he be familiar with drug reactions and interactions, patient hypersensitivities, expiration dates, label warnings, contraindications, precautions, and adverse reactions.

The current broad concept of drug interaction is that such action occurs whenever the absorption, distribution, biotransformation or excretion of one drug is altered by concomitant administration of another drug or other chemical in the food or environment. This applies to liquid oral medications as well as to solid dosage forms given concurrently. See Chapter 13.

Prescriptions

33

℞ Elixophyllin   120 ml
   Marax
   Actifed-C   aa   60 ml
   Sig: 5 ml q.i.d. for asthma

34

℞ Phenobarbital   100 ml
   Tr. Belladonna   12 ml
   Mft.
   Sig: Teaspoonful T.I.D.
   (Phenobarbital Elixir USP intended)

35

℞ KCl 10% in Wild Cherry Syrup   4 oz.
   Sig: 15 ml q.i.d.

36

℞ Ephedrine SO₄   0.3
   Benylin Exp., q.s. ad   120
   Sig: One teaspoonful q4h for relief of asthma

37

℞ Elixir Donnatal   3 oz.
   Liq. Dramamine q.s.   6 oz.
   Sig: Two teaspoons before bedtime

38

℞ Pbz. Expt.   60 ml
   Sudafed   60 ml
   Sig: teaspoonful 4 times a day

39

℞ Butibel
   Bidrox   aa   120 ml
   Sig: 30 min. AC. & HS

Although exactly as written, the pharmacist needs to tell the patient what dose.

40

℞ Deodorized Tincture of Opium   12 ml
   Elixir of Pamine   q.s. to   4 oz.
   Sig: Take one or 2 teaspoonfuls every 4 hours as needed for stomach

41

℞ Tylenol   90 ml
   Phenobarbital   30 ml
   Sig: Take one Tsp. every 4 hours for fever

Long-Acting Liquids

Most of the work in producing orally administered long-acting dosage forms has been in the development of encapsulated or tableted products; however, orally administered long-acting liquid preparations are also useful.

Smith, Kline & French Laboratories, besides providing capsules and tablets for sustained action based on slowed disintegration, markets a liquid preparation in which very fine microscopic particles of a drug are dispersed throughout slightly larger microscopic particles of a slowly disintegrating matrix. The resulting microscopic pellets are suspended in a viscous aqueous vehicle. The powdered drug marketed in such form is sulfaethylthiadiazole, which is rapidly excreted by the kidneys (when compared with other clinically-available sulfonamides), and is commercially available in the sustained-action liquid preparation known as Sul-Spansion *(SK&F)*.

Other pharmaceutical companies have described the use of either ion-exchange resins or tannates in long-acting liquid preparations; however, it has been stated that it is doubtful if a large enough particle size would be acceptable in a liquid preparation in order to allow reasonable prolongation of release. The use of either tannates or ion-exchange resins is discussed in Chapter 2.

External Liquids

Prescription orders for pharmaceutical formulations in liquid form for external application comprise a wide variety of ingredients, combinations, and physical characteristics. This type of formulation includes several different categories identified by intended therapeutic action or finished physical form. The more important types of dermatological formulations, especially those applied to the skin, are included in this section. Medications in liquid form intended for application to body orifices or cavities are also considered. General pharmaceutical products represented in this class include prefabricated aerosol sprays, aqueous and alcoholic solutions, collodions, emulsions, liniments, lotions, and tinctures.

Extemporaneous mixtures of drugs and other chemicals are called for in prescription orders and take the form of solutions, lotions, collodions, emulsions and suspensions. These preparations may be applied to the external surface or to body orifices with or without friction, by means of local wet dressings or compresses, sprayed on the surface, or applied by means of special apparatus such as aerosol spray containers, syringes, atomizers, nebulizers, or medicine droppers. Some are administered by the addition to bath water or by irrigation of a surface area. The objective of liquid pharmaceutical formulations for topical application is to alter some local surface condition that is abnormal or pathological.

There are certain pharmaceutical product classifications such as emulsions, aerosols, ophthalmic solutions, and suspensions that are important enough to be presented in a more extensive manner elsewhere in the text because of the special pharmaceutical technology and biopharmaceutics involved. Miscellaneous external liquid preparations such as bath oils, dental liquids, enemas, gargles and mouthwashes, jellies, and wet dressings or compresses are only briefly mentioned.

Some liquids for external use are clear solutions containing one or more ingredients, while others contain material in suspension as a coarse or colloidal dispersion. The formulation may consist of a combination of therapeutic ingredients individualized to suit the patient needs as determined by the physician. Adjuvants used are of many forms, including vehicles or solvents, suspending agents, stabilizers, surfactants, and preservatives, but not necessarily all of these are used in one formulation.

Table 13 lists a variety of topical therapeutic effects associated with ex-

Table 13—Therapeutic Effects of External Liquid Medications

Antibacterial	Demulcent
Antifungal	Drying
Anti-inflammatory	Emollient
Antipruritic	Keratolytic
Anesthetic	Protective
Astringent	Parasiticide
Counterirritant	Rubefacient

ternal liquid medications.

Hospital pharmacists and community pharmacists practicing in the vicinity of certain medical specialists such as dermatologists, dentists, ophthamologists, or podiatrists are called upon to dispense a variety of extemporaneous formulations. Certain physicians adhere to formulations long found successful in their individual practice and therefore individualized pharmaceutical technology may be required in compounding their prescriptions, to develop acceptable formulations.

42

R̲ Resorcin
   Boric Acid, aa   4
   Glycerin
   Zinc Oxide, aa   30
   Witch Hazel   60
   Aq. Dist, q.s. ad   180
   Sig: Apply q.i.d. and prn

Dissolve the resorcin and boric acid (crystalline) in the witch hazel and levigate the zinc oxide with the glycerin. Bring the two mixtures together and add sufficient purified water to make 180 ml. A shake-well label is required. The use of boric acid is being discouraged.

Many elegant formulations for external use are available as proprietary or tradenamed products, either restricted to prescription order only or for self-medication by OTC purchase. Physicians occasionally still write for a wide variety of drugs and chemicals to be included in a single formulation. This presents a challenge to the pharmacist to produce a stable preparation with the use of accepted pharmaceutical techniques. Indeed, the physician expects such performance as an essential element of good pharmaceutical practice.

43

R̲ Menthol   ¼%
   Cetaphil Lotion, q.s. ad   4 oz
   Sig: Apply to affected area of skin prn

To prevent the formation of a gummy mass, the menthol should first be dissolved in 5 ml of propylene glycol and this solution added to enough Cetaphil Lotion to make 4 fl oz.

Preparation

A knowledge of the physical and

chemical properties as well as therapeutic use of active agents is basic to the compounding of external liquid formulations. Pharmacists should understand the properties of solvents, vehicles, suspending agents, surface-active agents, preservatives, and other adjuncts, and properly utilize them. The multitude of drugs and chemicals encountered in liquid formulations for external use makes it impractical to formulate any organized specific set of instructions for this class of pharmaceuticals. However, a general procedure involves (1) determining proper order of mixing to insure a stable and uniform preparation, (2) noting any drug or therapeutic incompatibility, and (3) making certain the patient is properly instructed as to use.

The dispenser should indicate the specific compounding procedure on the prescription order so that renewals always conform to the original physical characteristics.

The pharmaceutical techniques used in the preparation of solutions for external use are essentially the same as those used for internal liquids. Solution, trituration, levigation and wetting are employed when necessary to prepare the ingredients. Clays such as bentonite need to be spread on the surface of water for hydration. Levigation with glycerin, liquid petrolatum, the glycols or polyglycols can be judiciously used.

44

℞	Calamine	8
	Zinc Oxide	8
	Carboxymethylcellulose Sodium (4000 c.p.s.)	2.2
	Dioctyl Sodium Sulfosuccinate	0.08
	Glycerin	4
	H₂O q.s., ad.	120

Sig: Apply to irritated areas prn

Glycerin is used to levigate the mixed powders. The sodium carboxymethylcellulose and dioctyl sodium sulfosuccinate are dissolved in 100 ml of purified water. The latter solution is added to the paste mixture and sufficient water added to bring the volume to 120 ml.

45

℞	Tween 20	½%
	Phenol	1.2 g
	Bacimycin Tab.	#4

Cetaphil Lotion, q.s. 120

Sig: Apply to affected areas 4 times a day and for discomfort

The methods used in the preparation of liquids for external use are essentially the same as for internal liquid formulations. Soluble active constituents are dissolved in ¼–½ the volume of solvent needed. Filtration is resorted to when required to effect clarity and uniformity without removal of active material. Final volumes are made up by addition of sufficient vehicle, measured in a graduated cylinder.

Order of Mixing—In some cases the order of mixing may be important as in the addition of methylcellulose to ½ the final volume of boiling water, followed by a period of maceration with agitation. The final volume is made up by the addition of cold water. Bentonite should be spread on the surface of water and allowed to become thoroughly hydrated before being used as a magma or suspension. Vigorous agitation hastens the process and aids in the production of a smooth product.

Order of mixing is significant in ℞ 46.

46

℞	Hydrocortisone	1%
	Menthol	⅛%
	Cetaphil, q.s. ad.	8 oz.

Sig: Label

The menthol should be dissolved in 5 ml of propylene glycol and the hydrocortisone levigated with a portion of the Cetaphil. The two portions are mixed and the volume made up with the lotion.

pH of External Liquids—The hydrogen-ion concentration has become an important factor in producing and maintaining optimum conditions for the stability and potency of external liquid preparations. Methods are available for development and control of the acidic or basic character of these formulations. The pharmaceutical manufacturer when necessary has taken care of this at the production stage, but the pharmacist should be aware of situations when the addition of other materials may effect a change in the acidity or basicity and thus the integrity of the product.

Aqueous External Liquids

The various types of aqueous pharmaceutical liquids that are used externally include aerosols, sprays, baths, dental liquids, douches, enemas, gargles and mouth washes, jellies, lotions, ophthalmic solutions, and wet dressings, including compresses.

Aerosols—Local anesthetics, antiseptics, germicides, dermatological products, nasal sprays, inhalants, first-aid films, dental anesthetics, and other preparations are available in a variety of pressurized containers with different types of delivery valves. Chapter 11 is devoted to the technology of this particular dosage form.

Sprays (Nebulae)—Sprays such as Afrin Nasal Spray (*Schering*) and Trisocort Spraypak (*SK&F*) are often ordered by the physician for his patient.

47

R   Trisocort Spraypak
    Sig: Use as directed

These are aqueous, buffered solutions intended for topical application to the nasal passage. The atomizer or nebulizer delivery system is employed. In this way, some control can be exercised over direction of the medication to the area, without injuring the patient by excessive pressure or concentration.

Some nasal solutions are administered with a dropper service container. Neo-Synephrine (*Winthrop*) is used in various concentrations from $\frac{1}{8}$–1%.

48

R   Neo-Synephrine Spray $\frac{1}{2}$%   15 ml
    Sig: Spray Nose 3 times in 10 min every 4
    hours

This solution is often diluted from a 1% concentration by use of normal saline solution in order to preserve the isotonic character of the product.

A true fog or mist is produced by a nebulizer which brings a jet of liquid and air together from a hand-operated, compressed bulb. For example, Isuprel (*Winthrop*), Adrenalin (*Parke-Davis*), Medihaler-Iso (*Riker*), are solutions which are applied to the nose, throat and lungs by means of an atomizer or nebulizer. The Medihaler device operates more on the aerosol principle.

Baths—A bath is any liquid or solid conductive medium such as mud, sand, water, or vapor in which the body is washed or wholly or partly immersed for therapeutic or cleansing purposes. The objective may be either the conservation or restoration of health. There are a number of different, special baths. Tepid sponge baths promote relaxation, relieve discomfort, stimulate circulation, and temporarily reduce high fever. Water at 80°F is used to sponge the body. A *Sitz bath* is intended to relieve urinary retention, local pain, congestion, and muscle spasm. Water (110°–120°F) is used in a tub at a depth of 6 in. in which the patient sits. Solutions or dispersions of ingredients are accomplished by use of solvents, oils, surface-active agents, soaps, and water. Potassium permanganate, sodium thiosulfate, sulfur, and coal tar (Coal Tar Solution USP) are sometimes prescribed as ingredients for baths. Up to 3 oz of coal tar solution is used in an adult bath. The patient is immersed for 20–30 min for the antipruritic effect.

Emollient Baths—These baths are given to relieve skin irritation. Water (at about 100°F), containing an emollient such as starch, bran, or oatmeal, is commonly used. One pound of cornstarch, made into a smooth paste with cold water, followed by hot water and boiled until thick, is added to a tub of water. Bran, enclosed in a muslin bag, is also used. The bag is soaked in hot water and used as a sponge by washing the skin and squeezing the bag against the surface. Cooked oatmeal, tied in a cheesecloth bag, is used as a washing sponge. Sodium bicarbonate (8 oz to about 30 gal of water) is used in conjunction with the emollient washes. Potassium permanganate (1–4 teaspoonfuls of crystals to two-thirds of a tubful of water) dries exuding surfaces and deodorizes lesions. Sulfur, as potassium sulfide (3 oz), zinc sulfate (5–10 teaspoonfuls), or Sulfurated Lime Solution, NF XII (5–7 oz) are added to $\frac{2}{3}$ of a tubful of water.

As a counterirritant to relieve congestion, 1–2 tablespoonfuls of mustard/gal of warm water is effective. In extensive burns, sepsis, or dermatitis, a hypertonic solution of sodium chloride (5–8 lb of ordinary table salt to 30 gal of water) is used.

A specially milled, colloidal oatmeal preparation, Aveeno (*Cooper*), contains 50% starch, 25% protein, and 9% oil. A cupful to a tub of water is effective as a demulcent and an antipruritic. This product is available as Aveeno Oleate (*Cooper*) for dry skin. Another specialty product is Surfactol-45, a thick liquid which is soluble in both oil and water. Ten per cent of Surfactol-45 in peanut oil or mineral oil is applied directly to the body. As a bath, 1 tablespoonful to 1 qt of warm water is added to the tub of bath water.

The application of baths is usually confined to hospitals or to the sick room. The patient, the nurse, or the home-care attendant usually receives instructions from the physician relevant to the preparation of the material for use as a bath. Ambulatory patients are directed to use pharmaceuticals of the type illustrated in ℞ 49.

49

℞	Menthol	0.12
	Surfactol	12
	Peanut Oil	120

Sig: ℥ ii to ½ tub of bath water

Mineral oil may be used instead of the peanut oil.

Dental Liquids—Prescriptions are seldom written for these medications and therefore the pharmacist is called upon to prepare only a limited number of these formulations extemporaneously. Dental supply houses provide the practicing dentist with most of the dental preparations he uses in his office. A few proprietary liquid dental products are sold over-the-counter, but the Council on Dental Therapeutics of the American Dental Association recognizes very few products in this category.

Ammoniacal Silver Nitrate Solution (Howe's solution) contains 29.5 g of silver in complex form in 100 ml of solution. Formerly official in the NF XII, it no longer appears in either the USP or NF. However, it still finds use and the dentist may obtain it in ampul form from the dental supply house, manufacturer, or pharmacist. One ampul as commercially available is more than enough for one patient. The silver nitrate, when reduced by eugenol or clove oil deposits free silver and is used in the treatment of root canal infection of the teeth, and for desensitization of dentin (on teeth cementum). It may also be employed when the patient complains of galvanic action between dissimilar metal tooth restorations. The pharmacist can prepare this solution by using the process given in the NF XII, page 354. The solution is somewhat unstable, may darken or show a deposit of silver oxide, and evaporates. The pharmacist can assist the physician in sealing the ampul following use, or prepare a fresh solution every time it is needed.

A substantial amount of investigative work has been carried out to determine the effect of fluoride solutions when applied to tooth surfaces for prevention of dental caries. A number of different fluoride preparations are commercially available for topical use, consisting mainly of sodium fluoride, stannous fluoride, or their aqueous solutions. Flavoring, coloring, and buffering agents are incorporated in the proprietary products available, but this practice is discouraged by the Council on Dental Therapeutics.

Sodium fluoride (2% *w/v*) became popular a few years ago as a routine office procedure for topical prophylactic treatment to prevent dental caries. The solution is still quite useful when applied to the teeth by a brush or dabbed on with cotton or gauze. A number of toothpastes, mouthwashes, gargles, and oral tablets with vitamins offer fluoride ion as a routine oral hygiene measure. In those communities with fluoridated drinking water, the need for dental office treatment has been reduced. However, in rural areas and in those communities that do not have the benefit of fluoridated drinking water, the practicing dentists use fluoride solutions in the office. The pharmacist should be aware of the safe and effective concentrations of fluoride ion to be used in the solutions and be able to make calculations to achieve the desired strengths.

Stannous fluoride solution (8%) is applied at 6-month intervals to reduce dental caries. The instability of the solution requires minimum exposure during preparation and use. For ease and simplicity, 0.8 g of stannous fluoride is placed in a No. 2 hard gelatin capsule by the pharmacist and stored in a tightly closed bottle. The contents of the capsule are emptied into 1 ml of purified water in a 25-ml Pyrex or plastic beaker, or other suitable container. Due to oxidation and hydrolysis of the stannous ion in aqueous solution, a fine, white precipitate of stannous hydroxide forms in time, even at a pH of 3. Stock solutions of stannous fluoride should not be prepared.

The following formulations represent typical fluoride treatment solutions and are mentioned as possible extemporaneous pharmaceuticals.

50

R   Sodium Fluoride   2 g
     Purified Water, to make   100 ml
     Sig: Dab on dried area with cotton

If stored for a long time in glass bottles, the above solution may form a sludge. This can be avoided by using polyethylene containers.

51

R   Sodium Fluoride   q.s.
     Purified water, q.s. ad   60 ml
     M. ft. sol. so that each drop contains sufficient sod. fluor. to provide 1 ppm of fluoride ion when added to 1000 ml of city water which contains 0.6 ppm of fluorine.
     Sig: One drop in 1000 ml of city water. Use as drinking water.

The calculations show the need for 950.4 mg of sodium fluoride in 60 ml.

52

R   Sod. fluoride   q.s.
     Purified water,   ad   50 ml
     Sig: Sod. fluoride sol., 12 drops to contain 0.5 mg. of fluorine.

By using a standard dropper, i.e., 20 drops = 1 ml, the number of doses in 50 ml can be determined.

Potassium fluorostannite (4% w/v) and sodium monofluorophosphate (6% w/v) in water are available under a variety of proprietary names. The sodium monofluorophosphate is marketed as a gel, but this is not accepted by the Council on Dental Therapeutics. Controlled studies generally indicate caries reduction as a result of the use of these fluorides.

Local anti-infective agents include Iodine Tincture USP and Povidone-Iodine Solution USP in solutions of 0.5–3%. Local anesthetic agents applied topically include tetracaine hydrochloride, 2%.

Oral moniliasis is treated with Nystatin Oral Suspension USP, 100,000 units/ml in a flavored vehicle. The solution is dropped in the mouth and held for some time before swallowing.

Douches—The word douche, as applied to pharmaceutical preparations, refers to an aqueous solution, used as an irrigation or wash, which is applied at low pressure to cleanse, deodorize, soothe, or medicate wounds, body orifices, or cavities. Douches may promote healing, or be astringent, antiseptic, or germicidal. In general, the pH is adjusted within a range of 3.8–4.4, although some have a pH as high as 5.5 when used in the vaginal tract. Sterile solutions are required when a douche is used following surgical procedures. Douches for the vagina are introduced by means of a suitable rubber syringe with a specially designed nozzle. Irrigations of the eye, ear, nose, throat, bladder, colon, or kidney are also carried out by means of douche solutions. Enemas may be considered a form of douche. Solutions for use in the eye, ear, nose and throat are discussed in more detail in Chapter 9.

A list of ingredients commonly found in a douche solution illustrates the types of materials used. Cleansing solutions commonly used include sodium chloride (0.9%; isotonic), boric acid (2%), sodium bicarbonate (1 or 2%), or saponated cresol (0.2–0.5%). Medicated solutions include mercuric chloride (1: 3000 to 1:10,000), vinegar (1 oz to 1 qt of water), potassium permanganate (0.1– 1%), green soap (1%), or lactic acid (0.5–3%). Tannic acid, acetic acid, alums, zinc sulfate, and zinc phenolsulfonate are employed as astringents. A deodorizing effect is accomplished by using peroxides, potassium permanganate, or perborates. Aromatics such as methyl salicylate, peppermint oil, thymol, menthol, and eucalyptol add fragrance and freshness to the preparations.

Specialty products, which are either prescribed or purchased over the counter, include Trichotine (*Reed & Carnrick*), Betadine Douche (*Purdue-Frederick*), Nylmerate Antiseptic Solution Concentrate and Jelly (*Holland-Rantos*), and Vagisec (*Schmid*). These are vaginal cleansers that contain antifungal and germicidal agents in addition to soothing, astringent, and aromatic materials. A product like Vagisec includes sodium ethylenediaminetetraacetate (EDTA).

53

℞ Vagisec Liquid   4 oz.
   Sig: One capful to one quart of water as douche

Betadine Douche offers a pleasantly scented solution clinically effective in nonspecific vaginitis and against moniliasis and trichomonas vaginitis. The active ingredient is Povidone-Iodine USP, an organic bound form of iodine which allows for a slow, continued release of a low but effective concentration of iodine, approximately 1% available I. Some formulations contain wetting agents such as sodium lauryl sulfate and dioctyl sodium sulfosuccinate; others contain kaolin and aluminum hydroxide gel. The availability and economy as well as the suitability of the prefabricated products decrease the use of individualized formulations prescribed by the physician.

54

℞ Betadine Douche   2 oz.

Sig: 3 teaspoonfuls in 1 qt. warm water to use as douche

55

℞ Nylmerate Douche   16 oz.
   Sig: 1 capful to 2 qts. warm H_2O douche

56

℞ Alum
   Boric Acid, aa   ʒ2
   Phenol   ʒ1
   Peppermint Oil   gtts. 3
   M. Ft.   Powder bulk
   Sig: ʒ ii in 2 quarts warm aq. as directed.

Mix powders in the usual way and then add to the peppermint oil in which phenol is dissolved with geometric dilution.

Enemas—An enema is a solution that is placed in the rectum or colon to cause evacuation or to bring about a local or systemic therapeutic action. The pharmacist may be called upon to furnish such medication. Dispensing requires a knowledge of proper concentration and method of application in order to instruct the patient in correct use of this form of medication. Among the chemicals commonly used in cleansing enemas that involve evacuation are magnesium sulfate, sorbitol (25%), normal saline, sodium bicarbonate, glycerin, castile soap, and sodium phosphate. Quantities of each as generally employed may be found in a standard reference such as *The Merck Manual* (see *Bibliography*). Enemas are classified as (1) cleansing or evacuating (tap water or weak soapsuds and saline), (2) carminative (milk and molasses, turpentine and soapsuds, or olive oil), (3) retention (chloral hydrate, paraldehyde, warm oil, starch, and water), (4) lubricating (vegetable oil or mineral oil), and (5) medicated (6–8 oz of coffee or 1 oz of whiskey/6 oz of normal saline). Specific amounts are prescribed by the physician.

Several plastic squeeze containers have been introduced for the administration of medication rectally as an enema. These contain formulations of sodium biphosphate (16%) and sodium phosphate (6%) in 130 ml amounts for adult use. A pediatric form and an oil retention form are available. The pediatric product contains a lesser amount of the two phosphates while the oil retention form contains Mineral Oil USP. ℞ 58 is a pediatric form.

57

℞ Rectal Emulsion   1 pt.
(½ raw linseed oil and ½ lime water)
Sig: As directed (agitation produces a water-in-oil emulsion)

58

℞ Fleet Enema   2¼ oz.
Sig: ii containers each of 2¼ oz.

Gargles and Mouthwashes—A mouthwash is generally regarded as a medicated liquid for cleansing the mouth or treating diseased states of the oral mucous membrane. It may be administered under the supervision of a dentist. Only superficial food particles and debris can be removed by mouthwashes and the germicidal or antibacterial effects are temporary. The Council on Dental Therapeutics does not recognize the claims that the use of a cosmetic mouthwash results in any real improvement in oral health. However, mouthwashes purchased over-the-counter are extensively used by the layman to rinse the mouth and to impart a refreshing sensation or pleasant odor. Also, rinsing or spraying the mouth after operative procedures adds to the comfort of the patient. A pH of 5–9.5 appears to be a safe range with 6.5–7 being optimum for liquids for oral use.

Gargles are also pleasantly flavored but they are more highly medicated than mouth washes. Antibiotics, antiseptics, local anesthetics, anti-inflammatory agents, antifungal agents, analgesics, and alkalinizing agents represent the major types of therapeutic agents found in both mouthwashes and gargles. Active ingredients include benzocaine, borax, eugenol, clove oil, phenol, potassium permanganate, creosote, chloroform, lidocaine, sodium chloride, sodium bicarbonate, and benzalkonium chloride in appropriate concentrations.

59

℞ Betadine Gargle   180
Sig: Use as mouth wash and gargle q3h

60

℞ Xylocaine Viscous   100 ml
Sig: Use as gargle q3h prn pain

61

℞ Sol. Mercurochrome 5%   30 ml
Sig: Swab mouth B.I.D.

62

℞ Glyoxide Drops   2 oz.
Sig: Gargle with 25 drops 4 times a day or every 4 hours as needed, then swallow.

Jellies—These are semisolid to thick viscous fluids that consist of submicroscopic particles in a somewhat rigid or plastic vehicle. The products are rich in liquid and have a mucilage-like viscosity. The formulations are either transparent or translucent. The consistency and appearance is that of a homemade jelly. Jellies, as pharmaceutical preparations, find use as effective lubricants for surgeons gloves, catheters, enema and douche nozzles, rectal thermometers, and hemorrhoids.

Substances commonly used to produce the gel state are alginates, carboxymethylcellulose, gelatin, glycerin, and tragacanth. Some are medicated or contain aromatics.

Xylocaine Viscous (*Astra*) finds use in the relief of pain and the discomfort of irritated or inflamed mucous membrane (see ℞ 60). Ora-Jel Liquid (*Commerce Drug*) is employed as a topical anesthetic for teething and for denture irritation. Tragacanth and glycerin form the base for these.

63

℞ Ora-Jel Liquid   15 ml
Sig: As directed

Surgitube (*Day-Baldwin*) is available in small sterile packages which are convenient for operating room use. K-Y Sterile Lubricant (*J&J*) is a long-time popular surgical lubricant with a vegetable gum base. The pharmacist does not prepare jellies on an extemporaneous basis and all have been deleted from the official compendia. Some formerly popular medicated jellies have been discontinued because of disappointing therapeutic results, or because better preparations have become available.

Lotions—Lotions are usually aqueous preparations containing insoluble solids held in suspension or dispersion, intended for external use by application to the skin without friction. Lotions may be completely inorganic or organic in composition. Combinations of these chemical entities are common. A few are clear solutions, but many are emulsions such as Benzyl Benzoate Lotion NF. Certain official lotions, such as White Lotion NF, are employed only when freshly prepared. Other lotions that are variations of the official formulations are manufactured commercially and have extended shelf-lives.

64

R̸ ZnO   6 g
  Boric Acid   5 g
  Menthol   1 g
  Alcohol   25 ml
  H₂O,   q.s. ad   120 ml
  Sig: Apply locally b.i.d.

Lotions with insoluble material in suspension are prepared by triturating the properly comminuted dry powders with a levigating agent to make a smooth paste. The desired volume is then prepared by cautious addition of the remaining liquid phase. High-speed mixers or hand homogenizers aid in better dispersion of the insoluble, or dispersed, phase. The viscosity can be controlled to some extent by judicious use of suspending agents, solution stabilizers, and surfactants. A uniform and smooth suspension is produced when the active ingredients are supported by adjunctive substances and blended by agitation at high speed. A Waring Blendor or fountain mixer serve very well for this purpose. These dispensing techniques are not difficult to apply, and cosmetically elegant preparations are easily obtained.

65

R̸ Sulfur, ppt   0.4 g
  Vanoxide Lotion   20 ml
  Sig: Apply to face t.i.d. after bathing

In some lotion formulations the insol-uble solids are formed by chemical interaction in the liquid, and are not filtered. No suspending agent is indicated since the precipitate is nearly colloidal. White Lotion NF illustrates this type.

Lotions may be employed for their local cooling, soothing, protective, drying or moisturizing properties, depending upon the ingredients used. Desired therapeutic uses include antifungal, antiinflammatory, antiinfective, antipruritic, scabicide, parasiticide, anhidrotic, and local anesthetic. Examination of the prescription illustrations indicates the variety of medications used to alter the pathology of body surfaces.

The skin-protective properties of silicone oils have been utilized in hand lotions to prevent irritation. There is an aerosol spray that contains 33% silicone (dimethicone) in a petrolatum base. Another version of a silicone formulation is Covicone Cream (*Abbott*) a 30% dimethyl polysiloxane with nitrocellulose and castor oil in a vanishing cream base. When applied to the skin, dimethicone imparts a coating effect that is resistant to removal by soap and water for a period of time. These preparations are most useful in preventing irritations caused by direct contact irritants.

Lubriderm (*Texas Pharmacal*) is an emulsion type lotion that contains refined derivatives of lanolin (a mixture of cholesterols), sorbitol, cetyl alcohol, mineral oil and cholestrin. Nivea is an emollient cream or oil in emulsion form containing neutral hydrocarbons in water with wool fat cholesterols.

Cetaphil Lotion (*Texas Pharmacal*) is widely used in some areas as a vehicle for medicinal agents (see R̸ 46). It is a lipid-free, skin cleanser consisting of propylene glycol, cetyl alcohol, stearyl alcohol, sodium lauryl sulfate, butyl and propyl parabens, and purified water. See R̸ 45 and R̸ 46.

Ophthalmic Solutions—Solutions for the eye are known as *collyria*. They are usually clear, aqueous liquids, sterile at the time of preparation, and adjusted to a suitable pH and osmotic pressure for comfort during irrigation or application to the eyes. The special importance of this class of pharmaceutical formulation is recognized by devoting a separate discussion in Chapter 9. It is sufficient here to point out that the pharmacist has available several simplified methods which permit quick, accurate preparation of buffered, isotonic solutions as a routine matter. Sterility is of special significance due to the danger of eye infection and damage of tissue because of contamination with bacterial organisms, especially *Pseudomonas aeruginosa (Bacillus pyocyaneus)*. Serious corneal ulcers may result. The formula given here has recently been prepared and thoroughly tested and found to be effective in the treatment of ophthalmic infections, particularly when due to *Pseudomonas aeruginosa.*

66

R   Sodium acid phosphate,

anhyd.	4.003 g
Disodium Phosphate,	
anhyd.	4.75 g
Sodium Chloride	4.30 g
Polymyxin B sulphate	5000 units/ml.
Thimerosal sol., 1:10,000	
q.s. ad.	1000 ml.

The solution is prepared under aseptic conditions. This basic ophthalmic solution is suitable to act as a vehicle for atropine sulfate, eucatropine, homatropine, ephedrine, and pilocarpine hydrochloride.

Medicaments used routinely in various conditions affecting the eyes include fluorescein, physostigmine salicylate, pilocarpine nitrate, scopolamine (hyoscine) hydrobromide, atropine sulfate, ethylmorphine hydrochloride, cocaine hydrochloride, dibucaine (Nupercaine), tetracaine hydrochloride (Pontocaine hydrochloride), cortisone, sulfonamides, antibiotics, sodium chloride, carbachol, diisopropyl fluorophosphate (DFP, Floropryl), nitrofurazone (Furacin), boric acid, and phenylephrine (Neo-Synephrine).

Wet Dressings—These are solutions of chemicals in an aqueous medium. Normal saline or slightly hypertonic saline solutions, boric acid solution (2–5%), Aluminum Acetate Solution USP, or prepared from such materials as Burosol Powder (*Oak*), potassium permanganate solution (1:10,000–1:4,000), magnesium sulfate solution (50% *w/v*), and quaternary ammonium solutions are applied directly by means of gauze packs. Incompatibilities of cationic and anionic agents need to be taken into account. Thus, soaps should not be used in conjunction with cationic germicides such as quaternary ammonium compounds.

Burosol Powder is prepared by adding 1 teaspoonful to 1 qt of water to produce a dilution equivalent to 1:15 dilution of Burow's solution. This is diluted frequently in a 1:20 or 1:40 dilution.

67

R   Burow's Sol.   ii
    Sig: Saturated ear pack q2h

68

R   Buro Sol Pwd.   16 oz.
    Sig: i → 40, compresses, legs ½ h, t.i.d.

Note: Burosol Powder is furnished as a solid mixture; ½ teaspoonful to 1 pt of water gives a 1:15 dilution of Burow's solution. Therefore, to obtain a 1:40 dilution, the patient is advised to measure out 6 fl oz of the 1:15 dilution and make up to 1 pt. This procedure may be repeated for the three daily applications.

Compresses—These are wet dressings. Solutions of the therapeutic agents mentioned above are applied to gauze pads and kept in contact with the appropriate dermatomucosal surfaces for extended periods of time. Inflammation is reduced and the dermatologic treatment can be followed with other local anti-inflammatory therapy.

Vleminckx' Lotion (Sulfurated Lime Solution NF XII) has been deleted from the NF. Vlem-Dome Liquid Concentrate (*Dome*), a similar formulation, is used as a hot wet dressing, soak, or compresses applied as directed by the physician to treat acute seborrheic dermatoses and pustular and fungal infections. One packet (teaspoonful) to 1 pt of hot water is equivalent to 4 teaspoonfuls of the old type Vleminckx' solution diluted to 1 pt and is used as a hot compress.

Betadine Skin Cleanser (*Purdue-Frederick*) is a povidine-iodine sudsing germicidal liquid. By covering the affected skin area with the solution, followed by a little water, a lathery suds is created. It is effective against pathogenic bacteria, particularly *Staphylococcus aureus,* and some fungi, yeasts, protozoa, and viruses. The iodine is available in a nonirritating form, and soap and water washes off any starched linen stain readily.

Nonaqueous External Liquids

Several types of nonaqueous liquids find application externally, including collodions, dental liquids, glycerites, and liniments. The liniments include certain tinctures and the dental liquids include toothache remedies.

Collodions—Official collodion is made up with ethyl oxide (3 parts), alcohol (1 part), and pyroxylin (4 parts *w/v*). Flexible collodion consists of 2 parts *w/w* camphor, 3 parts *w/w* castor oil in collodion sufficient to make the weight required. A protective film is formed on the surface and keeps any incorporated medication in contact with the skin for an extended period of time.

69

R̥   Lactic Acid   20%
     Salicylic Acid   20%
     Flexible Collodion   15 ml
     Sig: Apply to wart with toothpick twice a day

This can be dispensed in an applicator bottle and applied by the drop.

Dental Liquids—Chlorobutanol in combination with essential oils, such as clove oil, methyl salicylate, cinnamon oil, and cinnamic aldehyde is used as a local analgesic in toothache, or as a sedative dressing for pulpitis or nearly exposed pulps. Dentalone (*Parke-Davis*) is such a product. A 2–4% solution of lidocaine is employed as a topical spray to produce superficial anesthesia of the oral mucosa. A 10% Xylocaine Dental Spray (*Astra*) is available.

Parachlorophenol (35%) and camphor (65%) form a eutectic mixture with a penetrating odor, and the liquid is corrosive to the skin. The mixture is used as a disinfectant in root canal and periapical infections of the teeth. Dark-colored, well-stoppered containers are essential for storage if the mixture is to remain colorless. The solution is easily prepared by the pharmacist for use in the dentist's office.

Glycerites—These are viscous, hygroscopic liquids or semisolids that contain not less than 50% by weight of glycerin, along with dissolved medicaments. Glycerites as a pharmaceutical class are obsolete and have been dropped from the official compendia and find practically no use in pharmacy or medicine.

Liniments—Liquid or semisolid preparations of an alcoholic, saponaceous, or oily character, intended for external use and applied with massage, are called liniments. Liniments are the least desirable form of external liquid formulation from the patient's point of view.

Green Soap Tincture NF is a detergent solution. Calamine Liniment NF IX is still a formulary item in some hospitals. It consists of 80 g each of zinc oxide and calamine, 500 ml of olive oil, and sufficient limewater to make 1000 ml. This is a water-in-oil emulsion used topically as an emollient and protective.

A number of proprietary liniments are popularly used in rural areas as antipruritics, rubefacients, counterirritants, astringents, or analgesics. The pharmacist should be familiar with the contents of each in order to supply information in the event of accidental poisoning. One teaspoonful of camphor liniment (camphorated oil) has been fatal in children.

Methyl salicylate 50%, isopropyl alcohol 25%, and cottonseed oil 25% is used as a counterirritant for inflamed joints, sprains and rheumatism. However, creams and lotions appeal more to the esthetic interests and replace liniments to a certain extent.

Prescriptions

70

R̥   Salicylic Acid   20%

Flexible Collodion   20 ml
Sig: Apply small amount to affected area of
toes, b.i.d.

71

℞ HgCl₂ Sol (1–100)   8 ml.
Boric Acid   2 g.
Alcohol USP, q.s. ad   60 ml.

72

℞ Camphor   1
Menthol   1
Calamine Lotion, USP q.s. ad   100
Sig: Apply topically to affected area

73

℞ Tinactin Soln   10 ml
Sig: Apply gtts. ii or iii to affected area and
rub in

74

℞ Betadine for Vaginal Douche   240 ml
Sig: One tbsp. in one qt. of hot water to
douche

75

℞ Scadan Lotion   120 ml
Sig: Apply B.I.D.

76

℞ Loroxide Lotion   45 g
Sig: Apply to face and other affected areas
twice a day or more

77

℞ Roccal Solution   1 bottle
Sig: Use one oz. to one gallon of water, soak
diapers at least 12 hours

78

℞ Americaine Aerosol Spray   5 oz.
Sig: Apply sparingly to rash areas b.i.d.

79

℞ Banalg Liniment   4 oz.
Sig: Rub on painful muscle twice a day

80

℞ Kwell Liquid
Sig: Apply to skin by massage b.i.d.

81

℞ Lime Water   50%
Olive Oil   50%
Menthol ¼%   120 ml
Phenol   ¼%
Sig: Apply prn for itching

82

℞ Triamcinolone   0.025%
Aqua   20%
Aquaphor   1 oz.
Sig: to R hand as directed

83

℞ Menthol   0.12
Phenol
Camphor   aa   2.4
Witch Hazel, q.s.   120
Sig: Locally q.i.d.

84

℞ Fluorouracil   1%
In Propylene Glycol   2 oz.
Sig: Apply to face, neck, arms as directed.

Dispensing

Certain significant fundamental factors which must be considered during prescription compounding and dispensing are enumerated here.

1. Physical and chemical properties of the prescription ingredients
2. Order of mixing and use of adjuvants
3. Pharmaceutical techniques required
4. Incompatibilities in preparation and storage
5. Stability and potency of ingredients
6. Proper labeling, including accessory labels

Qualities of a good external liquid formulation are

1. Esthetic appearance insofar as possible.
2. Stable formulation with regard to permanency of color and absence of sedimentation.
3. Uniform distribution of active ingredients.
4. Ease of spreading and penetration according to intended activity.
5. Release and availability of medication, either rapidly or over a prolonged period of time on extended contact with dermatomucosal surfaces.

Therapeutically inactive constituents used in the development of pharmaceutically elegant external liquids consist of various relatively nontoxic solvents, suspending agents, surface-active agents, preservatives, and other adjuncts in addition to the active ingredients. Descriptions and discussions of the use of these materials are found elsewhere in this textbook.

References

1. Harned HS, Owen BB: *The Physical Chemistry of Electrolytic Solutions,* 3rd ed, Reinhold, New York, 161, 1958.
2. Becker P: *Emulsions: Theory and Practice,* 2nd ed, Reinhold, New York, 2, 1965.
3. Ibid: 11.
4. McBain JW, *et al: Kolloid-Z* 78: 1, 1937.
5. Gerding PW, Sperandio GJ: *JAPhA Prac Ed 15:* 356, 1954.
6. Colgan MT, Mintz AA: *J Ped 50:* 522, 1957.

7. Leonards JR: *Clin Pharm Ther 4:* 476–479, 1963.

8. Monte-Bovi AJ: *JAPhA 12:* 565, 1951.

Bibliography

Introduction

Ecanow B, Balagot R, Gold B, Ecanow C: *J Soc Cos Chem 23:* 681, 1972.

Ecanow B, Klawans H: In Klawans H, ed: *Models of Human Neurological Diseases,* Excerpta Medica, Amsterdam, Chap. 9, 1974.

Solution Technology

Spiegel AT, Noseworthy MM: *J Pharm Sci 52:* 917, 1963.

Discher CA: *Modern Inorganic Pharmaceutical Chemistry,* Wiley, New York, 31, 1964.

Hildebrand JH, Scott RL: *The Solubility of Nonelectrolytes,* 3rd ed, Dover, New York, 1964.

Kavanau JL: *Water and Water-Solute Interactions,* Holden-Day, San Francisco, 1964.

Jirgensons B: *Organic Colloids,* Elsevier, Amsterdam, 1958.

Martin AN, Swarbrick J, Cammarata A: *Physical Pharmacy,* 2nd ed, Lea & Febiger, Philadelphia, Chap. 9, 1969.

Emulsion Technology

Becker P: *Emulsions: Theory and Practice,* 2nd ed, Reinhold, New York, 1966.

Parrott EL: *Pharmaceutical Technology,* Burgess, Minneapolis, 1970.

Griffin WC: In Kirk RE, Othmer DF: *Encyclopedia of Chemical Technology,* vol 5, Interscience, New York, 692–718, 1950.

Osipow LI: *Surface Chemistry,* Reinhold, New York, 337–341, 1962.

Swarbrick J: In *Remington's Pharmaceutical Sciences,* 15th ed, Mack Publ. Co., Easton, PA, Chap. 22, 1975.

Schick MJ, ed: *Nonionic Surfactants,* vol 1, Dekker, New York, 1967.

Burlage HM, Lee CO, Rising LW, eds: *Physical and Technical Pharmacy,* McGraw-Hill, New York, 575–577, 1963.

Suspension Technology

Verwey EJW, Overbeek JThG: *Theory of Stability of Lyophilic Colloids,* Elsevier, New York, 1948.

Martin AN, Swarbrick J, Cammarata A: *Physical Pharmacy,* 2nd ed, Lea & Febiger, Philadelphia, Chap. 18, 1969.

Liquid Dosage Forms

Kutscher AH, Zegarelli EV: Dental services. In *Remington's Pharmaceutical Sciences,* 15th ed, Mack Publ. Co., Easton, PA, Chap. 105, 1975.

The Merck Manual, 12th ed, MSD Research Laboratories, Rahway, NJ, 1760, 1972.

Day RL: *Handbook of Non-Prescription Drugs,* 89–95, 1969.

Accepted Dental Therapeutics, 1969–70, American Dental Assoc., Chicago, IL, 196.

9

EENT
medications

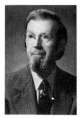

John D. Mullins, PhD
Director, Dermatology Dept.
Science and Technology Div.
Alcon Laboratories
Fort Worth, TX 76101

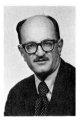

Donald E. Cadwallader, PhD
Professor of Pharmacy
School of Pharmacy
University of Georgia
Athens, GA 30602

Ophthalmic Medications

Products for use in the eye are classified as ophthalmic preparations and include sterile solutions, sterile suspensions, and sterile ointments. Such products may be instilled into the eye by a variety of means including drops, sprays, or mists; continuous streams for irrigation; and applied as ointments. The USP defines these products as follows:

Ophthalmic Solutions—Sterile solutions that are compounded and packaged for instillation into the eye.

Ophthalmic Ointments—Special sterile ointments for application to the eye. They are manufactured from sterile ingredients under rigidly aseptic conditions or are terminally sterilized.

Probably the most important single aspect of ophthalmic solutions is the requirement that such solutions be sterile; however, the requirement that an ophthalmic product be sterile is a surprisingly recent event. USP XV (1955) was the first to include sterility as a requirement. The Food and Drug Administration (FDA) adopted the position in 1953 that a nonsterile ophthalmic solution was adulterated. This is not to say that prior to 1955 all ophthalmic solutions were not sterile; however, it was not until 1955 that sterility was adopted as a requirement by the official compendium and thus acquired the force of law.

Prior to World War II and well into the 1940's only a few ophthalmic solutions were commercially available. Solutions to be used in the eye were usually compounded in the community pharmacy and were intended almost entirely for immediate use in the sense of a typical prescription usage. This situation is reflected in the pharmaceutical literature of that time. In the 1940's and even into the early 1950's the stability of ophthalmic solutions is often discussed in terms of immediate use, i.e., use within 30–60 days.

In the historical sense solutions for use in the eye can be traced to antiquity. Collyria are mentioned in the Ebers papyrus and in the Hippocratic Codex.

The word belladonna stems from the use during the Middle Ages of this plant to dilate female pupils for cosmetic reasons. Belladonna alkaloids are used today in solution form as mydriatics. A dilated pupil is no longer considered a cosmetic necessity by the ladies.

The use of solid material in the eye in the form of ophthalmic suspensions dates from the early 1950's when corticosteroids were first introduced. Cortisone acetate ophthalmic suspension was, for all practical purposes, the first liquid product containing insoluble suspended material recommended for use in the eye. At the time this represented a significant departure from the concept of solutions only for use in the eye. Clinical experimental work at the time revealed that with a particle size sufficiently small there was no discomfort and indeed no sense of solid particulate matter in the eye. This fact, the lack of sensation caused by insoluble solids, is partially a function of concentration as well as particle size. As the percentage of insoluble material increases, the sensation of foreign material becomes increasingly apparent.

The requirement for sterility of ophthalmic ointments is of even more recent vintage. Sterility requirements for ointments to be used in the eye were first included in the 3rd Supplement of USP XVIII (1972). Prior to that time— in part because of the low organism counts customarily found in ophthalmic ointments—and in part because of the difficulty of testing sterility of ophthalmic ointments, there was no formal legal requirement for a sterile product.

Anatomy and Physiology

The eye is the organ of sight. The spherical eyeball is positioned in the bony orbital cavity and cushioned by fat and connective tissue. The anterior aspect is exposed and is comprised superficially of the transparent cornea, the opaque sclera, and the conjunctival membrane. The eyeball itself is protected by the eyelids and eye lashes (Fig. 1).

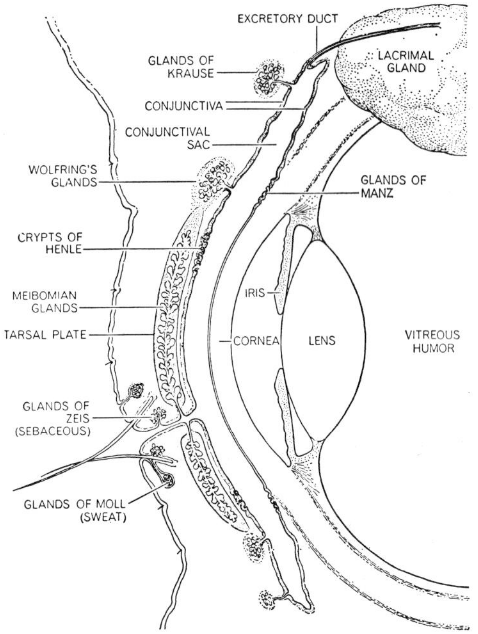

Fig. 1—The eye and eyelids.[1]

The skin of the eyelids is thinner than the skin on any other part of the body. This of course facilitates folding and the opening and closing of the lids. The internal surface of both lids is covered by an extension of the same conjunctival membrane covering the sclera.

The secretions of the eyelid glands contribute to eye protection by helping prevent the loss of tear fluid. The secretion of the meibomian glands is lipoidal and forms a part of the precorneal tear film. Meibomian secretions also help prevent the overflow of tears at the lid margins. The inner eyelid surfaces form the cul de sac, divided in turn into the superior and inferior fornix.

The cornea is the first lens in the optical system of the eye. Anatomically the cornea is a multilayer structure, avascular but rich in sensory nerves. Corneal tissue usually maintains a steady water content of 75–80%. Proper water equilibrium is critical to optical integrity of the cornea.

The normal cornea is entirely devoid of blood vessels. This lack of vasculari-

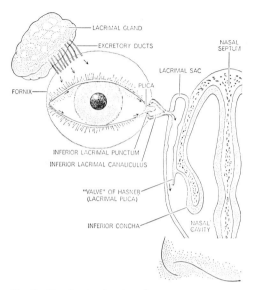

Fig. 2—Nasolacrimal system.[1]

zation is probably due to the compact arrangement of normal corneal tissue which is both dense and highly ordered. The cornea and also the conjunctiva, however, are abundantly supplied with nerve endings depicting pain. Indeed the cornea is one of the most pain-sensitive regions in the body.

The avascular cornea depends on permeability for much of its nutrition. Oxygen and other substances are absorbed from the tear film and other fluids. The permeability of the cornea is also a major factor in the absorption of drugs intended for ophthalmic use.

The remainder of the visible "white of the eye" is made up of the dense, opaque, fibrous sclera with its covering of conjunctival membrane. The conjunctival membrane covers the outer surface of the sclera and extends over the inner surface of the eyelids. The membrane is only loosely attached to the eyeball, permitting freedom of movement and, by lifting the membrane, the so-called subconjunctival injection of drugs.

Tear fluid is a rather complex mixture made up of electrolytes, protein, carbohydrates, enzymes (lysozyme), and organic acids. Solids total about 1.8%.

Lacrimal fluid is comprised of the lacrimal gland secretions and secretions of the mucous glands of the conjunctiva. The pH of the tears is about 7.4, ranging 7.3 to 7.7. The osmotic concentration is equal to 0.9% sodium chloride.

The surface of the eye is covered by the tear film. This is a three-layered film of distinctly different composition. The innermost layer of the tear film is made up of a mucoid material secreted from the goblet cells of the conjunctiva. The middle layer, some 6.5–7 μm thick, is made up of tear fluid. The outer or third layer is the superficial oily layer made up of lipoid meibomian secretions.

The total volume of eye fluids is small, but turnover rates are significant. Approximately 7 μl of lacrimal fluid is in contact with the cornea at any one time, while the turnover rate is about 1 μl/min in the human eye.

The lacrimal drainage system is shown in Fig. 2. Much of the volume of drug solution instilled into the cul de sac drains into the nasal cavity via the lacrimal drainage system, and the remaining solution is diluted by the continuous replenishment of tears, i.e., tear turnover. It has been shown in rabbits that instilled solutions are rapidly drained from the eye, up to 50% of a 50-μl drop being lost within 30 sec, and over 80% within 3–4 min.

Absorption

Drugs are normally instilled into the cul de sac of the eye and distributed into the precorneal tear film by the action of the lids and movement of the eye. Ophthalmic drug bioavailability is generally conceded to be poor from topically applied solutions. For most drugs, less than 1% of an instilled dose crosses the cornea to the anterior chamber.

Drugs intended for ophthalmic use other than local effects enter the aqueous humor or the anterior chamber by passive diffusion primarily through the cornea. A substance will be most readily absorbed through the cornea if it has both fat and water-solubility characteristics, i.e., biphasic solubility. Since the

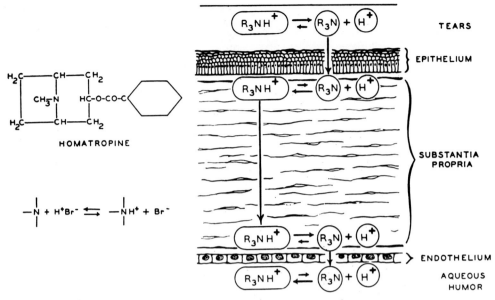

Fig. 3—Transfer of homatropine through the cornea, according to Kinsey.[2]

majority of ophthalmic drugs are the salts of weak bases, instillation into the tear fluid will normally convert such salts, at least in part, to the free-base form. This latter is readily absorbed by the lipoidal epithelial cells. Ionic substances will also penetrate the cornea although at rates significantly less than their lipid-soluble basic counterparts. Evidence suggests that ions can penetrate the cornea between cells; however, absorption may be erratic as in the case of carbachol.

Fig. 3 is a representation of a mechanism by which drugs may penetrate the cornea. Drugs intended for ophthalmic use are usually most rapidly available for absorption when administered in the form of weakly buffered aqueous solutions. Solution composition and/or solution additives can influence drug absorption by controlling the ionic form of the drug or by modifying tissue permeability or drug contact time.

The USP permits the addition of various substances to ophthalmic solutions in order to increase viscosity. Methylcellulose, hydroxypropylmethylcellulose, carboxymethylcellulose, and poly-

vinyl alcohol are commonly used for this purpose. The addition of such materials increases solution viscosity and increases the contact time of ophthalmic solutions in the eye. The addition of ionic materials may also be used to enhance drug absorption. The inclusion of benzalkonium chloride in carbachol solutions augments the miotic response attributable to direct corneal absorption.

Although the greatest amount of drug absorption does occur through the cornea, the sclera does not necessarily act as a differential solubility barrier. Injection of human serum albumin tagged with radioactive iodine in Evans blue into the subarachnoidal space of rabbits resulted in a rapid escape of the albumin across the sclera into the orbital tissues. Based on the visible location of dye, the albumin moved directly across the sclera toward the exterior of the eye, apparently driven by intraocular pressure. This indicates the sclera will allow the transfer of even relatively large molecules however the passage of these molecules was brought about by a relatively high intraocular pressure.

Dosage Forms

Solutions—Ophthalmic solutions comprise the overwhelming majority of products used in the eye. Ophthalmic solutions include the following categories:

> Solutions for therapeutic use—such as pilocarpine
> Solutions for diagnostic use—such as fluorescein
> Solutions for irrigation—such as balanced salt solution
> Unit dose solutions
> Special solutions for use with contact lenses
> Oil solutions—such as diisopropylfluorophosphate in peanut oil

Suspensions—Ophthalmic suspensions are not defined separately in the USP; however, they are accepted as a part of the general definition of ophthalmic products. Such suspensions require and meet the same specifications as ophthalmic solutions with the exception of clarity. In the place of clarity we are concerned with particle size and resuspendability of the suspension product. Insoluble solids for use in the eye must be microfine. Ophthalmic studies have reported that suspended particles having a diameter of 50 μm will be uncomfortable and irritating to most individuals. Corticosteroids comprise all of the insoluble solids used in suspension form in the eye and are either micronized or microcrystallized to assure a minimum particle size.

Ointments—Ophthalmic ointments are dispersions of medicinal substances in petrolatum or in a petrolatum-like vehicle. Only most recently has the concept of sterile ophthalmic ointments become a reality. A particular requirement of ophthalmic ointments is that of spreadability. Ideally the ointment inserted into the cul de sac will soften and spread due to the temperature and pressures obtained. Such temperature sensitivity in turn imposes formulation and storage limits to avoid melting and nonhomogeneity within the tube prior to its being used. The best general base for ophthalmic ointments is white petrolatum. A drug can be readily dissolved or dispersed in this bland base. White petrolatum can be sterilized by heating to 170°C for 2 hours, and mineral oil can be added to the petrolatum if a lower-melting base is preferred. As they are anhydrous, the petrolatum bases can be used for dispensing moisture-sensitive drugs such as antibiotics and isoflurophate.

Other Methods of Application—In addition to the comparatively well-known methods of administering drugs to the eye, the following are mentioned as useful, but less well-known means, of applying medication into or on the eye.

Subconjunctival Injection—This method is rarely used and should only be considered with drugs such as antibiotics where penetration is known to be poor. Subconjunctival injection is not a precisely accurate term. Such an injection should be given below Tenons capsule; thus the term sub-Tenons is probably more appropriate. The advantages of sub-Tenons injection are often overcome by the disadvantages such as patient apprehension, pain, and inconvenience.

Continuous Irrigation—Continuous irrigation has been used as a technique in which polyethylene tubing is passed through the lid by means of a surgical needle. With this tubing in place, the (usually) antibiotic solution is administered in much the same fashion as intravenous drip.

Ocular Therapeutic System—This method is a recent innovation. The system, comprised of four laminated elements, is known commercially as the Ocusert. The reservoir containing the drug (only pilocarpine is currently available) is encased in polymer membranes. The structure of the polymer membrane controls the passage of pilocarpine from the system into the eye. The ocular therapeutic system is placed in the cul de sac. Once in place it provides pilocarpine at a constant rate for 1 week. The "hills and valleys" typical of conventional eye-drop therapy are said to be avoided.

General Considerations

The human eye is a particularly sensitive organ. It reacts quickly to nearly any change in environment. For this reason, solutions for use in the eye as well as suspensions and ointments must be prepared with meticulous care. Requirements which must be considered in the preparation and in the control of ophthalmic products are:

Sterility
Clarity
Buffer
pH
Tonicity
Preservatives
Additives
Viscosity
Packaging
Stability

Many of these requirements are interrelated and cannot be regarded as isolated factors to be considered individually. Stability, for example, can be related to pH, to the buffer, and to packaging. The buffer system must be considered with tonicity in mind, with product comfort in mind, etc.

Sterility—The sterilization of eye products is a major factor in preventing serious eye infections and must be considered both the most important and most exacting procedure in the preparation of products for use in the eye. Failure to achieve sterility may cause serious eye injury, including the possibility of complete loss of vision.

The means of achieving sterility are varied and depend on the physical and chemical characteristics of the product and its components, equipment, and product packaging. General procedures include:

Dry heat
Steam under pressure
Sterilizing solutions
Gas, i.e., ethylene oxide
Filtration

The details of each of these procedures are given in USP XIX and in Chapter 10. In general, however, any eye solution may include several sterilization procedures rather than a single method. Equipment, packaging, materials, and finished product must be fitted to the most appropriate methods in order to achieve total product sterility.

Dry-heat sterilization is normally carried out at 160–170°C for 2–4 hours. Time and temperature schedules must be determined for the specific material to be treated. It is particularly important that warmup time, circulation, and other variables be compensated for in order to assure exposure of the material itself to the required temperature and time cycle.

Steam sterilization is carried out in an autoclave and is based on the sterilizing action of steam under pressure. Temperature is usually 121°C. To assure proper heat distribution, recording thermocouples sealed into representative containers are often recommended. Both the temperature and the time at a specific temperature should be recorded.

Materials in solution may be sterilized by filtration through a suitable sterilizing medium. Filtration media vary considerably in the means by which sterilization is effected as well as in composition. Sterile filtration by adsorption or by a physical sieving mechanism should yield a sterile, particle-free filtrate. The filter medium should not react with or remove components of the solution, i.e., preservatives, buffer, salts, etc.

Sterile filtration may be accomplished by the use of suitable-porosity membrane filters, filter pads, microporous porcelain, or specially sintered materials. A variety of each of these materials is available commercially, together with data on typical uses. Reactivity or a lack of reactivity of filter media should never be presumed. Specific products should be evaluated as a part of the process of selecting a suitable filtration medium.

Gas sterilization of heat-sensitive substances may be carried out by exposure to either propylene oxide or ethylene oxide. The latter is more commonly used and requires specialized, although not elaborate, equipment.

Table 1—Ethylene Oxide Mixtures Available Commercially

Trade name	Mixture	Manufacturer
Cry-oxide	11% Ethylene oxide 79% Trichloromonofluoromethane 10% Dichlorodifluoromethane	Ben Venue Labs. Bedford, OH
Benvicide	11% Ethylene oxide 54% Trichloromonofluoromethane 35% Dichlorodifluoromethane	The Matheson Co. East Rutherford, NJ
Pennoxide	12% Ethylene oxide 88% Dichlorodifluoromethane	Pennsylvania Eng. Co. Philadelphia, PA
Steroxide-12	12% Ethylene oxide 88% Dichlorodifluoromethane	Castle Ritter Pfaudler Corp. Rochester, NY
Carboxide	10% Ethylene oxide 90% Carbon dioxide	Union Carbide Corp. Linde Div. New York, NY
Oxyfume Sterilant-20	20% Ethylene oxide 80% Carbon dioxide	Union Carbide Corp. Linde Div. New York, NY
Steroxide-20	20% Ethylene oxide 80% Carbon dioxide	Castle Ritter Pfaudler Corp. Rochester, NY

Ethylene oxide for sterilization is commercially available, diluted either with carbon dioxide or with halogenated hydrocarbons. Ethylene oxide is a colorless flammable gas at standard temperature and pressure. The gas liquefies below 12°C and is highly irritating to the eyes and to mucous membranes. The chemical structure is

$$CH_2 \underset{O}{\diagdown \diagup} CH_2$$

The use of ethylene oxide as a sterilizing agent was at one time severely limited because of its flammable and explosive properties. The use of carbon dioxide as a diluent, however, greatly reduces this danger. The mixture known as Carboxide contains 10% ethylene oxide and 90% carbon dioxide. A list of the commercially available ethylene oxide mixtures is given in Table 1.

Ethylene oxide sterilization demands careful consideration of conditions required to effect sterility. Temperature and pressure requirements are somewhat low in contrast to wet or dry methods; however, a careful control of exposure time, ethylene oxide concentration, and humidity is essential to achieve sterility.

Ethylene oxide exerts its bactericidal activity by alkylating protein molecules. With the increased use of this method the potential for human toxicity has become obvious. In order to avoid harmful contact an aeration period should be included as a part of the total ethylene oxide sterilization cycle. The length of time necessary to dissipate possible toxic residues depends on the material being sterilized, packaging, sterilization cycle, and end-use of the article.

The USP refers to a procedure of sterilization by exposure to sterilizing gases such as ethylene oxide and indicates that gas sterilization requires the use of specialized, but not necessarily elaborate, equipment designed for the purpose.

So-called gas autoclaves may range from the large-scale elaborate equipment used in industry to quite-small portable units recommended for small hospitals, clinical laboratories, or pharmacies. One such unit effects sterilization in a cylindrical chamber (Fig. 4). The sterilizing gas diluted with an inert diluent is contained in a metal bulb which, after activation, delivers enough gas to effect sterilization in the exposure chamber. The manufacturer recommends a 5-hour sterilization cycle although materials may be kept longer in the chamber.

Gas sterilization can produce irritating byproducts of chemical reaction such as ethylene chlorohydrin and ethylene glycol. To minimize such materials particular care should be exercised in sterilizing halide-containing materials such as polyvinyl chloride.

After ethylene oxide sterilization the sterilized article(s) should be aerated for a minimum of 24–48 hours, which depends on the nature of the material sterilized. Ambient aeration time for polyethylene dropper-bottle units should be about 48 hours.

It should be noted that ethylene oxide sterilization is effective and recommended only for solid materials which will not withstand wet- or dry-heat sterilization, i.e., polyethylene dropper bottle caps and dropper inserts. Ethylene oxide cannot be used to sterilize solutions, ointments, or other product forms.

Clarity—As officially defined, ophthalmic products must be free from foreign particles. Clarity is usually achieved by filtration. The degree of clarity can be estimated by the use of light-scattering devices such as the Coleman Nephelo-Colorimeter. Nephelos units are numerical values on a 100 scale and are used to define the region between absolute clarity and visible turbidity; i.e., the nephelos unit then is a measure of departure from clarity.

Solution clarity is normally obtained by proper filtration, either as a part of sterile filtration or by the use of a clarifying filter. Nonfibrous filters such as clarifying membranes or in-line sintered glass are often effective in clarifying solutions. It must be realized, of course, that a clarified solution must be filled into a clean container. This implies both particle-free rinse water and a particle-free filling area.

Buffer and pH—Product pH and the buffer required to establish pH are a part of product design and are usual essentials for product stability. The pH of the tear fluid is generally accepted to be approximately 7.4, although this value may vary. The active ingredients

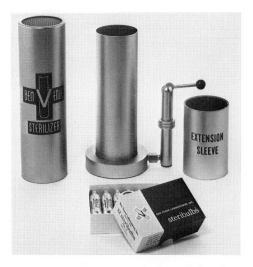

Fig. 4—Ethylene oxide sterilization unit (courtesy, Ben Venue Labs.).

commonly used in ophthalmic solutions are usually acid salts of weak bases; as such, these are most stable at an acid pH.

This, then is the dilemma in the formulation of eye products. Good product stability often requires an acid pH. Product comfort, on the other hand, should ideally be based on a pH of approximately 7.4. It is not possible to compromise product stability. On the other hand, some formulation latitude is permissible in choice of buffer salts and buffer capacity.

It is generally accepted that a low (acid) pH *per se* will not necessarily cause stinging or discomfort during use. Difficulties generally arise as a result of buffer capacity at a specific pH rather than the pH value itself.

Solution pH is, of course, a measure of acidity or alkalinity; it is defined as the negative log of the hydrogen ion concentration. "Buffer capacity" indicates the capacity or ability of a buffer system to resist change. A properly formulated eye product should include a buffer with a capacity sufficient to maintain product pH during the proposed shelf-life. At the same time, the capacity should be minimized in order to permit the tear fluid to readjust to pH 7.4 following instillation of the product into the eye. Discomfort is caused by the inability of the tear fluid to overcome the buffer and adjust pH.

Many buffer solutions have been recommended for use in ophthalmic products. The USP lists several together with suggested pH values. It should be emphasized that if product stability is considered a function of pH, stability should be verified by specific tests. Stability should never be accepted by reference.

Viscosity—During the 1950's increased viscosity was suggested as a means of increasing the contact time of ophthalmic solutions in the eye. Since that time the USP has permitted the use of additives such as methylcellulose, hydroxypropyl methylcellulose and polyvinyl alcohol to prolong contact time. Solution viscosity may be increased to approximately 25–50 cps by such additions; however, particular care must be exercised to be certain that solution clarity can be achieved in the presence of such viscosity-imparting agents.

Tonicity—The theory and practice of tonicity adjustment has been presented in Chapter 8. Tonicity refers to the osmotic pressure exerted by salts in solution. An ophthalmic solution is generally considered isotonic with another solution when the magnitudes of the colligative properties of the solutions are equal. As a convenience, an ophthalmic solution is said to be isotonic when its tonicity is equal to that exerted by a 0.9% aqueous solution of sodium chloride. Since isotonicity implies equivalent colligative properties, freezing-point depression is usually selected as the basis for determining sodium chloride equivalency.

As a general rule, ophthalmic solutions should be isotonic in order to minimize discomfort. Normally this is not difficult to achieve. As a practical matter, exact isotonicity is not a strict prerequisite for product comfort. The eye can usually tolerate solutions equivalent to a range of 0.5–1.8% sodium chloride.

Solution tonicity has been investigated extensively over the years. Since osmotic pressure is a function of particles in solution, it in turn depends on the use of electrolytes and nonelectrolytes, and on the degree of ionization in addition to concentration. One result of prior investigations has been the accumulation of a large number of sodium chloride equivalents. These values have been computed for many drugs, electrolytes, buffer salts, and preservatives and are available in Chapter 8 and also in *Remington's Pharmaceutical Sciences* (see under *Eye* in *Bibliography*).

Preservatives—With the single exception of unit-dose products, sterile ophthalmic solutions must contain a suitable antimicrobial preservative to prevent the growth of microorganisms inadvertently introduced during use. The need for adequate preservation of ophthalmic solutions was recognized and discussed during the 1930's. The possibility of contamination was realized at that time; however, means of preservation ranged from the use of preservatives such as chlorobutanol to daily sterilization by boiling. The early use of preservatives was, in fact, recommended for economic reasons and to obviate the tiresome daily boiling.

The selection of an adequate chemical preservative for ophthalmic solutions is by no means a simple procedure. Ideally a preservative substance should meet the following criteria:

Broad-spectrum antibacterial activity to include efficacy against both Gram-positive and Gram-negative organisms and fungi.
Satisfactory chemical and physical stability over a wide pH range.
Compatibility with chemical components and with packaging materials.
Safe and nonirritating during use.

Preservative substances must be evaluated for suitability as a part of the total product. *In vitro* bacteriological studies must be carried out against representative organisms present in adequate concentrations for specific time periods. Activity against several strains of *Pseudomonas aeruginosa* should be

Table 2—Ophthalmic Preservatives[a]

Type	Typical structure	Concentration range	Incompatibilities	Remarks
Quaternary ammonium compounds	R_1—$\overset{R_2}{\underset{R_3}{N}}$—$R_4$ Y^-	0.004%–0.02% 0.01% Most Common	Soaps Anionic materials Salicylates Nitrates	Benzalkonium chloride is the single most frequently used ophthalmic preservative. EDTA increases effectiveness.
Organic mercurials	SHgC$_2$H$_5$ / COONa (Thimerosal)	0.001%–0.01%	Certain halides with phenylmercuric acetate	Typically used as substitute for benzalkonium where latter is incompatible.
Parahydroxy benzoates	COOCH$_3$ / OH	Maximum 0.1%	Adsorption by macromolecules	Infrequently used; activity limited to bacteriostasis.
Chlorobutanol	CH$_3$—$\overset{CH_3}{\underset{OH}{C}}$—CCl$_3$	0.5%	Stability is pH-dependent; activity concentration is near solubility maximum	Will diffuse through low-density polyethylene container.
Aromatic alcohols	CH$_2$OH	0.5%–0.9%	Low solubility in water	As above; occasionally used in combination with other preservatives.

[a] From Brown MRW, Norton DA[3] and Mullen W, Shepherd W, Labovitz J.[4]

included in any preservative evaluation. This organism is recognized as a most dangerous eye pathogen. Detailed procedures for investigating the antimicrobial efficacy of preservatives are given in the USP.

An evaluation of the suitability of preservatives should include an indication of chemical stability. A lack of stability could result in the formation of decomposition products which may be irritating or which may be inactive as preservatives. Chlorobutanol typifies this situation. Although this substance has been used as a preservative for many years, its chemical stability is highly dependent on pH. Stability decreases sharply as the pH is increased above the pH 5–6 range.

Many preservative substances may be inactivated by binding with other formulation additives, in particular with macromolecular compounds. Studies have shown that inactivation by various substances is selective and generalizations are difficult to make. For example,

chlorobutanol and benzyl alcohol are inactivated by polysorbate 80 and polyvinylpyrrolidone, but not by methylcellulose. Cetylpyridinium chloride is inactivated by methylcellulose; benzalkonium chloride is not.

Preservative safety testing is normally carried out as a part of the general toxicological assessment of the ophthalmic product. It should be recognized, however, that preservatives are potent substances and can easily cause eye irritation or discomfort even in comparatively low concentrations.

There are relatively few classes of chemical compounds used as preservatives in ophthalmic solutions. In no class do we have the ideal preservative substance. The general classes together with specific examples are summarized in Table 2.

Compounding

Although many solutions, and indeed most of the important therapeutic preparations, are commercially prepared,

Table 3—Volume of Isotonic Solution Which Can Be Prepared Using 0.3g of Drug[a]

Drug (0.3 g)	Volume of isotonic solution (ml)
Atropine sulfate	4.3
Butacaine (Butyn) sulfate	6.7
Cocaine hydrochloride	5.3
Dibucaine (Nupercaine) hydrochloride	4.3
Ephedrine hydrochloride	10.0
Ephedrine sulfate	7.7
Epinephrine hydrochloride	9.7
Eucatropine (Euphthalmine) hydrochloride	6.0
Homatropine hydrobromide	5.7
Phenacaine (Holocaine) hydrochloride	6.7
Phenylephrine (Neo-Synephrine) hydrochloride	10.7
Physostigmine (Eserine) salicylate	5.3
Pilocarpine hydrochloride	8.0
Pilocarpine nitrate	7.7
Pipercaine (Metycaine) hydrochloride	7.0
Procaine hydrochloride	7.0
Scopolamine (hyoscine) hydrobromide	4.0
Sulfadiazine sodium	8.0
Tetracaine (Pontocaine) hydrochloride	6.0
Zinc sulfate	5.0

[a] Adapted from the NF XIV.[5] A more complete table is presented therein.

special prescriptions which require extemporaneous compounding are still presented to the pharmacist. A great deal of care must go into the proper dispensing of these prescriptions.

The specifications and requirements for ophthalmic solutions are many, varied, and rigid as indicated in the foregoing discussion. Nonetheless, individual ophthalmic prescriptions can be compounded to meet these specifications without undue time and expense following the acquisition of the basic equipment required.

Recommended Extemporaneous Procedures—The NF and USP recommend extemporaneous procedures for the preparation of two types of ophthalmic preparations. An outline of these procedures is presented below.

Type I.   Solutions Intended for Application to Traumatized Eyes (Accident or Surgery)

1. With the exception of sodium fluorescein and the sulfonamides, all drugs used in traumatized eyes should be compounded with 2% boric acid solution.

2. Sodium fluorescein and the sulfonamides should be compounded in distilled water.

3. 0.2% sodium bisulfite may be added to the boric acid solutions of physostigmine, phenylephrine, and epinephrine.

4. No preservatives are to be added to these solutions since all preservatives at bactericidal concentrations are irritating to the inner structure of the eye.

5. All solutions are to be filtered and then dispensed in small containers (5- to 10-ml glass bottles with screw caps) for single patient use only.

6. The closed bottle, plus a separate dropper, should be packaged in a container that can be autoclaved. See *Sterilizing Procedure No. 1* or,

7. The solution can be passed through a single-filtration, presterilized disposable unit into a sterile container (see *Bacterial Filtration*).

Type II.   Solutions Intended for Application to Eyes with Intact Corneal Epithelium

1. Solutions are prepared by dissolving the drug (acid salt) in a proper stock vehicle (See *Vehicles*).

2. Sterile solutions are prepared by autoclaving or bacterial filtration (See *Sterilizing Procedures*).

Vehicles

Sterile, isotonic (or isotonic and buffered) solutions containing a preservative are convenient for preparing ophthalmic solutions. To obtain an isotonic solution, the drug(s) is dissolved in a calculated amount of distilled water and the solution brought to the prescribed volume using an appropriate stock vehicle (see Table 3). In most cases where the concentration of active ingredient(s) does not exceed 3%, the drug(s) can be dissolved in an appropriate stock vehicle. The finished preparation will be slightly hypertonic.

Stock solutions of various vehicles can be prepared in advance so that they are conveniently available for the compounding of prescriptions.

Recommended stock vehicles are presented below.

Isotonic Solutions—

Isotonic Sodium Chloride Solution

Sodium Chloride USP	0.9 g
Benzalkonium chloride	1:10,000
Sterile distilled water, to make	100 ml

Commonly prescribed ophthalmic drugs can be dispensed in this vehicle.

Boric Acid Solution

Boric Acid USP	1.9 g
Benzalkonium chloride	1:10,000
Sterile distilled water, to make	100 ml

Since zinc salts form insoluble hydroxides at a pH above 6.4, this latter solution is ideal for solutions of zinc salts because of its lower pH and slight buffering action. Where nitrates or salicylates are used, benzalkonium chloride should be replaced with 0.002% phenylmercuric nitrate.

Sodium chloride cannot be used to adjust the tonicity of silver nitrate solutions because of the incompatibility which results in the precipitation of silver chloride. Sodium nitrate should be used as the adjusting substance and phenylmercuric nitrate as the preservative.

Isotonic Buffer Solutions—The commonly used ophthalmic drugs have been divided into two principal groups and a buffer system is recommended for each group.

Group I—Buffered to pH 5: Consists of drugs that should be maintained at pH 5 in order to retard the rapid formation of the irritating free base and thus allow a more gentle and prolonged action. Therefore, when these solutions are applied, the free base is not instantly liberated, but the lacrimal fluid slowly neutralizes the buffer solution and the base is liberated gradually. The main advantage is increased comfort to the patient.

Buffer Solution for Drugs in Group I

Boric Acid USP	1.9 g
Benzalkonium chloride	1:10,000
Sterile distilled water, to make	100.0 ml

Drugs included in Group I are salts of:

Amprotropine (Syntropan)
Cocaine
Dibucaine (Nupercaine)
Ethylhydrocupreine (Optochin)
Ethylmorphine (Dionin)
Neostigmine (Prostigmin)
Phenacaine (Holocaine)
Piperocaine (Metycaine)
Procaine
Tetracaine (Pontocaine)
Zinc

Group 1A—Buffered to pH 5: A modified boric acid buffer is used for salts of physostigmine, phenylephrine, and epinephrine. Because of an incompatibility, benzalkonium chloride is replaced with phenylmercuric nitrate. Sodium sulfite is added to prevent discoloration (oxidation) of physostigmine, phenylephrine, and epinephrine solutions.

Buffer Solution for Drugs in Group IA

Boric Acid USP	1.9 g
Sodium sulfite, anhydrous	0.1 g
Phenylmercuric nitrate	1:50,000
Sterile distilled water, to make	100.0 ml

Group II—Buffered to pH 6.5: Consists of drugs that have their greatest stability at pH 2–3, but at the same time have their minimum therapeutic action at this pH range. In order to provide a vehicle which would give the greatest stability commensurate with physiological action, a phosphate buffer with pH 6.5 is recommended.

Buffer Solution for Drugs in Group II

Sodium acid phosphate (NaH_2PO_4), anhydrous	0.560 g
Disodium Phosphate (Na_2HPO_4), Anhydrous	0.284 g
Sodium Chloride USP	0.50 g
Disodium ethylenediamine tetraacetate (Na_2EDTA)	0.10 g
Benzalkonium chloride	1:10,000
Sterile distilled water, to make	100.0 ml

This solution is isotonic with a 0.9% sodium chloride.

Drugs included in Group II are salts of:

Atropine
Ephedrine
Eucatropine
Homatropine
Penicillin
Pilocarpine

Sterile distilled water is readily available in the form of liter bottles of water for injection. For 500 ml of stock solution containing 1:10,000 benzalkonium chloride, 0.3 ml of 17% Zephiran Concentrate Buffered Aqueous Solution can be used.

The sealed bottles of stock solutions should be sterilized (*Sterilizing Procedure No. 1*). An alternative sterilizing procedure is to boil the preservative-containing stock solution for at least 30 min.

Sterilizing Procedures

Sterilizing procedures best suited for the extemporaneous preparation of ophthalmic solutions are as follows:

1. **Solutions in Final Container**
   a. Place the filtered solution in containers that have been washed and rinsed with distilled water.
   b. Seal dropper bottles with regular screw caps. The dropper assembly should be stapled into a stiff paper envelope.
   c. Sterilize 10 to 15 min at 15 psi (121°C).
   d. Do not assemble until ready to use.
2. **Dropper Bottles**
   a. Wash container thoroughly and rinse with distilled water.
   b. Loosen caps and place bottles in autoclave.
   c. Autoclave 10 to 15 min at 15 psi (121°C
   d. Partially cool autoclave.

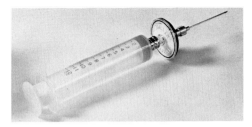

Fig. 5—Syringe and Millex filter unit (courtesy, Millipore Corp.).

e. Remove bottles from autoclave and immediately secure caps.
f. Store sterilized bottles in a clean, dustproof cabinet or under a bell jar.
    Note: Rubber bulbs on the dropper bottles should collapse because of the partial vacuum produced upon cooling.

3. Glassware and Equipment
a. Wrap adapters (containing filter), syringes, glassware, spatulas, etc. in autoclave paper and secure with masking tape.
b. Place articles in autoclave and sterilize in the manner decribed in section 2.
c. Store in separate cabinet until ready to use.

4. Bacterial Filtration
a. All equipment and glassware as well as stock solutions should be sterile. The prescription should be dispensed in a sterile container.
b. Unwrap sterile syringe and draw prepared solution into syringe.
c. Unwrap sterile adapter (Swinny or Gelman) containing bacterial filter and attach to syringe. These are available as single-filtration, presterilized disposable units and should be utilized whenever possible.
d. Force solution through filter directly into sterile container (dropper or plastic Drop-Tainer type).
e. By employing an automatic filling outfit, more than one container of the same prescription can be prepared.
f. Cap container immediately.

The above procedure for bacterial filtration does not eliminate the need for other aseptic conditions such as clean, secluded compounding areas, UV lights, and specialized hoods and chambers, i.e., laminar-flow hoods.

Bacterial filtration using a Millex filter unit attached to a Cornwall syringe (Figs. 5 and 6) is a convenient way to prepare sterile ophthalmic solutions. Adapters employing either 13 mm or 25 mm cellulose ester filter disks (0.45 μm) are used; however, the larger diameter

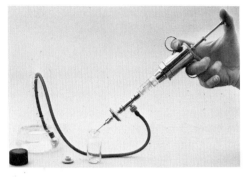

Fig. 6—Cornwall syringe with Millex filter unit (courtesy, Millipore Corp.).

adapter is more convenient since it is easier to force the solution through disks having a greater surface area. The solution to be sterilized is drawn into the syringe; then the adapter is attached to the end of the syringe. The solution is forced through the bacterial filter directly into a sterile container and an appropriate closure placed on the container. When filtering a solution into many containers, a continuous pipetting device (B-D Cornwall) can be attached between the syringe and adapter.

The Drop-Tainer type polyethylene bottle is a convenient container for ophthalmic solutions. Unfortunately, presterilized containers are available only in gross quantities and not as single, sterile units. These containers could be utilized in a small manufacturing program. However, since it is difficult to maintain sterility once the supplier's package has been opened, they are not convenient for the extemporaneous preparation of ophthalmic prescriptions. Polyethylene containers can be sterilized with ethylene oxide (see page 234).

The use of the above procedures is illustrated by the following prescriptions.

1

R̥ Atropine sulfate 30 ml.   1.5%
   M & Ft. Isotonic solution with saline
   Sig.   2–3 gtts. O.S. q. 6 h.

The amount of atropine sulfate needed for this prescription is 0.45 g. The volume of isotonic solution that can be prepared by adding distilled water to this amount of drug is 6.45 ml (Table 3). After dissolving the atropine sulfate to 6.45 ml, the solution is brought to 30-ml volume using a stock vehicle of isotonic sodium chloride solution. The solution is then passed through a 0.45-μm bacterial filter into a sterile container as previously described. The finished preparation is isotonic, sterile, and contains a suitable preservative.

2

R̸ Pilocarpine nitrate 30 ml.   1.75%
   M & Ft. Isotonic-buffered solution
   Sig. 2 drops ea. eye q. 4 h.

The amount of pilocarpine nitrate needed for this prescription is 0.53 g. By simple proportion (7.7 ml/0.3 g = x/0.53 g) it is calculated that this amount of drug will prepare 13.2 ml of isotonic solution. Dissolve the drug in distilled water up to 13.2 ml and qs to 30 ml using the stock pH 6.5 phosphate buffer solution for Group II drugs. Sterilize the solution as previously described. The finished preparation is isotonic, buffered to pH 6.5, sterile and contains a suitable preservative.

3

R̸ Pilocarpine nitrate   0.5%
   Physostigmine salicylate   0.5%
   Suitable vehicle q.s.   30.0 ml
   Sig. i–ii gtts. both eyes q. 4–6 hrs.

Equal amounts (0.15 g) of each drug are weighed and dissolved in distilled water up to a volume of 6.65 ml (4.0 ml for the pilocarpine and 2.65 ml for the physostigmine). Bring the volume to 30 ml using the special buffer for Group IA drugs. The solution is sterilized and placed in a sterile container. The finished preparation is isotonic, buffered to pH 5.0, sterile, and contains a suitable and compatible preservative.

Laminar Flow Principles and Equipment

A laminar air-flow work station is a convenient and highly useful adjunct for the preparation of sterile, particle-free ophthalmic solutions. Laminar flow is defined in *Federal Standards 209a* as "air flow in which the entire body of air

Table 4—Effectiveness of Laminar Flow in Reducing Bacterial Contamination[6]

Airborne contamination of work areas[a]
Colonies/plate

Hospital	Surgical	Medical	Pharmacy
A	630	445	424
B	326	615	174
C	520	600	300
D	684	788	186
E	246	298	135
F	407	574	164

Airborne contamination within laminar flow areas[a]

A	0.5	0	4.0
B	0	0	0.5
C	0	0	1.0
D	0	0.5	0
E	0.5	1.0	1.0
F	0.5	0.5	1.0

The use of a laminar flow work-station is not a substitute for sterility procedures. Laminar flow equipment does provide air essentially free from viable particles and does much to prevent the introduction of airborne contamination.

[a] After 2-hour sampling time.

within a confined area moves with uniform velocity along parallel flow lines with a minimum of eddies." Laminar flow minimizes the possibility of airborne microbial contamination by providing air free of viable particles and by its efficiency in preventing airborne microorganisms (and particulate matter) from entering the critical area. Laminar flow units are available in a variety of sizes and shapes and in two general categories.

1. Horizontal laminar flow in which the HEPA (high efficiency) filter forms the backwall of the work station.
2. Vertical laminar flow in which the air moves downward through a top positioned HEPA filter. The vertical unit takes advantage of gravity in addition to laminar flow to maintain a particulate-free atmosphere.

The effectiveness of laminar flow was investigated in hospitals in the Baltimore area; the results are shown in Table 4. In each of six hospitals three areas were selected for investigation: a surgical patient care unit, a medical patient care unit, and the pharmacy.

Therapeutic Use Categories

Ophthalmic products can be loosely grouped into two divisions of significance to the pharmacist; these include prescription ophthalmic products in either single- or multiple-dose products and nonprescription OTC products. Prescription ophthalmic products normally include the following therapeutic categories:

Anesthetics
Mydriatics
Miotics
Antiinflammatory agents
Antiinfective agents
Antibiotics
Diagnostics
Vasoconstrictors

The nonprescription OTC products include therapeutic categories such as vasoconstrictors and astringents but also nontherapeutic products such as those recommended for use with hard contact lenses. Some of this latter category products might be termed indirect ophthalmic solutions since they are recommended for cleansing or storage of contact lenses and may not be actually instilled into the eye in the normal sense of the use of ophthalmic products. Nonetheless, since these solutions do come in contact directly with articles which are used in the eye, they should be prepared and handled with the same general considerations applicable here as are employed for ophthalmic solutions with one or two exceptions. Sterility is very clearly a critical requirement; however, tonicity may not be a critical requirement, for example, in a storage or cleaning solution as long as this is not also recommended for instillation into the eye.

Patient Information

In dispensing ophthalmic prescription products the pharmacist should advise the patient (particularly the new patient) on the kinds of ophthalmic physiological activities that might be expected. For example, if a miotic is prescribed, the patient should be cautioned that some pupillary constriction will occur; conversely, a mydriatic may cause some pupil dilation. Since either of these effects can be startling, the pharmacist should caution the patient on which might be expected after instilling such products. Suspension products should be adequately shaken prior to use, particularly if such products are dispensed in opaque or translucent plastic containers. If the pharmacist is dispensing a solution that is known to be hypertonic, such as some of the antiinfective solutions, the patient should be cautioned against the stinging that may occur on instillation and why this sting is a part of the medication. Sting cannot be reduced without reducing concentration, which cannot be accomplished without reducing therapeutic effectiveness.

The patient should be cautioned against accidental contamination of ophthalmic products even though such solutions contain preservatives. The system cannot be relied upon to achieve sterility in each and every case without exception. It can be overpowered by the introduction of gross contaminants; therefore, the patient should be instructed in the proper care and handling of ophthalmic solution packaging to avoid accidental contamination either by touching, for example, the dispensing dropper tip to the infected eye surface or by careless handling in nonsterile areas.

In dispensing OTC ophthalmic medications to the patient the pharmacist should bear in mind that these products are intended to correct relatively minor ophthalmic disorders; if such is not the case, the patient should seek medical assistance. In the same fashion the pharmacist can advise the user on the characteristics of the various contact lens solution products and how these should be used in the care of contact lens whether for wetting, soaking, cleaning, or a combination of these.

The patient should be cautioned about proper medication storage. It is usually sensible to avoid a window ledge in bright sunlight as well as a shelf over

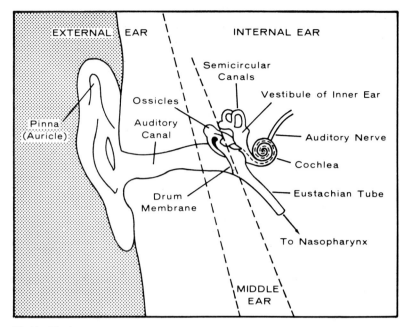

EXTERNAL EAR   INTERNAL EAR

Semicircular
Canals

Vestibule of Inner Ear

Ossicles

Auditory
Canal

Pinna
(Auricle)

Auditory Nerve

Cochlea

Eustachian Tube

Drum
Membrane

To Nasopharynx

MIDDLE
EAR

Fig. 7—The human ear.

a radiator. The patient should also be given some estimation of shelf life or recommended storage time. Prescriptions should neither be stored indefinitely nor used by more than one person.

Ear (Otic, Aural) Medications

Medications such as local anesthetics, peroxides, antibacterial agents and fungicides, as well as liquids for cleaning, warming, or drying the external ear are introduced into the ear canal for their local effect. These materials are usually instilled into the ear canal by means of ear drops; however, irrigating solutions, gauze wicks, ointments, and insufflations are sometimes employed.

Anatomy and Physiology—As shown in Fig. 7, the human ear is composed of three distinct parts: the external, middle, and inner ear. The external ear, the middle ear, and cochlea of the inner ear are parts of the hearing apparatus; the semicircular canals and other portions of the inner ear control equilibrium.

The external ear includes the auricle and external auditory canal; sound is funneled into the canal until it hits the eardrum. The auditory canal is the only cavity of the human body that is lined with epidermal tissue (skin), and many medical problems of the external ear are dermatological in nature. The external canal is approximately 2.6 cm long, and inflammations of the canal are extremely painful because there is no subcutaneous tissue or "padding" to relieve the tension and stretching of the skin.

The middle ear consists of the eardrum and tympanic cavity. The tympanic cavity is an air-filled pocket that contains the auditory ossicles, the malleus, incus, and stapes. The cavity is connected to the pharynx via the eustachian tube which allows air pressure on both sides of the eardrum to be equalized. Infections of the middle ear are usually concomitant with infections of the nasopharynx region via the eustachian tube. Inflammation of the middle ear (otitis media) is usually very painful, and symptomatic relief can be obtained by the instillation of remedies into the external auditory canal. Control of an acute infection is usually attained by systemic administration of antibiotics after proper diagnosis.

The inner ear, or labyrinth, is a complex series of fluid-filled channels that in a large part control a person's orientation in space. Diseases and symptoms associated with the inner ear are Meniere's disease, vertigo, nausea, and tinnitus.

Cerumen—Cerumen (ear wax) is a mixture of the secretions of the sebaceous and ceruminous glands. These glands are located in the lining of the outer 1 cm of the ear canal. Ear wax is a composite of lipids, fatty acids, mucoproteins, wax alcohols, and other lipophilic materials. It has some lubricating and protective functions and picks up dust, debris, and small foreign bodies that may enter the external canal. Normally it dries and falls out of the ear but it may accumulate, eventually become impacted and possibly block the canal.

Uncomplicated accumulations of cerumen usually can be removed by gentle irrigation of the ear with plain warm water, saline solutions, or sodium bicarbonate solutions using an ear syringe. Hard and tenacious impactions might require the application of a cerumenolytic agent to soften and mobilize the mass. A surfactant-propylene glycol solution (Cerumenex) facilitates the removal of ear wax by gentle irrigation by first softening and partially emulsifying the lipid material. Wax can be loosened by the mechanical action of effervescent oxygen after the application of 3% peroxide solution or a solution of carbamide peroxide in anhydrous glycerin (Debrox) into the ear canal.

Solutions and Suspensions—The vehicles most often employed for ear medication are glycerin, propylene glycol, and liquid polyethylene glycols. They are particularly suited for otic medication because they are viscous and will adhere well to the surface of the auditory canal. Mineral oil is used as a vehicle for terramycin-hydrocortisone acetate suspension. Vegetable oils, especially olive oil, are sometimes used as solvents, and are often used alone for their soothing and warming effect in the ear. Ethanol and isopropyl alcohol are useful solvents for medications and may be applied full-strength in the ear. Except for irrigating solutions, aqueous solutions are not recommended for otic preparations because in most disease conditions it is important that the ear canal be kept free of moisture. Moisture, macerated tissue, and a warm cavity provide ideal conditions for the growth of bacteria and fungi. External ear infections are most common during the hot, humid months and are a constant nuisance to swimmers. Practically all medicinal liquids for instillation in the ear are anhydrous solutions. The corticosteroid drugs are about the only medicinal agents applied to the ear as a suspension.

Solutions for the ear are usually dispensed in dropper bottles, and the patient is instructed to tilt the head to the side and place a specified amount or number of drops into the ear. If instructions call for the drops to be warmed before instillation, the pharmacist should give the patient some practical advice; e.g., individual doses of medication can be warmed by first heating a household teaspoon in boiling water or under the hot water tap, thoroughly drying the spoon with clean tissue, placing a dropperful of liquid in the spoon for 10–20 sec, drawing the liquid back into the dropper, and applying the proper amount of warmed liquid into the ear. Sometimes a cotton pledget is placed in the ear to prevent leakage.

When continuous contact of liquid medication with the inner canal surfaces is preferred, a gauze wick may be inserted by the physician or nurse. The wick can then be saturated with the ear solution and the patient instructed to add medication at intervals and leave it in place until removed or replaced by the physician.

Ear irrigations are aqueous solutions used to clean and wash out the external auditory canal. An ear syringe is used to gently direct a stream of warm solution (approximately 100°F) against the side of the auditory canal and not directly at the eardrum. Normal saline solution and weak sodium bicarbonate or boric acid solutions (0.5–1%) are used to remove ear wax, purulent discharges of infection, and foreign bodies from the canal.

Some typical prescriptions for the treatment and prevention of external ear diseases and the pain of otitis media are as follows:

4

℞   Phenol   3%
     Glycerin q.s.   30 ml
     Sig   5–10 gtts (warmed) q 2 h. in left ear

To minimize the amount of water in the prescription, pure phenol, not liquefied phenol, should be dissolved in glycerin. Since glycerin is very hygroscopic, the preparation should be prepared quickly to avoid undue exposure to the atmosphere.

5

℞   Benzocaine   0.3 g
     Antipyrine   1.2 g
     Glycerin q.s.   30 cc
     Sig.   Dropperful of warm liquid in right ear t.i.d.

The antipyrine is used as a solubilizing agent for the benzocaine and has no pharmacological action of its own in this prescription. The antipyrine and benzocaine are mixed together in glycerin, and gentle heat may be necessary to obtain a clear solution.

6

℞   S.S.B.A.   15.0 ml
     Alcohol q.s.   60.0 ml
     Sig.   One-half dropperful in each ear after swimming.

7

℞   Resorcinol   1.0%
     Olive oil q.s.   30 ml
     Sig.   3–4 drops in ea. ear for fungus infection

Resorcinol is readily soluble in olive oil but is not soluble in mineral oil.

8

℞   Mycostatin Oral Suspension   15 ml
     Sig.   3 gtts in ear QID

Apparently this serves as a good vehicle for the fungistatic agent even though it is an aqueous suspension.

Insufflations (Powders) — Fine powders can be insufflated into the ear canal as a means of inserting an antibacterial and/or antifungal agent in a dry form which would create a repository for the drug. A small rubber bulb insufflator (powder blower) is used to blow the powder into the ear. Examples of ear insufflations are:

9

℞   Polymyxin B   500,000 units
     Chloramphenicol   500 mg
     Mycostatin   1 g
     Mix and make powder.
     Sig.   1–2 puffs daily in infected ear

Mix 1 g of mycostatin, the contents of two chloramphenicol capsules, and the contents of a commercially available vial containing Polymyxin B sterile powder for injection, 500,000 units, in a mortar. Dispense in a small, amber glass square and provide the patient with a small rubber-bulb insufflator.

10

℞   Iodine   0.5 g
     Boric acid, q.s.   30.0 ml
     M & Ft. fine powder
     Sig.   1 puff in ea. ear b.i.d.

The iodine cannot be reduced to a fine powder by trituration. It should be dissolved in a small amount of chloroform or alcohol, and the solution dispersed in boric acid powder. Allow the solvent to evaporate and dispense in a tight glass container.

Ointments—Special ointments are not prepared specifically for treating ear ailments, however, ophthalmic and topical ointments (antibacterial, antifungal, corticosteroids) are sometimes prescribed for infections and inflammatory conditions. Ointments can be applied directly to the exterior portions of the ear or may be applied to the ear canal with a cotton wick.

Nasal Medications

Drugs most commonly used in the nose include vasoconstrictors, antibiotics, corticosteroids, antiseptics, and

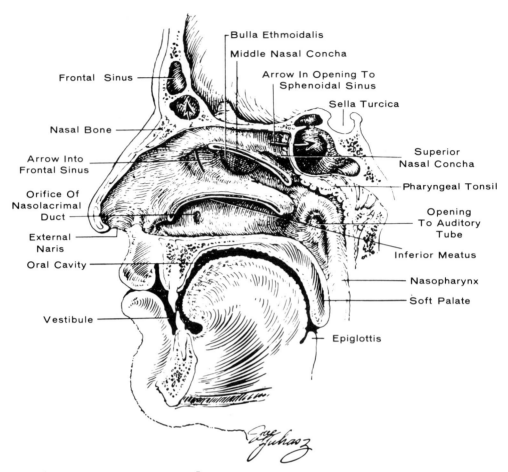

Fig. 8—Nasal passageways and pharynx.[7]

local anesthetics. The vasoconstrictors constitute the largest group of drugs for nasal use; all six monographs on nasal solutions in the USP are vasoconstrictors. Numerous prescription and OTC nasal preparations are available commercially to the physician and patient. Most nasal preparations are aqueous solutions to be administered as drops or sprays, or sometimes as douches or with nasal tampons. Drugs are sometimes applied intranasally as ointments or jellies. A few volatile drugs can be carried into the nasal passages by the movement of an air current through an inhaler.

Anatomy and Physiology—The nasal cavity is a long, narrow, high channel, divided into two halves by the nasal septum. The several cavities that open into the nose are called collectively the paranasal and include the various sinuses (see Fig. 8). Most of the nasal cavity is covered with a mucous membrane which has an extremely rich capillary network and contains numerous mucous glands. Mucus is continually being produced and secreted, and a film of mucus is continually being moved toward the pharynx by the beating action of the cilia, tiny hairlike projections that cover most of the nasal cavity. Proetz, an authority on nasal physiology, stated that "all infectious ailments of the nose stem somehow from a single source, namely the failure of the filter to cleanse itself." [8] Moisture is an essential element for the well-being of the chief defense mechanisms of the nose-ciliary movement, which is con-

Table 5—The Effect of Various Drugs on the Cilia of the Nasal Mucosa[a]

Substance	Concentrations studied	Ciliary response/activity
Sodium chloride	0.2–0.3%	Cilia activity ceases, difficult to reverse
	0.9%	Cilia remain active
	4.0–4.5%	Cilia activity ceases, readily reversible
Distilled water	—	Cilia activity ceases, difficult to reverse
Oils	100%	Interferes with ciliary motion
Mild silver protein	10%	Cilia activity initially retared, recovery is rapid
Silver nitrate	0.5%	Destroys cilia
Cocaine	2.5%	Paralyzes cilia
	less than 2.5%	Little effect on cilia
Ephedrine in 0.9% NaCl	0.5–1.0%	No effect
Camphor, thymol, eucalyptol, menthol	0.1% or higher less than 0.1%	Decreases activity Negligible effects
Penicillin in 0.9% NaCl	250–500 units/ml. 5000 units/ml.	No damage Decrease in activity
Atropine	oral administration	Drying and eventual cessation of ciliary motion
Benzalkonium chloride	1:1000–1:2000	Cessation of motion
Benzalkonium chloride in 0.9% NaCl	1:1000–1:2000	No effect

[a] Abstracted from the investigations of Proetz AW[9] and Riegelman S, Sorby DL.[10]

stantly pulling the blanket of mucus toward the nasopharynx.

Mucus is a moderately viscous, pseudoplastic, mucoprotein system that provides a protective cover to the mucosa as well as entrapping particulate matter that enters the nasal passages. Under normal conditions foreign bodies such as dust, pollen, bacteria, powder, and oil droplets are engulfed in the mucous film and carried out of the nose into the nasopharynx, where the mass may be swallowed or expectorated.

Effective ciliary action or beat depends on the viscosity of the mucus. If it is too viscous or too fluid, the cilia are unable to move the film of mucus. Many of the uncomfortable symptoms of nasal ailments are due to the increased viscosity and dehydration of the secretions. Many conditions can increase or decrease the production and/or viscosity of mucus. Among these are temperature and humidity effects, dust, pollenosis and other allergies, various

drugs (see Table 5), and bacterial and virus infections.

The normal pH of nasal secretions is about 5.5–6.5. The pH tends to shift more toward the alkaline side when conditions such as common cold, rhinitis, sinusitis, etc. exist. The nasal secretions appear to have very little buffer capacity, and the continuous application of preparations having pH values several units removed from the normal values may be irritating and possibly cause tissue damage. Alkaline nasal preparations should not be used for acute inflammatory conditions since this would only exacerbate the uncomfortable alkaline condition of the nasal passages. Although the nasal mucosa can tolerate a relatively large variation in tonicity, isotonic solutions (0.9% NaCl) seem to be compatible and nonirritating to the nose, while very hypo- or hypertonic solutions cause irritation (see Table 5).

Some drugs are absorbed systemically via the nasal vasculature after intranasal application. However, there is little evidence to show that intranasal administration would be a good routine method of obtaining significant blood levels of drugs.

Absorption of intranasally administered drugs can occur from the gastrointestinal tract after they have drained from the nasal passages. Fortunately, most drugs applied intranasally are administered in amounts which are less than their usual effective doses or are destroyed within the gastrointestinal tract. The potential for absorption via this route must be considered, however, especially if large amounts of solution are being used or administration is to infants or small children.

Solutions (Sprays, Nose Drops, Collunaria)—Most preparations for local application to the nasal passages are aqueous solutions. Although light liquid petrolatum was widely used several decades ago, oil solutions are infrequently prescribed, and in fact are not recommended for use in the nose. Oils, especially mineral oil, are dangerous and have been proved to cause lipoid or oil-inspiration pneumonia due to aspiration or inspiration of some of the liquid. They also interfere with normal ciliary action and do not efficiently release dissolved medication.

A vehicle for nasal solutions should:

1. Have a pH in the range of 5.5–7.5, preferably less than 7.
2. Have a mild buffer capacity.
3. Be isotonic or nearly so.
4. Not modify the normal viscosity of mucus.
5. Be compatible with normal ciliary motion and ionic constituents of nasal secretions.
6. Be compatible with the active ingredient.
7. Be sufficiently stable to retain activity upon long standing on the patient's shelf.
8. Contain a preservative to suppress growth of bacteria that may be introduced by the attached dropper.

Sodium chloride and/or dextrose are preferred for adjusting the tonicity of nasal solutions. Phosphate buffer systems are compatible with nasal secretions and most nasal medications. A suitable phosphate buffer for nasal use

(pH 6.5 and isotonic) can be prepared as follows:

$NaH_2PO_4 \cdot H_2O$	0.65
$Na_2HPO_4 \cdot 7H_2O$	0.54
NaCl	0.45
Benzalkonium chloride	0.05–0.01%
Distilled water q.s. ad	100 ml

An isotonic, buffered, and preserved nasal solution can be prepared using the same techniques previously discussed for ophthalmic solutions (see *Vehicles*, page 238).

Consider the following prescription.

11

℞ Ephedrine Sulfate	1.5%
Isotonic vehicle q.s.	60.0 ml

M & F Isotonic Nasal Soln.
Sig. 3–4 drops ea. nostril t.i.d.

The NF provides a table (see page 238 in this text) that gives the definite volume of isotonic solution that 1 g of drug makes. From the table note that 1 g of ephedrine sulfate requires sufficient distilled water to give a final volume of 25.7 ml to make an isotonic solution. In ℞ 11, 0.9 g of ephedrine sulfate is needed. By direct proportion it can be determined that 0.9 g requires enough distilled water to give a volume of 23.1 ml. The final prescription would be dispensed as follows:

12

℞ Ephedrine sulfate	0.9 g
Distilled water q.s.	23.1 ml
pH 6.5 Phosphate buffer (isotonic) q.s. ad ml	60

Some examples of nasal prescriptions requiring extemporaneous compounding are as follows:

13

℞ Decadron Inj. 4 mg/cc	1cc
Normal saline q.s.	15 cc

Sig. Use as nose spray 3–4 x's a day

Use 1 ml of the commercially available product and dilute with 0.9% sodium chloride. A 2-week expiration date should be put on the label since the actual stability of the preparation is not known.

14

℞ Neo Silvol	10%

Ephedrine SO$_4$ ¼%
Dist. water q.s.   30 ml
Sig. ½ dropper ea. nostril t.i.d.

Dissolve the ephedrine sulfate in 10 ml of water and disperse the Neo Silvol on 15 ml of water with gentle agitation. Combine the two solutions and qs to 30 ml.

15

℞ Premarin IV   25 mg
   Normal saline q.s.   30 ml
   Sig. Spray in nose for bleeding.

The Premarin IV is available as a powder for reconstitution. Dissolve the powder in the vehicle that comes in the package, then qs to 30 ml with 0.9% saline. Dispense in a flexible plastic spray container.

16

℞ KCl   0.2
   NaCl   2.0
   Distilled water q.s.   240 ml
   Sig. Use as nasal douche as instructed.

Most solutions for the nose are applied using a dropper, an atomizer or a spray package. The conventional amber glass bottle with a medicine dropper top should be used for drop medication. Plastic spray packages are available for dispensing prescriptions with "spray" instructions. Atomizers which produce a coarse spray rather than a fine mist are preferred for nasal application. Nebulizers which produce a fine mist are used when medication must penetrate into the respiratory tract. Drug manufacturers provide nasal solutions in a variety of containers including dropper bottles, squeeze spray packages, metered valve and pump devices, and aerosols. Whenever nasal preparations are to be used, they should be applied gently and directly to the affected area.

Tampons or packs are used when prolonged and intensive therapy is required. The cotton packs are moistened with solution and gently and carefully inserted in the nasal cavity.

Nasal douches should be applied using gentle pressure, preferably by gravity. These irrigating solutions or washes can be applied using an irrigating bag and tube or a glass nasal douche device (see Fig. 9).

Ointments and Jellies—Antibacterial, protective, and soothing topical ointments are sometimes used to treat inflammations, dermatological conditions, and fissures of the nasal vestibule. Water-miscible jellies are infrequently used to apply vasoconstrictors (Ephedrine Jelly NF XII) or local anesthetics (Pramoxine Jelly NF) higher in the nasal canal when prolonged action is desired. These jellies are composed of tragacanth, methylcellulose, and other water-miscible ingredients; oil-base preparations should not be used on a regular basis.

Inhalants—Inhalants are drugs or combinations of drugs which by virtue of their high vapor pressure can be carried by an air current into the nasal passages. Menthol, eucalyptol, and thymol are widely used in OTC inhaler products. Propylhexedrine, a volatile vasoconstrictor, is the active ingredient in a widely used nose preparation (Benzedrex inhaler). These preparations are not to be confused with inhalations which are drugs or solutions of drugs administered as a nebulized mist intended to reach the respiratory tree.

Precautions—A large number of proprietary and prescription products intended for nasal use are used by the public. The average patient suffering with a nasal disorder may procure his own medication, probably a highly advertised product. The pharmacist should be knowledgeable of the usefulness and potential harm concurrent with the use of nasal medications.

In general, frequent and long-term use of any nasal preparation containing decongestants, antiseptics, astringents, and volatile ingredients such as menthol and eucalyptol should be avoided.

The most commonly prescribed and most widely used OTC nasal preparations are those containing vasoconstrictors (sympathomimetics). The shrinking effect of the vasoconstrictor on the swollen nasal membranes of an acute head cold affords impressive, immedi-

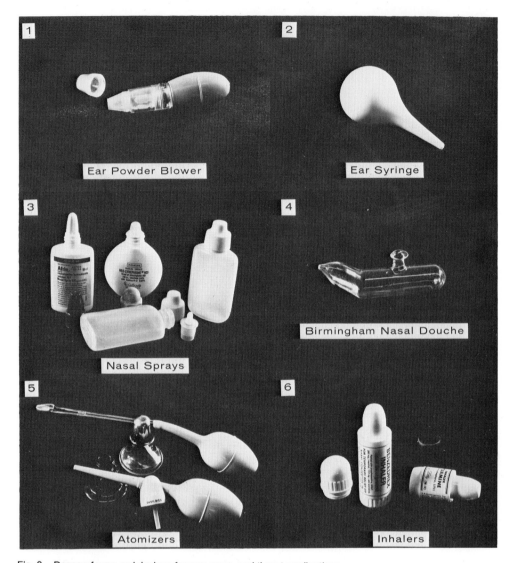

Fig. 9—Dosage forms and devices for ear, nose, and throat medications.

ate relief. However, excessive and/or repeated use of these preparations can result in a rebound hyperemia or congestion rebound. This secondary reaction may be worse than the original congestion, and an acute condition may progress to a chronic state. Sensitive persons (cardiac patients, hypertensives) may react adversely to certain preparations containing phenylephrine, epinephrine, or some other sypathomimetic drug.

The pharmacist, when dispensing nose preparations containing deconges-
tants, should advise the patient to use the drops or spray sparingly and as little as possible, preferably only 2 or 3 times a day. The results will be better and uncomfortable side effects will be minimized.

The patient should be cautioned not to use solutions in which a noticeable darkening or discoloration has occurred.

The frequent and continued use of silver preparations should be avoided since there is a chance of argyria occurring.

Mouth, Dental, and Throat Medications

Solutions are the most widely used dosage form for topical application of medicinal agents to the mouth, throat, and teeth. Mouthwashes, gargles, swabs, toothache drops, teething lotions, and dental solutions for office use are prescribed and used by licensed practitioners and widely used, in the case of mouthwashes, by the public. A large variety of medicinal substances are used in these preparations: local anesthetics for topical use, dyes for fungus infections, perborates and quaternary ammonium compounds for deodorizing and antibacterial action, volatile oils such as clove oil for relief of toothache, camphor and menthol for their pleasant cooling effect, and astringents such as zinc chloride and tannic acid.

Ointments and jellies are sometimes applied to the mucous membrane of the mouth and gums. Troches and pastilles are useful for obtaining a more prolonged release of medication in the mouth and throat.

Anatomy and Physiology—The oral cavity includes the mouth, gums, teeth, and tongue as well as the necessary structural units such as the hard and soft palate which form the roof of the mouth. The appendage of the soft palate that hangs down at the back of the mouth is the uvula. The posterior portion of the mouth opens into the pharynx, a wide, muscular channel that allows the passage of air and food. Both the mouth and pharynx are lined with mucous membranes. These are relatively thick membranes that are not as sensitive as other mucous membranes of the body. The mucosa in the mouth secrete copious amounts of mucus and some enzymes. Most mouth enzymes are produced by the salivary glands, sublingual, submandibular, and—the largest—the parotids. The floor of the mouth (sublingual) and the sides of the mouth (buccal areas) are richly supplied with blood vessels which are close to the membrane surface. Some drugs (nitroglycerin and hormones) are effi-ciently absorbed systemically by the sublingual or buccal route.

The tongue is covered by a mucous membrane and numerous projections called papillae. Some of these papillae contain specialized taste receptors or taste buds, which are chemoreceptors stimulated by molecules dissolved in the fluids of the mouth. Most taste buds are on the tongue but some are located on the buccal area, soft palate, and pharynx. Just behind the tongue attached to the walls of the pharynx are the tonsils, a pair of lymph glands frequently infected in children.

Teeth are supported by the bones of the jaw and the gingiva (gums). The entire structure is called the periodontium. Teeth consist of an external portion, the crown, and a root that is imbedded into the jaw bone. The crown is covered with enamel (the body's strongest and hardest substance) to the gum line. Directly underneath the enamel is the dentin, a softer material that extends throughout the entire structure of the tooth. Under the dentin is the tooth pulp, the tissue which contains the nerves and blood and lymph vessels that maintain life in the tooth.

The most common oral disease is dental caries or tooth decay. It is generally accepted that caries are caused by strong acids in the mouth, which are formed by the action of mouth bacteria on carbohydrates, chiefly sucrose.

The oral cavity is swarming with bacteria, both resident and transient microorganisms. The resident flora helps maintain the integrity and normal function of oral tissue. Normally, these organisms do not invade tissue and cause infections. Transient microorganisms invade the oral cavity via inspiration, dietary intake, and contact with fingers, foreign objects, etc., and they may be nonpathogenic and/or pathogenic. They may remain in the mouth and throat for hours, days, or weeks; however, the resident organisms keep the foreign microorganisms in check. Transient organisms usually do not proliferate or cause disease unless the resident flora is

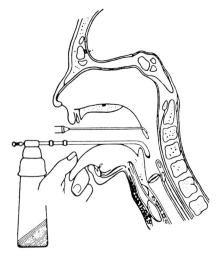

Fig. 10—Application of medication within trachea and pharynx.[11]

changed.

Various acute and chronic conditions occur in the oral cavity and throat as a result of bacterial, viral, or fungal invasion. Inflammations of various areas of the mouth and throat include stomatitis and glossitis, gingivitis, periodontitis, aphthous ulcers (canker sores), pharyngitis, and tonsilitis. The treatment of choice for infective diseases of the mouth and throat is usually systemic antibiotic therapy.

The pharmacist is often the first person a patient seeks for relief of pain for various oral ailments. Patients with toothaches and canker sores, fever blisters, or mouth and lip lesions of long durations (more than 2 weeks) should be referred to a physician or dentist. These may be symptoms of more serious diseases, including cancer.

Solutions for the Mouth and Throat—Simple solutions of antiseptics and astringents are frequently used by the public as mouthwashes and gargles. Strictly speaking, mouthwashes (collutoria) are used in the area in front of the uvula, while gargles are used in the posterior regions by agitating the solution with expired air. Most solutions are used simultaneously as mouthwashes and gargles. Objectionable breath (halitosis) is the primary motivating factor for purchasing and using

mouthwashes. OTC preparations are pleasantly flavored and colored solutions containing astringents, antibacterial agents (usually quaternary ammonium compounds), menthol, thymol, and other aromatics and 10–20% alcohol. The main benefit from the use of these solutions is the mechanical rinsing and swishing that helps to remove food and debris from the mouth, and there is also some transient deodorant effect. These preparations do not prevent caries, periodontal disease or other oral problems; in fact, they may mask offensive mouth odor that is sometimes a symptom of an oral or systemic disease. The Council on Dental Therapeutics of the American Dental Association does not believe the unsupervised use of medicated mouthwashes contributes to the oral health of the general public. Many dentists prefer to use a colored, flavored, nonmedicated solution such as the formula presented below.

Sodium chloride	2.0 g
Sodium bicarbonate	1.0 g
FD & C coloring solution	2.0 ml
Peppermint water q.s.	240.0 ml
M Ft. Solution	

Direct topical administration of drugs to the mouth and throat is possible by swabbing with a cotton-tipped applicator. Although mouth "swabs or paints" can be self-administered by the patient, throat medication would have to be applied by a physician, nurse, or an experienced individual. An atomizer can be used for direct application to the mouth, and a special applicator nozzle is preferred when medication must reach the throat (see Fig. 10).

Some prescriptions that would require extemporaneous compounding are as follows:

17

℞	Sodium borate	1.5
	Sodium bicarbonate	1.75
	Liquefied phenol	0.3
	Glycerin	3.5
	Distilled water q.s.	100.0 ml
	M & Ft. Soln.	
	Sig. Use as mouthwash and gargle	

18

℞	Tincture ferric chloride	6

Potassium chlorate	6
Peppermint oil	0.25
Glycerin	25
Distilled water q.s.	90

M & Ft. Soln.
Sig.   One tsp. in ½ glass of warm water q. 3–4 hrs as gargle.

Solutions containing ferric chloride and potassium chlorate are popularly known as "Golden Gargles," and are prepared by simple solution of the individual ingredients and admixture. Since the chlorate might be toxic if swallowed, an appropriate warning "do not swallow" should be affixed to the prescription bottle.

19

R Phenol	1.2
Glycerin	15
Listerine	45
Lavoris	180

M & Ft. Soln.
Sig.   Dilute with equal parts of hot water and gargle q. 3 h.

Dissolve the phenol in the glycerin, mix the liquids together, and place a "shake well" label on the prescription container in case the preparation does not remain clear.

20

R Gentian violet	1%
Alcohol	6 ml
Distilled water q.s.	30 ml

M & Ft. Soln.
Sig.   Swab on white patches on tongue and mouth.

Because of the strong staining properties of the dye, extreme care should be used in compounding the prescription. It is prepared by simple solution, adding alcohol to aid in dissolving the dye. This preparation is used to treat oral candidiasis (thrush) in infants.

21

R Iodine	0.2
KI	1
Glycerin	15
Distilled water q.s.	30

Prepare Solution
Sig.   Apply to back of mouth and throat with cotton swab.

22

R Elix. Benadryl	3 oz.
Xylocaine Viscous	½ oz.
Maalox	½ oz.

Sig.   Use full strength for sore throat.

Prepare by admixture of the three commercially available products. Dispense with a "shake well" label.

Dental Preparations—Dentists write only a small percentage of the total prescriptions dispensed each year and, of these, very few need to be compounded by the pharmacist. However, there are some interesting preparations prescribed by dentists that the pharmacist may be called on to prepare. The dentist uses many preparations in his office and usually purchases most of these supplies from dental supply houses. It is impractical for pharmacies to carry these items since dentists can purchase them at less cost than pharmacies can offer. However, there may be a few special formulations that are not readily available, and the pharmacist should offer to prepare and stock these preparations as a service to the dentist. Formulas for these preparations are usually available in *Accepted Dental Remedies* (see *Bibliography*).

In addition to using mouthwashes and similar solutions discussed in the preceding section, dentists may prescribe various preparations for local application to the mouth, gums, and teeth. Certain pains of dental origin may be treated by topical application of a local anesthetic directly to the involved area such as exposed pulp, cavity, an abraded area or lesion, or into a dry socket (alveolitis). The medication may be swabbed or dropped onto or packed as a medicinal paste into the affected area.

Examples of dental prescriptions to be compounded are:

23

R Clove oil	
Chlorobutanol aa q.s. ad	10 ml

M & Ft. Toothache drops
Sig.   One or two drops on cotton pledget and pack into cavity.

Clove oil is widely used in toothache preparations. The patient should be cautioned to avoid contact with oral tissue because of irritation and possible damage to tissue.

24

R̥ Benzocaine	3 g
Peppermint oil	0.3 ml
Alcohol	5 ml
Propylene glycol q.s.	30 ml

Sig.   Swab on sore gums prn pain.

Dissolve the benzocaine in glycerin; warm slightly to hasten solution. Dissolve the flavor oil in alcohol and mix the two solutions.

A few of the formulations for dental office practice are as follows:

Alveolar Analgesic
(Treat alveolitis)

Benzocaine	3 g
Guaiacol	3 g
Peruvian balsam	9 g

Triturate the benzocaine with the guaiacol to form a smooth paste and then incorporate the Peruvian balsam.

Socket Dressing

Tincture of iodine, strong	
Oil of clove	
Guaiacol	
Glycerin aa q.s. ad	240 ml
Chloroform	15 ml

Mix the oil of clove, guaiacol and glycerin together in a 12-oz bottle. Add the iodine tincture in small portions and shake. If the iodine precipitates, add some alcohol to obtain a solution. Last, add the chloroform.

Cavity Sanitation

Chloroform	10 ml
Alcohol	50 ml
Thimerosal tincture (1:1000) q.s.	100 ml

Topical Fluoride Solution

| Sodium Fluoride | 2% |
| Purified Water q.s. | 100% |

Prepare the solution using USP grade sodium fluoride. Store the solution in plastic or pyrex glass containers. The sodium fluoride will react with soft glass which may result in the formation of some sediment. This solution should be labeled "For Office Use Only" and "Poison."

References

1. Botelho SY: *Sci Am 211:* 80, 1964.
2. Moses RA: *Adler's Physiology of the Eye,* 5th ed, Mosby, St. Louis, 1970.
3. Brown MRW, Norton DA: *J Cos Chem 16:* 369, 1965.
4. Mullen W, Shepherd W, Labovitz J: *Survey Ophthalmol 17(6):* 460, 1973.
5. *National Formulary XIV,* APhA, Washington, DC, 936, 1975.
6. Lamy P: *Drug Cos Ind (Feb.):* 140, 1969.
7. Crouch JE: *Functional Human Anatomy,* 2nd ed, Lea & Febiger, Philadelphia, 391, 1972.
8. Proetz AW: *Proc Roy Soc Med 41:* 793, 1948.
9. Proetz AW: *Essays on the Applied Physiology of the Nose,* Annual Publ. Co., St. Louis, 1973.
10. Riegelman S, Sorby DL: EENT preparations. In Martin EW, ed: *Husa's Pharmaceutical Dispensing, 6th ed,* Mack Publ. Co., Easton, PA, 346–347, 1966.
11. *Progress in Allergy II,* S. Karger, Ltd., Basel, Switzerland, 1949.

Bibliography

Eye

   The United States Pharmacopeia, 19th rev, Mack Publ. Co., Easton,, PA, 702, 1975.
   Merck Index, 8th ed, Merck & Co., Inc., Rahway, NJ, 1281, 1968.
   Remington's Pharmaceutical Sciences, 15th ed, Mack Publ. Co., Easton, PA, 1408, 1975.
   Martin AN: *Physical Pharmacy,* Lea & Febiger, Philadelphia, 287, 1960.
   Moses RA: *Adler's Physiology of the Eye,* Mosby, St. Louis, 17–75, 1970.
   Havener WA: *Ocular Physiology,* 2nd ed, Mosby, St. Louis, 12–23, 1970.
   Ellis PP, Smith DL: *Handbook of Ocular Therapeutics and Pharmacology,* 4th ed, Mosby, St. Louis, 3–15, 159–240, 1973.

Ear, Nose, Mouth, Dental, and Throat

   Fabricant ND: *Modern Medicine for the Ear, Nose and Throat,* Grune & Stratton, New York, 1951.
   Fabricant ND. *JAMA 151:* 21, 1953.
   Proetz AW: *Essays on the Applied Physiology of the Nose,* Annual Publ. Co., St. Louis, 1973.
   Darlington RC: Topical oral antiseptics and mouthwashes. In *Handbook of Non-Prescription Drugs,* APhA, Washington, DC, 123–134, 1973.
   Martin EW, ed: *Husa's Pharmaceutical Dispensing,* 6th ed, Mack Publ. Co., Easton, PA, 340–358, 819–827, 1966.
   Martin EW: *Techniques of Medication,* Lippincott, Philadelphia, 74–79, 93–101, 1969.
   Accepted Dental Remedies (ADR), Am. Dent. Assoc., Chicago, IL, published annually.
   Grossman LI: *Dental Formulas and Aids to Dental Practice,* Lea & Febiger, Philadelphia, 1952.
   The Dentist and the Pharmacist (pamphlet), Am. Dent. Assoc., Chicago, IL, 1970.
   Kutscher AH, Zegarelli EV: Dental services. In *Remington's Pharmaceutical Sciences,* 15th ed, Mack Publ. Co., Easton, PA, 1886–1896, 1975.

10

Parenteral medications

Kenneth E. Avis, DSc
Professor and Director
Division of Parenteral
Medications
Department of
Medicinal Chemistry
College of Pharmacy
The University of Tennessee
Memphis, TN 38163

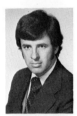

**William A. Miller, PharmD,
MSc** Associate Professor
and Director
Division of Clinical Pharmacy
Department of
Pharmaceutics
College of Pharmacy
The University of Tennessee
Memphis, TN 38163

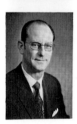

G. Briggs Phillips, PhD
Director
Becton, Dickinson & Co.
Research Center
Research Triangle Park, NC
27709

Dr. Avis coordinated the chapter and prepared, with **Dr. Miller,** the section on *Rational Parenteral Therapy.*

Dr. Phillips prepared the section on *Sterilization.*

Parenteral medications are sterile pharmaceutical dosage forms intended for administration by injection under or through one or more layers of skin or mucous membrane.

Injections may be conveniently grouped into two general classes: biological products and pharmaceutical products. Biological products include any virus, therapeutic serum, toxin, antitoxin, or analogous parenteral products. Pharmaceutical products include single- and multiple-dose small- and large-volume parenterals. Injections may be solutions, emulsions, suspensions (ready for injection), or dry solids which when mixed with a suitable solvent will yield a solution or suspension.

To aid the reader it has been deemed desirable to divide the subject matter in this chapter into two parts because, although closely interrelated, the parts logically can be divided. The first part will cover rational parenteral therapy and the involvement of the hospital pharmacist and the second part will cover quality characteristics of parenteral medications and the involvement of the industrial pharmacist.

Rational Parenteral Therapy

Rational parenteral medication therapy is conceived to encompass prescribing, compounding, dispensing, administering, and monitoring the effects of injectable drugs in patients. To assure safe and effective therapy an interdisciplinary team approach should be employed, particularly for total parenteral nutrition. Pharmacists and properly trained pharmacy technicians should carefully compound and dispense parenteral medications as prescribed by a physician. The role of nurses or other qualified personnel is to administer these medications to patients. Then, physicians, nurses, and/or pharmacists should carefully monitor patients for subjective and objective evidences of drug response. Based upon this response, therapy should be reevaluated and adjusted.

Prescribing

Physicians and primary care clinicians must carefully weigh the benefits versus the risks associated with parenteral drug therapy. Injections provide the most direct route for achieving the effect of a drug within the human body yet, by planned formulation of the dosage form combined with an appropriate choice of one of the injection routes, it is possible to vary the effect of a drug from an almost instantaneous onset with a few minutes duration to a delay of several hours onset and a duration of up to several weeks. This versatility of therapeutic effect, which makes the injection of therapeutic agents a very valuable route of administration, is being utilized because of recently acquired understanding of human physiology and biopharmaceutics, newer concepts in formulation, and developments in process technology.

The parenteral route circumvents the gastrointestinal tract, hence it is the route of choice for drugs which are degraded or are erratically or unreliably absorbed when administered orally. The parenteral route alone may be suitable if the patient cannot be given drugs by any gastrointestinal or dermatomucosal routes due to conditions that preclude the use of these routes.

The parenteral route provides a reliable dose-response relationship as well as a means for varying the dosage requirements for each patient. It also provides the prescriber with more control of therapy due to inhibitions for self-medication by the patient. The rapidity of action afforded by parenteral routes is often life-saving, as in the intracardiac use of epinephrine in cardiac arrest or of lidocaine in treating ventricular arrhythmias.

In addition to the administration of life-saving drugs, the intravenous route provides a means for the administration of whole blood, plasma, and other protein fractions in various disease and injury conditions. Intravenous solutions are used for the replacement of fluids and electrolytes, and to maintain acid-base balance in patients. Total parenteral nutrition is employed to provide the carbohydrate, protein, electrolyte, and vitamin needs of a patient over a prolonged period of time.

No dosage form is without disadvantages. For parenterals these include:

The necessity of aseptic technique in production, extemporaneous compounding, and administration.

The requirement of special skills for administration.

The real or psychological pain associated with an injection.

The relatively high cost.

These disadvantages can lead to various hazards or complications, namely:

Effects due to error in the selection or dose of a drug.
Allergic drug reactions.
Infection.
Pyrogenicity.
Particulation.
Thrombophlebitis.
Air embolism.
Fluid overload.
Filtration and extravasation.
Punctured vessels.
Breaking of catheters.

A study by the Boston Collaborative Drug Surveillance Program indicates that a significant percentage of patient deaths relate to the parenteral administration of various drugs, and to fluid and electrolyte abnormalities that occur subsequent to the administration of large volume parenteral solutions.[1] It is to be emphasized that these disadvantages or complications can be minimized through careful prescribing, production, extemporaneous compounding, dispensing, administration, and monitoring of the drugs utilized.

Pharmacists should review parenteral medication orders for problems pertaining to dosage, stability and compatibility of drug additions, route of administration (i.e., intramuscular, intravenous, subcutaneous, etc.), and rate of administration. Where necessary the pharmacist should be prepared to provide information to physicians about the safe and effective use of these dosage forms.

Compounding and Dispensing

The pharmacist usually begins the dispensing function with reputable products of high quality and purity produced by the pharmaceutical industry and packaged in either the unit of use (unit-dose) or the bulk system. In the unit-dose system the medication may be supplied in a prefilled syringe (properly labeled and ready for administration to the patient), a large-volume container up to 1000 ml in size, or in other single-dose containers. Special unit-dose additive units are available for use in preparing large-volume intravenous admixtures. In the bulk system the medication is supplied in ampuls, vials, or bottles and requires withdrawal into a syringe prior to administration to the patient.

The advantages attributed to unit-dose packaging are:

Positive identification of the medication until the time of administration.
Elimination of errors due to withdrawal of an incorrect medication or quantity into a syringe.
Elimination of the potential contamination problems associated with multiple dose vials.
A reduction in the time required to prepare the medication for administration.

In the bulk system there are basically two packaging units, the single-dose and the multiple-dose container. Single-dose containers have the advantages of:

A reduction in contamination because of one withdrawal only.
Accountability of quantity (which is useful in the control of narcotics).
Maintenance of the integrity of the product until the container has been irretrievably opened or entered.

Single-dose ampuls have disadvantages which include:

Difficult entry.
The possibility of injecting into the patient glass particles introduced during opening.
Breakage due to their fragility.

Single-dose vials may contain rubber particles, cut out as the needle penetrates the closure, that could be injected into the patient.

Multiple-dose vials have characteristics which are essentially the opposite of the advantages named above for single-dose containers, plus the risk of injecting rubber particles. Since there is a risk of introducing microbial contamination through multiple entries into these vials, it is essential to exercise strict aseptic procedural techniques. However, in practice, this is often not done. The particular advantage for multiple-dose containers is the flexibility of dosage provided the prescriber.

Patient safety and therapeutic efficacy must be the primary factors in determining the system to be utilized. Because of the advantages of patient safety and convenience, an increasing number of unit-dose parenterals are being used. Whenever possible the pharmacist should reconstitute and prepare parenterals in unit-dose form. However, in some hospitals pharmacists still merely supply parenterals to patient-care units for dosage, preparation, and administration by nursing personnel.

Nurses simply are not trained to perform compounding and dispensing functions. Therefore, it is not surprising that a high proportion of errors sometimes occurs in hospitals where nurses are given the responsibility for compounding intravenous admixtures, the sterile unit-dose parenterals compounded extemporaneously and consisting of large-volume parenterals to which one or more therapeutic agents have been added.

In one study of medication errors in a nurse-controlled intravenous admixture program a 21% error rate occurred.[2] This error rate is higher than those reported in published studies of nursing preparation and administration of other types of medication. Five of the 15 errors (33%) in this study were related to failure to follow procedures while the remainder could be classified as more general or varied in nature (wrong volume of diluent, wrong volume of drug, etc.).

It is the responsibility of the pharmacist to be sure that the right patient receives the right dose of the right drug by the right route at the right time. Because of their expertise in drug dosage forms, pharmacists are remiss in their obligation for patient care if they do not extend this expertise to include intravenous admixtures.

Intravenous admixture services were initiated by a few hospital pharmacists in the 1960's. The experience gained by these hospitals has demonstrated the inherent advantages of a pharmacy IV admixture service. These advantages are:

It centralizes the responsibility for the compounding, dispensing, and control of parenteral admixtures.

It reduces the need for nurses to compound admixtures, freeing them for other nursing duties.

It helps to standardize the labeling of admixture solutions and helps to reduce errors.

It helps to provide effective control over the use of unstable, deteriorated or outdated drugs in admixtures.

It helps to provide accuracy in the calculation of the quantity of ingredients and in the compounding process.

It helps to provide the proper controlled environmental conditions by using a laminar flow hood. Accepted standards of aseptic technique are facilitated.

It helps to provide for proper screening of physicochemical incompatibilities in drug admixtures.

It provides the nurses and physicians additional time for their professional responsibilities.

The Joint Commission on Accreditation of Hospitals has promoted the concept that the pharmacist should be involved in preparing intravenous admixtures. In the Pharmacy Section of the current standards for Accreditation of hospitals the following statement is made:

The director of the pharmaceutical service should be responsible for at least the following: . . . Admixture of parenteral products, when possible. Preparing and sterilizing parenteral medications that are manufactured in the hospital. . . . Written policies which are essential for the safe administration of drugs to patients, shall include at least the following . . . Acceptable precautionary measures for the safe admixture of parenteral products shall be developed. Whenever drugs are added to intravenous solutions, a distinctive supplementary label shall be affixed that indicates the name and amount of the drug added, the date and time of the addition and the name of the person who prepared the admixture.[3]

In the future it is apparent that increasing numbers of hospitals will develop pharmacy-based reconstitution, unit-dose, and intravenous admixture programs.

Assuming that the need for an admixture program exists, pharmacists becoming involved in such a program are required to successfully develop, implement, and operate it. The basic steps to be followed include:

Read and study the literature on intravenous admixture services.

Visit and observe established intravenous admixture services.

Prepare a proposal for approval by hospital administration, nurses, and the medical staff through the Pharmacy and Therapeutics Committee.

Develop a policy and procedures manual detailing how all involved health-care personnel will be affected by the service.

Establish a target date to start the service and conduct an orientation program for the staff, (i.e., pharmacy, nursing, and medical).

Start the pilot service.

Evaluate and modify the pilot service as needed over the first few weeks.

Extend the pilot service gradually hospitalwide.

Space limitation prevents a more comprehensive discussion of the administrative procedures involved in developing an intravenous admixture service, however, journals devoted to hospital pharmacy practice (i.e., *American Journal of Hospital Pharmacy, Drug Intelligence and Clinical Pharmacy,* and *Hospital Pharmacy*), contain numerous articles on intravenous admixture service programs.

Although pharmacists are the best prepared professionals to dispense parenteral medications, they should not accept such a role without a thorough awareness of the demanding standards required and without training in the specialized techniques involved. These dosage forms are unique, requiring freedom from viable microorganisms, pyrogens, and nonviable particles and to be of an exceptional level of purity. Even when so prepared there remains a risk associated with an injection into a patient. Therefore, the entire history of their preparation and administration must be under the supervision of specially trained and responsible professional persons.

Pharmacy technicians can be used to assist the pharmacist in the dispensing process. However, hospital pharmacy departments should conduct formalized training programs to prepare the technician to properly function as an assistant in the parenteral products area.

The dispensing of parenteral medications involves at least five basic activities:

Selection of reliable products of high purity which are sterile and pyrogen free.

Thorough inspection of the product and package for defects.

Aseptic compounding and dispensing of preparations into an appropriate administration container or device, or otherwise preparing for administration to the patient under carefully controlled, aseptic conditions.

Careful examination of all combinations for incompatibility or other defects.

Performing appropriate or required tests to provide assurance that the quality and safety of the preparation has not been compromised.

Selection of Reliable Products

The pharmacist has the responsibility to supervise and direct the procurement of reliable products for use in treating patients in the hospital. The reputable standing of the supplier should be confirmed for all pharmaceuticals but, particularly, for parenteral products. While cost must be given attention, reliable quality must have the preeminent consideration. Meeting USP quality standards alone is not enough to be assured of the quality needed, for there also must be the assurance that good manufacturing practices are meticulously followed in the manufacture of these products. Such attention also must be given to the devices used for administration of the product to the patient.

The pharmacist has the responsibility to become acquainted with the supplier's manufacturing reliability and the quality assurance program which will generate the confidence that the quality is present in each unit of every lot of all products. To this end the hospital phar-

macist should become familiar with good manufacturing practices, which are stated in general terms in the US Food and Drug Administration "Current Good Manufacturing Practice" (CGMP) regulations,[4] and visit or otherwise become informed of the actual conditions for manufacture of the products chosen for use in the hospital. In addition, after a supplier is selected, a careful record should be kept of all types of defects. These should be reviewed periodically and, if an adequate response to reports of rejects is not received, a change in supplier should be considered.

As a means of aiding the hospital pharmacist in evaluating the quality of available products, a review of the characteristics of such products and the good manufacturing practices essential to achieving such quality is given (see *Quality Characteristics of Parenteral Medications*, page 270).

There is no substitute for inherent quality in a product. Previous historical records confirm that such an attribute is only achieved as the manufacturer practices quality assurance throughout the manufacturing process.

Inspection for Defects

Occasionally a hospital pharmacist will begin the compounding of a product to be rendered sterile with the selection and incorporation of raw materials. The steps utilized would be comparable to those described beginning on page 270 of this chapter for products made by the pharmaceutical industry and should include planned quality-control steps to be assured that the substances to be used meet the quality standards previously determined to be necessary. Further, chemicals of even the highest available purity probably will contain particulate matter and microbial contaminants. Therefore, steps must be taken to eliminate such contaminants, as by filtration of solutions through a microbial retentive filter or by sterilization of the individual components prior to compounding.

More frequently, the hospital pharmacist uses products previously prepared to be sterile and free from contaminants. Although manufactured by a reliable producer of such products, the pharmacist assumes responsibility as soon as he uses them in a dispensing function. Therefore, at the least, he must carefully and thoroughly inspect them for defects. While visual inspection will not detect all possible defects, it will make possible the detection of defects most likely to occur as a result of aging and rough handling during shipment.

Initial inspection of outer shipping cartons should be for evidences of mishandling such as water marks from wet exposure or broken containers, mold growth from wet storage, or broken or deformed cartons from rough treatment. All of these may indicate damage to the primary containers or packages thereby jeopardizing their integrity.

The primary package is designed to prevent the entrance of contaminants into the product and leakage of the product to the outside; therefore, its integrity must be maintained until used. If an outer wrap is present, as with infusion bags or packaged devices, there should be no evidence of penetrating holes, cuts, or abrasions. This would be especially critical if the penetration was through the inner bag. Squeezing a flexible bag may help to detect small holes by making visible a stream of liquid. If the package is a glass container, there must be no evidence of cracks or other penetrating defects. Rubber closures and aluminum caps should show no distortion that might have permitted the entrance of contaminants. In short, the entire outside of the package should be carefully inspected for any indications that the integrity of the package seal might have been jeopardized.

In the case of solutions, the contents should be examined in good light against a black and a white background. This permits the discovery not only of any visible particulate matter of a nondescript nature but of microbial growth (if above approximately 10^5 organisms/ml), chemical precipitates, discoloration, and glass, rubber, or plastic particles. Normally such solutions should be discarded although small amounts of nondescript particulate matter may be removed by membrane filtration to render the solution usable.

Solids in sealed containers should be examined for discoloration, particulate matter, wetness, or other evidences of deterioration. Also, after reconstitution the solution should be examined, particularly for particles. In such cases, nondescript particles may be removed by membrane filtration to render the product suitable for use in a patient.

Devices should be examined for defects such as missing or defective port covers, torn filter membranes, loose connections, particles within tubing, and oily exudation of plasticizers. All such defects would require that the device be discarded or returned for credit.

Human errors may occur in the best of manufacturing plants. Therefore, the packages should be examined for matching labels; those between carton and primary package and from container to cap code, if present. The date of use should be within the expiration date on the label and the label should be intact and legible.

Should there be any suspicion upon visual inspection that the package or its contents is not the quality purported to be, it is the pharmacist's responsibility either to perform such additional tests as necessary to assure its quality and safety or to discard it.

Aseptic Compounding and Dispensing

As all pharmacists know, compounding includes the steps involved in combining two or more components to prepare a dosage form of a drug suitable for administration to a patient. The term "aseptic" means without sepsis or, without contamination that probably would cause an infection in a patient. A procedure that would keep microorganisms out of a product also would be likely to keep out particulate matter and many

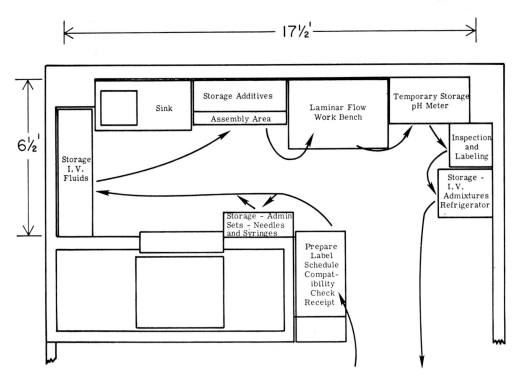

Fig. 1—Line drawing of facility for preparation of intravenous admixtures, showing work flow (courtesy, *University of Illinois Medical Center*).

other types of physical and chemical contaminants. Therefore, an aseptic compounding procedure is one designed to meticulously prevent contaminants from entering the product during compounding or to remove them during the process, with particular emphasis on microorganisms.

To accomplish this objective, aseptic compounding must be performed in a microbiologically controlled environment and the techniques employed must minimize the risk of introducing contaminants.

In addition, the arrangement of the adjacent area must provide for an efficient operation. It should include provisions for meeting the following needs and activities in essentially the sequence listed:

Receipt and review of the physician's order.
Scheduling of the filling of the order and preparation of the label.
Storage of administration sets, needles, and syringes.

Storage of fluids.
Refrigerated storage of additives and selected fluids.
Counter area for assembly of needed materials prior to mixing.
Environmentally controlled laminar flow workbench for preparation of product.
Temporary storage area for labeling.
Inspection facility to examine for particulate contamination.
Instrument to measure the pH of a portion of the finished product when required.
Refrigerated storage for products prior to delivery to the patient.

An example of such an arrangement is shown in Fig. 1.

Environmental Control—The normal hospital environment is heavily laden with microorganisms and other contaminants such as particulate matter. Especially when suspended in the air above work height, contaminants may enter a product, as by falling into an open bottle, being drawn into an evacuated container, or collecting on an exposed needle. Perhaps of even greater concern is contamination from people such as hairs falling from the head or contaminants from the hands being transferred to critical surfaces (touch contamination). Therefore, careful attention must be given to controlling the sources of contamination in the environment and from people. These factors will be discussed in part here and further in a later section of this chapter.

The development of HEPA (high efficiency particulate air) filters followed by laminar flow work enclosures, has vastly improved the achievable control over the work environment. HEPA filters are made of glass and paper or asbestos and are defined as capable of removing particles of 0.3 μm and larger with an efficiency of at least 99.97%. The efficiency rating of these filters is based on the DOP Test in which dioctylphthalate smoke, having a uniform 0.3 μm particle size, is generated upstream from the filter and the degree of penetration is measured downstream with a particle counter. Likewise, holes in the filter or unsealed joints at the margin can be detected by finding a stream of particles downstream of the defect. The useful life of these filters is extended by the frequent cleaning of prefilters and by the pleated design of the HEPA filter itself. Because of the sloping sides of the pleats, particles from the air collecting on the upper portion of the filter are pushed by the air stream toward the tip of the pleat; thereby, most of the filter surface remains clean.

Enclosed areas, such as workbenches or entire rooms, bathed with HEPA-filtered laminar flow air which is flowing either horizontally or vertically at a uniform velocity of 90 ± 20 fpm from the entire downstream side of the filter, provide an ultraclean environment. While the air cannot be considered to be sterile, it will approach that degree of cleanliness. Therefore, it is possible to perform aseptic procedures in such an environment, provided the filtration system is operating as it should, the surrounding area is arranged to preserve this degree of cleanliness, and the personnel using the facility follow proper procedures to prevent the introduction of contamination from their manipulations.

Laminar Flow Workbench—The following guidelines summarize the proper utilization of a laminar flow workbench for the preparation of sterile products in a hospital setting:

1. The laminar flow workbench should be located in an area which is clean, orderly, and free from strong air currents; an area which will buffer the workbench against the influx of contamination.

2. At the beginning of each workday, the beginning of each shift, and when spillage occurs, the workbench surface should be wiped thoroughly with a clean, nonlinting sponge dampened with a suitable disinfectant such as 70% ethyl or isopropyl alcohol.

3. The blower should be operated continuously. However, should there be a long period of nonuse, the blower may be turned off and the workbench opening covered with a plastic curtain or other shield. Before use all of the internal surfaces of the hood should be cleaned thoroughly and wiped with a disinfectant and the blower then should be operated at least 30 min.

4. Traffic in the area of the workbench should be minimized and controlled. The workbench should be shielded from air currents that might overcome the air curtain and carry contaminants into the work area.

5. Supplies entering the buffer area should be isolated in a remote place until they can be decontaminated by removing outer packaging. That is, outer cartons and packaging materials should not be brought near the workbench.

6. All supply items should be examined for defects prior to being introduced into the aseptic work area.

7. Supplies to be utilized in the workbench should be decontaminated by wiping the outer surface with 70% ethyl or isopropyl alcohol, or other suitable surface disinfectants, or by removing an outer wrap at the edge of the workbench as the item is introduced into the aseptic work area.

8. Personnel may enter the buffer area with street clothes or normal work uniforms but may not approach the workbench. Before approaching the workbench, personnel must thoroughly scrub hands and arms with a detergent followed by an appropriate skin antiseptic. They must then don a clean cap that provides complete coverage of head hair and a clean, nonlinting, long-sleeved coat with elastic or snaps at the wrist and, preferably, a solid front panel. A face mask must be worn if there is no transparent barrier panel between the operator's face and the aseptic work area. This is more critical if the operator has facial hair or an upper respiratory condition that promotes sneezing and coughing.

9. After proper introduction of supply items into the aseptic workbench, they are to be arranged in a manner such that operations can take full advantage of the direction of laminar air flow, that is, either vertical or horizontal. Supply items within the workbench should be limited to minimize clutter of the work area and provide adequate space for critical operations. A clean path of HEPA-filtered air must be provided directly from the filter to the critical work site. No supplies and no movement of the personnel should interpose a nonsterile item or surface between the source of the clean air and the critical work site. Therefore, no objects should be placed behind the critical work site in a horizontal nor over the critical work site in a vertical laminar flow workbench. Likewise, the hands and arms should not be moved into the airstream behind the critical work site in a horizontal nor above the critical work site in a vertical laminar flow workbench. Also, all work should be performed at least 6 in. within the workbench to avoid drawing in contamination from the outside and arms should not be moved in and out of the work area any more than absolutely necessary.

10. All supply items should be arranged so that the work flow will provide maximum efficiency and order.

11. It should be noted that the hands are clean but not sterile. Therefore, all procedures should be performed in a manner to minimize the risk of touch contamination. For example, the outside barrel of a syringe may be touched with the hands since it does not contact the solution, but the plunger or needle should not be touched.

12. All rubber stoppers of vials and bottles and the neck of ampuls should be cleaned, preferably with 70% alcohol and a nonlinting sponge, prior to the introduction of the needle for removal or addition of drugs.

13. Avoid spraying of solutions on the workbench screen and filter. This may cause cracking of the filter material or otherwise generate holes.

14. After every admixture, the contents of the container must be thoroughly mixed and then should be inspected for the presence of particulate matter or evidence of an incompatibility.

15. Filtration of solutions to remove particulate matter is frequently necessary, particularly where admixtures have been prepared. A small volume of solution may be filtered by attaching an appropriate membrane filter to the end of a syringe, using the plunger to force the liquid through the filter. *Note:* To avoid rupture of the membrane, force may be applied in one direction only through the filter, unless the membrane is adequately supported on both sides. Where larger volumes of solutions must be filtered, this may be accomplished by means of an appropriate inline filter and an evacuated container to draw the solution through the filter or, preferably, by means of a pressure tank of nitrogen, or other inert gas, to apply pressure to the liquid in the container to force it through the inline filter. In the latter sit-uation, the pressure must be maintained low enough to avoid the risk of explosion of the solution container (usually a maximum of 10–12 psig). There are at least two disadvantages of the vacuum system as compared with the pressure system: (1) any leakage draws contamination into the container and system and (2) the vacuum may be lost, thereby stopping the procedure.

16. The porosity of the appropriate membrane filter is determined by the objective of the filtration. To remove particulate matter a 1 μm porosity filter should be satisfactory. To sterilize a solution a 0.2 μm filter would be required.

17. The completed preparation should be provided with an appropriate tamperproof cap or closure to assure the user that the integrity of the container had been maintained until the time of use.

18. The workbench should be cleaned with a clean sponge, wet with distilled water, as often as necessary during the workday and at the close of the workday. This should be followed by wiping the area with a clean sponge wet with an appropriate disinfectant.

19. After each procedure, used syringes, bottles, vials, and other waste should be removed, but with a minimum of exit and reentry into the workbench.

Examination of Combinations

It is the responsibility of the pharmacist to prevent or correct incompatibilities in dosage forms of drugs. This is no less the case in parenteral preparations, and the consequences of failure can be very serious.

While it may be pharmaceutically ideal to administer one drug at a time, physicians often combine two or more drugs to reduce the multiplicity of injections received by the patient, or for other reasons. Therefore, the pharmacist must carefully review all orders for combinations of drugs to be given by injection, applying his knowledge to detect incompatibilities *before* compounding whenever possible. Many factors are known to affect the compatibility and stability of parenteral admixtures, including pH, particular formulation of a commercial brand, drug and/or excipient concentration, order of mixing, and temperature. Data in the form of compatibility charts from pharmaceutical manufacturers are available. However, most of these have been developed by observing visible changes only, following selected combinations. Therefore, their usefulness is limited. The space available here precludes detailed discussion of the subject but basic considerations of incompatibilities of therapeutic agents are given in Chapter 13.

Assuming that a careful attempt has been made to prevent an incompatibility, it remains essential that the product be carefully observed for insolubility, color change, or other evidences of incompatibility after compounding. This is particularly true when more than two preparations have been combined since the presence of multiple substances may make it almost impossible to predict all possible chemical and physical interactions. Wherever possible the period of observation should include immediately after compounding, throughout any storage period, and through the period of administration, particularly in the case of an IV infusion which will hang for 6–8 hours at room temperature during administration.

It also should be noted that storage in a refrigerator for an IV infusion prepared in advance of use is often practiced. At low temperatures reaction rates are normally reduced but solubility levels may be lower also, resulting in precipitation of some ingredients. Therefore, the product should be carefully observed for such changes and assurance be obtained that any precipitate returns to solution while being warmed prior to administration.

Quality Assurance

While the hospital pharmacist normally relies upon the quality assurance program of a reputable supplier to provide reliable products for dispensing, a limited but essential quality assurance program should be a part of a dispensing program for parenteral medications.

To begin with, the pharmacist must recognize that there is always present a possibility that the product quality required will not be achieved, either as provided by the manufacturer or as prepared for dispensing by the hospital pharmacist. While the risk of such an occurrence can be expected to be very low, it does exist. Therefore, the pharmacist must be alert and critically evaluative of the products used and of the dispensing techniques employed.

Since most products prepared in the hospital pharmacy are single products prepared for a single patient, it is not feasible to perform complete quality-control testing for each product unit. However, it is possible and feasible to establish a monitoring program whereby, in addition to individual observation of each unit prepared, samples of products from a selected group, such as one day's production by one person, are monitored for the quality required. The size of the sample and the composition of the group should be determined by a careful evaluation of the compounding program. For example, such an approach was recently reported for sterility monitoring of IV admixtures.[5] Following this careful study of the microbial load of the environment, an estimation of the probability of contamination of IV admixtures during processing, and a trial program, it was determined that sampling 5 admixtures/day 5 days a week would provide a valid sample for monitoring sterility. The samples used for direct inoculation into culture media were the last 50 ml in an administration unit. The upper acceptable limit was determined to be 4 positive samples/week. Such an approach can be used with other quality control parameters.

Monitoring Program—It is recommended that a quality-control monitoring program be developed, to include *at least* the following parameters:

Microbial Monitoring of the Environment— The laminar flow workbench and the buffer area should be monitored at least once a week by exposing nutrient agar plates perpendicular to the air stream in the workbench for 10 min at representative sites and in the buffer area to settling for 30 min. Rodac surface sampling also is desirable.

Leakage Checking of the HEPA Filters in the Workbench—Particle counts should be performed downstream of the HEPA filters at least every 6 months, but more frequently if the filter is splashed with solution or there is other suspected damage. In addition, new filters should be checked for leakage around the periphery immediately after installation.

The Aseptic Manipulative Technique of Each Operator—The ability of each individual operator to maintain asepsis during operations intended to be aseptic should be evaluated as a part of the initial training program and at regular subsequent intervals, such as quarterly. One method for such an evaluation is to perform all of the required manipulations using culture media instead of products, practicing until no contamination is introduced.

Testing for Sterility of Representative Samples—A method such as that described above may be employed using the last portion of the solution in the container or returned, unused solutions as the test samples.

Visual Inspection of Every Product—Every product prepared should be visually inspected in good lighting against a black and a white background for the presence of particulate matter or discoloration, and for such defects as cracks in glass bottles or pin holes in plastic bags, improper or defective labeling, and improperly sealed containers.

pH Changes—A pH meter, preferably, or pH test paper should be available to check the pH of solutions, particularly after compounding, as a means of indicating possible unexpected changes. This may be done on a monitoring basis for multiple units of a similar composition.

Pyrogen Testing—From time to time it may be desirable or essential to test products or a system, such as the distilled water system, for the presence of pyrogens. The services of an outside laboratory may be obtained for performing the official rabbit test, but the development of the Limulus Test may provide a simple *in vitro* method suitable for use in the hospital.

Proving the Effectiveness of Sterilizers—The effectiveness of steam, dry air, and gaseous sterilizers should be proven before initial use and at regular intervals, such as twice a year. This may be done under full-load conditions using biological indicators and, in the case of steam or dry air, thermocouples located in the most difficultly penetrated sites within the load. The objective is to be sure that all parts of the load within the chamber will be effectively penetrated by the sterilant during a normal sterilization cycle.

Additional Testing—Special situations may require additional testing from time to time, some of which may not be possible to carry out in the hospital. In such instances, the hospital pharmacist should secure the services of an outside laboratory. For example, it may be desirable to speciate the organisms found as contaminants in a parenteral solution, as a means of tracing the source of contamination.

In summary, the hospital pharmacist is responsible for the parenteral medications that he dispenses. He must do all that is required to fulfill this responsibility for the good of the patient, from the selection of quality components for compounding to the delivery of the final product for administration to the patient. This must be done in cooperation with other health professionals but only the pharmacist can adequately perform the duties associated with the proper preparation of a parenteral dosage form.

Administration

Parenteral medications to be administered to human patients may be conveniently categorized as small volume and large volume parenterals. Because of the difference in volume, differences exist in the techniques required for administering the injection as well as differences in formulation, the manufacturing process, and packaging. Therefore, distinctions will be made between these two categories of parenterals in the subsequent discussion.

Small-Volume Parenterals

Small volume parenterals may be classified as such either because of the volume of material to be injected into the body or the volume of medication within a container. These factors usually are closely related since a small package unit normally is appropriate when a small dose is required. The volume of medication in a container, when multiple withdrawals are intended from one package unit, is limited by the USP to 30 ml.

Routes of Administration—The four routes of administration most frequently used are intradermal, intramuscular, intravenous, and subcutaneous. These will be discussed, along with less frequently used routes, in the following paragraphs.

Intradermal—The term intradermal (ID) is derived from "intra," meaning within, and "dermis," the sensitive, vascular inner layer of the skin. While this anatomical site has a high degree of vascularity, the blood vessels are extremely small. Hence, absorption from the injection site is slow and limited, with comparable systemic effects. Because of the limited absorption, this route is usually employed for a local action in skin

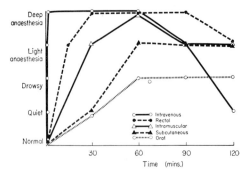

Fig. 2—Relation of onset, intensity and duration of hypnotic drug effect to route of administration.[6]

testing for drug sensitivity or to determine sensitivity to microorganisms as in the Tuberculin or Histoplasmin skin tests.

Intramuscular—The term intramuscular (IM) designates an injection within a muscle. The intramuscular route provides a speed of onset of action which is normally less than the intravenous route but greater than the subcutaneous route. Fig. 2 shows an example of the comparative onset, intensity, and duration of action of a drug given by the three parenteral routes, along with rectal and oral administration.

Medication injected IM forms a depot from which the drug is absorbed somewhat slowly, the peak concentration in the blood usually occurring within an hour. Several factors influence the rate of release of the drug from the depot, including, volume of the injection, concentration of drug in the vehicle, nature of the solvent, tonicity of the formulation, particle size, and particle-size distribution of the drug in solution or suspension in the vehicle.

The site selected for an IM injection should be located as far as possible from major nerves and blood vessels and should be capable of accepting the volume of fluid to be injected. Being an extravascular site the volume of fluid is limited. Suitable areas include the gluteal muscles (buttocks), vastus lateralis (lateral thigh), quadriceps (midanterior thigh), and deltoid (upper arm).

Intravenous—The term intravenous (IV) refers to an injection within a vein. Since no absorption is involved, the peak concentration in the blood occurs immediately, and the desired effect of the drug is obtained almost instantaneously. See Fig. 2.

Small-volume parenteral IV administration is also referred to as direct IV push administration. Direct push medications are usually given by performing a venipuncture for direct administration with a syringe and needle or by injecting the medication at the gum rubber flash ball site on an IV administration set. Drugs needed in emergencies are often administered by direct IV push. Also, most cancer chemotherapeutic agents used are best administered by direct IV push because of their highly toxic local effects if administered by continuous drip. Agents which are incompatible with other drugs are also infused by direct push.

Certain drugs should not be administered by direct IV push due to the local or systemic toxicity produced by rapid administration of the drug in high concentrations. For example, amphotericin is not recommended for administration by direct IV push because of the high incidence of phlebitis associated with the administration of concentrated solutions.

In selecting a site for an intravenous injection, the proximal veins, such as those in the antecubital area, are usually used. Distal sites such as the ankle or wrist region may be used. However, they should be avoided if a potentially irritating material is to be injected because the vascular stasis occurring in the distal regions may increase the risk of thrombosis. Provided large, proximal veins are utilized, the IV route may be used for administering drugs which are irritating or even caustic to tissue, such as mechlorethamine hydrochloride (Mustargen), because the vein walls are insensitive to pain and dilution by the blood occurs rapidly.

Subcutaneous—Subcutaneous (SC, sq, Sub Q) or hypodermic injections are given under the skin. Parenterals given by this route have a comparatively slow onset of action with less absorption than those given either IV or IM. See Fig. 2. Although this is an extravascular route it can be used to administer relatively large volumes of fluid because of the flexible nature of the tissue. The injected fluid forms a depot from which the drug is slowly absorbed, hence the peak concentration in the blood does not occur immediately.

This route is probably the most frequently used when patient self-administration is required, as for insulin. The sites suitable are numerous and include most portions of the arms, legs, and abdomen. When daily injections are necessary, as with the diabetic patient, the sites of injection should be rotated.

Other Routes of Injection—In addition to the four primary parenteral routes discussed, several other routes are used for specific effects, sometimes for a local rather than a systemic effect.

The *intra-arterial* route, that is, directly into an artery, is used in place of the intravenous route when immediate action is desired in a peripheral area of the body.

An injection into a joint (*intra-articular*) is usually made to obtain a local action of the medication, as for example, the anti-inflammatory action of steroids in treating arthritis.

The *intracardiac* route, that is, directly into the heart, is used when life is threatened in emergencies such as cardiac failure. In such cases, 0.5–1 ml of epinephrine solution 1:1000 may be used to stimulate the heart muscle.

An *intracerebral* injection, that is, an injection into the cerebrum, is used primarily for a local action as in the use of phenol in treating trigeminal neuralgia.

An injection into the spinal canal (*intraspinal*) results in a high concentration of drug in a local area within the canal. This site is generally used in counteracting infection or in treating certain neoplastic diseases, for example, treating leukemic meningitis with methotrexate.

Additional routes, such as, injection into the peritoneum (*intraperitoneal*) and injection into the pleural cavity or the lung (*intrapleural*) may be used to meet particular needs.

Space is not available here to discuss the procedures involved in administering parenteral medications, however, this information is available.

Syringes and Needles—Small-volume parenterals are usually administered by means of syringes and needles. The syringe is a graduated container for measuring the dose of liquid. The needle is a hollow tube, attached to the syringe on one end, sharpened on the other, and used to provide a passageway for the liquid to be forced from the syringe into the tissue.

The two types of syringes most frequently encountered by pharmacists are the tuberculin syringe and the hypodermic syringe. Tuberculin syringes are small, not exceeding 1 ml in capacity, and are graduated in 0.01-ml or 0.1-ml divisions. The use of this type of syringe is limited to the administration of small volumes of fluid such as those used for intradermal skin tests, or of small doses of medication that require a high degree of accuracy.

The hypodermic syringe usually has a capacity of from 2–50 ml and may be graduated in milliliters and subdivisions, or minims. Special hypodermic syringes, such as those graduated in units of insulin, are available also.

A syringe is composed of two elements, a graduated, hollow, tubular portion, the "barrel," and a solid portion, the "plunger." The plunger fits snugly into the barrel and, when pressure is applied, forces the liquid in the barrel out of the syringe. Traditionally, syringes have been made of glass and were intended to be reused. This necessitated careful cleaning, matching of plungers and barrels, wrapping, and sterilizing after each use. In recent years sterile disposable syringes have become available. Their use eliminates not only the chore of cleaning and re-sterilizing but also the risk of transmission of pathogenic viruses, such as infectious hepatitis, from ineffectively sterilized syringes. Today, in most hospitals and physicians offices, disposable syringes are used almost exclusively.

Disposable syringe barrels may be made of glass or plastic and the plungers of glass, plastic or metal with a rubber sealing tip attached. Disposable syringes may also be obtained with needles attached, thus eliminating the step of affixing the needle to the syringe at the time of use.

A needle is composed of two elements, a "hub" which locks on the tip of the barrel of the syringe and a "cannula," the pointed, hollow tube. The cannula of the needle is usually made of stainless steel and the hub of stainless steel, plastic or aluminum.

Needles have three dimensions: the length, measured along the cannula from the hub to the tip of the point (usual range, $\frac{1}{4}$ in. to $3\frac{1}{2}$ in.), the outside diameter (gauge) of the cannula (usual range, 13–27 gauge), and the cannula wall thickness (regular or thin wall). Hypodermic needles are sized as to diameter using the English Wire Gauge System. With this system the outside diameter of the cannula is inversely proportional to the gauge of the needle, that is, an 18-gauge needle is larger than a 22-gauge needle.

The sharpened point of the needle is designed to reduce pain and provide ease of penetration of tissue. Two bevels (angle of cut), long and short, are commonly available. The long bevel is generally used on needles for subcutaneous or intramuscular injection, the short bevel for intravenous and intradermal injection.

The selection of the proper gauge, length, and type of bevel is important for the comfort and safety of the patient and should be based on such factors as the viscosity of the liquid to be injected, the route and site of injection, the anatomic characteristics of the patient (obese, thin) and the age of the patient (pediatric, adult).

Sterile disposable needles are also used extensively. The problem of processing reusable needles to be sure that the lumen is completely clean and that the needle point is sharp, has thereby been eliminated.

Large-Volume Parenterals

Large-volume parenterals are classified as such due to the large volume of fluid to be injected and the volume of the liquid within each container. A large-volume parenteral is defined by the USP as a sterile solution of 100 ml or more, intended for intravenous injection. It is used in the diagnosis, cure, mitigation or treatment of disease or modification of physiological functions in human beings, but excludes blood.

Due to the large volume of fluid per container, facilities having large production capacities are required. This, combined with larger containers and increased handling, enhances the potential for contamination as compared with small volume parenterals. Since large volumes of fluid are to be administered, usually directly into the blood stream, the necessity for the assurance of a sterile, particle-free preparation is increased. Coupled with this is the need to utilize strict aseptic techniques in the administration of these fluids.

Large-volume parenteral fluids generally are intended to provide water, electrolytes, and nutrients to seriously ill patients. These include solutions, such as dextrose 5% in water for injection (D5W), which provides water and calories, dextrose 5% and sodium chloride 0.9% injection (D5S), which provides water, electrolyte, and calories and is used as a hydrating solution. These solutions may be formulated to be hypotonic, isotonic, or hypertonic to provide further flexibility for use in maintaining body fluid, electrolyte, and acid-base balance.

The electrolyte content is usually expressed as milliequivalents (mEq). This may be defined as $1/1000$ part of the equivalent weight in grams. Since the values expressed as grams are small

decimal fractions, for convenience they are usually expressed in milligrams. Such an expression provides a means for interrelating ionic activity which, in turn, is directly related to the physiological activity of an electrolyte solution.

Routes of Administration—Due to the large volume of solution administered, only the intravenous and subcutaneous routes are normally used. The intraarterial route is used occasionally. The intravenous route is preferred unless a suitable vein is unusually difficult to find or enter. This may occur in infants and geriatric or obese patients.

Since the IV and SC routes have already been discussed, only factors relative to administering large volumes of fluids will be considered below. Large-volume parenterals can be administered by intermittent infusion or by continuous intravenous drip. Continuous drip administration is the method of choice for drugs which are best given at a steady level of concentration. Regular fluid and electrolytes are administered most frequently by means of continuous drip. Certain drugs, e.g., oxytocin, are given by continuous drip to maintain a certain blood level of the drug during the entire period of administration.

Intravenous—The advantages of this route include (1) a wider variety of injectable fluids and additives can be used IV than via the subcutaneous route, (2) a large volume of fluid can be injected relatively rapidly, (3) a direct systemic effect is obtained, (4) a continuous blood level of drug is provided, and (5) direct access to an open vein for routine drug administration and use in the event of an emergency situation is provided.

The disadvantages of this route are largely preventable, but include (1) cardiovascular, pulmonary, and renal disturbances from the increased volume of fluid in the circulatory system following rapid administration of large volumes of fluids, (2) potential development of thrombophlebitis, (3) possibility of local or systemic infection from contaminated solutions or septic injection techniques, and (4) the limitation to administration of aqueous fluids.

Subcutaneous—Subcutaneous infusion (hypodermoclysis) provides an alternative when the intravenous route cannot be used. Relatively large volumes of fluid can be administered, but the injection must be given slowly. Absorption of the fluid is improved by prior injection of hyaluronidase. However, compared with the intravenous route, there is slower absorption, more pain and discomfort, a smaller variety of fluids that can be administered (usually limited to isotonic solutions), and a more limited variety of solution additives.

Administration Sets and Supplies—Since the injection of a liter of fluid normally requires 6–8 hours it is more convenient to provide a means of administration that can proceed unattended once it has been initiated. Gravitational force is utilized to keep the fluid flowing. The administration assembly usually consists of a glass bottle or plastic bag containing the fluid, an air filter and tube to admit air into the container to allow for an equilibration of internal and external pressure on the fluid, a tubular insert to affix the set to the container, a drip chamber for visually adjusting flow rate, a length of connecting tubing, a pinch or screw clamp to adjust or stop the flow rate, and a needle adapter to permit the connection of a needle or intravenous catheter.

Although the basic administration sets are similar, differences exist from one manufacturer to another. In addition, there are specialized sets, such as those with connections for multiple injection sites, sets which permit the connecting of two or more containers of fluid, intermittent drug administration sets, and those with microdrop drip chambers that permit more careful control of the administration rate.

Specialized Large-Volume Solutions—In addition to the large-volume fluids intended primarily to provide fluid, calories, and electrolytes, other large volume fluids with specialized uses are available. Several of these are prepared or dispensed by the pharmacist and warrant consideration here.

Hyperalimentation Solutions—Parenteral alimentation has, in the past, been possible through the use of carbohydrate, electrolyte, vitamin, and amino acid solutions. However, patients rarely, if ever, gained weight or passed into a significant and continuing anabolic state for prolonged periods with intravenous nutrition alone.

Total parenteral nutrition (hyperalimentation) is the intravenous administration of nutrients in amounts sufficient to achieve tissue synthesis, and an anabolic state in the severely ill when oral ingestion is not possible or is not adequate alone. Parenteral hyperalimentation has permitted the maintenance of a continuing anabolic state for prolonged periods of time, as evidenced by the maintenance of patients, exclusively by vein, for periods of 100–200 days with 2400–4500 calories/ day.

The solutions, which are infused continuously into the superior vena cava by means of an indwelling catheter, vary in their components but basically consist of 20% glucose and 5% protein or fibrin hydrolysate plus essential amounts of electrolytes, minerals, and vitamins.

Parenteral hyperalimentation now provides a means for giving life-sustaining nutrients to patients with conditions such as chronic complicated gastrointestinal disease, esophageal obstruction, gastric carcinoma, colonic carcinoma, and ulcerative colitis. This represents a totally new dimension for parenteral therapy.

Peritoneal Dialysis Fluids—Peritoneal dialysis provides a fairly simple means for removing toxic substances and metabolites from the body that would normally be excreted by the kidneys. The fluid is injected continuously into the abdominal cavity, bathes the peritoneum, and is continuously withdrawn. The peritoneum is a semipermeable membrane covering the viscera in the abdominal cavity. It has a filtering surface of 22,000 cm^2 and is an excellent dialyzing membrane.

Peritoneal dialysis is based on two principles, osmosis and diffusion. Dialysis fluids usually are formulated to contain glucose and an ionic content similar to normal extracellular fluid. Therefore, catabolites and other toxic substances diffuse into the dialysis fluid so that they can be removed. Concurrently, excess water can be withdrawn from the patient by osmosis because the glucose renders the fluid hyperosmotic.

Peritoneal dialysis is indicated in a number of conditions, the most frequent being acute renal insufficiency.

Irrigating Solutions—Irrigating solutions are sterile, pyrogen free, large volume fluids intended for irrigating body cavities and wounds. Although not intended for intravenous administration, they must be made with the same care, procedures and controls as with intravenous fluids.

Intravenous therapy is associated with an appreciable risk of life-threatening septicemia. However, infusion-associated infections can be minimized if physicians, nurses, and other hospital personnel adhere to established infection control procedures when administering intravenous fluids.

Monitoring Therapy

Physicians, nurses, and/or pharmacists should carefully monitor parenteral drug therapy. Patients should be observed for subjective and objective indication of drug response. Subjective data are obtained through patient interviews. Objective data are obtained through direct observation of the patient, clinical laboratory data, physical examination, and radiology. These data should be used to establish the effectiveness or ineffectiveness of parenteral therapy. The patient also should be observed for evidences of side effects, toxicity, allergic drug reactions, and drug interactions that may occur secondary to therapy. Inadequate monitoring may lead to fatal therapeutic problems including drug toxicity, infection and fluid, electrolyte and acid-base imbalance.

Quality Characteristics of Parenteral Medications

To achieve a quality product, every component and every process step must be carefully designed and controlled. The entire history of the product must reflect a planned and executed quality assurance program.

Since the pharmacist has the responsibility for selecting parenteral products for administration to patients from among those commercially available, a review of the required characteristics and the applicable good manufacturing practices (GMP's) will contribute to the making of an intelligent professional selection.

Product Components

The specifications for components of the product, both the ingredients of the formula and the constituents of the container intimately in contact with the product, must help to achieve the objective of a quality product. Requirements for the processing facilities and the process itself must, likewise, meet high standards. These parameters will be discussed in the following sections.

Vehicles

Since the transport systems of the human body are aqueous in nature, medications to be injected should normally be in an aqueous system. But, because of the solubility and stability properties of therapeutic compounds, it is not always possible to formulate drugs in such a system. The required solvent system may be miscible with water in some instances but immiscible in others. For all products, the vehicle must be nontoxic in the amount and by the route administered. Purity specifications also must be explicit and exacting.

Most parenteral products are preferably prepared as solutions, although suspensions and emulsions also may be used. The vehicles for such products must meet specifications similar to those for solutions.

Aqueous Vehicles—Water for Injection (WFI) is the most widely used and important vehicle for injectable preparations. The USP monograph states the specifications for this ingredient, including the requirements that it must contain only a limited amount of specific anions and cations and of total solids, it must be pyrogen free, and it must be made by distillation or reverse osmosis. Sterile Water for Injection also must be sterile, and is described as water packaged in a container to be used as a vehicle for a product just prior to administration.

The very stringent limitation for contaminants in WFI is necessary to minimize the possibility of toxic effects from its use and to minimize the risk of chemical reactions. For example, copper present at a level of only a few parts per billion may be sufficient to catalyze oxidation reactions for a drug such as ascorbic acid. The specification limits given by the USP are often not sufficiently stringent for a particular situation, since they are intended to serve as minimal limits and to be subject to more rigorous requirements where needed.

Water for Injection must be pyrogen free. This is readily achieved by proper distillation. Other aspects of pyrogens will be discussed later.

The USP monograph does not require WFI to be sterile when used as a vehicle in the manufacture of a bulk product but it may be required to be so by an in-plant product specification. The latter requirement serves to reduce the level of contamination in the final product, thereby increasing the effectiveness of terminal sterilization processes.

WFI must be prepared by distillation or reverse osmosis because these are the only methods adequate to provide the purity required. Ideally, distillation converts liquid water mixed with various impurities into pure molecules of water vapor by means of heat energy. The pure water vapor is condensed back to liquid water (distillate) by cooling. Actually, the water vapor is contaminated to varying degrees by:

Substances carried along with the vapor from the distillate.

Substances such as metal ions picked up from contact with parts of the still, the storage tanks or the pipes and other parts of the distribution systems.

Substances picked up from exposure to the environment, including gases, particulate matter, and microorganisms.

Therefore, the still must be designed to provide an efficiency equal to the quality level of water required, with minimal contamination pickup during the process, including storage and distribution.

Reverse osmosis (RO) is a relatively new process now recognized by the USP as an acceptable method for the preparation of WFI. As the name signifies it is a method by which the natural flow of water through a semipermeable membrane from a solution having a lower concentration is reversed. This is accomplished by applying pressure on the more concentrated solution, forcing the water through the membrane. The degree of selectivity and efficiency of the membrane in retaining ions and solute molecules while permitting permeation of water molecules determines the purity of the water produced. Suspended solids are also retained. The rate of water production is higher and the cost lower with available RO systems as compared with stills.

Deionization is a process widely utilized for the production of purified water. A mixed-bed resin deionizer functions by efficiently exchanging metallic cations and anions in the water for hydrogen ions and hydroxyl ions, respectively, on the resin. Suspended nonionized materials are physically entrapped but may migrate gradually through the bed and provide nutrients for any microorganisms also entrapped. Therefore, substantial microbiological and pyrogenic contamination of the effluent may occur, thereby rendering such water unfit for parenteral products. Although a much higher flow rate of water can be obtained than from a still, deionization cannot be used for the final step in the preparation of WFI.

The purity of water is most conveniently evaluated by means of conductivity measurement. This measurement is dependent upon ions (charged particles) in the water to conduct a current between two electrodes. The resistance in ohms or the conductivity in mhos is a measure of the number of charged particles in the water. It is not a measure of any noncharged substances present. A gravimetric test for total solids is necessary to determine the content of all dissolved or suspended particles. Other specific tests are required to detect specific anions or cations, pyrogens or microorganisms.

Other aqueous vehicles frequently used in place of WFI include dilute electrolyte and carbohydrate solutions, such as, Sodium Chloride and Dextrose Injections.

Nonaqueous Vehicles—Nonaqueous vehicles include both those which are miscible with water and those that

Table 1—Selected Preservatives Used in Parenteral Products

Purpose	Compound	Usual concentration (%)
Antibacterials	Benzalkonium chloride	0.01
	Benzethonium chloride	0.01
	Benzyl alcohol	2.0
	Chlorobutanol	0.5
	Chlorocresol	0.1–0.3
	Cresol	0.3–0.5
	p-Hydroxybenzoate esters	
	Methyl	0.18
	Propyl	0.02
	Phenol	0.5
	Phenylmercuric nitrate	0.002
	Thimerosal	0.01
Antioxidants	Ascorbic acid	0.02–0.1
	Sodium bisulfite	0.1–0.15
	Sodium formaldehyde sulfoxylate	0.1–0.15
	Thiourea	0.005
	Butyl hydroxyanisole	0.005–0.02
	Tocopherol	0.05–0.075
Chelating agents	Ethylenediaminetetraacetic acid salts	0.01–0.075
Buffers	Acetic acid and a salt	1–2
	Citric acid and a salt	1–3
	Acid salts of phosphoric acid	0.8–2
Tonicity adjustment	Dextrose	5.5
	Sodium chloride	0.9
	Sodium sulfate	1.6

are not miscible. Only a very limited number of vehicles have a sufficiently low level of toxicity or sensitizing property to be utilized for injection. Of these very few can be injected into the blood stream, but are limited to use in small volumes intramuscularly or subcutaneously.

The water immiscible vehicles are limited almost exclusively to fixed oils and their derivatives, such as, ethyl oleate. They are used for their solvent properties, as vehicles for suspensions having repository effects and, with selected fixed oils, for the preparation of intravenous emulsions having nutrient properties. These vehicles must be of vegetable origin so that they can be metabolized, they must be liquid at room temperature so that they can be injected, and they must be nontoxic to host tissue. Among the oils most commonly used are corn oil, cottonseed oil, and sesame oil.

Solutes

The solutes in parenteral formulations, either the medicinal agent or substances added for preservative or certain other effects, must be of exceptionally high quality. The commercial grades obtainable may require further purification to render them suitable for use in parenteral products. Purity specifications should be explicit and exacting for each ingredient and should include requirements for potency and purity of the substance, level of specific trace contaminants, solubility characteristics as determined by the physical form of the compound, freedom from microbial contamination, freedom from pyrogenic contamination, and freedom from gross dirt.

In addition to the medicinal agent, most formulations contain one or more added substances to preserve the product from degradation. These preservatives include antibacterial agents, antifungal agents, antioxidants, chelating agents, solubilizing agents, buffers, and agents to adjust tonicity. A number of these agents are listed in Table 1. Many of these agents are active chemical compounds, useful under proper circumstances but contributing to incompatibilities if used improperly. For example, the reducing agent, sodium bisulfite is an effective antioxidant, but if used with an organic mercurial compound in aqueous solution the compound may be reduced and elemental mercury released.

Antifungal or antibacterial agents must be included in the formulation of all multiple dose containers and may be included in products subjected to marginal methods of sterilization. They are used at relatively low concentrations which produce inhibition of growth (stasis) of any microorganisms introduced at the time of use. Because of potential direct or cumulative toxicity they may not be included in preparations to be given into nerve compartments, such as the spinal cord, or given in large volume as intravenous solutions. They must always be used with full recognition of their potential toxicity.

Antioxidants are used to protect drugs from the oxidative effects of oxygen or other substances in the environment. Chelating agents are often used to enhance the action of antioxidants by complexing metal ions that would otherwise catalyze oxidation. Buffers are usually included in formulations to stabilize the pH during processing and storage, thereby protecting drugs that are sensitive to variations in hydrogen ion concentration. They may also be used to help adjust the tonicity of the solution. The adjustment of tonicity to isotonic conditions is particularly important for preserving the integrity of red blood cells upon the administration intravenously of large volumes of solution or preventing pain upon injection subcutaneously or intramuscularly in the presence of nerve endings.

Containers

The most important requirement for a container is to maintain the integrity of the product as a sterile, pyrogen-free, high purity preparation until it is used. In addition, it should be attractive, permit inspection of the contents, be strong enough to withstand processing and shipping, and not interact with the product. With disposable administration units the container is often an integral part of the unit.

Most containers for parenteral products are made of glass and are closed by fusion of the glass or by the insertion of a rubber or plastic stopper. Plastic polymers are beginning to be used for containers of commercial parenteral products. Polyethylene has been used for some time for sterile ophthalmic preparations because the flexible walls make possible drop-dispensing containers. Plastic containers also have the advantage of less weight than glass.

Glass—Glass is composed of silicon dioxide combined with various additives that alter physical and chemical properties, such as melting point, thermal coefficient of expansion, color, transparency, and chemical reactivity. The addition of boric oxide lowers the melting point but does not markedly alter the other properties. The addition of oxides of sodium, potassium, calcium, magnesium and iron markedly lower the melting point, increase the thermal coefficient of expansion, and increase the degree of chemical interaction with the product. The latter is due to the fact that these oxides can be leached from the glass by liquids, particularly water, in contact with the glass.

The USP Glass Types are related to the chemical reactivity of the glass as measured by the alkalinity leached from the glass by water in one of the two glass tests. See Table 2. The borosilicate glass releases less alkaline substances to the leaching water than soda-lime glass which contains a relatively high proportion of sodium, calcium, and related oxides.

Containers of Type I glass are best for aqueous parenteral products.

Plastic—The basic structural unit of plastics is a linear polymer, usually a saturated hydrocarbon, sometimes having one or more hydrogens replaced with a halide, such as the chlorine in polyvinyl chloride. Most plastics selec-

Table 2—Glass Types and Tests

Type	General description[a]	Type of test	Size[b] (ml)	Limits ml of 0.02 N Acid
I	Borosilicate glass, highly resistant	Powdered glass	All	1.0
II	Treated soda-lime glass	Water attack	100 or less	0.7
			Over 100	0.2
III	Soda-lime	Powdered glass	All	8.5
NP	Soda-lime glass, general-purpose	Powdered glass	All	15.0

[a] The description applies to containers of this type of glass usually available.
[b] Size indicates the overflow capacity of the container.

tively permit passage of chemical molecules and most are permeable to gases. Since they melt at elevated temperatures only a few can be subjected to the heat of autoclaving. Many plastics contain additives, such as plasticizers, antioxidants, antistatic agents, and lubricants, which may subsequently be leached from the plastic into a product.

Because of such properties, the use of plastic containers for parenteral products has developed slowly. Improvements in plastic technology, increased purity of the polymer, and less extensive use of additives have increased the use of plastic containers for parenteral products. Plastics are being used extensively for components of administration sets, particularly disposable ones.

Chemical and biological toxicity testing procedures and limits for these materials have been developed as a means of determining the suitability of the test material for use. The biological tests utilize injection of extracts and implantation procedures in animals and the chemical tests include pH, heavy metals, and residue determinations. Such tests are included in the USP.

Rubber—The basic structural unit of natural (crepe) rubber is a linear unsaturated hydrocarbon, isoprene. Various synthetic rubber polymers are sometimes used to replace all or part of the natural polymer in a compound. These include neoprene, butyl and silicone polymers. Combined with the polymer are fillers, a vulcanizer, an accelerator, an antioxidant, and lubricants. A typical formula is given in Table 3. The accelerator and vulcanizer should be completely chemically consumed in producing cross linkage of the linear polymer chains during vulcanization, but may not be. The other ingredients are generally simply dispersed through the plastic mass of the polymer during the milling operation. Therefore, these substances can be leached from the rubber compound into a pharmaceutical product and may be the cause of chemical interactions. In an attempt to reduce the leaching, and also to reduce permeation, lacquer or plastic coatings are sometimes applied to the surface of the rubber closures in contact with the product. These coatings are at best only partial barriers.

Rubber closures are intended to provide a hermetic seal against the side of the opening of cartridges, vials and bottles. Therefore, they must be elastic but firm enough to:

Conform to minor dimensional irregularities but not to distort.
Permit the insertion of a hypodermic needle with minimal cutting of fragments by the hollow configuration of the needle.
Reseal upon withdrawal of the needle.

Table 3—Rubber Closure Type Composition

Ingredient	Content (%)	Purpose
Crepe rubber	43.5	Elastomer
Barium sulfate	52.0	Filler
Zinc oxide	1.7	Activator
Stearic acid	0.8	Lubricant
Sulfur	0.8	Vulcanizer
2-Mercaptobenzo- thiazole	0.4	Accelerator
Titanium dioxide	0.8	Colorant

They must be resistant to aging changes, to sterilization procedures, and to permeation of moisture and vapors. Butyl rubber compounds provide the best resistance to moisture permeation and should be used where such a property is required, although they have greater hardness and are more difficult to penetrate with a needle.

Physicochemical and biological toxicity tests were included for the first time in the *NF XIII*. They are intended to aid in the lot to lot quality control of rubber closures, but no limits have been given.

Other ingredients and components are sometimes used for products to be administered by injection but space limitations do not permit discussion of them. The general guidelines for purity and the necessity for adherence to critical specifications must apply equally to any other substances utilized.

Process Facilities

A parenteral product is exposed repeatedly to the environment during processing. Therefore, a low level of particulate matter in the environment must be maintained to prevent viable and nonviable contaminants from entering the product. To achieve low levels of particulate contamination the environment must be designed, maintained and operated in a manner conducive to reaching that objective.

Particles that are suspended in the air within an environment are those most likely to be introduced into a product.

Only relatively large particles tend to settle out of the air, even without the resuspending effect of air currents. Since there are resuspending effects, it is necessary not only to clean the incoming air, down into the submicron range, but also to eliminate particles from surfaces and other collecting points and to minimize the generation of particles.

In connection with the space exploration program, a classification of clean rooms has been developed, based upon the particulate level in the environment.[7] Aseptic processing areas for pharmaceuticals should meet the specifications for a Class 100 clean room, which is defined as having a particle count not to exceed a total of 100 particles/ft^3 of 0.5 μm and larger.

Production Areas

Clean rooms should be constructed to prevent inward air leaks and dirt collecting crevices, corners or projections. See Fig. 5. Ceiling and wall construction material should be low in particle shedding, easy to clean, and resistant to decontamination procedures. Floor surfaces should be similar, with the additional quality of wear resistance. For ceiling and walls, epoxy and vinyl polymeric continuous film coating materials have proven to be quite useful. Cement mixed with polymeric compounds has proven to be an effective floor material.

Furnishings and equipment should also be constructed of low particle shedding materials. Work counters should be suspended from the wall and the number of cabinets should be minimized in the most critical processing areas. Lights and other fixtures should be recessed into the ceiling or wall. Pipes, air ducts, and other supply lines should be recessed in the wall or run through chases or plenums outside of the critical environment, since this permits access by maintenance personnel without entering the aseptic area.

Housekeeping of the environment is a very critical operation. Janitorial personnel may not always be adequately motivated or trained to perform the kind of effective cleaning required, at least not without very careful and alert supervision. Operating personnel may be more reliable for housekeeping of aseptic areas. All surfaces must be adequately washed with an effective detergent in a manner that does not generate additional particulate matter from the cleaning equipment. Wet vacuum removal of cleaning solutions is the most effective procedure.

Surface Disinfectants—For maxi-

Table 4—Liquid Surface Disinfectants

Disinfectant	Bactericidal efficiency	Sporicidal efficiency	Fungicidal efficiency	Comments	Usual concentration
Alcohols, ethyl and isopropyl	Good	Not effective	Not reliable	Safe, evaporates completely, readily available	70%
Chlorine	Good	Fair	Good	Irritating, corrodes metal, inactivated by organic matter	Equiv. to 1–5% sod. hypochlorite
Formalin	Excellent	Good	Good	Toxic and irritating, effective in presence of organic matter, does not corrode metal	8%
Iodine and iodophors	Good	Fair	Good	Low tissue toxicity, corrosive, stains	1–2% and 75–100 ppm respectively
Mercurials	Fair	Not effective	Not reliable	Irritating, corrodes metal, activity reduced by organic matter	Varied, depending on compound
Peracetic acid	Excellent	Excellent	Excellent	Irritating, corrodes metal, surfactant required for maximum effect	1–3.5%
Phenolics	Excellent	Not reliable	Excellent	Mildly irritating to skin, odor, some discoloration	1–3%
Quaternary ammonium compounds	Fair	Not effective	Not reliable	Nontoxic, colorless, odorless, inactivated by anionic compounds	1:750

mum effectiveness when applied either by wiping or spraying, a disinfectant requires a thorough removal of dirt and other contaminants, an effective concentration level, and an adequate time to act. Table 4 lists some of the common disinfectants that are utilized and a general statement concerning their effectiveness. It must be remembered that the chemical surface disinfectants having sporicidal activity are generally too irritating or corrosive for general use. Therefore, the use of surface disinfectants at best can be considered to be only a supplement to good housekeeping.

Surface disinfection by means of ultraviolet (UV) irradiation also can be utilized as a supplement to good housekeeping. Toxicity of the radiation against microorganisms has been established but reactivation of organisms has been reported where insufficient exposure has occurred. Glowing mercury vapor produces a high proportion of the 253.7 nm wavelength of ultraviolet light, which is effectively germicidal. This wavelength can be transmitted through a high silicon content glass tube, although it gradually loses this capability with aging, provided these lamps are kept clean. Its effectiveness is essentially limited to exposed surfaces since penetration is poor and no effect is obtained in shadow areas.

Personnel

Personnel are the most difficult factor to control in a clean room because they are constantly discharging to the environment both viable and nonviable particulate matter. Therefore, where possible, a barrier must be placed between people and the product. This barrier may take the form of a glass panel, a curtain of clean air, or a uniform.

Professional and lay personnel must be given specialized training to be prepared to accept and fulfill the level of responsibility required for sterile product processing. This may be achieved by formalized course instruction or by on-the-job training. Personnel selected for such training should show personal qualities of neatness, orderliness and alertness, and they should be responsive to the training and to the responsibilities described. These people should show evidence of existing habits of good personal hygiene, freedom from nervous habits such as scratching parts of the body, and should have a good state of health.

Garments worn should provide not only a barrier but they should not contribute particles to the environment, as does short fiber cloth. Continuous filament synthetic fibers are preferred. In nonaseptic areas clean garments may simply be donned in place of outer street clothes. See Fig. 4. In aseptic areas garments should be sterilized and should provide as complete a barrier as possible.

Garments for the nonlaminar flow aseptic area include the following items (see Figs. 3, 7, and 8):

A mask made of nonlinting material, usually disposable, preferably deflecting the breath back along the cheeks.

A hood completely covering the head and neck and extending under the collar of the uniform.

A uniform preferably of a coverall type.

Footwear consisting of boots having a plastic sole and synthetic fiber tops extending about half way up the leg with a secure snap or tie at the top. These are normally worn over comfortable shoes that are used only within the clean area. Sometimes the shoes are worn alone because boots are awkward and may cause personnel to fall.

Sterile rubber or plastic gloves that may be worn over the hands. Because rubber gloves are easily contaminated, are clumsy, produce sweating and require dusting powder, it is sometimes considered to be better simply to wash and disinfect the hands. After thorough scrubbing of the hands the best skin disinfectant is probably 70% ethyl alcohol.

In vertical laminar flow facilities gowning requirements may be less restrictive, particularly below the knees, because particles liberated at this level will be carried away from the critical work areas.

Since the comfort and efficiency of personnel also must be considered, it is sometimes not possible to achieve ideal barrier characteristics with garments.

Handling of the Air

From 10–20 complete changes of air per hour are considered necessary where personnel are present. All of this air must be cleaned, conditioned, and distributed with minimum turbulence. Positive air pressure within an enclosed space is necessary to prevent outside unclean air from entering the environment through cracks or doors when opened.

The air is most frequently cleaned by filtration. Filtration cleans air by screening, entrapment, or electrostatic attraction, and frequently by a combination of all three. Several types of filters are used. Prefilters are made of spun glass, shredded polyethylene, or continuous filament cloth and are intended to screen or entrap large particles. The high efficiency particulate air filters (HEPA filters) provide the final, highly effective cleaning step, as discussed previously.

Electrostatic precipitators remove particles from the air stream by inducing a positive charge on particles and then attracting them to negatively charged plates. Particles are removed irrespective of size but, if the velocity of the air stream is too great the particles can be carried on through the unit.

A typical air cleaning installation for an aseptic processing area includes one or more prefilters followed by an electrostatic precipitator and then a HEPA filter as near the point of discharge as possible.

Laminar Air Flow—Laminar air flow may be defined as the flow of an entire body of air within a confined space moving with uniform velocity along parallel flow lines. HEPA filters are installed to occupy one complete side of the area to be maintained clean. The bank of filters is arranged to provide either a horizontal or a vertical airflow. Class 100 facilities are fully achievable with this type installation.

Laminar flow installations are possible and available in the form of work benches (Fig. 3 and 7), overhead modules, portable curtained rooms, entire

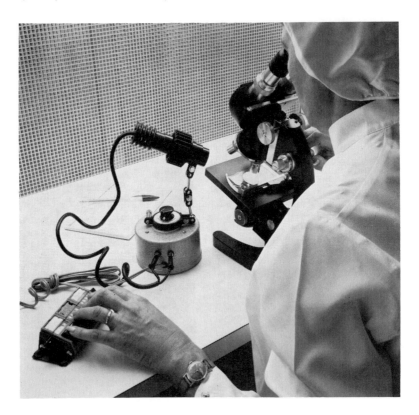

Fig. 3—Microscopic examination of a membrane filter for particulate matter in a laminar flow work bench (courtesy, *Millipore Corp.*).

rooms with fixed walls, and tunnels. HEPA filtered laminar air flow has made it possible to provide a much cleaner environment than was formerly possible. With the use of work benches or modules, it is possible to provide an aseptic environment almost anywhere, although the surrounding buffer area is a significant factor in the efficiency of operation.

Laminar flow units, however, are not without limitations. It is possible to overcome the established air flow velocity by a strong reverse current or projectile coughing or speaking of personnel. Turbulence or suck-back can be produced by objects placed in the area, particularly when close to the working edge of a work bench. Contamination introduced upstream from a piece of equipment, the operator's hands, or other items can be carried downstream to the critical work area. Leaks may

occur through or around the filter unit. Therefore, it is necessary to recognize not only the marked advantages of laminar flow environmental control but its limitations.

Evaluation of the Environment

Since no environment is perfectly free from viable and nonviable particulate matter, it is necessary to evaluate the level of effectiveness achieved. In general, environmental evaluation is performed by sampling the air or surfaces in the environment for viable and nonviable particles. Table 5 lists several methods used, with comments concerning their effectiveness.

Each of these methods of evaluating the environment has limitations. Most of those described are directed primarily toward the collection of viable microorganisms. Because of the limitations of each method it is normally necessary to

Table 5—Environmental Evaluation Techniques

Method	Equipment used	Effect	Comments
Air Sampling			
For viable particles			
Sedimentation	Nutrient or blood agar plates / Stainless steel settling strips	Microorganisms settle on agar or stainless steel strip	Simple, inexpensive, mainly collects large particles, strongly affected by air currents
Solid surface impactors	Slit samplers	Microorganisms deposited on rotating nutrient agar plate by high velocity, measured air flow	A measure of concentration with time, vegetative cells often killed by impact, drying effect may be lethal to cells
	Sieve samplers (Andersen)	Microorganisms deposited on fixed nutrient agar plates under six graded sieves by high velocity, measured air flow	A measure of size distribution of viable particles, vegetative cells often killed by impact, drying effect may be lethal to cells
Liquid impingement	Glass liquid impingers, intercepting membrane filter holder with 0.2 μm filter	Microorganisms washed from measured volume of air bubbled through sterile saline, nutrient broth, or other liquid, then collected on intercepting membrane filter and cultured	A measure of viable cells and spores in air sample because vegetative cells are more apt to survive in liquid, loss of liquid can occur from frothing
For viable and nonviable particles			
Filtration	Filter holder with 0.45 μm membrane filter	Particles screened from measured air sample, then cultured or counted directly (see Fig 3)	Simple, positive collection of all particles above a given size, vegetative cells killed by drying, quantitative analysis laborious
Electrostatic precipitation	Electrostatic precipitators	Particles collected on electrically charged surface	Complex equipment, high sampling rate, high efficiency, uncertain effect on survival of microorganisms
Electronic particle counters	Light scattering instruments, such as, Bausch & Lomb, Dynac, Royco	Particles in measured air sample detected by light scattered from its surface	Costly equipment, no differentiation between viable and nonviable particles, high sampling rate, total counts electronically computed
Surface Sampling			
For viable particles			
Agar contact	Rodac plate with nutrient agar	Microorganisms picked up from test surface by contact with convex agar surface	Flat, smooth test surfaces better, efficiency of recovery low
Swab-rinse	A moistened sterile cotton swab, tube with sterile diluting fluid, ultrasonic unit, plating medium	Microorganisms picked up from surface by rubbing swab over prescribed area, dislodged ultrasonically in diluent, and then plated in appropriate culture medium	Recovery of microorganisms from surface unreliable, release from cotton uncertain, easy procedure to perform
Rinse	Appropriate sterile fluid in an appropriate container	Rinsing microorganisms from surface with a sterile liquid by flushing, spraying or immersion. The rinse fluid is then assayed for viable particles	Several modifications possible, efficient method particularly from small surfaces
Vacuum probe	A probe tip attached to a vacuum source with an intercepting membrane filter between	Microorganisms are picked up by vacuum from a dry or wet surface and collected on intercepting membrane and cultured	Works well on flat surfaces only, good assay efficiency particularly with low contamination level

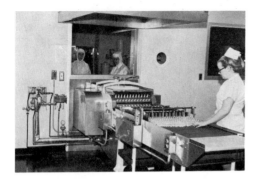

Fig. 4—Cleaning vials with pass-through washer into clean room used as the sterilizer loading area (courtesy, *Ayerst*).

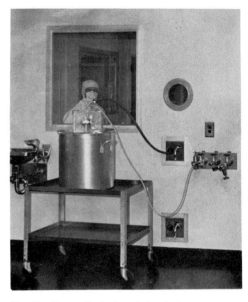

Fig. 5—Nonsterile bulk solution being pushed by compressed gas from bulk preparation area through porthole into aseptic processing area (courtesy, *Ayerst*).

use a combination of several of these methods for a critical evaluation of an environment.

Design and Traffic Flow Patterns

The design of an aseptic processing area must provide a series of effective barriers between progressively more secure areas. The risk of carrying contamination into the maximum security area is reduced by the use of buffer rooms, barrier walls, and controlled access through air locks with a very rigid control of the flow of supplies, equipment, product components, and personnel. Containers are often passed from the receiving area by means of through-the-wall washers to minimize the carrying of shipping debris into the clean area. See Fig. 4. Equipment and supplies normally are passed through sterilizers to reach the aseptic processing area. Bulk solutions (nonsterile) may be pumped through port holes to filters within an aseptic area to eliminate the necessity of conveying nonsterile bottles and carts into aseptic areas. See Fig. 5. Personnel must go through locker rooms and airlocks with prescribed entry procedures to minimize the risk of carrying contamination into aseptic areas. Normally a unidirectional flow of components and supplies must exist. The access of personnel to the aseptic processing area is rigidly controlled and limited to only those having a responsible reason for being there.

Manufacturing Processes

The steps required in the preparation of a small quantity of a product are familiar to all pharmacists. When a large number of product units are to be prepared, the manufacturing process becomes much more complex. Many problems are encountered in maintaining control of the process; in assuring the identity, quality and accuracy of ingredients incorporated; in measuring and handling the larger quantities of solid and liquid ingredients; in providing reliable transport from one step in the process to another; in maintaining control of the environment; in coordinating the personnel and processes involved; and in maintaining overall control of the process. These are the particular areas of expertise and responsibility of the industrial pharmacist. Because of limitations in space and the availability of discussions of these processes in detail elsewhere, only a general overview of the manufacturing processes will be given below. The flow diagram in Fig. 6 will be used as the basis for discussion.

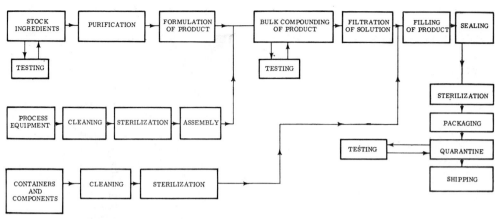

Fig. 6—The manufacturing process, proceeding in the direction of the arrows.

Planning

In the manufacturing process, advance planning is essential. As an early step, a lot number must be assigned to each product, to be used to identify the particular lot (batch) of that product. It is necessary for ingredients, containers and other supply items to be available and ready for utilization in the process when they are needed. Testing for identity and quality must be synchronized with the process in order that the components and the in-process product may be released for the next processing step. Some of this interrelationship can be seen in the flow diagram.

Stock ingredients, containers and other components which have been tested and released, as well as process equipment, must be available and ready to use when needed. In some instances, purification of stock ingredients may be required before they are of the quality required for formulation of the product. The process equipment must be cleaned, sterilized, and assembled, ready to receive the product at the time of formulation. This equipment may vary from a glass flask of a few liters to a stainless steel tank of several thousand gallons capacity. Regardless of size, the equipment must be thoroughly cleaned and sterilized or, in the case of a large tank, asepticized with the use of filtered steam, surface disinfectants, or ultraviolet radiation.

Compounding

Ingredients are combined in equipment designed for holding the bulk product. Mixing must be thorough and efficient to ensure rapid dispersion of individual ingredients and thus achieve a homogeneous condition. When a suspension is to be prepared it is necessary to wet and disperse the suspended material effectively, and then keep it uniformly dispersed while the product is being filled into individual container units. All of these steps must be carried out in containers which are covered and designed to prevent the introduction of contamination from the environment, operating equipment, or careless personnel. In-process testing of the bulk product for ingredient content is often desirable to assure that the compounding has been carried out properly.

Filtration

The next step in processing a solution is filtration. By means of filtration, solutions are rendered free from particulate matter to the required level. Normally, parenteral solutions are filtered to a high polish (high degree of clarity), that is, freed from particulate matter to a size of approximately 5 μm and larger. A solution having a high polish conveys to the user that it is a pure product. In addition, foreign particulate matter may be dangerous if injected. When a solution is filtered to render it free from

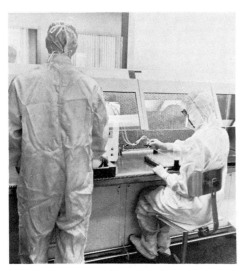

Fig. 7—Filling vials with measured quantities of liquid under aseptic conditions in a laminar flow workbench (courtesy, *Ayerst*).

viable microorganisms, the filter must remove particles as small as approximately 0.2 μm. Therefore, clarification or sterilization of a solution by filtration constitutes a difference in degree of particle removal.

Membrane filters are disposable filters used almost exclusively today for the filtration of parenteral solutions. They consist of very thin, delicate sheets of cellulose nitrate or acetate or of other polymeric material, such as polycarbonate, which must be handled carefully and supported smoothly and firmly in filter holders. They are manufactured to have quite uniform and controllable pore sizes and, therefore, are effective and reliable. Because of their inert character they have little or no adverse effect on solutions passed through them. They can be sterilized by means of steam under pressure or by ethylene oxide.

Filling

The completed bulk product is now ready for filling measured quantities into final unit containers. The containers and components, such as rubber closures, must have been previously cleaned, sterilized and made available for use at this point in the process. During the filling operation, the product is transferred from the bulk container by measuring devices, having a precision and accuracy appropriate for the particular product, and deposited in the individual unit containers. During this step it is possible for the product to pick up particulate matter and other contaminants if it is not adequately protected from exposure to the environment or, if the filling equipment or the containers themselves have not been adequately cleaned. In many processes this is the most critical step, particularly where the product is a solution that has been sterilized by filtration. See Fig. 7. Any inadvertent contamination from the environment renders the product unfit for use.

The filling operation may be accomplished by relatively simple equipment on a small scale, using essentially a hypodermic syringe attached to a motor driven cam. This moves the plunger and forces measured volumes of liquid into the unit containers. High-speed, automated equipment might fill as many as 300 or more containers a minute. Various types of filling equipment are also available for delivering measured quantities of powders. The operation of automated equipment requires careful and continuing attention to assure the accuracy and precision required, particularly where therapeutic agents of high potency are involved. The filling and sealing of ampuls under aseptic conditions using automated equipment may be seen in Fig. 8.

Sealing

As soon as possible after filling has been completed, the individual package units should be closed (sealed). For ampuls this involves high temperature fusion of glass to seal the opening in the container. For cartridges, vials, and bottles this involves the insertion of a rubber closure. This step may be achieved manually, or in large production processes by automatic machinery. To insure that the rubber closure does not

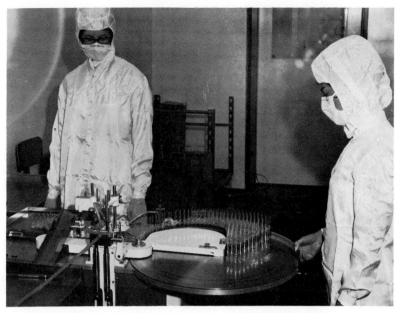

Fig. 8—Filling and sealing ampuls under aseptic conditions using automated equipment (courtesy, *McNeil*).

become dislodged from the container, an aluminum cap is normally crimped around the closure and the lip of the container to provide a tamper proof seal.

Sterilization

Once the container has been sealed, the contents are protected from contamination from the environment. However, at this point in the process the contents of the container normally would not be sterile. Therefore, it must be subjected to an effective sterilization process.

Sterilization classically has been defined as the complete destruction or removal of all forms of life. A more practical definition is that it is the process by which living organisms are removed or killed to the extent that they are no longer detectable by standard microbiological culture techniques.

Sterilization as an operational concept has as its aim the guaranty that the treated items are sterile without the necessity of testing each individual item. Certification of sterility is based upon: (1) adherence to a set of proven proce-dures known to produce sterile products, (2) microbiological control over preparation procedures prior to sterilization, and (3) a means of checking the sterility of each lot by sterility testing or by the use of biological indicators (spore controls).

Verification of Procedures—Conventional sterility tests alone cannot provide absolute confirmation of the sterility of a lot of treated items even if large numbers of samples are tested. This is illustrated by the relationship of the probabilities of acceptance of treated lots of items of varying assumed degrees of contamination with respect to the number of items tested. See Table 6. Thus, if 5 out of every 100 items in a lot are not sterile, the lot would be accepted as sterile 35% of the time when 20 items are tested. If the level of contamination is 1%, the lot would be accepted as sterile 82 out of 100 times with a 20-item test.

Two approaches can be used either separately or together to assure the sterility of processed materials. The first is to establish the rates of kill of the various types and quantities of microorga-

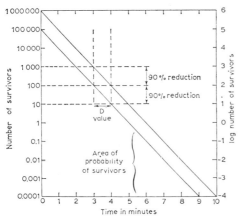

Fig. 9—Microbial death rate curves that illustrate concept of 90% reduction (*D* values) and probability of survivors.[9]

nisms on the product prior to sterilization. Such studies yield data from which the probabilities of survivors can be calculated. As a practical guide the lower the microbial content *prior* to sterilization, the greater will be the efficiency of the process and the confidence in its success. Although it may be impractical for the dispensing pharmacist to conduct microbial assays on all lots of items to be sterilized, he should remember that such assays are typical of the procedures used by industrial firms serving the health-care field. Industrial firms generally use presterilization assay data and kinetic destruction data in designing statistically based sterilization cycles.

The second approach is the use of biological indicators in each lot to be sterilized. Usually, the biological indica-

tor is a bacterial spore suspension which has been dried on a suitable carrier such as a small strip of filter paper. The destruction of all of the spores on the strips provides excellent evidence that sterilization has been achieved. The total numbers of spores in the biological indicators used in a sterilization run should be equal to or greater than the natural contaminants on the product.

Kinetics of Microbial Death during Sterilization—A term frequently used in industrial sterilization processes is the Decimal Reduction Value (*D* value). When a population of microorganisms is exposed to a sterilizing environment, the rate at which the organisms die can be described in mathematical terms. The death rates will usually follow first order reaction kinetics (logarithmic death rates).

The *D* value is usually defined as the time in minutes required to destroy 90% of the microorganisms exposed under any standard set of conditions. The simplest method is to plot the data on semilog paper. The number of initial and surviving organisms is plotted on the logarithmic scale against time in minutes on the linear scale and the best straight line determined.

Fig. 9 demonstrates the use of the *D* value in a situation where the destruction of each logarithmic unit of a population requires 1 min; the *D* value is 1 min. A population of 10^6 organisms is exposed to a given steam temperature and after a 1-min exposure, only 10^5 cells are viable. The remaining 10^5 cells are reduced to 10^4 after the 2nd min.

Table 6—Relationship of Probabilities of Acceptance of Lots of Varying
Assumed Degrees of Contamination to Number of Samples[a]

Number of samples	Contaminated items in lot (%)						
	0.1	*0.3*	*0.5*	*1*	*3*	*5*	*10*
10	0.99	0.98	0.96	0.91	0.74	0.60	0.34
20	0.98	0.94	0.90	0.82	0.54	0.35	0.11
50	0.95	0.86	0.78	0.61	0.22	0.08	0.005
100	0.91	0.74	0.61	0.37	0.05	0.01	
200	0.82	0.55	0.36	0.13	0.002		
300	0.74	0.41	0.22	0.05			
400	0.67	0.30	0.13	0.02			
500	0.61	0.22	0.08	0.01			

[a] From Ref. 8.

After 7 min the number would be 0.1 of an organism and at the end of 8 min, there would be 0.01 of an organism or 1 chance in 100 (10^{-2}) of a survivor. Treatment could be continued until the probability of 10^{-6} is reached. With sterile medical supplies it is recommended that the treatment result in a probability of 10^{-6} or less of a survivor being present.

For use in the sterilization of liquids the F and Fo values are of importance. The F value is the time required to inactivate an exposed microbial population at a specified temperature while the Fo value is the time to destroy a specified number of microorganisms. Both expressions derive from calculations of the Z value which represents the number of degrees increase in temperature needed to effect a 1-log increase in kill with no increase in exposure time.

Methods of Sterilization—

Moist Heat—Sterilization by saturated steam under pressure is the most practical and dependable method for the sterilization of medicaments. All known microorganisms are rapidly destroyed by this method.

Factors Affecting Sterilization—The general factors influencing the resistance of microorganisms to inactivation by steam include their chemical composition, genetic character and previous cultural history, the time and temperature of exposure, and the environment in which the organisms will be placed following thermal processing.

Various organic substances (e.g., peptone and albumin) increase the thermal resistance of microorganisms. Acid or alkaline solutions generally decrease the resistance of bacteria to moist heat destruction. Various cations (e.g., calcium and magnesium) and anions (e.g., phosphate) affect the thermal resistance of spores. For materials such as metals, plastics, rubber, cloth, and paper, the amount of moisture (steam) actually permeating to the microbial cell determines the rate of "die-off."

The exposure temperature and the total number of contaminants regulate the length of the sterilization cycle. Rather than measuring the actual D values of the most resistant microbial population contaminating the material, contamination with a heat-resistant bacterial spore former can be assumed. In this instance judgment is necessary because the heat resistance of bacterial spores varies considerably. As an example, in phosphate buffer at 250°F, spores of *Bacillus stearothermophilus* and *Clostridium sporogenes*

have D values of 3.0 and 1.3 min, respectively. If the total microorganisms contaminating a load is approximately 10^6 and if it is assumed that the heat resistance is equivalent to *C. sporogenes,* the rationale illustrated in Fig. 9 can be used to establish the time needed to sterilize with moist heat at 250°F. For a probability of a survivor being no greater than one chance in 10,000 the time is 13 min (10 × 1.3 min). If the D value for *B. stearothermophilis* spores is used, the time is 30 min (10 × 3 min).

Applications and Equipment—Moist heat is the most efficient and economical way to sterilize medical supplies. With solutions, heat transfer is by conduction and convection, and is usually much faster than the penetration of steam into nonliquid items. The factors that pose the greatest deterrent to steam sterilization are: difficult moisture penetration, poor air removal and entrainment, superheating, heat and moisture damage, and severe wetting of fabrics.

The basic apparatus is a jacketed chamber that is filled with saturated steam and held at a specific temperature and pressure for a stated time. The steam sterilizer used most commonly is the downward gravity displacement type. It takes advantage of the higher density of air relative to steam in displacing the air from a chamber through a drain at the bottom. This type generally has a lower initial cost as compared to sterilizers with automatic controls. The disadvantages of downward displacement chambers are: (1) the time required to remove air and to heat the load, (2) the time needed to dry the load after processing if an exhaust and vacuum drying portion of the cycle is not included, and (3) the time and care needed for proper loading and operation.

The high vacuum sterilizer is one in which the air is rapidly withdrawn by a vacuum to 15 mm Hg (absolute pressure) before the introduction of steam. This phase of the cycle makes it possible to remove air effectively from a porous load, thereby enhancing the subsequent penetration of steam. In turn, this significantly shortens the overall sterilization cycle. The practical advantage in the hospital is that one vacuum sterilizer can process 2–3 loads in the time one conventional sterilizer can process one load.

Another operational modification consists of the intentional introduction of air or some other gas into the chamber along with the steam to generate an overpressure to prevent bursting of packages, such as plastic LVP bags.

Monitoring Procedures—Sterilization with steam is so much more efficient than the other processes that routine product sterility tests should detect significant breakdowns in sterilization processes. The use of biological indicators to meet the sterility requirements for a sterilized product was formally introduced in USP XVIII. The organism most frequently used as a biological monitor for steam sterilization cycles is *B. stearothermophilus.* It is recommended that biological indicators or inoculated specimens of product carry at least 10^4 spores/item.

Table 7—*D* Values for Sterilization by Hot Air[a]

Temperature (°C)	D Value (Hours)
105	19
110	12
115	7
120	4.5
125	2.7
130	1.7
135	1.0
140	0.62
145	0.38
150	0.23 (13.8 min)
155	0.14 (8.4 min)
160	0.087 (5.2 min)

[a] Data taken from Ref. 10; these values represent the resistance of dry (washed) spores of *B. subtilis* var *niger* trapped in dental plastics. The resistance of these spores dried on paper or glass would be approximately 50% of these values.

Dry Heat—Although hospital and medical microbiologists routinely use dry heat to sterilize hospital and surgical supplies, little fundamental knowledge was available until the recent interest in dry heat for spacecraft sterilization.

Factors Affecting Sterilization—Hot air and gases, dry heat in a vacuum, superheated steam, and infrared lamps cannot be considered as equivalent sources for dry-heat sterilization. Recent research has demonstrated that the activity of water of microorganisms is a critical parameter in their destruction by dry heat. Dry-heat sterilization can require a range of conditions depending upon the moisture content of the microorganisms, since this affects their thermal resistivity, and the chemical and physical composition of the materials containing the microorganisms.

Considering these factors, it is obviously difficult to specify time-temperature relationships for dry-heat sterilization. To establish a dry-heat cycle it is best to make determinations of *D* values using a model of the dry-heat sterilization procedure and equipment that will be used in the processing of the materials. If this is not possible one should assume a worst case situation and use the *D* values presented in Table 7.

The calculation of a processing cycle for dry heat using *D* values is analogous to that presented in the section on moist heat. However, allowance must be made in the calculations for "come-up" and "cool-down" time. In any heat-processing cycle the integration of the kill occurring during come-up and cool-down time can significantly reduce total processing time.

Applications and Equipment—Dry heat can be used with those materials not compatible with steam or in instances where steam cannot reach the microbial contaminants. Dry-heat sterilization is used for many glass and metal objects, powders, and ointments. With fatty or oily substances, it is the method of choice.

There are two types of hot-air sterilizers: the *gravity convection type* in which cool air moves in a downward direction, is heated, and moves upward to establish a convection current, and the *mechanical convection type* which is fitted with a fan which assists in air circulation and heat transfer by convection. The gravity convection sterilizer is slower and less efficient. A longer period of time is needed to reach sterilization temperature, and there is more likely to be temperature variations due to air stratification. The increased cost of the mechanical convection sterilizer is usually justified because of the more rapid heating and better control over temperature. Sterilization by dry heat is slower and requires higher temperatures than does moist heat. Its principal advantages are its penetrating power and lack of corrosiveness.

Monitoring Procedures—Obviously there should be careful control over the temperature and exposure time for sterilization cycles and records should be maintained. Whenever possible biological indicators prepared from spores of *B. subtilis* var *niger* should be used to monitor the procedure.

Ethylene Oxide—Ethylene oxide (ETO) is a cyclic ether with a flashpoint of less than −29°C and a boiling point of 10.4°C. The explosive limits for ETO in air are from 3.6–100% by volume. The explosion hazard can be reduced by mixing it with such gases as CO_2 or dichlorodifluoromethane (fluorocarbon-12). When CO_2 is used, safety is achieved at considerable reduction of ETO concentrations for a given gas pressure since about 90% (by weight) of this mixture is CO_2. This loss of potency is less with fluorocarbon mixtures (12% ETO by weight) because the concentration of gaseous ETO in these mixtures at 1 atm of pressure is almost three times that in CO_2 mixtures. ETO is a toxic gas, and the industrial hygiene standard for ETO vapor is 59 ppm for an 8-hour exposure.

Factors Affecting Sterilization—Sterilization with ETO depends on the temperature, relative humidity, gas concentration, and time of exposure as well as the physical and chemical nature of the environment in which the microbial contaminants are located, and the number and species of microorganisms in the environment. When these factors are properly controlled, ETO is capable of the inactivation of all organisms against which it has been tested, including viruses. Microbial destruction occurs primarily through the alkylation of tertiary nitrogen groups and phosphoric acid esters of nucleic acid moieties.

The optimal relative humidity range for ETO sterilization is 30–60%. When microorganisms in large loads of materials have not been extensively prehumidified at the same RH which will be used in the sterilizer, the dynamic exchange of water is primarily toward microbial sites and increases proportionately with the difference in RH. Thus, more ETO is carried by the water molecules into the cells as the RH increases. Prehumidification is recommended for industrial loads with additional moisture being added during the cycle. Microorganisms which have been highly desiccated (chemicals or high vacuum) or are highly contaminated with organic materials acquire a resistance to ETO which is not completely overcome until they are essentially saturated with moisture. This then enables the ETO to permeate the cell and alkylate labile nucleophilic groups in nucleic acids and proteins.

Applications and Equipment—ETO is capable of sterilizing a wide variety of materials including ophthalmic and surgical instruments, bedding, blankets and pillows, surgical gloves, plastic syringes and disposable needles, inhalation equipment, electrical equipment, catheters, heart-lung oxygenators, and kidney dialysis units.. Plastic materials processed with ETO can absorb small quantities of this gas and by-products such as diethylene glycols and ethylene chlorohydrin can be formed. For this reason adequate aeration must be provided for processed materials to remove absorbed ETO.

The following aeration times are suggested:

1. Glass, paper, and thin rubber articles—24 hours at room temperature.
2. Gum rubber (thicker than ¼ in.) and polyethylene articles—48 hours at room temperature.
3. All other articles except PVC—96 hours at room temperature.
4. PVC items—7 days at room temperature.
5. Aerate any of the above at 50°C in a properly designed aerator for 12 hours or follow manufacturer's recommendations.

The successful use of ETO is associated with the ability of the gas to pass through plastic films and articles. Therefore, care must be exercised to select packaging or wrapping materials capable of transmitting ETO gas and water vapor. Polyethylene film readily transmits ETO, whereas most cellulose films, polyvinyl alcohol, and polyester films do not. Saran and Nylon films are very resistant to permeation by ETO.

Most commercial and medical uses of ETO employ sterilizer chambers with controls that automatically control pressure, temperature and other parameters. It is most important that a chamber with such controls be used and that the manufacturers recommended procedures for sterilization be followed carefully. Systems that employ prehumidification and the introduction of ETO gas heated through a heat exchanger have the highest probability of yielding successful results.

Monitoring Procedures—A successful ETO cycle requires the proper integration of gas concentration, temperature, relative humidity and time of exposure. Most modern ETO sterilizers are equipped with various forms of physical sensors to monitor many of these parameters. In addition, a number of color-change chemical indicators exist for ETO. These, however, are only qualitative and are not sufficient to indicate that sterilization has been achieved. The use of biological indicators provides the best method of certifying sterility because they test the interaction of all cycle variables. The biological indicators most widely used for ETO cycles contain spores of *B. subtilis* var *niger*. The indicator strips should have a minimum of 10^5 to 10^6 spores/unit.

Liquid Chemicals—Chemical solutions are widely used in hospitals and in industry to destroy, control or inhibit the growth of microorganisms. For the purpose of this discussion it should be emphasized that chemical solutions qualify as *sterilants* only in special, well-controlled situations although their ability to disinfect and control microbial growth is of enormous value. Also the corrosive, toxic or unstable nature of many solutions limits their usefulness in practical situations.

Among the chemicals considered for use as liquid sterilants are glutaraldehyde (2% in an alkaline buffer), formaldehyde (2–8% in methanol or 2-propanol), peracetic acid (1–3% in water), and ethylene oxide (0.5–2% in water and ethyl alcohol).

Other chemicals such as iodophors and hypochlorites can also sterilize materials under certain controlled conditions. A host of other chemicals have been used as germicides, disinfectants, and preservatives.

Factors Affecting Sterilization—The mechanical structure of devices is an important factor in regulating the effectiveness of liquid chemicals. Crevices and joints are penetrated with difficulty by the liquids and require long exposure times. Organic contamination on an item can react with the liquid and limit the concentration available for microbial destruction. If organisms are imbedded in materials, they may never be contacted by the chemical. Proper cleaning is necessary to reduce the number of contaminating organisms prior to immersion of items to be treated.

Effective use of liquid chemicals depends on the concentration and temperature of the chemical solution, the inactivation rate of the solutions by the objects being treated, and the types and numbers of bacterial contaminants. The length of time that an effective concentration of the chemical can be maintained must be known if repeated successful sterilization is to be achieved.

Monitoring Procedures—The proof that a liquid chemical is effective can be determined by tests in which instruments are contaminated with a known number of organisms, exposed to the solution and then tested for sterility. However, a better test is that required by the US Environmental Protection Agency for the registration of sterilant chemicals. These sporicidal procedures have been sanctioned by the Association of Official Analytical Chemists (AOAC) and are available in their book of official methods.

Liquid sterilants have been used to a limited degree with liquid drug products or with items such as sutures that can be immersed and held in the solution. Sterilization under these conditions is a terminal process, and the use of biological indicators is encouraged to confirm sterility.

Ultraviolet Radiation—

Factors Affecting Sterilization—The ultraviolet (UV) spectrum includes electromagnetic waves with wavelengths ranging from about 100–400 nm. The germicidal range is from 240–280 nm with maximum activity at about 260 nm. The fundamental germicidal reaction is thought to be regulated by photochemical excitations and appears to exhibit exponential kinetics. The inactivation process probably is a "one-hit process" in that only one photon has to hit the crucial target within the organism.

Because so many environmental factors limit the effectiveness of UV it has only minor application as a sterilizing agent. The practical ability of UV to destroy microorganisms is determined by the extent of its penetration into the organism. Any protective coating around the cell, such as a spore wall, acts as a barrier. Other factors that affect UV radiation include shielding by dust particles, the type of surface holding the microorganisms, the cell concentration, the layering of one cell upon another, the extent of pigmentation in the cells (particularly for fungal spores), and the relative humidity of the environment.

Applications and Equipment—In spite of its limitations, UV radiation can act rapidly against both spores and vegetative cells under proper conditions. Irradiation of clean solid materials can result in a substantial reduction of microorganisms on surfaces. In industrial applications UV radiation has been used for the surface treatment of food products, packaging materials, processing areas, and the destruction of air-borne organisms. The irradiation of water is generally practiced only to a small degree because of the limited penetration. Solutions containing proteins are difficult, if not impossible, to sterilize with UV radiation.

In hospitals UV radiation has been used to control the transfer of infection during and after surgical operations. The germicidal effect is dependent on the types of organisms present and the radiation dose absorbed. Under proper conditions and with good air circulation the airborne bacterial contamination level of a room can be reduced by 90% within 30 min. UV radiation has also been used to keep instruments sterile and to disinfect tables, walls, floors and other surfaces in hospitals, pharmacies, and various laboratories. However, the intensity of the radiation falls off inversely as the square of the distance from the lamp and proper intensities must be present for significant reductions of microorganisms to occur.

The most common artificial source of UV radiation is the low-pressure mercury vapor lamp. Most of the radiation (95%) from this lamp is emitted as the 253.7 nm resonance line of mercury.

Ionizing Radiation—Although radiation sterilization, other than UV radiation, is almost never used by the dispensing pharmacist, a brief discussion is included to illustrate a method used extensively by industrial firms in the sterilization of medical products.

Radiation sterilization may employ either electromagnetic radiation (photons, gamma, or x-radiation) or particulate radiation (beta particles or high-energy electrons). The interaction of charged particles with matter causes both ionizations and excitations. Ionization of matter results in the for-

mation of ion pairs, comprised of ejected orbital electrons (negatively charged) and their counterpart ions (positively charged). Charged particles such as electrons interact directly with matter causing ionization whereas electromagnetic radiation causes ionization through various mechanisms that result in the ejection of an orbital electron with a specific amount of energy transferred from the incident gamma ray. These ejected electrons then behave similarly to beta particles in ionization reactions. Thus, both corpuscular and electromagnetic radiation (i.e., high-energy gamma and x-rays) are considered as ionizing radiation and differ from UV radiation in this respect.

One theory of the mechanism by which high-energy radiation affects microorganisms is that orbital electrons are dislodged and reunited with ionized molecules to form unstable chemical intermediates. In the radiolysis of water the reactive free radicals can combine to form hydrogen peroxide, resulting in damage to the cell. Another theory involves the direct action of a vital structure of the cell, such as the chromosomal nucleoprotein. Probably a combination of both effects is present, causing complete and irreversible inactivation of microorganisms.

The penetrability of matter by ionizing radiation is a function of the type, energy and the density of the irradiated material. Beta particles have significantly shorter mean ranges than gamma rays of equivalent energy; i.e., a 1-Mev gamma ray has a range more than 80 times as great as a 1-Mev electron in water. Important parameters for radiation sterilization include absorbed dose, the energy level of the radiation and the power output available.

In radiation exposure, the "rad" is widely used in expressing dose; it is defined as the absorption of 100 ergs/gm of energy, independent of the nature of the irradiated substance. Sterilization doses, for convenience, are usually expressed in megarads.

Vegetative bacteria are the most sensitive to radiation inactivation, followed by molds, yeasts, spore formers, and viruses in that order. It is generally agreed that under most conditions a radiation dose of about 2.5 megarads is sufficient to kill the most resistant microorganisms with an adequate safety factor.

The source of gamma rays is radioisotopes such as cobalt-60 and cesium-137. Industrial sterilization facilities generally utilize cobalt-60 and are designed to hold up to 2,000,000 curies of radioactive material.

Electron accelerators may be of the electrostatic type such as the van de Graaff accelerator in which negative electricity is carried by a continuous belt to a hollow dome where the electrons are removed and accumulated. The electrons are then discharged through a vacuum column where they are accelerated by magnetic fields. The electron beam is then spread over a conveyor carrying the product. In the linear accelerator, electrons are emitted from a cathode source at the top of the column and accelerated by means of microwaves traveling down the accelerator tube.

Ionizing radiation has been used for the sterilization of vitamins, antibiotics, steroids, hormones, bone and tissue transplants, and medical devices such as plastic syringes, needles, surgical blades, plastic tubing, catheters, prostheses, Petri dishes, and sutures. Although there is no doubt of the effectiveness of this process, the cost and size of the installation makes it practical only for high volumes of materials such as processed by industrial firms.

Filtration—Filtration of liquids through bacterial retentive filters is widely used in the pharmaceutical industry where it is an acceptable means of sterilizing thermolabile solutions. This method of sterilization has been discussed previously in this chapter.

Packaging and Storage—An adequate sterilization process can be invalidated by inadequate packaging. If the sterile item is to be stored before use, the packaging must protect the material from deterioration and maintain sterility. The objective of proper packaging is to provide safe and effective medical supplies to the consumer.

Packaging materials generally include cloth, paper, plastic, and glass. Industrial firms frequently use a "surgical" grade paper (controlled porosity) and plastic films for packaging sterile items because these appear best for maximum maintenance of sterility at the lowest cost to the customer. Industrial packages have been shown to maintain sterility for at least 10 years under adequate storage conditions. Hospitals often use two thicknesses of muslin as a dust filter and protective wrapper for surgical supplies, towels, sheets, and laboratory packs. Materials wrapped with muslin should remain sterile in clean storage for approximately 2 weeks, after which resterilization should be considered. Occasionally, experience and laboratory data show sterility is maintained for longer periods.

Parchment papers, especially developed for use in steam and ethylene oxide sterilization are used because they are economical and are effective wrapping materials. If it is dry, such paper provides adequate protection, good transmission of vapors, and a reasonable shelf-life.

The use of special papers and plastics for packaging by industry was initially associated with nonheat sterilization processes. However, today plastic-coated papers and plastic films and containers are available that can be steam sterilized.

It is necessary to conduct stability studies on each particular sterilized drug-package combination to assure that the drugs maintain their identity and that they are not subject to deterioration. The testing must insure that leaching of toxic components does not occur during sterilization and storage of the drug. The storage stability characteristics of the plastic container must be evaluated with time to show that the passage of oxygen, carbon dioxide, and other gases through the plastic is not sufficient to cause stability problems. Furthermore, it is necessary to determine that sterilization does not increase the sorption of drug ingredients by the plastic container.

The storage conditions in the hospital for packaged sterile materials is obviously related to the maintenance of sterility. The cardinal rules are use of a clean, dry, ventilated area with even temperature and limited access; proper shelving for storage to achieve the above and keep stock off the floor; and proper inventory records and rotation of stock on a first-in-first-out (FIFO) basis. Cartons of sterile packaged goods purchased from manufacturers should be stored in the shipping containers, if practical, and marked for date of receipt to assure adherence to the FIFO principle.

Following sterilization, the product is either placed in quarantine, while testing is being performed, or passed directly into the packaging department and then into quarantine. In the packaging department labels are affixed to the containers which are then placed in cartons for distribution. A product may not be released from quarantine until all tests have been performed to insure that it meets the required quality specifications.

Labeling

At the time of packaging, the lot number assigned at the beginning of the process is applied to the label. This identifies the product lot and is the key to a disclosure of the complete history of the individual product unit.

Therapeutic agents intended for parenteral administration must be prepared under conditions which assure the highest quality standards technically achievable under accepted good manufacturing practices.[4] Only when such a goal has been achieved is it possible to be confident that the product is safe for clinical use in human patients.

Quality Control

As the name implies, quality control is the sum of all tests and procedures that are utilized throughout the entire history of a product to give assurance that the final product meets the standards desired. For parenterals this quality must exceed that of most if not all other pharmaceutical preparations.

In general, quality control may be divided into three areas:

Raw materials control—the evaluation of the components of the product.

In-process control—the tests and procedures used during the process to be assured that the specifications are being met.

Product control—the tests and assays performed on the finished product to give assurance that it meets the established specifications.

The individual responsible for quality-control decisions should be committed to the principle that a product may not be released for use unless it has met the established specifications. He must also be an individual distinct from the one responsible for meeting production goals.

Space here does not permit a thorough analysis of quality-control procedures, but only of ones which are particularly pertinent to sterile preparations. It should be realized that no amount of dosage form testing can assure product quality unless in-process and raw material controls have been practiced. Prod-

uct quality must be built into the product from the beginning of its production history.

Sterility Testing

The objective of sterility testing must be clearly understood. The test is not designed to *prove* that a product is sterile but to provide an estimate of the probable sterility of a lot of articles. The degree of contamination may be of such a low order of magnitude that it is not detected by the test. Therefore, confidence in the results from the sterility test must be based upon the knowledge that the lot has been subjected to a sterilization procedure of proven effectiveness.

The results of sterility tests must be made a part of the product record. However, to confirm the validity of the test results there also must be evidence that the culture medium was sterile, that it supports the growth of microorganisms, and that the personnel are qualified to carry out the test properly.

Two sterility test procedures have official status in the USP, the direct inoculation method and the membrane filtration method. In the direct method, an inoculum of the product is placed in culture tubes containing a measured volume of fluid thioglycollate (FTM) or soybean casein digest (SCD) medium. The tubes of FTM are incubated at 30–35°C and the SCD medium at 20–25°C for a period of 14 days, unless otherwise indicated. If the nature of the product or the sterilization procedure used is conducive to producing slow-growing organisms, a longer incubation period may be required. Positive and negative control tubes must be incubated concurrently to confirm the sterility and growth promoting properties of the medium. If a product has inherent antibacterial activity this must be neutralized or eliminated by dilution. The article or sample passes the sterility test if no growth is observed.

The membrane filtration technique is required for sterility testing of large volume infusions and may be used for other products. The sample is filtered through a bacterial retentive membrane filter, using a closed system in a controlled environment to minimize the risk of inadvertent contamination. The membrane filter is aseptically removed from the assembly, one half is placed in FTM, and the other half in SCD medium. Only 7 days of incubation is required, at 30–35°C and 20–25°C, respectively, for the samples from this method.

The principal disadvantage of the filtration method when compared with the direct method is an increased risk of inadvertent contamination from the environment. With adequate environmental control and a qualified analyst, this risk can be minimized. The advantages of this method include reduction in the amount of culture medium consumed, use of larger and pooled samples, and the opportunity to remove interfering substances, such as antibacterial agents and oils, from contact with the organisms thereby permitting them to grow in the culture medium. If no growth appears the sample passes the sterility test.

Sampling for both test procedures is critical, for the samples must be representative of the entire batch. The USP requires that 20 samples be tested from a batch subjected to a reliable method of sterilization, unless otherwise indicated, although as few as 10 and as many as 30 samples are required in certain instances. The samples must be selected on a planned basis from various areas in an autoclave load and from the beginning, the end and at planned intervals throughout an aseptic fill process. A similar representative selection must be used for other methods of sterilization.

Pyrogens

Pyrogenic substances are the products of metabolism of microorganisms. Chemically they are lipid in nature and are usually attached to a polysaccharide or an amino acid carrier. All microorganisms apparently produce pyrogenic substances, but there is variation in potency. The gram negative bacilli generally produce the most potent pyrogens.

In man, pyrogens produce chills and fever with headache and pain in the back and legs. They do not produce a true immunological effect but a temporary resistance. It is believed that pyrogens act on the temperature control center in the hypothalmus. Not all animals respond physiologically to pyrogens in the same way. Rabbits have a fever response closest to that in man, with a peak within 3 hours after injection.

Pyrogens, such as those produced in the fermentation process for the production of antibiotics, are inherently present in many pharmaceutical preparations. From such preparations pyrogens must be effectively removed. For most pharmaceutical preparations pyrogens should be prevented from entering the product. Pyrogens may be present wherever microorganisms have grown or are growing. Solvents such as water are one of the major sources, but water can be rendered free from pyrogens by effective distillation. Containers and equipment are another source of pyrogens although washing and final rinsing with pyrogen-free water markedly reduces the pyrogen content. A pyrogen-free container can be assured by hot air sterilization at 175°C for 3–4 hours, or the equivalent. Medicinal substances and other solutes may be a source of pyrogens if they have not been properly purified. In addition, improper storage of solutes may sometimes permit microbiological contamination and the subsequent formation of pyrogens.

Although pyrogens can be destroyed by heat, the heat of a normal autoclave cycle is not sufficient. Moderate heating in the presence of an acid, alkali or oxidizing agent is necessary to destroy pyrogens. One or a combination of these methods are often used to destroy the pyrogen produced during antibiotic fermentations. Pyrogens can also be adsorbed on substances such as charcoal, aluminum hydroxide gel, or asbestos fibers of a filter pad. The mechanism of adsorption often cannot be used for pharmaceutical preparations, since the medicinal substance or other solutes may also be adsorbed.

Pyrogen Testing—Testing for the presence of pyrogens is usually done by the fever response in rabbits. The USP test has been used with little modification for many years. The sample to be tested is injected into the marginal ear vein of the rabbit and the rectal temperature of the animal is taken during 3 hours. An elevation of more than 0.6°C in temperature above normal is the basis for failure to pass the test. The details of the test are given in the USP. However, it should be pointed out that the rabbit is very sensitive to outside stimuli. Therefore, exceptional care must be taken in the handling and housing of the animals, if the test is to give reproducible results.

A pyrogen which gives just a positive response in rabbits normally produces mild fever and chills in man. Therefore, the test is biologically valid. Pyrogenic reactions are rarely fatal in man. In fact, pyrogens are used in fever therapy. However, their presence in a pharmaceutical product is contraindicated because such presence is due to failure to maintain proper manufacturing control.

A simple method for the detection of pyrogen has recently been developed, known as the Limulus Test.[11] A test sample is incubated with the lysate of the blood of the horseshoe crab (*Limulus polyphemus*). A gel is formed if pyrogen is present. While not recognized by the compendia as yet, it is receiving wide study and use as an in-process control test.

Leakers

Containers for injections must be hermetically sealed in order to maintain the integrity of the product. It is obvious that if contents can escape, contamination can enter. The testing for a leaking container is relatively simply performed on an all-glass ampul. The usual procedure is to immerse the ampul in a water-soluble dye, such as 1% methylene blue solution, and then evacuate the chamber. If the container is not hermetically sealed, when the vacuum is released the dye is pulled into the container. After careful washing of the outside, the dye can be seen within.

This method does not lend itself to rubber stoppered containers because of the flexibility of the rubber. Bottles that have been sealed under vacuum can be tested by the sharp click of the "water hammer effect" when an evacuated bottle is struck with a rubber mallet or with the heal of the hand. In general, to seal containers with rubber closures, reliance is placed upon the elasticity of the rubber fitting snugly against the side of the opening of the container, without the use of a leaker test.

Particulate Matter and Its Evaluation

Particulate matter in injections has long been considered of significance primarily because it conveys to the user that the product is inferior—that it is not clean. However, more recently, during the 1960's, studies showed that emboli in the capillaries of vital organs can be caused by proliferation of cells around foreign particles such as lint, rubber, or chemicals.[12] Still more recent studies have shown that the incidence of phlebitis is reduced when IV infusions are filtered as they are injected into the patient, suggesting a relationship between this complication and particles.[13] Therefore, the significance of particulate matter has assumed a much more serious complexion. The level of contamination and the size of particles that may be considered to be toxic have not been established. However, the USP has established a limit of 50 particles of 10 μm and larger per ml for large-volume infusions.

Particulate matter may arise from the environment, including shedding from ceilings, walls, floors, and furniture, and from the body and garments of personnel; from containers, including

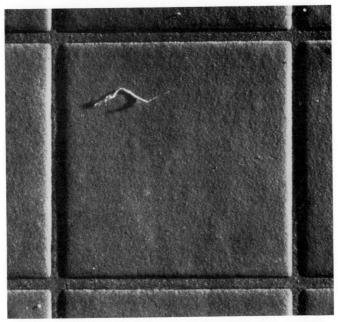

Fig. 10—Particles removed by membrane filtration from a parenteral solution, magnified 100X (courtesy, *Millipore Corp.*).

particles from glass, plastics, or rubber; and from processing, including deposits from unclean rinse water or as particles of metal, paint or other material from operating equipment. Particles from these sources may find their way into the parenteral product. See Fig. 10. Also, particles may be present in administration sets if these are not adequately cleaned and sealed during manufacture. Finally, particles may be introduced at the time of administration.

Before corrective measures can be taken to eliminate particles in a product, it is necessary to trace their source. Once the source has been identified, appropriate corrective measures can be taken.

A process technique which aids in the elimination of particulate matter from solutions is filtration of the solution at the last possible moment, that is, just before it enters the final container.

Methods of Evaluation—Human visual inspection with the aid of good direct lighting on the container of product against a black and a white background has been, and continues to be, the basic and traditional method of inspection. Visual limitations under such conditions are probably particles of about 40 to 50 μm in diameter. Visual inspection is subject to human limitations, including psychological effects, visual acuity, fatigue and environmental distractions. The advantage of visual inspection is that it is comparable with the inspection given by the user just prior to use, and all units of the product can be inspected in their final intact container.

A number of other methods of inspection have been developed, but most of these require the opening of the container, which may introduce particulate matter. One of the most widely used methods is that of collecting the particles on a membrane filter and examining them microscopically, as shown in Fig. 3. With this method it is not only possible to obtain a count of particles and to classify them according to size, but a preliminary identification may be rendered. However, this method is very time consuming. It is not suitable for process line evaluation, but can play an important role in the development of quality control procedures.

Certain instrumental methods have also been developed and are quite widely used.

These instruments detect particles in a sample by light reflected from their surfaces, by the shadow cast by the particle, or the alteration of resistance by a particle in an electrolyte solution. These instrumental methods require the development of skill by the analyst in handling the sample, even then reproducibility of results is often difficult to achieve.

The use of a video camera and viewer has shown some improvement over human visual inspection because of some magnification and a sharpening of the visual image of the particles. A challenge still exists, however, to the technologists in the field to find ways of eliminating particles from solutions and developing methods of evaluation which effectively determine whether or not a solution is clean.

Analytical Procedures

The assays designed to determine qualitatively and quantitatively the existence and purity of components in a parenteral preparation are as important or more so for parenteral preparations than for other dosage forms. As is well known, assays must be performed on raw materials to determine the purity of the compound and the possible existence of contaminating substances. It is often desirable and necessary to perform assays on bulk solutions in process to be sure that when distribution into final containers is performed the product will meet the potency and quality specifications required. Adjustments may be made in the bulk preparation to bring the product within specifications, if necessary, a procedure which is impossible in the final container.

These analytical results add substantiation to assays performed on the final product. It is not possible normally to perform assays only on the final prod-

uct and thereby determine all that needs to be known about the potency, freedom from contamination, and general quality of the product. The treatment of this topic has been brief due to space limitations, but this should not in any way suggest a minimization of the importance of analytical control.

An aspect of quality control which needs special emphasis is that of record keeping. Every test performed, every step in the process, and every factor which has a bearing on the control exercised to maintain assurance of quality should be made a written record. Each such record should be authenticated by the signature of the individual responsible. Only when a real sense of responsibility for the quality of the final product is recognized and fulfilled by each person involved in the process can there be real assurance that the product has met the quality specifications intended.

References

1. Shapiro S, Slone D, Lewis G, Jick H: *JAMA 216:*467, 1971.

2. Thur M, Latiolais C, Miller W: *Am J Hosp Pharm 29:*298, 1972.

3. Accreditation Manual for Hospitals, Joint Commission on Accreditation of Hospitals, Chicago, 1970.

4. *Drugs: Current Good Manufacturing Practice in Manufacturing, Processing, Packing, or Holding.* Part 133, Title 21. *Federal Register 34:* 13553, Aug. 22, 1969 (FR Doc 69–9980); 36:601–605, Jan. 15, 1971 (FR Doc 71–638).

5. Ravin R, *et al: Am J Hosp Pharm 31:*340, 1974.

6. Greenleaf JC, Hadgraft JW: *Chem Drug 173:*41, 1960.

7. *Clean Room and Work Station Requirements, Controlled Environment.* Washington, DC, Federal Standard No. 209B General Services Administration, 1973.

8. Brewer JH: Sterility tests and methods for assuring sterility. In Reddish GF: *Antiseptics, Disinfectants, Fungicides, and Sterilization,* Lea & Febiger, Philadelphia, 158–174, 1957.

9. Chick H: *J Hyg 10:*237, 1910.

10. Bruch CW: Spacecraft sterilization. In Lawrence CA, Block SS: *Disinfection, Sterilization, and Preservation,* Lea & Febiger, Philadelphia, 686–702, 1968.

11. Cooper J: *Bull Parenteral Drug Assoc 29:* 122, 1975.

12. Garvan J, Gunner B: *Med J Austral 2:*1, July 4, 1964.

13. DeLuca P, Rapp R, Bivins B, McKean E, Griffen W: *Am J Hosp Pharm 32:*1001, 1975.

Bibliography

National Coordinating Committee on Large Volume Parenterals. *Am J Hosp Pharm 32:*261, 1975.

Training Manual for Centralized Intravenous Admixture Personnel, Travenol Labs, Morton Grove, IL, 1972.

Martin E: *Techniques of Medication,* Lippincott, Philadelphia, 1969.

Trissel L, Grimes C, Gallelli J: *Parenteral Drug Information Guide,* Am. Soc. Hosp. Pharm. Washington, DC, 1974.

White P, Nagy M: *Total Parenteral Nutrition,* Publ. Sci. Group, Inc., Acton, MA, 1974.

Avis K: Parenteral preparations. In *Remington's Pharmaceutical Sciences,* 15th ed, Mack Publ. Co., Easton, PA, 1461–1487, 1975.

Avis K: In *The Theory and Practice of Industrial Pharmacy,* Lea & Febiger, Philadelphia, 563–604, 1970.

Turco S, King R: *Sterile Dosage Forms,* Lea & Febiger, Philadelphia, 1974.

Laboratory Manual for Food Canners and Processors, vol 1, AVI Publ. Co., Westport, CT, 1968.

Lawrence C, Block S, eds: *Disinfection, Sterilization, and Preservation,* Lea & Febiger, Philadelphia, 1968.

Phillips G, Miller W, eds: *Industrial Sterilization,* Duke Univ. Press, Durham, NC, 1973.

Benarde M: *Disinfection,* Marcel Dekker, New York, 1970.

AOAC sporicidal test. In *Official Methods of Analysis of the AOAC,* 11th ed, Assoc. of Off. Anal. Chem., Washington, DC, 1970.

11

Aerosols

Harvey Mintzer, MS
Vice President, Technical
Sales and Services
Armstrong Laboratories
Division
Aerosol Techniques,
Incorporated
West Roxbury, MA 02132

The pharmaceutical aerosol, or auto-dispensing medicinal package, first established itself as a distinct dosage form during the 1950's. It has attracted interest due to its unique and complex technology and because of its high degree of acceptance by both prescriber and user. This interest has manifested itself in the rapid growth of units produced annually since the 1950's, with the figure about 78,000,000 in 1974.

This rate of growth, and the basis on which it is predicated to continue, is associated directly with the ability of the aerosol to provide a group of advantages not fully available from any other form of administration.

While other available dosage forms perform an individual function in a manner similar to the aerosol, none of them is capable of duplicating the combined efficiencies of the aerosol in specific instances:

1. Provides enhanced drug stability.
2. Affords protection of active ingredients.
3. Provides unequaled ease and speed of application (in most instances directly to the intended site and with generally better control over the amount applied) as well as superior characteristics of deposition.
4. Provides increased therapeutic efficiency of the medicaments involved.

If the aerosol form can continue to make such contributions, it will maintain an important role in medicine and pharmacy.

Aerosol products do not lend themselves to extemporaneous preparation by the pharmacist because of the need for specialized and complex handling techniques and packaging equipment.

However, as a member of the health profession responsible for proficiency in all dosage forms, the pharmacist is called upon to display knowledge in the art and science of aerosols. An understanding of the complexities of this class of products is important in properly advising the patient at the time of dispensing. At the same time he can be an important source of information for the prescriber in this relatively new and unique dosage form area.

The NF includes a section on aerosols in its discussion of pharmaceutical dosage forms, monographs of the three most commonly used fluorocarbon propellants, and monographs for seven specific active ingredients in aerosol form. This listing will undoubtedly expand as more drugs appear in aerosol form and become commonly accepted by medical practitioners.

The aerosol today is a pressurized, self-propelling product, powered by means of a liquefied or compressed gas. It is recognized in its varied commercial forms as a package whose contents are expelled through an opened valve by means of the internal pressure of the materials contained within. Only a vague similarity remains between this modern adaptation of the term, and its classical definition employed by the colloid chemist.

The early use of the generic term aerosol was coined to describe fine aerial suspensions of arsenical smokes developed toward the end of World War I. Originally intended to define a system of particles small enough to be stable, relative to sedimentation, when dispersed in air, the word aerosol is used today in this field to refer to almost any dispersion in air. The three broad groups of modern pressurized packages are described as follows:

1. *Space sprays,* which are finely divided sprays, exhibiting particle sizes ranging up to 50 μm in diameter. Important as aerial disinfectants, room deodorizers, and insecticides, this class of products attempts to produce a dispersion of droplets of particles which remain airborne for prolonged periods.

2. *Surface coatings,* which are also sprays, but are coarser in size, "wetter," and designed for continuous film formation on a surface. Examples of such products are the hair sprays, personal deodorants, and topical medicinals. Powder sprays must be listed within this group, not necessarily because of the particle size exhibited but because of the residual effect intended.

3. *Aerated foams,* which are produced by the rapid expansion of certain propellants "through" an emulsion, give rise to numerous small bubbles. Examples in this class include shaving cream, whipped toppings, and topical and vaginal products. Foamed products may vary from those which come forth fully formed at the actuator to those which are delivered as a stream and foam

upon reaching a surface. In addition, foams may be described as stable or quick-breaking depending upon the design of the formulation.

History—A historical review of the aerosol packaging principle as it is known today can be summarized as follows:

1862   Lynde (US Pat. 34,894) developed a valve (with dip tube) for dispensing aerated liquids from a bottle.

1899   Helbin and Pertsch (US Pat. 628,463) used methyl and ethyl chloride within a sealed container equipped with a dispensing orifice.

1901   Gebauer (US Pat. 668,815); and

1902   Gebauer (US Pat. 711,045) developed means of containing and administering volatile liquids.

1903   Moore (US Pat. 746,866) developed perfume atomizer using carbon dioxide propellant.

1921   Mobley (US Pat. 1,378,481) developed method for applying liquid antiseptics using carbon dioxide propellant.

1931   Reidel and deHaen (DR Pat. 557,259) developed perfume atomizer using methyl chloride propellant.

1931   Rotheim (US Pat. 1,800,156); and

1933   Rotheim (US Pat. 1,829,750) helped to shape much of the theory of modern aerosol principles.

1933   Midgley, Henne, and McNary (US Pat. 1,926,396) synthesized fluorocarbon gases and employed them as fire extinguishers and as refrigerants.

1935   Bichowsky (US Pat. 2,021,981) developed self-pressurized fire extinguishers.

1942   Goodhue and Sullivan adapted dichlorodifluoromethane to propel insecticide materials which formed the basis in 1943 (US Pat. 2,321,023) for World War II insecticide "bombs."

The successful use of insecticide "bombs" by the Armed Services groups during World War II paved the way for the development, during the late 1940's, of aerosol components and materials for civilians.

A series of rapid advancements were made in this area. The heavy-walled, bulky, steel container which was expensive and, therefore, used as a refillable unit gave way to the lighter-weight, thin-walled, and more attractive container which we know today as a disposable aerosol "can."

The first commercial aerosols were pharmaceutical proprietaries, packaged in glass and relying upon condensed and compressed gases for propellant force. For a time, during the surge of growth of the commercial aerosol during the late 1940's and early 1950's, cosmetic items and insecticides appearing in metal containers and using the liquefied fluorocarbons almost exclusively, were given the greatest emphasis. Now, great interest has again been exhibited in the pharmaceutical area. The growth of pharmaceutical aerosols accelerated phenomenally during the 1960's and this class of products has most certainly benefited from the general advances in formulation and packaging technology made by the aerosol industry during this period. This growth rate will likely continue as the pharmaceutical industry expands current basic technology.

The Aerosol Principle

The aerosol mechanism is based upon the relatively simple principle that a compressed or liquefied gas exerts a force upon the internal surfaces of the container in which it is enclosed. This force per unit area (pressure) is expressed in the aerosol industry exclusively in terms of pounds per square inch gauge (psig). The use of the term "gauge" is a practical measure which refers to the pressure beyond atmospheric pressure, which is approximately 15 psi absolute. Because almost all pressure determinations are made under atmospheric conditions, most gauges used in aerosol work are arranged to read zero at atmospheric pressure. All pressure values referred to in this chapter as well as all those appearing in the literature of the aerosol industry assume the psig designation.

The pressure of an aerosol system refers to the pressure being exerted by the vapor within the container. A liquefied gas in a sealed container appears within the container in two phases. One is the liquefied gas itself and the other is composed of the gas vapor which has volatilized from a part of the liquid and fills the space above the liquid. It is the pressure of the vapor in equilibrium with the liquid which exerts the force against the internal walls, the liquid,

and all accessory packaging components within the container. These latter parts generally are the underside of the valve which seals the container and the eduction tube or dip tube, if there is one, which serves as a conduit for the liquid phase, leading it to the valve opening. As the valve is opened, and the contents of the container have access to the atmosphere, they are propelled out of the container by the higher than atmospheric pressure within. The vapor pressure referred to may also be supplied by a noncondensable gas which has been compressed within the container. The effect of temperature on the pressure of a given aerosol system is significant and will be discussed in the later section on propellants (page 301).

Liquefied Gas Systems

A propellant which can reside in the aerosol container in its liquefied form has advantages over a compressed gas, one of the more important of which is providing more constant pressure throughout the life of the container's contents.

Solutions—The system which includes a liquefied propellant miscible with a solution of active ingredients describes a "soluble" or "two-phase" (liquefied gas solution and its vapor) system. This system, owing to its simplicity, has been used more than any other for commercial products.

Most often the active ingredients are not soluble in the liquefied propellant and require a cosolvent material to support this combination; ethanol and isopropyl alcohol have been used extensively for this purpose due to their wide solvent properties, low cost, miscibility with liquefied gases in all proportions, lack of extreme toxicity and irritation effects, and degree of volatility which is complemented in combination with the more volatile propellants.

Two-phase liquefied gas systems (Fig. 1) have found wide usage because of their ability to provide constant delivery pressure as previously mentioned and, perhaps of greater importance to

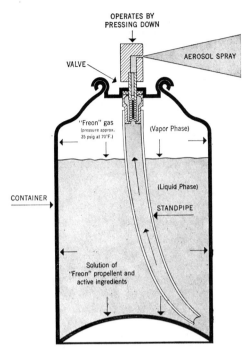

Fig. 1—Two-phase liquefied gas system.

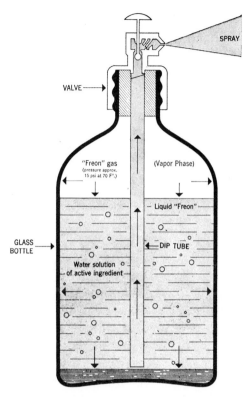

Fig. 2—Three-phase system with fluorocarbon propellant.

the formulator, because of their greater flexibility in providing desired effects upon release.

Products such as air sanitizers, space insecticides, room vaporizers, and locally acting inhalation products are designed to produce a droplet size distribution sufficiently small to remain airborne for prolonged periods.

The flexibility previously mentioned lies in the ability to vary the two-phase liquefied gas system to achieve the exact discharge properties desired. In addition, the constant pressure provision of liquefied gas solution systems has also lent much to consumer acceptance of aerosols. This property provides two benefits to the user. First, the spray characteristics designed by the formulator are maintained for the entire contents and secondly, the entire contents are available to the user with a much greater indwelling tolerance of misuse.

It may occur to the reader that mention has not been made of the universal solvent, water, in the discussion of the role of the cosolvent. This is because

the liquefied propellant gases currently used, almost without exception, are not miscible alone to any significant extent with this substance. Solubility of water in the fluorocarbons, for instance, is only a fraction of 1% by weight.

Water is considered not primarily for its low cost but because of its applicability as a vehicle as in the case of preparations imparted to sensitive areas such as mucous membranes and open wounds.

Despite the lack of miscibility with water alone, systems have been devised which include aqueous based solutions. These have been termed "three-phase" or "two-layer" and include as the name implies two immiscible liquid layers in addition to the vapor phase. This system is illustrated in Fig. 2 which shows the liquefied propellant layer below the aqueous layer. This system reacts during discharge very much the same as the soluble system, wherein constant pressure is maintained by the reservoir of liquefied gas. A very significant difference, however, involves the characteristics of the spray. Since the eduction tube, as pictured, is designed to reside in the aqueous phase, only this material is propelled from the container and it lacks the volatility to produce fine droplets. If a mechanical breakup configuration were not used as part of the spray adapter, the material issuing forth would take the form of a liquid stream.

Three-phase systems of this type have found little use among commercial products. Except for the opportunity for constant pressure, the use of a liquefied propellant as a piston is best replaced by a compressed gas as will be explained in a later section. The cost is lowered and the hazard of spraying liquefied propellant is eliminated and this more than offsets the absence of constant pressure dispensing.

Suspensions—When active substances resist solubilization in a propellant-cosolvent system, or more often, when it is desirable to dispense the active ingredients in discrete solid particle form, suspensions in liquefied propellant may be prepared. The suspended solids constitute a third physical phase and this combination is another type of "three-phase" system. The propellant mechanism is identical to that outlined for the two-phase solution system with its constant pressure and uniform spray characteristics.

Suspensions in liquefied propellants have been widely represented by pharmaceutical aerosols for topical and inhalation use. An apparent advantage of this system is that, at the option of the formulator, a powdered active ingredient may be finely deposited at the site, while the propellant vehicle evaporates upon release. To date, however, most powder aerosols have involved an auxiliary suspending agent or vehicle additive.

Emulsions—An additional system regarded as a three-phase system involves the incorporation of liquefied propellant in an emulsion.

The simplest emulsion system is represented by the aerosol shave creams that have become so popular.

Use of a high vapor pressure propellant or larger amounts of propellant yields stiff, dry foams whereas propellants with lower vapor pressure or smaller concentrations of propellant produce soft, wet foams. Other factors, including the type of emulsifier, the presence and nature of additives, especially those soluble in the propellant, and the type of valve and actuating device employed, all serve to affect the foam characteristics. While standard foam actuators are constructed to deliver an almost fully pre-expanded foam, the identical formulation actuated through a button with a mechanical breakup arrangement in the small orifice produces a finely dispersed stream which foams upon reaching a surface.

When water is antagonistic to active ingredient stability, the emulsion form can be retained by substituting various glycols for the water. In other instances, reduced stability of a foam has been achieved by addition of alcohol to the formulation. This produces a "quick-breaking" foam which collapses to a liquid pool soon after actuation. This latter effect has good potential for specific cosmetic and pharmaceutical applications.

Liquefied gases, when compared with nonliquefiable (or compressed) gases, have certain obvious disadvantages. These include a higher cost, more propellant material generally required, and greater change in pressure with temperature. The latter effects cause undesirable changes in the designed spray characteristics at wide temperature extremes, or far worse, can cause a container to be inoperable or to burst.

Compressed Gas Systems

Insoluble compressed gases serve as pistons to propel the contents of containers forward in totally unchanged form through large valve orifices or in subdivided form through restricted or "break-up" orifices. The gases which display some solubility in the product, (generally 1–3%) are capable of introducing some changes in the physical state of the product upon release from the container due to pressure, temperature, and viscosity changes.

Misuse of products with compressed gas propellants, in terms of tilting or shaking so as to allow the compressed vapor direct access to the valve orifice, results in greater acceleration of pressure drop or total loss of propellant power.

The insoluble compressed gases have found use in propelling products in stream form where physical change of the product is undesirable, as for cosmetic creams, ointments, vitamin syrups, and dental cream. In addition, where liquefied gases are felt to be contraindicated because they are incompatible with the product or potentially irritant to the site of deposition, the insoluble compressed gases have been useful. An interesting adaptation of compressed gas as propellant is the use of lowered dispensing pressure combined with a viscous solution and a restricted valve orifice to form a pressurized drop dispenser.

For spray products, a less coarse droplet distribution is available and for emulsions there is an opportunity for expansion to a foam which is impossible with insoluble compressed gases. Products which are used at temperatures which do not permit a liquefied gas system to function such as windshield deicers and whipped toppings have used partially soluble compressed gases to advantage. This has been possible because these systems do not react as radically to temperature changes as the liquefied gases. Until recently no liquefied propellants were suitable for edible products but the partially soluble compressed gases made possible the whipped toppings which have been available for several years. These also can be refrigerated to preserve the contents without undergoing drastic loss of dispensing pressure.

Propellants

There are very few aspects of aerosol design, packaging, and manufacture which do not, at least in part, depend on the propellant for their selection. The type and amount of propellant involves so many considerations that it is difficult to equate it in terms of importance to any other aerosol component.

A definition of the propellant in terms of its basic function hardly seems necessary, the term itself serving to imply its role. The aerosol industry, however, has officially evolved the following description: "A liquefied gas with a vapor pressure greater than atmospheric pressure at a temperature of 105°F."

Reed[1] has listed the following basic requirements of a propellant:

1. A vapor pressure in the range of about 15 to 100 psig at 70°F
2. A low order of toxicity
3. Chemical inertness
4. Nonflammability and nonexplosiveness
5. Freedom from odor and color
6. Good solvent power
7. Freedom from irritation
8. Practicable cost

While these describe an ideal material, the aerosol industry has progressed extremely well with a limited number of propellants, none of which fully comply with these properties. Those which come closest are the fluorocarbons and these have dominated the industry since their development.

The propellant materials which are currently used are as follows:

Fluorocarbons
  Methane series
    Trichloromonofluoromethane
    (Propellant 11)
    Dichlorodifluoromethane
    (Propellant 12)
    Monochlorodifluoromethane
    (Propellant 22)
  Ethane series
    Dichlorotetrafluoroethane
    (Propellants 114 and 114a)
    Monochlorodifluoroethane
    (Propellant 142b)
    Difluoroethane
    (Propellant 152a)
    Trichlorotrifluoroethane
    (Propellant 113)

Butane series
  Octafluorocyclobutane
    (Propellant C318)
Hydrocarbons
  Propane
  Isobutane
  Normal Butane
Compressed Gases
  Soluble
    Nitrous Oxide
    Carbon Dioxide
  Insoluble
    Nitrogen

A wide variety of other materials have been used to a limited extent as propellants, either alone or in combination with some of those listed previously. These include a group of chlorinated (nonfluorinated) compounds such as ethyl chloride, trichloroethane, methylene chloride, and vinyl chloride. In 1973, however, the Food and Drug Administration listed trichloroethane as a new drug when used in products intended for inhalation directly or indirectly. In addition, FDA directed in 1974 that vinyl chloride monomer no longer be used because of its potential health hazard via inhalation. An ether-type compound, dimethyl ether, has attracted interest because of its miscibility with large percentages of water and its vapor pressure of about 60 psig at 70°F. Although it is a liquefiable gas and as such would lend certain formulation flexibility, its flammability may limit its use.

Fluorocarbon Gases

This group of propellants has been used to the greatest extent in the aerosol products since the early 1950's. Their combined properties are most appropriate for pharmaceutical products, if they are judiciously selected and incorporated in the final formulation. Several of these fluorochloro-derivatives of methane, ethane, and butane have been made available. However, three in particular account for better than 90% of fluorocarbon consumption for aerosol products and are contained in probably 99% of pharmaceutical aerosols. These are propellants 11, 12, and 114. In this country, they are available from three major sources: Freons (*Du Pont*), Genetrons (*Allied*), and Ucons (*Union Carbide*). These were originally developed as refrigerants in the quest for materials less toxic than ammonia.

The choice of a propellant or a blend of propellants is based on consideration of the pressure required to achieve the product properties desired (i.e., particle size and rate of deposition): rate of spray, foam stability, compatibility with active ingredients, container and valve chosen (and regulatory limitations on pressure for that container), solvent ability of the blend, etc.

In 1974 it was reported that certain of the fluorocarbons could cause an abnormal depletion of ozone, a natural substance in the stratosphere, which acts to prevent most ultraviolet radiation from reaching the earth's surface. It has been theorized that these compounds are not removed from the lower atmosphere by natural means due to their chemical inertness, but are available to diffuse into the stratosphere where they decompose, releasing chlorine atoms. The theory continues that ozone is then destroyed by a series of catalytic chain reactions involving the released chlorine. This theory is based on hypothetical mathematical models only, and work on it is underway, funded by the National Academy of Sciences and other agencies, as well as by industry groups; it probably will be several years before the facts are known.

The fluorocarbons as a group are characterized by their nonflammability. This property has led to the use of some of them as fire-extinguishing agents alone or in combination with other materials which are propelled by these gases.

Toxicity—Most of the fluorocarbons are classified as gases or vapors which in concentrations up to at least about 20% by volume in air for durations of exposure of the order of 2 hours do not appear to produce injury. This determination has assisted their use in the inhalation products currently available.

Although the fluorocarbons are chemically stable under ordinary circumstances, they decompose at very high temperatures reacting with moisture in the air to form the toxic material phosgene, but this particular hazard appears to be extremely rare and unusual.

Investigations have shown the fluorocarbons not to be physiologically inert as had been previously assumed. Beginning in 1970 reports appeared of several deaths occurring as a result of teenagers "sniffing" aerosol products in an attempt to get "high." Many of these deaths were due to asphyxiation; however, some were found to be the result of cardiac sensitization inducing arrhythmia and cardiac arrest. Although one report linked fluorocarbons in bronchodilator aerosols to reports of increased mortality among asthma patients, subsequent investigations failed to confirm that they are unsafe in the normal, or even excessive, use of such inhalation aerosol products. These compounds, if abused, can increase the reactiveness of the mammalian heart to endogenous epinephrine and can cause fatal cardiac arrhythmias. As a result of recent investigations disclosing the mechanism of this activity, it is now mandatory that aerosol products bear a caution against deliberate concentration and inhalation of the vapors. Exempt from this requirement are those products with limited amounts of propellant (less than ½ oz of total contents or foam products using less than 10% fluorocarbons), or providing limited access (metered products of less than 2 oz of contents).

The topical toxicity effects involve the ability of fluorocarbon gases to freeze tissue with subsequent necrosis, owing to their low boiling points. This is possible with many aerosol products if they are held very close to the site or sprayed for prolonged periods. To date there are few recorded incidences of toxic or irritation effects attributable to the propellant alone, and several aerosol products have been available for a number of years which are used on both intact and broken skin as well as on mucous membranes.

A unique application of the tissue-chilling effects of fluorocarbons involves their use alone or in combination with ethyl chloride to freeze tissue during skin planing.

Hydrocarbon Gases

Usage of this secondary group of liquefiable propellants, including normal butane, isobutane, and propane and certain blends of these, has risen sharply since the early 1960's. This has been spurred by the desire to reduce costs wherever possible as the entire industry has grown and become progressively competitive. This applies to many household and chemical specialty aerosol products and certain cosmetic products wherein the lower-cost hydrocarbon propellants have been shown to be more compatible with the newer water-based formulations. As yet pharmaceutical products have not employed hydrocarbons except in a few isolated instances, perhaps because cost has not been a prime consideration for this group of products.

It is doubtful that hydrocarbons will ever become widely used for pharmaceutical products. Their flammability coupled with a somewhat objectionable odor and taste, leaves the field wide open for the more versatile fluorocarbons. In addition, the cost of propellant in pharmaceutical products is rarely a strong enough factor to warrant engaging the hydrocarbons.

Compressed Gases

The compressed gases which have been used in aerosol products include nitrous oxide, carbon dioxide, and nitrogen. There are wide differences in product form and dispensing characteristics resulting from the use of compressed gas propellants rather than liquefiable materials. While both nitrous oxide and carbon dioxide are capable of liquefaction at room temperature, their vapor pressures at that point are about 720 and 835 psig, well beyond those that available containers can withstand. Used, therefore, in the vapor state only, they cannot provide constant pressure, as they expand with increasing volume.

Containers

There are several critical requirements for containers which house products exerting a pressure greater than atmospheric. The major concern, perhaps, is that they be substantial enough to contain pressure safely throughout the anticipated shelf-life of the product and during various expected conditions of storage and use. Such considerations prompted the early use of heavy, thick-walled steel cartridges as the first fluorocarbon gases became available. Considerable progress has since been made in the reduction of formulation pressures and the simultaneous creation of light-weight tin-plate cans having a more functional design and well capable of withstanding maximum potential pressures. In addition to a continuous series of refinements for this type of metal container, the can industry has introduced aluminum and stainless steel as additional materials. A return to the use of glass as well as introduction of synthetic resins and plastics has broadened the selection of containers.

Tin Plate

The tin-plated steel container with which we are familiar today borrowed its design and methods and materials of construction from the beer industry and has become known as the "beer-can" container. These "low-pressure" units today constitute the image of the aerosol package for the consumer and are used for the majority of pressurized products currently marketed. They remain the least expensive and most durable of all aerosol containers.

Tin-plate containers are made in two basic forms, seamed (three-piece) and seamless (drawn). The three-piece unit consists of a seamed or welded cylindrical body open at both ends to which are joined, by seaming, a concave or flat bottom and a top shaped to form a 1-in.

diameter opening which is curled to accept a valve cup. This type of container is more widely used today than any other.

Both the three-piece and two-piece types of containers are available with a variety of internal linings made of epoxy, vinyl, and phenolic organic resins and combinations of these. Such coatings afford some protection to the container when the contents are potentially reactive. For the most part these coating materials are applied to the tin plate in the flat form prior to rolling or shaping. As a general rule, the formulator seeks to adjust the formulation so that adverse physical and chemical effects are eliminated or reduced and rarely relies upon an internal lining to provide complete protection for the container. When advisable, double coating is available.

Standard-sized three-piece tin-plate containers are available from three major suppliers: American Can Co., Continental Can Co., and Crown Can Co.

Recent advances include the welding of container side seams. The first commercial units employing the Sudronic process were introduced in 1966 in Europe. In 1969 the Conoweld process was introduced by the Continental Can Co. and these containers are finding broader commercial use in the US. Welded side seams are stronger than soldered seams and are less obtrusive. They also permit can shapes differing from the conventional cylinder and therein lies the most probable reason for their increased use in the future.

Two-piece or seamless units are made available by the Crown Can Co. and are known as "Spray-Tainers." Many early products and particularly the first shave cream was marketed in a 6-oz version of this type. The internal coating system devised then, a phenolic lacquer on the body and the bottom plus two additional coats of vinyl lacquer on the bottom, has endured to this day and is still referred to as a "shave cream specification." The two sizes available now are a "6-oz" size (having an overflow capacity of 7.3 fl oz) and a "12-oz size" (having an overflow capacity of 12.5 fl oz).

Other two-piece tinplate containers are available as Pressuremaster cans (*Continental Can*) and as Apachecans (*Apache Corp.*).

Aluminum

Although tin-plate containers are now available in a number of sizes ranging from a 2-oz up to a 24-oz size, these are all of the same basic design and shape. The method of manufacture and the cost of equipment involved prohibits the introduction of distinctive shapes. While new methods currently under investigation may change this in the near future, a wider variety of more functional and attractive shapes and sizes are available today in aluminum.

Aluminum aerosol containers are produced from a single slug of aluminum alloy by an impact extrusion process and have no seams, neither side, top, nor bottom. Major suppliers of such units are the Peerless Tube Co., Bradley-Sun Div. of the American Can Co., and the Virjune Mfg. Co.

The Alusuisse Metals Co. in Europe manufactures a broad range of sizes of monobloc aluminum containers. These Boxal containers are finding broader use in the US because of their excellent internal lining.

A unique set of aluminum tubes for aerosols has been made available by the Bradley-Sun Tube Div. of the American Can Co. These miniatures with capacities of ½ and 1 fl oz are pencil-shaped (½ to ¾ in. diameter and 4 in. high) and comparatively inexpensive and lend themselves well for use as promotional sizes or for single-dose pharmaceuticals.

Stainless Steel

Used for some perfume and inhalation pharmaceutical products, stainless steel vials permit the use of increased pressures more safely than glass which is the only other container material acceptable for so many of these products.

In many instances, pressures somewhat higher than those ordinarily allowed, are required to produce the small droplet size distribution which makes the product cosmetically acceptable or therapeutically efficient. Stainless steel is a logical choice for such products, especially for products containing about 15 ml or less. These containers provide the resistance to attack inherent in the material and for this reason are the only metal containers which are not made available with internal linings.

Glass

Although some of the early aerosol products were housed in glass, the aerosol industry while rapidly expanding with the development of fluorocarbons, reverted for several years to the exclusive use of metal containers. The introduction of fluorocarbons with relatively low-vapor pressures (propellants 11 and 114) permitted the widening of available containers to include both plain and plastic coated glass. This step contributed greatly to the advent of pharmaceutical aerosols, which almost seemed to wait for this classic drug packaging material to be made available. Glass aerosol containers, especially those that are plastic-coated, are now used perhaps as widely as any other material for pressurized medicinals.

While glass, whether plain or plastic coated, cannot match the strength, durability, and economic advantages of either tin plate or aluminum, certain important features are provided. These include, in order of relative importance to pharmaceuticals as a product group:

1. Nonreactive with active ingredients
2. Freedom from corrosion and deterioration
3. Distinctive design and shape
4. Greater patient acceptance

An advantage of glass containers not mentioned is the ability to view the contents. This can be important to the patient who can see the level of contents remaining and if prolonged aging or extreme climate conditions have adversely affected the product. For this purpose

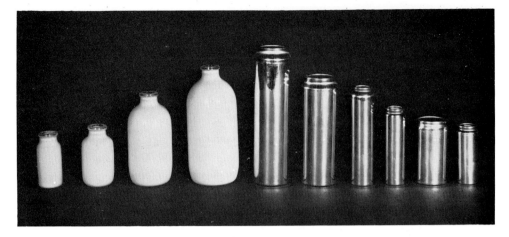

Fig. 3—Plastic-coated glass bottles and Peerless aluminum tubes frequently used for pharmaceutical aerosols.

both clear and tinted translucent plastic coatings are available.

Plastic-coated glass aerosol containers are available from both the Wheaton Glass Co. and the Owens-Illinois Glass Co. in a number of shapes and sizes. Some of these containers are shown in Fig. 3. The coating material is essentially polyvinyl chloride plastic, which is applied to the glass by a controlled-temperature dipping process.

The coating serves to protect the glass by cushioning during impact and preventing scratching and subsequent fracture. In addition, should the glass break when dropped, the plastic serves to contain the shattered glass fragments which could ordinarily be projected with great force due to the pressurized state of the contents. The Wheaton bottle jacket is a form-fitting separate covering which can be peeled away from the glass whereas Owens-Illinois prefers to bond the plastic permanently to the glass. Both types of coatings have been shown to afford protection adequately. In addition, the Wheaton coating has vent holes, ranging from slits along the side to larger round openings in the bottom, which serve to release propellant when the glass fractures before the resilient plastic can expand dangerously.

Plastic

Plastic containers will undoubtedly become a dominant factor in aerosol packaging in the near future. This material potentially combines the safety advantages of metal with the inert characteristics of glass. Materials such as Nylon, Polyethylene, Delrin, Melamine, Zytel, and Celcon have been used for aerosol containers. Problems involving permeation of propellants and actives, incompatibility of plasticizers, high-temperature instability and production problems among others, have been experienced. But new materials and production methods are currently being studied and may succeed in changing the status of this type of material for aerosol packaging. Such containers may be especially useful for packaging certain types of pharmaceutical products.

Valves

One of the more critical components of the aerosol package is the valve. It serves to seal the container hermetically and to regulate the passage of product from the container. In this regard, it influences the characteristics of the product and complements the design of the formulation. The valve, along with the actuating device, may be selected so as to produce a fine or coarse droplet distribution, a fully expanded foam, a slow or rapid rate of product release, a wide or narrow spray pattern, or a continuous or precisely measured amount of product.

A great variety of valve and actuator designs have been evolved by several manufacturers to meet the dispensing requirements of the many different types of aerosol products. A simple means of classifying aerosol valves depends on whether the valve delivers a continuous spray when actuated or releases only a measured amount. The former (conventional) are employed far more often than the latter (metering).

Conventional Valves

Valves in this broad group have acquired descriptive terms referring generally to either the form of product they dispense or to some characteristic design feature. The "product form" group includes spray valves, foam valves, stream valves, powder valves, and food valves, among others. This means of classification is weak and tends to be misleading and overly restrictive in that such valves each have a specific modification to suit a particular purpose but this alteration does not necessarily preclude their use for other types of products. These terms refer more to the type of actuator involved rather than the entire valve construction. The "valve design" means of classification appears to be more meaningful, if not all-encompassing:

1. "Toggle" or "vertical" action valves referring to the direction in which the valve stem is depressed to release product.
2. "Bottle" or "can" valves referring to the container with which the valve is used and differentiating between the standard 1 in. opening of tin plate and certain aluminum containers and the common 20 mm ferrule of glass, plastic, and some aluminum and stainless-steel containers.
3. "Vapor tap" or "vapor phase orifice" valves referring to the additional orifice in a valve housing which permits the simultaneous flow of liquid formulation and propellant vapor.

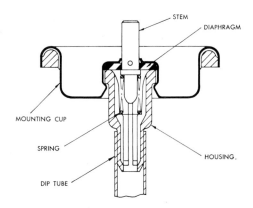

Fig. 4—Continuous action aerosol valve shown with 1-in. metal mounting cup.

4. "One-shot" valves referring to the type of construction which produces a continuous release of container contents once actuated.
5. "Low delivery rate" valves referring to certain restricted orifices which permit a reduced rate of product release.
6. "Pressure filling" valves referring to specialized valve constructions which permit the filling of liquefied propellant under pressure at relatively high rate through the valve into the container.

These terms provide a better understanding of the valve function and picture the construction more clearly, however limiting they may be in describing the overall features of a particular valve assembly.

The conventional aerosol valve is composed of several basic components assembled together (Fig. 4) and include:

1. The *actuator,* which is often referred to as the button or spout. This component is fitted onto the stem of the valve or is inserted into the valve body and serves as the final exit for product leaving the container as well as a means of easily depressing the valve stem to start that process.
2. The *valve stem,* which is the component actuated to bring product forth from the container.
3. The *diaphragm* or stem seal, which is made of rubber, functions to seal the product from the stem orifice.
4. The *valve cup* or ferrule, which is the external housing for the valve parts and is the component which is affixed to the container to hold the entire valve in place. The cup refers generally to the 1 in. metal valve exterior while the word ferrule is used to describe the same functional part for bottle valves.
5. The *valve spring,* which serves to return the valve stem to its rest position after actuation.
6. The *valve housing* or body, which serves to contain the stem and spring and to hold the top of the dip tube at its base, if one is used.

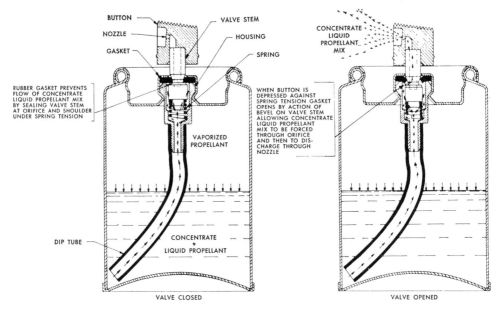

Fig. 5—A valve mechanism during actuation and at rest.

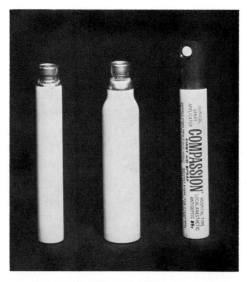

Fig. 6—Miniature aluminum aerosol tubes, ½ fl oz and 1 fl oz sizes.

7. The *dip tube* or eduction tube, which when used, conducts the product from the bottom of the container to the housing tail orifice. When not used, the container is held in the inverted position to release product.

Fig. 5 shows the assembly of these parts from an operational standpoint during actuation and at rest. Several valve-producing companies supply the industry with valves of this type and all have design similarities to the extent that they are almost interchangeable.

Some specialized valves have been developed which are worthy of separate discussion. One of these is the 1300 series valve made by OEL, Inc, which is shown in Fig. 6 on the Bradley-Sun aluminum tubes.

Metering Valves

The metering valve is constructed to deliver a prearranged measured quantity of product each time the valve is actuated. This is achieved by a valve design which isolates a given volume of product in a separate chamber and releases it when the valve is actuated, while simultaneously shutting off the flow of the remaining contents.

Most metering valves employ a molded plastic or machined stainless-steel chamber whose internal dimensions serve to determine the metered quantity delivered. This chamber is simply a valve housing of specific capacity. Fig. 7 shows a typical metering valve of this type and explains the delivery mechanism.

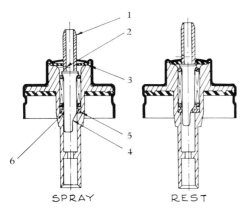

Fig. 7—Metered valve construction and operation in the spray and rest positions. *Spray position:* When the stem (1) is depressed, it allows the stem orifice (2) to go below the diaphragm (3); and, at the same time, the lower grooved section (4) of the stem travels through the seal (5) until the full diameter of the stem seals off at the lower tank opening (6); with the stem orifice below the diaphragm and the lower tank opening sealed off, the metered contents of the tank are discharged. *Rest position:* When the stem (1) is released, the stem orifice (2) comes above the diaphragm (3) and simultaneously the lower groove section (4) lines up with the seal (5), allowing the tank to refill for the next spraying.

Specialized Actuators

The actuator serves to determine the form of the sprayed product to a large extent. The actuator is the last component the product travels through on its way out of the container and there is an opportunity for this device to produce the total effect desired or to put the finishing touches on characteristics initially shaped by the formulation and inner valve orifices.

Standard spray buttons are available with a variety of internal groove arrangements and external orifice sizes to achieve various effects. They are available as single-piece units or with separate inserts containing the external orifice. A feature built into many provides a spray direction for the user that prevents application of product onto other than the intended site. Also, specialized designs permit delivery of product vertically, horizontally, and at a 45° angle. Foam spouts have larger internal areas which permit their use as pre-expansion

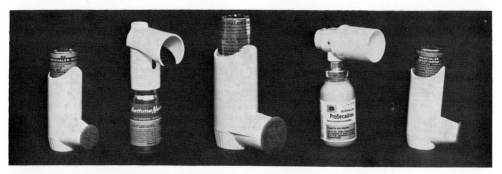

Fig. 8—Commercial inhalation aerosol products in suspension form.

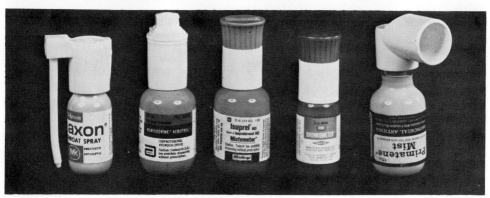

Fig. 9—Commercial inhalation aerosol products in solution form.

chambers so that the foam delivered is almost fully formed when dispensed. In combination with certain formulations, foam spouts have been made to deliver a circular puff, a flat ribbon, or a multiribbon comb effect of foamed product.

Oral adaptors, shown in Figs. 8 and 9, permit the evaporation of liquefied propellant and the intake of air to produce a fine dispersion of small droplets of particles for inhalation. A specialized adapter, pictured in Fig. 9, has a long barrel which permits placement of product onto the back of the throat.

For several types of products, an adapter with a mechanical breakup design in the orifice helps create finely-divided droplets. It is especially useful when the maximum amount of propellant or propellant pressure has been used and the spray requires further subdivision. See Fig. 10.

Most recently, specialized actuating devices have been introduced for inhalation products which eliminate problems associated with poor coordination of the valve. These devices actuate a metered dose in response to the vacuum created by the initial part of the inhalation process. A cocking device prepares the valve for this automatic form of dispensing. Working on the basis of diaphragm-lever-spring arrangements, these devices help greatly in reducing the incidence of overdosing, occasionally reported for conventionally actuated inhalation aerosol products.

Protective Caps

The essential function of this component is to insure that the valve/actuator assembly is neither damaged in shipment nor able to release product accidentally. Most overcaps are made of plastic, generally high-density linear polyethylene. Overcaps serve the secondary functions of keeping the valve and actuator dust-free and providing a decorative finish to the package.

A wide variety of "spray-thru" actuator caps have been developed which serve these same functions while providing the means to actuate the valve when desired, without removing the protective cap portion at each use. These are quite decorative as well as functionally convenient.

Additional designs provide a "tamper-proof" feature integral with the protective function. More recently "child-proof" and "child-resistant" designs have been devised, and some categories of aerosol products are now required to employ this capability as stipulated by the Poison Prevention Packaging Act of 1970.

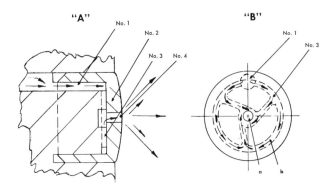

Fig. 10—Design and function of a mechanical breakup actuator. *A:* Cross section of the mechanical break and insert; *B:* Front view of the mechanical break, without an insert. *Function:* The material flowing from the valve stem first enters the inner orifice (1); its flow is then restricted by the insert (2) (plastic or metal); the construction of the rib section (3) channels the flow of material into the center swirl chamber forcing the breakup of material as it passes through the outer orifice (4). *Notes:* By varying the depth of the center swirl chamber (a) the rib section (b) and changing the hole size of the outer orifice (4), the consistency and width of the spray can be varied.

Pharmaceutical Applications

Pharmaceutical aerosol products currently marketed fall into two major groups, those intended for *internal* use which include inhalation, oral, nasal, rectal, and vaginal products and those intended for *topical* use on intact or injured skin, or on mucous membrane sites. As yet, products have not been developed to treat the eye or ear. These applications are presently considered too hazardous for current aerosol technology or have been shown to yield nothing more than other forms of administration can provide. An additional category encompassing *environmental products* might be included in a discussion of pharmaceutical aerosols, however, these products which include surface disinfectants, air sanitizers, diagnostic aids, and instrument lubricants approach the category of chemical specialties rather than pharmaceuticals, and are not included in the sections which follow. Several of them in fact, come under the auspices of the Environmental Protection Agency rather than the Food and Drug Administration. One exception is the room vaporizer which is not entirely an environmental product although it is sprayed into the atmosphere. Its vaporized actives are intended for inhalation to relieve nasal congestion.

Aerosols for Internal Use

Aerosol products applied in body cavities continuous with the dermatomucosal surfaces include inhalation therapy and medications for use in the nose, mouth, throat, rectum, and vagina.

Respiratory Medication

The pharmacist is called upon to dispense medication for the treatment of the lower respiratory tract in the form of vapors and aerosols. A true aerosol is a dispersion of solid or liquid particles in air. In the accepted, physical-chemical sense, an aerosol must be in the colloidal range (about 100 nm); however, none of the medically useful aerosols are in this size range. In fact, they would lose their effectiveness if they were colloidal.

Particle Distribution—Fig. 11 offers diagrammatic representations of size distribution of particles required to reach various sites within the respiratory tract.

Liquid and Solid Dispersion (Non-Aerosol)—*Atomizers* are frequently used to disperse liquids into spray form. The vacuum type is the most common in which a partial vacuum is created in a dip tube by forcing air across the T-tube. A modified pathway (baffle) appears to reduce the particles slightly, merely acting to capture the heavier particles.

Fig. 12 illustrates the use of an atomizer for large particle atomization of the trachea and bronchi. By the use of this form of administration, many special formulations can be applied to the upper respiratory passages.

A *nebulizer* is a special atomizer within a flask. The placement of the outlet, as well as the general dimensions, are such that the heavier droplets are caused to fall back into the reservoir. The commercial glass nebulizers are constructed for primary use with compressed air so that a high flow rate is achieved. A portable model with a rubber bulb is available.

The Vaponephrin and De Vilbis No. 40 nebulizer appear to be capable of producing aerosols in the effective particle size range, and probably others meet this criteria. Other modifications may be equally effective. Fig. 13 represents the fine mist produced by a nebulizer for aerosol treatment of lungs. Many of these particles are in the range of 1–5 μm. A relatively new nebulizer, the Nebhalent "touch action" Nebulizer is claimed to produce a large fraction of the aerosol particles in the effective size range. All of these three systems can be used with a formulation of the physician's choice.

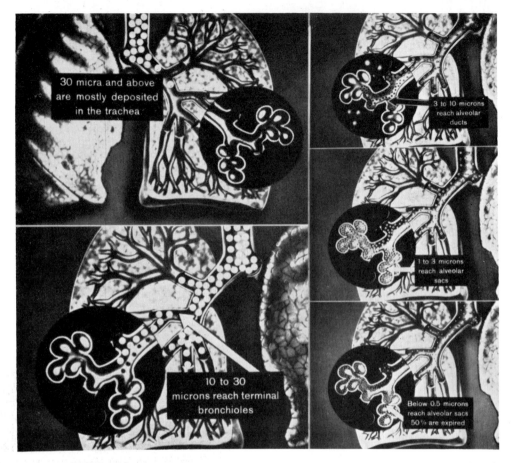

Fig. 11—Diagrammatic sketches, representing the anatomical sites of deposition within the lungs of particles of varying radii.[2]

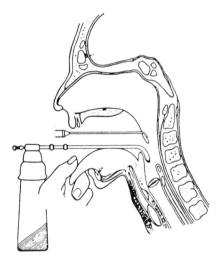

Fig. 12—The use of an atomizer to disperse large particles within the pharynx and trachea.[2]

Insufflators are special devices designed to disperse solid particulates into the respiratory tract. (Vitamin B_{12} can be administered in this manner.) The particle size of the solid is dependent on the original form of dispersion prior to packaging.

Vaporizers are used to humidify the atmosphere by dispersing water and certain volatiles into a gaseous form. They are a very inefficient means of humidifying the lungs relative to the use of "cold humidification" by employing water-based aerosols dispersed with the proper nebulizer.

A special form of a "vaporizer" is the *sublimator* (inhaler), which acts by sublimation of its volatile, sympathomimetic amine carbonates.

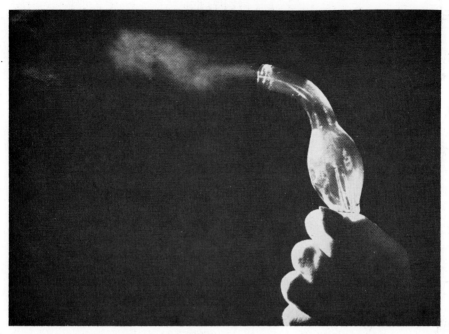

Fig. 13—The fine mist produced by a nebulizer suitable for aerosol therapy of the lungs.[2]

Vehicles for Non-Aerosol Respiratory Medication—Normal saline and other aqueous-based systems have been commonly used in such formulation. The nebulization of water creates a very fine mist, which evaporates rapidly under normal conditions of humidity. Propylene glycol, glycerol, and other additives have been utilized to stabilize the droplet so that the system does not reduce to a size so small as to be exhaled. Alcohol may be substituted for water in the above systems.

Surface-active agents have been incorporated in nebulizer vehicles to decrease the surface tension, which in turn affects the particle size pattern produced. These include anionic surfactants (Tergitol 08, Aerosol OT), nonionic surfactants (Triton A-20, X-100, and Tween 80), and quaternaries (e.g., benzalkonium chloride). All of these agents have been found useful in approximately a 1:1000 concentration. However, a recent report on a control series of a nebulizer vehicle minus the nonionic surfactant, claimed that both solutions were of value in enabling the sputum to be expectorated. Apparently, the use of plain water droplets is adequate to cause hydration of the viscid sputum. The alkalinity of sodium bicarbonate (2%) in proprietary aerosol vehicle (pH 8.5) has been suggested as a potential source of the irritation occasionally noted with its use.

Aerosol Inhalation Therapy

Inhalation therapy has been rapidly advanced by the adaptation of pressurized packaging for this mode of administration. For this purpose, the aerosol unit offers many advantages. It is compact and portable. The manner of use has been quite simplified, requiring only a few seconds for dosage delivery. Most inhalation products which have been offered in aerosol form have been packaged to deliver between 100 and 300 sprays, providing both convenience and economy for the user.

Products currently available in this area are pictured in Figs. 8 and 9 and include agents such as isoproterenol, epinephrine, and dexamethasone, for the symptomatic alleviation of bronchial asthma, pulmonary emphysema, bronchospasm, and related respiratory conditions. In addition to this principal category of treatment of the respiratory tract, other products using the same means of administration include ergotamine for the treatment of migraine and octyl nitrite for vasodilation effect.

To date, the inhalation aerosol has been utilized in only these few therapeutic areas, and most are concerned only with localized treatment for respiratory disorders. In the future it is likely that the inhalation aerosol form will be investigated for the delivery of antibiotics, enzymes, hormones, and other drug classes, not only for local activity but for systemic effect. The inhalation route is capable of providing speed of drug response approaching that associated with intravenous injection. Combining this aspect with the aerosol's features of self-administration and absence of time-consuming material or apparatus preparation, the potential for these other agents administered via aerosol inhalation is considerable.

Research directed toward replacement of the oral route by inhalation aerosol, for certain medicaments, may uncover methods to obtain equivalent response with smaller amounts of drug without the need for complex protective processes, owing to the absence of interaction with digestive enzymes.

Products currently available in this area have been either dissolved in alcoholic solution with the fluorocarbon propellants or suspended in them utilizing surfactants.

Oral and Nasal Therapy

Taking advantage of the aerosol's property of propelling its contents forward, this dosage form has been utilized to instill medication into body orifices and to reach mucous membrane areas in a manner more efficient than with conventional forms. In most instances, such as nasal and throat sprays, application is made directly from the aerosol via a valve-actuating device suitably adapted for the purpose. The early aerosol nasal sprays incorporated medication as solids suspended in propellant to avoid the irritative effects of alcoholic solutions. Most recently, advances in valve and propellant technology have made it possible to consider aqueous solutions for nasal application. Obvious advantages of the aerosol for nasal use include more accurate delivery by means of the metering valve, ability to penetrate the nasal cavity more deeply, and freedom from contamination of contents by replacement of the auxiliary applicator after use.

The development of unique aerosol adapters makes it possible for the first time to treat throat areas by direct placement of medication at the intended site. By means of these devices, a fine mist is directed onto surfaces inaccessible to lozenges and gargles. The discomforts of swabbing may also be eliminated in this way. A currently available product of this type is shown in Fig. 9, on the far left.

Vaginal Therapy

Contraceptive products in the form of an aerosol foam inserted within the vaginal tract are available. These products depend for activity both upon the concentration of spermicidal agent and the barrier effect of a stable foam produced by the expansion of volatile propellant through an emulsion containing the spermicide and the propellant. These products have not employed a metering valve, but are used in conjunction with a vaginal applicator which receives a definite volume of foam when operated with the aerosol container. The applicator is then detached from the aerosol and inserted in the vagina, its contents being deposited by depression of a plunger. Aerosol foam has also been employed to treat diseases of the vaginal tract. The antimycotic agent, gentian violet, has been incorporated in a water-washable emulsion as an aerosol, and still another product provides a foaming solution of a quaternary ammonium compound for cleansing and deodorizing the vaginal vault. Both products employ specially designed adapters for direct application of the aerosolized

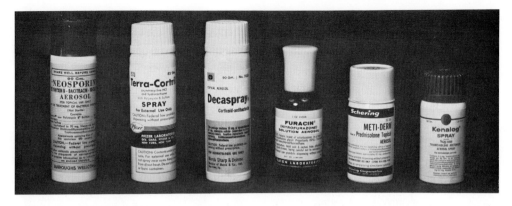

Fig. 14—Topical pharmaceutical aerosols for dermatological use employing solution or suspension systems.

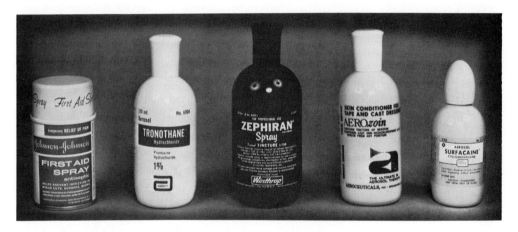

Fig. 15—Topical pharmaceutical aerosols incorporating anesthetics and antiseptics.

product. In addition to these vaginally applied products, the aerosol form may prove useful for rectal application, and some medicated foams have appeared on the market to treat anal and rectal irritation and swelling.

The compressed gas propellants are incapable of producing foams and are therefore not used for these products.

Aerosols for Topical Use

Aerosol products intended for topical administration as a solution, powder, or foam have appeared for a wide variety of applications. Some of these are shown in Figs. 14–17. For efficient treatment of external body surfaces, in addition to the advantages previously outlined, the aerosol adds the ability to cover large areas quickly and uniformly and without contact by auxiliary applicators. This latter advantage can be most critical in the treatment of painful or infected sites.

Certain three-phase systems may prove to be more valuable for topically applied pharmaceuticals than all other systems. These are the suspended powders and the emulsions which produce foams of varying stability. Powder sprays are prepared by suspending the active ingredients directly in the liquefied propellants.

The other three-phase system in which interest is advancing rapidly for pharmaceuticals is represented by the foam products. In this system, the active ingredients are solubilized in the selected vehicle, and this solution is emulsified with the propellant. A sys-

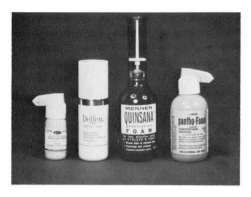

Fig. 16—Topical pharmaceutical aerosols employing foam systems.

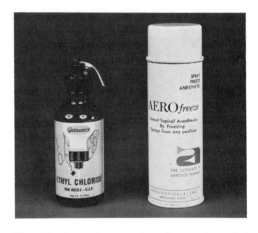

Fig. 17—An early aerosol package using ethyl chloride as both active ingredient and propellant, and its modern counterpart using liquefied fluorocarbon gases.

tem whereby propellant is combined with a preformed oil-in-water emulsion also produces a foam. Interesting innovations in this area are represented by (1) transparent foam-producing systems which are actually colloidal dispersions of propellant in the active solution which need no shaking and (2) anhydrous systems which employ a glycol base, should it be desirable to exclude water from the system.

Special Systems

A series of unique formulation and packaging innovations have appeared recently. These include co-dispensing valves, aspirator or venturi systems, and bag-in-can containers. While they bear no real relationship to each other, they collectively represent a distinct departure from aerosol container and valve systems previously used. Available by these means, for the first time, are products which are heated, or contain usually incompatible or reactive ingredients, or are too viscous for conventional dispensing.

Co-Dispensing—The co-dispensing method involves two compartments within the package which hold reactive phases. These phases are allowed to combine only at the time of use, and in a predetermined ratio, by the valve construction design.

The first and most notable commercial application for co-dispensing systems was heated shaving cream.

A second bag-in-can system is the Sterigard dispenser. This package differs in that its inner polyethylene bag occupies more inside container area than other bags and does not conform to any preformed shape.

Aspirator (Venturi)—These systems are also noted for the separation of product and propellant. However, in these instances a greater variety of spray characteristics is possible, from finely divided to coarse. The Preval (*Precision Valve Corp.*) and Innovair (*Geigy*) both employ an inner cylinder of high pressure propellant. When the valve is actuated, the propellant is discharged past the valve opening leading to the product, thus creating a partial vacuum. This causes the product to be drawn up the dip tube to mix with the vaporizing propellant.

Bag-in-Can—These are comparable with the co-dispensing systems in that two phases are kept separate from each other by inner physical barrier arrangements. They differ by permitting the extrusion of only one of the phases. In this system the product is maintained in a plastic bag whose upper portion is affixed to the mouth of the outer container. The propellant, whether liquefied or compressed gas, is held outside the plastic bag and exerts an external force on the bag, forcing the contents out via a conventional valve, without its dip tube.

Such package types are excellent for the extrusion of highly viscous materials as well as products which are extremely reactive with metals. Product is available having undergone very little physical change inasmuch as the propellant is always maintained apart from the concentrate. Premature loss of propelling force is thereby avoided and the containers may be held in any dispensing position.

The Sepro can (*Continental Can*) is an example of the bag-in-can system. Introduced in 1966, it has been used commercially for food products such as cheese spreads and cosmetics such as depilatory creams. Specialized equipment is employed for the filling of viscous concentrate into the pleated bag and for the injection of propellant through the bottom rubber valve plug.

Dispensing

The pharmacist can help insure the safe and effective use of aerosol products by reinforcing the handling cautions and usage directions supplied with each package at the time of dispensing. Most often the directions for use are either printed on each package label or furnished with the package in the form of an insert. These directions should be reviewed by the pharmacist and, if possible, discussed with the patient, to be sure that misuse is avoided. For some products, shaking prior to use is critical to uniform and accurate dosage delivery. For certain inhalation and foam products the container is held inverted rather than upright during use, and this, too, should be instructed. For spray products, the distance held from the site and length of spraying time are most important.

Equally important are the warnings pertaining to misuse hazards. The law requires printed caution statements on each package relative to safe storage and handling conditions, and these can be pointed out as part of the dispensing instructions.

Signs of adverse topical reaction should be explained as possibilities in certain cases, particularly with initial use, and the patient should be instructed to discontinue use and consult the physician. Most aerosol packages are opaque, and so the pharmacist can be helpful by advising the patient of the less-obvious signs of product depletion, and in this way help insure that a continuing supply of medication is available if intended by the prescriber.

References

1. Reed FT: *Propellents.* In Shepherd HR: *Aerosols: Science and Technology,* Interscience, New York, 221–223, 1961.

2. *Progress in Allergy II,* S. Karger, Ltd., Basel, Switzerland, 1949.

Bibliography

Shepherd HR: *Aerosols: Science and Technology,* Interscience, New York, 1961.

Sciarra JJ: Aerosols. In *Remington's Pharmaceutical Sciences,* 15th ed, Mack Publ. Co., Easton, PA, 1975.

Herzka A, Pickthall J: *Pressurized Packaging (Aerosols),* Butterworth, London, 1961.

Dautrebande L: *Microaerosols,* Academic, New York, 1962.

Hatch TF, Gross P: *Pulmonary Deposition and Retention of Inhaled Aerosols,* Academic, New York, 1964.

12

Radio-
pharmaceuticals

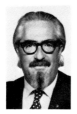

Walter Wolf, PhD
Radiopharmacy Program
School of Pharmacy
University of Southern
California
Los Angeles, CA 90033

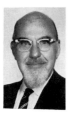

Manuel Tubis, PhD
Radiopharmacy Program
US Veterans Administration/
Wadsworth Hospital Center
Los Angeles, CA 90073

The radiopharmaceutical is a chemical material containing a radioactive element that is used for diagnosis, in an *in vitro* test or in therapy, because of the radiation emitted. The radiopharmaceutical may be the radioactive analog of a simple molecular species, such as sodium iodide I-131 or a complex mixture of technetium sulfide Tc-99m and sulfur in colloidal form.

The use of diagnostic radiopharmaceuticals may be predicated on the basis of active transport and/or metabolic conversion within an organ, e.g., the uptake of the radioiodide ion and its ultimate conversion to thyroxine by the thyroid gland. The uptake of the radioiodide ion serves diagnostically to evaluate the physiological and metabolic status of the thyroid and thus replaces the previously used basal metabolic rate test. A range has been established for the normal thyroid gland and thus this test defines the hypo-, eu-, and hyperthyroid states.

The use of a dose of sodium iodide I-131 ten times as large as the uptake dose results in sufficient radioiodide acquisition by the thyroid gland to permit delineation of the gland by the appropriate instrumentation so as to indicate a hyperfunctioning nodule or a nonaccumulating tumorous growth (Figs. 1 and 2).

In the therapy of hyperthyroidism, the goal is the selective destruction of some portion of the thyroid gland in order to decrease the excessive production of thyroxine and its physiological effects. To achieve this, the dose of radioiodide is increased 2000–5000 times the thyroid uptake dose. Further, in order to destroy an inoperable cancerous thyroid gland, the dose of sodium iodide I-131 is increased still further, namely to 100,000 times the uptake dose. The gland is thus ablated by the intense destructive and necrotizing radiation released in the radioactive decay of the radionuclide [131]I. The patient is then placed on a regimen of thyroid replacement medication.

The posology (dosage) of radiophar-

318

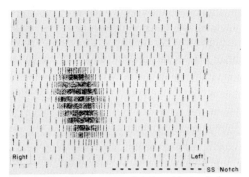

Fig. 1—Rectilinear scan of a thyroid gland showing a hyperfuctioning (autonomous) nodule.[1]

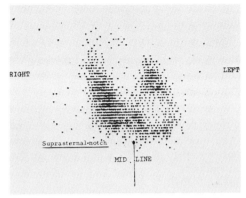

Fig. 2—Scan of a nonaccumulating thyroid tumor (nonfunctioning, cold nodule).[2]

maceuticals is calculated in terms of units related to the number of radioactive nuclear disintegrations with the concomitant release of electrons which are particulate beta energy and gamma radiation, which is electromagnetic and hence, similar to x-rays. The smallest unit commonly used is the microcurie (μCi), which is the quantity of radionuclide producing 37,000 disintegrations/sec. The next unit is 1000 times as large, namely the millicurie (mCi). The curie (Ci) is 1000 times as large as the millicurie and is a magnitude never used in either diagnostic or therapeutic medicine as a single dose.

In addition to the radiopharmaceuticals administered to the patient for diagnosis and therapy, there are a number used for *in vitro* tests in which the patient receives no radiopharmaceutical directly and therefore no radiation, but rather the diagnostic test is performed on the patient's serum, plasma, or other body fluid. This has led to the development of a number of "kits" which greatly simplify the *in vitro* tests and lead to the rapid performance of the test. Representative examples are presented in *Radiopharmacy*, Table 15.10.5 (see *Bibliography*).

Similarly, many test materials based on radioimmunoassays are now available in kit form which greatly simplify the procedures (see Table 15.10.6 of the above-mentioned text).

For a more extensive discussion on the nature of radioactivity and the physics involved, the reader is referred

to Chapter 29 of the previous edition of this text or to the above-mentioned text.

Energy is expressed in electron volts (eV), kilo-electron volts (keV) or million electron volts (MeV). One eV is equivalent to 23.4 kcal, and those γ emitters that are most useful in radiopharmacy have energies ranging from 25 keV (^{125}I) to 140 keV (^{99m}Tc) to 511 keV (positron emitters such as ^{18}F, ^{68}Ga, etc.).

Nuclear radiation can be corpuscular or electromagnetic. Particles include β^- radiation (electrons ejected from the nucleus), β^+ (positrons; these annihilate by collision with an electron producing two γ-rays of 511 keV energy), and α radiation (^{4}He nuclei). Electromagnetic energy emitted from the nucleus is gamma (γ) radiation and is produced at very narrowly defined energy levels. The total emission from a radioactive decay process is known as the decay scheme, and its knowledge is important to determine the potential usefulness of a given radionuclide. Radioactive decay is characterized by the nature of the emission, their energy, and the rate of decay.

The decay of a radioactive nucleus is a first-order exponential:

$$-dn/dt = \lambda N$$

where λ is the decay constant and N is the number of atoms. A practical unit is the biological half-life ($t_{1/2}$), defined as the time to decompose 50% of all radioactive nuclei originally present; it is related to λ by $t_{1/2} = 0.693/\lambda$.

The Biological Mechanisms Which Determine the Use of Radiopharmaceuticals

Simple Diffusion—Many diagnostic radiopharmaceuticals, irrespective of their molecular composition, introduced parenterally, penetrate the walls of the vascularity in the area of the lesion and thereby diffuse into the extravascular space. During their residence in the abnormal tissue, the position, size, shape, and frequently the pathology of the organ can be determined by external scanning, thus providing, nontraumatically, the necessary information for therapy.

Compartmental localization is a mechanism whereby a radiopharmaceutical is confined to a physiological compartment. For example, Indium-113m is injected in ionic form and combines with transferrin, the iron-carrying blood plasma protein, and thus distributes itself throughout the vascular compartment. Thus, by scanning in the area of the placenta, a large abnormal pool of blood in that location may delineate abnormal bleeding and aid in the diagnosis of placenta previa.

Phagocytosis and pinocytosis are mechanisms in which colloidal particles are sequestered by cells of the reticuloendothelial system, such as the Kupffer cells of the liver and spleen. If these colloids are labeled, the organs containing them may be scanned.

Cell sequestration is a similar mechanism in which labeled damaged red cells are sequestered by the spleen for destruction; thus, the radionuclide is deposited in the organ thereby permitting scanning.

Capillary blockade is another mechanism used as a means of scanning. The important characteristic of the agents employed is that of particle size which occlude a small proportion of the total number of capillaries in the specific organ to be scanned. The composition of the radiopharmaceutical is variable but should combine minimal radiation dose, short "effective" half-life, biodegradability, lack of toxicity, and ease of preparation. Examples are macroaggregated particles of human serum albumin labeled with ^{99m}Tc or ^{113m}In sulfide and gelatin denatured with glutaraldehyde, of particle sizes 10–75 micrometers (μm) for lung scanning.

Another macroaggregated form is that of the "microsphere" consisting of a sphere of heat-denatured albumin incorporating one of several radionuclides of uniform diameter, which are used for lung scintigraphy by reason of their capillary blockage.

Production of Primary Radionuclides

Radionuclides used in radiopharmaceutical work have half-lives ranging from that of a few minutes to days, or sometimes even weeks. In recent years the tendency has been to use mostly short-lived radionuclides, so as to reduce patient dose. This has led to the local development of radiopharmacies, by requiring "in house" or extemporaneous preparation of most radiopharmaceuticals in current use. The production of radionuclides is within the scope of nuclear chemistry, and makes use of two primary types of reactions. A nucleus can react with a neutron, absorb that neutron, emit some of the excess energy as electromagnetic radiation, and produce a radionuclide by the (n,γ) reaction. For example, the production of a clinically useful radionuclide such as ^{24}Na, $t_{1/2} = 15$ hours, is done by taking stable ^{23}Na and bombarding it with neutrons:

$$^{23}\text{Na} + \text{n} \rightarrow {}^{24}\text{Na} + \text{Energy (}\gamma \text{ radiation)}$$

This process is abbreviated as ^{23}Na(n,γ)^{24}Na. The device used to produce neutrons is the nuclear reactor and there are a large number of reactors throughout the country that are used in that process. In recent years, more and more emphasis has been placed on the use of another machine, the cyclotron, for the production of primary nuclides. A cyclotron is a device that accelerates charged particles such as nuclei of hydrogen, "heavy hydrogen" (deuterium), and helium and produces primary radionuclides by charged particle bombardments. For example, the medically useful ^{67}Ga can be produced by the bombardment of natural zinc with protons, where the useful reactions are

$$^{67}Zn(p,n)\ ^{67}Ga$$

and

$$^{68}Zn(p,2n)\ ^{67}Ga$$

The key issue is that reactors usually produce neutron-exceedant radionuclides, which are usually beta emitters and longer-lived than the neutron-deficient radionuclides produced in cyclotrons (usually gamma emitters). However, as hospitals do not usually have direct access to either a medical cyclotron or a reactor for in-house production of short-lived radionuclides for clinical use, it would have been unlikely that short-lived radionuclides could have become widely used had it not been for the full-scale development of a third type of system, the generator, which makes use of the fact that some radionuclides decay with the production of other radionuclides. A typical and extremely widely used system is that of the ^{99}Mo ^{99m}Tc generator ("the isotope cow"). ^{99}Mo is produced in a reactor by ^{98}Mo(n,γ)^{99}Mo. In turn, ^{99}Mo decays with a 67-hour half-life to ^{99m}Tc, which in turn decays to ^{99}Tc with a half-life of 6 hours. Inasmuch as ^{99}Mo decays continuously, a generator is now a system whereby an insoluble form of ^{99}Mo is periodically extracted ("milked") and the soluble ^{99m}Tc daughter is produced as sodium pertechnetate (NaTcO$_4$). Such a system (see Fig. 3) is an extremely simple and compact system and can be readily used in any nuclear medicine installation. This method for the primary production of the radionuclide together with the more sophisticated cyclotron and reactor production, constitutes the

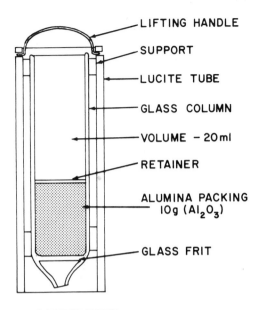

LIFTING HANDLE

SUPPORT

LUCITE TUBE

GLASS COLUMN

VOLUME – 20 ml

RETAINER

ALUMINA PACKING
10 g (Al$_2$O$_3$)

GLASS FRIT

GENERATOR

Fig. 3—Radionuclide generator system.

basis on which radiopharmaceutical practice has been made possible.

Nuclear Instrumentation

The use of radiopharmaceuticals for imaging normal and abnormal structures has already been discussed. The principal instruments used for scanning are the rectilinear scanners, previously referred to, and the stationary scintillation camera with a single large probe that provides for static and dynamic imaging. Fig. 4 shows such a camera and Fig. 5 is an image of a normal liver obtained with this instrument and technetium sulfur colloid (Tc-99m) as the radiopharmaceutical.

With this camera, dynamic functions such as the arrival and uptake of technetium-99m sulfur colloid by liver Kupffer cells or the removal and excretion of iodohippurate sodium I-131 by the nephrons can be studied. The scintillation camera also visualizes metabolic processes as for example the metabolism of a labeled amino acid such as selenomethionine Se 75, the analog of methionine, which is used by the pancreas to form zymogen granules, etc.

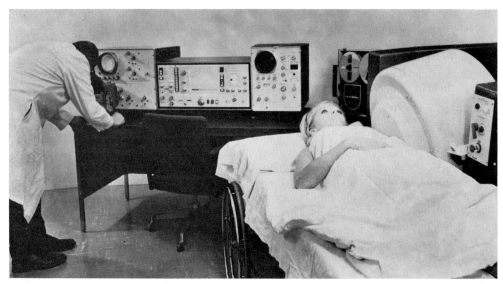

Fig. 4—Anger Camera with electronic controls. Patient is positioned for left lateral lung study (courtesy, *Picker Nuclear*).

Radiopharmaceutics

The scope of radioactive tracer methodology is summarized in Table 1. Appendix A includes the presently and generally used radiopharmaceuticals for diagnostic purposes. There are many others in less-common use and still others in various stages of acceptance which will be added to these lists at some later time. Some of the present ones will be deleted as new agents with superior properties are devised by radiopharmaceutical scientists and clinicians.

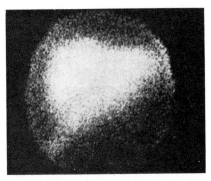

Fig. 5—Picture of a liver, obtained with an Anger Camera; time of exposure, 5 min (courtesy, *Picker Nuclear*).

Appendix B includes radiopharmaceuticals used in nuclear medicine for therapeutic purposes. These are designed to yield a definite quantity of radiation *in situ* for the purpose of destroying cells which are hypersecretory or neoplastic. The doses are variable and are calculated by the therapist so as to achieve a desired result.

Dosage Forms

These comprise the following physical forms:

1. Gases like ^{85}Kr and ^{133}Xe. These gases may also be dissolved in sterile apyrogenic normal saline solution, for injection.
2. Liquids, including solutions of radiopharmaceuticals for oral administration which may be sterile and contain a bacteriostat or consist of sterile, apyrogenic solutions for parenteral use, in single- or multiple-dose vials.
3. Colloidal solutions, which are suspensoids of particles in the range of 10–500 nm. Gold Au 198 colloid contains particles about 25 nm (nanometer) in size.
4. Suspensoids of particle size of 500 nm to about 1 μm (micrometer) properly referred to as "microaggregates."
5. Suspensoids of particles of sizes up to 50 μm or somewhat larger, referred to as "aggregates" or "macroaggregates," used for capillary blockade.
6. Microspheres which are spherical aggregates in a range of sizes of 0.5–50 μm, generally produced by heat denaturation of biodegradable sub-

Table 1—Scope of Radioactive Tracer Methodology

Isotope dilution	*Diffusion and flow*	*Metabolic studies*
The determination of total body water.	Various cellular membrane and tissue absorption and permeabilities	Normal and abnormal metabolism of endogenous and exogenous compounds such as amino acids, proteins, carbohydrates, lipids, and minerals
Estimation of body tritium contamination.	Simple diffusion	
Exchangeable sodium and potassium	Compartmental localizations	
Exchangeable anions such as chloride ion.	Active transport	Metabolism, conjugation, and excretion of drugs and hormones
Blood volume	Cellular sequestration	
Measurement of hormonal secretion	Cardiac output	
	Cerebral, hepatic, and renal blood flow	
	Spatial distribution (organ and wholebody scanning).	

stances. They are normally suspended in sterile normal saline for parenteral injection and used for specific capillary blockade.

7. Capsules of hardened gelatin either containing some solid in which is absorbed the radiopharmaceutical, or having the radiopharmaceutical evaporated on the inner surface, as in the case of sodium iodide I 123 or I 131. Oily liquid radiopharmaceuticals are dispensed in this manner.

8. Therapeutic radiopharmaceuticals in solid forms such as beads, seeds, wires and plaques, and applicators are used. The reader is referred to *Radiopharmacy* (see *Bibliography*) for a fuller description of dosage forms.

Pharmaceutics of Radioactive Solutions—Such solutions for parenteral use must be dispensed with regard to sterility, apyrogenicity, freedom from spicules, fibers and flakes, as are nonradioactive solutions. Since some solutions are "carrier-free," they must not contain more than a trace of the stable counterpart of the radioactive component or of a chemically similar element which may compete physiologically with the radioactive element.

All glassware used to contain the solution must be sterile, apyrogenic, and scrupulously clean to prevent adsorption of the trace quantities of the radioactive substance. In some instances, the surface of the glassware must be "saturated" with the nonradioactive analog to prevent adsorption of the radioactive constituent.

Sterility is most frequently obtained by membrane filtration using sterile, disposable, plastic filters to minimize metallic or siliceous contact.

Since many radiopharmaceuticals are light-sensitive, they must be stored in dark bottles or kept within their lead containers. Heat-sensitive substances should be stored in their lead containers at 4°C or frozen, as specified by the manufacturer.

All materials are to be used within the expiration date stated by the manufacturer on the label and stored as specified.

Doses are calculated with due regard to the half-life of the radionuclide as described earlier. Plastic, disposable, sterile syringes are most desirable for withdrawing doses. Forcing unsterile air into sterile multiple-dose vials is most undesirable since many solutions do not contain bacterial preservatives and, in addition, oxidation may be engendered.

Many of the newer radiopharmaceuticals are now available as "kits." These contain all the ingredients in a lyophilized form for greater stability and the avoidance of chemical interaction and require only the addition of the radionuclide and simple mixing or simple manipulation to form the radiopharmaceutical. Some are not heated or sterilized by filtration so that it is imperative that they be prepared aseptically. Sterility-testing of representative preparations should be performed to substantiate the technique. The final reconstituted product has a finite "shelf-life" and should be used within that time, according to the manufacturer's recommendations. These kits are used mainly to prepare radiopharmaceuticals for imaging or radioassays.

Quality Control—This is best illustrated by reference to two typical USP radiopharmaceuticals. In the case of Chlormerodrin Hg 197 Injection USP, part of the mercury contained is that of the radioactive nuclide ^{197}Hg. The monograph, in addition to other requirements, indicates that radioactive dosage is to be calculated with regard to the half-life of the radionuclide, namely 64.8 hours. The radiochemical purity is determined by paper chromatography. The radionuclidic purity is determined by gamma-ray spectrometry. The assay for radioactivity is conducted in accordance with recommendations of the USP.

The second example is the monograph for Sodium Pertechnetate Tc 99m Solution USP. The monograph discusses the nuclear preparation of the parent radionuclide, ^{99}Mo, from which the daughter radionuclide, ^{99m}Tc is formed by spontaneous decay. The "m" indicating metastability whereby the ^{99m}Tc with a half-life of 6 hours decays to ^{99}Tc. The radionuclide identification is given as well as the means of determination of other radionuclidic impurities. If the ^{99m}Tc is prepared by elution from the parent nuclide on an alumina column in a generator, tests are prescribed for the determination of aluminum and the presence of ^{99}Mo in the eluate.

The solution of Sodium Pertechnetate Tc 99m meets the requirements of sterility and other criteria for an injectable solution.

In the case of colloidal and particulate radiopharmaceuticals, particle size is an important requirement for their proper use.

The Radiopharmacy—The physical environment where the preparation, dispensing, and quality control of radiopharmaceuticals is to be performed is the Radiopharmacy, which must be developed, based on the following special areas for: receiving, storing, and compounding radioactive materials; quality control; dispensing; and bookkeeping and accounting.

It should be stressed that these six areas do not each represent a room but identified spaces for the tasks specified.

To test/meet its objectives, the location and equipment of a Radiopharmacy should consider the following parameters:

1. The environment where this work takes place needs to be properly ventilated so that radioactive materials cannot be airborne from this environment to other nonoccupationally unrestricted areas.

2. The environment must be properly shielded so that radiation cannot be impinging upon persons and/or objects in surrounding environments.

3. The environment must be properly located so that the receipt and dispersal of radioactive materials will not result in inadvertent and undesired contamination of other nonoccupationally labeled areas.

4. The area must be designed in such a manner that radioactive materials can be contained in given areas to ensure adequate safety and protection to personnel working in them and to ensure proper operation of the corresponding assay equipment.

5. The environment must be constructed, operated and designed in such a manner that no one radioactive material can contaminate another material and therefore vitiate and adulterate other potential drugs or drug ingredients, radioactive or not.

Certain equipment is necessary and desirable, e.g., proper hoods, including a laminar flow hood, to properly contain and handle radioactive material and protect the personnel. A chemical hood is only necessary when handling volatile products or material that can become airborne, while a small laminar flow hood is desirable for the dispensing and product preparation process (Fig. 6).

Quality-control equipment should include a microscope for particle size determination, chromatographic tools for assessing radiochemical purity, a scintillation counter for quantitation and determination of radionuclidic purity, a dose calibrator for verification of the quantity of activity dispensed, and adequate health physics instruments for evaluating any spillage and contamination.

One key to success of a Radiopharmacy is the development of a good system and organization. Forms should be preprinted for all routine procedures, with a minimum of information to be filled in. Inasmuch as most radiopharmaceuticals are normally prepared between 7 and 10 a.m., to be dispensed throughout the day, the late morning and afternoon are ideal to prepare all needed materials for the next day.

Regulatory Aspects

According to the Food, Drug, and Cosmetic Act, any agent intended for the diagnosis, mitigation, or treatment of disease in humans or other animals is labeled a drug. When, in 1963, the Congress adopted the Kefauver-Harris amendment to the Act, there were very few radiodiagnostic agents that were in use at that time, and the Food and Drug Administration (FDA) made an agreement with the Atomic Energy Commission (AEC) to exempt for a short period of time, those radiodiagnostic agents from the full implementation of the Act, provided the AEC undertook full regulation both of the pharmaceutical as well as the radiation safety aspects. This exemption has been completely lifted as of 1975, and radiopharmaceuticals are now under the same jurisdiction of the FDA as are any other drugs. As with any specialized drug, special considerations do apply. From a regulatory point of view, persons working in radiopharmacy have to consider their responsibility and involvement with the following federal and state regulatory bodies:

1. All aspects concerning radiological health and safety must obey the corresponding regulations on radiological health and safety developed by the Nuclear Regulatory Commission and the corresponding state agreement agencies, in those states which are agreement states.
2. All radiopharmaceuticals must comply with the regulations specifically developed for radiopharmaceuticals by FDA and the corresponding

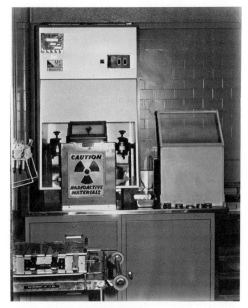

Fig. 6—Laminar flow hood for preparing and dispensing radiopharmaceuticals.

State Bureaus of Food and Drug (usually part of a state Department of Health).
3. Transport of radiopharmaceuticals and radioactive materials must comply with Department of Transportation regulations of transport of radioactive materials for medical use, as well as with the corresponding regulations of the Nuclear Regulatory Commission.

One of the unique aspects of radiopharmaceuticals is that radiopharmaceuticals are in general agents prepared extemporaneously in a hospital and administered to the patient within minutes or at most a few hours after preparation. It is therefore incumbent upon the pharmacist to satisfy himself that the material administered to the patient meets the highest standards of quality, safety, and efficacy.

Dispensing

Training of a Radiopharmacist

Radiopharmacy is a relatively new specialty and formal training of such individuals was developed at the University of Southern California in 1968 in a graduate program leading to the Master of Science in Radiopharmacy degree. Such training involves the acquisition of knowledge in radiation physics, radiological health, safe operation of radioisotope laboratories, radiation chemistry, radiation biology, radiochemistry, synthesis and metabolism of labeled compounds, radiopharmaceutics, dosimetry, and elements of nuclear medicine, as well as practical experience in the synthesis of labeled compounds, operation, and handling of radiation-detection instrumentation, preparation and use of radiopharmaceuticals, and operation of a radiopharmacy service. Since 1968, other programs have developed and several alternatives exist according to the intensity in which a pharmacist will be dedicated to radiopharmacy. Most schools of pharmacy now provide some introduction to radiopharmacy as part of the overall curriculum in pharmacy. Other institutions provide a short-term intense specialization for pharmacists in radiopharmacy with limited objectives, while a few institutions provide specialized training towards an advanced degree. Full information of those activities can be obtained either from the American Association of Colleges of Pharmacy or from the authors.

References

1. Blahd, WH, ed: *Nuclear Medicine,* 2nd ed, McGraw-Hill, New York, Fig. 10-11(a), 232, 1971.
2. *Ibid,* Fig. 10-9, 231.

Bibliography

Andrews GA, Kniseley RM, Wagner HN Jr, eds: *Radioactive Pharmaceuticals,* USAEC, Oak Ridge, TN, 1966.
Blahd WH, ed: *Nuclear Medicine,* 2nd ed, McGraw-Hill, New York, 1971.
Freeman LM, Johnson PM, eds: *Clinical Scintillation Scanning,* Hoeber (Harper & Row), New York, 1969.
Hahn PF, ed: *Therapeutic Uses of Artificial Radioisotopes,* Wiley, New York, 1956.
Lawrence JH: *Polycythemia: Physiology, Diagnosis and Treatment,* Grune & Stratton, New York, 1955.
Silver S: *Medicine,* 3rd ed, Lea & Febiger, Philadelphia, 1968.
Silver S: *Radioactive Nuclides in Medicine and Biology: Medicine,* 3rd ed, Lea & Febiger, Philadelphia, 1968.
Tubis M, Wolf W, eds: *Radiopharmacy,* Wiley-Interscience, New York, 1976.
The United States Pharmacopeia, 19th rev, Mack Publ. Co., Easton, PA, 1975.

Appendix A—Radiopharmaceuticals Used in Diagnostic Procedures

Radio-nuclide	Radiopharmaceutical form[a]	Nuclear medicine use	Dose[b] (μCi)
^{82}Br	Sodium bromide Br 82	Extracellular water measurement, exchangeable chloride	20—50
^{131}Cs	Cesium chloride Cs 131	Myocardial scanning, peripheral circulation studies, tumor localization	1250
^{51}Cr	Chromated Cr 51 serum albumin	Gastrointestinal protein loss studies	30—50
	Sodium Chromate Cr 51 USP	Red cell mass and volume	10—25
		Red cell survival studies	100—200
		Spleen scanning	100—300
		Placental scanning	10—20
^{57}Co	Cyanocobalamin USP	Pernicious anemia and malabsorption syndromes	0.25—1
^{58}Co	Cyanocobalamin	Same	0.25—1
^{60}Co	Cyanocobalamin	Same	0.25—1
^{64}Cu	Cupric acetate Cu 64	Copper metabolism	1000 (orally) 100—1000 (IV)
	Cupric acetate Cu 64	Wilson's disease	
^{67}Cu	Ceruloplasmin Cu 67	Enteric protein loss	20
^{18}F	Sodium fluoride F 18	Bone scanning	1000
^{67}Ga	Gallium citrate Ga 67	Staging of Hodgkin's disease Tumor localization Tumor scanning	1500—3000
^{198}Au	Gold Au 198 (colloidal)	Liver scanning	100—150
^{113m}I	Indium DTPA In 113m	Brain scanning	10,000
	Indium "stabilized" at pH 3.5	Cardiac scanning	2000
		Placental scanning	1000
	Indium In 113m-iron hydroxide colloid	Liver scanning	1000
		Spleen scanning	3000
^{113m}I	Indium sulfide macroaggregate In 113m ("In SMA")	Lung scanning	3000
^{111}In	Indium phosphate In 111	Cerebrospinal fluid scanning	200—1000
^{111}In	Indium chloride In 111 sterile solution	Scintigraphy of bone marrow and localization of soft tissue tumors	2000—5000
^{111}In	Indium 111 bleomycin	Detection of soft tissue tumors	5000
^{123}I	Sodium iodohippurate I 123	Renal function	1000
		Renal imaging	2000
^{125}I	Insulin I 125	Determination of bound and free insulin	—
	Iodinated I 125 Serum Albumin USP	Blood volume	3—20
		Cardiac output	20—40
	Sodium iothalamate I 125	Glomerular filtration rate and renal plasma flow	50—100
^{131}I	Iodinated I 131 serum albumin	Blood volume	3—20
		Brain tumor scanning	300—500
		Cardiac output	10—30
		Cardiac blood pool scanning	300—400
		Placental localization	3—5
		Albumin metabolism	100
	Iodinated I 131 serum albumin aggregated	Liver and spleen scanning	300—1000
	Iodinated I 131 serum albumin macroaggregated	Lung scanning	300—500
	Oleic acid I 131	Fat absorption studies	25—50
	Sodium Iodide I 131 Capsules USP	Thyroid uptake studies	2—20
	Sodium Iodide I 131 Solution USP	Thyroid gland scanning	25—200
	Iodohippurate Sodium I 131 USP	Kidney function studies	10—50
	Rose Bengal Sodium I 131 USP	Liver function test	20—50
		Liver scanning	100—300

Appendix A—*Continued*

Radio nuclide	Radiopharmaceutical form[a]	Nuclear medicine use	Dose[b] (μCi)
	Sulfobromophthalein sodium I 131	Liver function	10–25
		Liver scanning	70–200
	Triolein I 131	Fat absorption	25–50
^{59}Fe	Ferrous citrate Fe 59	Iron absorption and metabolism	5–20
^{85}Kr	Krypton 85	Cardiac and extracardiac shunts	100–400
^{28}Mg	Magnesium chloride Mg 28	Magnesium metabolism	60–80
^{197}Hg	Chlormerodrin Hg 197 USP	Brain scanning	700–1000
^{203}Hg	Chlormerodrin Hg 203	Kidney scanning	100–200
^{32}P	Sodium Phosphate P 32 USP	Detection of eye tumors	250–500
^{42}K	Potassium chloride K 42	Distribution and metabolism of potassium	100–300
^{75}Se	Selenomethionine Se 75	Pancreas scanning	100–250
^{22}Na	Sodium chloride Na 22	Distribution and metabolism of sodium	3–10
^{85}Sr	Strontium chloride or nitrate Sr 85	Bone scanning	50–100
^{87m}Sr	Strontium nitrate Sr 87m	Bone cancer studies	1000–4000
^{99m}Tc	Serum albumin Tc 99m	Cardiac blood pool scanning	2000–5000
		Placental scanning	500–1000
^{99m}Tc	Technetium pyrophosphate Kit form containing lyophilized stannous pyrophosphate under nitrogen to which is added sodium pertechnetate Tc 99m solution	Bone scanning	to 15,000
	Serum Albumin Tc 99m Aggregated USP	Lung scanning	1000–3000
	Serum albumin microspheres	Lung scanning	2000–4000
	Technetium-penicillamine-acetazolamide complex Tc 99m (TPAC)	Renal imaging	3000–15,000
	Technetium penicillamine Tc 99m	Cholescintigraphic agent	3000
	Sodium Pertechnetate Tc 99m USP	Brain scanning	5000–15,000
		Thyroid scanning	1000–3000
	Technetium Tc 99m Sulfur Colloid USP	Liver and spleen scanning	1000–3000
^{3}H	Tritiated water	Measurement of body water	150–300
^{133}Xe	Xenon Xe 133 as a gas or in solution in 0.9% NaCl solution	Lung scanning, perfusion, and ventilation studies	1000
		Cerebral blood flow	1000
^{169}Xe	Ytterbium DTPA Yb 169	Cisternographic agent	1000
		Brain scanning	10,000

In this tabulation are listed the most frequently used radiopharmaceuticals for diagnostic nuclear purposes, arranged in the alphabetical order of the radionuclide. There are included some which have been used experimentally and which may not be in general use.

[a]USAN names are used where available.

[b]The doses are variable and only approximate and are determined according to the equipment and technique used.

Note: Other tables of radiopharmaceuticals used for special organ imaging (see *Clinical Scintillation Scanning* in the *Bibliography*) and an extensive table listing a great variety of agents, some of which have been used previously and many which have been used experimentally (see *Nuclear Medicine* in the *Bibliography*) are suggested to the reader.

Appendix B—Radiopharmaceuticals Used in Therapeutic Nuclear Medicine[a]

Radio-nuclide	Radiopharmaceutical Form [b]	Therapeutic Use or Nuclear Medical Use	Dose (mCi)
[125]I	Sodium iodide I 125	Hyperthyroidism	2.5–6.0
[131]I⁻	Sodium iodide I 131	Cardiac disease	25–50 in divided doses
		Hyperthyroidism	2–10
		Thyroid cancer	75–150
[32]P	Sodium phosphate P 32	Chronic leukemia (lymphatic or myeloid)	1–2/week
		Polycythemia vera	3–8
		Metastatic bone cancer	10–15 in divided doses
	Chromic phosphate P 32	Treatment of peritoneal effusions	9–12
		Treatment of pleural effusions	6–9
[198]Au	Gold Au 198	Treatment of peritoneal effusions	50–150
		Treatment of pleural effusions	35–75
	Gold Au 198 seeds or wires	Interstitial implantation into tumors	Variable
[60]Co	Cobalt Co 60 needles, wires, or seeds	Interstitial implantation into tumors	Variable
[90]Sr	Strontium 90 applicators	Treatment of ophthalmological lesions	Variable
[192]Ir	Iridium 192 seeds	Interstitial tumor irradiation	Variable
[182]Ta	Tantalum Ta 182 needles	Bladder tumors	Variable

[a]Arranged in order of their probable frequency of use.
[b]USAN names used where applicable.

13

Compounding and dispensing information

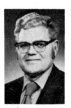

Jack K. Dale, PhD
Vice President/Quality
Control
Carter-Glogau Laboratories-
Chromalloy Pharmaceuticals
Glendale, AZ 85301

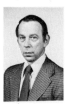

Roger E. Booth, PhD
Manager, Control Records
and Services
The Upjohn Co.
Kalamazoo, MI 49001

The vital importance of educating the physician, pharmacist, and even the patient to the hazards and confusion which may arise from multiple drug therapy has been pointed out by many authors. Investigators have found instances where the same patient over a relatively short period of time took as many as 24 different prescriptions, sometimes prescribed by the same physician and even dispensed by the same pharmacist. In many cases the prescribed drugs were contraindicated or were simultaneously additive or antagonistic among themselves and various over-the-counter (OTC) preparations also being taken. This situation can be corrected if the pharmacist involved has access to proper compounding and dispensing information.

In the past, prescription ingredients were considered to be incompatible (undesirable) in a combination prescribed if they adversely affected appearance, elegance, safety, or therapeutic efficacy. Modern usage recognizes that in addition to the physical, chemical, and therapeutic incompatibilities which may occur in compounding and dispensing prescriptions, other types of drug interactions may also occur with untoward results as for example when a patient takes a pharmaceutical preparation which interacts with another drug or other exogenous chemical already present in the body. Actually, these and other pharmaceutical interactions may occur at any stage during the formulation, manufacture, packaging, prescribing, compounding, dispensing, or administration of drugs, and may be complicated further by drug interactions in the patient.

In this discussion background information and theory helpful in compounding and dispensing the more common drug types or families will be presented first. This will be followed at the end of the chapter by individual monographs containing more specific information on the official USP and NF items and on the top 500 drugs. These monographs are arranged alphabetically by official name where available. Drug combinations are usually listed by the most common trade name. Other important entries can be located through the index.

Compounding Theory

Since the previous chapters have covered the principles of compounding each dosage form or type separately, this discussion will be limited chiefly to problem-type prescriptions and their solutions.

Physical and chemical incompatibilities are less common in prescriptions presented today since the bulk of current prescriptions are for manufactured products. Almost ninety-eight per cent (97.7%) of all prescriptions have been estimated to be "count out or pour out" items which require no compounding. The wide-spread use of single unit packages has also contributed to a reduction in incompatibility difficulties. When the physician wishes to add a second or third item to the therapy, he frequently writes additional prescriptions. Even when the prescriber does add several items to a manufactured product, he frequently follows a sample prescription supplied by the manufacturer or reported in the literature.

Despite this trend the pharmacist must still be prepared to handle any combination which is prescribed. He should accordingly become familiar with each new product as it is introduced and learn the pharmacologic activity of each ingredient and the potential physical, chemical, and therapeutic incompatibilities. The manufacturer's representative should be consulted for information that is not available either in the current literature or on the package or insert. Keeping up-to-date is vital since the pharmacist should be able to point out to the physician any therapeutic or other incompatibility, even if two or three different prescriptions are involved.

Drug interactions and incompatibilities are easier to prevent than to correct. Recognizing a potential incompati-

bility before it is compounded may save time, material, and money. On the other hand, it is just as important not to imagine incompatibilities which do not exist.

In cases of real doubt it is usually best to check the suspected incompatibility or interaction in a reference work and then, if still in doubt, to fill the prescription as written. This procedure is suggested since it is often possible to correct an incompatibility after it appears. This may be done, for example, by increasing the volume and dose, by adding a suitable solvent and increasing the dose, by adding an appropriate suspending agent and dispensing with a "Shake Well" label, or by adopting another procedure acceptable to the physician. Where very expensive or very scarce drugs are involved, it may be preferable to prepare a small trial prescription. See Table 1.

Some prescriptions which contain obvious drug incompatibilities may be intended by the physician. For example, in R 1 the white precipitate of zinc polysulfides which occurs when solutions of zinc sulfate and sulfurated potash are combined is an expected or intentional incompatibility.

1

R	$ZnSO_4$	4 g
	Sulfurated Potash	4 g
	Water qs. ad	100 ml
	M. Ft. lotion	

In other cases a precipitate may form which the physician did not anticipate, e.g., in R 2 the precipitation of free phenobarbital due to the acidity of the elixir lactated pepsin is very likely an unintentional incompatibility since it may produce erratic dosage unless dispensed with a "shake well before use" label.

2

| R | Sodium phenobarbital | gr. vi |
| | Elixir lactated pepsin   q.s. ad fl. oz. | 1 |

Most types of intentional incompatibilities are so common that there is no question as to the intent of the physician. These prescriptions are usually

Table 1—Summary of Common Incompatibilities with Recommended Corrections

Consult the physician if incompatibility appears to be unintentional. Fill "secundum artem" if incompatibility is intentional. These recommended corrections apply only to dispensing where the prescription will be used in a short time (i.e., about 1 month). Incompatibilities in manufactured products are handled differently.

Recommended Procedure:	Therapeutic		Physical						Chemical				
	Overdosage, underdosage, wrong drug, etc. (c)	Incomplete solution	Precipitation (a)	Separation of immiscible liquid	Liquefaction of solid ingredient	Gelatinization or solidification	Unpalatable	Precipitate or "oil" formation (a)	Effervescence (a)(b)	Color change (a)	Decomposition or oxidation or reduction (b)	Hydrolysis or other delayed incompatibilities (a)	Production or toxic substances
1. Consult physician (c)	●	—	—	—	—	—	○	○	○	●	●	●	●
2. Use special pharm. technique													
a. ▲ Modify order of mixing	—	●	●	●	●	—	—	—	—	●	○	○	—
b. ▲ Dispense with "shake well" label	—	○	○	○	●	○	—	—	—	—	—	—	—
c. ▲ Dispense with "store in refrigerator" label	—	—	—	—	—	—	○	○	—	—	●	●	—
d. ▲ Allow to react then package	—	—	○	—	—	—	—	—	○	●	○	○	—
e. ▲ Protect from air, light, or moisture	—	—	—	—	—	—	—	—	○	○	○	○	—
3. Addition of an ingredient (c)													
a. ▲ Add suspending agent	—	○	●	—	—	—	○	○	—	○	○	○	○
b. ▲ Add emulsifying agent	—	○	—	●	—	—	—	○	—	—	—	—	—
c. Add solubilizer or miscibility agent	—	●	○	○	—	—	—	○	—	—	—	—	—
d. Add diluent and correct dose	—	●	—	—	—	—	—	○	—	—	—	—	—
e. ▲ Add stiffener or softener	—	—	—	—	●	○	○	—	—	—	—	—	○
f. ▲ Add stabilizer (buffer, antioxidant, preservative, etc)	—	—	○	—	—	—	—	—	○	—	●	●	—
g. Add dye, flavor, perfume	—	—	—	—	—	—	○	—	—	—	—	○	○
4. Omission of an ingredient (c)													
a. Leave out troublesome ingredient	—	○	○	○	—	—	○	○	—	—	—	○	—
b. Filter off inactive sediment	—	○	○	—	—	—	○	○	—	—	—	—	—
c. Divide into two prescriptions	—	○	○	—	—	—	○	○	—	—	—	—	—
5. Change of vehicle (c)													
a. Increase volume, increase dose	○	○	○	○	—	—	○	○	○	—	—	—	—
b. Decrease volume, decrease dose	○	○	○	○	—	—	○	○	—	—	—	—	—
c. Change solvent, same dose	○	○	○	○	—	—	○	○	○	—	—	—	—
6. Change of ingredient (c)													
a. ▲ Use form most compatible with other ingredients	—	●	●	●	●	●	○	●	●	●	●	●	●
b. ▲ Use form soluble in vehicle	—	●	●	●	—	○	—	○	○	—	○	○	○
c. ▲ Use form stable in vehicle	—	●	●	●	—	○	○	○	○	○	○	○	○
7. Change in dosage form (c)													
a. Use more suitable dosage form	—	○	○	○	○	○	○	○	○	○	○	○	○
b. Use different brand	—	○	○	○	○	○	●	○	○	○	○	○	○

(a) Slow changes in appearance and gas formation may be due to growth of microorganism (i.e., yeasts, molds, etc).

(b) Beware of explosions!

(c) Consult physician if therapeutically significant drug or dosage change is required. ▲ "Secundum artem" procedure usually not requiring physician's prior approval.

● = Preferred procedure. ○ = Acceptable procedure. — = Procedure not applicable.

dispensed as written. Unintentional incompatibilities, on the other hand, must always be corrected. The ability of the pharmacist to interpret the doctor's intentions properly is thus fully as important as his ability to correct an incompatibility. The pharmacist can often gain insight as to the prescriber's intent by adroit questioning of the patient and by a careful study of the directions in both the subscription and the signature as they apply to the formula prescribed. If there is still any doubt, he should call the physician.

Incompatibilities of the physical and chemical types may be either instantaneous or delayed. Most instantaneous incompatibilities are recognized by visible changes such as effervescence or precipitation. Complexation and other reactions may occur which are not readily visible. The same considerations apply concerning visibility relative to delayed incompatibilities. Commonly, the timing of a recognizable change classifies the incompatibility.

In 1962 it was estimated that 4,200,000 incompatibilities occurred among the 800,000,000 prescription orders that were filled each year. Since that time, however, more and more prescription orders have been written for dosage forms prefabricated by pharmaceutical manufacturers and, therefore, incompatibilities have declined. Nonetheless, it is still obvious that one of the responsibilities of the pharmacist is to recognize and to properly handle all types of incompatibilities so that only safe and effective medications are dispensed to the patient.

Physical Incompatibilities

Physical incompatibilities usually cause nonuniform, unsightly, or unpalatable mixtures which possess the potential danger of nonuniform dosage. The proper application of the principles described should help the pharmacist predict possible incompatibilities and to transform such prescriptions into safe, pharmaceutically elegant preparations.

Physical or pharmaceutical incompatibilities may be classified into the following types.

Incomplete Solution—When two or more substances are combined, they may not give a homogeneous product due to immiscibility or insolubility. Thus, silicones are immiscible with water, gums are insoluble in alcohol, and resins are insoluble in water. Sometimes the physician may prescribe the wrong or insufficient solvent or vehicle. The use of heat is usually objectionable, except to make slowly soluble substances dissolve more rapidly, because there is danger of forming a clear solution (at a high temperature) which will deposit crystals on cooling. If the undissolved material is not beneficial or is definitely objectionable, it may be permissible to remove it by filtration, but in all doubtful cases the physician should be advised regarding the situation and his approval secured before any radical steps are taken.

3

Ŗ Terpin Hydrate   3 g
    Simple Syrup   q.s. ad   120 ml
    M. Sol.

The terpin hydrate is not soluble in this vehicle. Half of the syrup may be replaced by alcohol, or isoalcoholic elixir (40%) may be used as a solvent. This low potency drug may also be suspended with acacia, tragacanth, or Methocel and dispensed with a shake label.

4

Ŗ Phenobarbital   250 mg
    Elixir Phenobarbital   q.s.   30 ml
    M. Soln.
    Sig: Teaspoonful at bedtime.

The excess phenobarbital is not all soluble in the elixir. Approximately 10 ml of the elixir must be replaced with alcohol to give a clear solution. This necessitates adding 40 mg more of phenobarbital as a solid so as to obtain the phenobarbital potency prescribed.

Precipitation—A substance is generally precipitated from its solution in one solvent if another solvent in which it is insoluble is added to the solution.

Thus, resins are often precipitated from alcoholic solution when water is added. Mucilaginous and albuminous substances and some metallic salts are frequently precipitated from aqueous solution when alcohol is added. Many substances may precipitate from a saturated solution when some other substance is dissolved in the solution; e.g., camphor and volatile oils are often "salted out" of aromatic waters when salts or metals are dissolved in the liquid. Boric acid is precipitated from a saturated solution when tragacanth is dissolved in the liquid. Colloidal solutions frequently show precipitation on the addition of electrolytes.

Separation of Immiscible Liquids— Oils dissolved in alcohol separate on the addition of water. Ethyl nitrite spirit separates and floats as a layer when a substantial proportion of potassium citrate is present in the prescription.

Such "salting out" and solubility phenomena are illustrated as follows:

5

℞	Chloral hydrate	15 g
	Sodium bromide	11.25 g
	Elixir Aromatic q.s. ad	60 ml

A mixture of chloral alcoholate, chloral, and alcohol is said to be salted out in such prescriptions by soluble bromides, etc. These appear as an immiscible layer and are dangerous if taken as one dose. Since clear solutions are formed above 50% alcohol or below 10% alcohol, this type of incompatibility can be solved by adding either water or alcohol. Since the sodium bromide is not soluble in 50% alcohol it is preferable to replace the elixir with water and syrup or add sufficient water (about 1 oz) to dilute the prescription below 10% alcohol. The physician should be informed.

Liquefaction of Solid Ingredients— Mixtures of solids sometimes liquefy due to the formation of eutectic mixtures or the liberation of water of hydration.

6

℞	Aminopyrine	0.3 g
	Codeine Sulfate	15 mg

	Belladonna extract	10 mg
	Acetylsalicylic acid	0.2 g
	M. ft. caps #1 D.T.D. #12	

This formula liquefies and becomes green within a few days. The liquefaction is due to a eutectic mixture formed by aminopyrine and acetylsalicylic acid. The green color is an intensification of the green color of the extract as it becomes wet. These changes can be avoided by incorporating one grain of light magnesium oxide or magnesium carbonate in each capsule. This diluent should be divided between the reacting ingredients, these combined with gentle trituration, and the remainder of the ingredients incorporated. Another method of filling such prescriptions is to allow the liquefaction to take place and then absorb the liquid on sufficient kaolin or magnesium carbonate to give a suitable capsule fill. Such prescriptions should be triturated until homogeneous, then encapsulated and placed in tightly-stoppered containers.

Incorrect Form Prescribed—A physician may prescribe an incorrect form for the most efficient preparation of the prescription. An alkaloidal salt to be dissolved in liquid petrolatum is an example. In such cases the free alkaloid should be prescribed since the free alkaloids are usually soluble in liquid petrolatum and the alkaloidal salts are insoluble in this solvent.

Chemical Incompatibilities

Chemical incompatibilities usually occur as a result of chemical interaction among the ingredients of a prescription. The usual chemical incompatibility occurs immediately upon compounding and is thus sometimes called an immediate incompatibility. Such incompatibilities are usually readily apparent due to effervescence, precipitation, or color changes. The incompatible mixtures should not be dispensed without correction, unless so intended by the physician.

Other mixtures which react to such a slight extent or at such a slow rate that no appreciable visible change occurs have been termed delayed incompatibilities. These may occur without immediate physical evidence of change. The delayed incompatibility may or may not result in loss of therapeutic activity.

A prescription containing a delayed incompatibility may be dispensed if the prescription will be used up before about 10% of the therapeutic activity is lost. The use of a "Store in a Refrigerator" label will often help decrease the rate of loss of activity in a product of this type. Such storage slows down hydrolysis, oxidation-reduction, or other chemical reactions which occur more rapidly at room temperature. A "Shake Well" label should be used where applicable to promote uniform dosage. If a potentially dangerous product results, the prescription should not be dispensed and the physician should be consulted.

It is possible to generalize by saying that ingredients with chemically similar active groups are usually compatible, while ingredients with different active groups will sometimes react. Drugs react like other organic and inorganic compounds. This is especially true if a high-energy system can form a more stable, low-energy system. Such reactions usually manifest themselves through the formation of precipitates, evolution of gas, addition or elimination of water, absorption or evolution of heat or formation of complexes or chelates.

A summary of the class reactions which monofunctional drugs commonly undergo in prescriptions are given in Tables 2 and 3. An understanding of these basic reactions will usually make it possible to predict the compatibility and stability of the active ingredients in simple mixtures. The compatibility of these ingredients is also discussed under the individual compound. This may help where the individual ingredients have several reactive groups and, hence, either do not fit a single general class pattern or may react in a number of ways. It is sometimes impossible to predict incompatibilities which may occur as a result of chemical interaction

of these official drugs with buffers, preservatives, suspending agents, stabilizers, and other ingredients which are not required by law to be disclosed on the label of manufactured drug products.

Chemical incompatibilities may be classified into the following types.

Oxidation—Although oxidation is chiefly a problem with stock solutions or inadequately formulated manufactured products, certain prescription mixtures may also oxidize if exposed to air, excessive storage temperatures, light, overdilution, incorrect pH adjustment, or presence of catalysts. Common catalysts include heavy metal ions such as ferric, ferrous, cupric or chromium, excess hydrogen or hydroxyl ions, bacterial or mold enzymes. Adrenalin (epinephrine), phenylephrine, isoproterenol, apomorphine, diamorphine, menadione sodium bisulfite, morphine sulfate, phentolamine, procainamide, noradrenaline (levarterenol), atropine, sodium aminosalicylate, sodium antimonyl tartrate, sodium aminohippurate, dextrose, sodium glutamate, procaine hydrochloride, and related compounds undergo oxidations activated by heat. These usually require special precautions against trace metal ion catalysts and/or use of an antioxidant such as ascorbic acid, sodium metabisulfite, or sodium sulfite for maximum stability. Sulfacetamide eye drops, sulfonamide injections, sodium aminohippurate, and phenylephrine oxidations may be activated by light and catalysts. Metal ion complexing agents such as disodium edetate and sodium calcium edetate are frequently useful here since they act as catalyst poisons or negative catalysts.

Oils and fats, phenolic substances, aldehydes and vitamins commonly undergo auto-oxidation, a chain-reaction type of oxidation, hence are sometimes used as antioxidants themselves. Auto-oxidation may be controlled by addition of still more reactive inhibitors to provide electrons and receive the excess energy possessed by the activated molecules. Propyl gallate, thymol, phenyl α-nap-

Table 2—Chemical Reactions Which May Occur in Prescriptions (Aqueous or Hydroalcoholic Type Vehicles)

Drug class	Oxidation	Photolysis	Hydrolysis	Addition	Polymerization	Cleavage	Reduction	Double decomposition	Esterification	Substitution	Neutralization
Hydrocarbons—saturated[l]	…	…	…	…	…	…	…	…	…	…	…
Hydrocarbons—unsaturated[l]	xx[a]	x	…	xx[b]	x	x	x	…	…	…	…
Halogenated hydrocarbons[l]	…	x	…	xx[c]	…	…	…	xx[e]	…	x[d]	…
Alcohols[l]	x	…	…	…	…	…	…	…	x	…	…
Halogenated alcohols[l]	x	…	…	…	…	…	x	…	x	…	…
Phenols[l]	xx[a]	x	…	…	x	…	…	…	x	x[n]	xx[h]
Aldehydes[l]	xx[a]	…	…	xx[f]	xx[g]	…	x	…	…	…	…
Ketones[l]	x	…	…	xx[f]	x	…	x	…	…	…	…
Carboxylic acids[l]	…	…	…	…	…	…	…	…	x	x	xx[h]
Esters[l]	xx[a]	x	xx	…	…	xx[i]	…	…	…	…	…
Ethers[l]	…	…	x	…	…	…	…	…	…	x	…
Amines—alkyl[l]	x	…	…	…	…	…	…	…	…	x	xx[m]
Amines—aryl[l]	xx[a]	x	…	…	…	…	x	…	…	x	xx[m]
Nitro compounds[l]	xx[a]	xx	…	…	x	x	x	…	…	x	…
Quaternary ammonium bases	…	…	…	…	…	…	…	…	…	…	xx[o]
Amino acids	…	…	…	…	x	…	…	…	…	…	xx[m]
Amides[l]	…	…	xx[j]	…	…	…	…	…	…	…	…
Sulfonic acids[l]	…	…	x	…	…	…	…	…	…	…	xx[k]
Carboxylic acid salts[l]	…	…	x	…	…	…	…	xx	…	…	xx
Amine salts	x	…	x	…	…	…	…	xx	…	…	…
Quaternary ammonium salts	…	…	…	…	…	…	…	xx	…	…	…

x, Possible reaction—doubtful under usual dispensing conditions.

xx, Common reaction—requires proper reactants and conditions.

[a] Cold dilute alkaline permanganate, chlorine, bromine, iodine in alcohol, ozone (air very slowly).

[b] HBr, HI, H_2SO_4, Hypohalous acid.

[c] Ammonia, amines.

[d] Alcoholic alkali forms alcohols.

[e] Aqueous alkali, sodium alcoholate, sodium or potassium salts of fatty acids, sodium nitrates.

[f] HCN, sodium bisulfate, ammonia.

[g] Calcium hydroxide, dilute NaOH, $ZnCl_2$.

[h] Hydrogen ion may be substituted by Na^+.

[i] Saponified by alkalies.

[j] Dilute acids, bases or nitrous acid replace NH_2 groups.

[k] Forms unstable salts with some acids, e.g., HCl.

[l] Usually immiscible or insoluble if over 4–6 carbons per hydrophilic group.

[m] Add acids to form acid salts.

[n] Substitution on para position possible with nitrous acid.

[o] Quaternary ammonium compounds are strong bases.

Table 3—Interreactions of Drug Classes

	Hydrocarbons, saturated	Hydrocarbons, unsaturated	Organic halogenated compounds	Alcohols	Phenols	Aldehydes	Ketones	Carboxylic acids	Esters	Ethers	Amines, aliphatic	Amines, aromatic	Quaternary ammonium bases	Nitro compounds	Amino acids	Amides	Carboxylic acid salts	Amine salts	Quaternary ammonium salts
Hydrocarbons, saturated																			
Hydrocarbons, unsaturated																			
Organic halogenated compounds											x	x					x		
Alcohols						x			x										
Phenols				x										x					
Aldehydes									x		x	x		x	x				
Ketones						x		x			x	x							
Carboxylic acids						x	x				x	x	x						
Esters				x		x	x												
Ethers																			
Amines, aliphatic			x																
Amines, aromatic			x		x														
Quaternary ammonium bases				x															
Nitro compounds				x		x									x				
Amino acids																			
Amines			x					x	xx									xx	
Carboxylic acid salts								x											
Amino salts		x															xx		
Quaternary ammonium salts																	xx		xx
Acids (pKₐ −2 to +2)						x		x	x		xx	xx	xx	x	x	xx	xx	xx	xx
Bases (pKᵦ −2 to +2)			xx		x			xx	xx	I	I	I		x	x	xx		xx	xx
Water	I	I	I	I	I	I	I	I	I	I	I	I		I		I			

x, Possible reactions—doubtful under usual dispensing conditions.
xx, Common reaction, may not always be obvious (or undesirable).
I, Usually immiscible or insoluble if drug has more than 4–6 carbons per hydrophilic group.

thylamine, butylated hydroxyanisole, butylated hydroxytoluene, hydroquinone, or similar antioxidants usually act in this way in oily solutions.

Reduction—Reduction reactions are less common in prescriptions although silver, mercury, and gold salts may be reduced by light to the metallic form.

Racemization—Racemization, the conversion of an optically active form to an optically inactive form without changing chemical constitution, usually produces reduced pharmacological activity. Such reactions have been reported with adrenaline, dextroamphetamine, methamphetamine, norephedrine, ephedrine, methylephedrine, noradrenaline, etc.

Precipitation—When two or more pharmaceuticals are combined, a chemical change may take place with the formation of an insoluble substance which precipitates from solution. Flocculent precipitates which develop several days after a stock solution or prescription is prepared may be due to delayed incompatibilities but more frequently are evidence of the growth of yeasts, molds, or bacteria. Such growth may be due indirectly to a chemical incompatibility if the preservative system is inactivated by a chemical reaction.

Evolution of a Gas—A gas may be formed by chemical reaction between ingredients. Examples are the effervescence caused by the liberation of carbon dioxide resulting from the reaction of carbonates and acids in aqueous media, and decomposition of syrups of paraaminosalicylic acid.

Color Changes—Various types of chemical changes may result in alterations in color. For example, the laxative phenolphthalein is colorless in acid solution but purple in alkaline mixtures.

Explosive Combinations—Oxidizing agents are chemically incompatible with reducing agents (oxidation-reduction reactions). Serious explosions may result from certain combinations. In some cases an explosion may not be likely, but the chemical change may not be in accord with the intent of the physician.

Cementation—In some cases all or part of the ingredients of a prescription may set into a mass of cement-like hardness. This sometimes occurs when compounds form hydrates (e.g., plaster of paris), polymerize, or convert to new crystal forms.

Separation of Immiscible Liquids—Immiscible liquids not soluble in the prescription may form as a result of chemical reaction. For example, chloral hydrate may separate as a layer of insoluble chloral alcoholate in vehicles containing 10–50% alcohol and large amounts of certain soluble salts.

Gelatinization—Solutions may form a gel when combined with certain substances. Thus, acacia solutions are gelatinized by ferric salts since acacia possesses carboxyl groups which may be cross-linked by trivalent ferric ions to form polymer chains. Collodion is gelatinized by phenol, probably by a related bonding reaction. Generally speaking, this type of incompatibility is rarely encountered.

Development of Heat or Cold—Some chemical reactions take place with either the liberation or absorption of considerable amounts of heat. Prescriptions undergoing such reactions should be carefully studied to determine if the activity is affected.

It is important to notice that most chemical reactions which take place spontaneously at room temperature do so with evolution of heat. Note also that systems tend to change spontaneously to another system of greater stability (although the more stable end product may be inactive as a drug). Stable systems can be changed to unstable systems by transfusions of free energy. Thus, compounds which are formed with evolution of heat tend to decompose when the temperature is raised, i.e.:

$$A + B \rightleftarrows C + \text{Heat (law of chemical equilibrium)}$$

Conversely compounds requiring heat for their formation are more stable at higher temperatures.

Hydrolytic Changes—Many substances tend to hydrolyze in water and the change may be hastened by heat, catalysts, hydrogen ions, and hydroxyl ions. Especially susceptible are esters, amides, certain metals (Zn, Fe), etc.

Invisible Changes—Chemical change may occur without formation of a precipitate, evolution of a gas, a color change, or any other visible evidence of the reaction. If such changes destroy or change the therapeutic effect, they are just as undesirable as visible changes. Naturally, such incompatibilities are the most likely to be overlooked. Therefore, adequate training of the pharmacist is needed.

Development of Poisonous Substances—Chemical reaction between two substances may produce products which are much more toxic than the original substances; thus, potassium iodide and calomel in presence of moisture react to form a toxic mercuric salt as one of the products.

Implosion—Weak bottles having thin spots or flaws may break inwardly due to development of a slight vacuum. In one such case, bottles of a syrup were broken by implosion due to removal of oxygen from the air in the bottle by oxidation of the syrup.

Other Types of Chemical Change—In some cases incompatibility may be due to other types of chemical change such as polymerization, double decomposition, substitution, addition, etc.

Correction of Incompatibilities

Consult the Physician

Many physical and chemical incompatibilities can be handled "secundem artem," i.e., using pharmaceutical knowledge. It is usually unnecessary to consult the physician before dispensing such mixtures, but it is often wise to note the method used on the prescription and discuss the matter with the prescriber and your co-workers when

convenient. Examples of such acceptable corrections might be: the use of modified mixing order, dispensing with a "shake" label, suspension or emulsification with official agents, the use of the most appropriate form of the drug for the vehicle prescribed, or other procedures where no therapeutically important change is made in the dosage or ingredients of the formula.

Other procedures may involve borderline cases which will depend on the prescription itself or on the relationship between the pharmacist and the physician. These include the addition of inert ingredients such as diluents, stabilizers, solvents, buffers, stiffening agents, preservatives, and the like or other procedures in which the dose or activity is not altered appreciably.

Procedures which usually require the approval of the physician might be: addition of materials requiring a change in the dose; addition of unofficial suspending agents, emulsifiers, chelating agents, or other materials which may interfere with therapeutic effectiveness; changes which may adversely affect the stability; omission of troublesome ingredients having little therapeutic activity; filtering out inactive sediments; dispensing a troublesome ingredient separately; changing a brand from that specified; changing the dosage forms, e.g., substituting capsules for powders, pills, tablet triturates, etc.; and other important changes.

If the cause of the incompatibility is not known, it is often possible to determine the specific ingredients involved by combining small quantities of the ingredients, two at a time. Some incompatibilities may not become apparent until three or more ingredients are mixed together.

Once the cause, type, and physical manifestation of the incompatibility are determined, several solutions to the problem can usually be derived from a study of the following sections. The physician's appreciation of the pharmacist's interest at this point is usually worth many times the cost of the drugs involved. This is true even if several products must be discarded in finding alternative methods of filling the prescription.

Use Pharmaceutical Knowledge

Most of the above-mentioned problems can be corrected using proper pharmaceutical skills and knowledge.

The following procedures should be considered first.

Modify the Mixing Order—Incompatibilities are often avoided by diluting the incompatible substances with inert ingredients before mixing. Dissolution of potentially incompatible salts separately in the maximum amount of solvent may minimize or prevent precipitation on mixing. This procedure is generally recommended for filling liquid prescriptions since precipitates formed through combination of concentrated solutions are frequently slow to dissolve, even though they may eventually be soluble in the final prescription. It is recommended that water-soluble salts be dissolved in the maximum quantity of water before diluting with alcoholic vehicles. Likewise, it is best to dissolve alcohol-soluble drugs in the maximum amount of alcohol before diluting with aqueous preparations. Precipitation can sometimes also be avoided by mixing glycerin or syrup with the incompatible ingredients before they are combined. If precipitates do form under these conditions, they may be of a diffuse type suitable for dispensing with a shake label.

When three or more ingredients in a prescription may react in several different ways (depending on the order of mixing), the intent of the prescriber must be determined. Thus, in ℞ 7, either a solution or suspension may be obtained since there is insufficient citric acid to neutralize and solubilize both of the carbonates.

7

℞	Magnesium carbonate	3.75 g
	Sodium bicarbonate	7.5 g
	Citric acid	7.5 g
	Distilled water q.s.	250 ml

If the citric acid is reacted first with the sodium bicarbonate, some magnesium carbonate will be insoluble, and a suspension will result. On the other hand, if the magnesium carbonate is solubilized with the citric acid, the sodium bicarbonate is soluble in the reaction mixture, and a solution will be obtained. The sequence selected in such cases will depend on the directions given in the prescription or requested by the physician.

8

℞	Menthol	1.25 g
	Camphor	0.8 g
	Phenol	1.25 g
	Salicylic Acid Powdered	1.8 g
	Boric Acid, Powdered	25 g
	Talc, q.s.	120 g

This particular prescription is best prepared by making an eutectic mixture with the menthol, camphor, and the phenol and absorbing this with the talc. The powdered salicyclic acid can be thoroughly mixed with the boric acid and the two mixtures combined and sieved. If one mixes each of the ingredients, menthol, camphor, and phenol separately with the talc, there is the risk of not getting them powdered finely enough. Eutectic mixtures make an excellent method of getting these materials incorporated as finely as possible. This eutectic mixture should then be taken up with some inorganic adsorbent if possible, talc in this case. By mixing the salicyclic acid with the boric acid one can disperse it more thoroughly. If it were mixed with the menthol-camphor-phenol, a pasty mass would be formed which would be difficult to incorporate.

9

℞	Menthol	0.06 g
	Spirit of Camphor	0.6 ml
	Hydrocortisone	0.15 g
	L. C. D.	2 ml
	Water	15 ml
	Aquaphor q.s.	60 g

The best way to get an elegant product with this prescription is to use the principle of dividing the amount of base (Aquaphor) into two parts. In the one portion, take up the alcohol-soluble ingredients and in the other, the water-soluble ingredients. Thus, mix the spirit of camphor with the liquor carbonis detergens (alcohol conc about 85%) and dissolve the menthol in this. Take this up with about ½ of the amount of Aquaphor needed in the prescription. Levigate the hydrocortisone thoroughly with a very small portion of Aquaphor, then add increasing amounts of Aquaphor until the other half has been used. Incorporate the water into the portion of Aquaphor which contains the hydrocortisone. Lastly, thoroughly mix the two portions.

Any separation is going to take place within the whole body of the base and can be easily dispensed. Mixing of the LCD with the water, before incorporating into the base, will cause a tar-like substance to separate which is difficult to incorporate.

Dispense with a "Shake Well" Label—If precipitation will do no particular harm other than necessitating a "shake" label, the precipitate may often be obtained in the lightest and most diffusible form by diluting the reacting ingredients to the fullest extent which is practical and mixing them cold. The addition of a protective colloid-suspending agent before mixing may also help. Acacia and tragacanth are frequently added either before or after the precipitate is formed.

The pharmacist should consider the nature of the precipitate formed since precipitates with little or no potency can be safely dispensed as "shake" preparations. Precipitates containing highly potent drugs may be dangerous, however, since the patient may fail to shake the bottle sufficiently and then get overdoses in the last few doses. Likewise, if the precipitate cakes on the bottom of the container, the patient may get little or no therapeutic activity from the prescription. It is best in such cases to give oral instructions to the patient as well as to affix a prominent shake label.

Dispense with a "Store in a Refrigerator" Label—Prescriptions which will not retain at least 90% of their therapeutic activity for the intended life of the prescription should be dispensed with a label: "Store in a refrigerator. Discard after (date)." This especially applies to prescriptions which show no change in appearance, yet hydrolyze, oxidize, or otherwise change greatly in potency. Prescriptions which change color on standing, taste bad, or tend to grow yeasts and molds are also good candidates for this label.

Complete the Reaction Before Packaging—Many prescriptions undergo rapid chemical reactions accompanied by the evolution of gas, precipitate formation, color changes, or production of heat or cold. With the prescribers consent, these may be allowed to react to completion in open containers, using ice, agitation, or careful addition of reactants to control the reaction. If the reaction is not desired or if it occurs too slowly to make this procedure possible, it may be necessary to change or omit an ingredient, dispense the prescription in two parts, or employ some other solution to the problem acceptable to the prescriber. Salts which slowly hydrolyze (e.g., zinc sulfate and bismuth subnitrate) are among the chief offenders here.

10

R̵ Zinc Sulfate — 24 g
Sulfurated Potash — 24 g
Ether — 16 g
Alcohol — 54 ml
Distilled Water   q.s. ad. — 180 ml

This is a variation of the age-old white lotion. It is best prepared by dissolving the zinc sulfate and the sulfurated potash separately in 50 ml of distilled water. The sulfurated potash solution, after filtering, is added slowly and with stirring to the zinc sulfate solution. It is best to then cool the prepared lotion to just below room temperature. Holding under the cold water tap works very well. Next, the ether is mixed with the alcohol and this mixture is added slowly to the prepared and cooled white lotion. Add sufficient distilled water to make up to volume where necessary.

When the ether-alcohol solution is added to the prepared white lotion soon after its preparation, there may be sufficient heat still present to cause the ether to boil. This may also be the case where the finished preparation is shaken unduly—heat from the hand and shaking encourages the volatilization of the ether. Several pharmacists and some of their customers have complained that, "it foams all over the place."

While the preparation should of course be dispensed with a "Shake Well" label, it is the duty of the pharmacist to inform the patient that undue shaking and heat might cause problems. A cool place should be recommended for storage.

Protect from Air, Light, and Moisture—Some liquid vitamin products and solutions of a barbiturate or sulfonamide are light and oxygen-sensitive and may darken or form precipitates on exposure to light and air. The use of green or amber glass containers (filled as full as possible) with tight-fitting screw caps will usually solve this problem. If colored glass containers are not available, the use of ordinary flint glass inside cardboard containers may be satisfactory. A warning label should be affixed, e.g., "Protect from light."

If extreme protection from moisture is required (as with many deliquescent or effervescent products which may soften, liquefy, or effervesce unless protected from moisture, the pharmacist may place dried silica gel, anhydrous calcium sulfate, or other desiccants in the bottom of a screw-capped container and cover the desiccant with a small amount of cotton. The prescription in capsules, powder papers, tablets, etc., is then placed inside and the cap is tightly closed. A prominent label such as "Protect from moisture," or "Keep tightly closed" should be used. Commercially available desiccant capsules (Dricaps, Humicaps) and desiccant bags (Drypaks) might be stocked by the pharmacist for this purpose. These contain dried silica gel and are harmless if swallowed. However, the patient should be advised of their presence and purpose.

Add an Ingredient

Substances may be added to prescriptions to correct or prevent certain types of incompatibilities: suspending agents, emulsifying agents, inert solubilizing or miscibility increasing ingredients, diluents, and stiffening or softening agents.

Suspending Agents—Insoluble powders or precipitates can usually be adequately suspended in a formula with small quantities of acacia, tragacanth, methylcellulose, carboxymethylcellulose, or bentonite. These are satisfactory for either internal or external use as long as they are compatible with the other prescription ingredients. In preparing such suspensions, it is well to use drugs as finely powdered as possible. Micronized forms of many drugs are commercially available for prescription use (e.g., sulfacetamide, hydrocortisone, and salicylamide). The addition of compatible wetting agents may also prevent caking and facilitate resuspension.

Suspensions can usually be prepared most easily by suspending the insoluble drugs in a magma or mucilage and then adding the remainder of the formula. If it is necessary to use dry suspending agents, these should be diluted with the maximum amount of the other dry ingredients before adding any liquids. This will help to evenly wet the suspending agent and may reduce the number of lumps which might otherwise result.

11

℞ Compound Tincture of Benzoin 2 ml
   Phenergan Expectorant   q.s. 60 ml
  Sig: i dr q. i.d.

The pharmacist states that this "gums up to such an extent that he is ashamed to dispense it."

Compound benzoin tincture contains a fairly high concentration of gums and resins which are exceptionally insoluble in water. A suitable preparation may be made by adding the compound benzoin tincture, dropwise and with thorough trituration, to about 4–5 ml of glycerin in a mortar. This causes a fine dispersion in the presence of the glycerin. To this, sufficient of the expectorant syrup is added, with thorough stirring, to make the final volume. The gums and resins may come to the top upon standing but are completely resuspendable upon shaking. Dispense with a "Shake Vigorously" label.

Emulsifying Agents—If the prescription calls for two immiscible phases such as oil and water, an emulsifying agent will normally be required even though none is specified. It is the pharmacist's responsibility in such cases to select an emulsifier system which will be safe, compatible with the other ingredients, and produce the type of emulsion required (e.g., oil-in-water or water-in-oil). The decision as to the type of emulsion to prepare may require consultation with the physician unless previous knowledge dictates the choice.

Very potent drugs which are insoluble in the vehicle prescribed are sometimes first dissolved in a suitable solvent which is immiscible with the vehicle and then emulsified. Since the potent drug is greatly diluted with a readily dispersed phase, the danger of overdosage is thus minimized.

A pharmacist compounded the following prescription which appeared satisfactory when prepared but was returned after about a month because it had separated.

12

R Oil of Cade   3 ml
   Precipitated Sulfur   1.5 g
   Salicylic Acid   1 g
   Rose Water Ointment   q.s.   30 g
   Sig: apply to the scalp as directed.

Note here that rose water ointment is a water-in-oil emulsion which owes its stability to the emulsifying agent, sodium cerotate, formed from beeswax and sodium borate. If acids are intimately mixed with this base, the alkalinity

needed for the existence of this soap is upset and free cerotic acid is formed. Where insufficient agent is left, the preparation will separate.

A reasonably stable preparation can be made by mixing the salicylic acid with a little white petrolatum (1 g) or heavy mineral oil, incorporating it into the rose water ointment. Thus, the best way to prepare this prescription would be to levigate the salicylic acid and the precipitated sulfur with one gram of heavy mineral oil. Incorporate the oil of cade into the rose water ointment followed by the addition of the sulfur-salicylic acid-mineral oil mixture.

Recently, emulsions have been recommended for increasing the absorption and prolonging the blood levels of sulfadiazine and reducing the irritating effect of ferrous gluconate on the gastrointestinal tract.

Inert Solubilizing or Miscibility-Increasing Ingredients—The addition of a small amount of an inert wetting agent or complexing agent will often make an incompatible prescription more elegant or less dangerous. For example, potassium iodide may be used to solubilize iodine in water. Frequently, a drop or two of acetic acid or lactic acid is used to inhibit the hydrolysis of basic metallic acetates or lactates. Sodium citrate is likewise used to prevent the precipitation of iron, bismuth, or lead salts by alkalies and to prevent color changes in combinations of iron salts with tannic acid, salicylic acid, etc. Soluble citrates are likewise effective solubilizers for many organic compounds such as salicylic acid, aspirin, benzoic acid, and the like.

Polyethers (e.g., Tweens, Spans, Myrjs, Pluronics, Carbowaxes, polyethylene glycol esters, and methylcellulose) are frequently recommended as solubilizing, dispersing, or complexing agents in incompatible prescriptions.

It has been pointed out that the physician should usually be consulted before using these materials since complexes, chelates, etc., may be formed which will not give the desired therapeutic response. Further, the use of solubilizing agents is not always the best answer to an incompatibility problem since drugs in solution are often less stable than those in suspension. A common example is aspirin, which hydrolyzes only 1–5% in 7–14 days as a suspension in chloroform water (Mixture of Acetylsalicylic Acid—*British Pharmaceutical Codex*, 1954), but when solubilized in water with potassium citrate, it may not be acceptable after the first day or two. One investigation reported 6% and 25% hydrolysis after 1 day and 1 week in such solubilized aspirin solutions.

Addition of a material soluble in both phases of a two-phase system will increase mutual solubility of the phases. Thus, soap or succinic acid will increase the miscibility of phenol-water systems.

The addition of a material soluble in only one of the phases will frequently produce a "salting out" effect and decrease miscibility. An example is the two-phase system which may occur in certain prescriptions containing ethyl alcohol-water-potassium carbonate, or phenol-water-potassium chloride mixtures. These considerations should be kept in mind when selecting solubilizers and other inert ingredients.

Diluents—Changes in volume are sometimes made in powders, capsules, tablets, pills, and other dosage forms in order to prevent contact of materials which form eutectic mixtures, to protect against oxidation-reduction reactions, or to protect the ingredients from the atmosphere. Lactose, starch, sucrose, magnesium oxide, calcium sulfate, glycyrrhiza, and similar materials have been most widely used for this purpose. In selecting the diluent to use, it should be noted that magnesium oxide is an alkaline material, while calcium sulfate is usually slightly acid. The dose will have to be adjusted if two capsules are required instead of one.

Changes in liquid prescriptions in which the volume is doubled or tripled in order to solubilize the active ingredients are often the best solution to in-

compatible prescriptions, especially if the dose is small or could be more conveniently measured if increased.

Stiffening or Softening Agents— Suppositories, ointments, creams, and lotions frequently are unacceptable as prescribed and it may be necessary to add stiffening or softening agents or agents which improve miscibility. Thus, polyethylene glycol 400 monostearate or castor oil are frequently added to improve preparations containing balsam of Peru. Paraffin, starch, wax, or spermaceti are sometimes added to stiffen ointments and suppositories. The increase in volume can usually be ignored if the volume is not changed significantly (i.e., less than 10%).

Remove an Ingredient

If one of the troublesome ingredients is of little therapeutic value, it may be best to secure the physician's consent to omit the item. ℞ 13 is a common example.

13

℞	Phenol	0.5 g
	Menthol	0.1 g
	*Tragacanth	0.5 g
	Olive Oil	50 ml
	Limewater q.s.	100 ml

The physician should be informed that the calcium oleate formed by the fixed oil and limewater provides sufficient emulsifier and that the tragacanth is incompatible with the W/O emulsion which is formed. In the event that the prescriber wishes an O/W emulsion, the prescription can be filled as written by substituting water for the limewater.

Discard the Inactive Sediment— Many tinctures, fluidextracts, wines, and similar alcoholic preparations may precipitate albumins, tannins, gums, sugars, and similar inactive sediments on standing. These may be filtered from the preparation without consulting the physician if the drug is reasonably fresh.

When similar inactive precipitates form during the compounding of a prescription, e.g., on diluting tinctures or fluidextracts with small amounts of water, the prescriber should be consulted, advised, and permission requested to remove these unsightly precipitates by filtration, decantation, etc. The possibility of precipitation of actives should be considered here too, as active alkaloids, etc. may be insoluble also.

Separate into Two Prescriptions—With the consent of the physician, one of the ingredients causing an incompatibility may be dispensed as a separate prescription with appropriate directions to the patient. This procedure was formerly considered a last resort, but with the ready availability of most drugs as tablets or capsules it will probably find increasing favor with the busy pharmacist faced with a problem prescription. This method is always recommended where an explosion could occur or a container could break as a result of a chemical reaction; for example, oxidation-reduction reactions or slow effervescing liquids, tablets, capsules, or powders.

It should be noted that most of these combinations can be safely dispensed as aqueous solutions if the reaction is carefully controlled and allowed to go to completion before the preparation is packaged. Such combinations may however, be potentially dangerous if milled, triturated, or heated together as powders, or if combined with flammable solvents such as alcohol, petroleum ether, and diethyl ether.

Change the Vehicle

Increase Volume of Mixture and Increase Dose—This has already been partially considered under a previous section. If the vehicle concerned is therapeutically active in itself, it may not be possible to double or triple the volume and dose without running the risk of an overdose of vehicle. In aqueous preparations this is an acceptable procedure. As with all changes in dose, the physician and patient should be notified.

Decrease Volume of Mixture and Decrease Dose—When a higher concentration of alcohol, glycerin or, in

some cases, water is needed to solubilize the drugs prescribed, it is often possible to omit part of the vehicle so as to obtain a higher concentration of solvent. For example (in certain hydroalcoholic prescriptions), if a higher alcohol strength is needed, it is often possible to use less water, thereby reducing the volume and dose. Both patient and prescriber should be informed of this change since the physician may have discussed the dosage with the patient.

Change Solvent and Use the Same Dose—In some cases incompatibilities due to insoluble crystals, precipitates, etc., may be corrected by the addition of glycerin or alcohol in place of some of the water.

14

R̜	Mercuric iodide	0.15 g
	Thymol	0.3 g
	Distilled Water q.s. ad	30 ml

In R̜ 14 it is impossible to dissolve all of the thymol or mercuric iodide in water, but a solution may be obtained by replacing most of the water by alcohol.

Likewise, in some cases it may be necessary to replace alcohol or glycerin with water since the latter has a greater solvent action on both organic salts. Note, however, that alcohol is a suitable solvent for many organic salts and deliquescent acetates, benzoates, nitrates, salicylates, bromides, iodides and chlorides. Water, on the other hand, is the preferred solvent for sugars, gums, proteins, inorganic acids, inorganic bases, and salts. Thus, in prescriptions containing these latter ingredients, the addition of alcohol or alcoholic preparations may produce an incompatibility. Most sugars and salts have appreciable solubility in up to about 40% alcohol, but gums, mucilages, albumins, and other proteins may precipitate when the alcoholic content exceeds 25%.

Alcohol is very useful for dissolving alcohols, aldehydes, ketones, ethers, esters, phenols, resins, organic acids, organic bases, glycosides, volatile oils, balsams, etc. It is usually also a good sol-

Ak

vent for barbiturates, local anesthetics, antihistaminics, sulfonamides, and alkaloids. When adding these to aqueous solutions, it is preferable to dissolve such ingredients first in alcohol (or in an ingredient containing alcohol) if it is present in the prescription. If alcohol must be added to the prescription for solubility purposes, these ingredients should be dissolved in the alcohol. Where mixtures of water-soluble and alcohol-soluble ingredients are prescribed, a careful balance must be maintained in certain cases. It is usually safe to judge the necessary or permissible alcohol content of a prescription from the USP, NF, or PRB mixtures, elixirs, solutions, etc. The alcohol content required to maintain compatibility and stability in a commercial preparation may be judged from that given on the product label or may be determined by looking up the product in a company catalog or in references listing ingredients of such products, e.g., *Modern Drug Encyclopedia, Physicians' Desk Reference,* or *Veterinary Drug Encyclopedia.*

Glycerin, polyethylene glycols, and propylene glycol frequently have solvent properties between those of alcohol and water. They are especially good solvents for phenols, cresols, iodine, tannins, borates, phosphates, volatile oils, and parabens.

15

℞	Potassium Iodide	40 g
	Ephedrine Sulfate	1.2 g
	Phenobarbital Sodium	9 g
	Glycerin	30 g
	Syrup of Glycyrrhiza	50 g
	Syrup of Wild Cherry q.s. ad.	240 g
	Sig: t.i.d.	

The proper method of preparation is to dissolve the ephedrine sulfate and the phenobarbital sodium, separately, in a minimum amount of water. Mix 100 ml of the syrup of wild cherry with the phenobarbital sodium solution and add the glycerin. To this add the syrup of glycyrrhiza and the ephedrine sulfate solution. Mix well. Lastly, add the potassium iodide, dissolved in a minimum amount of water and q.s. with the syrup of wild cherry.

If the acid salt (ephedrine sulfate) and the alkaline salt (phenobarbital sodium) were mixed in concentrated solutions a precipitate would result. Potassium iodide, a very soluble salt, would further reduce the solubility. The presence of glycerin and the syrups aid in preventing the precipitation.

Change an Ingredient

Use the most compatible form. The pharmacist usually employs the form of the drug most compatible with the vehicle specified, even though the prescription does not so indicate. This implies that if the drug mixture is not compatible as written he may select another common or official form of the drug. These must be adequately stable during the use time of the prescription and must permit therapeutically effective, uniform doses of a pharmaceutically elegant preparation to be administered. The amount of the drug used should of course be corrected so that the dose is equivalent to that prescribed. Such changes should be noted on the prescription and discussed with the physician when convenient. Examples of these changes might be the substitution of salts with compatible ions for those with incompatible ions, e.g., the substitution of nitrates for chlorides where insoluble chlorides would precipitate.

The question is frequently asked: Is it permissible to use tablets as a source of hydrocortisone or other steroid hormones in the extemporaneous compounding of ointments and lotions?

16

℞	Hydrocortisone	0.3 g
	Water to levigate q.s.	
	Aquaphor q.s. ad.	30 g

This prescription and variations thereof are quite common today. It is not generally acceptable to use tablets as the source of hydrocortisone. Unless the physician has specifically indicated that tablets may be used, the prescription should be prepared from the micronized bulk powder. The reasons for this are: first, the bulk powder has been micronized and hence is of finer particle size—more easily dispersed, more effective, and there is less chance of irritation. Secondly, the tablets contain extraneous material which is not necessary in the prescription and may even be undesirable. Since the micronized powder is readily available, there is no excuse for not using it.

Use the Most Soluble Form—If an alkaloid or other water-insoluble nitrogenous base is prescribed in aqueous solution, it is usually acceptable to use an equivalent amount of a water-soluble salt. If the vehicle prescribed is oily in nature, the more oil-soluble alkaloidal base would be used.

Use the Most Stable Form—The stability of the prescription may dictate the preferred method of compounding. For example, oral sulfonamides are usually prescribed as suspensions rather than solutions because most of their soluble sodium salts are unstable, unpalatable, and highly alkaline. A notable exception is sodium sulfacetamide.

If the prescription is reasonably stable as written, no change should be made.

Change the Dosage Form

Use a More Suitable Dosage Form—Prescriptions which slowly effervesce, gradually change color, slowly yield a precipitate, or present some other obvious reaction may undermine the patient's confidence in the pharmacist or physician. Such prescriptions should be corrected or changed to more suitable dosage forms which obviate the difficulty. Thus, with the physician's approval effervescent powders or tablets that are directed to be added to water might be substituted for an effervescing solution which is allowed to react to completion prior to packaging. Separation of the incompatible ingredients into powders, capsules, tablets, or solutions with proper directions on each container may also be the answer to certain prescriptions.

If cachets, extemporaneously prepared soft elastic capsules, tablet triturates, or other time-consuming or hard-to-obtain dosage forms are prescribed, the physician may permit the substitution of other equivalent dosage forms. Thus, tablets, capsules, powders, etc., may be approved by the physician if he is made aware of the difficulty.

Sometimes an emulsion or lotion cannot be prepared due to an incompatible ingredient which will break the emulsion. In this case it is often possible to prepare compatible mixtures of the active ingredients in acceptable nonemulsified forms such as alcoholic solutions, grease-base ointments, aqueous lotions, polyethylene glycol ointments, etc. This procedure should always be approved by the physician before dispensing since the substituted product may not meet the therapeutic requirements of the patient.

Use a Different Brand—Occasionally pharmacists may wish to substitute another brand for the one specified if they do not have the prescribed brand in stock or if the patient complains of the taste, side effects, or other properties of a commercial product. The physician should be consulted here. Occasionally, the notation "ARB" will be found on a prescription calling for a commercially manufactured item. In this case "any reliable brand" *can* ethically be dispensed.

If no manufacturer is specified for a generic name product, the pharmacist is free to select the brand to be used; however, he is still expected to dispense only "high quality and efficacious material," and if possible at a reasonable cost to the patient.

Read the Literature

Further suggestions for handling problem prescriptions may be found in Table 1. This summarizes the previous discussion and indicates some of the methods which retail pharmacists use to solve the various types of prescription problems.

Other types of incompatibilities very familiar to the manufacturing pharmacist occasionally become a problem for the community pharmacist. These so-called "delayed incompatibilities" include caking of suspensions or development of particles too large to inject or use topically due to crystal growth, improper drug release in enteric tablet coatings due to changes with age, loss of preservative due to absorption by rubber stoppers, loss of potency due to hydrolysis, oxidation, racemization and the like, and so on. Many of these problems are discussed in the following sections under the appropriate drug.

The graduate pharmacist would do well to resolve to purchase and study modern pharmacy textbooks and to keep one or more continually revised reference works handy to peruse when he has a spare moment. Subscriptions to professional journals and abstract journals are certainly indicated, as is the avid reading of new and old product inserts and advertising brochures.

Lest the reader be concerned about the infrequent occurrence of some of the prescription examples cited in this chapter it should be noted that a study of the common incompatibilities of the past and present aids in training the pharmacist to recognize and solve the formulation and compatibility problems of the future for several reasons: (1) many new drugs are simple chemical modifications of older drugs whose structure, properties, compatibilities, incompatibilities, doses, uses, contraindications, etc., usually appear in the literature and (2) more and more information is becoming available as to the effect of structure and structural changes on physical properties, chemical properties, and pharmacological activity. In addition, if examples can be found of the way in which the addition or subtraction of certain organic chemical groups has affected the solubility, chemical reactivity, and pharmacology of related drugs, useful deductions can often be drawn about the physical, chemical, and therapeutic compatibili-

ties of the new drug. This latter postulate presupposes that the pharmacist will keep up-to-date as new drugs are introduced and will maintain a current file on their structure, solubilities, compatibilities, and adverse reactions.

Actual data on drug compatibility are rather scarce. Occasionally, articles on this subject appear in the various professional journals.* Articles that apply to compatibility may be gleaned from the abstract journals listed in this chapter.

All prescription legend drugs now carry product inserts and other labeling which list the active ingredients, indications for use, recommended dosages, contraindications, side effects, recommended storage conditions, expiration date (if required), and other valuable information. Compatibility data may or may not be included although warnings of drug potentiation or inactivation are common. The FDA is currently requesting manufacturers to furnish compatibility data for mixtures likely to be compounded in disposable intravenous equipment.

It is imperative that a complete collection of inserts and labeling be made and continually revised. It is also recommended that the pharmacist retain this information even after the inserts are changed or the product disappears from the market since prescriptions may be kept and used over a period of years.

Many pharmaceutical manufacturers also publish either trade journals, brochures, new product file cards, or catalogs directed to the pharmacist. It should perhaps be noted that some manufacturers do not publish compati-

---

* In an effort to stimulate publication of such data, the former APhA Section on Pharmaceutical Technology sponsored a pioneering series of symposia on "Incompatibilities of Manufactured Pharmaceuticals." These symposia, chaired by one of the present authors, were held in 1961, 1962, and 1963. The papers presented have appeared in numerous journals, chiefly the *Journal of the American Pharmaceutical Association, American Journal of Hospital Pharmacy,* and *Journal of Pharmaceutical Sciences.*

bility information but prefer that the pharmacist contact their product development or control departments with problem prescriptions.

Most of the professional pharmacy journals publish data on the structural formulas, properties, uses, cautions and contraindications, and dosage forms available as new drugs are introduced.

Many reference books are issued annually or supplemented frequently so as to help the pharmacist keep abreast of current prescription legend and proprietary drugs, their uses, and their properties. It is recommended that the pharmacist have current copies of several of these publications available for use in determining therapeutic incompatibilities and potential adverse drug reactions.

It is unfortunate that none of these books contain any significant amount of physical or chemical compatibility data, although they are very helpful in describing contraindications, toxicity, and other therapeutic incompatibilities.

Several frequently revised publications are especially helpful in predicting compatibility of the newest drugs since they contain structural formulas which make it easier to spot potentially reactive groups and structures. These may require close inspection and interpretation since the structural formulas are usually depicted as two-dimensional structures which do not always demonstrate the three-dimensional possibilities. A useful publication here is *Remington's Pharmaceutical Sciences.*

It should be emphasized that even where published compatibility data are available, a statement that two products are compatible usually does not imply endorsement of the therapeutic value of such combinations. The pharmacological activity of these mixtures is determined only rarely. Actually, many combination prescriptions are discouraged by the pharmaceutical manufacturer because he has delicately balanced the preservative, antioxidant, suspending agent, buffer, and other ingredients of the product for maximum effective-

ness and stability, freedom from irritation, and sterility. Moreover, compatibility is frequently a function of concentration, pH, solvents present, etc., and the combination prescribed may not fit the test conditions.

Despite these and other complications, freedom to prescribe is the perogative of the physician, and the pharmacist must do the best he can with the resulting prescription. He is greatly aided in this effort by several observations:

1. Most prescriptions written today are for manufactured dosage forms and do not require compounding. Accordingly, incompatibilities are the exception, not the rule.

2. Most extemporaneously compounded prescriptions will be used before they have time to deteriorate excessively.

3. The mild conditions normally present in a prescription (slightly acid to slightly alkaline aqueous or oily vehicles at room temperature or below) do not favor many of the classical chemical reactions usually taught in organic chemistry.

Tables 2 and 3 give useful generalizations based on these points. Since there are exceptions to all rules, these should be looked upon solely as helpful first approximations. Most drug descriptions which follow give condensed incompatibility and compatibility data available in greater detail in the *Parenteral Drug Information Guide, USP, NF,* Martindale's *The Extra Pharmacopeia, Merck Index,* previous editions of this text, and other reference books. These are collected here as an illustration of the type of data which will aid in predicting compatibility. Although some indication of compatibility can be obtained by comparing a new drug with only one similar old drug, a much closer approximation can be obtained by comparison with a series of known compounds.

It may be seen from the foregoing discussion that the chief difficulty in predicting incompatibility is the large number of potential incompatibilities which may occur. Given hundreds of drug preparations, an almost inconceivable number of combinations may be made. For example, 500 drugs or preparations will make 257,838,552,475 different combinations using from 1 to 5 items in each combination. It is evident at once that the subject of incompatibilities cannot be presented by discussing any appreciable percentage of the individual incompatibilities which may occur. General principles must be learned and practice obtained in the application of these theoretical principles to actual prescriptions. This should be done, as far as possible, in dispensing and refresher courses using current and commonly occurring examples which illustrate the points to be made.

The pharmacist should try to devise as many additional ways as possible of filling the sample prescriptions given in this textbook. It is safe to say that different physicians will prefer different solutions to each problem.

Dispensing Theory

Various types of *in vivo* drug actions and interactions, both intended and unwanted, are covered in introductory form in this section.

Drug Reactions and Interactions

Table 4 defines the more common clinical problems, cites typical examples, and suggests corrective measures.

Specific examples of important drug interactions are arranged alphabetically by generic name and/or drug type in Table 5.

Table 6 lists alphabetically some of the more clinically significant drug-interacting pairs and gives references to further discussions of mechanisms of interaction effects, etc. Since full treatment is outside the scope of this chapter, it is recommended that pharmacists prepare drug profiles for their patients and that the components of prescriptions and OTC drugs taken be checked against such tables as a means of avoiding drug treatment problems. Further, such tables should be continually expanded and brought up-to-date by the pharmacist's reading and abstracting articles as they appear in the medical and pharmaceutical literature. The col-

lection of original papers or even the addition of *International Pharmaceutical Abstract* reference numbers to these or similar tables will serve as a useful means of storing and recovering necessary knowledge in this field.

It should be noted that undesired *in vivo* drug interactions can usually be corrected by proper dosage adjustment provided the suspected interaction is recognized by the pharmacist. However, the ubiquitous possibilities for desirable and undesirable interactions to occur simultaneously must always be recognized. In practice full correction is sometimes difficult since common substances such as alcohol (beer, wine, cocktails), caffeine (coffee, tea, cola beverages), nicotine (cigarettes, cigars), salicylates (aspirin, APC, other headache, pain and cold medicines), some foods (strong cheeses, Chianti wine, fava beans), certain proprietary (OTC) drugs, or even the same or different prescription drugs may cause drug interactions. Since most patients, some physicians and a few pharmacists are not familiar with the composition of many trademarked prescription or proprietary drugs, the possibilities for addition, antagonism, potentiation, and other possibly hazardous interactions are not always recognized. This is even further complicated by the fact that manufacturers are not required to list on their labels ingredients to which many people are already sensitized (e.g., chocolate, corn starch, wheat, milk sugar, etc.).

Of course, some drug actions that are closely related to drug interactions, such as the enzyme induction actions of diphenylhydantoin in Cushing's Syndrome or of alcohol or barbiturates in neonatal hyperbilirubinemia, may be clinically advantageous.

An *in vivo* drug interaction may involve an instantaneous chemical reaction, a delayed equilibrium reaction, adsorption, or another physical or mechanical interaction, depending on whether the substances involved are capable of interaction, and whether they are present simultaneously in the stom-

Table 4—Common *In Vivo* Drug Reactions and Interactions

Clinical problems	*Corrective measures*	*Typical examples*
Adverse reaction (nonallergic) Unwanted direct toxic action of drug on cytoplasm, usually not involving an immune reaction (see *Side Effects* and *Extension Effects* below).	Withdraw all medication immediately. Start suitable corrective treatment. Warn patient and medical team of future danger.	Cytopenia (antipyrine, chloramphenicol). Gastrointestinal ulcer (antiflammatory steroids, indomethacin, reserpine, salicylates). Kidney damage (phenacetin).
Allergic reaction Undesirable immune response to antibody-antigen (drug) reaction.	Withdraw medication immediately. Start symptomatic treatment; possibly desensitize. Warn patient, family, and medical team of future danger.	Cholestatic jaundice (halothane, hydrazines. MAO inhibitors, phenothiazines). Cutaneous eruptions (novobiocin, penicillins, sulfonamides). Hematologic cytopenias (chloramphenicol, chloroquine, nitrofurantoin, penicillin, PAS, sulfonamides). Hepatitis (methyldopa).
Blood dyscrasia Blood disorder, often drug-induced (e.g., anemia, leukopenia, etc).	Monitor blood of persons taking dyscrasia-causing drugs. Withdraw drug immediately if problem arises. Warn patient and medical team of future danger. Start appropriate treatment.	Anemia (benzene, carbutamides, chloramphenicol, chlordane, chlorothiazide). Hemolytic anemia (acetanilid, phenacetin, aminopyrine, nitrofurantoin, pamaquine, PAS). Leukopenia (dipyrone, imipramine, meprazine, meprobamate, phenylbutazone). Pancytopenia (streptomycin, sulfamethoxypyridazine, tolbutamide, trimethadione). Thrombocytopenia (acetazolamide, arsphenamine, carbutamide, phenytoin).
Chemical carcinogenesis Unrestrained proliferation of somatic cells due to carcinogen.	Monitor patient taking potential carcinogenic drugs. Withdraw drug immediately if problem arises. Warn patient and medical team of future danger. Start appropriate treatment.	Polycyclic hydrocarbons (covalent-bonding methyl and cyclomethyl cholanthrenes). Aromatic amines (those metabolizing to covalent bonding carcinogens). Azo dyes (those metabolizing to N-hydroxy derivatives). Nitrosamines and urethanes (those metabolizing to alkylating agents by N-hydroxylation). Alkylating agents (busulfan, ethionine, mechlorethamine).
Chemical mutagenesis Permanently inheritable change in germ cells to mutagenic effects.	Further study needed. Possibly avoid use of these by children and adults of child-bearing age.	Not well established in humans. Potential mutagens may include aflatoxins, benzopyrene, captan, caffeine, cyclamates, nitrites, LSD, etc.
Chemical teratogenesis Abnormalities in fetus due to teratogens.	Further study needed. Avoid all drug use during first 3 months of pregnancy, especially those crossing placenta. Study suspected infants thoroughly. Avoid use of known teratogens.	Thalidomide. Potential danger from any drug, virus, etc. that crosses the placental barrier during first trimester of pregnancy, especially those causing teratogenesis in animals (e.g., alkylating agents, azo dyes, anoxia-inducing agents, cytotoxic drugs, heavy metals, purine or pyrimidine analogs, etc).
Contraindication Pre-existing condition potentially aggravated by drug.	Study drug labeling, including package insert, closely. Withdraw drugs or treatments indicated. Warn patient and medical team of future danger. Study patient closely.	Glaucoma-closed angle type (parasympatholytics). Jaundice-newborn (chloramphenicol). Peptic ulcer (corticosteroids, indomethacin, reserpine, salicylates). Porphyria (barbiturates).
Drug addiction	(See *Drug Dependence* below)	

Table 4—*Continued*

Clinical problems	*Corrective measures*	*Typical examples*
Drug dependence Undesirable condition induced by drugs involving tolerance, physical dependence, or psychic craving.	Withdraw medication carefully under medical supervision. Institute psychotherapy and other support.	Caffeine, cocaine, nicotine, opiate narcotics.
Drug interaction Increase or decrease in pharmacological response due to drug, food or treatment interactions.	Determine if the interaction is desirable or undesirable. Monitor drugs, proprietary products, foods, beverages, clinical tests, or other suspected interactants. Correct drug or drug ratios as required.	Alcohol with barbiturates and other CNS depressants. Coumarin type anticoagulants with phenylbutazone, salicylates, etc. Folic acid with hydantoins. Thiazide diuretics with digitalis, calcium injections, etc.
Drug resistance Acquired insensitivity or reduced sensitivity of pathogens (protozoa, bacteria, fungi, etc.) to drug therapy.	Test for sensitivity of the pathogen to the various drugs. Treat with specific antipathogenic drug. Avoid combination drugs where possible.	Antibacterial resistance (penicillins, serine, sulfonamides). Antimalarial resistance (chloroquine). Antineoplastic resistance (5-fluorouracil, methotrexate).
Drug tolerance Reduced pharmacologic response due to prior administration of drug or congener.	Increase the drug dosage or frequency. Change to a more effective drug.	Acute tolerance (acetylcholine, amphetamines, atropine, ephedrine, histamine, nicotine, nitrites). Equilibrium adjustments in the body (adrenal hormones, ammonium chloride, thyroid). Modification in circulation, binding, metabolism, excretion (alcohol, barbiturates).
Extension effect Unwanted effect due to overdosage, etc. (excessive action).	Decrease the drug dosage or frequency. Titrate to minimal effective dose.	Acidosis (paraldehyde). Cardiac arrhythmias (digitalis). Convulsions (local anesthetics). Gastrointestinal distress (digitalis). Hemorrhage (anticoagulants-dicumarol, etc.).
Hypersensitivity Undesirable toxic or excessive pharmacogenetic drug response, caused by unusual susceptibility.	Withdraw the medication immediately. Institute suitable corrective treatment. Avoid future exposure. Warn patient, relatives, and medical team. (May often be avoided by full family case history and sensitivity testing.)	Apnea (succinylcholine). Anemia, hemolytic (primaquine). Acute porphyria (barbiturates).
Idiosyncrasy Rare, abnormal, undesirable, and unexpected genetically determined drug effect (phenotypic).	Withdraw the medication immediately. Treat symptomatically. Avoid future exposure. Warn patient, medical team.	Adverse reactions, wide variety (adrenal steroids, aminopyrine, *p*-aminosalicylic acid, amitriptyline, amphotericin, ampicillin, antipyrine, atropine, azepinamide, caffeine, carbutamide, chlordiazepoxide, chlorpromazine, cinchophen, colistimethate, colistin, demeclocycline, demecolcine, dimercaprol, ectylurea, ergotamine, erythromycin estolate, ethionamide, ethanol, ethyl norepinephrine, fluoxymestrone, fluphenazine, folic acid, glutethimide, gold salts, guanethidine, halothane, hydralazine, imipramine, iothiouracil, isocarboxazid, licorice, mebanazine, mepazine, meralluride, methandrostenolone, methylphenidate, MAO inhibitors, nicotinic acid, etc.).

Table 4—*Continued*

Clinical problems	Corrective measures	Typical examples
Iatrogenic disease Complication or disease induced by the physician's treatment (usually undesirable and unintentional drug reaction).	Withdraw the medication or treatment immediately. Treat symptomatically.	Drug-induced adverse reactions (allergies-penicillin, novobiocin, streptomycin, etc.; addiction morphine, codeine, etc.). Treatment-induced adverse effects (X-rays, electroshock, etc.).
Physical dependence Continued need for a drug which may have lost much of its usual biologic effect but is still necessary for the individual to function normally.	Withdraw the medication preferably under medical supervision, gradually.	Alcohol, barbiturates, caffeine, cocaine, nicotine, meprobamate.
Side effect Usually an unavoidable, secondary pharmacological effect of the usual drug dosages.	Monitor treatment carefully. Treated symptomatically. Withdraw or reduce dosage of medication where indicated.	Constipation (astringent antacids, codeine, morphine). Diarrhea (antibiotics suppressing normal intestinal flora, e.g., tetracycline, novobiocin). Gastric bleeding (aspirin, butazones, salicylates). Methemoglobinemia (nitrites). Nausea (cardiac glycosides, iron salts). Xerostomata (atropine, belladonna, propantheline).
Therapeutic incompatibility Combination of drugs or treatments producing unexpected *in vivo* results. These may be desirable but are commonly undesirable, and sometimes fatal.	Withdraw one or more incompatible or interacting drugs, when indicated.	Alcohol with disulfiram, certain sulfonylureas, nitroglycerin, furazolidone, etc. Digitalis with calcium injections, potassium, etc. MAO inhibitors with reserpine, sympathomimetics, tyramine-containing foods, etc.
Withdrawal syndrome Symptoms characteristic for each drug producing a drug dependence which disappears on readministration of the drug.	Withdraw the dependence-producing medication carefully and gradually under medical supervision.	Alcohol, barbiturates, heroin, meprobamate, morphine.

ach, blood, lymph, or urine, or at a receptor site, or some other place where they can interact in the body.

Drugs already in solution (e.g., solutions for injection, syrups, elixirs, tinctures, fluidextracts, infusions, etc.) should be available for rapid action if the drug is not precipitated, adsorbed by other substances or otherwise inactivated. On the other hand, less soluble drugs (e.g., suspensions for injection, oral suspensions, time-release capsules, slowly dissolving tablets, etc.) must first go into solution in body fluids. Some dosage forms such as nondisintegrating tablets or even undissolved drug parti-

cles may not enter into drug interactions as such, and may produce no drug action other than possibly a placebo effect. Of course any situation that causes a drug to be noneffective is just as undesirable as a mixture demonstrating an obvious chemical reaction.

Drug interactions and other incompatibilities therefore depend on such factors as the potential for *in vivo* or *in vitro* physical or chemical interaction, the rates of adsorption, distribution, or penetration of each individual drug; the speed, degree and site of attachment of the drugs to their receptors; the possibilities of redistribution or displace-

Table 5—Selected Drug-Drug Interactions[a][1]

Drug A	plus	Drug B	=	Potential Reaction
Analgesics				
Acetaminophen		Anticoagulants		Potentiation of anticoagulant
Aspirin		Anticoagulants		Potentiation of anticoagulant
		Penicillin and sulfonamides		Potentiation of anti-infectives
		Probenecid		Decreased uricosuric effect
		Tolbutamide		Hypoglycemia
Antibiotics				
Penicillin		Anticoagulants		Potentiation of anticoagulant
Tetracyclines		Antacids		Delayed absorption
Anticoagulants		Butazolidin		Potentiation of anticoagulants
Antidepressants				
Tricyclic Agents		Guanethidine		Inhibition of guanethidine
		Phenothiazines		Additive effect
Anti-inflammatory Agents				
Phenylbutazone		Antacids		Inhibition of phenylbutazone
		Aspirin		Urate retention
		Oral hypoglycemics		Potentiation of hypoglycemic
Steroid derivatives		Antihistamines		
		Barbiturates		Inhibition of steroid
		Diphenylhydantoin		
Antinoplastics				
Methotrexate		Salicylates		Bone marrow depression
6-Mercaptopurine		Allopurinol		Potentiates the 6-mercaptopurine
Anticonvulsants				
Diphenylhydantoin		Anticoagulants		Diphenylhydantoin toxicity
		Phenobarbital		Decreased plasma levels of diphenylhydantoin
Barbiturates				
Butisol sodium		Anti-inflammatory agents		Inhibition of anti-inflammatory
Phenobarbital		Anticoagulants		Inhibition of anticoagulants
		MAO inhibitors		Potentiation of barbiturate
		Antihistamines		Inhibition of both
		Phenothiazines		Additive effect
Decongestants				
Sympathomimetics		Guanethidine		Blocks uptake of guanethidine
		Hypoglycemics		Increased blood sugar levels
		MAO inhibitors		Enhances action of decongestants
Sedatives and Tranquilizers		Anticoagulants		Inhibition of anticoagulants
Chloral hydrate		MAO inhibitors		Potentiation of chloral hydrate
Major tranquilizers		Antihistamines		Additive effect
Minor tranquilizer				
Chlordiazepoxide		CNS depressants		Additive effect
		Alcohol		Enhanced sedation
		Reserpine		Potentiation of reserpine

[a] Cross referencing between Drug A and Drug B can serve to expand the scope and usefulness of this type of table.

ment from binding sites; any significant stimulation or depression of general metabolism or of drug-specific biotransformation; any changes in enzyme mechanisms; any addition, potentiation, synergism or depression in pharmacologic or toxic action; any change in rate or mechanism of excretion; or any combination of these. Related considerations such as reactions between drugs and endogenous enzymes, hormones or other physiological chemicals, (i.e., monoamine oxidase inhibitors, epinephrine, etc.) are also important, although they are not true "drug interactions."

When compounding and dispensing, all of these many possibilities for interactions have to be considered in the light of the physical, chemical, biochemical, geometric, pharmacologic and toxic properties of each of the materials involved, including such structurally related factors as reactivity, solubility, permeability, ionization, pH, etc.

One source of confusion which must be especially noted by the hospital and consulting pharmacist is the *in vivo* and

Table 6—Drug-Pair Interactions Believed Clinically Significant[a]

Acetaminophen–Warfarin, B 401
Acetohexamide–Phenylbutazone, **A 1**
  Alcohol–Amitriptyline, A 4
  Alcohol–Aspirin, A 13
  Alcohol–Chloral Hydrate, A 15
  Alcohol–Chlordiazepoxide, A 18
  Alcohol–Diazepam, A 35
  Alcohol–Guanethidine, B 372
  Alcohol–Meprobamate, A 103
  Alcohol–Metronidazole, A 109
  Alcohol–Pargyline, A 117
  Alcohol–Phenformin, A 121
  Alcohol–Propoxyphene, B 394
  Alcohol–Tolbutamide, A 144
  Alcohol–Warfarin, B 402
Allopurinol–Aminophylline, **A 3**
  Allopurinol–Chlorpropamide, A 25
  Allopurinol–Mercaptopurine, A 105
Allopurinol–Probenecid, **B 359**
  Aluminum Hydroxide–Quinidine, A 128
  Aluminum Hydroxide–Warfarin, A 153
  Aluminum Ions–Tetracycline, A 136
  Aminophylline–Allopurinol, A 3
Amitriptyline–Alcohol, **A 4**
Amitriptyline–Chlordiazepoxide, **A 6**
Amitriptyline–Pargyline, **A 7**
Amobarbital–Chlorpromazine, **A 10**
  Amphetamine–Chlorpromazine, A 21
Amphetamine–Furazolidone, **A 12**
  Amphetamine–Guanethidine, A 70
  Amphetamine–Propoxyphene, A 123
  Ascorbic Acid–Ferrous Sulfate, B 369
  Ascorbic Acid–Warfarin, B 404
Aspirin–Alcohol, **A 13**
  Aspirin–Chlorpropamide, A 26
  Aspirin–Indomethacin, A 87
  Aspirin–Penicillin, A 118
  Aspirin–Sulfinpyrazone, A 135
  Aspirin–Warfarin, A 155
  Butabarbital–Hydrocortisone, A 83
  Calcium–Digitalis, A 37
  Calcium Ions–Tetracycline, A 136
  Carbenicillin–Gentamicin, A 67
Chloral Hydrate–Alcohol, **A 15**
Chloral Hydrate–Furazolidone, **B 360**
  Chloral Hydrate–Warfarin, A 157
  Chloramphenicol–Chlorpropamide, A 28
  Chloramphenicol–Penicillin, B 389
  Chloramphenicol–Tolbutamide, B 399
Chlorcyclizine–Pentobarbital, **A 17**
Chlordiazepoxide–Alcohol, **A 18**
  Chlordiazepoxide–Amitriptyline, A 6
  Chlordiazepoxide–Warfarin, A 159
  Chlorothiazide–Chlorpropamide, A 29
  Chlorothiazide–Digitalis, A 38
  Chlorothiazide–Probenecid, B 393
  Chlorpheniramine–Propranolol, A 124
Chlorphentermine–Phenelzine, **A 20**
  Chlorpromazine–Amobarbital, A 10
Chlorpromazine–Amphetamine, **A 21**
Chlorpromazine–Piperazine, **A 23**
  Chlorpromazine–Thiamylal, A 139
Chlorpropamide–Allopurinol, **A 25**
Chlorpropamide–Aspirin, **A 26**
Chlorpropamide–Chloramphenicol, **A 28**
Chlorpropamide–Chlorothiazide, **A 29**
Chlorpropamide–Warfarin, **A 31**
  Chlorthalidone–Digitalis, A 40
  Chlorthalidone–Tubocurarine, A 149

Cholestyramine–Phenylbutazone, B 391
Cholestyramine–Thyroid, A 143
Clofibrate–Warfarin, B 405
Cortisone–Tolbutamide, A 146
Cyclopropane–Epinephrine, A 59
Desipramine–Guanethidine, A 71
Desipramine–Propranolol, A 126
Dexamethasone–Phenytoin, **A 32**
Dexamethasone–Secobarbital, **A 34**
  Dexpanthenol–Succinylcholine, B 396
  Dextran–Heparin, B 374
Diazepam–Alcohol, **A 35**
  Diazepam–Gallamine Triethiodide, B 371
Digitalis–Calcium, **A 37**
Digitalis–Chlorothiazide, **A 38**
Digitalis–Chlorthalidone, **A 40**
Digitalis–Phenytoin, **B 361**
Digitalis–Reserpine, **A 42**
Digitoxin–Spironolactone, **A 45**
Digoxin–Ethacrynic Acid, **A 47**
Digoxin–Furosemide, **A 49**
Digoxin–Propantheline, **B 363**
  Diphenhydramine–Warfarin, A 161
  Phenytoin–Dexamethasone, A 32
  Phenytoin–Digitalis, B 361
  Phenytoin–Insulin, A 90
Diphenylhydantoin—see *Phenytoin*
Ephedrine–Reserpine, **A 57**
Ephedrine–Tranylcypromine, **B 366**
Epinephrine–Cyclopropane, **A 59**
  Epinephrine–Halothane, A 76
  Erythromycin–Lincomycin, B 383
  Ethacrynic Acid–Digoxin, A 47
  Ethacrynic Acid–Gallamine Triethiodide, A 63
  Ethacrynic Acid–Kanamycin, A 93
Ether–Neomycin, **A 61**
Ferrous Sulfate–Ascorbic Acid, **B 369**
  Ferrous Sulfate–Tetracycline, B 397
  Furazolidone–Amphetamine, A 12
  Furazolidone–Chloral Hydrate, B 360
  Furosemide–Digoxin, A 49
Gallamine Triethiodide–Diazepam, **B 371**
Gallamine Triethiodide–Ethacrynic Acid, **A 63**
Gallamine Triethiodide–Kanamycin, **A 65**
Gentamicin–Carbenicillin, **A 67**
  Glutethimide–Warfarin, A 162
Griseofulvin–Phenobarbital, **A 68**
  Griseofulvin–Warfarin, A 163
Guanethidine–Alcohol, **B 372**
Guanethidine–Amphetamine, **A 70**
Guanethidine–Desipramine, **A 71**
Guanethidine–Hydrochlorothiazide, **A 73**
Guanethidine–Methylphenidate, **A 75**
Halothane–Epinephrine, **A 76**
Halothane–Phenelzine, **A 78**
  Halothane–Reserpine, A 131
Heparin–Dextran, **B 374**
Hexobarbital–Propranolol, **A 80**
Hydralazine–Nialamide, **A 81**
  Hydrochlorothiazide–Guanethidine, A 73
Hydrocortisone–Butabarbital, **A 83**
  Imipramine–Meprobamate, B 385
  Imipramine–Reserpine, A 133
Imipramine–Thyroid, **A 84**
Imipramine–Tranylcypromine, **B 376**
Indomethacin–Aspirin, **A 87**
Indomethacin–Probenecid, **A 88**
Insulin–Phenytoin, **A 90**

Table 6—*Continued*

Insulin–Propranolol, **B** 378
Insulin–Tranylcypromine, **B** 380
Iproniazid–Meperidine, A 101
Isocarboxazid–Tyramine, **A** 91
Isoniazid–Phenytoin, A 51
Isoniazid–Pyridoxine, **B** 381
Kanamycin–Ethacrynic Acid, **A** 93
Kanamycin–Gallamine Triethiodide, A 65
Kaolin–Lincomycin, A 98
Leucovorin–Methotrexate, A 106
Levodopa–Phenelzine, **A** 95
Levodopa–Pyridoxine, **A** 96
Lincomycin–Erythromycin, **B** 383
Lincomycin–Kaolin, **A** 98
Magnesium Ions–Tetracycline, **A** 136
Meperidine–Iproniazid, **A** 101
Meprobamate–Alcohol, **A** 103
Meprobamate–Imipramine, **B** 385
Meprobamate–Warfarin, A 165
Mercaptopurine–Allopurinol, **A** 105
Methandrostenolone–Oxyphenbutazone, **B** 387
Methandrostenolone–Warfarin, A 166
Methotrexate–Leucovorin, **A** 106
Methotrexate–Sulfisoxazole, **A** 108
Methoxyflurane–Tetracycline, A 138
Methylphenidate–Phenytoin, A 53
Methylphenidate–Guanethidine, A 75
Metronidazole–Alcohol, **A** 109
Neomycin–Ether, A 61
Neomycin–Tubocurarine, **A** 111
Nialamide–Hydralazine, A 81
Nitrofurantoin–Probenecid, **A** 114
Orphenadrine–Propoxyphene, **A** 115
Oxyphenbutazone–Methandrostenolone, **B** 387
Pargyline–Alcohol, **A** 117
Pargyline–Amitriptyline, A 7
Penicillin–Aspirin, **A** 118
Penicillin–Chloramphenicol, **B** 389
Penicillin–Probenecid, **A** 119
Pentobarbital–Chlorcyclizine, A 17
Phenelzine–Chlorphentermine, A 20
Phenelzine–Halothane, A 78
Phenelzine–Levodopa, A 95
Phenformin–Alcohol, **A** 121
Phenobarbital–Phenytoin, A 54
Phenobarbital–Griseofulvin, A 68
Phenobarbital–Warfarin, A 168
Phenylbutazone–Acetohexamide, A 1
Phenylbutazone–Cholestyramine, **B** 391
Phenylbutazone–Warfarin, A 171
Piperazine–Chlorpromazine, A 23
Probenecid–Allopurinol, B 359
Phenytoin–Isoniazid, **A** 51
Phenytoin–Methylphenidate, **A** 53
Phenytoin–Phenobarbital, **A** 54
Probenecid–Chlorothiazide, **A** 393
Probenecid–Indomethacin, A 88
Probenecid–Nitrofurantoin, A 114
Probenecid–Penicillin, A 119
Propantheline–Digoxin, B 363
Propoxyphene–Alcohol, **B** 394
Propoxyphene–Amphetamine, **A** 123
Propoxyphene–Orphenadrine, A 115
Propranolol–Chlorpheniramine, **A** 124
Propranolol–Desipramine, **A** 126
Propranolol–Hexobarbital, A 80

Propranolol–Insulin, B 378
Propranolol–Quinidine, **B** 127
Propranolol–Tubocurarine, A 150
Pyridoxine–Isoniazid, B 381
Pyridoxine–Levodopa, A 96
Quinidine–Aluminum Hydroxide, **A** 128
Quinidine–Propranolol, A 127
Quinidine–Reserpine, **A** 130
Quinidine–Tubocurarine, A 152
Quinidine–Warfarin, A 173
Reserpine–Digitalis, A 42
Reserpine–Ephedrine, A 57
Reserpine–Halothane, **A** 131
Reserpine–Imipramine, **A** 133
Reserpine–Quinidine, A 130
Reserpine–Thiopental, A 141
Secobarbital–Dexamethasone, A 34
Spironolactone–Digitoxin, A 45
Succinylcholine–Dexpanthenol, **B** 396
Sulfaphenazole–Tolbutamide, A 147
Sulfinpyrazone–Aspirin, **A** 135
Sulfisoxazole–Methotrexate, A 108
Tetracycline–Aluminum Ions, **A** 136
Tetracycline–Calcium Ions, **A** 136
Tetracycline–Ferrous Sulfate, **B** 397
Tetracycline–Magnesium Ions, **A** 136
Tetracycline–Methoxyflurane, **A** 138
Tetracycline–Warfarin, B 408
Thiamylal–Chlorpromazine, **A** 139
Thiopental–Reserpine, **A** 141
Thyroid–Cholestyramine, **A** 143
Thyroid–Imipramine, A 84
Thyroxine–Warfarin, A 174
Tolbutamide–Alcohol, **A** 144
Tolbutamide–Chloramphenicol, **B** 399
Tolbutamide–Cortisone, **A** 146
Tolbutamide–Sulfaphenazole, **A** 147
Tranylcypromine–Ephedrine, B 366
Tranylcypromine–Imipramine, B 376
Tranylcypromine–Insulin, B 380
Tubocurarine–Chlorthalidone, **A** 149
Tubocurarine–Neomycin, A 111
Tubocurarine–Propranolol, **A** 150
Tubocurarine–Quinidine, **A** 152
Tyramine–Isocarboxazid, A 91
Vitamin K–Warfarin, A 177
Warfarin–Acetaminophen, **B** 401
Warfarin–Alcohol, **B** 402
Warfarin–Aluminum Hydroxide, **A** 153
Warfarin–Ascorbic Acid, **B** 404
Warfarin–Aspirin, **A** 155
Warfarin–Chloral Hydrate, **A** 157
Warfarin–Chlordiazepoxide, **A** 159
Warfarin–Chlorpropamide, A 31
Warfarin–Clofibrate, **B** 405
Warfarin–Diphenhydramine, **A** 161
Warfarin–Glutethimide, **A** 162
Warfarin–Griseofulvin, **A** 163
Warfarin–Meprobamate, **A** 165
Warfarin–Methandrostenolone, **A** 166
Warfarin–Phenobarbital, **A** 168
Warfarin–Phenylbutazone, **A** 171
Warfarin–Quinidine, **A** 173
Warfarin–Tetracycline, **B** 408
Warfarin–Thyroxine, **A** 174
Warfarin–Vitamin K, **A** 177

[a] Indented italic entries represent the inverted order of Drug-Pair titles. The designation "A 1" refers to page one in the APhA Handbook *Evaluations of Drug Interactions—1973,* While "B 401" refers to page 401 in the *1974 Supplement* of this handbook. This table is included here to provide a handy cross-index to both lists of significant drug interactions. The original references must be consulted for clinical details.

in vitro interactions now recognized between clinical or diagnostic test reagents (and procedures) and common foods (e.g., avocado, Metrecal, certain vitamins, etc.) or OTC or prescription drugs. Many materials have been shown to influence and confuse the interpretation of clinical tests of blood, serum, plasma, urine, hormones and miscellaneous tissues.

The dispensing picture is further complicated by various pharmaceutical problems and errors in drug therapy. These are discussed below in modest detail since they must be eliminated if undesired drug interactions are to be separated from the fairly common errors in diagnosis, prescribing, labeling, packing, storage, and administration of drugs, or for that matter, from allergic reactions, idiosyncrasies, or other adverse drug reactions (see Table 4).

Since the knowledge available in some of the pertinent areas is still rather limited, a complete system for predicting and resolving all drug interactions and incompatibilities remains to be developed in the future. A partial system given below provides the pharmacist with an overall view of the types of problems which may be encountered and the sources of information which may aid in their solution. It is hoped that he will also see the necessity for learning as much as possible about biochemistry, chemistry, enzymology, molecular biology, pharmacology, physiology, and the other medical sciences interrelating pharmacy and medicine. Such knowledge will enable him to render valuable consultation services to the prescribing physician.

The number of visits to private physicians for adverse drug reactions has increased in recent years. Although oral contraceptives and antimicrobials have accounted for 40% of these visits, other medications such as anticoagulants, antidepressants, enzyme inhibitors, steroids, and tranquilizers have also been involved.

Patients should usually be advised not to take medications which poten-

Table 7—Bronchial Asthma, Cough, Cold, Hay Fever and Rhinitis Remedies with Drug Interaction Potentials[a,b]

Key-product content	Product name
2, 3, 4	Coldene
1	Creo-Terpine (25% alcohol)
2, 4	Noscomel
2, 4	Novahistine, Novahistine-DH
4	Orthoxical
2	Robitussin-AC
2, 4	Romilar CF
4	Sudafed
2	Super Antihist Cough Syrup
1	Terpin Hydrate
1	Terpin Hydrate with Codeine
	Terpin Hydrate with Dextromethorphan
2, 4	Triaminic
2, 4	Triaminicol
4	Trind

[a] 1-alcohol; 2-antihistamine; 3-aspirin-salicylates; 4-sympathomimetics.
[b] Reproduced in part from Ref. 2.

tiate or inhibit the specific action of a drug being administered at the same time. For example, diphenhydramine (Benadryl) has an atropine-like (anticholinergic) effect. This should be considered during dispensing, particularly if the patient has glaucoma or is taking other medication with a similar effect. Also, excessive central nervous system depression (drowsiness, dizziness, etc.) may be experienced due to an additive effect when diphenhydramine is used along with barbiturates and other CNS depressants. This problem should be recognized by the pharmacist. There are hundreds of useful publications on this subject.

Selected categories of liquid pharmaceuticals available as OTC products that have potential for drug interactions are listed in Table 7 which is reproduced here in part from a lengthier one.

Self-medication advice is a serious responsibility of the pharmacist. The patient needs instruction as to safe use of OTC drugs alone or in combination with prescription products. The contraindication of sympathomimetic amines for patients on antidiabetic medications is a case in point. Only six pharmacists out of 36 contacted gave satisfactory information about this precaution when it was sought by one prospective patient. Self-medication is here to stay and the public needs the guidance of the pharmacist in the proper use of such OTC medications.

The pharmacist has the obligation not only to dispense the proper drug product but to make sure that the patient understands the safe use of the medication. Consultation with the patient should be at the point of dispensing. The alert pharmacist takes every opportunity to review the literature available and to prepare himself to relate accurate drug information to the patient when necessary, as long as he does not preempt the physician's prerogatives.

Recognition of the prevalence of adverse drug interactions and patient hypersensitivities is essential. This involves knowledge of the potential effect of one drug on another, the side effects known to occur, the multiple drug formulations used by the patient, the potentiating or inhibiting effects of one drug on another and the drug actions that are possible at various dosage levels of individual medications.

The effectiveness of a patient record system and the need for alertness of the pharmacist to drug interactions can be emphasized by the failure of 11 pharmacists of 12 surveyed to recognize the contraindications of Parnate (tranylcypromine hydrochloride), a monoamine oxidase inhibitor. When each was confronted with a prescription 1 week later for Tofranil (imipramine hydrochloride), only one pharmacist gave any warning regarding the potential drug interaction.

Cogent examples of the pharmacist's role in detecting potential adverse drug reactions may be cited. He may observe a patient purchasing an OTC sleep aid or a prescribed hypnotic while at the same time being treated with reserpine for hypertension. The patient may be experiencing early symptoms of depres-

sion and insomnia. The pharmacist should know that diabetics may be subject to aggravation of the disease in the presence of thiazide diuretics (Diuril, Hydrodiuril, etc.). He should be aware that oral steroids, sulfonamides, coumarins, anticoagulants and pyrazolones have been known to potentiate the action of sulfonylureas, and thereby bring on hypoglycemia. Thirst, frequency of urination, and hunger may be significant patient complaints.

One of the most frequent adverse drug effects is the drowsiness caused by certain antihistamines. Many nasal and chest decongestants and cold preparations contain these drugs and the patient should be warned of the hazards if he is known to be susceptible; however, for psychological reasons the pharmacist should not routinely attempt to warn patients that a drug may cause a reaction. The judgment of the pharmacist must be based on the merits of the situation, the particular patient involved, and other appropriate factors.

A request for an antacid like Maalox (*Rorer*), Amphojel (*Wyeth*), or milk of magnesia by a patient already taking phenylbutazone, aspirin, indomethacin, or an oral steroid may mean an ulcer is developing. Heartburn that occurs when these drugs are taken may be avoided by taking milk along with each dose of the medication. Such a request should, of course, trigger an alarm bell in the pharmacist's mind when tetracycline antibiotics are also being dispensed.

A particular area of caution is associated with the concurrent administration of sympathomimetic drugs such as amphetamines, phenylpropanolamine, and phenylephrine (in liquid cough, cold and nasal decongestant preparations) and MAO (monoamine oxidase) inhibitors. Sympathomimetic drugs are effectively deaminated by the monoamine oxidase in the body. If this reaction is interfered with by the presence of a MAO inhibitor (e.g., pargyline, nialamide or tranylcypromine) the amines can accumulate and therefore cause ex-

Table 8—Selected Adverse Reactions

Drug	Potential reactions
Ampicillin	Pruritic maculopapular rash
Aspirin	Ulcerogenic effect
Chloramphenicol	Aplastic anemia, optic neuritis, retards metabolic transformation of tolbutamide, diphenylhydantoin and dicoumarol
Demeclocycline	Photodynamic reaction (allergic response) on exposure to natural or artificial sunlight, dental staining
Diphenhydramine	Atropine-like action
Furazolidone	MAO inhibitor after 4–5 days; hemolysis in glucose-6-phosphate deficient patients
	Pruritic maculopapular rash
Methotrexate	Cirrhosis, hepatic fibrosis in psoriatic patients
Phenylbutazone	Edema, fever, sore throat, gastrointestinal irritation (ulcerogenic effect)
Reserpine	Depression, insomnia, weight gain
Tetracyclines	Action antagonized by antacids containing calcium magnesium, aluminum and bismuth; gastrointestinal irritation; dental staining; photodynamic reaction
Tolbutamide	Metabolized twice as fast in alcoholics (requires increase in hypoglycemic dosage); thiazide diuretics aggravate diabetic state (increase dose of hypoglycemic)

cessive stimulation of the sympathetic nervous system. The action may be prolonged or potentiated, resulting in headache and severe hypertension which is sometimes fatal.

Pharmacists generally are aware of the mounting evidence of drug sensitivities and potential drug-drug interactions. However, a continuous flow of such information is not usually provided or sought at the community pharmacy level. The objective here is to cite a few of the more frequently occurring specific patient drug reactions. The reactions pointed out for each drug are by no means exhaustive and new patient sensitivities are constantly being observed as medications are administered over extended periods of time and concurrently with other therapeutic agents. See Table 8.

Prescription Drugs in Drug Interactions

Unexpected increases or decreases in drug action with prescription drug therapy may be due to actions taken anywhere along the chain of events that take place in the medicopharmaceutic system: manufacturing, packaging, storage, distribution, diagnosis, prescribing, dispensing, administration, absorption, transport, metabolism, reaction on the receptor, and excretion.

Some of the effects of altering route and frequency of administration; absorption site and rate of intake; degree of alimentary motility; rate of intestinal blood flow; volume of digestive secretions; protein binding; receptor blocking; metabolism, by microsomal enzymes, of drugs, their metabolites and other substrates; storage in fat, bone, muscle, liver, kidney, lung, and other sites; rate of attachment and release at binding sites; rate of resorption from bile, kidney tubule, and elsewhere; and similar factors have been discussed in Chapter 2. Some of these are reconsidered in subsequent paragraphs as they affect multiple drug therapy and drug interactions. Obviously, the same considerations apply to OTC drugs. However, since most of these latter drugs are ten or more years old, the pharmacy, chemistry, pharmacology, toxicity, pathology and medical effects are usually well known, whereas many of the data on prescription drugs, especially new drugs, are locked in the files of the originating company and of the Food and Drug Administration. The latter agency usually does not release this information even after they have declared the compound "no longer a new drug" unless special label warnings are issued.

Some helpful information on prescription drug interactions and adverse reactions is given in the insert accompanying the original package. Additional information may be found in the references given in the package insert. *International Pharmaceutical Abstracts* condenses most of the medical articles on this subject and pertinent references can be found in the semi-annual and annual indexes of this journal listed under the generic name.

Many tables list the more common interacting drugs by generic name, classify them as to usual type of activity, and give the more common trade names. Some list by a decimal reference number or other system the more important drugs or drug classes which are additive, antagonized by, potentiated by, or which potentiate the drugs listed. They indicate which drugs are habit forming, excreted in mother's milk, or which may cross the placenta; also those drugs causing allergy, blood dyscrasias, hypersensitivities, or occasional idiosyncrasies. They caution against uncontrolled use in patients with cardiovascular problems, eye conditions such as glaucoma, gastrointestinal disease, joint and bone problems, kidney disease, liver disease, and nerve problems. They warn of possible adverse effects on the oral membranes, respiratory organs, skin, and urogenital, venous, and other systems. When any of these designations appear it is advisable to read the product insert carefully or look up the drug in the *Physicians' Desk Reference* which is a compilation of the 2500 most frequently used package inserts.

For best use of any table designed to predict possible drug interactions or adverse drug reactions, it is helpful to know the full medical history of the patient and what prescription drugs, OTC drugs, or chronically or occasionally taken preparations or foods may be present to interact. By listing the active ingredients of all medications taken and looking them up it is possible to see if any have been reported as additive, potentiating or antagonistic to any of the other ingredients. Interactions noted

can be looked up in cited references where available or the pharmacist may study the product inserts and discuss possible temporary or permanent changes in therapy with the physicians involved.

Common prescription drugs which have been reported as interactants with other prescription drugs, OTC drugs, and common foods should be considered in evaluating each prescription or therapeutic regimen.

Proprietary (OTC) Drugs in Drug Interactions

The significance of many over-the-counter (OTC) products in drug interactions has been emphasized. There are widespread interactions of legend drugs with such common proprietary products as:

Analgesics—Contain aspirin, salicylates, etc., e.g., ASA Compound, Alka-Seltzer, Anacin, Ascriptin, Aspirin, BC, Bufferin, Cope, Doan's Pills, Ecotrin, Empirin Compound, Excedrin, Fizrin, Measurin, Midol, Pabirin, PAC Compound, Pamprin, Phensal, Pre-Mens Forte, Stanback, Vanquish, Zarumin.

Antacids—Contain aluminum, calcium, magnesium, bicarbonate, citrate, hydroxides, oxides, silicates, e.g., Alglyn, Alkets, Alka-Seltzer, Aludrox, Alzinox, Amitone, Amphojel, AMT, Bellans, Bisodol, Calcium Carbonate, Soda, Chooz, Dicarbosil, Di-Gel, Gelusil, Gelusil-Lac, Krem, Kudrox, Maalox, Malcogel, Mucotin, Phosphaljel, Riopan, Rolaids, Robalate, Soda Mint, Syntrogel, Titralac, Tricremalate, Trisomin, Wingel.

Antihistamines (cold tablets and capsules)—Contain antihistamines, aspirin, belladonna alkaloids, etc., e.g., Allerest, Bronitin, Bromo-Quinine, Bronkaid, Cheracol cold capsules, Chexit, Colchek, Contac, Coricidin, Coricidin-D, Coryban-D, Dondril, Dristan, Fedrazil, Pyrroxate, Triaminicin, Tussagesic, Ursinus Inla Tabs, 4-Way Cold Tablets.

Antihistamines (liquids)—Contain antihistamines, alcohol, sympathomimetic amines, etc., e.g., Coldene, Creo-Terpin, NTZ, Novahistine, Novahistine-DH, Orthoxicol, Robitussin-AC, Romilar-CF, Sudafed, Super-Anahist, terpin hydrate preparations, Triaminic, Triaminicol, Trind.

Antihistamines (nasal sprays and nose drops)—Contain antihistamines, sympathomimetics, etc., e.g., Alconefrin, Contac, NTZ, Neo-Synephrine, Paredrine, Privine, Sinex, St. Joseph's Nose Drops, Super Anahist, Vasoxyl.

Anti-Asthma Preparations—Contain sympathomimetics, e.g., Adrenline Chloride, Asthmanefrin, Breatheasy, Bronkaid Mist, Epinephrine solution, Medihaler-Epi, Orthoxicol, Primatine Mist.

Antimotion-sickness Preparations—Contain antihistamines, e.g., Bonine, Dramamine, Marezine, Mothersill's Remedy.

Diarrhea Remedies—Contain attapulgite, bentonite, charcoal, colloidal antacids, kaolin and other clays, etc., e.g., Charcoal, Diabismul, Donnagel, Donnagel-PG, Kao-Con, Kaopectate, Paocin, Parepectolin, Quintess.

Laxatives—Contain surfactants, etc., e.g., Ceo-Two, Colace, Dialose, Doxan, Doxinate, Milkinol, Peri-Colace, Polykol, Rectalad, Regutol, Senocaps, Surfak.

Sleeping Aids—Contain antihistamines, belladonna or related alkaloids, etc., e.g., Dormin, Nytol, Relax-U Caps, San-Man, Sleep-Eze, Sominex.

Tonics—Contain alcohol, quinine, etc., e.g., Adenocrest, Betacrest, Cenalene, Feosol Elixir, Metalex-P, Fellows Syrup, Glytinic, Peruna, SSS, etc.

Other information as to the composition of these products may be found in the *APhA Handbook of Non-Prescription Drugs, Martindale's Extra Pharmacopeia,* or *Clinical Toxicology of Commercial Products* which give many tabulations of active ingredients of the more popular formulas and often point out potential drug interactions or toxicity. Prediction of drug interactions or adverse reactions can usually be accomplished by looking up the proprietary product in one of these handbooks and then looking up the known interactions of each active ingredient.

Foods in Drug Interactions

Drugs are often taken with foods to reduce gastric irritation. While such combinations may decrease gastric irritability they frequently delay gastric emptying time or affect passage through the gut and hence may affect absorption and rapidity of action. Often, chemical interactions or adsorption of drug onto food substances may also delay adsorption. The reduced activity of penicillin taken orally with foods, for example, is probably an acid-instability problem due to stimulation of gastric juice by the food.

Many common foods have been reported to interact with legend drugs. Some of the more important are:

Alcohol—May react with antianginal agents, antibacterial agents, antibiotics (penicillins), antifungal agents (furazolidone), antidiabetic agents (insulin, tolbutamide), antihistamines, antihypertensive agents, phenothiazine derivatives, monoamine oxidase inhibitors, sedatives, and hypnotics (barbiturates).

Fruits and Vegetables (*Brassica sp*) Brussels sprouts, cabbage, cauliflower, kale, turnips, soy bean preparations, peaches, pears, spinach, and carrots—(May interact with thyroid or affect the thyroid gland).

Leafy Green Vegetables—May interact with anticoagulants.

Licorice—May interact with oral diuretics, antihypertensive agents, and cardiac glycosides.

Milk and Dairy Products—May interact with cardiac glycosides, novobiocin, and tetracyclines.

Foods Containing Pressor Amines (histamine, tyramine, tryptamine, octopamine or serotonin)—In aged cheeses, broad or fava beans, beer, chicken livers, chocolate, pickled herring, some wines, bananas, passion fruit, pineapples, tomatoes, lemons, yeast extracts—May interact with antidepressants (monoamine oxidase inhibitors) and antihypertensive agents.

Beverages—Drug interactions may occur with a wide variety of alcoholic beverages (beer, wine, gin, vodka, whiskey, etc.) and caffeine containing beverages (coffee, tea, cola drinks).

Other Factors in Drug Interactions

Metabolic transformations, hereditary factors, allergies and psychosomatic situations are also well established as important factors in many drug interactions. In some cases, patients may have previously taken high or too frequent drug dosages or received certain drugs with prolonged action, or may have been exposed to toxic materials which adversely affect drug receptors or modify metabolizing enzymes or kidney, lung, and liver tissue. Decreased or increased action may take place in these tissues even if only one active ingredient is actually taken at a time.

In other cases, variations in body enzyme systems with age, high or low body temperatures, disease, nutritional state, physical condition, posture or heredity may make individuals, families, or even races sensitive or sometimes resistant to certain drugs or combinations of drugs. This may result in drug inactivity, toxicity or other unexpected action (idiosyncrasies, mutagenesis, carcinogenesis, teratogenesis, etc.).

Drug interactions and incompatibilities can also cause allergic reactions to a previously prescribed drug, a closely related compound, or an OTC product. It has been estimated that 10–12% of all persons are allergic to some kind of drug. Some authorities have estimated that as many as 10% of hospitalized patients are in the hospital due to iatrogenic (drug induced) diseases.

Apparently a great number of drug reactions are not allergic in nature but manifestations of individual overdosage or secondary pharmacologic action. Frequently, the drug absorption, transport, excretion, and metabolizing enzyme systems vary with age, sex, size, weight, race, temporary conditions (e.g., pregnancy, lactation, menstruation, nausea, vomiting, diarrhea, etc.), chronic conditions (e.g., diabetes, colitis, peptic ulcer, kidney disease, etc.), species, family, and individual. These factors, not always considered by the busy physician, are undoubtedly responsible for many unexpected drug actions and interactions. These again may produce either more or less or different actions than anticipated.

A drug interaction is commonly produced when a patient taking medication for a chronic condition is given other prescriptions for an acute illness which contains an additive, antagonistic, or potentiating drug. This therapeutic incompatibility usually takes place when two different physicians are prescribing for the same patient. It may also occur in psychosomatic situations (drug addiction, habituation, hypochondria, suicide, or murder) where the patient takes unintended or secret medication. Of course it probably occurs most often when the same doctor or pharmacist is untrained in the field of drug interactions or has an incomplete record of the prescribed drugs that the patient may still be taking. Such interactions are also common when the patient also takes interacting over-the-counter products, or when he takes medicine prescribed for another person. The latter may be either accidental or deliberate. Drug interactions and other therapeutic incompatibilities may be further complicated by placebo effect, doctor-patient relationships, and other psychosomatic considerations which sometimes potentiate, sometimes reduce drug actions, or produce bizarre effects. The complex nature of this entire problem is just beginning to be recognized in the literature on biopharmaceutics, enzymology, pharmacodynamics, pharmacogenetics, molecular pharmacology, clinical evaluation, and other disciplines.

All of these possibilities for drug interactions and incompatibilities among prescription drugs, OTC drugs, and foods, are convincing arguments for selection of both a family pharmacist and a physician who keep proper records for each member of the family, e.g., a pharmaceutical index of new prescriptions, prescription refills, proprietary drugs used chronically or occasionally, known drug reactions, food and pollen allergies, and the like. Such records should of course include the patient's name, address, age, telephone number, and information on chronic diseases (e.g., diabetes, asthma, hypertension, hyperthyroidism, kidney or liver problems, etc.), plus the names, addresses, and telephone numbers of other prescribing physicians, dentists, etc.

Pharmacogenetics (i.e., the study of the influence of heredity on drug action), is becoming a very important discipline in the study of drug interaction problems. Also, such studies as the AMA Council on Drugs *Registry on Adverse Reactions* and the FDA attempts to develop an adverse reaction reporting system, are playing an increasingly more important role in warning family medical consultants of potential adverse drug reaction and drug interaction problems.

Interferences in Clinical Laboratory Tests

Certain OTC products and prescription drugs may positively or negatively interfere with clinical diagnostic tests sufficiently to mislead the physician. The potentially confusing effect of many common drugs on laboratory diagnostic procedures has been noted. It has been shown that many such drugs influence clinical tests for constituents of blood, serum, plasma, urine, and various tissues. In similar extensive compilations, such interferences can be grouped into two general categories, pharmacological and chemical. In the first instance the drug interferes with the test through its toxicity or pharmacologic action on the body and perhaps distorts such normal indicators as blood sugar level, white or red cell counts, etc.

These interferences are, of course not true clinical *in vivo* drug interactions as previously defined, but they are frequently dose related and are very common. Examples are the short term alteration of the renal secretion of phenolsulfonphthalein (PSP) by sulfinpyrazole, the alteration of serum levels of chloride, potassium, and sodium ions by thiazide diuretics and the glycosuria produced by bismuth salts, nicotinic acid, isoniazid or large doses of epinephrine.

Some compounds may give false positive reactions in some tests and false negative reactions in others. For example, thiazide diuretics give false positive glucose tests in urine by either the Ames or Benedict methods and yet give false negative tests for calcium, creatinine, PSP, and uric acid in urine.

Drugs, other chemicals, and their metabolites may also interfere with clinical tests by coloring the urine or other body fluid or perhaps by combining chemically with the test reagents. Compounds which add their own color to urine, for example, include acriflavine, aminosalicylic acid, amitriptyline, anthraquinone derivatives, chloroquine, and phenazopyridine. Penicillin, streptomycin and ascorbic acid are examples of drugs which may affect test reagents; these may, for example, react with the copper sulfate in Benedict's test solution to produce invalid false positive tests for sugars.

Physical and Chemical Factors Influencing Drug Interactions

An obviously simplified concept of drug action and interaction may be introduced by considering man to be an integrated system of chemical molecules which, as he develops from fertilized egg to adult human, successively form more and more complex structures. Vertical integration accordingly produces an expanding system here in the following order: molecules → enzyme systems → cells → tissues → organs → total man. Now if a sufficient number of molecules are affected anywhere along this integrated chain by drugs or other chemicals, a change of response or function at higher levels is to be expected. Such chemical action may result in the production of a familiar drug effect or a less familiar drug interaction.

This oversimplified approach is, of course, based on conceptional reactions and interactions of even smaller units of atomic construction, e.g., electrons, protons, neutrons, positrons and other postulated subatomic components which make up the 105 currently known elements or atoms. The positively charged nucleus of protons, neutrons and positrons, surrounded by a cloud of activated negative electrons are believed to combine with other suitable activated atoms to form not only chemotherapeutic agents but also the proteins, minerals, fats, carbohydrates, water, and other constituents of human cells and tissues. Thus the same basic starting materials make up both drugs and those macromolecules which form polymolecular systems (cells), polycellular systems (tissues), polytissue systems (organs), and polyorgan systems (man). It is not surprising, therefore, that drugs and other chemicals can produce profound effects on man.

Drug actions requiring chemical reactions may occur if the outer shell electrons of a substrate atomic radical become suitably activated so as to interact with the outer shell electrons of another activated drug atom or radical which comes in contact with it. Often activation is produced by absorption of thermal or photoelectric energy in the presence of a catalyst (e.g., an enzyme). Interaction usually results in the formation of new molecules, possibly with the liberation of the enzyme catalyst and enough energy to continue a chain reaction. Such chemical reactions usually continue until structures of optimum stability are formed or until equilibrium conditions exist.

An even more complex process is one in which the newly formed molecules are immediately used as substrates by other enzymes present to form even more complex macromolecules which are then used as substrates for still other enzyme reactions. Cells, tissues, organs and even the individual person may be affected in turn by simple subatomic and atomic interactions. This is especially true when enzymes themselves are affected since these important biochemicals may speed up biochemical reactions many thousands of times.

Assuming that normal biochemical reactions are modified by chemical reactions of drugs, pharmacologists may go a step further and predict that administration of a different drug might produce a modified drug action by using up substrates by precipitating or adsorbing or otherwise modifying them chemically, or perhaps by interacting with the second drug when it appears. Drug interactions might also result from changes in physical properties, e.g., solubility, ionization, pH changes, etc., which one drug might induce in another and which might thereby affect pharmacodynamic functions such as absorption, distribution, biotransformation, and excretion.

Structural Factors

In regard to drug interactions, structurally related drugs producing the same pharmacological type of activity are likely to be exactly additive in effect. Potentiation through synergism is sometimes more apparent but it may involve different sets or types of receptors. Drug antagonism by structurally related compounds however is more likely to be due to competition for the same kinds of active receptor sites on key enzymes, cell membranes, or other specialized cell components.

Solubility and Related Factors

Drug interactions seem to frequently involve the more lipid-soluble drugs (alcohol, ether, etc.). This probably happens because these drugs are readily absorbed and reabsorbed into cells and tissues and frequently require extensive metabolism before they can be excreted. Their more prolonged contact with receptor sites, longer presence in the circulation and in the tissues, and prolonged reactions with normal body enzymes, not only increase the likelihood of clinical interactions but also creates certain difficulties in projecting pharmacological data from animals to man. This is especially true for animals whose liver microsomes have enzymatic processes which metabolize drugs differently from man.

On the other hand, highly ionized electrolytes, ionic compounds and other poorly lipid-soluble drugs, e.g., antibiotics, ganglionic blocking agents, and the like are frequently poorly absorbed; and since they are rapidly excreted with minimum metabolism, they are less likely to upset enzyme systems, produce drug interactions, incompatibilities, or toxic reactions. The action, toxicity and pharmacology of these drugs is thus easier to extrapolate to man from animals. Although a lipid-soluble drug might sometimes be expected to be absorbed, act and perhaps be excreted before a second ionic drug potentially incompatible with it has a chance to contact it, in actuality where multiple doses of each are taken both drugs are likely to be present in body fluids simultaneously.

Most active drugs are weak organic acids or bases which are often soluble in body fluids both as nonionized and ionized species. The nonionized portion may cross cellular membranes by preferential solubility in the lipid membrane (simple diffusion), while the ionized portion usually is low in lipid solubility and often is unable to penetrate the lipid membranes unless it sufficiently resembles normal substrates (specialized transport). Of course both ionized and nonionized molecules can filter through pores and spaces between cells if the molecular size is small enough. This usually requires a molecular weight less than 100.

Since simple diffusion seems likely to be the most important transfer mechanism with the transfer rate dependent on the lipid-water partition coefficient, solubilities of many drugs in water, alcohol and other organic solvents have been compiled so that partition coefficients may be approximated. Changes in acid-base balance may also have profound influences on the absorption and activity of drugs. The pK_a and pH values are accordingly listed where available so that the proportion of drug in the nonionized lipid-soluble form can be estimated.

A useful equation for estimating the percentage of ionization of a basic drug at any pH value is: 100/1 + antilog $(pH-pK_a)$; conversely, the per cent ionization of an acidic drug can be approximated by the equation 100/1 + antilog (pK_a-pH). The percentage of nonionized drug can then be calculated by subtracting the percentage ionized from 100%.

Whereas the nonionized form of a drug penetrates cells best it is usually the ionized form which exerts the specific biologic effect. The action of alcohol in potentiating aspirin, barbiturates and other drugs may arise then from the solvent action of alcohol as well as its effect on drug ionization.

pH and Related Factors

The pH value of drugs and their mixtures are often valuable in interpreting or predicting drug interactions. If unknown, the pH of a drug can frequently be approximated from the known values of close relatives or similar compounds. Adequately useful approximations can often be made by recalling that acids ionize to form positive ions similar in charge to the familiar hydrogen ion, H^+. Since such drugs are positively charged they tend to attract both negative electrons and negatively charged ions such as hydroxyl ions, OH^-. Of course, acids in the body may range in pH from the acid in gastric juice (approximately pH 1) up to the essentially neutral pH 6.99. Compounds which can either ionize to give a hydrogen ion (e.g., phenols, carboxylic acids, minerals acids) or can accept negative electrons or hydroxyl ions (e.g., enolizable ketones such as barbiturates) are considered to be acidic. These are often central nervous system depressants or compounds that are additive with these in their side effects.

Bases on the other hand are negative in charge and hence may attract hydrogen ions or donate electrons to an acceptor acid. Bases may range in pH from the essentially neutral pH 7.01 up to pH 14, although most useful drugs probably do not exceed pH 10.5 due to physiological intolerance at higher ranges. Common bases include primary, secondary and tertiary amines (e.g., amphetamines, nicotine) and nonenolizable ketones (e.g., camphor). These often are central nervous system stimulants or possibly compounds that are additive with these in their side effects.

Drugs with both acidic and basic groups may be neutral, slightly acidic, or slightly basic depending on their ability to ionize H^+ or OH^- groups or to accept or donate electrons. Nicotinic acid, for example, has both a basic heterocyclic nitrogen and an acidic carboxyl group, hence it is expected to be neutral and to have little additive effect with either central nervous system stimulants or depressants. Of course, drugs which are metabolized in the body so that new acidic or basic groups are formed may undergo changes in the intrinsic pH values of their solutions and in their central nervous system activity. Codeine for example becomes intrinsically more depressant as it is O-demethylated to more acidic morphine.

pH values of common inorganic compounds are given in Table 12 (page 406) as an aid in estimating the pH of prescription mixtures.

Additional pH values of USP and NF drugs and of the "Top 500" drugs and their dosage forms are given at the end of the chapter in separate alphabetically listed monographs.

Pharmacodynamic Mechanisms Influencing Drug Interactions

Pharmacodynamics has been defined as the study of the biochemical and physiological actions of drug and their mechanisms of action.

To produce its characteristic effects, a drug must achieve adequate concentration at its sites of action. It has been pointed out that the biological activity of a compound is not only a function of its impact at a locus of action, but also its ability to get to and be removed from the active site (i.e., pharmacokinetics). The speed of action, duration, relative toxicity, and possible routes of administration may then depend not only upon drug dosage but also upon the physicochemical properties* or biopharmaceutical properties† which in turn influence absorption, distribution, metabolism, and excretion.

Since drug action depends upon reaction of the drug with an active site, and since the drug attached to this site is in equilibrium with the free drug in the adjacent body fluid (plasma, lymph, cerebrospinal fluid, tears, nasal secretion, saliva, gastric juice, intestinal juices, urine, vaginal secretions, etc.) and with drug bound to plasma proteins, amino acids, fats, enzymes, cells, etc., calculations of drug kinetics become quite

---

* Hydrogen bonding or other weak chemical bonds, water and lipid solubility, thermodynamic action, dissociation constants, intramolecular distances, oxidation-reduction potentials, metal catalysts or complexes, shapes, etc.

† Particle size, crystal form, ester or salt form, tablet formulation factors, fillers, etc.

complex. These become even more complex when more than one drug or other potential interactant is present.

Absorption, Transport, Storage and Excretion

The important pharmacodynamic factors in drug interactions have been discussed previously in this chapter; hence, comments below will be restricted to a few points which may need further emphasis from the standpoint of drug interactions.

Preceding discussions noted that drugs which are weak acids follow the law of mass action and are driven by the high hydrogen ion concentration of the gastric juice principally to the nonionized form. Since this form is best absorbed across lipid membranes, it is better absorbed from the stomach than from other portions of the gastrointestinal tract where the higher pH tends to ionize them. Furthermore, weak acids tend also to maintain their blood levels with an acid urine because of increased reabsorption in the cells of the kidney tubules while they tend to have diminished blood levels with a more alkaline urine because of decreased reabsorption.

This theory, of course, assumes no significant changes in pK_a caused by metabolism of the drug in the body or by interaction with other compounds. Actually, simultaneous administration of several weakly acidic drugs usually does not significantly change gastric absorption or renal excretion of any one of them, although strong acids if they produce a sufficient increase in the acidity of the stomach contents, may improve absorption of weak acids. Conversely, the simultaneous administration of a sufficiently alkaline material with a weakly acidic drug should tend to reduce gastric absorption, and if the alkalinity affects the pH of the urine, may also promote excretion.

On the other hand, drugs which are weak bases (e.g., ephedrine, morphine, quinidine) should equilibrate rapidly in the intestinal contents to nonionized base forms and hence be better absorbed there than from the stomach where they are highly ionized. Weakly basic drugs are also likely to maintain their blood levels better with an alkaline urine than with an acid urine because of greater reabsorption in the kidney tubule, provided pK_a changes due to chemical interaction with other drugs or to metabolic effects do not interfere. These considerations suggest the possible value of alkaline buffers in promoting initial absorption and reducing excretion of weak bases.

Theoretically, lowered pH in the gastrointestinal tract and the urine should potentiate acidic drugs and inhibit basic drugs and vice versa, since acidic drugs tend to migrate across membranes to regions of higher pH and basic drugs do the opposite. All general rules seem to have exceptions, however, and the reported improvement in the speed of action of buffered aspirin over plain aspirin seems to contradict the above theory. Other factors may be the rate limiting ones in this instance. Since insoluble aspirin must first go into solution before it can be absorbed, transported or produce its effect, the apparent differences here may actually be due to differences in drug dissolution rate as influenced by formulation, disintegration time, active drug particle size, and other biopharmaceutic factors. Other important considerations such as drug binding, metabolism or excretion factors may also play a part, as is discussed later.

Apparently, unless a drug goes into solution (before or after administration) it does not produce its intended action. Drug interactions which reduce solubility (precipitation, complexation, adsorption) usually adversely affect drug activity, while those that increase solubility (formation of soluble ions, complexes, salts, esters, etc.) usually promote drug action. The choice of vehicle or diluent may therefore be important. Oral drugs are usually administered in or with hot or cold liquids (water, milk, juices, carbonated beverages, teas, wines, cocktails, elixirs, spirits, syrups, emulsions, suspensions, etc.). Those containing alcohol may sometimes be contraindicated due to the many drug interactions that occur with alcohol. Those containing oils sometimes delay absorption if the drug is very soluble in the oily phase. On the other hand hot beverages may promote absorption due to increased blood circulation in the oral or gastrointestinal areas. Carbonated beverages may be advantageous if their pH, carbonic acid, organic acids, and other ingredients promote solubility as is sometimes noted with drugs such as caffeine, theophylline, and theobromine.

Once absorbed into the blood a drug may have to cross several lipid type membranes to reach intended sites of action. During transport, the drug may be vulnerable to interactions with plasma proteins or other drugs or inactivating or detoxifying substrates of the body such as sulfate ions, glucuronic acid, etc., or it may be absorbed into fatty droplets, blood cells, and other storage areas.

Most ionized drugs are excreted through the glomerulus or tubule of the kidney where special transport mechanisms are available to assist their passage into the urine. Drug interactions may occur in the nephron if a drug interferes with these excretion mechanisms by altering the pH of the tubular urine, or interacting in other ways already discussed. For example, penicillin excretion can be delayed and blood levels maintained by coadministration of probenecid which interferes with these transport mechanisms. Salicylates antagonize the uricosuric activity of probenecid and sulfinpyrazone by competing for tubular secretion in the kidney while the latter may displace organic ions such as salicylates from plasma proteins and thus influence their distribution and excretion. Methenamine and its compounds which release antiseptic formaldehyde in acid urine can affect excretion of sulfonamides; the formaldehyde may react to form an insoluble precipitate capable of causing blockage.

Some sulfonamides crystallize as free acids in the kidney tissues when the concentration is optimum and the pH of the urine is sufficiently low. This latter possibility is one of the reasons for administering sodium bicarbonate or sodium citrate and large quantities of water with sulfonamides.

Some lipid soluble drugs (alcohol, ether, chloroform, nitrous oxide, etc.) can be excreted in limited amounts through the lungs in the expired air, through the apocrine glands in the sweat, or through the liver in the bile which passes into the intestines and is excreted in the feces. Some drugs (thyroid type drugs) are conjugated as glucuronates and sulfates by the liver but these complexes are often destroyed again by the digestive processes so that the drug is reabsorbed in the intestine and principally excreted by the kidney. This enterohepatic cycling continues until all the available drug and its metabolites are excreted fecally or in the urine.

It should be noted that the blood usually has enough proteins, amino acids, phosphate ions and other buffers to enable it to maintain a pH value of about 7.4, even in the presence of weak acids or bases which are buffers in their own right. Thus, to evaluate drug interactions in blood and some of its filtrates such as the tears, lymph, and cerebrospinal fluid, values for the ionization of drugs in water or aqueous solutions at pH values near neutrality can usually be utilized. This approach does not hold true of course for urine since the pH of this blood filtrate commonly varies widely from pH 4 to 8.5, depending on the metabolites and other solutes present, buffers taken, ions reabsorbed, and related factors.

The activity of certain drugs may depend upon their concentration within certain cells. Since intracellular fluids are often more acidic than pH 7.4, bases which are less ionized in plasma tend to migrate into cells and usually show greater intracellular concentrations than acids of comparable molecular weight. Changes in extracellular pH can therefore change the concentrations of drugs within cells and affect their activity. For example, a slight decrease in plasma pH may decrease the plasma concentration of a weak acid like phenobarbital, concomitantly increase its intracellular concentration, and thereby increase its sedative action. Administration of bases such as sodium bicarbonate after phenobarbital increases the alkalinity of the plasma, favors passage of the drug out of the cells, and reduces its sedative potency.

Other drug activity may be a function of plasma level rather than intracellular level, as for example, mecamylamine blocking activity in ganglia. An increase in plasma acidity, perhaps by infusion of certain acidic injectables, tends to favor plasma concentration of this weak base, and thus to potentiate it.

In summary, to predict the absorption, transport, storage, or excretion of a drug and its activity or its chances of drug interaction, one must first know whether it is a lipid or an electrolyte, whether it is a weak acid, base or neutral compound, whether its action is of an intracellular or extracellular type, and also its probable response to changes in acid-base balance.

It has been repeatedly pointed out that some of the available published information on drug interactions or incompatibilities may actually be misinformation since formulations vary from company to company and from time to time. Thus the pharmacist and physician may need to study the original references to determine date of publication, actual brands and dosages of products used, clinical circumstances, applicability of any statistical evaluation, and other pertinent information.

Multiple Interactions

When more than one mechanism is involved in a drug interaction, prediction becomes difficult. For example, accepted theory regarding acetylcholinesterase inhibitors points to two types of anticholinesterase (cholinergic) drug action, e.g., drugs which compete with acetylcholine for the enzyme (competitive inhibition) and those which inactivate acetylcholinesterase by combining with the enzyme (noncompetitive inhibition).

The incidence of multiple types of drug action and interaction is rather high. Several types of enzyme mechanisms may operate simultaneously in the more complicated drug therapies and thus make adequate explanation difficult. The anticancer drug methotrexate, for example, is highly toxic because it is a folic acid antagonist; but it also interferes in the essential functions of all cells through chemical blockage of endogenous synthesis of thymidine, purines, and glycine. Such complex toxicities are best regarded as drug interactions since they can often be overcome by administration of the normal end products of the metabolism blocked or depressed.

Many of these multiple mechanisms are too complicated or too imperfectly understood to consider fully in this brief introduction to drug interactions, hence the original literature should be searched and studied for further details.

Clinical Factors in Drug Interactions

The many clinical factors that cause drug interactions are discussed below under the headings: diagnostic errors, prescribing errors, and drug administration and patient care.

Diagnostic Errors

Several types of incompatibilities are caused by errors in diagnosis made either by the physician about to write a prescription or by a customer who has made a self diagnosis and is planning to purchase a certain OTC drug.

Errors of this type include those made during the first visit to the physician when the accurate history of the patient is not obtained, as when a hypochondriac or other emotionally disturbed patient gives inadequate, inac- curate or exaggerated information, or when the symptoms are covered up by drugs previously taken, e.g., fever reduced by aspirin or other OTC analgesics. Diagnostic problems can also arise if the patient is an infant or otherwise unable to communicate, if the patient or his family has failed to have a previously prescribed prescription filled, if he has taken too much or too little of the medication, or if he has concurrently taken other drugs which produce adverse interactions.

The patient or his family may often make errors in self diagnosis after watching television commercials or perhaps asking a neighbor with a home medical encyclopedia what could cause their symptoms. Further, enthusiastic drug articles in such popular publications as *Time, Reader's Digest,* or *Parade* may actually generate problems for their more suggestive readers. This is especially true for hypochondriacs. The family pharmacist can often render a valuable service by making sure the customer understands the full purpose, use, and dosage of OTC items.

The confusion which can be caused by interferences in laboratory tests has already been discussed.

Prescribing Errors

The rationale for prescribing more than one ingredient at a time, either in the same or in simultaneous prescriptions, is hopefully to ameliorate the disease and discomfort of the patient without creating additional disease and discomfort. This sometimes involves prescribing an active ingredient to eliminate the etiology of the disease plus other ingredients to relieve discomfort, and possibly a third group of ingredients to reduce the undesirable effect of the first two. Since every patient is an individual case with differing age, weight, body surface, metabolism, and other characteristics, the desired effect is seldom perfectly achieved with the prescription of a single manufactured product (i.e., a rigid dosage combination).

In hypertension, peptic ulcer, allergy, diabetes, tuberculosis or other chronic disease, it is usually possible for the physician, by experimenting with combinations of ingredients and titrating dosages, to achieve the best medication for that particular patient. He may treat less chronic situations such as infections with heroic doses of broad spectrum or "shotgun" antibiotic combinations in hopes of overcoming the infection before the causative agent develops resistance or the patient dies. He may also prescribe additional medication to ease discomfort. He is often guided in his selection of treatment by his knowledge of the infectious agents currently endemic, epidemic or pandemic and the antibiotic or combination treatment currently effective. When the symptoms suggest that a new etiologic agent is present, the physician may gamble on a broad spectrum antibiotic while testing a specimen for sensitivity to more effective agents. Drug interactions often arise in prescribing such combinations because the physician overlooks the fact that the second or third group of ingredients (even excipients, preservatives, etc.) may alter the degree of absorption or penetration, may change the rate of degree of action, metabolism or excretion, or perhaps produce drug synergism, potentiation, or antagonism. These possibilities are discussed in later paragraphs. Many prescribing errors evolve when prescriptions are written in a hurry or the practitioner is inexperienced in prescription writing. The pharmacist, with a friendly call, can assist in correcting the errors.

Insufficient Study of the Patient—Based on his observations of the OTC products purchased by a customer, the questions asked, the prescriptions filled in the past, friendly conversation, and other bits of information, the pharmacist is frequently in a position to assist the busy or new physician who may not have the complete case history of a patient. Thus where the prescription tendered indicates that the physician is not aware of chronic disease, hereditary defects, previous idiosyncrasies, and drug toxicities, drug tolerances, habituation, addiction, alcoholism, allergy, hypochondria, pregnancy, or other contraindications it becomes the professional duty of the pharmacist to diplomatically bring this to the attention of the prescriber. This is especially true in cases of hypersensitivity and idiosyncrasy where the safety and welfare of the patient or an unborn child requires it. This is a matter of judgment and experience and no firm rules or suggestions can be made which will fit every situation. Of course the efficacy of medicine often depends on the confidence of the patient in the physician and the medication, so the pharmacist must be extremely careful not to upset critical doctor-patient relationships.

Contraindicated Drugs—Consult with the physician if the prescription calls for a drug to which the patient is known to be allergic; also check with the patient if it is suspected that he is still taking a previously acquired medication which may be contraindicated for use with the new one. Thus, the pharmacist should watch for prescriptions which might neutralize another drug, potentiate it to a dangerous level, or be incompatible with the patient's chronic conditions. For example, epinephrine and other vasoconstrictors usually cannot be given safely to a person receiving treatment for hypertension, while certain sulfonamides should not be given to patients receiving urinary acidifiers. Morphine, barbiturates, and similar drugs are frequently dangerous in severe asthma or in pulmonary congestion complicated by respiratory infection. Violent reactions to penicillin have also occurred with these respiratory conditions, and the physician's attention should be directed to known cases of drug sensitivity. Chlorpromazine, chlorothiazide, probenecid, prochlorperazine, and arsenicals have been responsible for jaundice in certain patients and certainly should be contraindicated in patients known to be subject to this condition. Likewise, adrenal steroids,

ACTH, and rauwolfia compounds are contraindicated in ulcer patients, and tetracycline antibiotics and chloramphenicol are dubious treatments for anemia. Tables 6 to 8 list other drugs which should be used with caution.

Reports of pharmacological incompatibilities arising from adverse interactions between drugs used simultaneously are increasing in the literature. For example, a number of cases are reported in which one of the offending substances was one of the newer antidepressant drugs belonging to the class termed monoamine oxidase (MAO) inhibitors. Members of that group of drugs, which includes phenelzine (Nardil) sulfate, isocarboxazid (Marplan), nialamide (Niamid), and tranylcypromine (Parnate) sulfate, have been shown to produce a number of severe, and often fatal, reactions when given with certain foods and drugs. For instance, other antidepressant drugs such as imipramine (Tofranil; Presamine) hydrochloride or amitriptyline (Elavil; Etrafon; Triavil) hydrochloride should not be given to patients who are being treated with one of the monoamine oxidase inhibitors until 2 or 3 weeks after the cessation of such treatment. To give the two types of antidepressants simultaneously may cause sweating, salivation, excitement, greatly raised temperature, coma, and in some cases, death.

There are other drugs and even certain amine-containing foods, (e.g., cheddar cheese) which should not be administered to patients while they are being treated with MAO inhibitors (nor within 2 or 3 weeks of discontinuing such treatment) because of the possibility of potentiating the effect of the drug. Many of these are indicated in published tables. Reactions may not occur in every patient to whom such combinations are given, but in view of their severity when they do occur, it is best to avoid them.

The pharmacist has a responsibility, when dispensing a prescription for two or more drugs for the same patient, to be on the lookout for possible pharma-

cological incompatibility. If he suspects a combination of drugs is likely to produce toxic reactions, he should so inform the prescriber. To do that he can be guided only by a knowledge of reactions that have been reported previously for the same or chemically related substances. However, a little knowledge can be dangerous and pharmacists must have knowledge of drug interactions in more depth and in better perspective than many practitioners have demonstrated. While charts such as Table 6 are useful as an initial screening mechanism to detect possible drug interactions, these cannot substitute for the full reports in the original publication. It is important for the pharmacist to study actual reports and to have an accurate reference which he can give to the physician when needed. For such knowledge, both the doctor and the pharmacist must rely on the prompt publication of reports of toxic effects in the professional journals. Manufacturers should therefore be made aware of the contribution which both physicians and pharmacists can make toward the prevention of toxic effects arising from drug interactions and should keep them fully informed of any new developments.

It is generally held that therapeutic incompatibilities are the responsibility of the physician rather than of the pharmacist, but the pharmacist can do much to promote professional relations with the physician if he is informed, yet diplomatic, in his attempts to eliminate any possibility of error in filling the physician's prescriptions.

The pharmacist who keeps abreast of the pharmaceutical and medical literature can obviously do a great deal to eliminate therapeutic incompatibilities and undesired drug interactions.

17

R	Sulfadiazine	250 mg
	Sulfamerazine	250 mg
	Ammonium chloride	500 mg
	M. Cap. D.T.D.	xxxvi
	Sig: 2 cap. q. 4 hours for cough.	

This is a contraindicated combination since urinary acidifiers such as ammonium chloride may cause deposition of sulfonamide crystals in the kidney. The physician should be consulted.

18

℞ Alba-Penicillin Capsules (Upjohn)   xxiv
  Sig: 2 caps. t.i.d.

The community pharmacist called the physician and recommended changing the prescription to "Albamycin capsules 250 mg." (Upjohn) since the patient had previously been treated by another physician for a suspected penicillin reaction.

Excessive Single Doses—Check with the physician if more than two to three times the usual dosage is prescribed. Use a suitable rule to calculate a child's dose.

19

℞ Atropine sulfate   0.006 g
  Phenobarbital   0.36 g
  M. Capsules D.T.D. #12
  Sig: One t.i.d.a.c.

This represents 12 times the dose of atropine and phenobarbital. The physician undoubtedly intended that the prescription be divided into 12 doses but wrote the wrong directions. It is necessary to call the prescriber and request permission to correct the directions, e.g., "M. Div. cap. #12."

20

℞ Strychnine sulfate   0.02 g
  Iron and ammonium citrate   0.5 g
  Ft. Caps tal ds. xx.
  Sig: One capsule tid pc.

This prescription calls for a 10 times overdose of strychnine and probably represents a decimal point error, i.e., the physician intended to prescribe 0.002 g but misplaced the decimal. He should be called for permission to change the dose.

21

℞ for Neil   Age 4
  Elixir phenobarbital   90 ml
  Simple syrup   q.s. ad   120 ml
  Sig: One teaspoonful q.i.d.

This represents an overdose of phenobarbital for a child. Using Young's rule, the usual dose would be 5 ml × [4/(4 + 12)] = 1.25 ml of phenobarbital elixir per dose. This prescription will give 3.75 ml per dose. Even though children tolerate large quantities of barbiturates, it is advisable to check with the prescriber.

22

℞ Fld. ext. Belladonna   12 cc.
  Elixir Phenobarbital   q.s.   100 cc.
  M. Sol.
  Sig: Teaspoonful t.i.d.

This called for an overdose of belladonna. The fluidextract is prescribed, but the tincture is probably intended, as the individual dose would give 10 times the accepted dosage. The prescriber should be consulted.

Excessive Daily Dose—Check with the physician if the prescription dosage exceeds the permitted daily dose given on the label or in official references.

23

℞ Codeine phosphate   15 mg.
  Ammonium chloride   500 mg.
  M. Caps. D.T.D. #24
  Sig: Two caps q.h. for cough.

This represents an improper frequency of dosage for codeine. The USP recommends the prescribed dose every 4 hours, not every hour. The physician probably intended to write "q. 4 hr for cough" and should be consulted.

24

℞ Amobarbital   200 mg.
  Acetylsalicylic acid   300 mg.
  M. Chart #1. D.T.D. #12
  Sig: One chart q.4. hours

This prescription calls for an improper frequency of dosage for amobarbital. The USP notes that the usual dose is 200 mg at bedtime. The physician should be called.

Additive and Synergistic Combinations—Check with the physician if several drugs having the same pharmacological action are prescribed together near their full or maximum individual dose. Drugs of such combinations usually should be prescribed in reduced amounts since the sum of their therapeutic activity may be too great. This is especially true if the combination is synergistic; i.e., the combined action is greater than would be expected from the sum of their individual actions.

Either additive or synergistic action is a desirable property if the toxicity or side effects are reduced by the lower dosages used, the activity is increased, or the prescription becomes less expensive. As examples, combinations of sulfonamides often show less nephrotoxicity than a single sulfonamide; bromide-barbiturate combinations reduce the bromide content, hence the danger of brominism; neomycin-erythromycin combinations have a broader spectrum than either antibiotic alone; and aspirin-prednisolone or aspirin-codeine combinations may reduce the amount of prednisolone or codeine required.

Prescriptions with more than one ingredient may sometimes produce both rapid and prolonged action if a rapid acting drug is prescribed with a drug having a prolonged action. For example, combinations of procaine penicillin and penicillin or secobarbital and phenobarbital give such an effect.

Sometimes superior activity with less tendency toward side effects and drug resistance can be obtained by the use of several drugs which produce a similar effect in a different way. One drug may act through one mechanism, while others act by a second or third mechanism; e.g., penicillin with sulfonamides for infections, combinations of aspirin, phenobarbital, and extract of hyoscyamus as an analgesic, or digitalis and an organomercurial diuretic for treating congestive heart failure. The addition of ammonium chloride to this latter therapy may also help since the acidifying effect of the ammonium salt may contribute to the ionization of the mercury.

Occasionally, toxicity may be increased by either additive or synergistic actions. For example, it has been reported that epinephrine and cocaine increase each other's toxicity. The simultaneous administration of santonin and alkaline carbonates or hydroxides results in the formation of soluble and toxic santoninates. Castor oil and other fixed oils also should not be given with santonin or aspidium as the oil increases the absorption of the active principles and thus increases their toxicity.

Numerous examples of possible overdosage due to drug combinations may be found in the PDR or published tables. Full doses of several stimulating drugs, i.e., drugs having the same positive type of action in a given direction, or several depressing drugs, i.e., drugs having the opposite type of action, may constitute an overdose due to additive action, i.e., $(+1) + (+1) = (+2)$ (additive stimulation), or $(-1) + (-1) = (-2)$ (additive depression). Potentiation may more closely resemble the situation: $(+1) + (+1) \cong (+3)$ (potentiated stimulation) or $(-1) + (-1) \cong (-3)$ (potentiated depression). A full dose of a stimulating drug plus a full dose of a depressing drug may give no therapeutic effect due to neutralization or antidotal action, e.g., $(+1) + (-1) = 0$.

It is obvious that careful study should be made of prescriptions containing several similarly acting drugs. For example, in the following discussion drugs from the same family, with the same group title or with equivalent action, may be additive. Thus, sympathetic stimulants may be additive in overall effects (but sometimes only in selected effects) with parasympathetic depressants as well as with other sympathetic stimulants. Likewise, parasympathetic stimulants may be additive with other parasympathetic stimulants or with sympathetic depressants.

25

℞	Amphetamine sulfate	0.2 g
	Ephedrine sulfate	0.5 g
	Syrup Orthoxine q.s. ad.	100 ml

Here, three sympathetic stimulants are prescribed in full dosage. Since the prescription represents a potential additive overdose, the physician should be consulted.

Antagonism in Combinations— Check with the physician if the full doses of two antagonistic drugs are prescribed together as this may be an unintentional error. In such cases, it is possible that the resulting prescription will have no therapeutic effect if the drug actions cancel each other. The prescribing of stimulants with sedatives, demulcents with irritants, sympathomimetics with sympatholytics, sympathetic stimulants with parasympathetic- stimulants, purgatives with antidiarrheals, acidifiers with alkalizers, or pyretics with antipyretics are examples which might fall under this heading. An interesting example of antagonism is seen when aspirin is prescribed together with probenecid (Benemid) in the treatment of gout. Each of these drugs is an effective uricosuric agent in itself, but the combination is antagonistic.

Pharmacologic antagonism may vary with the biologic system involved. Thus, while theoretical neutralization may occur with regard to gross central nervous system stimulation and depression, it has been found that the simultaneous administration of amphetamines with amobarbital usually produces a euphoric response with little sedative action. This combination does not affect all people in the same way or even the same person the same way at all times. This variation emphasizes the need for rational individualized therapy and especially close medical supervision of the patient.

In many cases the prescribing of antagonistic combinations is beneficial. For example, if one drug has some desirable effects and some undesirable effects, it may be prescribed with drugs which oppose the unwanted actions but do not interfere with the desired effects. Thus, in prescribing morphine as an analgesic, a physician may use atropine to prevent an excessive depressant effect of morphine on the respiratory center.

In treating congestive heart failure, a combination of opposite-acting quinidine and digitalis is sometimes used. In these cases, it is common for the drug which is used to neutralize the side effects to be prescribed only in partial doses. As an example, in R 26 a partial dose of caffeine is intended to overcome the cerebral depressant action of the acetophenetidin. Note also that the acetophenetidin and aspirin are prescribed only in partial doses since they are both analgesics.

26

R	Acetophenetidin	2½ gr.
	A.S.A.	3½ gr.
	Caffeine	½ gr.

Other examples include the use of mild laxative antacids to overcome the constipating action of astringent antacids (e.g., magnesium hydroxide with aluminum hydroxide) and the addition of central nervous stimulants to overcome the drowsiness of antihistaminics [e.g., Plimasin (*Ciba*)].

In rare cases, antagonistic combinations may be prescribed for their placebo effect.

27

R	Dexedrine	5 mg.
	Ergonovine maleate	0.5 mg.
	M. Caps. D. T. D. #6	
	Sig: As directed	

This is a potential antagonistic combination. Dexedrine, a sympathetic stimulant, and ergonovine, a sympathetic depressant, are both prescribed at full dosage. The prescriber should be consulted.

28

R	Methamphetamine HCl	5 mg.
	Pilocarpine Nitrate	5 mg.
	M. Ft. Capsule D.T.D. 12	
	Sig: One capsule on arising	

This may be intended as an improved analeptic. Methamphetamine is both a CNS and sympathetic stimulant and pilocarpine is a parasympathetic stimulant. Consult the prescriber.

29

R	Benemid	500 mg
	Aspirin	300 mg
	M. capsule äl D.T.D. XII	
	Sig: One capsule a day for gout.	

This prescription calls for an antagonistic combination. Although both drugs are effective uricosuric agents separately, the combination is reportedly ineffective. The physician should be consulted.

Prescription Writing Errors—Check with the physician if the amount of drug prescribed is only $\frac{1}{10}$ to $\frac{1}{1000}$ of that which is usually prescribed as it is likely that an error in placing the decimal point has been made or that milligrams were written when grams were intended.

Frequently, the physician writes the formula for a single dose and specifies that a certain number of such doses be dispensed. Errors can then occur if the prescriber uses incomplete or incorrect directions or the pharmacist misinterprets them to mean that the single dose is to be divided into the specified number of doses.

The pharmacist should calculate the actual dose prescribed for each potent drug and in this way can often determine the intent of the prescriber. However, he should consult the prescriber if there is any doubt.

30

R	Hyoscyamus Tincture	1.67 ml
	Potassium Citrate	1.67 g
	Comp. Cardamom Tr. q.s. ad	100 ml

M. Soln.

Sig: One teaspoonful as directed.

Prescription 30 probably represents a decimal point error since the dose of hyoscyamus and potassium citrate are only about $\frac{1}{10}$ of that normally prescribed.

Nomenclature Error—Check with the prescriber if the drug specified does not match the use or directions of the prescription, especially if there is danger involved.

The expanding number of manufactured products with very similar names and the occasional difficulty of deciphering difficult handwriting make it imperative to determine the physician's intent; e.g., the close, written similarity between "Alphaden" (*Alphaden Co., Inc.*), a mineral supplement, and "Alphalin" (*Lilly*), a vitamin A product. Confusion might also result, when receiving an oral prescription via the telephone, between the latter product and "Alphyllin" (*Massengill*), a diuretic and coronary vasodilator.

In order to assist him in the determination of the physician's intent, the pharmacist usually maintains an up-to-date card file on new products, professional journals which publish the latest information on new drugs, and the latest reference books.

Nomenclature errors should also be considered such as the prescribing of barium sulfide for barium sulfate, sodium sulfite for sodium sulfate, or mercuric chloride for mercurous chloride.

31

R	Barium sulfite	350 g
	C.M.C. Low visc.	30 g
	Aerosol OT	1.6 g
	Sorbitol Soln. 70%	150 ml
	Water, to make	1000 ml

M. Susp.

Sig: To be used as a retention enema before coming to office.

This prescription calls for the wrong drug. The physician intended nontoxic barium sulfate but prescribed a toxic dose of soluble barium sulfite. He should be consulted.

32

R   C.T. Mannitol with Phenobarbital #24
Sig: One tab. q.i.d.

This is a wrong title. "Mannitol Hexanitrate with Phenobarbital" (*Fellows* or *Squibb*) is probably intended. Call the physician.

33

R   Sedaco (Massengill)
Sig: P.r.n. for cough

This is undoubtedly a wrong trademark. "Sedaco" is a *Strasenburgh* trademark for a cough syrup, but since the physician specified Massengill, he probably intended "Sedacof." He should be consulted.

34

R	Aminopterin	300 mg.
	M. Ft. Caps D.T.D. #12	

Sig: One capsule for Headache

This is a very serious and dangerous generic name error. The physician undoubtedly meant to specify "Aminopyrine" which is safe at this dosage. This is more than a 300 times overdose as written. Contact the physician.

Dosage Form Error—Check with the physician if a potentially toxic topical preparation is prescribed internally, a drug known to be destroyed in the digestive tract is prescribed orally, skin preparations are prescribed for the eye, etc. Examples here are Goulard's Extract (lead subacetate solution) prescribed as an internal preparation; directions to swallow testosterone propionate buccal tablets; Neo-Delta-Cortef Lotion (Upjohn) prescribed as an ophthalmic drop, etc. The latter is a good example of the application of one trademark to a family of dosage forms since it is applied to a topical ointment, eye-ear ointment, eye-ear drops, and nasal spray, as well as to the topical lotion. Other examples cited in the literature as potentially confusing are Theominal, Theominal-M, and Theominal-RS; Novahistine, Novahistine-LP, Novahistine with Penicillin, Novahistine Syrup, Novahistine Expectorant, and Novahistine-DH; Dimetane, Dimetane Extentabs, Dimetane Elixir, Dimetane Expectorant, and Dimetane-DC. The pharmacist should be alert when such trademarks are prescribed so that the proper dosage form is dispensed.

Some pharmacists are tempted to "counter prescribe" when an epidemic is in progress, the symptoms are unmistakable, or the customer is known to be out of work or otherwise unable to afford medical or hospital care. Many rural and small-town pharmacists seem to have a working arrangement with their close physician friends so they can call their offices and obtain permission to refill prescriptions when appropriate. Since the law varies from state to state and from time to time, no general advice can be given.

Drug Administration and Patient Care

Errors in drug administration have been attributed to physicians, nurses, hospital pharmacists, family members and even to the patient himself. It has been pointed out that medication errors are already among the leading causes of accidents in hospitals and that each of the professions involved in the prescribing and administration of drug preparations (medicine, nursing and pharmacy) makes its own characteristic mistakes. Studies have shown that the pharmacist is less likely to make a medication error than the physician or nurse, probably because he is a specialist in handling drugs and is not ordinarily preoccupied with other aspects of the patient's care.

It has been reported that a total of 1461 errors were detected in one hospital alone during a five day study involving 32 registered nurses. While this study may not be typical, it indicates an average of 8.3 errors per nurse per day. After elimination of wrong time errors, the greatest number of mistakes were found to be due to miscalculation or mismeasurement of the dose (especially liquids) given to the patient. These authors suggested that similar errors occur in the home and that the possibility of dispensing all prescription medications in premeasured doses (i.e., unit-dose) should be seriously considered.

It has been claimed that "the utilization of a unit-dose drug distribution system allows the pharmacist to supervise drug distribution and at the same time project himself into the patient care area."[3] Smith foresees here the role of the hospital pharmacist in the patient care area of the future as that of a consultant to the medical team, especially in the areas of pharmacology and toxicology and thus recommends that he be responsible in the future for interviewing and preparing a pharmaceutical service record for each patient. This record would contain the patient's drug history, clinical laboratory tests, allergies and sensitivities to drugs, intravenous drug therapy, prescribed drugs and time of administration, plus selected medical history facts.

A very common error of administration is the failure to "Shake Well" or otherwise follow label directions. Most of the compounded liquids and many manufactured ones are suspensions, emulsions, and other dispersed systems which may produce underdosage followed eventually by overdosage unless such label warnings are heeded. Prescriptions packaged in containers made of opaque or dark-colored glass or entirely covered by labeling are especially subject to this error. The pharmacist should always discuss this problem with the customer when dispensing such prescriptions. Special separate "Shake Well" labels should always be attached in a conspicuous place.

Still another common source of danger is the administration of the wrong prescriptions. Medicines taken at night are especially subject to this error. Many pharmacists use different style bottles or distinctive caps for pediatric and adult medications or for "His" and "Hers" to help avoid this difficulty. Expiration dating the prescription to encourage throwing away old bottles or giving a "trade in" on old prescriptions may also help.

It has been pointed out that "improper dosage with the proper drug is at least as common a reason for therapeutic failure as the application of an improper drug," and "the dosage must be tailored to suit the patient as well as the disease."[4] If the latter statement is true the safety and efficacy of a particular dose and drug can only be determined by exposing the patient to the drug. There is usually not time in acute illnesses for the physician to titrate doses, check the mode and speed of elimination, and the many other factors required to obtain activity without side effects. Accordingly minor side effects after an average dose may need to be explained to the patient as indications that adequate dosage is being taken. It may be wise to discuss the dosage actually taken, however, since patients, parents, *et al,* have mistaken the capacity of various spoons, droppers, and other measuring devices or used them at the wrong time or too frequently. The philosophy that "if a little does good, a lot more will do a lot better" is sometimes applied by the patient to drugs—especially those with a pleasant taste or an alcoholic vehicle. This increased dosage or increased frequency of use should of course be discouraged unless the physician agrees to the change once it is discovered.

All such changes should be noted on the pharmacist's records for obvious reasons. Of course, an overdosage may not always be clearly established since children often consume dangerous quantities of flavored aspirin or chewable vitamins because of their appealing color, shape or taste.

Drugs which cause gastric irritation or undesirable aftertastes are usually most acceptable if taken with meals or diluted with water, milk, juices, soft drinks, honey, applesauce, etc.; unless, of course, their action is adversely affected by such diluents. Tetracyclines, for example, are usually contraindicated with antacids such as milk of magnesia since these drugs may interact in the gastrointestinal tract to reduce antibiotic adsorption. In this example several interactions are possible, e.g., the magnesium ions freed by the gastric juice may allow formation of a firmly complexed magnesium tetracycline which is likely to produce slow and irregular absorption, or the magnesium hydroxide may act as a solid adsorbent to tie up chlortetracycline base.

The rate of drug administration which can be tolerated depends on the rate of metabolism and excretion and on the tissue irritation threshold. If the drug is administered faster than it can be destroyed or eliminated, it may accumulate in the blood or other tissues and produce irritation or other toxic effects.

Prolonged action may also result if a drug is given to a patient who cannot metabolize or excrete it. Infants are a case in point since they typically lack drug-metabolizing enzymes and drugs should be administered only under exceptional circumstances—unless excreted unchanged in urine.

Toxicity and death have been reported to occur because trade names obscured the fact that the same drug was present in two prescriptions taken simultaneously or in a prescription taken with an OTC drug. Aminophylline, for example has been given to infants by suppository and also in an oral tradenamed mixture which the physician did not realize contained this drug. The pharmacist should be alert in pointing out this situation wherever it may occur.

One potential danger which should be recognized is that the patient may not take (or be given) the proper amount or frequency of drug prescribed. If the physician then increases the dose, frequency, concentration, etc., thinking more drug is required, the increased amount may constitute a toxic dose.

Placebo and Psychosomatic Factors—Perhaps one of the most important errors which the pharmacist (and nurse) may make is the failure to build confidence in the physician and his medications. It has been stated that 35% or *more* of a drug's activity may reside in its placebo effect. For example, 77% of the effect of morphine on severe pain is believed to be placebo action. Thus if the pharmacist, nurse, mother, grandmother, *et al,* add their faith and enthusiasm to the true pharmacologic action, the total action will be maximal and the side effects minimal. Conversely, a skeptical pharmacist, nurse, or parent may create doubt, mistrust, and fear in the patient's mind with resultant poor effect. It may be wise to dispense each prescription with proper confidence and professional dignity.

It has been pointed out that too many physicians write their prescription directions for use in language that is negative in psychological effect. Thus, he recommends fortifying the pharmacologic action of the drug with the power of positive suggestion. For example, the directions, "one teaspoonful before meals for spasm" could better become, "one teaspoonful before meals to *prevent* spasms;" and "one at mealtime for indigestion" could well read, "one at mealtime to *improve* digestion." He also recommends addition of other positive phrases to the directions when appropriate, e.g., "for relief," "to ensure sleep," "to settle stomach," "to regulate bowels," "to build blood," "for relaxation," "to strengthen back." This may be a suggestion which pharmacists could use in detailing physicians. Although it is doubtful that the Fair Trade Commission (FTC) would allow a salesman for a pharmaceutical house to make such positive statements without full disclosure of negative warnings about possible side effects.

Actually the confidence of the physician in a specific drug or course of treatment may greatly contribute to the therapeutic benefits and the pharmacist must therefore be careful in his comments to the physician regarding such matters.

The beliefs, attitudes, and behavior of the whole medical team (physician, pharmacist, nurse, parent, patient) may thus color drug and placebo effectiveness. It has been reported that "the placebo is probably the most widely employed therapeutic device at the physician's disposal—and one to be used with profound respect. Perhaps as many as 40% of all prescriptions written represent placebos." [5] This statement is supported by an editorial in a 1961

British Medical Journal. "At the present time many of the medicines commonly administered are placebos."

It has also been pointed out that "Generally the unsophisticated use of sugar pills has been supplanted by the subtle prescription of unnecessary (but harmless) agents such as vitamins, or the prescription of active agents in doses too small to produce any medical effects." [6] The low doses of tranquilizers typically given psychiatric out-patients have been described as "the triumph of the impure placebo." [7]

Many dosage forms and procedures are apparently capable of placebo action. In addition to capsules, placebo effects can be obtained with injections, powders, suppositories, lotions, inhalations, supportive "talking" sessions, and even sham surgery (for angina pectoris) or sham electroconvulsive therapy (for chronic schizophrenics). Honigfeld believes that the "two useful components of the placebo situation are first, an element of mystery, and second, a bit of discomfort to the patient. [6]

Placebo actions are said to rival or in some cases surpass active drugs in apparent effectiveness. Researchers have reported symptomatic improvement followed placebos in 92% of peptic ulcer patients and in over 80% of patients suffering from both rheumatoid and degenerative forms of arthritis.

Placebos may also produce adverse drug reactions. In psychiatric treatment, placebos appear to produce depressant or stimulant action depending on the conditions of use and even "dependency and addiction" or other undesirable reactions may occur.

In a review of 67 placebo-controlled drug studies, the frequent occurrence of some 38 different types of placebo side effects were recorded. The most common complaints were drowsiness, weakness, fatigue, and other manifestations of central nervous system depression. Headache and such apparent symptoms of central nervous system stimulation as nervousness, tension, and insomnia were also frequent.

Psychological or organoleptic incompatibilities may exist only in the mind of the patient. For example, it has been pointed out that the Japanese dislike any flavor compounded with oil of wintergreen while most Americans do not like oral liquid preparations which are dark blue, green, or purple in color. These authors also noted that many people do not like suspension mixtures in which the insoluble material floats instead of settling to the bottom. Such floating white particles, possibly suggestive of mold growth, appear in mixtures containing equal parts of Ilosone for Oral Suspension with Robitussin, Robitussin AC, or Histadyl EC among others. These incompatibilities and others can be dispensed without the pharmacist being aware that an "incompatibility" may be recognized and disliked by the patient.

An incompatibility may exist only in the mind of the compounder, yet might be the source of an unjustified complaint, e.g.:

35

℞ Calcium glucoheptonate Injection   1 cc
   Streptomycin Sulfate Injection   1 cc
   Mix and use for intramuscular injection.

Most pharmacists and others trained in chemistry assume there is an incompatibility in this mixture since calcium sulfate usually precipitates when calcium ion and sulfate ion are present in aqueous solution in these concentrations. No such precipitate has formed after several years of observation of several different combinations. Apparently these solutions contain sufficient hydrogen-bonding sugar residues to prevent significant inorganic ion combination since these solutions can be mixed in any proportions without the formation of a calcium sulfate precipitate; there is a noticeable color change to a darker tone as mixing takes place, however.

Unpalatability—In a sense, unpalatability is a form of incompatibility since, if the prescription is unpalatable, the patient may fail to take the medication as required; the medication, therefore, does not accomplish its intended purpose.

36

℞ For Joan, Age 6
   Iron and ammonium citrate   10 g
   Water   5 ml
   Simple syrup   q.s.   120 ml

M.S. Teaspoonful in water t.i.d. pc.

Prescriptions containing unpleasant drugs are frequently more acceptable to the patient if administered in a compatible flavored syrup or elixir. Syrup of cherry has been recommended for this prescription.

Combinations of Factors

Sometimes more than one error or drug interaction problem may occur in a clinical situation. In such cases the cause is sometimes never determined although it is the joint responsibility of the physician and pharmacist to attempt to find the cause and eliminate any further similar situations. The pharmacist can best use his training to investigate the pharmaceutical aspects of these problems (possible drug instability, physical, chemical, therapeutic incompatibilities) while cooperating with the physician in exploring clinical aspects (possible drug interactions, adverse drug reactions, diagnostic prescribing or administration errors, etc.). The alert pharmacist can make invaluable contributions by helping to detect pertinent physical, chemical, pharmacodynamic, pharmacological, and pharmaceutical factors.

Pharmaceutical Factors Influencing Drug Interactions

The prescribing errors described above (overdosage, underdosage, etc.) can become dispensing or drug usage errors if the community pharmacist, hospital pharmacist, dispensing physician, or nurse fail to recognize that a mistake has been made in writing or telephoning a prescription. Although the incidence of such errors is rather small they may be so serious in consequence when they do occur that the drug dispenser should be alert to the various possibilities and look for them in every drug order.

It has been established by legal precedent that a pharmacist is justified in refusing to prepare a prescription order when the physician has erred. If he fails to question a dangerous prescription and damage occurs, the pharmacist may be held jointly responsible with the physician. On the other hand, the pharmacist need not refuse a prescription merely because it is out of the ordinary, provided he inquires of the physician to make sure there has been no error. This does not mean that a pharmacist can safely fill prescriptions calling for doses that are obviously fatal. The pharmacist obviously must exercise a degree of care commensurate with current knowledge, skills and dangers involved in his profession. It has been suggested that the hospital pharmacist, perhaps with an MSc or PharmD degree might legally have to provide care of a higher degree and skill than a community pharmacist with a BSc degree. For example, if a toxic dose of a drug is prescribed and the physician refuses to change the dose, and if withholding the drug might possibly harm the patient, the community pharmacist might be absolved of liability by dispensing the drug to the physician rather than to the patient. The hospital pharmacist on the other hand might be required to consult hospital authority at a higher level than the prescribing physician in order to protect both himself and the hospital. In the court case of Darling vs Charleston Community Memorial Hospital the court held a hospital liable for the the adverse effect of treatment approved by the physician in charge because of what was found to be negligent failure of the hospital to review the treatment approved by the physician. Bernzweig has noted that under no circumstances should a pharmacist dispense a medication or combination of medicaments which in his professional judgment he knows to be potentially harmful to the patient. He has the moral and legal obligation to attempt first to persuade the physician that the medication should be changed, citing appropriate examples of drug interactions, physiological contraindications, pharmacological incompatibilities, or other harmful effects of the drugs ordered. If he fails in this, and he is a hospital pharmacist, he should bring the matter to the immediate attention of proper hospital authorities for appropriate resolution.

The pharmacist himself may originate errors if he misreads or misinterprets prescriptions, mislabels them or knowingly supplies drugs of poor quality. He is fully responsible for such mistakes. It is his responsibility to bring such errors, as soon as he discovers them, to the immediate attenton of appropriate medical personnel, so that any necessary remedial measures may be instituted at once. The willful concealment of an error which proves harmful may not only result in the pharmacist's tort liability to the patient, but once established, may prompt state licensing authorities to suspend or revoke his license.

A serious error which the pharmacist can correct is the dispensing of nonsterile solutions intended for the eye or for injectable use. Such prescriptions are often filled without special precautions even though the physician specifies "sterile," "isotonic," "buffered," etc. Such carelessness borders on pharmaceutical malpractice. The pharmacist should definitely refer such prescriptions to another location where they can be properly filled if he is unable to follow the prescriber's request. Directions for the proper filling of these prescriptions are given in Chapters 9 and 10.

Manufacturing Factors

Many dispensing problems have their origin in the choice of product with which the prescription is filled. Of course if the physician specifies the brand of drug to be used, the pharmacist must honor this request in most states unless he is aware of a drug recall, a brand-related incompatibility, or other reason for change. In such a case he should of course discuss any recommendation of proposed change with the physician and obtain his permission before dispensing a product with which he may be totally unfamiliar.

Although under ordinary circumstances the pharmacist is only held liable for his own negligent conduct, a pharmacist can indeed be held liable for negligent acts committed by nonprofessional pharmacy personnel working under his direction. This emphasizes the need for the closest possible supervision of assistants.

This point may become very important if the function of the hospital pharmacist shifts to include drug-use control also. It has been proposed that the hospital pharmacist assume the responsibility for controlling the process by which the ordered dose is measured or otherwise made ready for administration. It has been estimated that the number of doses requiring compounding is in excess of one dose every other day per hospitalized patient—or about 700,000 compounded doses per day in the US. More than 9 out of 10 of such doses apparently involve sterile dosage forms demanding the highest degree of sterility and accuracy of techniques. This emphasizes the current and future importance of pharmacists learning about the preparation and control of proper parenteral solutions and the compatibilities of IV mixtures.

Very likely, many therapeutic problems of the past had their origin in the choice of product with which the prescription was filled. This is not intended to imply that the pharmacist picks the cheapest available acceptable generic drug with which to fill a prescription, although this may be the policy of many stores in situations of cut-throat competition. It is well known that many large retail operations, hospitals and clinics buy on a competitive quotation basis, often without personally investigating the source of drugs, or checking out the manufacturing and quality control facilities and procedures used in their production. While it may seem impossible for the purchasing agent to visit personally the source of each product, some progressive buyers have developed plant evaluation questionnaires which they send to each prospective supplier. If expertly worded and truthfully answered, such questionnaires can do much to eliminate questionable sources. Also many questionable supply sources are being improved by the current FDA

intensive drug inspections (IDI) which place one or more resident inspectors in a manufacturing or repackaging operation to find and point out any areas which do not meet current good manufacturing practices (CGMP). It is anticipated that this FDA activity will raise the quality of mass produced products to at least a minimum acceptable level since products which are produced under conditions which do not meet current good manufacturing practices or fail to meet the required assay and other quality control standards are embargoed or recalled from the market.

This further suggests that purchasing agents might do well to buy from companies which have completed their IDI if they are concerned about drug quality. Products produced or packaged on a smaller scale, as in the hospital pharmacy or by some manufacturers, drug repackers and wholesalers, may continue to pose serious problems for some time. Many common difficulties can be taken care of if proper research and development, competent quality control personnel, and adequate facilities are available and if certain key procedures are personally handled or properly supervised by adequately trained pharmacists, technicians, chemists, and other specialists.

A 1969 workshop on subprofessional hospital personnel pointed out the need for properly experienced pharmacists to prepare master formula cards (i.e., the exact manufacturing formulas and processing procedure) for a hospital produced product before manufacture begins. While this step can likely be done by an outside consultant where necessary, a pharmacist should personally release the finished product from quarantine only if it meets all required quality control standards. Predictably, this workshop suggested that a pharmacist should supervise the manufacturing, packaging, sterilizing, labeling and quality control work although much of this could be carried out by specially trained technicians. Properly trained technician specialists and technician trainees were apparently believed adequate to handle many of the inventory, records and supply details with only an occasional audit by the pharmacist, and indeed can themselves supervise aides in many cleanup operations. These suggestions emphasize the need for selected pharmacists to be trained in formulation theory, physical pharmacy, stability testing, bulk compounding, packaging and labeling, quality controls and analytical procedures, incompatibilities and intravenous additives as well as pharmacy administration, personnel planning, drug administration, drug distribution, communications, etc.

Since the legal liability for the quality of finished products is identical regardless of whether they are manufactured by a pharmaceutical company or by the hospital pharmacy, increased emphasis should be placed on the research and quality control departments and programs in the hospitals. If the hospital does not have the resources to equip its own research and control laboratory, or if the pharmaceutical or analytical staff is too busy with other duties, an outside consultant or independent laboratory may be the answer. Since time is usually of the essence in manufacturing and releasing a batch of product it seems logical to select several nearby analytical laboratories which specialize in the particular areas of analytical interest and are competitive in service cost. These can be used alternately so that rapid dependable service is always available in times of emergency. It is usually advisable to request a copy of the raw data and assay calculations so that the assay reports can be double checked by the responsible pharmacist.

Lists of suitable independent laboratories are published in various buyer's guides and directories or may be located through the directory published by the American Council of Independent Laboratories, Washington, DC.

In general, most physical, chemical and pyrogen tests can be completed in two or three days after entering the laboratory schedule. Sterility, Pseudomonas, yeast, mold and similar bacterial contamination tests may require seven to fourteen days.

It has been predicted on the other hand that the hospital pharmacy of the future may become less of a production center and more of a professional center in the hospital. Regarding the changing nature of the drugs dispensed, it has been pointed out that the adoption of unit dosage may make it impractical for the hospital pharmacy to produce very much of what it uses. The hospital pharmacy will probably become increasingly less self-sufficient and therefore turn to outside manufacturers for readymade, prepackaged items and disposables. Hospital pharmacists as an organized group will then need to become more active and influential in determining standards and specifications for the pharmaceutical industry.

Stability, Storage, and Supply Factors

Although many of the delayed incompatibilities (physical or chemical instabilities) formerly noted in manufactured products have been eliminated it is still necessary to follow closely the recommendations of the manufacturer as to storage conditions and expiration dates. Products which are stored for prolonged periods outside of the recommended ranges may be lacking in potency or may have developed decomposition products which can produce undesirable drug actions or interactions, unexpected precipitates, or other signs of unsatisfactory drug mixtures.

The pharmaceutical manufacturer thus has a vital interest in incompatibilities and research to reduce possible interactions as they pertain to his products. This interest can be divided into three parts.

1. Basic research (i.e., chemical synthesis, screening, toxicity testing, pharmacology, pharmaceutical and clinical studies) lead to the formulation of stable, safe, and effective new medicaments free of incompatibilities.

2. The manufacturer develops procedures for manufacturing, packaging, labeling, shipping and storage of products so that they do not develop delayed incompatibilities.

3. The manufacturer maintains deep concern as to what will happen when one of his specialties is prescribed alone or with other products. All of these interests may require extensive physical, chemical, animal, and therapeutic studies.

In order to attain the desired 2- to 5-year shelf-life, manufacturers often deliberately formulate with so-called induced "incompatibilities." These include, for example, conversion of a medicament to a very slightly soluble but perhaps more active or more stable derivative or polymorph which is then prepared as a suspension in water, non-solvent oil or synthetic ester. In most cases these require a "Shake-Well" label.

It has been pointed out that when Neotrizine Suspension was first marketed, it was made with bentonite as a suspending agent. Since it was frequently prescribed in combination with alkaloids, such as atropine, codeine, etc., it became necessary to change the suspending agent to sodium carboxymethylcellulose. This was required because the alkaloids usually increased the viscosity of the mixture to the point where it would not pour out of the bottle. Perhaps even more important, the bentonite adsorbed the alkaloids so strongly that they were only slightly effective.

Of course, formula changes in some cases may make formerly compatible mixtures incompatible. This is illustrated by the following prescription in which the vitamin elixir made with glucose was compatible with Lugol's solution, but when the formula of the elixir was revised to use sucrose, a precipitate developed.

37

| ℞ | Lugol's solution | | 2 cc |
| | Betalin S Elixir | q.s. ad | 100 cc |

Investigation of this incompatibility also led to the finding that iodine and potassium iodide had no deleterious effect on thiamine hydrochloride stability in this mixture. This discovery contradicted a widely held opinion and at the same time indicated one of the values of incompatibility studies.

Other examples of related formulation technique may be located in Chapters 3 to 12 by looking under the appropriate dosage form. The drug producer, however, cannot forsee all of the problems which may arise involving his products and their combinations, hence incompatibilities may still occur.

Complaints—The results of compatibility studies or complaints about incompatibilities, ineffectiveness, safety or instability may induce a manufacturer to make formula, packaging, label or expiration date changes to eliminate these problems. All manufacturers are currently required by the Food and Drug Administration to keep a separate file of customer complaints. Such files include complaints from patients, pharmacists and physicians together with the action which the manufacturer took to resolve the complaint. Such complaints are all important to the manufacturer since they are the basis for many of the drug recalls which have been made for pharmaceutically inelegant products (unpalatable, nauseating, contaminated by insects or other filth, unstable color or flavor, precipitate formation, crystal growth, cementation in container, painful on injection, sterile abscess formation, hemolysis of blood cells, etc.). Recalls reported and summarized in the *Journal of the American Pharmaceutical Association, FDC Reports* (Pink Sheets), *FDA Papers*, etc. have also been made for overpotency, underpotency, lack of sterility, contamination with *Salmonella*, molds, *Pseudomonas*, *Staphylococcus*, and other organisms, pyrogenicity, incorrect labeling, instability and such packaging problems as swollen rubber stoppers, glass particles, floaters, loss of preservative, change in pH, metal particles in ophthalmic ointments, cracked containers or closures, leaking plastic or glass bottles, and for other reasons.

Nearly every pharmacist has encountered complaints where a refilled prescription is not the "right medicine" because the pharmacist has changed brands or perhaps has intentionally used a generic drug to reduce the cost of medication. It is important to mention such changes to the customer as a part of good customer relations, as well as being important therapeutically in removing a cause of patient concern.

Complaints may also come about because the manufacturer has changed the color, viscosity, taste or other obvious property. Or perhaps the shipper, wholesaler, pharmacist, or patient had stored the medicine where sunlight or heat gradually faded the color, changed the flavor, etc. Many preparations will likely be the subject of similar complaints in the future since the FDA has recently decertified or removed from the GRAS (generally recognized as safe) list a number of colors, flavors and sweetening agents.

Less obvious or dramatic drug interactions or "incompatibilities," e.g., reduction in expected effect from decomposition of drugs through improper storage, or poorly formulated tablets which may change in disintegration or dissolution time to release the desired ingredient at unknown rates, may delay recovery of the patient and should be avoided. Although tablets may sometimes show definite physical signs of decomposition (such as cracking, build up of gas pressure, softening, darkening or other color changes, unpleasant odors, sublimation onto bottle walls, *et al*) decomposition frequently occurs without any physical evidence of change. Here only actual analytical assays plus full clinical pharmacology will give an absolute answer. Fortunately, a basic knowledge of chemistry, incompatibilities, and stability plus a careful following of storage directions and expiration dating as given on the label will usually solve the storage problem.

Nonetheless, inadequate research and development work on the formulation by the manufacturer does not always show up in the physical appearance of the product. Thus, it is important that the pharmacist have confidence in the integrity and the research, control, and manufacturing facilities of the manufacturer.

Many manufacturers farm out part of the production of their generic drug products to "Custom Manufacturers." This may be done in times of great product sales growth or to insure production capacity in times of future need, as during sales promotions, strikes, or epidemics. This possibility can usually be determined by a close study of the product label because products manufactured by other manufacturers must be labeled "manufactured for," "distributed by" or other wording to show the true situation. Conversely those products made by the original company (or its subsidiaries) bear only name, address, and zip code.

It is becoming increasingly obvious from the growing drug recall list that not all drug products containing the same active ingredients give the same clinical effectiveness. This will likely be corrected in time since the FDA is cooperating with special drug product committees of the National Research Council to classify drugs as "effective," "probably effective," "possibly effective," or "ineffective." The ineffective drugs are removed from the market and the second and third classes must be shown to give blood levels or clinical effects equal to a standard effective drug if they are to be allowed to continue on the market.

An early FDA manual for pharmacists says: "The licensed pharmacist has an ethical and legal responsibility to maintain a stock of therapeutically reliable drugs. Only in this way can he dispense the drugs specified by the prescriber. This assurance to doctors and patients can be given only if prescriptions are filled from drugs received by the pharmacist from authentic sources. Drugs should be purchased only in the original, labeled, and sealed manufacturer's packages. Pharmacists should be alert for any unusual packaging or labeling on the part of the drug suppliers, and should report to their Board of Pharmacy or the Food and Drug Administration whenever drugs are offered to them on suspicious terms or circumstances." [8]

The above paragraph points up the need for wholesalers and pharmacists to keep a stock of fresh, properly stored drugs. Since it is not always possible for the pharmacist to determine the age of a product unless it is expiration dated, he should deal only with reputable wholesalers, manufacturers, etc., who will replace any questionable stock with fresh stock. Frequently the wholesaler's or manufacturer's salesmen can interpret the date of manufacture from the lot number or package date code. The pharmacist should be aware that outdated or soon-to-be-outdated goods are frequently recalled by the supplier for reworking or destruction. Such products are sometimes reassayed, repackaged and redated with a new expiration date, or in some cases the active ingredients may be recovered and used to prepare a new batch of product. While such products are usually satisfactory it is well to check out the source of any material offered at attractive discount prices since the merchandise may be short-dated or in extreme cases may be highjacked or counterfeit goods. Some products are not actually short-dated in the usual sense but may have been exposed to excessive temperatures. These may then have a lowered potency or contain decomposition products which can produce an incompatibility or drug interaction. This danger of course especially applies to fire, heat, or water damaged goods.

It is especially advisable for the wholesaler and pharmacist to carefully read the label of medications so they can advise their employees and customers of proper handling. The storage conditions recommended on the packaging have not always been followed at the wholesale, retail and consumer level in the past. Some products (e.g., antibiotics, vaccines, insulin etc.) are especially heat or light sensitive and should be refrigerated or kept in the dark for maximum stability. Manufacturers usually label a product with the highest temperature consistent with acceptable stability since a refrigeration or other special storage label may detract from sales.

Adverse Drug Reactions

The desirable effects of a drug are those which the physician hopes to attain in a particular patient at a particular time. Undesirable effects (adverse drug reactions) may be either *side effects or extension effects.*

Types of Adverse Drug Reactions

Side effects are normally troublesome, secondary pharmacological effects—usually not very dangerous. They are sometimes useful in determining when the effective dose is reached (e.g., methantheline, dry mouth indicates the ulcer patient is receiving adequate dosage), and rarely may even be beneficial as with the sedative effects of antihistamine syrups given children. Unwanted side effects can sometimes be minimized and the desired activity still retained by fractionally reducing the dosage or using the proper combination of drugs.

Extension effects are excessive pharmacologic actions, normally dose-related. These will probably show up in any patient given enough drug. Such toxic effects usually develop rapidly; however, some drugs may produce a delayed toxic effect through cumulative build-up. For example, yellowing of teeth in the young child given tetracycline, ataxia after chlorpromazine, or yellowing of skin from quinazine are cumulative toxic effects which are undesirable.

An occasional patient may develop a drug *hypersensitivity* or *idiosyncrasy.* These reactions, which are unrelated to the usual pharmacologic action of a drug, occur only in certain individuals (likely those with an inherited tendency) and usually after common doses of drugs.

Hypersensitivity reactions have also been said to represent overdosage of the exquisitely sensitive individual given a normal size dose, or may be due to allergies or other immune reactions which require prior sensitization. Of course after sensitization has taken place, only a fractional dose is required to produce anaphylaxis.

Some of these adverse reactions have been associated with inheritable disorders, some of which are related to race. It has been found that such reactions are more common in Caucasians than in Negro patients and more common in women than in men.

Idiosyncrasies, for example, are totally unexpected the first time, and are qualitatively different pharmacological actions which probably occur in individuals with hereditary, genetic or induced metabolic enzyme problems. These bizarre effects may be brought about by too little or too much enzyme.

It has been reported that some enzyme deficiencies may result from a genetic variation in which either no enzyme is made, or if made, is defective, or perhaps made in insufficient amounts. Individuals showing slow inactivation of Isoniazid may fall in one of these categories.

On the other hand, an example has been described of enzyme overproduction (hepatic porphyria) in which the liver in response to ordinary doses of barbiturates, etc., goes berserk in manufacturing the enzyme α-aminolevulinic acid synthetase. This may bring about a chain reaction type synthesis of porphyrin precursors which produce nervous system disorders (e.g., severe abdominal pain) or skin sensitivity to light.

An interesting example of deficiency-type idiosyncrasy is the defect in erythrocyte glucose-6-phosphate dehydrogenase action which is sex-linked and dominant and it has been found that approximately 11% of Negroes in the US have a deficiency of this enzyme in their red blood cells. Individuals with this inherited metabolic abnormality may show a dose-related hemolytic crisis after several doses of primaquine,* certain sulfonamides, and many over-the-counter analgesics, or after eating fava beans. Families suspected of having this idiosyncrasy or similar genetic ones should be examined for the defect

and those family members found susceptible should be given a list of contraindicated foods and drugs.

Other idiosyncrasies may be related to enzyme deficiencies caused by certain chronic diseases such as cirrhosis of the liver, coronary artery disease, peptic ulcer, glaucoma, etc. For example, ulcer patients may show bleeding or increased ulceration after adrenal steroids, aspirin, imipramine, para-aminosalicylic acid, rauwolfia.

The need for caution in the administration of drugs in the presence of one or more diseases of the kidney, liver, or lung should be emphasized since these serve as the principal means of drug excretion or destruction.

Predicting and Resolving Adverse Drug Reactions

Some of the more troublesome adverse drug reactions are defined in Table 4 while some causative drugs and drug pairs and classes are listed alphabetically in Tables 5, 6, and 7. *International Pharmaceutical Abstracts* and other journals summarize important cautions and contraindications in the use of drugs (i.e., idiosyncrasies, hypersensitivities, side effects, habit-forming properties, ability to cross the placental barrier, excretion in breast milk, and the like). It should be emphasized that not all dosage forms of drugs produce adverse reactions, and indeed a few of the listed drugs have not been clearly established as giving such reactions in humans. The drug families are usually included for consideration in such tables as it is better to be oversuspicious of close structural or pharmacological

---

* A more complete list includes: acetanilid, acetylphenylhydrazine, acetophenetidin, acetylsalicylic acid, antipyrine, aminopyrine, N⁴-acetylsulfanilamide, ascorbic acid, diaminodiphenyl sulfone, fava beans, furazolidone, methylene blue derivatives, naphthalene, nitrofurantoin, *para*-aminosalicylic acid, pamaquine, pentaquine, primaquine, phenylhydrazine, probenecid, quinidine, sulfanilamide, sulfacetamide, sulfamethoxypyridazine, salicylazosulfapyridine, sulfoxone, thiazosulfone, tolbutamide, trinitrotoluene, and vitamin K.

relatives than to overlook possible danger. Note also that not all drugs have been examined for all adverse reaction possibilities, thus the absence of an adverse report does not necessarily mean these cannot occur. Many adverse reactions observed also have never been reported in the literature.

Note also that there is considerable confusion in the literature as to the proper classification of certain adverse reactions. For example, whereas the term hypersensitivity usually refers to an allergic type of reaction and the term idiosyncrasy ordinarily points to hereditary origin nonallergic reactions, a few workers in this field believe any lesion in any organ may have an allergic origin. It has been concluded that drug reactions such as asthma, urticaria, angioneurotic edema, and certain types of dermatitis are usually allergic in origin (thus are listed here as "hypersensitivities"), while jaundice, acute yellow atrophy, and optic neuritis are nonallergic (hence listed as "idiosyncrasies"). Anemia, granulocytopenia, thrombocytopenia, and polyneuritis may belong in one or the other category and usually are listed as "blood dyscrasias" or "side effects." In other cases the classification used follows the classification given in the product insert or assigned by the tabulator cited. In any event, the significant thing to note here is that a particular drug sometimes has a particular problem and that a complete study of label and insert is indicated where this could be a problem. This is especially true for drugs listed as *habit forming, crossing the placenta,* or *excreted in milk,* since these situations are particularly hazardous.

Several instructive comments were made regarding adverse drug reactions at a conference of professional and scientific societies sponsored by the Commission on Drug Safety. One speaker noted that some investigators are reluctant to furnish information of this type since there is a certain fear they may be held legally or professionally responsible for the reaction; on the other hand, some may find it convenient to explain away as drug reactions those developments which suggest the original diagnosis was in error.

One of the biggest problems mentioned was that there is insufficient background data on the population as a whole to determine if reported reactions really represent an increase over the incidence normally expected. The use of blind comparisons may help here in the future.

Another problem mentioned was that the most widely used drugs (e.g., penicillin, chloramphenicol, etc.) have a greater chance to be blamed for coincidental reactions. Further, most drugs are marketed before sufficient cases are collected in any one country (e.g., 100,000 or more) to really determine the likelihood of reactions, thus it is important to keep track of international developments. Finally, it was pointed out that although thalidomide reactions were first reported in the correspondence columns of British and German medical journals, such early sources (perhaps based on insufficient or prejudiced observations) may be erroneous and may lead to false assumptions of danger. This type of reporting may be especially misleading if picked up by a sensation-seeking lay press; thus such reports should be carefully confirmed before and after they appear in print. This may present an increasing problem since reports of adverse drug reactions are currently being collected by a number of noncoordinated groups (e.g., FDA, AMA, ASHP, etc.).

Because of the above problems, it is recommended that the latest insert copy of prescription legend drugs be studied carefully. Current FDA regulations require drug manufacturers to report adverse drug reactions and update label and insert copy when significant reactions are observed.

It may be wise for the pharmacist to keep an up-to-date file of *International Pharmaceutical Abstracts* and product inserts in the prescription area, ready for telephone conferences with physicians. Adverse drug reports will also be found in various FDA reports (e.g., *Monthly Report—Adverse Reactions to Drugs and Therapeutic Devices; MLB Journal of Literature Abstracts; Reports of Suspected Adverse Reactions "FDA Papers," et al*), *Journal of the American Medical Association, British Medical Journal, Journal of the American Pharmaceutical Association, Canadian Medical Association Journal, Lancet, American Journal of Clinical Pathology, Journal of Investigative Dermatology, New England Journal of Medicine, Anesthesia, Anesthesiology, Anaesthesist, Circulation, Journal of Clinical Investigation, Pediatrics,* etc., to mention only a few published in English. The weekly drug news sources such as *FDC Reports, Drug Trade News, Drug Topics,* or their successors may be helpful in early reports on problem drugs. The FDA reports and *International Pharmaceutical Abstracts* are especially valuable.

Clinical Factors in Drug Reactions

In further explanation of clinical reports, hypersensitivity reactions most often involve the reticuloendothelial system and the skin, nerves, blood, bone marrow, and liver. These allergic reactions usually appear immediately in a previously sensitized patient but quite commonly appear after a week or 10 days of continued administration of certain drugs to hypersensitive individuals. As an example, some extremely long-acting penicillins or biologicals containing horse serum given as a single injection have remained in the body long enough first to sensitize the patient and then to produce the allergic reaction. *Caution:* Individuals who have shown drug reactions in the past are likely to react to members of the same drug family and to develop hypersensitivity to new drugs which work through the same mechanisms. Patients with an active infection also tend to develop these reactions.

Skin reactions are among the most common hypersensitivity reactions and may vary in severity from mild rashes (sometimes produced by phenobarbital), fixed drug eruptions (sometimes produced by phenolphthalein, barbiturates, thiazides), and urticaria (penicillin) to the more severe exfoliative dermatitis (occasionally produced by hydantoins, phenothiazines, phenylbutazone) and erythema multiforme (sometimes due to certain antibiotics, antihistaminics, and sulfonamides). The latter has been known to cause death.

Systemic allergic reactions, e.g., anaphylaxis or serum sickness, often develop after intravenous or intramuscular drugs (e.g., arsenicals, barbiturates, heparin, insulin, mercurials, penicillin, etc.) but rarely develop from oral dosage. The more serious of these allergic reactions such as periarticular nodosa (sometimes produced by iodides, mercurials, thiouracil) or shock (which may follow aspirin, anesthetics, sulfobromophthalein) have led to arterial lesions, kidney failure, and death.

Blood dyscrasias such as granulocytopenia (agranulocytosis), hemolytic anemia, thrombocytopenia purpura, and aplastic anemia are hypersensitivity reactions which require prior sensitization although bone marrow depression due to drug toxicity may also cause similar manifestations. These latter reactions are very serious and fortunately not too common. Since they may appear rapidly and unexpectedly, they do not always respond to discontinuance of therapy, and death may occur before blood transfusions and other emergency therapy can be instituted. Such reactions have been noted with quinidine, chloramphenacol, sulfonamides, phenylbutazone, phenindione, thiouracils, phenothiazines, nitrofurans, and tolbutamide.

Jaundice and hepatitis are symptoms of liver necrosis sometimes found with erythromycin estolate, monamine oxidase inhibitors, isoniazid, sulfonamides, phenothiazines, methyl testosterone, indandione, thiazides, triacetyloleandomycin and others.

The best drug in its class may produce hypersensitivity less often than others, but when reactions do occur they will probably be the same type as noted for close relatives. It has been suggested that hypersensitivity reactions in most instances can best be handled by complete withdrawal of the drug producing the reaction and substitution with drugs of similar therapeutic effect but different chemical structure. Adrenal hormone administration is frequently helpful. These procedures will of course require consultation between pharmacist and physician.

Toxicity, including side reactions and extension effects such as idiosyncrasies, can often be controlled by titration of the dose, substitution of another drug of the same class, or even prescribing a second drug to overcome the undesired effects of the first.

Many adverse drug reactions may be avoided if proper care is taken in collecting the patient's past history, keeping adequate records, giving required warnings, recommending test dosage, selecting the correct dose, and the like. These situations are of course vital to the patient and offer an opportunity for the alert pharmacist to earn his proper reputation as "drug consultant to the medical profession."

Inorganic Incompatibilities

The inorganic compounds discussed in this chapter are divided into several groups: metals and their salts, nonmetals, acids, and alkalies. Certain incompatibilities are characteristic of the positive metallic ions and apply in general to all of the salts of a given metal, while other incompatibilities are characteristic of the acid radical and apply in general to all salts of a given acid.

Many incompatibilities of salts are the result of insolubility. Additional solubility data may be obtained from the USP, NF, or other reference books. However, a general knowledge of solubility relationships is useful in understanding and predicting incompatibilities. With each incompatibility, a decision must be reached as to whether the prescription could be dispensed as such or whether the available means of correcting it are acceptable to the physician.

General Solubility Principles

In general, sodium, potassium, and ammonium salts are soluble in water. Nitrates, acetates, chlorates, and chlorides of all common metals are water soluble with the exception of a few basic nitrates and acetates and silver, lead, and mercurous chlorides. The solubilities of salts of the other halogens, except the fluorides, are comparable to the chlorides and vary only in degree. Mercuric iodide and the basic halides of antimony and bismuth (BiOI) are insoluble. Phosphates, carbonates, sulfides, and hydroxides—other than sodium, potassium, and ammonium—are insoluble in water. Phosphates and carbonates are usually soluble in mineral acids. Many inorganic salts are insoluble in alcohol; most of them are insoluble in nonpolar solvents such as benzene, chloroform, and ether (Table 9).

Hydrolysis

Although a salt may be sufficiently soluble to be free of incompatibilities in itself, it may hydrolyze on standing to form solutions which are neutral, acidic, or alkaline, depending on the salt. Many salts, on hydrolysis, form precipitates of basic salts or hydroxides. Such hydrolysis is greatest in the case of elements such as arsenic, bismuth, antimony, tin and mercury; less marked for lead, aluminum, chromium, and iron; and still less marked for zinc, copper, and manganese. Hydrolysis occurs to an appreciable extent when one of the products of hydrolysis is insoluble, volatile, or only slightly dissociated.

When both the acid and base formed by hydrolysis are highly dissociated, there is very little hydrolysis because the hydroxyl ions and hydrogen ions unite to form undissociated water. When either the acid or base is weak, appreciable hydrolysis occurs. When

Table 9—Water Solubility^a of Inorganic Salts

Cations	Na	K	NH_4	Mg	Ca	Sr	Ba	Al Mn^{2+}	Cr^{3+} Cu^{2+}	Fe^{3+} Bi^{3+}	Zn^{2+} Hg^{2+}	Ni^{2+} Co^{2+}	Cd^{2+}	Ag	Pb^{2+}	Hg^+
Anions—NO_2	S	S	S	S	S	S	S	S	S	S	S	S	S	S	S	S
—Ac	S	S	S	S	S	S	S	S	S	S	S	S	S	S	S	S
—Cl	S	S	S	S	S	S	S	S	S	S	S	S	S	I	I	I
—SO_4	S	S	S	S	I	I	I	S	S	S	S	S	S	I	I	I
—CO_3	S	S	S	I	I	I	I	I	I	I	I	I	I	I	I	I
—PO_4	S	S	S	I	I	I	I	I	I	I	I	I	I	I	I	I
—S	S	S	S	I	I	I	I	I	I	I	I	I	I	I	I	I
—OH	S	S	S	I	I	I	I	I	I	I	I	I	I	I	I	I

^{a} S—soluble. I—insoluble. Soluble in this table includes the USP designations of *very soluble* (1 part of solute in less than 1 part of solvent), *freely soluble* (1 in 1 to 10), *soluble* (1 in 10 to 30), and *sparingly soluble* (1 in 30 to 100). Insoluble includes the USP designations of *slightly soluble* (1 in 100 to 1000), *very slightly soluble* (1 in 1000 to 10,000), and *practically insoluble*, or *insoluble* (1 in more than 10,000).

both the acid and base are weak, hydrolysis is very extensive because both the hydrogen ions and hydroxyl ions are removed from the solution to form the weakly dissociated acid and base.

Solutions of the salts of a strong acid and a strong base are neutral in reaction; a sodium chloride solution is an example of this type. Solutions of the salts of a weak base and a strong acid are acid in reaction. Thus, when ferric chloride is dissolved in water, slight hydrolysis occurs according to the equation:

$$FeCl_3 + 3HOH \rightleftarrows Fe(OH)_3 + 3HCl$$

The HCl formed by hydrolysis is highly ionized, while the $Fe(OH)_3$ is only feebly ionized. The resulting hydrogen ions predominate over the hydroxyl ions and the solution is acid in reaction. Other salts of a weak base and strong acid behave similarly.

Solutions of the salts of a strong base and weak acid are alkaline in reaction. Thus, when sodium carbonate is dissolved in water, there is a slight hydrolysis as follows:

$$Na_2CO_3 + 2HOH \rightleftarrows 2NaOH + H_2CO_3$$
$$\updownarrow$$
$$H_2O + CO_2$$

In this case a strong base and a weak acid are liberated by the hydrolytic change, and the solution is alkaline. Salts of a weak base and a weak acid, for example, $Al(OCOCH_3)_3$, are hydrolyzed to a considerable extent, and the resulting solutions may be either acid or alkaline, depending on the relative strength of the acid and base.

Hydrolysis is retarded by increasing the concentration of either or both of the products of hydrolysis. Thus, the addition of free acid in sufficient quantities decreases the hydrolysis of salts such as $Bi(NO_3)_3$ and prevents the precipitation of basic salts such as $BiONO_3$.

An increase in the concentration of both products of hydrolysis is equivalent to increasing the concentration of the salt solution, and it follows that hydrolysis is lesser on a percentage basis in concentrated solutions than it is in dilute solutions.

Incompatibilities of Metals and Their Salts

The incompatibilities of metals and their salts are considered according to the occurrence of the metals in the Periodic Chart of Elements. Elements of particular interest in pharmacy are discussed by groups in the following pages.

Group I A (Li, Na, K, Rb, Cs, Fr)

The members of this group that are of pharmaceutical interest are the alkali metals—lithium, potassium, and sodium (the ammonium ion will also be discussed, although it is not a metal and forms a weaker hydroxide). These metals react violently with water to liberate hydrogen and simultaneously form the

$$Li, K, Na + H_2O \rightarrow NaOH + H^+$$

hydroxides of the metal. These hydroxides are stable to heat. The chief incompatibilities of this group are due to precipitation of the anions by other metals since nearly all the common salts of this group are soluble in water. Many sodium salts are soluble in glycerin, but as a rule they are nearly insoluble in alcohol.

Sodium—Sodium bicarbonate (soluble 1 in 10 in water) and sodium perborate (soluble 1 in 40 in water), are among the least water soluble sodium salts. These may be precipitated if sodium and bicarbonate, or perborate, ions are present in a prescription in a concentration excess of their solubility. When concentrated solutions of sodium salicylate and potassium bicarbonate are mixed, for example, sodium bicarbonate forms and is precipitated because of its limited solubility. The solution will also darken on standing as is usual with alkaline solutions of salicylates.

Potassium—Practically all potassium salts are soluble in water. A few of its salts, including potassium bitartrate (soluble only 1 in 165 in water), form precipitates. This precipitation may occur in mixtures of potassium salts with acid solutions of tartrates.

$$K^+ + HC_4H_4O_6^- \rightarrow KHC_4H_4O_6\downarrow$$

This salt dissolves freely in solutions containing boric acid and borax. Its saturated aqueous solution is acid to litmus.

Sulfurated potash is essentially a mixture of the thiosulfates and polysulfides of potassium. It is brown when fresh but absorbs moisture, oxygen, and carbon dioxide from the air, turning greenish yellow and finally gray. It is incompatible with acids, hydrogen sulfide being liberated. It is almost completely soluble in water (1 in 2), and its solutions are alkaline in reaction. It reacts with zinc sulfate to form insoluble zinc sulfide and various polysulfides.

Lithium—Lithium hydroxide, carbonate, orthoarsenate, fluoride, and phosphate are less soluble than the corresponding sodium and potassium salts.

In this respect the chemical properties of lithium compare with those of the alkaline earth metals. Lithium is precipitated as the carbonate or phosphate from alkaline or neutral solutions. Lithium carbonate is soluble in a solution of ammonium chloride; it is insoluble in alcohol. Lithium bromide, however, is soluble in alcohol, ether, and water.

Ammonium—Ammonium salts will form a white precipitate with tartaric acid. Sodium acetate speeds this reaction. In the presence of moisture, fixed alkalies liberate ammonia from ammonium salts. Many ammonium salts are volatilized without decomposition on heating. Most ammonium salts liberate ammonia on decomposition except for ammonium nitrate, which decomposes to nitrous oxide, and ammonium nitrite, which yields nitrogen.

$$NH_4^+ + OH^- \xrightarrow{\Delta} NH_3\uparrow + H_2O$$

$$NH_4NO_3 \xrightarrow{\Delta} N_2O\uparrow + 2H_2O$$

$$NH_4NO_2 \xrightarrow{\Delta} N_2\uparrow + 2H_2O$$

Free chlorine and iodine tend to form explosive substances with some ammonium compounds due to the instability of nitrogen chloride and nitrogen iodide. Ammonium salts of strong acids are acid in reaction; for example the pH of a 0.5% solution of ammonium chloride is 4.6.

Group I B (Cu, Ag, Au)

The coinage metals—copper, silver, and gold—are of limited importance medicinally, but some generalizations can be made. All of these metals occur free in nature and are relatively inactive. Their hydroxides and oxides, except those of silver, are weakly basic. Halides of each (except the cupric salts) are insoluble in water; they form water soluble complexes such as $Cu(CN)_2^-$ and $Ag(NH_3)_2^+$.

Copper—Cupric acetate, nitrate, and sulfate, in addition to the chloride, are soluble in water; most other cupric salts are insoluble in water but are readily soluble in acids. Soluble copper salts give precipitates with solutions of tannic acid, arsenates, arsenites, alkalies, carbonates, and phosphates. The precipitation by alkali hydroxides is prevented by glycerin, tartrates, citrates, and similar organic hydroxy compounds. Solutions of cupric salts with iodides give a precipitate of cuprous iodide, and iodine is liberated. Cupric salts in alkaline solution are reduced to cuprous oxide by glucose and other reducing agents. Cupric acetate, only sparingly soluble in water, is readily soluble in solutions of alkali citrates.

Silver—Silver nitrate and silver chlorate are soluble in water; the acetate and sulfate are slightly soluble; and the chloride, bromide, iodide, arsenate, arsenite, borate, carbonate, and phosphate are practically insoluble. Grayish-brown silver oxide is precipitated by alkalies from solutions of silver salts. Yellowish-white silver carbonate, which may be contaminated with silver oxide if the solution is alkaline, is precipitated by the carbonates and bicarbonates of the alkali metals. Many silver salts are decomposed by light with the formation of metallic silver.

Silver nitrate is a strong oxidizing agent, being reduced to metallic silver by some organic compounds; this accounts for the black stain which is formed when silver nitrate comes in contact with the skin. Silver oxide (Ag_2O) is a powerful oxidizing agent which may cause explosions when triturated with reducing agents. Silver is precipitated by sulfides, tannin, alkaloids, and proteins from solutions of its soluble salts.

Gold—Gold salts are unstable, being reduced to the metal by even the weakest reducing agents such as organic matter or by heat alone. Gold hydroxide, a brown precipitate, forms on the addition of fixed alkalies to solutions of gold salts. An excess of alkali quickly solubilizes the precipitate by converting it to the aurate ($NaAuO_2$). Gold tribromide gradually decomposes in aqueous solution yielding free bromine. Gold sodium thiomalate and gold thiosulfate are very soluble in water but practically insoluble in alcohol and most other organic solvents.

Gold sodium thiosulfate darkens slowly on exposure to air or light. Aqueous solutions, neutral to slightly alkaline, turn yellow on standing. Sterile solutions must be freshly prepared from sterile powder.

Gold injections are administered intramuscularly, at a level of 40 to 50 mg/week, for arthritic treatments. Gold toxicity, associated with this therapy, is managed by use of steroids and a chelating compound such as dimercaprol.

Group II A (Be, Mg, Ca, Sr, Ba, Ra)

The alkaline earth group—magnesium, calcium, strontium, and barium—in general forms water soluble salts of the halides and nitrates. Insoluble salts occur, for the most part, with carbonates, phosphates, sulfates, hydroxides, bicarbonates, borates, oxalates, and arsenates (Table 9). The halides and nitrates of this group are deliquescent and are quite soluble in alcohol and glycerin. Such powders often must be dispensed with an absorbing agent.

Magnesium—Magnesium trisilicate ($Mg_2Si_3O_8$), in the hydrated form, is a white, odorless, tasteless powder which is insoluble in water. It has the property of neutralizing hydrochloric acid in the stomach with the formation of soluble magnesium chloride and a gelatinous mass of hydrated silica. It has marked adsorptive properties for alkaloids, dyes, and toxins.

Magnesium sulfate, an exception to the solubility generalities previously mentioned, is soluble 1 g in 1 ml of water or slowly soluble in 1 ml of glycerin. Its solutions form precipitates on the addition of soluble phosphates, carbonates, hydroxides, and silicates, e.g.:

$$3MgSO_4 + 2Na_3PO_4 \rightarrow Mg_3(PO_4)_2 \downarrow + 3Na_2SO_4$$

Magnesium oxide absorbs moisture and carbon dioxide when exposed to air. It readily dissolves in acids. Due to its

Table 10—pH of Precipitation of Hydroxides and Basic Salts

Metals	Hydroxides or basic salts	Basic chromates	Basic borates	Basic carbonates	Basic silicates	Phosphates
Magnesium	10.5	...	None	10.5 T^a	9.5	9.8
Silver	7.5—8.0	...	...	...	...	...
Manganous	8.5—8.8	...	8.8 T^a	8.7	7.4	5.8
Calcium	None	...	...	...	10.1	7.0
Cerous	7.4	...	...	...	...	...
Mercuric (Cl)	7.3	...	...	...	...	...
Zinc	7.0	5.5	5.3	7.0	5.3	5.7
Cobalt	6.8	7.0 T^a	...	...	...	...
Cadmium	6.7	...	...	...	...	...
Nickel	6.7	6.8 T^a	...	...	...	...
Lead	6.0	...	...	...	...	...
Ferrous	5.5	...	...	...	...	...
Cupric	5.3	...	...	...	...	...
Chromium	5.3	5.2	5.2	5.3	...	5.1
Aluminum	4.1	4.2	4.2	4.2	4.0	3.8
Mercurous	3.0	...	...	...	...	...
Ceric	2.7	...	...	...	...	...
Mercuric (NO$_3$)	2.0	...	...	...	...	...
Stannous	2.0	...	...	...	...	...
Zirconium	2.0	...	4.0	4.0	4.0	1.6
Ferric	2.0	...	...	...	...	...

^{a} T—turbidity or opalescence only.

hydration properties magnesium oxide forms a cement-like mass with a small proportion of water. The finer the particle size, the more this occurs. The use of magnesium oxide in capsules sometimes causes the contents to fuse into a hard, insoluble mass. Its alkalinity (pH $\cong$ 10) may also cause destruction of certain drugs such as aspirin and prednisolone. In liquid mixtures containing sodium bicarbonate and magnesium oxide the insoluble powder is likely to form an indiffusible mass that cannot be broken by shaking the bottle. The reaction which first takes place is the hydration of magnesium oxide to form magnesium hydroxide. The insoluble magnesium hydroxide then slowly reacts with sodium bicarbonate to form a cement-like mass while the crystalline, basic magnesium carbonate (Mg$_2$(OH)$_2$CO$_3$) is being produced. Light magnesium oxide is more reactive here than heavy magnesium oxide. Since the latter is more dense with a larger particle size, it reacts more slowly.

Numerous antacids contain various magnesium salts alone or combined with alkaline salts, e.g., calcium carbonate or sodium bicarbonate. Bromide preparations added to these antacids for sedation may cause difficulty due to liberation of ammonia if ammonium bromide is present. Magnesium salts also have laxative properties.

Calcium — Calcium compounds which are sparingly soluble or insoluble in water generally are soluble in acids, with the exception of calcium sulfate. Thus, calcium salts in general are incompatible with hydroxides, citrates, arsenates, carbonates, oxalates, tartrates, and phosphates except in acid solution and are incompatible with sulfates except in sufficiently dilute solutions (Tables 9 and 10). Calcium hydroxide is soluble in syrup, forming soluble sugar compounds with the sucrose; it is also soluble in glycerin, but not in alcohol. Calcium iodobehenate is insoluble in water and very slightly soluble in alcohol. Soluble calcium salts react with fatty acids to form insoluble soaps. Calcium chloride is very deliquescent, and its aqueous solutions are acid in reaction. It is soluble in alcohol. Calcium *d*-saccharate is used as a sequestering agent to increase the solubility of calcium gluconate in sterile solutions. Glycerin is similarly used to maintain calcium glycerophosphates in solution in the elixir.

Prescription combinations of calcium bromide with ingredients such as sodium citrate, sodium salicylate, and ammonium carbonate will produce precipitates respectively of calcium citrate, calcium salicylate, and calcium carbonate. Replacement of the calcium bromide with sodium bromide will overcome these difficulties.

Strontium—The properties of strontium are almost identical to those of calcium.

Strontium bromide has been used only for its bromide effect. More appropriate bromide salts, such as sodium bromide, should be prescribed.

Barium—Barium sulfate ($BaSO_4$) is less soluble than either calcium or strontium sulfates. It is even essentially insoluble in dilute acids. Soluble barium salts are *extremely toxic*. Solutions of barium chloride and iodide will form insoluble precipitates from solutions when combined with soluble sulfates, carbonates, tartrates, oxalates, phosphates, and tannic acid. Barium sulfate is usually administered alone as an aqueous suspension.

Group II B (Zn, Cd, Hg)

Zinc and mercury are the only members of this group which are of interest in pharmaceutical compounding. They differ sufficiently in solubility properties and incompatibilities and are, therefore, described separately.

Zinc—Soluble zinc salts such as the chloride, nitrate, sulfate, and acetate are converted by solutions of alkali hydroxides, carbonates, and phosphates to the corresponding insoluble basic zinc compounds (Tables 9 and 10). Zinc hydroxide exhibits amphoteric properties by dissolving in acids to form salts and also in alkalies to form zincates. Sulfides such as sulfurated potash precipitate white zinc sulfide from solutions of zinc salts; in such combinations the incompatibility is generally intended in order to produce a lotion of zinc sulfide.

Solutions of zinc salts undergo partial hydrolysis, e.g.:

$$ZnCl_2 + HOH \rightarrow Zn(OH)Cl + HCl$$

The basic salt may precipitate, especially in weak aqueous solution, forming a cloudy solution, particularly with samples of zinc chloride which contain basic impurities. The basic salt will dissolve in HCl, but in most cases the addition of HCl is not permissible. In eye washes the precipitation may be prevented by replacing part of the water by saturated solution of boric acid. Filtration removes part of the zinc and is, therefore, not very acceptable. Zinc iodide frequently gives similar cloudy solutions. Ordinarily, the degree of hydrolysis of zinc salts in aqueous solutions is less than 1%.

Solutions of zinc salts of moderate concentration have a pH range of 5–6.9. Heating for one hour at 100°C increases the pH slightly, probably driving off carbon dioxide, but heating for ten hours at 100°C lowers the pH of a 0.1 M solution of zinc sulfate from 5 to 4.8 by increasing the hydrolysis of the salt.

Zinc phenolsulfonate is soluble in water (1 in 1.6) and alcohol (1 in 1.8) and exhibits the incompatibilities of zinc salts. It also turns pink on exposure to light and air. Its solutions are acidic.

Zinc salts precipitate fatty acids such as caprylic, undecylenic, and stearic and such substances as acacia, proteins, and tannins.

Mercury—There are two series of mercury salts: mercurous (Hg^+) and mercuric (Hg^{2+}). Mercurous salts are very insoluble. They are easily reduced to the free metal by light, moisture, and trituration. Mercurous oxide and the chloride are the normally used mercurous salts. Mercuric salts are reduced to mercurous salts by hypophosphorous acid, arsenites, ferrous salts, alcohol, and numerous organic substances. Solutions of mercuric salts are acid in reaction due to hydrolysis, and except in the case of the chloride, an excess of acid is necessary to prevent precipitation of basic salts. Alkaline media speed this hydrolysis.

$$Hg(NO_3)_2 + HOH \rightarrow Hg(OH)NO_3 + HNO_3$$

Mercuric chloride slowly decomposes

in aqueous solution but is more stable in the presence of excess chloride such as ammonium chloride. Mercuric salts are soluble as follows: the acetate, chlorate, cyanide, succinimide, and nitrate are soluble; the chloride, bromide, benzoate, oxycyanide, and sulfate are slightly soluble; and the arsenate, arsenite, carbonate, iodide, oxalate, salicylate, and phosphate are insoluble (Tables 9 and 10). Mercuric iodide is solubilized by the addition of potassium iodide.

$$HgI_2 + 2KI \rightarrow K_2HgI_4$$

Solutions of mercuric salts precipitate alkaloids, proteins, tannins, and many organic acids. Fixed alkali hydroxides precipitate yellow mercuric oxide from solutions of mercuric salts; if the mercuric salt is in excess, red-brown precipitates of basic salts are formed. The combined use of ammoniated mercury and salicylic acid in ointments frequently causes severe skin irritation due to the formation of mercuric salicylate.

Mercurous nitrate is soluble but hydrolyzes and gives a precipitate of a basic salt unless nitric acid is added; mercurous acetate is slightly soluble, but other mercurous salts such as chloride, bromide, iodide, arsenate, arsenite, carbonate, phosphate, and sulfate are insoluble. The mercurous halides are less soluble, and correspondingly less toxic, than the mercuric halides. Since the mercurous halides are given in correspondingly larger doses, any incompatibility in which mercurous salts are changed to mercuric salts is dangerous. Most of the mercurous compounds are stable in air but are oxidized to mercuric compounds by oxidizing agents such as iodine. Iodides and bromides in the presence of water convert mercurous chloride or iodide into mercuric compounds and metallic mercury.

$$Hg_2Cl_2 + 4KI \rightarrow Hg + K_2HgI_4 + 2KCl$$

An ointment containing calomel and potassium iodide is irritating because of the formation of a mercuric salt. Calomel tends to decompose into mercuric chloride and free mercury if exposed to sunlight or if triturated excessively. Some reducing agents reduce calomel to metallic mercury, e.g.:

$$Hg_2Cl_2 + Sn^{2+} \rightarrow 2Hg \downarrow + Sn^{4+} + 2Cl^-$$

Calomel is converted into either the black, insoluble oxide (HgO) or basic salts on addition of alkalies. Ammonia water with calomel gives a black mixture, the reaction being as follows:

$$Hg_2Cl_2 + 2NH_4OH \rightarrow Hg + HgNH_2Cl + NH_4Cl + 2H_2O$$

Mercury toxicity occurs and is associated with acrodynia, a disorder of skin and limbs in children. The absorption of mercury is followed by measurements of urinary mercury concentrations. Treatment consists of removing the mercury source and administering a chelating agent such as dimercaprol.

Group III A (B, Al, Ga, In, Tl)

Aluminum — Aluminum chloride, sulfate, phosphate, and hydroxide are the most widely used salts of aluminum. Solutions of aluminum salts have an acid reaction due to hydrolysis and have the incompatibilities of dilute acids, e.g., effervescence with carbonates. Most inorganic aluminum salts are soluble in water, with the exception of the phosphate and carbonate. Aluminum salt solution will precipitate insoluble salts or complexes when mixed with many soluble organic salts, e.g., aluminum penicillin, aluminum sulfonamides, and aluminum-penicillin-sulfonamide complexes. Aluminum and potassium sulfate (alum) has the incompatibilities of the soluble sulfates and is also a protein precipitant. Aluminum ion is precipitated as the hydroxide by alkali hydroxides, carbonates, and borax (Tables 9 and 10). These precipitates are soluble in an excess of an alkali hydroxide through the formation of the aluminate salt. The amphoteric nature of aluminum hydroxide is further illustrated by its solubility in acid to form aluminum salts. The phosphates, arsenites, and arsenates of the alkali metals precipitate the corresponding aluminum salt.

Aluminum hydroxide gel is a suspension of aluminum hydroxide in water. The gel is destroyed by heat, freezing, electrolytes, acids, fixed alkalies, and dehydration. Incompatibilities of the aluminum silicates should be mentioned. Bentonite, represented as a mixture of

$$[H_2O \cdot (Al_2O_3 \cdot Fe_2O_3 \cdot 3MgO) \cdot 4SiO_2 \cdot nH_2O] \text{ and } (K_2O \cdot Al_2O_3 \cdot 6SiO_2)$$

in water suspension has a pH of 8.5 to 10. It swells in water up to fifteen times its bulk. Bentonite suspensions are thixotropic. Kaolin ($Al_2Si_2O_7 \cdot 2H_2O$ or $Al_2O_3 \cdot 2SiO_2 \cdot 2H_2O$) is insoluble in all common solvents. It does not swell in suspension but has adsorptive properties. It may not only adsorb toxins and bacteria but, in mixtures, may adsorb drugs to inactivate them (e.g., strychnine and atropine).

Group III B (Sc, Y, La Series, Ac Series)

None of the rare earths is widely used in pharmacy.

Cerium—Cerium, the least typical of the group, may be encountered as cerous oxalate. It is insoluble in water and alcohol and incompatible with oxidizing agents.

Group IV A (C, Si, Sn, Pb)

Soluble tin and lead salts are precipitated from aqueous solution by alkali hydroxides (Table 10). They are then dissolved in an excess of the precipitant due to their amphoteric nature. They are also precipitated by sulfides, carbonates, tannins, phenols, many organic acids, and plant extracts.

Tin—Stannous fluoride is water soluble but unstable due to oxidation and hydrolysis. Hydrolysis yields insoluble stannous hydroxide; therefore, only freshly prepared solutions should be used in dentistry. Extra care should be taken even with the dry powder to prevent contact with moisture during storage.

Lead—Of the compounds of bivalent lead, the acetate, subacetate, chlorate, and nitrate are soluble. The chloride and bromide are slightly soluble, and the arsenate, arsenite, borate, carbonate, iodide, oxide, phosphate, sulfate, and tannate are insoluble (Tables 9 and 10). On exposure to air, solutions of lead salts absorb carbon dioxide and become cloudy due to the precipitation of basic lead carbonate.

Group IV B (Ti, Zr, Hf)

Titanium—Titanium dioxide is used as a refractory material in sun creams and in tablet coatings. Aqueous suspensions are neutral in reaction. Titanium dioxide is stable and does not react with sulfides. The important caution in its use is to obtain material of extremely fine subdivision.

Zirconium—Zirconium carbonate and its oxides are insoluble in water. They are used in ointments or suspensions for external application and usually present no serious incompatibilities. Dextrose added to zirconium chloride solution prevents the precipitation of zirconium by alkali.

Group V A (N, P, As, Sb, Bi)

The chemical properties of arsenic, antimony, and bismuth are similar with bismuth having the most pronounced metallic properties. Antimony in its pentavalent form is nonmetallic and acid forming, but in its trivalent form it is base forming and acts like a metal. Arsenic is strictly acid forming and, thus, nonmetallic. None of these three elements replace hydrogen in dilute acids.

Arsenic—The incompatibilities of arsenic are centered around two forms—arsenous acid solution and potassium arsenite solution. These are prepared by solubilizing arsenic trioxide by the addition of HCl with heat in the former case and $KHCO_3$ in the latter case. Thus, incompatibilities may occur depending on the pH of the solution which is added (see Table 10). The arsenites and arsenates of the alkali metals are soluble, but their solutions form precipitates with the salts of practically all the other common metals in neutral or slightly acid solution. These precipitates are soluble in mineral acids. Arsenous chloride, bromide, and iodide are almost completely hydrolyzed in dilute, aqueous solutions, forming arsenous acid and the halogen acid. Arsenites are oxidized to arsenates by oxidizing agents and are slowly oxidized by oxygen of the air in alkaline but not in acid or neutral solution. Both arsenites and arsenates are reduced to metallic arsenic by hypophosphites in acid solution. Arsenic triiodide is hydrolyzed in solution to arsenous acid and hydriodic acid. On standing, the solution becomes yellow due to liberation of iodine.

$$AsI_3 + 3H_2O \rightarrow As(OH)_3 + 3HI$$

$$4HI + O_2 \rightarrow 2I_2 \uparrow + 2H_2O$$

Antimony—Antimony salts hydrolyze in aqueous solution, and free acid must be added to avoid the precipitation of basic salts. Antimony potassium tartrate, $K(SbO)C_4H_4O_6$, is insoluble in alcohol but its aqueous solution is clear. Antimony potassium tartrate (tartar emetic) forms precipitates with aqueous solutions of the salts of most metals and forms a precipitate of potassium bitartrate with mineral acids.

$$K(SbO)C_4H_4O_6 + 3HCl \rightarrow KHC_4H_4O_6 \downarrow + SbCl_3 + H_2O$$

It also has the incompatibilities of antimony salts; e.g., the precipitation of antimony oxide by alkalies and the formation of a precipitate with tannic acid.

Bismuth—Many bismuth compounds are insoluble in water, and most of the soluble salts hydrolyze to form insoluble basic salts. Alkali hydroxides precipitate bismuth hydroxide from aqueous solutions of bismuth salts (Table 9).

$$Bi^{3+} + 3OH^- \rightarrow Bi(OH)_3$$

Also precipitated will be bismuthyl hydroxide from the product of the hydrolysis of the bismuth salts.

$$Bi^{3+} + 3H_2O \rightarrow BiO^+ + 2H_3O^+$$

$$BiO^+ + OH^- \rightarrow BiOOH$$

The addition of citric acid or sodium citrate to solutions of bismuth salts prevents precipitation in the presence of excess alkali. Bismuth sulfide is precipitated from acid solutions of bismuth salts by sulfides.

Bismuth subnitrate leads to the most common incompatibilities of all bismuth salts. If suspended in water, bismuth subnitrate undergoes hydrolysis to yield a suspension which is acid in reaction.

$$2BiONO_3 + HOH \rightarrow (BiO)_2(OH)NO_3 + HNO_3$$

Repeated washing with water will convert bismuth subnitrate to the normal hydroxide and also liberate nitric acid. Thus, these aqueous suspensions have the incompatibilities of acids such as effervescence with carbonates and precipitation of salicylic acid from aqueous solutions of salicylates. The use of bismuth subcarbonate avoids these incompatibilities.

Hypophosphites and other reducing agents slowly reduce bismuth salts to metallic bismuth. Under varying conditions iodides convert bismuth salts into the dark brown iodides (BiI_3) or the red basic iodide ($BiOI$). Bismuth salts form precipitates with gallic and tannic acids. Bismuth subcarbonate differs from the subnitrate in that it does not have an acid reaction; it effervesces with acids.

Group VII B (Mn, Tc, Re)

Only manganese requires mention here.

Manganese—Manganese hypophosphite and other manganous salts give a precipitate of manganese hydroxide with alkali hydroxides, manganese carbonate with soluble carbonates, and manganese phosphate with alkali phosphates (Table 10). These precipitates soon darken due to absorption of oxygen and conversion to hydrated manganic hydroxide. Manganese hypophosphite also has the incompatibilities of the hypophosphites.

Manganese dioxide is a strong oxidizing agent and is likely to cause explosions if triturated or heated with reducing agents such as phosphides, hypophosphites, and organic substances. Manganese citrate is solubilized by sodium citrate, and manganese glycerophosphate is solubilized by citric acid. Soluble manganous salts are precipitated by sulfides in neutral solutions.

Group VIII (Fe, Ru, Os, Co, Rh, Ir, Ni, Pd, Pt)

Iron, cobalt, and nickel are closely related chemically, and their typical incompatibilities can be described as a group under the most common member, iron.

Iron—Solutions of iron salts have a slightly acid reaction due to hydrolysis yielding ferric hydroxide plus the free acid.

$$FeCl_3 + 3HOH \rightarrow Fe(OH)_3 \downarrow + 3HCl$$

The incompatibilities of iron are concerned with the insolubility of the hydroxides and various oxidation-reduction situations.

Ferrous salts in aqueous solution are unstable when exposed to air, being oxidized to the ferric state, usually with the precipitation of a basic ferric salt, e.g.:

$$4FeSO_4 + 2H_2O + O_2 \rightarrow 4Fe(OH)SO_4 \downarrow$$

The oxidation is prevented by iodides and hypophosphites in acid solution and is retarded by other reducing agents which function as antioxidants to prevent reduction of the ferric ion to the ferrous ion. Nitric acid and other oxidizing agents hasten the oxidation. The addition of alkali hydroxides to solutions of ferrous salts precipitates ferrous hydroxide (Table 10), which is white when pure. It is generally green due to partial oxidation and may be further oxidized to brown ferric hydroxide. Soluble carbonates, arsenites, arsenates, oxalates, and phosphates precipitate the corresponding ferrous salt from solutions, e.g.:

$$Fe^{2+} + CO_3{}^{2-} \rightarrow FeCO_3 \downarrow$$

Ferric salts are reduced to the ferrous state by iodides or hypophosphites in acid solution, iodine being liberated in case of the iodides.

$$2Fe^{3+} + 2I^- \rightarrow 2Fe^{2+} + I_2$$

Solutions of ferric salts give a precipitate of ferric hydroxide on addition of alkali carbonates or hydroxides, a precipitate of basic ferric borate on addition of borax, and a precipitate is also formed with alkali phosphates (Table 10). Precipitation of ferric hydroxide is prevented by the presence of organic hydroxy acids or their salts; e.g., tartrates, citrates, or polyhydric alcohols such as glycerin and sugars. Tannic acid and preparations which contain it give a blue-black solution or precipitate with ferric salts; the color is diminished by phosphoric acid. Acetates give a red color with solutions of ferric salts, the color being due to basic ferric acetate. Solutions of ferric salts give a violet color with salicylates and a red color with antipyrine. Some insoluble iron salts such as ferric phosphate are soluble in solutions of an alkali citrate. Solutions of ferric ammonium citrate support mold growth on standing.

Incompatibilities of Nonmetals

The nonmetallic elements have the incompatibilities of the acids they form and they are, therefore, discussed in the acid section. Certain additional characteristics of carbon, sulfur, and iodine are discussed in this section.

Carbon—The form of carbon that is of interest here is activated charcoal. Charcoal is easily oxidized and should not be triturated with oxidizing agents. Because of its adsorptive properties it should not be dispensed with potent drugs such as alkaloids since they may be inactivated. Fluid preparations tend to cake and become physically unacceptable.

Sulfur—In pharmacy three forms of sulfur are encountered: precipitated, sublimed, and washed. These forms are fine, yellow, essentially odorless and tasteless powders. They are soluble in carbon disulfide but insoluble in most common solvents. Sulfur is oxidized in the presence of water to yield sulfuric acid. On heating with fixed alkali hydroxides, sulfur is solubilized, forming the metal thiosulfate and sulfides, e.g.:

$$14S + 12KOH \xrightarrow{\Delta} K_2S_3 + 2K_2S_2O_3 +$$

$$2K_2S + K_2S_5 + 6H_2O$$

Iodine—Iodine is an oxidizing agent, especially in alkaline solution in which it is reduced by arsenites, hypophosphites, and other reducing agents (excepting the nitrites).

$$I_2 + H_3AsO_3 + H_2O \rightarrow 2HI + H_3AsO_4$$

Iodine reacts strongly with volatile oils such as turpentine oil by substitution and oxidation. Explosions may result from such combinations. Preparations in which iodine is dissolved with the aid of potassium iodide precipitate most alkaloids. Iodine is soluble in water (1 g in 2950 ml), alcohol (1 in 13), carbon disulfide (1 in 4), and glycerin (1 in 80). Iodine is also oxidized by strong oxidizing agents such as chlorates or nitrates to yield iodates.

(a) $3I_2 + 5KClO_3 + 3H_2O \rightarrow 6HIO_3 +$
$$5KCl$$

(b) $I_2 + 10HNO_3 \rightarrow 2HIO_3 + 10NO_2 \uparrow +$
$$4H_2O$$

Incompatibilities of Acids

All acids have incompatibilities due to their acidity, but there are some differences because some acids are highly ionized in aqueous solutions (strong acids), others are only slightly ionized (weak acids), some are oxidizing agents, and some are reducing agents. The following is a list of some common acids from each of the above categories:

Categories of Acids

Strong—Perchloric ($HClO_4$), Sulfuric (H_2SO_4), Hydrobromic (HBr), Hydrochloric (HCl), Nitric (HNO_3), Hydronium ion (H_3O^+), Phosphoric (H_3PO_4).

Weak—Acetic (CH_3COOH), Carbonic (H_2CO_3), Hydrogen Sulfide (H_2S), Hydrocyanic (HCN), Boric (H_3BO_3).

Oxidizing—Nitric (HNO_3), Nitrohydrochloric (mixture of $HCl + HNO_3 + NOCl + Cl_2$), Permanganic ($HMnO_4$), Chromic ($H_2CrO_4$), Perboric ($HBO_3$), and Nitrous ($HNO_2$).

Reducing—Hypophosphorous (HPH_2O_2), Sulfurous (H_2SO_3), Hydriodic (HI), Thiosulfuric ($H_2S_2O_3$), Thiocyanic (HSCN), Hydrosulfuric (H_2S).

The acids shown under "strong" and "weak" are listed in the approximate order of decreasing acid strength. An additional group of compounds, not normally thought of as acids, are capable of giving up a proton and thus function in certain reactions as very weak acids, for example: phenol (C_6H_5OH), water (H_2O), ethyl alcohol (C_2H_5OH), methylamine (CH_3NH_2), methane (CH_4). The ability of an acid to react may be predicted from the relative strengths of the acid component and its position in reference to its conjugate base.

All acids which are stronger than carbonic acid liberate carbonic acid from carbonates. Acids that are stronger than hydrosulfuric acid liberate H_2S from sulfides, e.g.:

$$FeS + 2HCl \rightarrow FeCl_2 + H_2S \uparrow$$

Metallic salts of weak acids act as buffers toward stronger acids. Insoluble acids such as salicylic and benzoic are precipitated when aqueous solutions of soluble salicylates or benzoates are acidified, e.g.:

Sodium benzoate + H^+ →
$$\text{Benzoic acid} \downarrow + Na^+$$

Strong Acids

Strong acids are those which are highly ionized and which give up a proton easily with the reaction proceeding essentially to completion. The products of such proton transfers are relatively weaker acids and bases:

$$HCl + H_2O \rightleftharpoons H_3O^+ + Cl^-$$

Heat is generated when concentrated strong acids are mixed with water and certain other liquids. The proper method of mixing is to pour the acid in a thin stream with constant stirring into the liquid contained in a shallow dish. Sulfuric acid chars many organic substances by dehydration, forming carbon. An example of this is the charring of sugar.

$$C_6H_{12}O_6 \rightarrow 6C + 6H_2O$$

Hot, concentrated sulfuric acid exhibits an oxidizing action on (1) metals, (2) nonmetals, and (3) many compounds.

(1) $Hg + 2H_2SO_4 \rightarrow HgSO_4 + SO_2 \uparrow + 2H_2O$

(2) $S + 2H_2SO_4 \rightarrow 3SO_2 \uparrow + 2H_2O$

(3) $2HBr + H_2SO_4 \rightarrow SO_2 \uparrow + Br_2 + 2H_2O$

Orthophosphoric acid (H_3PO_4) gives precipitates with salts of lead and silver, but in neutral or alkaline solution the phosphate ion forms insoluble compounds with almost all other metallic ions except those of the alkali group. Sodium phosphate ($Na_2HPO_4 \cdot 12H_2O$) is alkaline in reaction and thus precipitates alkaloids. It gives a soft mass when triturated with some substances such as phenol, chloral hydrate, and acetanilid.

Weak Acids

Weak acids are those which are only slightly ionized and which give up a proton only to a limited extent. The products of such reactions are relatively stronger acids and bases, thereby controlling the equilibrium.

$$CH_3COOH + H_2O \rightleftharpoons H_3O^+ + CH_3COO^-$$

Carbonic acid is a very weak acid and is very unstable, existing only in dilute solution in equilibrium with carbon dioxide. Owing to hydrolysis, aqueous solutions of the alkali carbonates are alkaline in reaction. Carbonates are decomposed with the liberation of carbon dioxide by all except the weakest acids such as boric and hydrocyanic.

Boric acid (H_3BO_3, boracic acid) is a weak acid. Sodium borate ($Na_2B_4O_7 \cdot 10H_2O$, borax, sodium tetraborate, sodium biborate) is slightly alkaline in reaction and, hence, has the incompatibilities of alkalies such as the precipitation of alkaloids from solutions of alkaloidal salts. The addition of glycerin or honey changes the reaction of borax solutions from alkaline to acid and thus prevents the incompatibilities due to alkalinity. In the presence of water, glycerin reacts with borax, forming sodium glyceroborate and glyceroboric acid, the latter being responsible for the acid reaction.

$$Na_2B_4O_7 \cdot 10H_2O + 8C_3H_5(OH)_3 \rightarrow$$
$$2[C_3H_5(OH)_2]_2BO_3Na +$$
$$2[C_3H_5(OH)_2]_2BO_3H + 13H_2O$$

The addition of glycerin (20 to 25%) is required to make a 2 to 10% solution of borax neutral in reaction. Mannitol, glycerin, and a number of other organic compounds having two adjacent hydroxyl groups increase the acidity of boric acid, usually by the formation of complex compounds. Concentrated solutions of borax gelatinize acacia mucilage unless the alkalinity is reduced by the addition of glycerin or an acid. Borates, except those of the alkali metals, are only sparingly soluble in neutral and alkaline solutions, but they dissolve in acid solution. Hence, borax gives precipitates of borates or basic borates with solutions of metals other than those of the alkali group (Table 10). Borax yields a moist mass when triturated with some compounds due to liberation of water of crystallization; e.g., alum, zinc sulfate, tartaric acid, and benzoic acid.

Oxidizing Acids

Strong oxidizing acids and oxidizing agents are incompatible with organic substances. Reaction occurs in some cases with explosive violence. See Table 11 for a summary of potentially dangerous mixtures. The following discussions and prescriptions illustrate the oxidiz-

Table 11—Summary of Potentially Dangerous Mixtures

Oxidizing agents	*Reducing agents*
Nitric acid (HNO_3)	Alcohol
Nitrates (NO_3^-); e.g., KNO_3, $NaNO_3$	Glycerin
Nitrohydrochloric acid	Lactose
Hypochlorous acid ($HClO$)	Sugar
Hypochlorites (ClO^-); e.g., $KClO$, $NaClO$	Charcoal
Chloric acid ($HClO_3$)	Volatile oils
Chlorates (ClO_3^-); e.g., $KClO_3$	Tannins and other extracts
Permanganic acid ($HMnO_4$)	Bisulfites (HSO_3^-); e.g., $NaHSO_3$
Permanganates (MnO_4^-); e.g., $KMnO_4$	Sulfur (S)
Hydrogen peroxide (H_2O_2)	Sulfurous Acid (H_2SO_3)
Peroxides (O_2^{2-}); e.g., ZnO_2	Sulfites (SO_3^{2-}); e.g., Na_2SO_3
Chromates (CrO_4^{2-}); e.g., K_2CrO_4	Thiosulfates ($S_2O_3^{2-}$); e.g., $Na_2S_2O_3$
Dichromates ($Cr_2O_7^{2-}$); e.g., $K_2Cr_2O_7$	Sulfides (S^{2-}); e.g., H_2S, FeS, ZnS
Perborates (BO_2^-); e.g., $NaBO_3 \cdot H_2O$	Hypophosphorus Acid (H_3PO_2)
Nitrous acid (HNO_2)	Nitrites[a] (NO_2^-)
Nitrites[a] (NO_2^-); e.g., $NaNO_2$	Hypophosphites ($H_2PO_2^-$)
Spirit of ethyl nitrite (in acid soln.)	Bromides (Br^-); e.g., $NaBr$
Trinitrophenol	Iodides (I^-); e.g., KI
Chlorine (Cl_2)	Hydriodic acid (HI)
Bromine (Br_2)	Phosphorus (P)
Iodine (I_2)	Lower valence salts of multivalent metals
Silver salts; e.g., $AgNO_2$, Ag_2O	e.g., Fe^{2+}, Hg^+, Sb^{2+}, As^{2+}, Cu^+
Higher valence salts of multivalent metals; e.g., Fe^{2+}, Hg^{2+}, As^{5+}, Sb^{5+}, Bi^{5+}, Cu^{5+}, Pb^{4+}	

[a] Nitrites in acid solution act as oxidizing agents toward some compounds, e.g., hypophosphites, and as reducing agents toward others, e.g., mercurous salts.

ing properties and some other incompatibilities of oxidizing agents.

Oxidizing and Reducing Agents— Mixtures of many of the oxidizing and reducing agents listed in Table 11 should not be triturated or mechanically processed either as dry powders or as concentrated solutions since explosions may result. Dilute aqueous solutions usually may be combined if the reaction is controlled by careful addition and cooling. A small trial combination is recommended where dispensing is necessary.

Nitric Acid—Nitric acid reacts with some alkaloids to form colored compounds. It forms explosive nitroglycerin when reacted with sulfuric acid and glycerin. Ferrous, arsenous, and mercurous salts are oxidized to a higher valence by nitric acid. Explosions may occur if nitrates are triturated with reducing agents such as charcoal, sulfur, sucrose, and glycerin.

Hypochlorous Acid—Hypochlorites are decomposed by acids, even carbonic acid, with the liberation of unstable hypochlorous acid ($HClO$). Solutions of hypochlorites must be prepared at room temperature since heat converts them into chlorates and chlorides. Chlorates are also powerful oxidizing agents.

Permanganic Acid — Explosions have occurred when permanganates have been placed in tightly closed, dirty bottles, which have previously contained a volatile oil or other substances yielding carbon dioxide on oxidation. Potassium permanganate solutions may turn brown if filtered through paper, but such solutions can be filtered through a sintered glass filter or glass wool.

When permanganates act as oxidizing agents in acid solution, the valence of manganese is reduced from $+7$ to $+2$. For example, the oxidation of ferrous sulfate in acid solution takes place as follows:

$$2KMnO_4 + 10FeSO_4 + 8H_2SO_4 \rightarrow$$
$$2MnSO_4 + K_2SO_4 + 5Fe_2(SO_4)_3 + 8H_2O$$

During oxidation by permanganates, in neutral or alkaline solution, the valence of Mn drops from +7 to +4, the manganese separating as MnO_2. In acid solution, permanganates oxidize sulfides, sulfites, hypophosphites, chlorides, bromides, iodides, arsenites, ferrous salts, and most organic substances. Many substances are also oxidized in neutral or alkaline solution. The paraffin hydrocarbons are rather inactive chemically; hence, pills of potassium permanganate may be made with an excipient of kaolin, paraffin, and petrolatum.

Hydrogen Peroxide—Peroxides of the metals react with acids, forming hydrogen peroxide. Sodium peroxide reacts with water to form sodium hydroxide and hydrogen peroxide.

$$Na_2O_2 + 2H_2O \rightarrow 2NaOH + H_2O_2$$

Zinc peroxide is a mixture of zinc carbonate, hydroxide, and peroxide. Its bacterial power depends on the slow liberation of oxygen.

Zinc peroxide powder may be sterilized before use by heating in an oven for 4 hours at 140°C; this heat treatment also activates the evolution of oxygen. Acids decompose zinc peroxide.

Hydrogen peroxide solution slowly decomposes with the evolution of oxygen; heat increases the rate of decomposition. In general, it is decomposed by alkalies, potassium permanganate, organic matter, and reducing agents.

Chromic Acid—Chromic acid (chromic anhydride, chromium trioxide) is reduced by alcohol, glycerin, and other organic solvents, in some cases violently. When chromium trioxide is mixed with hydrogen peroxide, both substances lose oxygen, which is liberated in gaseous form. Potassium dichromate, potassium chromate, and other chromates are powerful oxidizing agents.

Perboric Acid—Sodium perborate ($NaBO_3 \cdot 4H_2O$) decomposes in warm or moist air with the evolution of oxygen. It is incompatible with reducing agents.

In aqueous solution sodium perborate reacts with water to form hydrogen peroxide and sodium metaborate.

$$NaBO_3 + H_2O \rightarrow H_2O_2 + NaBO_2$$

This reaction is greatly accelerated by acids and acid salts. An aqueous solution of sodium perborate is alkaline because of the hydrolysis of the sodium perborate and sodium metaborate. Oxygen is gradually evolved from a solution of sodium perborate due to decomposition of the hydrogen peroxide. The alkalinity of sodium perborate can be effectively reduced by the addition of monocalcium phosphate, thereby removing a common objection to its use.

Nitrous Acid—Nitrites in solution are slightly hydrolyzed since nitrous acid is a weak acid. Nitrites in acid solution are very reactive, behaving as oxidizing agents toward some substances and as reducing agents toward others. Thus, hypophosphites are oxidized to phosphates, and mercurous salts are reduced to metallic mercury. Nitrates are much less reactive in neutral or alkaline solution. Ethyl nitrite spirit, on standing, gradually decomposes with nitrous acid as one of the products; the resulting incompatibilities may be retarded by neutralizing the spirit. Nitrous acid causes color changes with some alkaloids and certain other substances, e.g., a green color with antipyrine, a yellow color with acetanilid and acetophenetidin, and a reddish-brown color with phenolic compounds. Ethyl nitrite spirit liberates iodine from iodides. Amyl nitrite has similar incompatibilities. Acids convert sodium nitrite into nitrous acid, which decomposes with the evolution of brown fumes of the oxides of nitrogen.

Nitrous acid and nitrites do not liberate bromine from bromides. However, ammonium bromide is incompatible with nitrites because the ammonium nitrite formed decomposes with the liberation of nitrogen, particularly when the solution is warmed giving an explosive package.

$$NH_4Br + NaNO_2 \rightleftarrows NH_4NO_2 + NaBr$$

$$NH_4NO_2 \rightarrow N_2 + 2H_2O$$

Reducing Acids

Strong reducing acids are incompatible with oxidizing agents. Refer to Table 11 for a summary of potentially dangerous mixtures. Explosions may occur if reducing agents are triturated with oxidizing agents. Relatively low concentrations of some reducing agents are added to preparations to maintain the reduced state of another component. Specific examples are included in the succeeding discussions.

Hypophosphorous Acid—Hypophosphorous acid and hypophosphites are oxidized to phosphorous and phosphoric acid by the oxygen of air and other oxidizing agents. Hypophosphorous acid acts as a preservative in diluted hydriodic acid syrup and ferrous iodide syrup by its capacity to reduce free iodine back to iodide.

$$2I_2 + HPH_2O_2 + 2H_2O \rightarrow 4HI + H_3PO_4$$

Hypophosphorous acid reacts with metal hydroxides to form the corresponding hypophosphite salts which are water soluble, except for ferric hypophosphite. This iron salt is solubilized by the presence of free hypophosphorous acid or concentrated solutions of alkali citrates.

Sulfurous Acid—Air slowly oxidizes sulfurous acid and sulfites to sulfuric acid and sulfates. Solutions of normal sulfites are weakly basic, while those of the hydrogen sulfites are slightly acid. Both types of salts are decomposed by heat.

$$4Na_2SO_3 \rightarrow Na_2S + 3Na_2SO_4$$

$$2NaHSO_3 \rightarrow Na_2SO_3 + H_2O + SO_2 \uparrow$$

Some organic coloring agents are bleached by acid solutions of sulfites. Most of the metallic sulfites are insoluble except the alkali sulfites.

Thiosulfuric Acid — Thiosulfuric acid ($H_2S_2O_3$) occurs only as salts, the thiosulfates. These salts are water soluble except those of Ag, Pb, and Ba. They are only slightly soluble. Aqueous solutions of the alkali salts are slightly basic. The addition of acid (HCl) liberates thiosulfuric acid, which decomposes into sulfur, sulfur dioxide, and water.

$$Na_2S_2O_3 + 2HCl \rightarrow H_2S_2O_3 + 2NaCl \rightarrow$$
$$S \downarrow + SO_2 \uparrow + H_2O + 2Na^+ + 2Cl^-$$

Thiosulfates will reduce oxidizing agents such as ferric salts, silver salts, mercuric salts, iodine, and permanganates.

$$2Na_2S_2O_3 + I_2 \rightarrow$$
$$\text{(colored)}$$

$$Na_2S_4O_6 + 2NaI$$
$$\text{(colorless)}$$

Hydriodic Acid—Hydriodic acid and iodides in acid solution turn brown on standing, free iodine being liberated according to the following equations:

$$2HI \rightarrow H_2 + I_2$$

$$4I^- + O_2 + 4H^+ \rightleftarrows 2I_2 + 2H_2O$$

The first of these reactions indicates why free iodine appears even if all air is excluded; in presence of air the oxidation reaction predominates. The second equation indicates that hydrogen ions are necessary in the oxidation of iodide ions, and this is in accord with the fact that neutral and alkaline solutions of iodides are so much more stable than acid solutions. Many iodides, when stored in crystalline form, gradually decompose with liberation of free iodine; to retard this change, iodides are generally crystallized from alkaline solution. This accounts for the fact that some samples of iodides give alkaline solutions when dissolved. Such alkaline iodides have the incompatibilities of weak alkalies such as causing the precipitation of alkaloids. Some alkaloids are also precipitated as alkaloidal iodides by concentrated solutions of iodides. When strychnine sulfate solutions are treated with an alkali iodide or hydriodic acid, strychnine hydriodide is formed, having a solubility of 1 g in about 345 ml of water at 25°C, but much less soluble in the presence of an excess of soluble iodide. When small amounts of iodine are liberated in iodide solutions containing strychnine salts, strychnine periodide, having a low solubility in both water and alcohol, is formed. Similar reactions are noted with codeine and dihydrocodeinone.

To delay the appearance of free iodine in iodine solutions, a substance which decolorizes free iodine may be used; e.g., hypophosphorous acid is used in preparations of hydriodic acid and 0.05 g of sodium thiosulfate is used in 100 ml of saturated potassium iodide solution.

Ferric salts oxidize the iodide ion to free iodine, the iron being reduced to the ferrous form

$$Fe^{3+} + 2I^- \rightarrow 2Fe^{2+} + I_2 \uparrow$$

Cupric salts similarly liberate iodine and are thereby reduced to the cuprous form. Ethyl nitrite spirit liberates iodine from iodides, but the reaction may be delayed by previously neutralizing the spirit with sodium bicarbonate. Silver, lead, mercurous, mercuric, cuprous, and basic bismuth iodides are insoluble; other common metallic iodides are soluble.

Mercuric iodide is readily soluble in solutions of other iodides, forming the complex ion (HgI_4^-), and the resulting solution is a general alkaloidal precipitant. In the presence of moisture and a soluble iodide, mercurous iodide decomposes as follows:

$$2HgI + 2KI \rightarrow Hg + K_2HgI_4$$

Calomel, in the presence of moisture and a soluble iodide, forms some mercurous iodide, which then decomposes as shown in the preceding equation. Mixtures of mercurous salts and iodides are dangerous to dispense, even in the form of powders, since the mercurous salt is converted in part into mercuric compounds which are more soluble and more poisonous.

Hydriodic acid behaves like a strong acid (comparable to hydrochloric and hydrobromic) but is the least stable of the hydrohalide acids. Iodine is liberated from HI by both chlorine and bromine.

$$2HI + Cl_2 \rightarrow I_2 \uparrow + 2HCl$$

Hydriodic acid reacts with all metallic oxides and hydroxides, except Cr_2O_3, to form a halide of the metal.

Preparations Having an Acid Reaction

The pharmacist should be on the alert for incompatibilities which occur because of the acidity of pharmaceutical preparations, as well as those caused by the acids or acidic compounds that were previously described. Gas-producing compounds such as carbon dioxide formers (e.g., carbonates and bicarbonates), chlorine formers (e.g., chlorates and hypochlorites), and nitrous oxide formers (e.g., nitrates) should not be combined with acidic preparations unless the reaction is carefully controlled and/or is allowed to go to completion before packaging. Screw capped bottles have been reported to explode when such reactants have been combined without precaution. Fluidextracts generally have a slightly acid reaction. Various company specialties are acid in reaction. When a question arises, an approximate pH of the preparation can be quickly determined with litmus or pH paper. The following list includes many preparations which are acid in reaction.

Acid Preparations

Fluidextracts—ergot, ipecac, nux vomica, aconite.
Elixirs—compound pepsin, compound glycerophosphates, lactated pepsin.
Solutions—ammonium acetate, ferric chloride, ferric subsulfate, iron and ammonium acetate, ferric sulfate, hydrogen peroxide, magnesium citrate, arsenous acid.
Syrups—citric acid, hydriodic acid, cherry, ferrous iodide, orange, raspberry, squill, ipecac, hypophosphites.
Glycerites—boroglycerin, pepsin.
Tinctures—aconite, ferric chloride, camphorated opium, nux vomica, cinchona.
Miscellaneous—squill vinegar.

Typical pH values of inorganic salts are given in Table 12.

Incompatibilities of Alkalies

Inorganic alkaline compounds of interest to pharmacists include the hydroxides of certain metals falling in Periodic Groups I through VI. Examples of strongly alkaline compounds are the hydroxides of lithium, sodium, and potassium (Group I); of weakly alkaline compounds are the hydroxides not only of magnesium, calcium, strontium, and barium (Group II) but also of the ammonium ion; and examples of amphoteric alkaline compounds are the hydroxides of zinc (Group II), aluminum (Group III), tin and lead (Group IV), bismuth (Group V), and chromium (Group VI). The incompatibilities of these inorganic groups of hydroxides fall into three general classifications according to solubility, reaction with acids, and precipitation due to pH.

The solubilities of metallic hydroxides have been mentioned under the various metal groups; however, it may be reemphasized that strong alkali hydroxides are soluble in water and weak alkali hydroxides are insoluble in water. Amphoteric alkali hydroxides are insoluble in water or in weakly alkaline solutions but are solubilized by the addition of acid.

This leads to the second type of incompatibility, reaction with acids. Alkalies react with acids to form salts. A precipitation will occur if the salt formed is insoluble in the solution. Conversely, an alkali may be solubilized (sometimes to the detriment of the product) by the addition of an acidic solution.

The third type of incompatibility encountered with these groups is associated with the pH of pharmaceutical preparations. Because pH affects compatibility, a basic understanding of this factor is essential to the pharmacist (Table 12).

It is useful in predicting compatibility since it describes the exact amount of hydrogen ion which may be present to form undissociated (hence, less soluble) acids or to combine with hydroxyl ions which may otherwise precipitate metallic hydroxides or neutralize amine acid salts.

The stronger the base, the more soluble it is in water and thus the higher the pH at which the hydroxide precipita-

tion begins. It is not only in the elements of the same periodic series that this sort of parallelism exists. Aqueous solutions of the chlorides of Sn^{2+}, Sb^{3+}, and Fe^{3+}, for example, are strongly acid, testifying to the extremely low ionization of the respective hydroxides. The latter hydroxides are formed at a solution pH of about 2-3. The aqueous solutions of chlorides of Cd^{2+}, Ni^{2+}, and Co^{2+}, on the other hand, are practically neutral, and the respective hydroxides precipitate at about pH 7. See Tables 10, 13, and 9.

Approximate pH values at which insoluble precipitates form when NaOH, K_2CrO_4, $Na_2B_4O_7$, Na_2CO_3, or Na_3PO_4 is added to dilute solutions of the salts are given in Table 10.

Thus, the lower the solubility the weaker the base, and the lower the pH at which precipitation begins. This does not mean, however, that the converse is true, inasmuch as not all readily soluble bases are strong electrolytes.

Preparations Having an Alkaline Reaction

Comparable to the acidic preparations previously discussed, there are a number of pharmaceutical preparations which are alkaline in reaction and therefore have the general incompatibilities of alkalies such as neutralization of acids, precipitation of alkaloids, precipitation of hydroxides or oxides of heavy metals from solutions of the salts, and liberation of ammonia from ammonium salts. Among pharmaceutical preparations having an alkaline reaction are those shown in the following list.

Alkaline Preparations

Fluidextracts—senega.

Ointments—rose water.

Elixirs—ammonium valerate, hydrastis compound.

Solutions—alkaline aromatic, lead subacetate, potassium arsenite, compound sodium borate, sodium hypochlorite, calcium hydroxide, soda and mint.

Spirits—aromatic ammonia.

Syrups—senega, ginger, rhubarb.

Waters—ammonia.

Table 12—Approximate pH Value of Aqueous Solutions of Inorganic Compounds

Compound	pH value (concentration 1% except as noted)	Compound	pH value (concentration 1% except as noted)
Aluminum acetate, basic	4.2; 5.2 (saturated)	Calcium chloride	7.5
Aluminum ammonium sulfate	4.2; 3.5; 4.6 (0.05 M)	Calcium citrate	6.0–6.2 (10% suspension)
Aluminum chloride	3.8 (0.01 M)	Calcium gluconate	6.7–6.9
Aluminum dihydroxyaminoacetate	7.4 (4% suspension)	Calcium glycerophosphate	9.4
Aluminum hydroxide	8.2–8.5 (10% suspension)	Calcium hydroxide	12.3 (saturated)
		Calcium hypophosphite	5.0
Aluminum lactate	3.7	Calcium iodide	9.9
Aluminum nitrate	3.6	Calcium lactate	6–7
Aluminum phenolsulfonate	4.0	Calcium levulinate	Neutral
		Calcium nicotinate	Neutral to sl. acid
Aluminum phosphate	3.6 (saturated)	Calcium oxide	12.4 (saturated)
Aluminum potassium sulfate	4.2; 3.6	Calcium pantothenate	7.2–8.0 (5%)
Aluminum silicate	6.0 (saturated)	Calcium phenolsulfonate	6.8
Aluminum sulfate	3.6 (0.01 M)	Calcium phosphate, dibasic	7.1–7.2 (10% suspension)
Ammonium acetate	Sl. acid	Calcium phosphate, monobasic	3.0
Ammonium bicarbonate	7.8 (0.1 M)	Calcium phosphate, tribasic	11.5 (saturated)
Ammonium bromide	4.6	Calcium salicylate	6.4 (saturated)
Ammonium carbonate	8.5	Calcium stearate	8.4 (saturated)
Ammonium chloride	4.8 (10%); 5.3 (1%)	Calcium sulfate	7.1 (saturated)
		Cobalt gluconate	6.0
Ammonium citrate, dibasic	5.1	Cobalt sulfate	4.5
Ammonium glutamate	4.9	Cobalt chloride	5.6
		Cupric acetate	5.0 (0.0033 M)
Ammonium iodide	4.6 (0.1 M)	Cupric nitrate	5.5 (0.0033 M); 4.4
Ammonium nitrate	5.5		
Ammonium phosphate, dibasic	7.9	Cupric sulfate	5.2 (0.0033 M); 4.5
Ammonium phosphate, monobasic	4.4	Ferric ammonium citrate	6.5 (0.05 M); 4.4
Ammonium salicylate	4.6	Ferric ammonium sulfate	4.7 (0.0033 M); 2.8
Ammonium sulfate	5.5		
Ammonium thiocyanate	5.7	Ferric chloride	2.7 (0.0033 M)
		Ferric citrate	2.5 (0.0033 M)
Antimony potassium tartrate	Sl. acid	Ferric nitrate	2.9 (0.0033 M)
		Ferric phosphate	3.5 (saturated)
Antimony trichloride	1.5	Ferric pyrophosphate	4.6
Arsenic triiodide	1.1 (0.1 N)	Ferric sulfate	2.6 (0.0033 M)
Barium chloride	6–7; 5.9	Ferric tartrate	6.8 (0.05 M)
Barium hydroxide	12.0	Ferrous gluconate	4.8 (0.0033 M)
Barium sulfate	10.5 (saturated)	Ferrous lactate	3.6
Bismuth glycol arsanilate	2.8–3.5 (saturated)	Ferrous sulfate	4.7 (0.0033 M); 3.8
Bismuth potassium tartrate	8.5	Lead acetate	6.2; 5.5–6.5 (5%)
		Lead nitrate	5.0–5.3; 3–4 (20%)
Bismuth salicylate	2.9 (saturated)	Magnesium acetate	7.5
Bismuth sodium triglycollamate	7–8 (2%)	Magnesium carbonate	9.8 (saturated)
		Magnesium chloride	6.1–7.8
Bismuth subbenzoate	8.2 (saturated)	Magnesium glycerophosphate	9.7
Bismuth subcarbonate	Neutral		
Bismuth subnitrate	4.6 (saturated)	Magnesium glycerinate	8.8–10.2 (saturated)
Boric acid	5.1 (0.1 M)		
Cadmium bromide	4.5	Magnesium hydroxide	9.8 (saturated)
Cadmium chloride	4.5	Magnesium hypophosphite	Neutral to sl. acid
Cadmium iodide	4.0		
Cadmium nitrate	4.5	Magnesium phosphate, tribasic	8.1 (saturated)
Cadmium sulfate	4.5		
Calcium acetate	7.4	Magnesium stearate	8.5–9.0 (saturated)
Calcium bromide	6.3–6.6	Magnesium sulfate	6–7; 6.5
Calcium carbonate	9.4 (saturated)	Magnesium trisilicate	9.5–9.7 (saturated)·

Table 12—*Continued*

Compound	pH value (concentration 1% except as noted)	Compound	pH value (concentration 1% except as noted)
Magnesium nitrate	6.7	Sodium cacodylate	8–9
Manganese chloride	4.0; 6.3	Sodium caprylate	7.5
Manganese hypo-phosphite	5.0 (saturated)	Sodium carbonate	11.6
Manganese iodide	Sl. acid	Sodium carboxy-methylcellulose	7.0
Mercuric acetate	6.5 (0.0033 M)	Sodium cellulose sulfate	6.2
Mercuric chloride	4.7; 3.0–4.6; 6.1 (0.001 M)	Sodium chloride	6.7–7.3; 6.2
Mercuric cyanide	5.7	Sodium citrate	8.0; 6.5 (20%); 7.0 (6%)
Mercuric iodide, red	6.3 (saturated)		
Mercuric nitrate	2.7 (saturated)	Sodium fluorescein	7.9
Mercuric oxide, red	7.8 (saturated)	Sodium formate	7.0; 7.3
Mercuric oxide, yellow	7.0 (saturated)	Sodium gentisate	6.5–6.9
Mercuric succinimide	8.7 (0.0033 M)	Sodium glutamate	7.0 (0.2%); 6.9
Mercuric sulfate	1.8	Sodium glycerophos-phate	9.5; 8.8–9.0
Mercurochrome	9.3, (0.0033 M); 8.8 (0.5%)	Sodium hydroxide	12–14 (0.05–5%)
Penicillin G potassium	5.9	Sodium hypophos-phite	Neutral; 6.9
Potassium acetate	8.3; 9.7 (0.1 M)	Sodium iodide	8–9.5; 7.1 (1%); 9.2 (4.5%)
Potassium bicarbonate	8.2	Sodium lactate	6.3 (3.4%); 7.0 (50%)
Potassium bromide	6.6		
Potassium carbonate	11.6; 11.1	Sodium laurylsulfate	Neutral; 7.2
Potassium chlorate	5.2	Sodium metabisulfite	4.3
Potassium chloride	7.0; 6.5	Sodium nicotinate	8.7–8.9; *circa* 7
Potassium citrate	8.5; 7.1–7.5	Sodium nitrate	Neutral; 6.4 (2%); 5.1–5.7
Potassium dichromate	4.3		
Potassium ferricyanide	6.0	Sodium nitrite	9.0
Potassium gluconate	5.3–6.2	Sodium phenolsulfo-nate	Neutral; 5.6–6.0
Potassium guaiacol-sulfonate	Neutral	Sodium phosphate, dibasic	9.5; 9.1–9.2 (0.1 M)
Potassium hydroxide	13.5 (0.1 M)	Sodium phosphate, monobasic	4.0; 4.5
Potassium hypophos-phite	7.4	Sodium phosphate, tribasic	12.1 (6.7%); 11.5 (0.1%)
Potassium iodide	7–9; 7.8	Sodium propionate	Neutral: 7.9–8.2
Potassium nitrate	7.0; 5.9	Sodium psylliate	8.7–9.2
Potassium *p*-amino-benzoate	7.0 (1%)	Sodium salicylate	5–6; 5.9 (5%); 6.2
		Sodium silicate	10.4
Potassium phosphate, dibasic	8.9	Sodium stearate	10.8
		Sodium sucaryl	5.5–7.5 (10%); 8.1
Potassium phosphate, monobasic	4.4–4.7; 4.7	Sodium sulfate	6–7.5; 6.3 (7.9%)
		Sodium sulfite	9.2
Potassium phosphate, tribasic	11.8	Sodium tartrate	7.0; 7.0–9.0
Potassium salicylate	5.2–6.3	Sodium thiocyanate	Neutral; 6.6
Potassium sodium tartrate	7–8; 7.0	Sodium thiosulfate	6.5–8; 6.4 (6%); 7.3
		Sodium undecylenate	7.5
Potassium sulfate	7.0; 8.8	Stannic chloride	1.2
Potassium tartrate	7–8; 7.0	Strontium bromide	Neutral
Potassium thiocyanate	4.9–5.9	Sulfadiazine sodium	9–11; 9.6
Silver nitrate	7.0; 5.6	Zinc acetate	5–6; 6.5–6.7 (0.001–0.1 M)
Silver sulfate	5.7		
Sodium acetate	8.3 (4%), 7.7; 8.9 (0.1 M)	Zinc bromide	4.0; 6.2–6.4 (0.001–0.1 M)
Sodium alginate	6.5	Zinc chloride	4.0; 6.1–6.5 (0.001–0.1 M)
Sodium *p*-amino-benzoate	7.2; 7.85 (2%)	Zinc iodide	5.0; 5.5–5.9 (0.001–0.1 M)
Sodium arsenate, dibasic	9.8	Zinc nitrate	4.0; 5.6–6.9 (0.001–0.1 M)
Sodium arsenite	9.5–9.7		
Sodium ascorbate	5–6; 7.1–7.5	Zinc oxide	8.4 (saturated)
Sodium benzoate	8.0; 7.2–7.5	Zinc phenolsulfonate	4.0; 6.0
Sodium bicarbonate	8.2; 8.1	Zinc stearate	9.0 (saturated)
Sodium bisulfate	1.4 (0.1 M)	Zinc sulfate	4.5; 5.2–6.0 (0.001–0.1 M)
Sodium bisulfite	5.2		
Sodium borate	9.5; 9.1		
Sodium bromide	6.5–8.0; 6.0 (13.3%)		

Table 13—Effect of Solubility on Precipitation pH and Basic Strength

Hydroxide	Solubility (moles/liter) [5]	pH at which precipitation begins	Strength of base
$Be(OH)_2$	8×10^{-6}	~6.5	Weaker base
$Mg(OH)_2$	1.1×10^{-4}	~11	
$Ca(OH)_2$	2×10^{-2}	>12	
$Sr(OH)_2$	6.7×10^{-2}	Does not precipitate	
$Ba(OH)_2$	2.2×10^{-1}	Does not precipitate	Stronger base

Magmas—magnesia.

Tinctures—guaiac ammoniated, valerian ammoniated, iodides.

Organic Incompatibilities

It is obvious from the previous discussion that most types of physical and chemical incompatibilities involve solubility, chemical reactivity, or stability in some way or other. For example, physical incompatibilities usually include one or more solubility problems (i.e., incomplete solution, precipitation of immiscible phases, incorrect selection of drug form, or even eutectic mixtures). Chemical incompatibilities frequently include a combination of solubility, reactivity, and stability phenomena (i.e., formation of precipitates, evolution of gases, caking, crystal growth, separation of immiscible reaction products, and the like). Even the less obvious chemical reactions—hydrolysis, oxidation, reduction, or racemization—which are important in stability, often require simultaneous consideration of solubility and reactivity.

Accordingly, this section first briefly considers solubility factors. Then other important factors are discussed, such as, structural factors and the chemical reactions which can occur under dispensing conditions, the interactions of drug classes, cationic-anionic-nonionic relationships, and, of course, more specific organic incompatibilities. It should be especially noted that much of the theory involved with "delayed incompatibilities" and other stability problems has been covered in previous editions (qv).

Compounds will usually be considered by drug family, classified according to the functional (reactive) groups present. Polyfunctional items may be classified by pharmaceutical use (e.g., gums, preservatives, etc.) or therapeutic use (e.g., antibiotics, sulfonamides, etc.). This should be useful where the compound has a number of potentially reactive groups or when it is desired that the possibility of therapeutic incompatibility be emphasized.

Solubility Factors

As mentioned above, solubility is involved in many organic and inorganic physical and chemical incompatibilities. The appearance of precipitates, insoluble "oils," or evolution of gases may be manifestations of solubility changes produced by chemical reactions, pH changes, temperature variation, dilution of solvents with nonsolvents, use of improper vehicles or drug forms, addition of substances which depress solubility, and the various related causes.

Since the dissolution of a drug involves the distribution of the solute ions or molecules more or less randomly among those of the solvent, it has been pointed out that the solubility of a drug depends upon the chemical and physical properties of the drug and the vehicle, plus or minus the effects of temperature, pressure, pH, and sometimes particle size. Such theoretical predictions of solubility require consideration of such structural, electrical, and chemical factors as hydrogen bonding, polarity, dielectric constant, solvation, internal pressures, acid-base interactions, and others. The calculations are quite complex and usually require use of certain simplifying approximations. Accordingly, it will usually be time-saving for the pharmacist to look up those solubility values which are readily available in the literature. Many solubility values are to be found in these chapters, the *USP, NF, Remington's Pharmaceutical Sciences, Merck Index, Lange's Handbook of Chemistry,* or Chemical Rubber Company's *Handbook of Chemistry and Physics.* Where exact values are not available, useful approximations can often be made from closely related compounds using the methods discussed briefly in this chapter.

There is incomplete agreement among authorities as to the relative importance of the various factors which may affect solubility. Since most drug preparations involve aqueous or other hydrogen-bonded vehicles, emphasis will be placed here on temperature effects and such hopefully important factors as chemical reactivity, chemical bonds, hydrogen bonding, polarity, ratio of polar to nonpolar groups, pH and pK factors, ionization, molecular weight, and other factors believed operative in such systems.

Temperature Solubility Effects

When a drug is dissolved in a solvent, solution may occur with a rise, fall, or no change in temperature.

If there is little or no interaction between drug and solvent, the addition of heat will be required to separate the drug and solvent into ions or molecules (endothermic reaction). Solubility usually increases with increasing temperature and decreases with decreasing temperature.

Normally, the more heat which must be applied to bring about solution, the less soluble the compound.

In some cases the interaction between solvent and solute produces an excess of heat, and the temperature rises (exothermic reaction). Frequently, the greater the rise, the greater the reaction between solvent and solute and the greater the solubility. In such cases, additional heat will drive the equilibrium reaction in the opposite direction so that the solubility is decreased (e.g., calcium sulfate-water mixtures, which exhibit lower solubility when heated).

If heat is neither given off nor absorbed, the solubility will not be appreciably affected by temperature; e.g., sodium chloride, which has a solubility of about 35% *w/v* from 0° to 100°C.

These considerations are important since insoluble material may separate from prescriptions requiring heat when these prescriptions cool to room temperature. This separation may be further accentuated if the prescription requires a "Store in a Refrigerator" label. Such separations do not always occur immediately; hence, it is usually wise to add a "Shake Well" label to refrigerated prescriptions.

It might be well at this point to note that many of the structures and mechanisms which will be suggested as explanations of observed phenomena are really ideas rather than proved facts. For example, the question has been raised: Do electrons inhabit matter or do electrons exist essentially as ideas in our heads? Future scientists may well shake their heads in amazement at some of our current explanations of observed data, especially structural units of substances, noble gas type structures as the determinants of the direction of reaction, oxidation and reduction mechanisms, minimum energy and the direction of equilibrium reactions, etc. Nevertheless, many such "explanations" will be used here if they appear to organize laboratory observations into a system which helps predict reactions, helps the student remember useful data, or provides useful approximations for new situations.

Structural and Chemical Factors

Depending on how the atoms are arranged, packed, and held together, we can identify several states of matter with different physical properties; such as, crystalline solids, liquids, gases, glasses, liquid crystals, or rubbers. The first two of these states are most important in incompatibilities and will be emphasized.

Chemical Reactions

Catalysts were once defined as substances which change the rate of reaction without being changed or used up. We currently recognize that many catalysts are consumed or "poisoned." These materials probably act by opening up new reaction pathways which have lower energies of activation.

Hydronium (H_3O^+) and hydroxide (OH^-) ions; aluminum, ferric, stannic ions, and other Lewis acids; and sulfuric and other Brönsted acids are among the inorganic catalysts common in prescription incompatibilities and drug decompositions. Sometimes only trace amounts present as impurities in water, rubber closures, drugs, etc., are sufficient to cause trouble. Organic enzyme catalysts such as oxidase, dehydrogenase, and penicillinase may be active in drug decompositions; while such enzymes as cholinesterase, monamine oxidase, and many others may be responsible for therapeutic incompatibilities and adverse drug reactions. Inactivation of these catalysts (e.g., by adjustment of pH to eliminate hydroxide or hydronium ions, addition of sequestering agents to tie up metal ions, heating or adding chemicals to destroy enzymes, or administering appropriate drugs to inactivate or compete with biochemical and metabolic catalysts and the like) may play an increasing role in the medication of the future.

Chemical Bonds—Chemical bonds may be divided into binding forces between atoms and binding forces between molecules.

The binding forces between atoms include: ionic bonds, nonpolar (covalent) bonds, and polar bonds (covalent with partial ionic character), while the common binding forces between molecules include: hydrogen bonds, van der Waals forces, and ion dipoles.

Ionic Bonds—Ionic bonds are coulombic forces which exist when the individual atoms are present as closely packed positive and negative ions and attract each other electrostatically.

These bonds are very common in pharmaceuticals since they occur in electrolytes (e.g., Na^+Cl^-), metal salts of organic acids (e.g., $CH_3—COO^-Na^+$), metal salts of phenols (e.g., sodium phenolates) and the acid salts of amines (e.g., $C_6H_5—CH_2—NH_3^+Cl^-$). Here it should be observed that the organic ions themselves (e.g., the acetate, phenolate, and amine ions) are largely made up of atoms held together by polar covalent bonds (qv).

sodium phenolate

Nonpolar Covalent Bonds—These bonds are less common in pharmaceuticals since they occur with equally shared and equally contributed electrons in compounds such as hydrocarbons (e.g., propane) or completely halogenated symmetrical hydrocarbons (e.g., carbon tetrachloride).

propane   carbon tetrachloride

Polar Covalent Bonds—These bonds occur in most drug compounds. They possess some actual or potential separation of positive (+) and negative (−) centers because the equally contributed electrons are not equally shared. Polar centers usually contain oxygen or nitrogen (e.g., OH, CHO, COH, CHOH, CH_2OH, COOH, NO_2, NH_2, and SO_3H) as may occur in alcohols, incompletely halogenated hydrocarbons (e.g., chloroform), nitro compounds, phenols, or acids.

Hydrogen Bonds—Although it has been suggested for some time that enzyme activity, muscle contraction, and many of the basic structural materials of man and animals (e.g., protein, collagen) depend on the presence of hydrogen-bonded water for their structure and activity, the potential importance of hydrogen bonding in pharmaceutical and therapeutic systems is just beginning to be realized. Certainly the solubility and compatibility of drugs in aqueous and hydroalcoholic systems should be influenced by hydrogen bonding since all of the physical and chemical properties of water are determined or influenced by the degree of association and bonding. Water at room temperature has been described as "one constantly changing, branched polymer."

Hydrogen bonding is a dipole-dipole interaction which requires the presence of special positive and negative groups in the same or adjacent molecules. One group serves as an acidic proton donor (e.g., the "positive" hydrogen in —COOH, —OH, etc.) while the other acts as a basic electron donor (e.g., the "negative" oxygen in —OH, —O—, etc.). Since water, alcohol, carboxylic acids, primary and secondary and tertiary amines, ketones, aldehydes, ethers, esters, olefins, and those halogenated compounds with sufficient halogens to activate the hydrogens are included here, it is obvious that hydrogen bonding is of great importance in pharmacy. It should perhaps be pointed out that hydrogen bonding takes place at the hydrogen already bonded to the proton donor, with the negative part of one molecule attracted to the positive portion of another. Thus, water molecules may form hydrogen bonds through either oxygen or hydrogen atoms since negatively polar oxygen may bond to the positively polar hydrogen of hydroxyl, amine, imine, etc., while the positively polar hydrogen may bond to negatively polar nitrogen or oxygen atoms of ketones, aldehydes, amides, amines, etc. This phenomenon may account for the excellent solvent action of water, alcohol, glycerin, or ethanolamine on many substances which contain

dipoles or charge-separation with hydrogen on the positive end. Such substances may interact with water; e.g.,

or

and cross-link as follows:

Intermolecular Hydrogen Bonding (Association)—Intermolecular hydrogen bonding by definition involves association of two or more bondable molecules. These may be the same compounds or different materials. Thus water in a hydro-alcoholic prescription may hydrogen-bond either to other water molecules or to the alcohol or even to the drugs present if these have either (or both) proton and electron-donor groups. The associations formed may be only dimeric linkages (e.g., acetic acid) or they may be enlarged to form rings, chains, or larger three-dimensional networks. The latter type associations commonly include enzymes, proteins, polypeptides, and inorganic hydroxide gels.

Intermolecular hydrogen-bonded compounds tend to have low solubility in compounds without proton or electron donor groups. Thus water is not very soluble in carbon tetrachloride or hexane. The intermolecular bonded substances may be more or less soluble in compounds with one or both types of reactive groups depending on whether the pressure for solute-solvent interaction is stronger than the mutual attraction already present. Thus water with both acidic (—OH) and basic (—O—) groups is miscible with methyl, ethyl, or isopropyl alcohols which also have these groups. It is not miscible with hexanol even though this higher alcohol has the required groups because the attraction of water for water is greater than it is for the hydrophobic six-carbon chain and the hexanol is literally "squeezed out" of solution. Molecular structure and the ratio of hydrophobic/hydrophilic groups are also a factor here as will be discussed later.

Unassociated substances which have the required acidic or basic groups usually dissolve in a solvent which can supply the opposite type. Thus chloroform ($CHCl_3$) with a hydrogen activated by the three halogen atoms is miscible with ethers, esters, ketones, aldehydes, and other solvents which have basic oxygen groups (—O—). This type of hydrogen bonding probably accounts for the tenfold greater water solubility of $CHCl_3$ (1:200) over that of CCl_4 (1:2000).

Intramolecular Hydrogen Bonding (Chelation)—Intramolecular hydrogen bonds are always found between appropriately reactive groups in the same molecule. This presupposes that the chain length, valence angles, lack of steric hindrance, and other structural features are suitable also. Salicylic acid, for example, is believed to form this type of hydrogen bond with itself by associating the —COOH and ortho —OH groups. Citric acid and *o*-nitroaniline may also bond in this way. Meta- and para-hydroxybenzoic acids on the other hand, are unable to form intramolecular rings due to their structural deficiencies, but they can and do form intermolecular bonds. Intramolecular bonded compounds or chelates are generally similar in solubility to nonbonded "normal" compounds since their reactivity has been largely self-satisfied (*cf,* water solubility of self-chelated salicylic acid (1:460) to that of *p*-hydroxybenzoic acid (1:125)).

Other Bonds—Other low-energy bonds (1–10 kcal/mole) may play a part in compatibility, solubility, etc. These include dipole-dipole interactions (orientation effect of Keesom force), dipole-induced dipole interactions (induction effect of Debye force), induced dipole-induced dipole interaction (dispersion effect or London force), ion-dipole interactions, and ion-induced dipole interactions. These interactions are believed associated with certain biological processes and drug actions as well as with the formation of some metal complexes and molecular addition compounds (e.g., the complexation of caffeine with esters such as benzocaine, tetracaine, and procaine, etc.), the solubility of certain drugs (e.g., alkaloidal bases in nonpolar solvents, ionic crystals in water, iodine in aqueous potassium iodide, etc.) and the condensation of gases. It should be noted that many of these interactions are so weak that the complexes, *et al,* cannot be isolated from their solutions as definite compounds, yet they may add sufficient stability to a system to permit dispensing. Further examples are cited elsewhere in this chapter.

Solubility Parameters

Solubility is probably most frequently thought of as the distribution of the molecules of a solid among those of a liquid. Actually more than 36 types of "solution" may occur if we consider these to be homogeneous mixtures of molecules producing a single observable phase. Thus we can have solutions of crystalline solids in liquids, gases, glasses, liquid crystals, rubbers, or other crystalline solids; liquids in crystalline solids, gases, glasses, liquid crystals, rubbers, or other liquids, etc. While the most common situations in dispensing probably involve solubility of solids or liquids in liquids, examples of the other types exist. Some products may contain three or more states in mutual solution, e.g., aerosols—gases, liquids, and solids; or ointments—solids, liquids, and liquid crystals.

Common Types of Liquids—Liquids can be broadly classified into three groups depending on their polarity and their ability to hydrogen bond:

1. *Nonpolar, Nonhydrogen-Bonding Liquids*—For example, benzene, carbon tetrachloride, heptane, hexane, mineral oil, mineral spirits, naphtha, toluene, turpentine, and xylene. These are usually miscible with other members of the group at ordinary temperatures.

2. *Medium Polar, Hydrogen-Bonding Liquids*—For example, alkyd resins, cellosolve, dioctyl phthalate, epoxy resins, polyglycols, polyester resins, and vegetable oils. These liquids are usually soluble in other members of the group but may separate on standing if the solubility limit is exceeded (e.g., Carbowax or Plurionics are soluble less than 1% in certain vegetable oils).

3. *Highly Polar, Hydrogen-Bonding Liquids*—For example, acetic acid, acetone, butanol, ethyl acetate, ethyl alcohol, ethylene glycol, glycerin, isopropyl alcohol, methyl alcohol, methyl ethyl ketone, methyl isobutyl ketone, propylene glycol, and water. These liquids are mutually miscible or at least adequately soluble for most pharmaceutical uses.

Polar—Nonpolar Structural Effects

Drugs are most likely to be soluble in these solvents which most resemble the drug (i.e., "like dissolves like"). Thus nonpolar drugs are most soluble in nonpolar solvents, and polar drugs are most soluble in polar solvents. Further, hydrocarbons are most likely to be miscible with other hydrocarbons, alcohols with other alcohols, ethers with other ethers, and so on; e.g., mineral oil, petrolatum and paraffin are soluble in deodorized kerosene, methyl alcohol is miscible with ethyl alcohol and many higher alcohols, and hydrochloric acid is miscible with acetic, sulfuric, and nitric acids.

Polar drugs or solvents have positive and negative centers which attract the negative and positive centers of other molecules, both ionic and polar. If sufficient attraction exists between solute and solvent, the charged centers interact and solution occurs. Hence water (HO^-H^+) dissolves both salt (Na^+Cl^-) and alcohol (RO^-H^+) by entering between the charged ions or molecules so that the charges are neutralized and the system stabilized.

Where there is little or no interaction, hydrogen bonding, intermolecular attraction, or similarity in structure, the solute and solvent molecules may be more attracted to their own kind than to the nonrelated molecules, and solubility will not occur. Nonpolar compounds are thus insoluble in, or poor solvents for, ionic and highly polar compounds. Hence, oils do not dissolve in, or dissolve, water or salts. Nonpolar solvents can, however, dissolve other nonpolar and slightly polar drugs, especially those which are structurally similar or not too highly associated; e.g., benzene dissolves phenol, aniline, ethanol, and methanol; also, ether is miscible with alcohols, chloroform, benzene, petroleum ether, and fixed and volatile oils. It should perhaps be noted that benzene can hydrogen bond to some extent due to pi electron activation.

Water, with a dielectric constant (ϵ value) of about 80, is considered to be highly polar (i.e., its molecules form strong dipoles with positive and negative centers). Glycerin and related polyhydroxy compounds, with ϵ values of about 56, fall between water and ethyl alcohol ($\epsilon = 26$) in polarity. Ethyl alcohol and similar monohydroxyl compounds have weaker dipoles and are considered semi-polar since they are miscible with some polar and some nonpolar compounds.

Normally, highly polar inorganic and organic salts, e.g., both ammonium chloride (NH_4Cl) and butylamine hydrochloride

$$(CH_3—CH_2—CH_2—CH_2—NH_2 \cdot HCl)$$

are increasingly soluble as the polarity of the solvent increases, and decrease in solubility as the polarity decreases. This may partially explain why water is a better solvent for these salts than is methyl alcohol ($\epsilon = 33$), while methyl alcohol is a better solvent than is peanut oil ($\epsilon = 3.0$). Typical ϵ values of common pharmaceuticals are given in Table 14.

Note that while a high dielectric constant is favorable it is not of itself suffi-

Table 14—Dielectric Constants
(ε Values) at 20°C[9]

Hydrogen cyanide	95.4
Water	80
Glycerin	43
Ethylene glycol	41
Methyl alcohol	33
Ethyl alcohol	25
Acetone	21
Paraldehyde	14.5
Benzyl alcohol	13
Methyl salicylate	9
Copper sulfate	7.8
Ammonium chloride	7.0
Calcium carbonate, sodium chloride	6.1
Chloroform	5.0
Castor oil	4.6
Ethyl ether	4.3
Phenol	4.3
Sulfur	4.0
Sucrose	3.3
Cocaine	3.1
Olive oil	3.1
Cottonseed oil	3.1
Peanut oil	3.0
Sesame oil	3.0
Acetanilid	2.9
Benzene	2.2
Turpentine oil	2.2
Mineral oil	2.1
Octane	1.9

cient for solubility of electrolytes and other highly ionized materials in polar solvents.

Hydrogen cyanide has an ε value of 95.4 and can form hydrogen bonds yet is still not as good a solvent for sodium chloride as is water in which ε = 80. The excellent solvent properties of water are probably due to a combination of factors, *viz:* dielectric constant, hydrogen bonding, and acid-base reaction.

While it is true that materials with low dielectric constants (i.e., nonpolar) are generally better solvents for other nonpolar materials, it is obvious that dielectric constants do not tell all of the solubility story for nonaqueous systems since highly hydroxylated sucrose (ε = 3.3) is not soluble in castor oil (ε = 4.6) or sesame oil (ε = 3.0). Ionized copper sulfate (ε = 7.8) is not soluble in nonionized chloroform (ε = 5.0) or methylsalicylate (ε = 9). However, nonionized cocaine (ε = 3.1) is soluble in nonionized olive oil (ε = 3.1), mineral oil (ε = 2.1), or sesame oil (ε = 3.0). Apparently then, ionization and hydrogen bonding play a very important part in the rather low solubility of hydroxylated or ionized compounds in nonpolar vehicles.

Polar–Nonpolar Ratios

Most organic drugs have both polar and nonpolar structures in the molecule. It may be expected that the solubility and other physical properties depend on the balance or ratios of these structures. By assigning arbitrary numerical values to various "organic" and "inorganic" structural groups and components, it appears that compounds with the same "organic/inorganic" ratio are indeed comparable in their physical properties. This proposal seems to merit further study and comment.

Nonionic drugs will usually not dissolve in water to any great extent unless they can form hydrogen bonds with the water molecules, while the water solubility of a polar organic drug, may also depend upon the relative proportions of polar "inorganic" hydrophilic groups (e.g., —OH, —NH$_2$, —SO$_3$Na) to nonpolar "organic" hydrophobic groups (e.g., CH$_3$—, C$_2$H$_5$—). The proportion of hydrophilic groups must be sufficient for the electronic attractiveness to break enough hydrogen bonds between water molecules to permit solubility. If too great a proportion of the molecule is hydrophobic, solubility will not occur. The usually accepted rule is that the drug will be soluble in water (≥3%) if there is at least one polar group to every four carbons in a normal chain, or to every five carbons in a branched chain. Actually, when there is more than one polar group present, the ratio drops to three and four carbons per hydrophilic group. This rule of thumb apparently applies to alcohols, aldehydes, ketones, acids, ethers, and esters. The tendency here for greater solubility of branched chain compounds should be noted (although in certain branched compounds steric hindrance may reduce solubility). Acid anhydrides and acyl halides are not very soluble as such in water, but they hydrolyze to form water soluble acids.

Highly basic amines are slightly more soluble in water. Here, the upper limit of water solubility is about six carbons to each polar group. This higher solubility is probably a function of both hydrogen bonding and ionization.

Less basic amides which do not ionize are less soluble since the three-carbon straight-chain compound propionamide ($CH_3CH_2CONH_2$) and the four-carbon branched-chain compound isobutyramide [$(CH_3)_2CHCONH_2$] represent the upper limit of water solubility. Unsubstituted amides (with the exception of these low molecular weight aliphatic compounds) probably have high melting points and low solubility in water because of the high degree of hydrogen bonding between the amine molecules themselves. These compounds can form tightly-bonded association complexes since the amide groups act as both acceptors and donors in forming hydrogen bonds. Substitution of alkyl groups for the acidic *N*-hydrogens interferes with the mutual attraction of the amines and permits interaction with water. For example, phthalamide has a solubility in water of 5.9 g/liter at 30°C, while the tetraalkylated *N,N,N',N'*-tetramethylphthalamide has a solubility of 710 g/liter.

phthalamide   *N, N, N', N'* -tetramethylphthalamide

Certain common substituents which increase the molecular weight such as phenyl (C_6H_5—) or a halogen (Cl—, Br—, F—, I—) apparently decrease water solubility unless they also increase the ionization of the compound. The phenyl group is roughly equivalent to four carbons in a chain as can be seen from a comparison of the water solubility of benzyl alcohol ($C_6H_5CH_2OH$) approx. 4% and *n*-amyl alcohol ($C_4H_9CH_2OH$) approx. 2% or, hydrocin-

namic acid ($C_6H_5CH_2CH_2COOH$) approx. 0.6% and *n*-heptanoic acid ($CH_3(CH_2)_5COOH$) approx. 0.24%.

When a halogen or other hydrophobic group is substituted for a hydrogen, the increase in molecular weight, together with the increase in hydrophobic properties, usually causes a decrease in water solubility; e.g.,

$$2CH_3CH_2CH_2OH \xrightarrow{Cl_2} 2ClCH_2CH_2CH_2OH$$

miscible   sol., 50 g/100 ml

or

soluble   soluble only 0.8%

On the other hand, if the hydrophobic group is substituted on the molecule so that the compound becomes a stronger acid, the increased ionization will increase water solubility since solvated anions have high solubility as previously noted.

$$2CH_3CH_2CH_2COOH \xrightarrow{Br_2}$$
sol., 5.62 g/100 ml

$$2CH_3CH_2CHBrCOOH$$
sol., 6.7 g/100 ml

Molecular Weight Effects—It has been pointed out that, in general, an increase in molecular weight leads to an increase in intermolecular forces in a solid. Thus, polymers and other compounds of very high molecular weight generally exhibit low solubility in both water (polar) and ether (nonpolar). Formaldehyde, for example, is readily soluble in water, but its polymer (paraformaldehyde) is insoluble. Glucose is soluble in water but its higher polymers (starch, glycogen, and cellulose) are insoluble. Many amino acids are soluble in water, but the proteins condensed from them are insoluble. Part of the decreased solubility here is probably due to the reduction in hydrogen bonding sites.

Table 15—Effect of Melting Point on Solubility

Compound	m.p. (°C)	Solubility (gm in 100 gm of solvent) Water	Benzene
meso-tartaric acid	140	125 (15° C)	...
d- or *l*-tartaric acid	170	139 (20° C)	...
dl-tartaric acid	206	20.6 (20° C)	...
m-dinitrobenzene	90	...	130 (50° C)
o-dinitrobenzene	116	...	47.5 (50° C)
p-dinitrobenzene	170	...	6.9 (50° C)

The tendency for some polymers like dextrins, starches, and proteins to form colloidal dispersions rather than true solutions should be noted. Methylcellulose and the polyethylene oxide derivatives, (e.g., polyethylene glycol 4000) are examples of high molecular weight materials which are readily soluble in water. Water appears able to separate the molecules of these compounds from each other, coordinate with them through hydrogen bonding of the oxygens of the polymer chains, and then dissolve the coordination complexes. In the case of methylcellulose, the coordination complex appears to be thermolabile since the compound will dissolve in cold water, but precipitate when heated.

Melting Point Effects—Generally, solids are less soluble than liquids of similar or closely related structures. This is probably because solids have stronger intermolecular cohesion than liquids. The melting point of a nonionic solid may be used as a rough guide in predicting solubility of a new drug from physical data available on older similar compounds since the melting point is generally a criterion of the forces holding the molecule together. Since heat is required to overcome these forces and change the solid to a liquid, usually the higher the melting point, the greater the intermolecular attraction and the less the solubility. Melting points are given for this reason in many of the drug monographs at the end of this chapter.

In the following prescription this theory suggests that the materials which form a eutectic mixture should be mixed so that the eutectic liquid forms, then this liquid should be dissolved in the vehicle.

38

℞	Menthol	0.3 g
	Camphor	0.3 g
	Mineral Oil q.s. ad.	30 ml

It has been noted that prescriptions containing various combinations of eutectic materials (e.g., chlorobutanol, menthol, campho phenol, eucalyptol, methyl salicylate, thymol, ephedrine, and chloral) will still show cloudiness when made by this procedure if any moisture or water of hydration is present in the ingredients.

The coincidence of high melting point and low solubility is illustrated by the *cis* and *trans* isomers, maleic and fumaric acids:

maleic acid (*cis*)   fumaric acid (*trans*)

Maleic acid melts at 130°C and is water soluble (78 g/100 g), while fumaric acid sublimes at 200°C and is insoluble in water (0.72 g/100 g).

Among *cis* and *trans* isomers, the *cis* form is usually the more water soluble. This may be related to a generalization that the more compact the structure, the greater the solubility, provided that comparisons are made of compounds of the same type.

Similar high solubility-low melting point relationships can be seen in the meso, active, and racemic tartaric acids and the meta, ortho, and para position isomers of the dinitrobenzenes (Table 15).

Presence of Other Substances

The solubility of a drug may also be dependent on the types and concentrations of other drugs and ions in the solution.

Solubility Product—If a prescription contains ions which may interact to form an insoluble salt, precipitation will occur when the solubility product of the salt is exceeded. Thus, in a prescription containing calcium chloride and sodium tartrate, insoluble calcium tartrate will separate if the molar concentrations of the calcium ion and tartrate ion multiplied together is greater than 0.77×10^{-6}, the solubility product.

Solubility products may also be used in other ways. Assuming the molar concentration of tartrate present in a prescription is $0.1 M$ ($= 10^{-1}$), then the calcium ion in the prescription cannot exceed $0.77 \times 10^{-5} M$ if a precipitate is to be avoided.

Further, if calcium tartrate is prescribed at its solubility limit in an aqueous prescription containing calcium ion, the calcium ion present will prevent the calcium tartrate from dissolving to its usual extent since the higher molarity of calcium ion will allow less tartrate ion to be present:

$$(Ca^{2+}) (Tartrate^{2-}) = 0.77 \times 10^{-6} =$$
$$(\text{more } Ca^{2+}) (\text{less } Tartrate^{2-})$$

For other type compounds, the solubility product assumes other forms:

$K_{sp} = (M^+)(A^-)$; where M^+ is a monovalent cation and A^- is a monovalent anion.

$K_{sp} = (M^{2+})(A^-)^2$; where M^{2+} is a divalent cation and A^- is a monovalent anion.

$K_{sp} = (M^+)^2(A^{2-})$; where M^+ is a monovalent cation and A^{2-} is a divalent anion.

Salting In—It is possible to effect some increase in the solubility of slightly soluble salts by the addition of a neutral salt without a common ion. This effect is due to an ionic strength increase and a decrease in the molecular "activity" of the ions. This explains why prescriptions containing a number of ingredients at their saturation point can still be compatible.

Salting Out—It should be noted that addition of a neutral salt may "salt in" some ingredients while simultaneously "salting out" others. While gases are most often liberated in this way, liquids and occasionally solids will sometimes separate when an added electrolyte (such as sodium chloride) or a nonelectrolyte (such as sucrose) attracts water molecules away from the ingredient which then separates.

Complex or Chelate Formation—Another method used to increase the solubility of sparingly soluble ionic substances is to complex the ions so that their ionic concentrations are lessened and the solubility product is not exceeded. Sodium, potassium, or ammonium citrates prevent the precipitation of iron and copper salts from neutral or alkaline solution. These likely act by forming chelate complexes with the metals so that the solubility products of their metallic hydroxides are not exceeded. This hydrogen-bonding technique may also apply to certain organic drugs since the solubility of drugs such as acetanilid, acetophenetidin, antipyrine, ethyl aminobenzoate, etc., is improved by sodium citrate.

Similar soluble complexes have also been reported as forming between caffeine and several aromatic amines.

On the other hand, less soluble complexes have been reported for caffeine and such drugs as sodium benzoate, sodium salicylate, sulfonamides, and barbiturates. These insoluble complexes are believed to be squeezed out of the aqueous phase due to the great internal pressure of water on the complexes which interact not only between the polarized carbonyl groups of caffeine and the hydrogen of the acid but also form secondary interactions between the nonpolar portions of the molecules. Similar hydrogen-bonded complexes between esters and amines, phenols, ethers and ketones have been studied, and insoluble complexes have been reported forming between polyethylene glycols and aromatic acids, phenols, phenobarbital, etc.; between polyvinylpyrrolidone and selected aromatic acids, sulfathiazole, phenobarbital, and chloramphenicol; and between sodium carboxy methylcellulose and quinine, procaine, tripelennamine, and diphenhydramine. Tetracycline and oxytetracycline have also been found to form complexes with sodium *p*-aminobenzoate, sodium salicylate, saccharin sodium, caffeine, and others.

Effect of pH on Organic Incompatibility

The absorption, excretion, metabolism, and action of drugs may be affected by the pH and pK_a of the medications into which they are compounded. These values play a role with the organic ingredients of a prescription. In addition to the possible liberation of insoluble free acids (e.g., sulfonamides or barbiturates), hydrogen ions may also:

1. Produce color changes in compounds having the proper chromophore groups (e.g., phenolphthalein).
2. Produce effervescence with organic carbonates, bicarbonates, nitrites, etc.
3. Promote hydrolysis of certain esters (e.g., acetylsalicylates).
4. Promote oxidation of compounds such as ascorbic acid.
5. Promote hydrogen ion catalyzed degradation of some antibiotics (e.g., penicillin G).

Hydroxyl ions, on the other hand, may liberate free bases (e.g., alkaloids, ammonia), produce color changes as with phenols and phenolphthalein or promote hydrolysis of lactones, esters, etc.

Whether or not the free acids and bases liberated in these reactions will form precipitates, "oils," etc., depends on their solubility in the total mixture at the final equilibrium pH value. Sometimes apparent incompatibilities are noted initially but disappear on agitation, dilution, or on standing. In such cases the reaction may be due to a temporary or local excess of hydrogen or hydroxyl ion.

Liberation of Acids

The addition of hydrogen ions (i.e., acids) to prescriptions containing salts of weak organic acids will usually liberate the free organic acid according to the following typical reactions:

Na salt of weak organic acid + $H^+ \rightarrow$
$$\text{free acid} + Na^+$$

Na sulfadiazine + HCl →
$$\text{sulfadiazine (free acid)} \downarrow + Na^+ + Cl^-$$

Na phenobarbital + HCl →
$$\text{phenobarbital (free acid)} \downarrow + Na^+ + Cl^-$$

Na novobiocin + HCl → novobiocin (free
$$\text{acid)} \downarrow + Na^+ + Cl^-$$

This type of reaction is noted with the alkali salts of many anionic type pharmaceuticals, e.g., acidic antibiotics, acid dyes, aromatic organic acids, barbiturates, synthetic detergents, synthetic acidic gums, acidic mercurial antiseptics, soaps, soluble penicillins, etc.

These reactions may occur either when solutions of low pH or ingredients with pK_a values sufficiently below 7 are added to susceptible ingredients. Here the quantity of free acid liberated must of course exceed the amount soluble in the vehicle, e.g., novobiocin free acid usually precipitates from novobiocin solutions as the pH of the final mixture falls below pH 6.8 since the solubility of the free acid is only 0.05 mg/ml in water.

In some cases an undissociated acid precipitate may form even when the pH value of the mixture is quite alkaline. Thus, if sodium pentothal solution (pH about 10.5) is lowered to pH 9.8 by the addition of dilute acids, buffer salts, or other prescription items yielding sufficient hydrogen ions, a precipitate of pentothal free acid develops. Similar reactions occur with solutions of sodium sulfonamides, which may even precipitate the free sulfonamide above pH 7.

Liberation of Bases

In prescriptions containing a water-soluble salt of an organic base, the addition of sufficient hydroxyl ion will neutralize the acid portion of the salt and liberate the organic base. This may occur according to the following typical reactions:

amine HCl + OH⁻ → free amine +
$$Cl^- + H_2O$$

phenacaine HCl + NaOH → phenacaine
(free base) ↓ + Na⁺ + Cl⁻ + H₂O

If the amine free base is sufficiently insoluble an incompatibility results.

Any ingredient having a pH or pK_a greater than 7, or which hydrolyzes to form hydroxyl ions, may act to liberate part or all of the free amine. Thus, a knowledge of typical pH values of common drug ingredients is valuable. The pharmacist will do well to memorize the approximate pH or pK_a values of various drug types or keep appropriate reference works at hand. Table 16 gives approximate values for many drug types. More exact values are given throughout these chapters.

Precipitation by hydroxyl ion is a property of many cationic type pharmaceuticals. These include many water soluble acid salts of alkaloids, alkaloid-like bases, amphetamine, basic antibiotics, basic antihistamines, antimalarials, basic dyes, epinephrine-like compounds, basic tranquilizing drugs, basic vitamins, basic narcotics, basic water soluble local anesthetics, and other high molecular weight basic compounds. Such precipitation by hydroxyl ion may or may not occur in the presence of citrates, tartrates, acetates, or other compounds which can form soluble chelates or hydrogen-bonded complexes. Precipitation by hydroxyl ion does not occur with quaternary ammonium compounds.

It has been noted that prescription mixtures containing combinations of salts of weak acids and salts of weak bases should be assumed to be incompatible until tested. It was found that precipitates slowly form in sodium phenobarbital solutions containing calcium chloride, magnesium sulfate, Benadryl Hydrochloride, or codeine phosphate at pH values above that required for precipitation of the free phenobarbital. Likewise, sodium sulfathiazole solutions similarly form precipitates with calcium chloride or magnesium sulfate.

Calcium and magnesium salts may form poorly absorbed calcium or magnesium tetracyclines when these ions are present with tetracycline hydrochloride.

It has been reported that precipitates were also formed in prescriptions containing Benadryl or codeine phosphate when approximately equimolar quantities of potassium iodide were added. The latter has been confirmed since it has been found that codeine phosphate, dihydrocodeinone bitartrate, Cheracol (*Upjohn*), or Mercodal (*Merrell-National*) formed precipitates with potassium iodide or hydrogen iodide if the proper concentrations were mixed.

Many of these problems can be minimized by mixing likely reactants in as dilute a form as possible or by adding pH adjusting ingredients or 10–20% alcohol.

Ionization and pK_a Values

Organic compounds containing an ionizable group show a great variation in solubility with pH and solvent system. In general, the salt of a carboxylic acid or the salt of an amine will be quite soluble in water but less soluble in alcohol or hydroalcoholic vehicles. The free acid or amine on the other hand, has the opposite solubility, so these are usually insoluble in water and more soluble in alcohol or aqueous alcohol.

Generally, a drug will be soluble in water if it can form hydrogen bonds, if it is ionic, or if it can be converted into ions by an acid-base reaction (Brönsted type included). Since the water molecule is both a Brönsted acid and a base, it can ionize many acids by accepting a proton from the acid, e.g., R—COOH + H₂O → R—COO⁻ + H₃O⁺. The carboxyl ion (R—COO⁻) then may form hydrogen bonds with water (+H—OH⁻). Water may also ionize an amine by donating a proton to the amine:

$$R—NH_2 + HOH \rightleftharpoons RNH_3^+ + OH^-$$

The negative oxygen anion and the pos-

Table 16—Approximate pKₐ Values for Common Drug Types

Acids[a] (pKₐ)			Ampholytes[b]
Strong (−2–+2)	Intermediate (2–7)	Weak (7–12)	
Acid anhydrides	Acid anhydrides	Alkyl formates	Amino acids
Dicarboxylic acids	β-Keto lactones	α-Hydroxy aldehydes	Amino phenols
Acid halides	Carboxylic acids	and ketones	Aromatic aminosul-
Nitro acids	Cyclic β-diketones	α-Keto aldehydes	fonamides
Polynitro phenols	Esters (easily hydro-	β-Diketones	Primary salts of di-
Alkyl acid sulfates	lyzed)	β-Keto esters	amines, dibasic
Bisulfates of bases	Phenolic aldehydes,	Cyclic-diketones	acids, dihydric
Sulfate salts of weak	ketones, and esters	Esters of phenols and	phenols, and phe-
bases	Triacyl methanes	weak acids	nolic acids
Sulfonic acids	α-Chloro esters	Phenols	Sulfadiazines
Sulfonamides	Halogen-acids	Quinones	
Sulfonimides	Polyhalophenols	Acylamino phenols	
Sulfonyl halides	Salts of weak bases	Aliphatic hydrox-	
	Nitramines	amic acids	
	Nitro- and cyano-	Amides	
	phenols	Imides	
	Nitrogenous acids	Oximes (except ali-	
	Ureides	phatic ketoximes)	
	Dialkyl sulfates	Pri- and sec-Nitro	
	Thiophenols	compounds	
	Aromatic aminosul-	Salts of intermediate	
	fonic acids	bases or ampho-	
	Sulfonamides	lytes	
	Sulfonhalides	Ureides	
		Thiols (mercaptans)	
		Aliphatic amino sul-	
		fonic acids	
		Aryl isothiocyanates	
		Aryl thioureas	
		Salts of intermediate	
		bases of ampho-	
		lytes	
		Sulfonamides	
		Thioamides	
		Thioureides	

itive hydrogen cation, i.e., RNH_3^+, formed in these reactions can then form hydrogen bonds with water (H^+OH^-) as previously discussed. These equations explain why some water solutions of drugs are acid in reaction and some are alkaline, i.e., note the free hydronium ion H_3O^+ (which is equivalent to H^+ plus H_2O) or hydroxyl ions (OH^-) liberated.

Water insoluble acids and bases are similarly converted into soluble ions which hydrogen bond with strong bases and acids, respectively; e.g., NaOH and HCl may react:

$$C_6H_5COOH + NaOH \rightarrow C_6H_5COO^- +$$

benzoic acid   benzoate ion

$$Na^+ + H_2O$$

whereas

$$C_{17}H_{23}NO_3 + HCl \rightarrow C_{17}H_{23}NO_3H^+ +$$

atropine   atropinium ion

$$Cl^- + H_2O$$

Here, the stronger the acid, the weaker may be the base required to react and dissolve it. Thus, bicarbonates (pKₐ 6.36) will solubilize acids with pKₐ values of 1–5 (e.g., some carboxylic, sulfonic, and sulfinic acids and acid halides) but will not dissolve weaker acids such as phenol with pKₐ values of about 9. For example:

$$phenol (pK_a\ 9.95) + NaHCO_3 \rightleftharpoons$$
$$undissolved\ phenol + Na^+ + HCO_3^-$$

whereas

$$HCOOH (pK_a\ 3.77) + NaHCO_3 \rightleftharpoons$$
$$HCOO^- + Na^+ + H_2O + CO_2$$

Also, the weaker the acid, the stronger must be the base that is required. Hence, sodium hydroxide (pKₐ 12–16) is required to solubilize weak acids with pKₐ values >9.

Table 16—*Continued*

Weak (2–7)	Bases[d] (pK_a) Intermediate (7–12)	Strong (12–16)	Neutrals[c,d]	
Aliphatic ketoximes	Aliphatic amines (*pri-, sec-, tert-*)	Alkyl guanidines	Acetals	Alkyl nitrates and nitrites
α-Oxides		Quaternary ammonium compounds	Alcohols	Amides .
Aryl alkyl amines	Aliphatic hydrazines		Aldehydes	Azo, azoxy, and hydrazo compounds
Aryl dialkyl amines	Amidines		Alkyl esters (not of phenols)	Di- and triaryl amines
Aryl hydrazines	Aryl Guanidines		Carbohydrates	Hydrazones
Azomethines	Imidazoles		Ethers (not diaryl	Nitriles
Betaines	Salts of Weak Acids and Ampholytes		Ketones	Nitro and nitroso compounds
Heterocyclic amines (benzenoid)			Lactones	Polyhalogenated aromatic amines
Primary aryl amines			Aryl alkyl ethers (a few)	Guanidinium and quatenary ammonium salts of strong acids
Salts of intermediate acids or ampholytes			Diaryl ethers	Ureas and urethanes
			Furanes	Alkyl sulfites and sulfates
			Halogenated hydrocarbons	Aryl sulfonates
			Triaryl methanols	Salts of alkyl sulfates and sulfonic acids

Neutrals continued:
- Sulfides and disulfides
- Sulfoxides and sulfones
- Thio Esters
- Thiophenes
- Alkyl isothiocyanates
- Alkyl thioureas
- *N,N*-Dialkyl sulfonamides
- Guanidinium and quaternary ammonium sulfates
- Thiocyanates
- Phosphates
- Phosphites

Important Equations

$$K_a = \frac{[H^+][A^-]}{[HA]}$$

$$K_b = \frac{[NH_4^+][OH^-]}{[NH_3]}$$

$$pK_a = \log \frac{1}{K_a}$$

$$pK_b = \log \frac{1}{K_b}$$

$$pH = \log \frac{1}{[H^+]}$$

$$pOH = \log \frac{1}{[OH^+]}$$

$$pK_a + pK_b = pK_w = 14$$

[a] Halogens may occur as extra elements in all divisions. The listing of a class in a division does not imply that all homologs of that class will necessarily fall in that division. The word "salt" in these tables refers to compounds of amines with acids.

[b] Ampholytes contain both acidic and basic groups (weak to intermediate types).

[c] Neutral to indicators. Usually contain both feeble acidic and basic groups.

[d] Halogens may be present as substituents.

Naturally, sodium hydroxide and other strong bases will react with both strong and weak acids.

The reverse is also true, and strong bases will be solubilized by either weak or strong acids. Both insoluble weak bases with $pK_a > 8$ or stronger bases with a pK_a of 12–16 will be solubilized by acids with pK_a values of −2–+8.

Many amphoteric compounds such as amino acids, amino phenols, amino thiols, and the oximes of low molecular weight ketones are water-soluble. However, even those members which are not water-soluble, will usually dissolve in both acids and bases since they possess both acid (—COOH), phenolic (—OH,

—SH, —NOH) groups and basic (—NH$_2$ —NH) groups which can react with bases and acids.

The dissociation constant, K$_a$, of any compound, HA, that give up a proton or a hydrogen ion (i.e., HA $\leftrightarrows$ H$^+$ + A$^-$) can be defined by the expression: K$_a$ = (H$^+$) (A$^-$)/(HA). K$_a$ is thus the fraction of the compound present in the ionized form.

This applies either to acids or bases as previously discussed. Then

$$pK_a = -\log K_a = -\log 10^{-pK_a}$$

just as the

$$pH = -\log (H^+) = -\log 10^{-pH}$$

From these relations, the higher the degree of dissociation of the acid HA, the stronger the acid and the higher the K$_a$, but the lower the pK$_a$. Most carboxylic acids and aromatic amines have pK$_a$ values in the range 3–6; most aliphatic amines and phenols have pK$_a$ values in the range 8–11. Typical pK$_a$ values are given throughout this chapter where data are available (Table 16).

A simplified approach to calculating solubility as a function of pH is to assume the solubility of the nonionized molecule to be independent of pH, if this is constant (i.e., in buffered solutions). The solubility of the ionized molecule can then be considered as infinite for simplified calculation purposes (although it actually has a finite solubility). The approximate solubility at any desired pH value can then be estimated using the Henderson-Hasselbach equation from the pH and from a knowledge of the pK$_a$ and the known solubility in water of the un-ionized molecule. In the case of a carboxylic acid the expression is:

$$pK_a = pH + \log \frac{(HA)}{C - (HA)}$$

where C represents the apparent solubility of ionized material and (HA) is the intrinsic molar solubility at high acidities where no salt (A$^-$) is assumed to be present.

Most acidic drugs may be estimated adequately using the simplified form:

$$pK_a = pH +$$
$$\log \frac{\text{molar conc. of un-ionized acid}}{\text{molar solubility}}$$

To find the solubility of aspirin at pH 4 and 26°C, substitute the appropriate values in the previous formula: e.g., aspirin (HA) has a solubility of 1.89 × 10^{-2} moles/liter at pH 1.0. The pK$_a$ is 3.62 at 25.6°C. Substituting these values in the previous expression, we have 3.62 = 4.0 + log (1.89 × 10^{-2}) whence C = 11.6 g/liter. This equation can be rearranged to estimate the pH below which a weak free acid (e.g., barbiturates, sulfonamides) will begin to precipitate from aqueous solutions of the soluble salt, i.e.,

$$pH = pK_a + \log \frac{\text{molar concentration of salt}}{\text{molar solubility of acid}}$$

Thus, to determine the pH at which phenobarbital (pK$_a$ 7.4) will precipitate from an acidified 10% solution of the sodium salt, calculate:

1. The molar concentration of the salt by dividing the weight of the salt in 1 liter by the molecular weight (254.22), i.e., 100/254.22 = 0.393 (since 10% = 100 g/liter).
2. The molar solubility of the acid by dividing the solubility in mg/ml or g/liter by the molecular weight, i.e., 1.0/232.22 = 0.0043 (since phenobarbital is soluble 1 g/liter and the molecular weight is 232.22). Then:

$$pH = 7.4 + \log \frac{(0.393)}{(0.0043)} =$$
$$7.4 + \log (90.4) = 7.4 + 1.96 = 9.36$$

and the pH of the solution would have to be greater than about pH 9.4 to avoid precipitation.

Similarly, the pH mentioned previously at which a weak base (alkaloids, antihistamines) will begin to precipitate from aqueous solution can be estimated from the equation:

$$pH = pK_a +$$
$$\log \frac{\text{molar solubility of free base}}{\text{molar concentration of the salt}}$$

These equations give only very rough approximations if solvents other than water are present in the prescription since the strength of an acid or base varies with the solvent. Combinations of solvents then may greatly affect the pK values in an unpredictable fashion.

Table 17—Effect of Solvent on the Dissociation Constant of Acids and Bases[10]

	pK_a (25°C) in water	pK_a' (25°C) in 50% ethanol
Benzoic acid	4.20	5.73
Phenol	9.95	11.28
Pyridine	5.17	4.38
Aniline	5.01	3.92
Methylamine	10.70	9.80

This is illustrated in Table 17 which gives the pK_a values in water and in 50% alcohol for several compounds.

When the pK_a values are not known but the pK_b values are available, the pK_a can be approximated from the equation $pK_a = pK_w - pK_b = 14 - pK_b$ (for aqueous solutions at 25°C). Conversely, pK_b values can be calculated when the pK_a values are known, e.g., $pK_b = 14 - pK_a$.

The pK_a can also be estimated in most cases as the pH value observed when the acid is half neutralized since $pK_a = pH + \log (HA)/(A^-)$. When half of the acid is neutralized to salt, the $(HA) = (A^-)$ and $pH = pK_a$. The pK_a value is also the pH value of maximum buffer capacity since buffer systems require the presence of a slightly dissociated acid or base and its salt. Maximum buffer capacity occurs when these are present in equal amounts.

A rough approximation of the pH value of a salt can be made using the calculations in Table 18. Similarly, the pH of a solution of a weak base or weak acid can be calculated from pK values:

Solution of weak acid:

$pH = \frac{1}{2} pK_a - \frac{1}{2} \log C$ (where C = molar concentration)

Solution of a weak base:

$pH = pK_w - \frac{1}{2} pK_b + \frac{1}{2} \log C$ or $pH = 14 - \frac{1}{2} pK_b + \log C$ (where pK_w (25°C) = 14)

pK values and molecular weights are given liberally throughout this chapter to facilitate these calculations. The pK_a is also a measure of the free energy of the dissolution reaction:

$$HA + S \rightarrow HS^+ + A^-$$

where S = solvent, and HA = acid; e.g.,

$$HAc + H_2O \rightleftarrows H_3O^+ + Ac^-$$

A substituent which favors formation of the dissociated ion over the undissociated acid or base will increase ionization (i.e., lower the pK_a). One which favors formation of the undissociated acid or base will cause a decrease in ionization (i.e., raise the pK_a).

As may be noted in Table 19, the introduction of a methylene group in formic acid (pK_a 3.77) to produce acetic acid (pK_a 4.76) brings about a marked decrease in acid strength (i.e., $\Delta pK = 1$, a 10-fold decrease). A further increase in length of the chain or branching of the chain has relatively little effect upon the pK_a and most of the fatty acids have pK_a values around 4.8, as may be seen from Table 19.

Similarly, the introduction of the first methyl group into the ammonia molecule (pK_a 9.25) to form methylamine (pK_a 10.64) results in a consider-

Table 18—Calculation of Approximate pH Value of a Salt[a]

Type of salt	Calculation	Approximate pH value
Salt of strong acid (pK_a −2−+2) and strong base (pK_b −2−+2), e.g., NaCl	$pH = pOH = \frac{1}{2}pK_w$	7 ($\approx$6 if CO_2 is present)
Salt of strong acid (pK_a −2−+2) and weak base (pK_b 3−8), e.g., atropine sulfate	$pH = \frac{1}{2}pK_w - \frac{1}{2}pK_b - \frac{1}{2} \log c$	3−5.5
Salt of weak acid (pK_a 3−8) and strong base (pK_b −2−+2), e.g., sodium barbital	$pH = \frac{1}{2}pK_w = \frac{1}{2}pK_a + \frac{1}{2} \log c$	8.5−11
Salt of weak acid and weak base, e.g., chlorpheniramine maleate	$pH = \frac{1}{2}pK_w + \frac{1}{2}pK_a - \frac{1}{2}pK_b$	4.5−9.5

[a] Adapted from Ref. 11.

Table 19—pK$_a$ Values for Acids and Bases Containing Strongly Polar Substituents

X=	—H	—NH$_3^+$	—CO$_2^-$	—SO$_2^-$	—CO$_2$H	—NH$_2$
		Aliphatic compounds				
X—COOH	3.77	. . .	4.19	. . .	1.23	. . .
X—CH$_2$—COOH	4.76	2.31	5.69	4.05	2.83	. . .
X—(CH$_2$)$_2$COOH	4.88	3.60	5.48	. . .	4.19	. . .
X—(CH$_2$)$_3$COOH	4.92	4.23	5.42	. . .	4.34	. . .
X—(CH$_2$)$_4$COOH	4.86	4.27	5.41	. . .	4.42	. . .
X—NH$_3^+$	9.25	0.88	. . .	~1	. . .	8.12
X—(CH$_2$)NH$_3^+$	10.64	. . .	9.77	5.75	. . .	. . .
X—(CH$_2$)$_2$NH$_3^+$	10.67	6.97	10.19	9.20	. . .	9.98
X—(CH$_2$)$_3$NH$_3^+$	10.58	8.59	10.43	10.05	. . .	10.65
X—(CH$_2$)$_4$NH$_3^+$	10.61	9.31	10.77	10.65	. . .	10.84
		Aromatic compounds				
o-X—C$_6$H$_4$COOH	4.20	. . .	5.41	. . .	. . .	. . .
m-X—C$_6$H$_4$COOH	4.20	. . .	4.60	4.15	. . .	. . .
p-X—C$_6$H$_4$COOH	4.20	. . .	4.82	4.11	. . .	. . .
o-X—C$_6$H$_4$NH$_3^+$	4.58	1.3	. . .	. . .	. . .	. . .
m-X—C$_6$H$_4$NH$_3^+$	4.58	2.65	. . .	3.80	. . .	. . .
p-X—C$_6$H$_4$NH$_3^+$	4.58	3.29	. . .	3.32	. . .	. . .
o-X—C$_6$H$_4$OH	9.95	. . .	. . .	. . .	. . .	. . .
m-X—C$_6$H$_4$OH	9.95	. . .	9.94	9.29	. . .	. . .
p-X—C$_6$H$_4$OH	9.95	. . .	9.35	8.95	. . .	. . .

able increase in the strength of the base (i.e., ΔpK = 1.4, a 25-fold increase) but further lengthening of the chain or branching does not significantly affect the pK$_a$ values since these generally agree within 0.1 pK$_a$ value (Table 19).

Table 19 also shows the effect of other common substituents on the pK$_a$ of aliphatic and aromatic acids and amines and indicates the somewhat varied effect which the addition of substituents may have.

Table 20 gives the pK$_a$ values of acetic acid and substituted acetic acids. This table may be helpful as a rough guide to the way substituents may affect the pK$_a$ of an acid. It should be noted that the greater the distance between the parent group and the substituent group, the less will be the effect on the pK$_a$. This is also illustrated in Table 19 by the small changes in pK$_a$ of the dicarboxylic acids as the chain length increases between carboxyl groups.

Dibasic acids and amino acids are usually described by two pK$_a$ values which might seem to imply ionization occurs in two sharply distinct steps. Such may be the case if the pK$_a$ values are farther than 4 pH units apart; e.g., simple amino acids such as glycine

where pK$_{a1}$ = 2.35 (—COO$^-$) and pK$_{a2}$ = 9.78 (—NH$_3^+$). When the values are closer than 4, there is some overlapping of the two stages (i.e., succinic acid where pK$_{a1}$ = 4.2 and pK$_{a2}$ = 5.63).

Polar but uncharged groups adjoining the ionizing group have a very marked effect on the pK$_a$ values. Table 20 demonstrates that chloroacetic acid (pK$_a$ = 2.86) is nearly 100 times as strong an acid as acetic (pK$_a$ = 4.76 whence ΔpK$_a$ = 1.9). Hydroxyacetic acid (pK$_a$ = 3.83) is about ten times acetic acid (ΔpH = 0.93).

There is a general parallelism between the dipole moment of the substituent group and the ΔpK$_a$ value (Table 20). There is also general qualitative agreement with the generally expected order of decreasing electronegativities of common substituent groups. Table 20 may thus be used to explain or predict the physical and chemical properties of molecules as described by Ferguson.

Note that phenols have pK$_a$ values near 10; however the introduction of an ortho carboxyl group gives the pK$_{a2}$ value of 13.4 for salicylic acid (ΔpK$_a$ = 3.4). This unusual value is probably due to intramolecular hydrogen bonding be-

Table 20—Effect on pK_a When Various Groups (R) Are Substituted
on Acetic Acid (R—CH$_2$COOH)

R	Observed pK_a	ΔpK_a*	Dipole moment of R—CH$_3$
O$_2$N	1.68	−3.08	3.0−3.8
(CH$_3$)$_3$N$^+$	1.83	−2.93	. . .
(CH$_3$)$_2$NH$^+$	1.95	−2.81	. . .
CH$_3$NH$_2$$^+$	2.16	−2.60	. . .
NH$_3$$^+$	2.31	−2.45	. . .
CH$_3$SO$_2$	2.36	−2.40	. . .
N≡C	2.43	−2.33	3.1−3.5
C$_6$H$_5$SO$_2$	2.44	−2.32	. . .
HOOC	2.83	−1.93	1.7
C$_6$H$_5$SO	2.66	−2.10	. . .
F	2.66	−2.10	. . .
Cl	2.86	−1.90	1.8−1.9
Br	2.86	−1.90	1.8
H—O—N≡	3.01	−1.75	. . .
I	3.12	−1.64	1.6
C$_6$H$_5$—O	3.12	−1.64	. . .
C$_2$H$_5$—$\overset{\text{O}}{\overset{\|}{\text{C}}}$—O	3.35	−1.41	1.7
C$_6$H$_5$—S	3.52	−1.24	. . .
CH$_3$—O	3.53	−1.23	. . .
N≡C—S	3.58	−1.18	. . .
CH$_3$—C≡O	3.58	−1.18	. . .
C$_2$H$_5$—O	3.60	−1.16	. . .
n-C$_3$H$_7$—O	3.65	−1.11	. . .
n-C$_4$H$_9$—O	3.66	−1.10	. . .
sec-C$_4$H$_9$O	3.67	−1.09	. . .
HS	3.67	−1.09	1.39
C$_3$H$_7$O	3.69	−1.07	. . .
CH$_3$—S	3.72	−1.04	. . .
C$_6$H$_5$CH$_2$—S	3.73	−1.03	. . .
C$_2$H$_5$—S	3.74	−1.02	. . .
HO	3.83	−0.93	1.65
—O$_3$S	4.05	−0.71	. . .
C$_6$H$_5$	4.31	−0.45	0.39
CH$_2$=CH	4.35	−0.41	0.34
H (Acetic Acid)	4.76	. . .	. . .
C$_2$H$_5$	4.82	+0.06	. . .
CH$_3$	4.88	+0.12	0.00
C$_4$H$_9$	4.88	+0.12	. . .
—O$_2$Se	5.43	+0.67	. . .
—OOC	5.69	+0.93	. . .

* ΔpK_a indicates here change in pK_a from that found for acetic acid (4.76).

tween the positive acidic hydrogen (—OH) and the negative charge on the neighboring ortho carboxyl ion (—COO$^-$). The meta and para hydroxybenzoic acids which can form intermolecular hydrogen bonds have pK_a values near phenol.

The exact effect of other substituents becomes quite complex due to the effect of hydrogen bonding, resonance, etc.

The not always predictable chemical equilibria illustrated in the previous pK_a tables has indicated that the equilibria, heats, and rates of individual reactions are not identical for members of the same chemical class, and the variations may be so great that a general class reaction may not hold for every member. Thus, the chemical reactions of a compound are not always exactly predictable by analogy from those of structurally related compounds. In dealing with most incompatibilities, however, we do not have to predict a chemical reaction "exactly" in order to be able to correct it; hence, "rules of thumb" are often used which do not always hold but will usually hold the great majority of the time. The chances of predicting compatibility or incompatibility are greatly increased when it has been established empirically that a relationship between structure and properties exists and that the structural modifications involved are not outside the range in which the relationship holds.

Therapeutic pH Considerations

One of the most important pH effects in prescriptions is the manner in which it may affect therapeutic activity and the response to drugs. The long duration of the oral muscle relaxant zoxazolamine has been ascribed to the precipitation of the drug in the gastrointestinal tract where it was then slowly absorbed over a period of many hours. Drugs which are unstable in gastric juice (e.g., benzylpenicillin) do not give this effect and buffers are sometimes necessary to give satisfactory blood levels.

It is also recognized that the optimum pH for stability is not always the optimum pH for pharmacological activity. It has been shown, for example, that several local anesthetics are more stable at an acid pH (*ca* pH 5) but for maximum activity they should be neutral or slightly alkaline. It has been pointed out that alkaloids applied to the eye are absorbed through the cornea as the free base. Unfortunately, such bases are frequently irritating and are not very stable. Isotonic buffered vehicles have been developed which satisfactorily compromise activity, irritation, and stability. Several drugs (e.g., atropine, scopolamine, and dibucaine) have been found more stable in solutions adjusted to the optimum pH with hydrochloric acid than when buffers are used. The pharmacist will have to consider all of the factors involved in such cases and

work out the best compromise. Several additional points should perhaps be emphasized. Apparently, all tissues of the body will accept products whose pH has been adjusted to approximately that of the blood (pH 7.4). Certain products may work best at higher or lower values, however. Nose drops, for example, have been suggested as being most physiological at pH 5.5–6.5 for adults and 5–6.7 for children since in this range the normal cilia beat is not interrupted, and lysozyme is most active.

It has been pointed out that death will occur if the pH of the blood varies outside the range 7–7.8, thus caution is necessary in preparing injectables (especially the intravenous type) to see that they are not strongly buffered outside this range. Intravenous injections are commonly made with products ranging in pH from 3.5–11 but they are weakly buffered (if at all), usually added to large volumes of infusion, and given so slowly the blood buffer system is able to neutralize them to pH 7.4.

Some intramuscular injectables of about pH 3–4 are injected into the deep gluteal muscle or other muscles where pain is less intense. Even so, these low pH values are quite irritating to the tissues, and some tissue degeneration should be expected.

Since the pharmacist may have no way of determining the pH value of his prescriptions, typical pH values of many drugs are included in these chapters. It will be safe to assume that if none of the ingredients prescribed fall in the irritating range, the finished prescription pH will be acceptable. If no buffer substances are present in the prescription, the pH value will usually fall near the proportional average of the pH values for the individual ingredients. Thus, in a prescription calling for two parts of A and one part of B, the pH value of the mixture can be roughly approximated by adding twice the pH of A to that of B and dividing by 3. Strongly buffered solutions may be assumed to take on the pH value of the buffer used; e.g., collyria dispensed in a phosphate buffer of pH 6.8 will usually measure about 6.8. In some cases the addition of appropriate buffers or the use of a less acid or less alkaline material is indicated to avoid irritation, promote activity, etc. The pharmacist should be encouraged to use pH test papers or a pH meter as a guide to therapeutic incompatibilities whenever possible.

Factors Affecting Chemical Reactions

The prediction of incompatibilities by general class reactions has been proposed as a solution to the problem of keeping up with the incompatibilities of new drugs. This approach will be stressed in this chapter, although actual compatibility data are presented where available. It can be assumed that a drug containing a number of active groups will probably be subject to the reactions of each group independent of the other groups present, unless the reactivity of the group is modified by the electron charge distribution, steric hindrance, etc. of the molecule (*cf* reactions of alcohols and phenols), and provided the groups are not so close together that they interfere with each other. In some cases the latter does occur; e.g., when hydroxyl (—OH) and carbonyl (—C=O) form carboxyl (—COOH) groups.

The more important reactions which a class of organic drugs may undergo in prescriptions will be discussed under the appropriate drug class; e.g., hydrocarbons, alcohols, acids, etc. A general chart showing the reactivity of these classes is given in Table 2 (page 336). This chart considers the reactions which would be likely to occur at room temperature in aqueous solutions in a matter of several weeks' time. Since it is almost impossible to make such generalizations that are wholly valid, this chart should be considered as a first approximation useful in eliminating certain reactions from consideration. A number of possible chemical classes which are heterocyclic or polyfunctional are not directly covered in this discussion or the following tables but may be adequately predicted in most cases by considering the reactions of the separate active functional groups. Such compounds are occasionally discussed under the most active of the functional groups or in some cases in special sections. These include: acetals (*cf,* esters, ethers); amidines (*cf,* amides, guanidines); amino alcohols (*cf,* amines, alcohols); amino ethers (*cf,* amines, ethers); amino ketones (*cf,* amines, ketones); enols (*cf,* ketones, phenols, quinones); guanidines (*cf,* amides, amidines); lactones (*cf,* acids, alcohols, ketones); metal containing compounds (*cf,* inorganic incompatibilities); pyrones (*cf,* ethers, ketones, lactones); quinones (*cf,* ketones, phenols); semicarbazides, semicarbazones, thiosemicarbazones, stilbenes (*cf,* amidines, phenols); sulfonamides (*cf,* amides, amines, sulfones); sulfones (*cf,* amines, sulfonamides); thioamides, thioureas (*cf,* thiosemicarbazones, ureides); ureas, ureides (*cf,* amides, amines, thioureas) and urethanes or carbamates (*cf,* amides, amines).

A second chart, Table 3 (page 337) considers the effect of the various organic classes (e.g., hydrocarbons, alcohols, etc.) on other classes. This chart also considers only those reactions that would be likely to occur at room temperature in aqueous or low hydroalcoholic solutions in several weeks' time if the class of compound at the top of the chart were combined with the class given at the side. If more than two classes of compounds are present in the prescription, or more than two types of reactive groups are present in a molecule, it will be necessary to check each one individually against the other types present. If any are incompatible, the total mixture will probably be incompatible. It should be recognized that conditions usually present in a prescription are usually not ideal for many of the reactions learned in organic chemistry. For example, an aqueous type pre-

Table 21—Ionic Type Classification of Organic Pharmaceuticals

Cationic (+)	Anionic (−)	Nonionic (0)
Alkaloids (e.g., atropine sulfate)	Acid dyes (e.g., fluorescein sodium, amaranth)	Benzocaine
Alkaloid-like bases (e.g., chloroguanide HCl)	Aromatic organic acids (e.g., sodium Salicylate)(Sodium p-amino salicylate)	Benzyl benzoate
Amphetamines (e.g., amphetamine sulfate)	Barbiturates (e.g., secobarbital sodium)	Carbowaxes
Antibiotics, basic (e.g., erythromycin HCl)	Detergents, synthetic (e.g., sodium lauryl sulfate)	Glycerol monostearate
Antihistamines, basic (e.g., diphenhydramine HCl)	Gums, synthetic acidic (e.g., sodium CMC, sodium alginate)	Methylcellulose
Antimalarials (e.g., quinacrine HCl)	Mercurial antiseptics, acidic (e.g., thimerosal)	Parabens
Basic dyes (e.g., methylrosaniline chloride)	Soaps (e.g., sodium stearate)	Gums
Epinephrine-like compounds (e.g., phenylephrine HCl)	Other organic acids and their sodium, potassium, ammonium, calcium or other salts (e.g., saccharin sodium)	Spans and Tweens
Local Anesthetics, soluble (e.g., phenacaine HCl)	Penicillin, soluble (e.g., penicillin G, potassium V, etc.)	Starches
Other organic bases and organic chlorides, hydrochlorides, sulfates, phosphates, acetates, citrates, tartrates, etc. (e.g., thiamine HCl)		Sugars
Quaternary ammonium compounds (e.g., benzalkonium chloride)		Other nonionizing esters, ethers, and alcohols

scription containing an organic acid and an alcohol will usually not produce any appreciable quantity of ester since the hydrogen ion concentration is not at the appropriate value and water may be present in excess. Similarly, drugs made into ointments will usually not react because the ointment base coats the particles of drug and prevents contact.

Cationic-Nonionic-Anionic Relationships

A related scheme for prediction of certain incompatibilities is based on a suggestion that drugs which ionize in solution can be classified by their structure into cationic, nonionic, or anionic types. Common examples are given in Table 21.

According to this theory, the anionic and cationic substances are usually compatible with compounds of their own type and with nonionic substances but are often incompatible with each other. This seems logical since the oppositely charged high molecular weight ions should interact to form still higher molecular weight compounds or complexes which are insoluble, pharmacologically inactive, etc. Low molecular weight compounds are not included in

this postulate because their greater solubility reduces the likelihood of incompatibilities.

A typical example is the double decomposition reaction of quaternary ammonium compounds with soap:

benzalkonium chloride + sodium stearate →
   benzalkonium stearate ↓ + NaCl

The benzalkonium stearate formed is insoluble; hence, it is inactive and will appear as a precipitate unless dispersed in colloidal form by an excess of one of the reactants, by another surface-active agent, or by other solubilizers.

"Whether or not precipitation occurs in such combinations is dependent on such factors as the hydrophobic nature or insolubility of the two combining ions, the strength of each as an acid or base, the concentration of each, the presence of substances such as sugars which inhibit crystal formation, and the presence of surface-active agents or protective colloids which tend to produce colloidal solutions and delay visible evidence of precipitation, but which do not eliminate the possibility of partial or complete inactivation."[12]

It has been noted that a reduction in biological activity may have occurred in

Table 22—Compatibility of Anionic vs Cationic Drugs[12]

Anionic drugs ＼ Cationic drugs →	Acriflavine HCl (mol wt 224)	Benzalkonium chloride (mol wt 263)	Meperidine (mol wt 283.79)	Methapyrilene HCl (mol wt 297)	Antazoline HCl (mol wt 301.83)	Thiamine chloride (mol wt 337.29)	Phenacaine (mol wt 337.75)	Methyl rosaniline chloride (mol wt 408)	Quinacrine HCl (mol wt 508.91)	Streptomycin sulfate (mol wt 581.58)
Sodium p-aminosalicylate (mol wt 211.16)	x	...	...	...	...	...	x	x	x	...
Saccharin sodium (mol wt 241.2)	...	x	...	...	...	...	...	x	...	...
Sodium lauryl sulfate (mol wt 288.4)	x	x	x	x	x	x	x	x	x	x
Secobarbital sodium (mol wt 260.28)	...	x	x	x	...	...	...	x	x	...
Penicillin G potassium (mol wt 372.49)	x	x	...	...	...	...	...	x	x	...
Fluorescein sodium (mol wt 376.28)	x	x	...	...	...	x	x	x	...	...
Thimerosal (mol wt 404.8)	...	x	...	x	...	...	x	x	x	...
Amaranth (mol wt 604.5)	x	x	...	...	x	...	x	x	x	x
Sodium alginate (mol wt 28–32,000)	x	x	...	...	...	x	...	...	x	x
Sodium carboxymethylcellulose (mol wt 50,000–500,000)	x	x	...	...	...	...	...	...	x	x

x, Indicates incompatibility.

some of these mixtures even though there is no physical evidence of change. This points up the need for biological or pharmacological testing when anionic and cationic drugs are combined. This potential inactivation may not apply to oral drugs since the acidity, buffers, enzymes, and other components of the gastrointestinal tract would be expected to reverse the reaction. The latter may occur at a very slow rate, however.

On the other hand, topical preparations containing such complexes will probably be inactive if the concentrations normally used are prescribed. For example, a prescription calling for acriflavin 1% in Hydrophilic Ointment USP may seem quite sound unless we remember this ointment base contains 1% sodium lauryl sulfate. Since there is also 37.5% water present, a reaction should occur although this may not be detected. Since sodium lauryl sulfate is one of the most widely incompatible anionic materials, it was replaced in Hydrophilic Ointment USP XV by polyoxyl 40 stearate, a nonionic agent, but was returned in USP XVI, et seq.

This ionic system of forecasting incompatibilities can be very helpful in selecting ingredients which may be combined without danger of incompatibility and in explaining those incompatibilities which may be observed. It cannot always be depended upon to predict immediate incompatibilities. It has been reported that only 52 out of 100 theoretically incompatible mixtures produce immediate precipitation at the concentrations normally used. More concentrated solutions usually gave either immediate incompatibilities or, in some instances, delayed incompatibilities. Several incompatibility studies have shown similar results.

Table 22 presents the results of a study with the compounds tested in approximate order of molecular weight. This type of chart may be useful to the pharmacist in learning to forecast incompatibility since the compounds tested are representative of many compounds in the same family (i.e., those having similar structures, molecular weights, pH and pK values, etc.). Thus, if the pharmacist wishes to predict the compatibility of a new drug with one or more ingredients listed on the chart (or a related compound), he can select a compound having close similarity in ionic type, structure, etc., and determine the probable incompatibilities by inspection.

The pharmacist may wish to prepare his own charts using the drop method previously advocated. This simple test may be especially helpful where only the tradename or generic name is known and where the ionic type, reactive groups present, structural formula, etc., are unknown or incompletely known. It is carried out by using standard droppers to mix various ratios of products on a spot plate or in tiny vials. Where laboratory facilities are available, the use of graduated centrifuge tubes for the mixing followed by centrifuging for several minutes will usually permit collection of any insoluble material for a better appraisal of compatibility (i.e., identification of precipitates by microanalysis, UV or IR spectrophotometer, melting point, etc.).

Nonionic materials have not been considered to any extent up to this point. These materials, with the exception of the polyhydroxyl types, are usually insoluble in water because they are not appreciably ionized. They are usually chemically and physically compatible with cationic, anionic, and other nonionic compounds. In certain instances they may interfere with the biological activities of each other, however. For example, Tweens and other nonionic surfactants have been reported to interfere with the preservative action of the parabens when the ratio of surfactant to preservative exceeded certain critical values. The pH value of the mixture or the pH value at the site of use may be very important considerations here since it has been reported that nonionic emulsifiers form hydrogen-bonded complexes with *p*-hydroxy-

benzoic, sorbic, and benzoic acids at pH values between 4 and 6. This should not affect the absorption of oral mixtures since they would likely be subjected to lower pH values during digestion which should break the complexes. On the other hand, preservative activity might be depleted to the point where "Keep in a Refrigerator" labels or addition of other compatible preservatives may be indicated.

It might be noted that there is still some confusion as to the exact conditions required for these interactions as illustrated by the report that sorbic acid, phenylmercuric borate, phenylmercuric nitrate, phenylmercuric acetate, methyl carbitol, hexylene glycol, benzalkonium chloride, and combinations of these are effective preservatives for solutions and dispersions of nonionic surfactants of the fatty acid ester type. It has also been reported that such cations as chlorpromazine, promethazine, tetracaine, methylrosaniline, and dodecylpyridinium and such anions as naphthalene sulfonate and methyl orange will bind to Tween 80 under certain conditions. Inactivation of quaternary ammonium germicides by nonionic surface-active agents has been noted, and also that methylcellulose forms complexes with many preservatives, e.g., *p*-hydroxybenzoic acid, *p*-aminobenzoic acid, methylparaben, propylparaben, and butylparaben in decreasing order of degree of interaction. On the other hand, it has been reported that there is a strong binding tendency for butylparaben, followed by propylparaben, ethylparaben, and methylparaben with nonionic macromolecules. These investigations showed that the parabens interacted to a greater extent with polyoxyethylene ester type macromolecules such as Tween 80 or Myrj 52 than with the hydrophilic types such as polyethylene glycol 4000 or 6000 or polyethylene polypropylene glycol. The actual practical significance of these interactions (chiefly hydrogen bonding) will require further research.

General Organic Incompatibilities

In the following sections of this chapter typical organic pharmaceutical compounds are categorized according to chemical structure, and the important incompatibilities and corrective measures are described for individual compounds. Numerous additional compounds may be represented by some categories and similar incompatibilities could be anticipated for them. It should be noted that compounds with only one reactive group (i.e., monofunctional) will be more predictable with regard to chemical reactivity than compounds with several reactive groups (i.e., polyfunctional).

Generally only those drugs believed to be in common use are included in this edition (i.e., those listed in *Drugs in Current Use, Drugs of Choice, USP, NF,* etc.). Drug monographs giving the appropriate compounding and dispensing information for as many USP, NF, and the most commonly prescribed drug items for which data could be obtained appear in alphabetical order at the end of this chapter. Specific incompatibilities of less common or obsolete drugs are included in some cases where they may serve to teach the reactions of possible future drugs, or serve as examples to teach the reading of prescriptions or the calculation of dosage. Other less common drugs will be found in earlier editions of this text, *Remington's Pharmaceutical Sciences,* the *Merck Index,* etc.

Products mentioned in this section of the text for which specifications have been established by current USP or NF monographs are intended to meet those specifications.

Hydrocarbons

Hydrocarbons include both saturated and unsaturated compounds of carbon and hydrogen.

Caution: Overexposure to volatile hydrocarbons may cause damage to the heart, liver, or kidneys. All hydrocarbons are solvents for vitamins A, D, E, and K and may cause vitamin deficiencies on prolonged exposure or use.

Saturated Hydrocarbons (Alkanes)—The saturated hydrocarbons used in pharmacy are not reactive under conditions of prescription usage; hence, their incompatibilities are chiefly those of physical immiscibility with water, alcohol, castor oil, salts, and other ionic and polar compounds. They are physically compatible with other hydrocarbons, lanolin, cetyl alcohol, cholesteryl esters, and chemically compatible with all solid drugs, although they probably will not dissolve the latter.

It has been pointed out that white petrolatum will dissolve the following quantities of drugs: salicylic acid, 0.03–0.06%; ethyl para-aminobenzoate, 0.05–0.1%; atropine, 0.02–0.04%; cocaine, 0.25–0.5%; camphor, 14–15%; ephedrine, 0.75–1.0%; iodine, 0.8–1.0%; menthol, 18–20%; naphthol, 0.1–0.13%; phenol, 0.5–0.75%; sulfur (ppt), 0.25–0.5%; thymol, 5.8–6.0%.[13] These solubilities also hold approximately true for these same drugs in liquid petrolatum.

Examples of saturated hydrocarbon mixtures frequently used in pharmacy include petroleum ether (ligroin) (C_5–C_7), deodorized kerosene (C_9–C_{15}), light mineral oil (C_{15}–C_{20}), mineral oil (C_{18}–C_{24}), petrolatum (C_{18}–C_{30}), white petrolatum (C_{18}–C_{30}), and paraffin (C_{24}–C_{30}).

Antioxidants such as *dl*-alpha tocopherol are sometimes added to prevent oxidation of unsaturated hydrocarbon impurities which may be present.

Unsaturated Hydrocarbons—Unsaturated hydrocarbons and other compounds containing double (alkenes) or triple (alkynes) bonds may add various groups (e.g., Br_2, HBr, H_2, H_2SO_4) or be oxidized or reduced at their unsaturated linkages:

The reactivity and poor stability of the double bond has been explained by the Bayer strain theory. This theory is based on the concept of the carbon atom as a tetrahedral arrangement of valence bonds where the carbon is located in the center of a regular tetrahedron and the four bonds are distributed in space symmetrically. The angle between any pair of bonds will then be 109°28′. Where several carbon atoms form a chain the arrangement will probably be a zigzag shape rather than the straight line usually depicted. If no double bonds are present the form of the chains may vary since the free rotation of the single bond does not fix the shape. Five- and six-carbon compounds will frequently form shapes in which the end carbons are near each other. Ring formation can then occur in those with a strain on the valence angle of only 0° to 5°. Three carbon chains will theoretically require a strain or distortion of about 24° to form rings while four carbon chains require only about 9°. Two carbon chains (i.e., double bonds) would have the greatest strain hence the greatest tendency to open up and react to reduce the strain. Thus the ease of formation and stability of the rings is in the general order C_5, C_6, C_4, C_3, C_2.

The substitution of sulfur, oxygen, or nitrogen in these chains and rings does not change this theory very much since the bond angles of those atoms are also about 100°. Thus large heterocyclic chains and rings can be formed and will be stable if the bonds fold back and forth to sufficiently relieve the distortion. For example, macrolide antibiotics (e.g., erythromycin) are stable yet apparently have 13 carbon atoms and one oxygen atom in a single ring. As many as 34 members in one ring have been reported.

Unsaturated hydrocarbons are not used in prescriptions at the present time. The only common example is ethylene ($CH_2{=}CH_2$), an inhalation anesthetic.

Cycloparaffins—These compounds are not found in prescriptions.

Aromatic Hydrocarbons—The aromatic hydrocarbons themselves are not used in prescriptions. Since they form the nucleus of many drugs, we should note that they may substitute or add various groups on strong chemical treatment but are less reactive than straight chain unsaturated compounds. The common examples are:

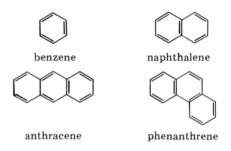

benzene   naphthalene

anthracene   phenanthrene

When such structures form the core of a drug they will be more reactive than aliphatic hydrocarbons, but will not exhibit the usual reactions of unsaturated compounds. They may substitute various groups on the aromatic ring on strong chemical treatment, but the ring itself will be resistant to oxidation or reduction.

Since the benzene ring has excess electrons, it acts as a negative group which can increase the acidity of acids or reduce the basicity of bases. It is perhaps worth noting that the presence on the ring of certain substituents (e.g., —OH, —NH$_2$, —NHR, —NR$_2$, —NH—CO—CH$_3$, —Cl, —Br, —I, and alkyl) directs a second added group to the ortho and para positions while the more negative and unsaturated substituents (e.g., —NO$_2$, —COOH, —SO$_3$H, —CHO, or —C≡N—) will direct the second group to the meta position.

The reactions of naphthalene resemble those of benzene as would be expected. The derivatives are also closely related (e.g., the alpha- and beta-naphthols resemble the phenols in chemical reactivity). Anthracene and phenanthrene also produce stable ring systems which resemble benzene in their reactions and stability.

Their incompatibilities are about the same as the hydrocarbons (i.e., chiefly physical immiscibility or potential toxicity) although they may undergo addition or double decomposition reactions.

Halogenated Hydrocarbons

Halogenated hydrocarbons are generally insoluble in water and soluble in alcohol and organic solvents. Their prescription incompatibilities are about the same as the hydrocarbons (i.e., chiefly physical immiscibility).

Saturated Halogenated Hydrocarbons—The halogenated alkanes are used to some extent in dispensing, and their chief incompatibilities are: (1) they are immiscible with water and (2) they usually have such low boiling points that they are hard to keep in the prescriptions. Under prolonged storage or at high temperatures they may react with hydroxyl ions to form alcohol or with ammonia to form amines:

$$C_2H_5Br + OH^- \longrightarrow C_2H_5OH + Br^-$$

$$C_2H_5Br + NH_3 \longrightarrow C_2H_5NH_2 + HBr$$

These reaction products would probably not be noticed in mixtures since they form to such a slight extent and are miscible with the starting materials.

Examples of halogenated saturated hydrocarbons include chloroform ($CHCl_3$), carbon tetrachloride (CCl_4), iodoform (CHI_3), ethyl chloride (CH_3CH_2Cl), butyl chloride (CH_3CH_2-CH_2CH_2Cl), mitotane ($C_{14}H_{10}Cl_4$), and chlorinated paraffin.

Unsaturated Halogenated Hydrocarbons—The halogenated alkenes are less stable since they will decompose in the presence of air, moisture, and light to liberate acids, phosgene, etc.:

$$Cl_2C{=}CCl_2 + H_2O \xrightarrow[\text{light}]{O} Cl_2C{=}O + 2HCl$$

These may be stabilized to some extent with ethanol (0.5–1%) or ammonium carbonate (0.02%).

The instability observed with unsaturated halides, dicarboxylic acids, *et al*, is sometimes intensified by certain structural factors. Geometrical isomerism (or two isomers with the same formula and reactive groups but differing slightly in geometry) may occur in double-bonded compounds which cannot rotate freely due to the more rigid structure. The isomer with the reactive groups on the same side of the molecule (i.e., the *cis* isomer) is normally more dense, more reactive, less stable, and lower melting than the isomer with reactive groups on opposite sides (i.e., the *trans* isomer). The *cis* or reactive isomer often may be converted by heat and acid or halogen to the more stable *trans* isomer. Conversely the *trans* isomer can often be converted to the unstable *cis* isomer by ultraviolet light. This is frequently the reason light must be excluded in the storage of drugs (i.e., use of carton or amber bottle).

Geometrical isomerism is also noted with compounds possessing the —C=N— bond (e.g., oximes, semicarbazones, and phenylhydrazones of aldehydes and ketones). For some such compounds the stability of the *trans* isomer may be so much greater than the *cis* isomer that only one isomer is known.

The number of possible isomers is usually increased exponentially by the number of double bonds. Compounds with triple bonds on the other hand do not form geometric isomers.

Examples of unsaturated halogenated hydrocarbons are trichloroethylene:

and tetrachloroethylene:

Caution: High concentrations are irritating to eyes and mucous membranes.

Saturated Cyclic Halogenated Hydrocarbons—These are quite stable in neutral or acid prescriptions but may form hydrochloric or other halogen acids in alkaline media. For example, gamma benzene hexachloride (lindane) will react in limewater (or other alkali):

$$2 \text{ (lindane structure)} + 3\,Ca(OH)_2 \longrightarrow$$

$$2\,Cl \text{(trichlorobenzene ring)} + 3\,CaCl_2 + 6\,H_2O$$

(or other trichloroethylenes)

Caution: Local sensitivity reactions or hepatic damage may result from prolonged or repeated application.

Aromatic Halogenated Hydrocarbons—The common members of this group are chlorophenothane (DDT), chlordane, aldrin, dieldrin, and toxaphene. These compounds are soluble in common organic solvents but insoluble in water. *Caution:* These compounds may be absorbed through the skin producing liver damage.

These compounds are useful as insecticides but find limited utility in prescriptions. Halogens linked directly to the ring are essentially inert thus these compounds are stable in mixtures with talc and even in aqueous acid, neutral, or alkaline solutions. Iron and aluminum salts should be avoided.

Other polyfunctional halogen derivatives where several reactive groups may be involved in degradation reactions, incompatibilities, etc. include brompheniramine, chlortetracycline, hexachlorophene, hydroxyzine, and tribromoethanol.

Alcohols

Alcohols are found among the most common prescription solvents and vehicles. The general formula for an alcohol is R—OH; however, the valence bond between the radical and the —OH group is a shared pair of electrons (i.e., nonpolar) hence the alcohols do not ionize and are neutral not basic. Their physical incompatibilities have been previously described (i.e., their immiscibility with salts, gums, proteins, etc.). Since an alcohol is present in many commercial products which may stand several years before use, the alcohol reactions which can take place at room temperature will be discussed. These include:

1. Oxidation with strong oxidizing agents to form aldehydes, ketones, and/or acids:

$$Primary \underset{alcohol}{\overset{(O)}{\rightleftharpoons}} aldehyde \overset{(O)}{\rightleftharpoons} acid$$

$$C_2H_5OH \longrightarrow CH_3-\overset{O}{\underset{H}{C}} \longrightarrow CH_3-\overset{O}{C}{\underset{OH}{}}$$

ethyl alcohol   acetaldehyde   acetic acid

$$Secondary\ alcohol \overset{(O)}{\rightleftharpoons} ketone$$

$$CH_3CH(OH)CH_3 \qquad CH_3COCH_3$$

isopropyl alcohol   acetone

$$Tertiary\ alcohol \overset{(O)}{\rightleftharpoons} \begin{array}{l} ketones, \\ aldehydes \\ or\ acids \end{array}$$

$$CH_3CH_2C(CH_3)_2OH \qquad CH_3CH_2COCH_3,$$

amylene hydrate   HCOOH, etc

2. Reaction of hydrogen of hydroxyl group with other drugs:

alkyl alcohol + organic acids $\longrightarrow$
C_2H_5OH CH_3COOH

alkyl esters + H_2O
$CH_3COOC_2H_5$

alkyl alcohol + acid anhydrides $\longrightarrow$
C_2H_5OH $CH_3COOCOCH_3$

alkyl esters + alkyl acids
$CH_3COOC_2H_5$ CH_3COOH

3. Replacement of hydroxyl group by another group:

alkyl alcohol + HI $\longrightarrow$ alkyl iodide + H_2O
C_2H_5OH C_2H_5I

alkyl alcohol + $H_2SO_4 \longrightarrow$ alkyl sulfate + H_2O
C_2H_5OH $C_2H_5OSO_3H$

alkyl alcohol + HNO_3 ⟶ alkyl nitrate + H_2O

C_2H_5OH $\qquad\qquad$ $C_2H_5ONO_2$

Some of the incompatibilities formerly ascribed to alcohols have been shown to be due to the presence of aldehyde, ketone, acid or ester impurities formed by the above reactions. These include: (1) the development of a dark color with alkalies, (2) the reduction of mercuric chloride to mercurous chloride, and (3) the formation of explosive mixtures with silver salts plus nitric acid.

Monohydric Alcohols—The most common alcohols containing only one hydroxyl group are ethyl alcohol (95% C_2H_5OH by volume), dehydrated alcohol (99+% C_2H_5OH by volume), isopropyl alcohol ($CH_3CHOHCH_3$), amylene hydrate ($CH_3CH_2C(CH_3)_2OH$), cetyl alcohol ($CH_3(CH_2)_{14}CH_2OH$), and stearyl alcohol (chiefly $CH_3(CH_2)_{16}CH_2OH$).

The lower alcohols are incompatible with acacia, albumins, and oxidizing agents such as chlorine, bromine, permanganate, and chromic acid.

See *Alcohol,* page 472.

Aromatic Monohydric Alcohols— Two examples of this group are benzyl alcohol and phenylethyl alcohol. These alcohols retain the chemical properties of the monohydric alcohols except that they may resinify with sulfuric acid rather than form sulfuric esters.

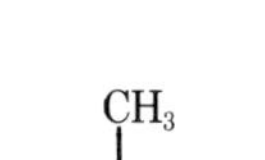

benzyl alcohol 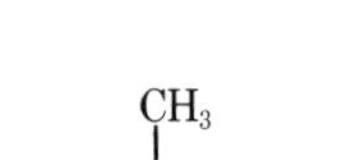 $\qquad$ phenylethyl alcohol

Terpene Alcohols—The chief examples are menthol and terpin hydrate (see index).

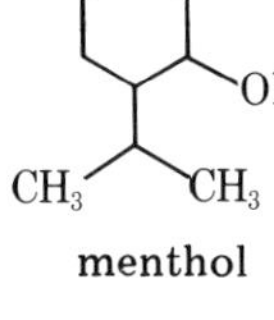

menthol 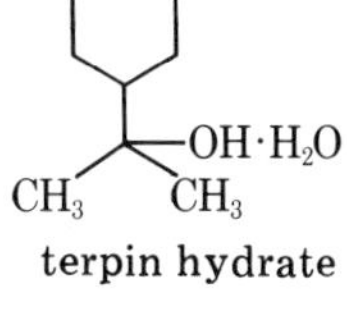 $\qquad$ terpin hydrate

Dihydric Alcohols (Glycols)— These pharmaceutical vehicle and solvent alcohols have two hydroxyl groups per molecule, and accordingly may be more polar than the corresponding monohydric alcohol. The low molecular weight members (i.e., less than C_5) are miscible with water and will not only dissolve some salts and gums but also volatile oils, some dyes, and resins. Chemically, they react like the monohydric alcohols hence are normally quite stable. Examples are propylene glycol ($CH_3CHOHCH_2OH$), ethohexadiol ($CH_2OHCH(C_2H_5)CHOHCH_2CH_2CH_3$), mephenesin ($CH_3C_6H_4OCH_2CH$-$(OH)CH_2OH$), polyethylene glycol 400 ($H(OCH_2CH_2)_{8-10}CH_2OH$), and polyethylene glycol 4000 ($H(OCH_2CH_2)_{70-86}$ CH_2OH).

The Pluronics ($HO(C_2H_4O)_n$-$(C_3H_6O)_n(C_2H_4O)_nH$) are similar to the polyethylene glycols.

Trihydric Alcohols—See *Glycerin,* page 535.

Polyhydric Alcohols—These stable, solid compounds are mannitol and sorbitol, q.v.

Halogenated Alcohols

These drugs are not very stable, and aqueous solutions deteriorate on standing or heating. The halogenated alcohols have sedative value if three bromine or chlorine atoms are attached to a single carbon atom. Examples are tribromoethanol and chlorobutanol.

Phenolic Compounds

Phenols are compounds in which one or more hydroxyl groups are attached directly to an aromatic ring. Being hydroxyl compounds, phenols undergo many of the chemical reactions characteristic of alcohols; however, these compounds also possess tautomeric "enol" structures i.e.,

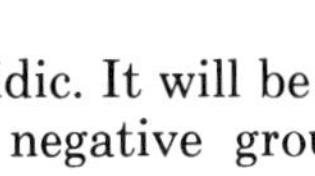

which are acidic. It will be recalled that unsaturated negative groups attached to a hydroxyl (as in —COOH, —SO$_2$OH, —NO$_2$OH) form weak to strong acids (i.e., carboxylic, sulfuric, and nitric). The hydrogen of the hydroxyl group has some acidic properties; it is replaceable by metals. This is shown by the fact that some phenols form salts on treatment with alkali hydroxides. The resulting salts, known as phenolates, are only slightly hydrolyzed by water.

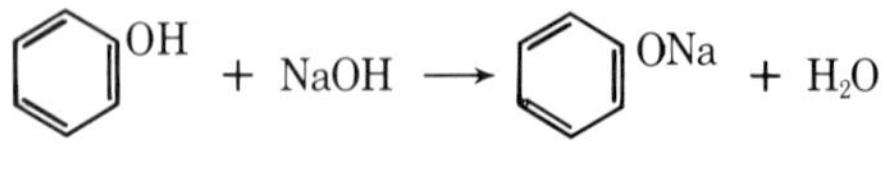

In the common examples below, the upper figures represent solubility in g/100 ml water and the lower figures the pK$_a$ for each phenol.

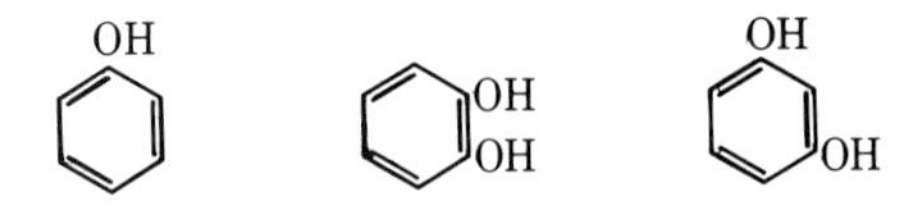

phenol
Sol. 6.6
pKa 9.94

catechol
45
9.48

resorcinol
123
9.44

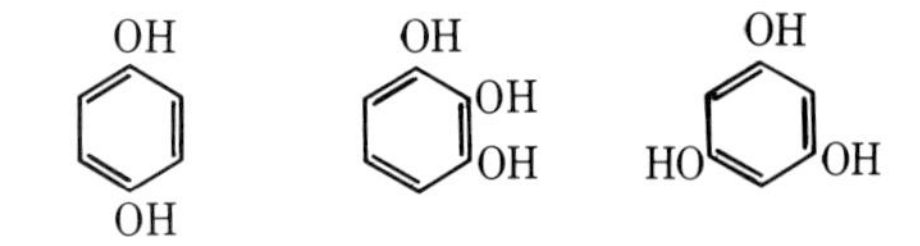

hydroquinone
Sol. 8
pKa 9.96

pyrogallol
6.2
—

phloroglucinol
7.7
—

One or more of the hydrogens remaining in the aromatic ring of phenols can be replaced by other groups. When the phenolic hydroxyl stays on the ring and remains reactive, these polyfunctional phenols will then usually show chemical reactivity in several places. Compounds of phenol with one or more ring hydrogens replaced by other groups leads to several useful pharmaceutical compounds. Thus, replacement with the proper alkyl group will give thymol; replacement with other substituted groups gives neosynephrine or perhaps even stilbestrol; replacement of a hydrogen with a carboxyl group will give salicylic acid, replacement with an aldehyde group will give salicylaldehyde, while proper replacement with

a chlorine will give parachlorophenol, etc. Similarly, dihydroxybenzene substituted by these groups can give eugenol, epinephrine, vanillin, hexylresorcinol, etc.

The phenols with pK$_a$ values around 9 are weak acids and will form salts with sodium hydroxide or potassium hydroxide, but not with alkali carbonates or bicarbonates. The pH of a 1% aqueous solution of these phenols is about 5. Other substituents which attract electrons (e.g., nitro groups) increase the acidity of phenols depending on the number of groups introduced (e.g., o-nitrophenol, pK$_a$ 7.23; m-nitrophenol, pK$_a$ 8.35; p-nitrophenol, pK$_a$ 7.14; 3,5-dinitrophenol, pK$_a$ 1.62; and 2,4,6-trinitrophenol (picric acid), pK$_a$ 0.80). The latter is nearly as strong an acid as hydrochloric acid and will decompose carbonates:

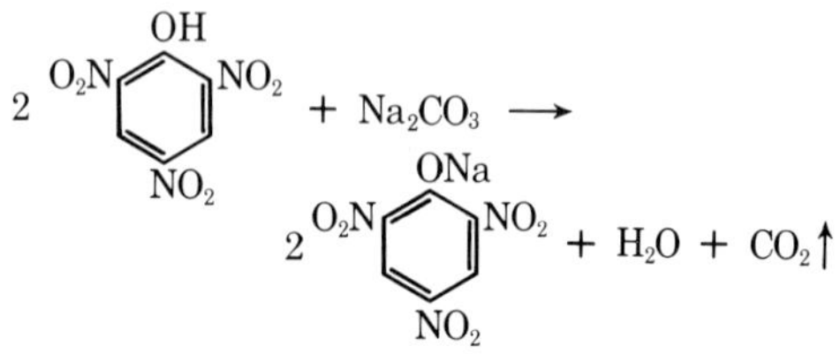

Many phenols precipitate albumin. Phenols are reducing agents, some more so than others. Most phenols react with ferric salts in neutral or slightly acid solution to form complex compounds which are colored blue, violet, green, red, or brown, according to the nature of the phenol. On reducing other materials they are themselves oxidized to quinone type compounds. This may occur in air or with oxidizing agents such as ferric chloride, chromic acid, permanganate, etc. The presence of a second or third hydroxyl ion greatly accelerates oxidation, and this occurs in a few minutes with catechol or pyrogallol. Compounds with ortho- or para-hydroxyl groups are especially susceptible to oxidation:

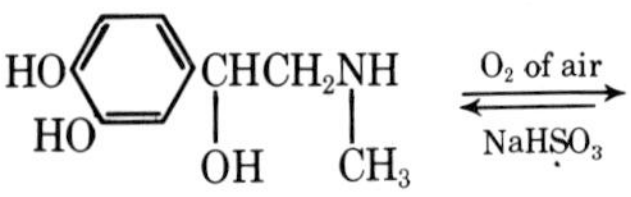

epinephrine

$$O=\text{(ring)}\ \overset{|}{\underset{OH}{C}}HCH_2NH\ \overset{|}{\underset{CH_3}{}}$$

oxidized epinephrine (quinone)

Thus, epinephrine may be stabilized by bisulfites or hydrosulfites. Other general reactions are discussed under the official compounds. Important monofunctional and polyfunctional phenols include epinephrine, hexylresorcinol, phenol, parachlorophenol, resorcinol, and thymol. Phenols react with iodine in aqueous solution to form insoluble compounds. *Caution:* Many phenols are toxic and ingestion of even small amounts may produce symptoms suggesting renal and nervous system toxicity. Phenols are also reducing agents and may cause explosions if improperly mixed with strong oxidizing agents.

Other polyfunctional phenols include acetaminophen, folic acid, and levallorphan tartrate.

Quinones

Quinones may be considered as oxidation products of *o*- or *p*-dihydroxy derivatives of aromatic hydrocarbons. Oxidation results in removal of two phenolic hydrogens, thus producing, theoretically, an aromatic peroxide which, through rearrangement, assumes the structure of an unsaturated alicyclic diketone. Quinones are thus derivable from various aromatic ring systems; e.g., benzoquinones from benzene, naphthoquinones from naphthalene, anthraquinone from anthracene, etc.

Quinones may develop then in prescriptions on oxidation of phenols, aminophenols, or amines. They are readily reducible to dihydrophenols, and they display various other properties also characteristic of ketones, e.g., formation of oximes and imines. The presence of the unsaturated alicyclic nucleus is abundantly evident through numerous addition reactions with such agents as halogens, amines, mercaptans, etc.

The quinones are colored compounds, and many naturally occurring principles such as alizarin in the root of the madder plant have been characterized as quinones or quinone derivatives. The quinoid grouping is the characteristic chromophore of the triphenylmethane, indophenol, indamine, azine, and certain other classes of dyes.

An example of a monofunctional quinone is phytonadione; examples of polyfunctional quinones are danthron, menadione sodium bisulfite, menadione, and menadione sodium diphosphate.

Aldehydes

Aldehydes include some of the most reactive organic compounds. They have the structure:

$$R-\overset{O}{\underset{}{\overset{\|}{C}}}-H$$

and are the first oxidation products of primary alcohols. The major incompatibilities which are likely to occur in prescriptions include:

1. Aldehydes are readily oxidized by air or oxidizing agents to form acids:

$$R-\overset{O}{\overset{\|}{C}}-H + \tfrac{1}{2}O_2 \longrightarrow R-\overset{O}{\overset{\|}{C}}-OH$$

In so doing they function as reducing agents.

2. Aldehydes add compounds having an active hydrogen to form hydroxylated compounds:

$$R-\overset{O}{\overset{\|}{C}}-H + H:H \longrightarrow R-\overset{H}{\underset{H}{\overset{|}{C}}}-OH$$

$$R-\overset{O}{\overset{\|}{C}}-H + H:NH_2 \longrightarrow R-\overset{H}{\underset{OH}{\overset{|}{C}}}-NH_2$$

$$R-\overset{O}{\overset{\|}{C}}-H + H:SO_3Na \longrightarrow R-\overset{H}{\underset{OH}{\overset{|}{C}}}-SO_3Na$$

$$R-\overset{O}{\overset{\|}{C}}-H + HOH \longrightarrow R-\overset{H}{\underset{OH}{\overset{|}{C}}}-OH$$

3. Aldehydes polymerize with hydrogen ions as a catalyst to form polymers:

$$3CH_3—C\overset{O}{\diagup}\hspace{-0.3em}\diagdown H \xrightarrow{H^+} (CH_3—C\overset{O}{\diagup}\hspace{-0.3em}\diagdown H)_3$$

acetaldehyde   paraldehyde

$$nCH_2O \longrightarrow (CH_2O)_n$$

formaldehyde   paraformaldehyde

All are very susceptible to oxidation (exposure to air is often sufficient), forming the corresponding acids. Several of the characteristic reactions involve rupture of the C=O linkage. Reaction with various reducing agents thus results in the formation of primary alcohols. $NaHSO_3$ adds mole for mole to form readily crystallizable solids; NH_3 adds to give α-hydroxyamines which usually polymerize. Condensation reactions resulting in replacement of the carbonyl oxygen atom are also characteristic. Such condensation with hydroxylamine, hydrazine, and semicarbazide produces, respectively, oximes, hydrazones, and semicarbazones. Under the influence of alkali, many aldehydes, especially the aromatics, undergo self-oxidation-reduction to produce equimolar quantities of the corresponding alcohol and acid.

Examples of monofunctional aldehydes are benzaldehyde, formaldehyde, and paraldehyde (trimer of acetaldehyde); examples of polyfunctional aldehydes are chloral hydrate, nifuroxime (oxime of 5-nitro-2-furaldehyde), pralidoxime chloride (oxime of 2-formyl - 1 - methylpyridinium chloride), streptomycin, and vanillin.

Halogenated Aldehydes

Chloral hydrate (page 496) and butyl chloral hydrate are examples of halogenated aldehydes which show some of the reactivities of both functional groups.

Ketones

Ketones are the first oxidation products of secondary alcohols; hence they are isomeric with aldehydes. For simple ketones the radicals are identical; for mixed ketones, they are different. Cyclic ketones comprise an additional type in which the C of the =CO group is part of a ring, thus they have the general formula:

$$R\,\lfloor\quad C\rfloor=O$$

e.g., cyclohexanone:

$$\overline{CH_2}—(CH_2)_4—\overline{CO}$$

On reduction, ketones give rise to secondary alcohols. Oxidation is much more difficult than with aldehydes; also, it requires a more drastic type of oxidation resulting in fission of the ketone molecule and conversion of its fragments into a mixture of acids. For this reason, ketones, unlike aldehydes, are not prone to polymerization. Ketone reactions with alcohols, mercaptans, hydroxylamine, hydrazine, and semicarbazide are similar to those of aldehydes, qv. Acetone and other aliphatic ketones in which one of the R's is methyl, and cyclic ketones having up to 8 carbon atoms yield addition products with $NaHSO_3$ as per aldehydes; however, aromatic ketones (e.g., acetophenone) do not.

Ketones, although possessing a carbonyl group:

$$R—\overset{\overset{\displaystyle O}{\|}}{C}—R'$$

are somewhat less reactive than the aldehydes because they do not have the labile hydrogen.

It should be noted that aromatic ketones are generally less reactive chemically than aliphatic ketones.

Examples of monofunctional ketones are acetone, anisindione, camphor, diphenadione, methylisobutyl ketone, and progesterone; examples of polyfunctional ketones are acenocoumarol, betamethasone, estrone, griseofulvin, hydrocodone, methadone, propiomazine, testosterone, and warfarin.

Fluocinolone and triamcinolone acetonide are examples of acetals of the reference ketone, acetone.

Organic Acids and Their Salts

The term organic acid as applied in this section includes molecules with one or more carboxyl groups (i.e., COOH). Saturated monocarboxylic acids, unsaturated acids, polycarboxylic acids, hydroxy acids, keto acids, halogenated acids, and aromatic carboxylic acids will be considered here since all have carboxyl groups which can ionize to form hydrogen ions: $RCOOH \rightarrow RCOO^- + H^+$. Although these compounds may show esterification, substitution, and neutralization reactions in prescriptions, their chief incompatibilities are probably formation of insoluble metal salts (e.g., aluminum monostearate) or precipitation of insoluble free acids (e.g., stearic acid).

Since most organic acids ionize only slightly, they are generally weak electrolytes. They usually react with alkalies to form water soluble salts: $RCOOH + NaOH \rightarrow RCOONa + H_2O$. The ammonium, potassium, and sodium salts are water soluble or dispersible even above 18 carbons per carboxyl group. Other salts such as those of aluminum, barium, calcium, magnesium, strontium, or zinc are usually insoluble when the carbon chain is over 5 carbons per carboxyl, hydroxyl, or other hydrophilic group. The soluble salts, e.g., acetates and citrates, act as buffers toward stronger acids. Salts of insoluble acids may precipitate the insoluble free acid when acidified. The water solubility of saturated and unsaturated carboxylic acids decreases with increasing chain length and over C_5 are usually insoluble unless other hydrophilic groups are present. All are soluble in alcohol or organic solvents. *Caution:* Organic acids and their salts are reducing agents and are thus incompatible with strong oxidizing agents.

Saturated Monocarboxylic Acids— Examples of monocarboxylic acids are acetic acid, formic acid, propionic acid, stearic acid, and valeric acid.

Saturated Polycarboxylic Acids— These have two or more carboxyl groups per molecule, but usually resemble the monocarboxylic acids in reactivity. The first carboxyl group to react is usually much more active than the second, and so on as may be noted from the pK_a values. Examples are oxalic acid and succinic acid.

Unsaturated Acids—Unsaturated acids and their salts have about the same incompatibilities as the corresponding saturated acids. In addition, because of their unsaturated bonds, they will add various groups as previously noted in the section on unsaturated hydrocarbons (i.e., addition of I_2, Br_2, HI, etc.). Examples are oleic acid and undecylenic acid.

Hydroxy Acids—Organic acids bearing one or more hydroxy groups often cause compounding difficulties. Examples are citric acid, gluconic acid, lactic acid, and tartaric acid (and their salts potassium citrate, sodium citrate, calcium gluconate, ferrous gluconate, and potassium gluconate).

Halogenated Acids—Only one or two organic acids bearing halogen atoms are encountered in routine prescription compounding. The most common is trichloroacetic acid.

Aromatic Acids—Certain aromatic acids and their salts are responsible for a wide range of organic chemical incompatibilities. These have been discussed at considerable length in previous editions of this text and include benzoic acid, salicylic acid, aspirin, nalidixic acid, and tannic acid.

Soaps

Soaps are usually considered to be ammonium, potassium, or sodium salts of fatty acids containing eight or more carbon atoms. Thus, the caprylates and stearates already discussed plus the laurates, oleates, undecylenates, etc., may be considered to be soaps. Other types of compounds are also considered to be soaps. Amine soaps (e.g., triethanolamine stearate) are widely used as washable ointment bases, and calcium fatty

acid soaps are the bases in lime lina-
ment.

Soap solutions are generally alkaline
and may produce some of the incompatibilities of the hydroxyl ion (pH values
= 10–11).

Aqueous solutions of soap are decomposed by acids, which liberate the free
fatty acids. Salts of heavy metals (e.g.,
zinc, aluminum, lead, mercury, and copper) will precipitate insoluble heavy
metal salts (e.g., zinc stearate, aluminum stearate, lead oleate, mercuric oleate, copper undecylenate, etc.).

Esters

An ester is a compound consisting of
a positive organic group joined to an
acid function. Since the acid may be either organic or inorganic, esters may be
thought of as salts of alcohols. As a rule,
esters are insoluble in water but are soluble in organic solvents. In the presence
of water most esters are gradually hydrolyzed to the corresponding acids and
alcohols, the change being hastened by
acids and alkalies; i.e., the hydrolysis
may proceed slowly in the near neutral
pH range 5.5–7 but accelerate greatly
with pH values above and below this
range; e.g.,

$$R-\overset{\overset{O}{\parallel}}{C}OH + R'OH \underset{OH^-}{\overset{H^+}{\rightleftharpoons}}$$
$$\text{acid} \quad \text{alcohol}$$

$$R-\overset{\overset{O}{\parallel}}{C}-O-R + H_2O$$
$$\text{ester} \quad \text{water}$$

In general, esters have the incompatibilities of the corresponding alcohols.

Many of the most commonly prescribed drugs are esters. Aspirin (already discussed), fats, and fixed oils,
many local anesthetics, alkaloids, synthetics, etc., are esters.

Esters may be categorized as:

1. Esters and partial esters of inorganic acids
(e.g., amyl nitrite and echothiophate iodide). See
also *Halogen Derivatives, Thiols,* and *Thio
Ethers.*

2. Monofunctional esters of carboxylic acids
(e.g., benzyl benzoate and estradiol dipropionate).
See also *Fixed Oils and Fats* and *Waxes.*

3. Esters of hydroxy acids (e.g., methylparaben
and scopolamine hydrobromide).

4. Esters of amino (NH₂) acids (e.g., benzocaine and meprobamate).

5. Polyfunctional esters of carboxylic acids
(other than 3 and 4 above) (e.g., aspirin and hydrocortisone acetate).

6. Esters of noncarboxylic acids (e.g., busulfan
and spironolactone).

Ester local anesthetics (e.g., benzocaine, procaine, tetracaine, and similar
esters) plus ester alkaloids (such as atropine, cocaine, physostigmine, *et al*)
are covered in later sections. Many of
these can be stabilized by complexation
with xanthines.

Some of these esters have a pH value
where minimum decomposition occurs;
e.g., procaine (pH 3.6), cinchocaine (pH
5), benzocaine (pH 4.9), atropine (pH
5). Unfortunately their values of maximum stability may differ from the pH
of maximal therapeutic effect. This is
due to the fact that the basic form of
these compounds seems to be the active
one, probably due to their solubility in
lipoids. A compromise is then necessary
with the desired pH of the prescription
being a mean between the ideal "pharmaceutical" pH value and the ideal
"medical" value. Such pH adjustments
are best done with strong hydrochloric
acid or sodium hydroxide rather than
buffers so as not to interfere with the
buffer capacity of the tissues.

Fats and Fixed Oils—The fats and
fixed oils are triglycerides of fatty acids.
Important esters include ethyl acetate:

$$CH_3-\overset{\overset{O}{\parallel}}{C}-OC_2H_5$$

spermaceti, chiefly

$$CH_3(CH_2)_{14}-\overset{\overset{O}{\parallel}}{C}-O-(CH_2)_{15}-CH_3$$

glyceryl triacetate (triacetic acid ester
of glycerin), cocoa butter (stearin, palmitin, olein, and laurin mixture), lard
(chiefly olein), benzoinated lard, olive
oil (70% olein–30% palmitin), and other

similar vegetable oils; e.g., corn oil, cottonseed oil, sesame oil, linseed oil, expressed almond oil, peanut oil, coconut oil, persic oil, castor oil (80% glyceride of ricinoleic acid), and halibut liver oil. On exposure to light and air, or in contact with metals in the dark, these become rancid. Rancid fats liberate iodine from potassium iodide due to the presence of peroxides. Unsaturated triglycerides take up iodine by addition at the double bond. Fats and fixed oils are insoluble in water and, with the exception of castor oil, are pratically insoluble in alcohol.

Salicylate Esters—See *Analgesics,* page 451.

Other Esters—A few additional esters are encountered in compounding work; e.g., benzyl benzoate, butylparaben, ethyl paraben, methylparaben, and propylparaben.

Ethers

Ethers are generally considered to be one of the most chemically inert classes of organic drugs. They are commonly assigned the structure R—O—R, in which R is an alkyl, alicyclic, heterocyclic, or aryl group. Thus, they may be considered as anhydrides of alcohols or phenols. Ethers are useful in drug extraction and assay procedures because they will not react at room temperature with strong acids or bases, oxidizing agents, sodium, or other active reagents. They are not found to any extent in prescriptions.

Solvent ether is a constituent of the following formerly official preparations (per cent present in parentheses): aspidium oleoresin (solvent), collodion (75%), flexible collodion, ether spirit (32.5%), compound ether spirit (32.5%), and salicylic collodion (75%).

Monofunctional Ethers—Solvent ether is similar in every respect to Ether USP (ether for inhalation), except that it is not required to be of such high purity, and does not contain ethanol to minimize peroxide formation. *Caution:* On long standing, especially in sunlight or ultraviolet light, ether produces per-

oxides which may be very explosive if heated:

$$C_2H_5\text{—}O\text{—}C_2H_5 \xrightarrow{O}$$

$$CH_3CH\text{—}O\text{—}CH_2CH_3 \xrightarrow{O}$$
$$| $$
$$O\text{—}OH$$

$$CH_3\text{—}CH \overset{O\text{—}O}{\underset{O\text{—}O}{\diagup \diagdown}} CH\text{—}CH_3$$

Peroxides may form after standing about 6 months but disappear after about a year if the alcohol present as a stabilizer in Ether USP is oxidized to aldehyde.

Ether groups—i.e., alkoxy groups such as propoxy (C_3H_7—O—)—are present in many drug compounds but are so inert that the drugs are usually classified by the more reactive groups. Thus, the hydroxy ethers—e.g., cellosolves (C_2H_5—O—CH_2CH_2OH, etc.), carbitols (C_4H_9—O—CH_2CH_2—O—CH_2CH_2—OH, etc.), polyethylene glycols ($HOCH_2(CH_2$—O—$CH_2)_n(CH_2$-OH)), methylcellulose (cellulose (—O-$CH_3)_n$), guaiacol, eugenol, creosote, mephenesin, etc.—are discussed under alcohols , and the phenols.

Other ether-type compounds containing alkoxy groups include benztropine mesylate, methoxsalen, and reserpine.

Benzyloxy and other complex "oxy" groups also occur in polyfunctional ethers, e.g., monobenzone, orphenadrine citrate, and trioxsalen.

Carbohydrates

This category includes aliphatic polyhydroxy aldehydes and polyhydroxy ketones along with their condensation polymers.

Examples of items which are carbohydrates, manufactured carbohydrate derivatives, or natural products useful because of their carbohydrate or carbohydrate-derivative content are dextrose, methylcellulose, and tragacanth.

Aurothioglucose, meglumine diatrizoate, and glucosulfone sodium are examples of synthetics which contain a carbohydrate (D-glucose) moiety. Carbohydrate residues are always present in glycosides and are frequently present in antibiotics (e.g., erythromycin, kanamycin, and novobiocin) and in various other biologically active substances (e.g., enzymes, coenzymes, glycoproteins, and vitamins).

Nitrogen Compounds

Amines and Amine Salts

Amines are organic compounds in which one or more of the hydrogens of ammonia are replaced by organic groups. Primary (R—NH$_2$, e.g., amphetamine), secondary (R$_2$NH, e.g., desoxyephedrine), or tertiary (R$_3$N, e.g., tripelennamine) amines are thus formed depending on the number of organic substituents (i.e., R = 1, 2, or 3). The groups may be aliphatic, aromatic, alicyclic, or derived from a heterocycle. Amines are also sometimes classified according to the number of nitrogen atoms in the molecule (e.g., C$_2$H$_5$NH$_2$) as monoamines (e.g., C$_2$H$_5$NH$_2$—ethylamine), diamines (e.g., NH$_2$CH$_2$CH$_2$NH$_2$—ethylene diamine), or triamines (e.g., NH$_2$CH$_2$CH$_2$NHCH$_2$-CH$_2$NH$_2$—diethylene triamine).

Polyamines are sometimes mixtures of primary, secondary, and tertiary types.

    1. Monofunctional amines—e.g., amphetamine, pheniramine, and tuaminoheptane.
    2. Amine derivatives of alcohols and phenols—e.g., cyclopentolate, ephedrine, and thiamine.
    3. Amino acids.
    4. Amino acid, esters of.
    5. Amino acids, salts of.
    6. Amine derivatives of amides (with or without other functional groups)—e.g., chlortetracycline, folic acid, and methotrexate.
    7. Amine derivatives of sulfonamides.
    8. Polyfunctional amines (other than 2 through 7 above)—e.g., aminophylline, cyclophosphamide, and oxophenarsine.

Many heterocyclic compounds, including the alkaloids, contain =N— or —NH— (or —NR—) in the ring and therefore display properties of amines

although they are not classified as such here. Synthetic heterocycles having nuclei of the:

$$\overline{C \cdot C_n \cdot NH} \text{ or } \overline{C \cdot C_n \cdot NR}$$

type are presented under *Imines,* page 444.

Amines of low molecular weight (C$_1$–C$_3$) are usually gases (e.g., (CH$_3$)$_3$N). Those of higher molecular weight are liquids or solids soluble in ether. The C$_1$–C$_5$ compounds are soluble in water.

Caution: Amines are sometimes irritating to skin and mucous membranes. Allergic reactions have been reported.

The simple amines are not used to any extent in medicine, but their ionic and organic reactions are very important since the amino groupings occur in many important drug classes; e.g., alkaloids, amino acids, aniline derivative, basic dyes, cinchophen derivatives, imides, purine bases, pyrazolon derivatives, proteins, sulfonamides, and in local anesthetics, antihistaminics, antibiotics, tranquilizers, sympathetic amines, parasympathetic amines, etc.

The ionic reactions of these compounds are identical with those of ammonia; e.g., they interact with water to form alkaline solutions:

$$NH_3 + HOH \longrightarrow NH_4^+ + OH^-$$

$$RNH_2 + HOH \longrightarrow RNH_3^+ + OH^-$$

$$NH_3 + HCl \longrightarrow NH_4^+ + Cl^-$$

$$RNH_2 + HCl \longrightarrow RNH_3^+ + Cl^-$$

The three classes of amines form salts with all strong organic and inorganic acids.

The amine salts formed are highly ionized, generally crystalline and are usually soluble in water or alcohol. On addition of stronger bases or excess alkali or hydroxyl ions the amine bases are again liberated and may separate out as "oils" or crystals if the free amine is not soluble in the vehicle: e.g.,

$$RNH_3Cl + OH^- \longrightarrow RNH_2 + HOH + Cl^-$$

amphetamine HCl amphetamine↓

Generally, aqueous solutions of the aliphatic amines, e.g., CH_3NH_2 ($pK_a = 11.7$), are more basic than ammonia ($pK_a = 9.24$), but solutions of the aromatic amines, e.g., aniline or phenylamine, $C_6H_5NH_2$ ($pK_a = 4.58$) are weaker. The basicity is due to the unshared pair of electrons on the nitrogen atom which hydrogen bond with the hydrogen ion (proton) of water-forming polar associations and free hydroxyl ions: i.e.,

$$R:\overset{R}{\underset{\dot{R}}{N}}: + H:OH \rightleftarrows R:\overset{R}{\underset{\dot{R}}{N^+}}:H + OH^-$$

The aromatic amines are weaker because of the additional negative character added by the aromatic ring. Usually one negative group (e.g., phenyl, nitro, carbonyl, amide, ester, or other unsaturated group) held directly on the nitrogen of the amine is sufficient to eliminate the basicity while two such substituents may decrease the basicity to such an extent that feeble acidic properties occur. Organic reactions are not too common in prescriptions containing amines. Primary amines may react with aldehydes:

$$RNH_2 + R'CHO \rightleftarrows R'—\overset{H}{\underset{}{C}}=N—R + H_2O$$

Amines are usually stable in acid media even in the presence of strong oxidizing agents.

Amines may also react with nitrous acid (present in decomposed ethyl nitrite spirit or in mixtures of nitrites in acid solution).

Primary amines may react with mineral acids and nitrites (i.e., nitrous acid) to form alcohols and alkenes.

$$RNH_2 + Na—O—N=O + 2HCl \rightarrow$$

$$ROH + N_2 + Na^+ + Cl^-$$

Secondary amines treated with these reagents form water insoluble *N*-nitrosoamines.

$$R_2NH + Na—O—N=O + HCl \rightarrow$$

$$R_2N—N=O + H_2O + Na^+ + Cl^-$$

Tertiary amines do not react but may form salts with the acid present.

$$R_3N + Na—O—N=O + 2HCl \rightarrow$$

$$R_3N·HCl + Na^+ + Cl^- + H—O—N=O$$

Amine salts are usually more stable than the corresponding free amine base; however, incompatibilities due to the acid anions present (e.g., sulfate, phosphate, etc.) are common.

Aryl Substituted Amines—Aryl substituted amines occur in numerous therapeutic classes, e.g., sympathomimetic amines, analgesics, alkaloids, synthetics, *et al.* Aryl amines are resistant to changes by hydrolysis or reduction but are frequently sensitive to oxidation with production of colored products (quinones, qv). As noted before, the negative nature of the aromatic ring in these amines greatly reduces the basicity of the amine group. Thus their tendency for salt formation is reduced.

Aryl amines with additional negative groups (i.e., Class II —COOH, —NO2, etc.) are such weak bases they do not form salts (e.g., acetanilide, acetophenetidin, etc.).

The attachment of certain aryl groups to the beta carbon of an aliphatic amine is correlated with stimulating action on the sympathetic nervous system in such compounds.

Typical aryl amines and amine salts encountered in dispensing include the following adrenergic, bronchodilator, and vasopressor polyfunctional amines:

Adrenergic—e.g., ephedrine and tuaminoheptane.

Bronchodilator—e.g., epinephrine and isoproterenol; *nasal:* naphazoline and xylometazoline; *ophthalmic:* phenylephrine and epinephryl borate.

Vasopressor—e.g., levarterenol and mephentermine.

Aniline Derivatives (*see also* Analgesics)

Most of these amine derivatives are both aniline (amine) derivatives and amides (qv). Some resemble aniline in their metabolism.

Imines

Quite a number of official drugs contain saturated or unsaturated residues from the cyclic polymethyleneimines (often referred to as cyclic imines) which may be represented by the formula:

$$\overline{CH_2(CH_2)_n NH}$$

The simplest of these cyclic imines is ethyleneimine (aziridine),

$$\overline{CH_2CH_2NH}$$

which, due to ring strain, is a highly reactive chemical. As the number of C atoms in the ring increases, however, this reactivity subsides. The result is that these higher members display essentially the properties of secondary amines and are, indeed, often considered as such.

These cyclic imines are true heterocyclic compounds, and they and their derivatives are often so named. For example, tetramethyleneimine,

$$\overline{CH_2CH_2CH_2CH_2NH}$$

is the familiar pyrrolidine. Like the amines (qv) they add acids to form (-iminium) salts, and the imino hydrogen is readily alkylable to give *N*-alkyl derivatives which resemble chemically the tertiary amines.

Examples of polyfunctional compounds containing the imine function are derivatives of methyleneimine (e.g., nitrofurantoin), derivatives of monocyclic imines (e.g., meperidine), and imine derivatives containing fused ring systems (e.g., dextromethorphan).

Amides

Amides are neutral compounds derived from ammonia by replacement of one or more hydrogen atoms by acyl residues:

$$-NO_2, \; -SO_3H, \; or \; -\overset{\displaystyle O}{\overset{\|}{C}}-R$$

Like the amines these may be subdivided into primary, secondary, and tertiary amides depending on the number of acyl groups linked with the nitrogen atom. Certain primary amides:

$$R-\overset{\displaystyle O}{\overset{\|}{C}}-N\overset{\displaystyle H}{\underset{\displaystyle H}{<}}$$

can theoretically form from the dehydration of organic ammonium salts (e.g., by heat in the presence of free acid), by the reaction of esters with ammonia (i.e., with the formation of the amide and alcohol), etc., however it is doubtful if these reactions occur normally in prescriptions.

Carboxylic acid amides being neutral compounds show little salt formation with acids. At higher temperatures these amides may hydrolyze in water in the presence of hydrogen ion catalysts to form acids and ammonium salts. The hydrolysis is even faster with hydroxyl ion catalysts with the formation of alkali salt of the organic acid and free ammonia, i.e.:

$$R-\overset{\displaystyle O}{\overset{\|}{C}}-NH_2 + HOH \xrightarrow{(H^+)}$$

and

$$R-\overset{\displaystyle O}{\overset{\|}{C}}-OH + NH_4^+$$

$$R-\overset{\displaystyle O}{\overset{\|}{C}}-NH + HOH \xrightarrow{(-OH)}$$

$$R-\overset{\displaystyle O}{\overset{\|}{C}}-O- + NH_3$$

These amides are stable toward mild oxidizing agents but strong reducing agents may produce primary amines and water:

$$R-\overset{\displaystyle O}{\overset{\|}{C}}-NH_2 \xrightarrow{(H)} R-\overset{\displaystyle H}{\underset{\displaystyle H}{\overset{\displaystyle |}{\underset{\displaystyle |}{C}}}}-NH_2 + H_2O$$

Such amides may also undergo tautomerization of the active hydrogen to form imino compounds:

$$R-\overset{\displaystyle O}{\overset{\|}{C}}-NH \rightleftarrows R-\overset{\displaystyle OH}{\overset{\displaystyle |}{C}}=NH$$

The latter may then form salts with metals.

Examples of amides are monofunctional (e.g., diethyltoluamide) and polyfunctional (e.g., cyanocobalamin).

Urea is an example of an amide which produces important secondary amides (i.e., ureides) on acylation. These may be useful as sedatives (e.g., bromural, adaline, *et al*). The cyclic ureides of malonic acid are discussed under barbiturates (qv). Many of the esters of amides (urethanes or carbamates):

$$R-O-\overset{\displaystyle O}{\overset{\|}{C}}-NH_2$$

are useful as hypnotics and insecticides. Ergonovine, and related ergot alkaloids; procainamide, dibucaine, and related local anesthetics; caffeine and other xanthine derivatives; saccharin and other imides; and salicylamide are also important amides. Sulfonamides (see separate entry) are especially important amides with sulfuric acid as the acyl group.

Polyfunctional Nitrogen Compounds

Ureides (*Urea Derivatives, Excepting Barbiturates*)

See *Phenytoin Sodium,* page 582.

Purine Bases (*Xanthines*)

Caffeine, theobromine, and theophylline are feebly basic substances related to amides such as purine and uric acid. Caffeine is 1,3,7-trimethylxanthine, theobromine is 3,7-dimethylxanthine, and theophylline is 1,3-dimethylxanthine. These compounds resemble the alkaloids in that they have weak basic properties but differ from the latter in that they are not precipitated by potassium mercuric iodide and some of the other general alkaloidal precipitants. The basic properties of the purine bases are so weak that they are scarcely able to form salts with acids, and the so-called salts are very weak combinations or mere mixtures. Guarana, coffee, and kola contain purine bases.

Other important xanthine derivatives include aminophylline, oxtriphylline, and theophylline sodium glycinate.

Imides

The diamides of dicarboxylic acids, $R(CONH_2)_2$, may lose ammonia on strong heating, resulting in the formation of imides,

$$\overline{R.CO.NH_2CO}$$

The imido hydrogen is acidic, thus the imides form well defined salts with alkalies; it is also readily substituted by chlorine and bromine, thus forming the strongly oxidizing *N*-haloimides, e.g., *N*-chlorosuccinimide.

Examples of imides include ethosuximide, glutethimide, and saccharin.

Hydrazides

This term is commonly restricted to the *mono*acyl derivatives of hydrazine; i.e., amide type compounds of the type $RCO \cdot NHNH_2$ (e.g., acetic acid hydrazide or acetohydrazide, $CH_3CO \cdot NHNH_2$). Hydrazides are thus closely related to the primary amides (*mono*acyl derivatives of *ammonia*). Hydrazine derivatives containing more than one acyl group are commonly named as acylated hydrazines; e.g., $CH_3CO \cdot NHNH \cdot COCH_3$ is 1,2-diacetylhydrazine.

Hydrazides are conveniently prepared by hydrazinolysis of esters, the procedure being simply to heat a mixture of the ester and 40% aqueous hydrazine hydrate. The reaction is analogous to the ammonolysis of esters to produce amides.

Examples of hydrazides are isoniazid and isocarboxazid. Other compounds such as phenylbutazone and sulfinpyrazone may be looked upon as acylated hydrazine derivatives.

Alkaloids and Their Salts

Alkaloids are naturally occurring amines which are sometimes also esters or amides. They usually are of vegetable origin and have a powerful physiological action. They will be classified in this chapter as derivatives of several nitrogen ring systems; i.e., pyridine, tropine, quinoline, isoquinoline, phenanthrene, indole, and miscellaneous synthetic systems.

Salts of the alkaloids with acetic, citric, and mineral acids are generally soluble in water but insoluble in ether, chloroform, and oils. The free alkaloids, as a rule, have just the opposite solubility relations, being soluble in ether, chloroform, and oils but insoluble in water. Usually, several thousand milliliters of water are required to dissolve 1 g of alkaloid, but there are some exceptions, e.g., atropine is soluble in water (1 in 460 parts), cocaine (600), colchicine (25), and codeine (120). Alcohol occupies a unique position since it is generally a good solvent for both the free alkaloids and the alkaloidal salts.

The precipitation of alkaloids in liquid prescriptions is a dangerous incompatibility because the alkaloid may settle to the bottom and concentrate in the last dose. The important general alkaloidal precipitants are as follows:

1. Alkalies and alkaline reacting substances such as borax, sodium phosphate, potassium citrate, etc., when added to aqueous solutions of alkaloidal salts in sufficient quantities to make the reaction alkaline, cause precipitation by converting the soluble alkaloidal salt into the insoluble free alkaloid.
2. Tannin and preparations containing tannin precipitate alkaloids as insoluble tannates. Most other organic acids, with the exception of acetic and citric acid, cause a similar precipitation.
3. Picric acid, a solution of iodine and potassium iodide, potassium mercuric iodide, mercuric chloride and gold chloride precipitate most alkaloids.

If the prescription contains a substantial proportion of alcohol or glycerin, the precipitation of alkaloids will usually not occur. In many cases the danger may be eliminated by securing the consent of the prescriber to increase the proportion of alcohol or to change the ingredients so that the alkaloid will not be precipitated. In all cases in which there is a possibility of alkaloidal precipitation it is advisable to attach a "shake" label, and in some cases it may be feasible to add some acacia mucilage or other suspending agent to retard the settling of the precipitate.

As a rule, alkaloids are incompatible with oxidizing agents.

Ester alkaloids are rather easily hydrolyzed by acids or alkalies, e.g., aconitine, atropine, cocaine, colchicine, and hyoscyamine. Amide alkaloids (e.g., ergonovine) are also subject to hydrolysis but are generally more stable than esters.

Color changes occur in aqueous solutions of some alkaloidal salts. Apomorphine hydrochloride solution rapidly becomes green, the change being hastened by alkalies and retarded by slightly acid solutions. A red color develops in aqueous solutions of physostigmine salts; sodium bisulfite, boric acid, and carbonic acid retard the change.

The more soluble alkaloids, e.g., codeine and coniine, are alkaline enough in some cases to cause precipitation in solutions of salts of the heavier metals.

Aqueous solutions of alkaloidal salts frequently show a precipitate due to mold growth. The addition of chlorobutanol (0.5%) for its preservative effect is often advantageous in such cases.

Alkaloids Derived from Pyridine— The free alkaloids derived from pyridine differ from most other alkaloids in two important respects:

(1) they are usually liquids, and
(2) they are more or less soluble in water.

Generally, the salts are crystalline solids which are soluble in water and alcohol. Alkaloids of this group are usually precipitated by the general alkaloidal precipitants, with the exception of alkalies. Alkaline substances do not ordinarily cause precipitation in this group because of the solubility of the free alkaloids in water.

See *Pilocarpine,* page 583.

Alkaloids Derived from Tropine— Several official alkaloids are esters of the hydroxy compound, tropine, with various organic acids. These alkaloids are solids that are very sparingly soluble in water but readily soluble in alcohol. In this group the usual incompatibilities with alkaloidal precipitants are encountered. Since these alkaloids are esters, they are more easily decomposed (being readily hydrolyzed) than most other alkaloids. Scopolamine, a tropic acid ester of scopine, is a liquid which is slightly soluble in water.

The free alkaloids in this group are fairly strong bases; thus, aqueous solutions of the free alkaloids are alkaline, and aqueous solutions of the alkaloidal salts are neutral or only very slightly acid.

Examples include atropine, hyoscyamine, and cocaine.

Alkaloids Derived from Quinoline—The free alkaloids derived from quinoline are solids which are practically insoluble in water but soluble in alcohol. The normal salts of the cinchona alkaloids are neutral or slightly alkaline in aqueous solution. The normal salts are not soluble in water as are the salts of alkaloids derived from pyridine and tropine. Acid salts such as quinine bisulfate are more soluble in water than the normal salts. The alkaloids derived from quinoline are precipitated by the general alkaloidal precipitants. Since the free alkaloids are practically insoluble in water, they are readily precipitated from solutions of alkaloidal salts by alkalies; however, the alkaloids are soluble in alcohol which, if present in sufficiently high concentration, thus corrects the incompatibility with alkaline substances.

Quinine and its salts (page 594) are useful antimalarials, analgesics, and antipyretics. *Caution:* Idiosyncrasies, hypersensitivities and other side effects may occur, especially with IV use.

See also quinidine and its salts, page 594.

Alkaloids Derived from Isoquinoline—The free alkaloids derived from isoquinoline are solids which are insoluble or sparingly soluble in water. Aqueous solutions of the salts are usually slightly acid. The alkaloids of this group are precipitated by the general alkaloidal precipitants.

Alkaloids Derived from Phenanthrene—Morphine, its salts, and its derivatives are useful narcotic analgesics. It has been pointed out that the incompatibilities of such analgesic-narcotic drugs should correspond to those of the organic cationic drugs due to the presence of tertiary nitrogen. Colchicine is also a related phenanthrene derivative. A related narcotic is fentanyl.

Alkaloids Derived from Indole—The free alkaloids in this group are solids which are soluble in alcohol but insoluble or only slightly soluble in water. Aqueous solutions of the salts are neutral or faintly acid.

Examples include physostigmine and ergotamine. Other useful compounds include strychnine and ergonovine.

Synthetics Similar to Alkaloids—Examples include chloroquine, eucatropine, and naphazoline.

Pyrazolon Derivatives

These synthetic derivatives are chiefly nonnarcotic analgesics. They produce colors when mixed with oxidizing agents or ethyl nitrite spirit. They are precipitated from aqueous solutions by alkaloidal precipitants. The solid compounds have a tendency to liquefy or form a soft mass when triturated with a number of hydrogen-bonding substances.

Examples include antipyrine and aminopyrine.

Aliphatic Amino Acids and Derivatives

Amino acids are carboxylic acids which contain an amino (NH_2) group attached to any carbon atom in the radical that is attached to carboxyl. The amino group may thus be attached to an aliphatic, alicyclic, or aromatic moiety. The aliphatic variety is by far the most important.

Amino acids, in general, are solids soluble in water and insoluble in alcohol. Although possessing both amine and carboxyl groups which will react in the normal way, their physical properties differ from the amines and acids since the free amino acids exist largely as internal salts formed between the amino and carboxyl groups. They are amphoteric, forming, for example, either hydrochlorides or sodium salts.

Examples of aliphatic amino acids are aminoacetic acid, dihydroxyaluminum aminoacetate, and methionine. Some derivatives are also important, e.g., acetylcysteine.

Aromatic Amino Acids

Examples include aminobenzoic acid, aminohippuric acid, and aminosalicylic acid.

Quaternary Ammonium Compounds

The quaternary ammonium compounds have the general formula R_4NX in which R represents alkyl or aryl groups, and X represents a monovalent acid radical or a hydroxyl group. The salts are usually prepared by reacting tertiary amines with organic halides: e.g.,

$$(CH_3)_3N + CH_3Cl \longrightarrow (CH_3)_4NCl \longrightarrow$$
$$(CH_3)_4N^+ + Cl^-$$

The quaternary ammonium bases can be prepared from the salts: e.g.,

$$2(CH_3)_4{-}N^+Cl^- + Ag_2O + H_2O \longrightarrow$$
$$(CH_3)_4NOH + 2AgCl$$

As there is no hydrogen atom in the positive R_4N^+ ion, these compounds do not liberate a free amine when treated with an alkali. The quaternary ammonium hydroxides (pK_a = 12–14) are strong, highly ionized, amorphous bases comparable to sodium hydroxide (pK_a = 12–16) and considerably more basic than ammonium hydroxide (pK_a = 9.26). This property is probably due to the fact that quaternary ammonium compounds cannot form hydrogen bonded, undissociated molecules (which would tend to reduce the basicity) as do the amines and ammonia.

$$H:\overset{H}{\underset{\overset{\cdot\cdot}{H}}{N}} + H:\overset{\cdot\cdot}{\underset{\cdot\cdot}{O}}:H \rightleftarrows H:\overset{H}{\underset{\overset{\cdot\cdot}{H}}{N}}:H:\overset{\cdot\cdot}{\underset{\cdot\cdot}{O}}:H \rightleftarrows$$

$$H:\overset{H}{\underset{\overset{\cdot\cdot}{H}}{N}}:H^+ + :\overset{\cdot\cdot}{O}:H^-$$

Quaternary ammonium bases are very soluble in water and readily absorb carbon dioxide from the air.

Quaternary ammonium salts are usually crystalline salts. These are highly ionized, and in aqueous solution the highly charged cation will react with the anions of weak acids (e.g., fatty acids, acidic dyes, certain antibiotics, and barbiturates) to form slightly dissociated and frequently insoluble complexes, i.e.,

$$(R_4N)^+Cl^- + Na^+(O\overset{\overset{O}{\|}}{C}{-}R')^- \rightleftarrows$$

benzalkonium   sodium
  chloride   stearate

$$(R_4N)(-O\overset{\overset{O}{\|}}{C}{-}R') + Na^+ + Cl^-$$

benzalkonium
  stearate

The addition of inorganic or organic salts (e.g., NaCl) will solubilize such complexes as would be expected from the equation. The failure of the precipitate to form in some theoretically incompatible mixtures can often be explained on the basis of salt content or on the hydrophilic groups present in the complex.

The inactivation of quaternary germicides by soaps and other anionic surface-active agents is explained by the previous equation. This may also explain the reduced effectiveness of quaternary germicides in combination with nonionic surface-active agents if the latter contain any free fatty acids or anions. It has been shown that the antibacterial effect of quaternary ammonium compounds is largely due to an anti-enzyme effect. The reaction of positive quaternary cations with negative groups (i.e., R—SH) in the enzyme may explain this action.

Examples are monofunctional (e.g., benzalkonium chloride) and polyfunctional (e.g., denatonium benzoate).

Choline and Its Salts—See *Choline,* page 503.

Curariform Drugs (Muscle Relaxants)—*Warning:* Overdoses may produce loss of diaphragmatic activity and asphyxia. Patients must be watched until normal respiration has returned. Antidote: neostigmine.

Curariform Antagonists—See *Edrophonium Chloride,* page 521.

Parasympathomimetic Agents (Cholinergic Agents)—See, e.g., *Bethanechol Chloride,* page 488.

Parasympathomimetic Agents (Cholinesterase Inhibitors)—See, e.g., *Neostigmine,* page 564.

Ganglionic Blocking Agents—These compounds are autonomic blocking agents with both parasympatholytic and sympatholytic actions.

Parasympatholytic (Cholinergic Blocking) Agents—See, e.g., *Atropine,* page 482.

Other quaternary ammonium compounds having similar properties will be discussed under *Preservatives* (e.g., benzalkonium chloride, etc.), *Surface-Active Agents, Dyes,* and *Vitamins* (qv).

Organic Halogen Derivatives

Examples of these polyfunctional halogen compounds include diiodohydroxyquin and iodochlorhydroxyquin.

Chloramine Derivatives

These chlorine-releasing agents are occasionally used as deodorants and antiseptics.

Organic Sulfur Compounds

There are several types of official organic sulfur compounds. The thiols, thio ethers, sulfonium compounds, and thioureides are sulfur analogs of corresponding oxygen compounds. The others (e.g., disulfides, sulfonamides) are distinctively sulfur compounds which do not have oxygen analogs.

Thiols or Mercaptans—These sulfhydryl compounds are the sulfur analogs of alcohols and phenols. They may also be considered as acid esters (bisulfides). The thiols are weakly acidic and dissolve readily in NaOH solution, forming R·S·Na compounds (*mercaptides*), the sulfur analogs of alkoxides and phenoxides. Mild oxidizing agents such as iodine convert mercaptans into dialkyl disulfides (RS·SR), while strong oxidants such as nitric acid convert them into sulfonic acids.

Examples include thiols (e.g., dimercaprol), mercaptides (e.g., methimazole), and disulfides (e.g., disulfiram).

Sulfones

Sulfones are compounds with the structure:

$$R - \overset{\overset{\displaystyle O}{\uparrow}}{\underset{\underset{\displaystyle O}{\downarrow}}{S}} - R'$$

They are related to the sulfonamides in both structure and activity. They are believed to act through their structural resemblance to para-aminobenzoic acid but may also be metabolized to diaminodiphenyl sulfone (DDS) which can chain two microorganisms together (assuming each ingests the amino portion). Sulfones are more active than sulfonamides but due to their toxicity (dermatitis, hemolytic anemia, etc.) are usually limited to treatment of leprosy and tuberculosis. Sulfones may appear in the urine for as long as 2–3 weeks due to recirculation in the bile. The more complex sulfones (e.g., promin) are poorly absorbed and must be injected for full activity.

Examples of polyfunctional sulfones include dapsone and sulfoxone. Phenolsulfonphthalein may be looked upon as a cyclic sulfone derived from 2,1(3*H*)-benzoxathiole, but it is more revealingly classed as a type of phthalein. Similarly, saccharin may be considered as a sulfone derivative of 1,2-benzisothiazole, but its properties are more evident if it is classed as a sulfonamide.

Glycosides

Glycosides are compounds formed by condensation of sugars with other organic molecules containing hydroxyl (occasionally sulfhydryl) groups. The pharmaceutically important ones are of natural origin.

In the presence of water, glycosides are hydrolyzed by heat, enzymes, or acids but are fairly stable toward alkaline hydrolysis. Most glycosides are precipitated by tannic acid or lead subacetate. A few of the drugs containing glycosides are aloe, cascara sagrada, digitalis, gentian, glycyrrhiza, jalap, strophanthus, and squill. Included among the useful glycosides are digitoxin, digoxin, lanatoside C, ouabain, rutin, and sennosides A and B. These are usually dispensed as solid dosage forms (capsules, tablets, powders) or as freshly reconstituted solutions because of their instability.

Also, various antibiotics and other biologically active substances contain carbohydrate residues in glycosidic union but are not commonly classed as glycosides (e.g., neomycin sulfate).

Proteins

From a chemical viewpoint, the term protein is commonly employed to embrace the following:

(1) naturally occurring condensation polymers of α-aminoacids and of derivatives of these acids,

(2) naturally occurring conjugates of these polymers with other (nonprotein) substances, and

(3) products formed from naturally occurring proteins by hydrolytic and coagulative processes.

Examples of items commonly categorized as proteins are fibrinogen, gelatin, and protamine.

Many other items are, or contain, proteins but are usually classed in more specific use-categories such as enzymes, some hormones, various biological products, surgical sutures, and mild silver protein.

Colistin, oxytocin, and vasopressin are polypeptides.

Solutions of gelatin and other similar proteins are coagulated by tannic acid, formaldehyde, and trinitrophenol, in addition to mercuric, ferric, and certain other heavy metal salts.

Silver-protein preparations are discussed separately.

Enzymes

Many of the enzymes are proteins, or, are so closely associated with proteins that separation is difficult. Thus, many enzymes have the incompatibilities of proteins, e.g., precipitation by alcohol, tannic acid, and salts of heavy metals. Strong solutions of salts may precipitate enzymes by a "salting out" effect. The activity of most enzymes in solution is destroyed by heating at 80°C; however, oxidases must usually be heated at 100°C for a few minutes to destroy their activity.

Organic Peroxides

See, e.g., *Benzoyl Peroxide,* page 487.

Resins

Natural resins generally form soluble resin soaps with alkalies. Resins are precipitated from alcoholic solutions on addition of water. Drugs which contain resins, e.g., guaiac, benzoin, jalap, and ipomea, have the incompatibilities of resins.

Organic Antimony Compounds

Examples include antimony potassium tartrate and stibophen.

Organic Arsenicals

Arseno Compounds—These R·AS:O compounds are analogous to the nitroso compounds in the nitrogen series. Instead of being named as arsenoso compounds, e.g., arsenosobenzene, they are often named as alkylarsenic oxides and as alkyl arsinoxides. Oxidizing agents readily convert the arsenic in arsenoso compounds into its maximum oxidative state.

The only common *arsenoso compound* is oxophenarsine.

Arsonic Acids—These are the arsenic analogs of the phosphonic acids. They may be looked upon as orthoarsenic acid with *one* of its OH groups replaced with a hydrocarbon radical; i.e., R·As(:O)(OH)$_2$. Either the name of the hydrocarbon or the name of its radical is used in naming the acids; e.g., C$_6$H$_5$-AsO(OH)$_2$ is known both as benzenearsonic acid and phenylarsonic acid. Arsonic acids are frequently prepared by *arsonation;* i.e., heating the parent hydrocarbon (or derivative) directly with concentrated orthoarsenic acid. They also result when diazonium salts are reacted with sodium arsenite in the presence of alkali and cuprous chloride. The salts of arsonic acids are termed arsonates.

Examples of marketed pharmaceuticals in this class include the arsonic acid, carbarsone, and the arsonates tryparsamide, drocarbil (an arecolinium salt), and glycobiarsol (a bismuthyl salt).

Arsinic Acids—Like the arsonic acids, these are also derivatives of orthoarsenic acid, but in this case *two* of the OH groups are replaced with hydrocarbon radicals, thus giving the general formula, R$_2$As(:O)OH. The best-known is dimethylarsinic acid, (CH$_3$)$_2$AsO$_2$H, usually called cacodylic acid. Similarly, its salts, the dimethylarsinates, are commonly referred to as cacodylates. Cacodylic acid is easily produced from cacodyl oxide [(CH$_3$)$_2$AsOAs(CH$_3$)$_2$] by oxidation with mercuric oxide in the presence of water. Cacodylic acid is a weak acid and is readily reducible, e.g., with hypophosphorous acid, forming cacodyl (tetramethyldiarsine). Sodium and ferric cacodylates were official for many years prior to 1960.

Organic Bismuth Compounds

Bismuth compounds used as adjuncts to arsenicals in the treatment of syphilis are usually administered intramuscularly, thus permitting the use of insoluble substances as well as soluble substances. Some bismuth compounds are administered in true solution in water, oils, or glycols, while others are used in the form of colloidal solutions or as suspensions in water or oil; e.g., bismuth subnitrate suspension (milk of bismuth). The most common organic bismuth compound is probably the polyfunctional bismuth arsphenamine sulfonate.

Organic Mercury Compounds

Examples include meralluride, nitromersol, and phenylmercuric nitrate.

Polyfunctional Compounds Classified by Use

Analgesics

These drugs are among the most widely used compounds. Examples are aspirin, propoxyphene, and pentazocine.

Antibiotics

Antibiotics hold first place among ingredients used in prescriptions. They occur in about one out of every seven prescriptions.

The stabilities of antibiotics have been reported by several workers. Antibiotics found stable at room temperature (25°C) and refrigerator (5°C) in therapeutically useful concentrations in intravenous solutions of 0.9% saline or 5% dextrose for 60 days were: chloramphenicol 0.5%, gentamicin sulfate 0.16%, kanamycin sulfate 0.5%, lincomycin HCl 0.24%, oleandomycin phosphate 0.2% and vancomycin 0.5%. In addition the following were less stable (i.e., stable for 60 days) in 0.9% saline at refrigerator temperature (5°C) but not at room temperature (25°C): ampicillin sodium 0.5%, carbenicillin disodium 4%, cephalothin sodium 1%, cephaloridine 1%, erythromycin lactobionate 0.5%, methicillin sodium 1.8%, nafcillin sodium 0.5%, penicillin G potassium buffered 20,000 u/ml, tetracycline HCl 1%. Dextrose 5% injection usually gave less (25°C) stability with these antibiotics although the refrigerator stability values (5°C) were the same at 60 days except for ampicillin sodium 0.5% stable only 14 days and nafcillin sodium 0.5% stable 21 days.

Other useful formulation and stability information may be located in the following general discussions of antibiotics by chemical families.

Polypeptides—These antibiotics may be neutral, acidic, or basic in nature. Examples include bacitracin, colistin, and polymyxin B sulfate.

Macrolides—The macrolide antibiotics include erythromycin, oleandomycin, and troleandomycin.

Cephalosporins—These antibiotics are produced by species of the fungus Cephalosporum and from synthetic processes. Examples include cephalothin, cephaloridine, and cephaloglycin.

Polyenes—These antibiotics are so named since they contain a conjugated polyene system. Several have useful antifungal activity; e.g., amphotericin, candicidin, and nystatin.

Penicillins—Penicillins are strong, monobasic carboxylic acids which are derivatives of the double-ring thiazolidine β-lactam structure commonly known as 6-aminopenicillanic acid. The differences in the physical, chemical, and biological properties of the 30 or more penicillins are due to their side chains. It has been pointed out that the β-lactam ring is quite labile, the relative stability of the penicillin depending on the side chain. The natural penicillins are produced by *Penicillium notatum, Penicillium sp.,* and *Aspergillus sp.* Different forms of penicillin may be obtained by growing these molds in special media. For example, phenoxymethyl penicillin (penicillin V) is grown in a medium containing phenoxyacetic acid. The various penicillins isolated so far (with their side chains indicated in parentheses) have been designated as "F" (2-pentenyl), "G" (benzyl), "K" (*n*-heptyl), "O" (allyl mercapto methyl), "V" (phenoxymethyl), and "X" (*p*-hydroxybenzyl). These penicillins vary slightly in their chemical stability and in their antibacterial potency on different organisms. Since 1958 it has become possible to selectively hydrolyze penicillin enzymatically at the amide linkage to produce 6-aminopenicillanic acid. Theoretically any side chain can now be linked to this nucleus to form a new penicillin. Table 23 gives a comparison of some of the old and new penicillins.

Penicillin is a strong acid. The free acid form is relatively insoluble in water and soluble in most organic solvents. Benzylpenicillin (penicillin G) is hydrolyzed at the lactam ring in neutral or alkaline medium to penicilloic acid. The reaction at constant temperature and pH is first order and is directly proportional to the hydroxyl ion concentration. In strong acid solution penicillin is rearranged to penicillic acid. This also is a first-order reaction at constant temperature and pH, and here depends on the hydrogen ion concentration. The pH profile indicates that the pH of minimum degradation is about pH 6.5, thus citrate and phosphate buffers are frequently used to formulate solutions at this pH value. Penicillin forms salts with inorganic and organic bases. It reacts with certain alcohols and amines to form the esters and amides respectively of penicilloic acid. A number of esters have been described in the literature but are not in current use.

In solid dosage forms the most critical factor in the stability of penicillin is moisture. It has been shown that when the moisture content in vials of crystalline sodium penicillin G was above 4%, significant loss in potency (40–80%) occurred after 6 months at 25°C. The effect was much less pronounced at refrigerator temperatures. The stability of many lots of commercial crystalline sodium and potassium penicillin in dry vials have shown only slight losses (1.5–2%) after three years at 25°C. The relatively insoluble amine salts of penicillin (e.g., procaine) are even less sensitive to moisture.

In addition to the incompatibilities noted with acids, bases, and water, a number of other incompatibilities have been determined. It has been pointed out that any material which changes the pH away from the neutral region will be incompatible with penicillin in solution. Specific incompatibilities mentioned include: oxidized cellulose, chlorocresol, glycerin, and glycols, heavy metals,

Table 23—Various Characteristics of Penicillins

Generic name	Trade names	Chemical name	Prosthetic group formula	Relative availability (unbound)	Blood level[a]	Activity Gram-positive sensitive	Activity Gram-positive resistant	Activity Gram-negative sensitive	Half-life[b]
Penicillin G	Many	Benzyl-		++++	+	++++	−	+++	+
Phenoxy-methyl-penicillin	Compocillin V (*Abbott*) Pen-Vee (*Wyeth*) V-Cillin (*Lilly*)	α-Phenoxy-methyl (Penicillin V)		++	++	+++	−	++	++
Thiphen-cillin	. . .	Phenylmercap-tomethyl-		++	++	+++	−	++	++
Phenethi-cillin	Alpen (*Schering*) Broxil Chemipen (*Squibb*) Darcil (*Wyeth*) Maxipen (*Roerig*) Syncillin (*Bristol*)	α-Phenoxyethyl-		++	+++	++	+	+	+++
Propyl-cillin	Brocillin Ultrapen	α-Phenoxy-propyl-		++	+++	++	+	+	+++
Phenbeni-cillin	Penspek	α-Phenoxy-benzyl-		++	++++	++	+	+	++
Methicillin	Celbenin Dimocillin (*Squibb*) Staphcillin (*Bristol*)	2,6-Dimethoxy-phenyl-		+++	+	+	+++	−	+
Oxacillin	Prostaphlin (*Bristol*) Resistopen (*Squibb*)	5-Methyl-3-phenyl-4-isoxazolyl-		+	++	+	++++	−	++
Ampicillin	Penbritin (*Ayerst*)	α-Aminobenzyl-		+++	++++	++	−	++++	++++

[a] Oral administration.
[b] Values at pH 2.0. Penicillin G and methicillin are buffered.

amines, resorcinol, zinc oxide, thiamine hydrochloride, procaine, ephedrine, iodine and iodides, alcohols, oxidizing agents, thiols, sugars, acids, aminoacridine hydrochloride, thimerosal, and certain flavors. Generally alcohols, glycols, polyglycols, glycerin, and some sugars appear to react with penicillin, probably by esterification of the acid group of the β-lactam ring forming biologically inactive penicilloates. Thiols act in a similar manner; however, thiosulfate and metabisulfite have no deleterious effect. Sulfite, bisulfite, and heavy metal traces catalyze the hydrolysis. Amines may form insoluble "oils" or crystals (if the salt formed is insoluble) but others may react to form a penicilloamide.

Tablets and troches containing most of the various penicillin salts can be made with various ingredients such as acetyl-*p*-aminophenol, most of the antihistamines, aluminum stearate, benzocaine, caffeine, calcium carbonate, calcium stearate, codeine, various dyes (such as FDC Red #1, FDC Red #3, FDC Yellow #1, and FDC Yellow #5), many flavoring agents (such as peppermint oil, lemon oil, spearmint oil, anethole, and cherry), lactose, magnesium stearate, magnesium trisilicate, phenacetin, salicylamide, sodium bicarbonate, sodium gentisate, starch, all of the sulfa drugs, and talc. Soluble effervescent tablets of sodium or potassium penicillin also are made with anhydrous citric acid, sodium benzoate, and sodium bicarbonate. If the moisture content of products containing the above is kept low, the products are stable for at least three years at room temperature and many months at summer temperatures. It is possible to make tablets or capsules containing an antihistamine, aspirin, caffeine, phenacetin, and procaine penicillin.

In the preparation of powders or granules for oral use containing potassium, procaine, or sodium penicillin one can use buffers (such as aluminum hydroxide, citrates, and phosphates), the parabens, acetyl-p-aminophenol, many of the antibiotics, Benemid, bismuth subcarbonate, caffeine, cocoa, codeine, dyes (such as FDC Red #2, FDC Red #4, FDC Green #2, and FDC Yellow #5), kaolin, phenacetin, salicylamide, sodium gentisate, sodium salicylate, preservatives (such as sodium benzoate), soluble and insoluble saccharin, Sucaryl, sugar, sulfa drugs (regularly available), and thickening agents (such as carboxymethylcellulose, gum acacia, gum tragacanth, and pectin). Flavors such as anethole, anise oil, clove oil, lemon oil, lime oil, and various cherry, strawberry, and raspberry flavors have been found acceptable. Vanillin and coumarin have been reported to cause inactivation of penicillin after extended storage, however. Antihistamines such as Bristamin and several of the vitamins such as B_1, B_2, B_6, B_{12}, calcium pantothenate, and niacinamide appear compatible. If these products are made with a low moisture content, the dry powder will be stable for two to three years at room temperature. After reconstitution with water, they will be stable for approximately 1 week under refrigeration.

Penicillin suppositories can be made with cocoa butter and spermaceti. Benzocaine, urea, various sulfa drugs, and some other antibiotics are compatible. The carbowax or glycerin type of suppository is not satisfactory for penicillin.

Penicillin ointments are of the grease type in which penicillin is stable for long periods of time. Petrolatum, bees-

wax, and mineral oil can be used. Lanolin can also be used if the peroxide content is very low. If lanolin with a high peroxide content is used, deterioration rapidly occurs. It has been pointed out that penicillin ointments made with peroxide bleached bases lose about 30% potency in seven months. If the peroxide value of petrolatum is kept below 0.06, stability is much greater. Penicillin is stable for only a few days in hydrophilic ointment base. A carbowax type, water miscible base can be made, but the penicillin is stable for 1–2 months under refrigeration and for only a few days at room temperature. Oil-in-water or vanishing cream type ointments are satisfactory for only a few days under refrigeration.

Ophthalmic ointments, very similar to the regular ointment described, can be made.

Dry powders for reconstitution with water can be made containing parabens, potassium chloride, potassium dihydrogen phosphate, sodium chloride and disodium phosphate. The reconstituted solutions are isotonic and are stable in the reconstituted state for 1 week under refrigeration. The dry ingredients are stable for long periods of time.

Dry powders for reconstitution with water can be used for nasal solutions. In this type of product penicillin is compatible with amphetamine, some of the various antihistamines, dl-desoxyephedrine HCl, ephedrine sulfate, FDC Yellow #5, FDC Green #2, lactose, phenylephrine HCl, sodium chloride, and sodium citrate. The dry powders are stable for 1–3 years at room temperature, and after reconstitution they are stable for about a week under refrigeration.

In the parenteral field, sodium, potassium, procaine, and many other penicillin salts can be suspended in injectable oils such as peanut oil and sesame oil. These products are stable for long periods of time, and at elevated temperatures. On gelling these oils with aluminum monostearate and suspending the same penicillin salts in them, improved products are obtained. These are stable for many years at room temperature and are also stable for at least 1–2 years at temperatures of 37° and 56°C. Edible oils such as corn oil, cottonseed oil, and soya bean oil are also useful and compatible. The oils used should have a moisture content of less than 0.1% and a free fatty acid content of less than 0.1%. Penicillin is stable also in mineral oil suspensions.

Aqueous suspensions for parenteral use are widely used. These aqueous suspensions of sparingly soluble amine salts (e.g., procaine, N,N′-dibenzylethylene diamine, N,N′-bis(dehydroabietyl)ethylenediamine) preferably contain buffers such as sodium citrate and suitable suspending and dispersing agents such as carboxymethylcellulose, lecithin, polysorbate, and polyvinyl pyrrolidone. Preservatives such as benzyl alcohol, the parabens, and the quaternaries are used. Quaternary ammonium compounds, e.g., 0.01% centrimide, appear as the best preservatives for many injectable suspensions (300,000 to 600,000 U/ml). These are both effective as preservatives and compatible with penicillin. Phenol (0.5%) or benzyl alcohol (1.5%) partially solubilize the antibiotic and affect the viscosity and color. The parabens slowly form a precipitate with procaine penicillin. Phenylmercuric nitrate (0.001%) is apparently partially inactivated. Procaine HCl (2%) is frequently used as a stabilizer. Considerable attention must be paid to particle size in order to have products which are acceptable in physical characteristics such as fluidity, ease of injectability, ease of resuspendability, etc. These suspensions are stable for 1 or 2 years either under refrigeration or at room temperature.

In the parenteral field there are also products which are dry powders for reconstitution with sterile water or physiological saline solution. Practically all compatibilities mentioned for the other parenteral products hold true for this type of product. Although these products are stable for several years in the dry state they are stable for only 1–2 weeks under refrigeration after reconstitution.

Streptomycin and Related Antibiotics—A number of important antibiotics are produced by *Streptomyces sp.* These include streptomycin, neomycin, and kanamycin. Note that gentamycin, a closely related antibiotic, structurally speaking, is obtained commercially from *Micromonosporo purpurea.*

All of these antibiotics are sulfates; hence, they usually show the incompatibilities expected of sulfate ions in dilute solutions although in some cases the expected insoluble sulfate may not precipitate, e.g., antibiotic mixtures theoretically yielding insoluble calcium sulfate.

Tetracyclines—Because these broad spectrum antibiotics are used in a wide range of topical, oral, and parenteral prescriptions, the pharmacist will often need the following compatibility information.

The tetracyclines are derivatives of an octahydronaphthacene hydrocarbon which is made of a system of four fused rings:

Tetracycline

A number of these compounds are in current use, all of which have the specific tetracycline activity and are similar in physiochemical and antibiotic properties. Differences are mainly found in the stability in acid and alkaline medium, the rate of absorption and excretion, and the degree of gastrointestinal disturbances produced. Certain minor changes in the molecule can take away antibacterial activity completely and structure-activity relationships are not fully understood. The active members are used orally, intramuscularly, or intravenously for both Gram-positive and Gram-negative organisms, *Brucella,* etc. They apparently act to block protein synthesis. Their chief toxicity problem is one of superinfection or overgrowth of resistant organisms. This may produce intestinal irritation, diarrhea, etc.

Examples are demeclocycline, methacycline, and tetracycline.

Barbiturates

Barbiturates are widely used sedatives and hypnotics. They are chemical derivatives of barbituric acid, a cyclic compound prepared from urea and malonic acid; hence, they are special polyfunctional amides sometimes described as hydropyrimidine derivatives or malonyl-ureas. Barbituric acid may exist as a "keto" form [1] or as an "enol" form [2].

[1]   [2]

The "enol" form is acidic in nature and can ionize at position 5 to produce a free hydrogen ion and a barbiturate ion. The latter may form metallic salts.

Barbituric acid itself has no hypnotic activity but is highly active when substituted at the 5,5 or the 1,5,5 positions with saturated, unsaturated, aromatic, and/or heterocyclic organic radicals. The resulting sedatives and hypnotics vary in length of activity from "ultrashort" to "long," usually depending on the rate at which they are inactivated by the liver or stored in the body fat. The substitution of a sulfur for the oxygen in the 2 position produces an "ultrashort" type barbiturate. These ultrashort acting compounds (e.g., thiopental) begin their action in seconds and last only for minutes hence are useful for intravenous anesthesia. The short acting (e.g., secobarbital or pentobarbital) or intermediate acting (e.g., amobarbital or butabarbital) types begin their action in minutes and may

last up to 8 hours, hence are useful in preoperative sedation and insomnia.

The long-acting types (e.g., phenobarbital, mephobarbital) usually begin acting after an hour and may last 10–12 hours thus are used for epilepsy, hypertension, and psychoses. The addition of bromine to the substituting groups may increase the sedative nature of the compound (e.g., butallylonal).

Usually, saturated solutions of the relatively insoluble 5,5-disubstituted barbiturates are only slightly acid. This is because the solid is probably present chiefly in the keto form and, hence, only slightly ionized. Addition of alkali (e.g., NaOH) to the insoluble "acid" produces a very soluble salt by replacement of the hydrogen of the NH group by sodium. Such salts are amides thus usually not very stable in solution and readily decompose under the influence of heat, light, and air. Carbon dioxide, for example, may liberate the insoluble free acid, unless buffers such as sodium carbonate are present. The degradation of various barbiturates in the presence of sodium hydroxide at room temperature has been studied and found increasing instability with an increase in methyl groups. Hydrolysis through autoclaving, boiling, or prolonged storage may produce insoluble precipitates of disubstituted acetyl carbamides and other inactive compounds. Such hydrolysis can be reduced by storage of the solutions in a refrigerator. The derivatives of barbituric acid are soluble in alcohol but only sparingly soluble in water.

Solutions of soluble barbiturates are quite alkaline, with pH values around 10 or above. The addition of any material which will lower the pH value to about 8.8 or below will usually precipitate at least part of the barbiturate as the free acid; thus, alkaloidal salts, acid buffers, acidic vitamins, acid syrups, and other acidic substances may produce precipitation. This does not apply to dilute solutions of barbital or other water-soluble barbiturate acids. A more complete list of incompatible substances may be obtained from a study of the sections of this chapter on "pH" and "Commercial Products Used as Vehicles." It should be recognized that buffer substances which may be present in commercial products make difficult an absolute prediction of compatibility or incompatibility based on the pH of the single components.

In the above mentioned incompatibilities, alcohol, glycerin, or propylene glycol may be added to solubilize the liberated barbiturate. Polyethylene glycol 400 is sometimes used as a stabilizing solvent in parenteral barbiturate solutions.

It is preferable to use the free acid form of the barbiturate in certain combinations, e.g., with thiamine HCl, since the alkalinity of the soluble barbiturate may decompose the other ingredients.

Soluble barbiturates are incompatible with ammonium salts and will liberate ammonia according to the reaction:

Sodium Barbiturate + $NH_4Cl \longrightarrow$

Barbiturate +

$$Na^+ + Cl^- + NH_3$$

Insoluble Barbiturates—The derivatives of barbituric acid are soluble in alcohol but only sparingly soluble in water. Soluble barbital and similar water-soluble derivatives are made by replacing the hydrogen of one of the NH groups with sodium. Aqueous solutions of the soluble barbital derivatives are alkaline in reaction; if they are acidified, the Na group is replaced with hydrogen, and the resulting insoluble barbiturate compound is again precipitated.

Other Compounds Similar to Barbital—Among other derivatives of barbituric acid having solubilities and chemical properties similar to those of barbital are the following:

Aprobarbital
Cyclobarbital
Cyclopentenyl allylbarbituric acid
Diallylbarbituric acid
Heptabarbital
Hexobarbital

Methabarbital
Mephobarbital
Narconumal
Talbutal
Phenobarbital
Allylbarbituric acid

Soluble Barbiturates—A number of water soluble salts of barbituric acid derivatives have been described. These readily hydrolyze in water to give alkaline solutions (pH 9–10). Buffering apparently has no real practical value in preventing hydrolysis.

Other Soluble Barbiturates—Among other compounds having properties similar to soluble barbital are the following:

Sodium Alurate (*Roche*)
Sodium Amytal (*Lilly*)
Sodium Butisol (*McNeil*)
Sodium Cyclopal (*Upjohn*)
Sodium Delvinal (*MSD*)
Sodium Evipal (*Winthrop*)
Calcium Ipral (*Squibb*)
Sodium Ipral (*Squibb*)
Sodium Luminal (*Winthrop*)
Sodium Nembutal (*Abbott*)
Sodium Ortal (*Parke-Davis*)
Sodium Pentol (*VanPelt & Brown*)
Sodium Seconal (*Lilly*)
Sodium Surital (*Parke-Davis*)

Psychotherapeutic Drugs

Psychotherapeutic drug is the term used by the Council on Drugs of the American Medical Association to describe those polyfunctional medications which have been known by a variety of names, including antidepressant, antipsychotic, ataraxic, tranquilizer, normalizer, calmative, neurosedative, psychic energizer, pacific, anticonfusion, and antihallucination drugs.

Examples are antidepressant (e.g., amitriptyline), antipsychotic (e.g., mesoridazine), and tranquilizer (e.g., meprobamate).

Tranquilizers may be divided chemically into:

(a) Phenothiazine derivatives,
(b) Reserpine derivatives,
(c) Diphenylmethane derivatives,
(d) Benzodiazepine derivatives,
(e) Mephenesin derivatives, and
(f) Other tranquilizers.

Psychic energizers may be characterized as

    (g) Diphenylmethane derivatives and related compounds,
      (h) Monoamine oxidase inhibitors,
      (i) Dibenzazepine derivatives, and
      (j) Other psychic energizers.

The phenothiazine tranquilizers resemble the phenothiazine antihistaminics except that the tranquilizers have a three-carbon chain between the nitrogen of the nucleus and the dimethylaminoalkyl side chain. The members with an aliphatic side chain (e.g., chlorpromazine, promazine, etc.) generally show less extrapyramidal tract symptoms but more jaundice and agranulocytosis than members whose side-chain nitrogen is included in a piperazine ring (e.g., prochlorperazine, perphenazine, etc.). Members whose side-chain nitrogen is included in a piperidine ring are still less toxic (e.g., thioridazine, mepazine).

Hormones

Hormones are commonly classified as follows:

Adrenal hormones and related compounds (e.g., desoxycorticosterone).
    Glucocorticoids (e.g., cortisone).
    Progestogens (e.g., progesterone).
    Progestogen-estrogen combinations (ovulation control) (e.g., dimethisterone and estinyl estradiol).
    Ovarian hormones and related estrogenic compounds (e.g., estradiol).
    Nonsteroid estrogens and derivatives (e.g., diethylstilbestrol).
    Thyroid-type compounds (e.g., levothyroxine).
    Antithyroid drugs (e.g., methimazole).
    Testicular hormones and related androgenic compounds (e.g., methyltestosterone).
    Hormone, posterior pituitary, antidiuretic (e.g., vasopressin).

Most prescriptions for hormones still call for manufactured dosage forms; however, an increasing number of prescriptions necessitate compounding hormones with other drugs such as prescriptions for cortisone with vitamins, aspirin, and the like. A number of finely powdered hormones (e.g., micronized cortisone acetate, hydrocortisone, and hydrocortisone acetate) are now available as bulk powders for dispensing use in ointments, suspensions, capsules, powders, or other dosage forms.

    The solubilities of the hormones are discussed under the appropriate drug title. These generally follow the rule that like dissolves like. Thus, steroid hydrocarbons are freely soluble in light petroleum or benzene but sparingly soluble in hydroxylic solvents. On the other hand, steroids having two or more hydroxyl groups are appreciably soluble in ethanol, virtually insoluble in light petroleum or benzene. Steroids having ionized groups—e.g., salts of carboxylic acids, glucuronides, or sulfate conjugates—are generally soluble in water, less soluble in alcohols, and (usually) insoluble in lipid solvents. Some salts formed by steroid anions with organic cations are soluble in lipid solvents.

    It might be noted that oil solubility decreases with an increasing number of hydroxyl groups and increases as these are esterified. Table 24, together with

Table 24—Solubility of Steroid Hormones in Pharmaceutical Solvents[1a]

Type of Compound[a]	Solvents		
	Good	Medium	Poor
No hydroxyls	Light petrolatum Ether Chloroform	Acetone	Ethanol
One hydroxyl	Ether Chloroform Acetone	Light petrolatum Ethanol	
Two hydroxyls	Ether	Acetone Ethanol Chloroform	Light petrolatum
Three hydroxyls		Ethanol Ether Acetone	Chloroform
Conjugates (sulfates or Glucuronides)	Water	Ethanol Acetone	

[a] Very roughly speaking, ester groups (acetoxyl, benzoyloxyl, methoxycarbonyl) or keto groups are each equivalent to $1/2$ or $1/3$ of a hydroxyl group on this scale.

the solubility data given under the particular compound, may be helpful in estimating solubility in pharmaceutical vehicles of which the solubility is unknown.

Most hormones possess more than one reactive group and, accordingly, may be considered in several chemical classes, e.g., alcohols, ketones, etc. The pharmacy of hydrocortisone and cortisone, for example, can be discussed in terms of their three functional groupings: the dihydroxyacetone side chain at carbons 17, 20, and 21; the α,β-unsaturated ketone at carbons 3, 4, and 5; and the secondary alcohol group of hydrocortisone (or the ketone group of cortisone) at carbon 11.

The C-17, 20, 21 side chain reacts like a reducing sugar. Thus, it reduces alkaline silver salts under mild conditions and tetrazolium salts in the presence of tetramethylammonium hydroxide. It also reduces alkaline copper salts. The side chain can be readily oxidized by strong oxidizing agents. Chromic acid oxidation removes the side chain and leaves a ketone group at carbon 17. In alkaline solution (above pH 8) the side chain is readily oxidized by contact with air. Strong acids cause rearrangement or cleavage of the side chain.

The α,β-unsaturated ketone at carbons 3, 4, and 5 is the chromophore responsible for the characteristic ultraviolet absorption exhibited by hydrocortisone and cortisone. This ketone group reacts with bisulfites, certain amines, hydrazines, and other substances which normally react readily with α,β-unsaturated ketones.

The secondary alcohol at carbon 11 in hydrocortisone is relatively inactive, but it can be oxidized to a keto group with chromic acid. In general, hydrocortisone, hydrocortisone acetate, and cortisone acetate have been found to be chemically stable in a wide variety of formulations prepared by conventional procedures. These include compressed tablets, dry-filled capsules, hydrophilic and lipophilic ointments, jellies, lotions, water soluble and oleaginous supposito-

ries, aqueous suspensions, and other pharmaceutical forms.

Although the solubility of the steroids in water is limited, the compounds are stable in neutral or weakly acidic solutions at or near room temperature. They are not stable in alkaline or strongly acidic solutions.

It has been observed that preparations of cortisone and hydrocortisone can be heated for two hours at 130°C without decomposition. Stability to pH changes was also very good; e.g., heating at pH 9 affected cortisone only very slightly.

No incompatibilities have been observed in experimental lots of pharmaceutical formulations containing hydrocortisone and each of the following substances:

In Dry Combinations (*Tablets, Capsules, Powders*)
Cornstarch
Lactose
Magnesium stearate
Aspirin
Pyrilamine maleate
Dibasic calcium phosphate
Potassium chloride
Acacia
Gum tragacanth
Talc
Sucrose

In Lipophilic Ointments
Anhydrous lanolin
Liquid petrolatum
White petrolatum
White wax
Lanette wax
Glyceryl monolaurate
Bacitracin
Polymyxin B sulfate
Chlortetracycline
Gramicidin
Tyrothricin
Neomycin sulfate
Sulfadiazine
Sulfathiazole
Sulfacetamide sodium

In Jellies, Lotions, Creams and Hydrophilic Ointments
Glycerin
Isopropanol
Propylene glycol
Polyethylene glycol 1500
Polyethylene glycol 4000
Cetyl alcohol
Stearyl alcohol
Spermaceti

Titanium dioxide
Sodium alginate
Zinc stearate
Polysorbate 80
Menthol
Camphor
Thymol
Stearic acid
Methyl salicylate
Eucalyptol
Methylcellulose
Diethylene glycol stearate
Veegum
Carboxymethylcellulose
Sodium lauryl sulfate
Methylparahydroxybenzoate
Propylparahydroxybenzoate

Antihistamines (and Related Antiemetic Drugs)

These are usually polyfunctional amines.

Most of the antihistamine prescriptions call for tablets or capsules as supplied by the manufacturer. Some are supplied as injection solutions, suppositories, nasal sprays (e.g., antazoline), topical creams (e.g., promethazine and hydroxyzine), and oral syrups or elixirs (e.g., pheniramine, tripelennamine, and diphenhydramine). The last four dosage forms are sometimes used as vehicles for other drugs, e.g., bronchodilators, analgesics, vasoconstrictors, antibiotics, etc. Occasionally, the pharmacist may be expected to empty capsules or grind tablets in the preparation of compound prescriptions where the bulk drug is not available. The procedure should not be applied to injection or ophthalmic prescriptions. Since antihistamines frequently cause drowsiness, caution should be exercised in administering sedatives or hypnotics with these drugs.

The antihistamines are commonly classified as derivatives of the general formula:

$$R—Z—\overset{\displaystyle |}{\underset{\displaystyle |}{C}}—C—N$$

where Z represents nitrogen, oxygen, or carbon, connecting the side chain to the nucleus. When Z represents oxygen, such derivatives may be classified as "ethanolamine derivatives" (e.g., Benadryl, Decapryn, Bristamin, or Clistin). When Z represents nitrogen, such derivatives are often classified as "ethylenediamine derivatives" (e.g., Antergan, Diatrin, Neo-Antergen, Pyribenzamine, Histadyl, Tagathen, Thenfadil, Neohetramine, Zolamine, Phenergan, Pyrrolazote, or Antistine), and when it represents carbon, such derivatives are classified as "miscellaneous derivatives" (e.g., Trimeton, Chlortrimeton, Pyronil, Thephorin, or Di-Paralene).

The antihistamines are all tertiary amines which form salts with mineral acids and with organic acids (e.g., succinic, fumaric, maleic, malic, tartaric, and citric acids).

$$R_3N + HOOC—CH\text{=}CH—COOH \longrightarrow$$
$$R_3N{\cdot}HOOC—CH\text{=}CH—COOH$$

The organic acid salts may be more stable in air (i.e., less hygroscopic), less toxic, or more potent.

Antihistamine salts may be converted to the water insoluble free amine when the acid group is neutralized by bases such as ammonium hydroxide, sodium hydroxide, etc.

$$R_3N{\cdot}HCl + NaOH \longrightarrow R_3N +$$
$$H_2O + Na^+ + Cl^-$$

As a general rule, antihistamine salts are bitter substances that are freely soluble in water or alcohol. The free bases are usually insoluble in water. Exposure to light usually causes darkening.

The motion sickness drugs are considered here as special-use antihistamines. Their structures, compatibilities, and properties are closely related.

Antihypertensives

Examples include guanethidine, methyldopa, and reserpine.

Vitamins

Vitamins are usually sold as manufactured dosage forms, primarily as mixtures. Multicomponent mixtures may exhibit stability problems even though most of the individual vitamins are stable and may be prepared as reasonably stable products by themselves. Interactions between thiamine and pantothenic acid, thiamine and cyanocobalamin, thiamine and riboflavin, cyanocobalamin and ascorbic acid, niacinamide and ascorbic acid and cyanocobalamin with folic acid, etc., may occur in all types of dosage forms (including dry-filled and oil-filled capsules, tablets, oral liquids, or injection liquids) unless these are properly formulated. It has been noted that even inert formulation additives and diluents may be involved in poorly stable products if they supply moisture, alter pH, introduce trace metals, or other reactive contaminants. Expiration dating of multivitamin products based on room temperature studies of actual formulas seems indicated.

Vitamin A—See *Vitamin A,* page 629.

Vitamin B Complex—The mixture of substances which was originally known as water soluble vitamin B has been separated into a number of components, including vitamin B_1 (thiamine), nicotinic acid (P-P or pellagra preventive factor), vitamin G (B_2 or riboflavin), pyridoxine (vitamin B_6, acrodynia factor), pantothenic acid, biotin, inositol, choline, *p*-aminobenzoic acid, folic acid, and vitamin B_{12}. The existence of other components appears to have been established biologically, but these substances have not yet been identified chemically.

Folic Acid and Citrovorum Factor—See *Folic Acid,* page 532, and *Leucovorin Calcium,* page 547.

Niacin and Niacinamide—See *Niacin,* page 564, and *Niacinamide,* page 564.

Vitamin C—See *Ascorbic Acid,* page 479.

Vitamin D—See *Vitamin D,* page 630.

Vitamin E—Vitamin E occurs in various foods such as wheat germ oil, cottonseed oil, green leafy vegetables, meat, and eggs. Three different compounds showing vitamin E activity have been isolated from natural sources. Alpha-tocopherol, $C_{29}H_{50}O_2$, is the most active substance known at present. Less activity is shown by the beta and gamma tocopherols, which are homologs of the alpha tocopherol, containing one less methyl group attached to the benzene ring.

vitamin E

Vitamin K (Prothrombogenic Vitamin)—See, e.g., *Menadiol Sodium Diphosphate,* page 552.

Multivitamin Products—It has been pointed out the interactions which occur between thiamine and pantothenic acid, thiamine and cyanocobalamin, thiamine and riboflavin, cyanocobalamin and ascorbic acid, niacinamide and ascorbic acid, and cyanocobalamin with folic acid. These are previously mentioned briefly under the first-named vitamin.

A number of other factors are involved in altering the stability properties of multivitamins. Where one factor such as pH may enhance the stability of one vitamin, that same factor may cause the instability of another vitamin. Ten different liquid multivitamin preparations were recently developed and prepared and four of these were formulated with a solution vehicle of 20% water, 40% glycerin, and 40% propylene glycol and a second series of four with a solution of 20% water and 80% propylene glycol. Some formulations contained a sequestering agent (disodium calcium ethylenediamine tetraacetate) to stabilize the oxidative decomposition of ascorbic acid by metals; some contained thiamine mononitrate instead of thiamine hydrochloride since the mononitrate form was reported to be more stable than the hydrochloride; another was formulated with the antioxidant, ethyl-cafferate, to study the antioxidant effect on the stability of vitamin A. Each formulation was initially assayed for ascorbic acid, nicotinamide, pyridoxine, riboflavine, thiamine, and vitamin A and then assayed again after a storage period of 30 days at 47°C.

The experimental results indicated the following: pyridoxine and thiamine, whether in the form of the mononitrate or hydrochloride, are more stable in formulations containing a minimum of water. The stability values for riboflavin ranged from 65 to 92% in all of the formulations. The sequestration phenomenon was effective in increasing the stability of ascorbic acid, which was further enhanced in those preparations containing both the antioxidant and sequestering agent. Relatively low stability was exhibited by nicotinamide but its highest stability values were shown in formulations containing the higher concentrations of water. The stability of vitamin A was increased by the antioxidant. Generally, it was concluded that formulations containing low amounts of water possessed higher stability values than formulations containing larger amounts of water.

In a recent study, seven different oral liquid multivitamin preparations were developed and tested. Three types of vehicles were used:

(1) sorbitol, 45% *w/v*, with the formulation adjusted to pH levels of 3.5, 4.0 and 4.5,
(2) glycerin, 24% *v/v*, propylene glycol, 24% *v/v*, and sorbitol, 25% *w/v;* and
(3) glycerin, 10% *v/v*, propylene glycol, 50% *v/v*, and sorbitol, 18.75% *w/v*.

The pH for the latter two vehicles was 3.4. In all of the formulations antioxidants and chelating agents were used. Each formulation was assayed initially for vitamin A, thiamine hydrochloride, riboflavin, ascorbic acid, nicotinamide, pyridoxine, folic acid, and vitamin B_{12}, and then stored in amber colored bottles at room temperature and at 37°C. The vitamins were assayed after an aging period of 30, 60, and 90 days. Thi-

amine hydrochloride and ascorbic acid were more stable in the formulations containing less amounts of water. Thiamine was more stable at a low pH. The variation of the pH between 3.5 to 4.5 had little effect on ascorbic acid; the stability of vitamin B_{12} increased as the pH became greater. Vitamin A, riboflavin, nicotinamide, and pyridoxine hydrochloride had high stability values in all of the formulations.

Narcotics and Related Drugs

Approximately one out of every 16 prescriptions contains a narcotic. The naturally occurring narcotics and their derivatives are discussed under "Alkaloids" (*viz*, morphine, Pantopon, Dilaudid, codeine, Dionin, cocaine, *et al*). Apomorphine, nalorphine and papaverine, which are nonaddicting but also come under the Controlled Substances Act of 1970 as derivatives of opium, are likewise considered under "Alkaloids." Some of the more commonly prescribed synthetic analgesics are closely related. These generally resemble the alkaloid type narcotics in incompatibilities (e.g., liberation of the insoluble free base on addition of sufficient hydroxyl ions, etc.).

Sulfonamides

Some polyfunctional sulfonamides are valuable even though they have little or no antibacterial activity. This group includes the antidiabetic drugs acetohexamide, chlorpropamide, tolazamide, and tolbutamide. Useful carbonic anhydrase inhibitors and diuretics include acetazolamide, chlorothiazide, and furosemide. Other useful sulfonamides include the antipsychotic agent thiothixene.

Other sulfonamides are antibacterial agents (chiefly bacteriostatic) which are effective against most Gram-positive bacteria (streptococci, staphylococci, pneumococci) many Gram-negative bacteria (gonococci, meningococci, influenza bacilli, and other bacilli), plus Actinomyces and certain large viruses.

They are believed to act against bacteria which require PABA for the synthesis of folic acid (since sensitive bacteria are impermeable to folic acid while insensitive bacteria are probably permeable).

Antibacterial sulfonamides include sulfadiazine, sulfisoxazole, and sulfasalazine.

Sulfonamides have weak acidic properties, due to the —SO$_2$NHR amide group, and form water soluble salts with strong bases. The pK$_a$ values vary from 4.8 to 10.4, with most of them between 6 and 8. The pH values of the sodium salts are usually in the range of 7.5 to 12.5, with most of them around pH 10. These salts have high water solubility, but the free sulfonamides have such low water solubility that only slight neutralization will produce a copious precipitate. Thus, the absorption of CO$_2$ from the air is frequently sufficient to precipitate the free sulfonamide. Typical drugs which may cause precipitation of the free sulfonamides are the mineral acid salts of local anesthetics (tetracaine HCl and procaine HCl), and sympathomimetic amines (Paredrine HBr, and ephedrine HCl). In some cases such precipitation reactions are intended by the physician, i.e., nasal suspensions may be formed by combining 5% sulfathiazole sodium and 2% ephedrine hydrochloride.

If the acidic substance causing the precipitation is present in low concentrations, the solubility of the free sulfonamide in the vehicle may not be exceeded and no precipitate will form. For example, it has been noted that clear, stable solutions can be formed by heating certain dilute aqueous solutions of sympathomimetic amines and sulfonamides and adjusting the pH to 8.7 with 3.6 N HCl:

39

℞	Sodium sulfathiazole	2.5%
	d,l-desoxyephedrine HCl	0.125%
	Sodium sulfite	2.0%
	Glycerine	1%
	Distilled water	q.s.
	HCl q.s. to adjust pH to	8.7

Local Anesthetics

These useful drugs may be divided into two groups based on their solubility.

Slowly Soluble Local Anesthetics— These polyfunctional alkyl esters of aromatic acids are almost insoluble in water and, hence, are unsuitable for injection but are used in the form of dusting powders, ointments, etc., on wounds of the skin or accessible mucous membranes.

Examples are local anesthetics (e.g., benzocaine), topical anesthetics (e.g., lidocaine), dental anesthetics (e.g., procaine), narcotic anesthetics (e.g., cocaine), and ophthalmic anesthetics (e.g., benoxinate).

Soluble Local Anesthetics—These are chiefly polyfunctional amine or amino ester salts which may produce incompatibilities due to their pH, the acids present (e.g., HCl, HNO$_3$, H$_2$SO$_4$, etc.) or in some cases due to the hydrolysis of the ester.

Examples are lidocaine, procaine, and tetracaine.

Dyes

Most of the dyes used in pharmacy may be classified as cationic, anionic, or nonionic. The first two groups usually produce the most problems in compounding since they may interact with oppositely charged components to form insoluble complexes. These are discussed under the ionic type. The pH values, chemical structures, and general properties of many FD&C and D&C dyes are given in Table 25.

Dyes and other colored compounds usually contain certain unsaturated color bearing groups known as chromophores:

The presence of any one of these groups on an aromatic nucleus is usually suffi-

Table 25—Stability of the FD&C Certified Dyes to Various Factors Which May Influence Their Color Stability in Pharmaceutical Preparations

FD&C certified dyes	Acid	Alkali	Light	Reducing agents	Oxidiz- ing agents	pH value[a]
Water-Soluble Dyes						
FD&C Blue #1 (Brilliant Blue)	Moderate	Moderate	Good	Good	Poor	4.9–5.6
FD&C Blue #2 (Indigo Carmine)	Good	Moderate	Poor	Moderate	Poor	8.5
FD&C Green #1 (Guinea Green)	Good	Poor	Poor	Good	Poor	3.2
FD&C Green #2 (Light Green SF Yellowish)	Good	Poor	Poor	Good	Poor	3.5
FD&C Green #3 (Fast Green FCF)	Good	Poor	Good	Good	Poor	4.2–5.8
FD&C Orange #1 (Orange 1)	Moderate	Moderate	Moderate	Poor	Fair	...
FD&C Red #1 (Ponceau 3R)	Good	Good	Good	Poor	Fair	7.3
FD&C Red #3 (Erythrosine)	Poor	Good	Fair	Moderate	Fair	7.7
FD&C Red #4 (Ponceau SX)	Poor	Good	Fair	Moderate	Fair	6.4
FD&C Yellow #1 (Naphthol Yellow)	Good	Good	Moderate	Fair	Fair	7.5
FD&C Yellow #2 (Naphthol Yellow (K salt))	Good	Good	Moderate	Fair	Fair	...
FD&C Yellow #5 (Tartrazine)	Good	Good	Good	Poor	Fair	6.8
FD&C Yellow #6 (Sunset Yellow FCF)	Good	Good	Good	Poor	Fair	6.6
Oil-Soluble Dyes						
FD&C Orange #2 (Orange SS)	...	...	Fair	Poor	Poor	...
FD&C Red #32 (Oil Red XO)	...	...	Fair	Poor	Fair	...
FD&C Yellow #3 (Yellow AB)	...	...	Poor	Poor	Poor	(6.6)
FD&C Yellow #4 (Yellow OB)	...	...	Poor	Poor	Poor	(6.3)

[a] pH values of 1% aqueous solutions (or suspensions).

cient to produce color (e.g., nitrobenzene). Reduction of the radical to the saturated state results in the loss of color (e.g., aniline). Other unsaturated groups, e.g.,

$$-\overset{\overset{\text{O}}{\|}}{\text{C}}-,\ -\overset{\overset{\text{S}}{\|}}{\text{C}}-,\ \overset{}{>}\text{C}{=}\text{N}{-},\ -\text{C}{=}\text{C}{-}$$

may also act as chromophores if they are conjugated: *cf*,

$$\text{CH}_3-\overset{\overset{\text{O}}{\|}}{\text{C}}-\overset{\overset{\text{O}}{\|}}{\text{C}}-\text{CH}_3\ \textbf{(yellow)}$$

$$\text{CH}_3-\overset{\overset{\text{O}}{\|}}{\text{C}}-\text{CH}_2-\overset{\overset{\text{O}}{\|}}{\text{C}}-\text{CH}_3\ \textbf{(colorless)}$$

The type of changes in drugs which decompose with color formation (e.g., neomycin, streptomycin, procaine, *et al*), or with loss of color or change in shade (e.g., amaranth) are believed due to appearance or disappearance of such chromophore groups under the effect of light, acid, alkali, reducing agents, oxidizing agents, catalysts, etc. Of course, in some cases the color change may be due to chromophore formation in an impurity present in the drug. Thus, discoloration does not always suggest loss of potency (e.g., neomycin sulfate). The mere presence of chromophore groups does not make a compound a dye and other polar groups (auxochromes) such as $-\text{OH}$, $-\text{NH}_2$, $-\text{NHR}$, or $-\text{NR}_2$; COOH or SO_3H are also required. The latter groups, however, are frequently added to change an oil-soluble dye into a water-soluble dye. Thus dyes with $-\text{SO}_3\text{Na}$, $-\text{CO-ONa}$ and sometimes $-\text{OH}$ groups are increasingly soluble in water (and insoluble in oil) as the number of these groups increase. For example, FD&C Red #8 with one $-\text{SO}_3\text{Na}$ is soluble less than 2% in water while similar FD&C Red #2 with 3 $-\text{SO}_3\text{Na}$ groups is soluble at 17.2%.

Azo dyes (i.e., most FD&C and D&C dyes which contain the $-\text{N}{=}\text{N}-$ group with one or more aminoalkylated amino, nitro, or phenolic hydroxyl groups) increase or deepen in color with the addition of nitro or methyl groups; with the substitution of hydroxyl groups for amino groups; or with the introduction of more azo groups. Thus the addition of a methyl group to FD&C Yellow #3 to form FD&C Yellow #4 gives a redder shade; while the substitution of hydroxyl for the amino group of the latter gives FD&C Orange #2 and the addition of one more methyl gives FD&C Red #32.

The positions occupied by substituent groups may affect color and solubility. The addition of a nitro group either ortho or para onto oil-soluble orange gives a red color. However the para position gives a deeper red and greater oil solubility. Similarly the introduction of a $-\text{SO}_3\text{Na}$ group in the para position on uncertifiable water insoluble CI #82 Pigment Bordeau gives water soluble Ext D&C Red #8 but introduction in the ortho position gives very slightly soluble D&C Red #10. Many such ortho substituted sulfonates are used as pigments due to their low solubility in both water and oil. Conversion of ortho substituted dyes to oil and water-insoluble calcium, barium, or strontium salts (i.e., alkaline earth salts) further improves their utility as pigments in cosmetics, etc., and also influences their shade. For example, D&C Red #10 (a sodium salt) is orange red, D&C Red #12 (its barium salt) is medium red, D&C Red #13 (its strontium salt) is medium red while D&C Red #11 (its calcium salt) is deep red.

Azo compounds oxidize easily with agents such as hydrogen peroxide and peroxyacetic acid to form azoxy compounds. More drastic oxidation yields nitro compounds. The hydrazo compounds readily undergo isomerization under the influence of strong mineral acids to yield commercially important benzidine-type compounds. Examples of polyfunctional azo compounds are amaranth and evans blue.

Basic Dyes (Cationic)—The basic dyes (R^+X^-) vary considerably in chemical structure, but they have many similar properties. Basic dyes usually contain amine or quaternary ammonium groups. Basic dyes form salts with acids, the colored ion being positively charged as in methylrosaniline chloride. In aqueous solution their particle size is large, and solution is facilitated by use of boiling water. With the exception of methylene blue and bismarck brown, the basic dyes are readily soluble in alcohol. Basic dyes may be mixed together without fear of incompatibility, but they give precipitates with substances having a large, negatively charged ion, such as soaps, tannins, or tartar emetic. They are precipitated by many salts and also tend to precipitate on negatively charged surfaces such as are often provided by filters and glassware. Cationic dyes are incompatible with concentrated mercuric chloride. Solutions of basic dyes should be stored in the dark as they are rapidly decolorized in sunlight. Precipitation results when basic dyes are mixed with acid dyes.

Acid Dyes (Anionic)—Acid dyes usually contain $-SO_3H$ or $-COOH$ groups which form salts with bases, e.g., $-SO_3Na$ and COONa. The colored ion is accordingly negatively charged as in scarlet red sulfonate. All of the water soluble FD&C dyes belong to this class. In aqueous solution, the particle size of acid dyes (Na^+R^-) is usually distinctly smaller than that of basic dyes. As a class, acid dyes are less soluble in alcohol than basic dyes and are insoluble in oils and fats. Acid dyes are not precipitated by tannins or other acid dyes but are incompatible with all basic dyes.

Vegetable Colors

See *Caramel,* page 493.

Carbohydrates

See, e.g., *Dextrose,* page 514.

Gums

Gums are defined here as carbohydrates or carbohydrate-like materials which dissolve or swell in water yielding a viscous liquid, from which they are precipitated on addition of sufficient alcohol. Gums are incompatible with strong oxidizing agents. The incompatibilities common to gums such as acacia, tragacanth, and agar are shared by mucilaginous drugs, e.g., althea, elm, malt, manna, and honey.

Gums dissolve in water very slowly. For quick extemporaneous preparation of mucilages, the powdered gum is triturated with a small proportion of alcohol or glycerin, and water is added with rapid trituration. Alcohol or glycerin facilitates wetting of the gum and aids in preventing lumping; thus, the mucilage may be prepared in less time than by the use of water alone.

Examples are acacia , carboxymethylcellulose, and tragacanth.

Surface-Active Agents

Substances which lower the surface tension of a liquid or the interfacial tension between two liquids are called surface-active agents. Such compounds are used as wetting agents, emulsifiers, dispersing agents, detergents, and foaming agents. Surface-active agents or interfacial modifiers consist of two component parts—a hydrophilic group which tends to make the compound water soluble and a lipophilic group which tends to make it oil soluble. There are three classes of surface-active compounds, designated as anionic, cationic and nonionic agents.

Anionic agents are those in which the negative ion contains the lipophilic group, which is usually a long-chain hydrocarbon or other oil soluble group. An example of this type is sodium lauryl sulfate, which has the following structure:

$$\left[CH_3(CH_2)_{10}CH_2-O-\underset{\underset{O}{\|}}{\overset{\overset{O}{\|}}{S}}-O \right]^- Na^+$$

_____lipophilic_____hydrophilic

In cationic agents the lipophilic

group is part of the positive ion, as in quaternary nitrogen compounds. An example is diethylmethyloctyl ammonium chloride, which has the following structure:

lipophilic   hydrophilic

Nonionic agents consist of two or more nonionizable groups. Usually, they are esters of fatty acids with polyatomic alcohols or polymerized glycols. An example is glycol monolaurate:

$$CH_3(CH_2)_{10}-CO-O-CH_2CH_2-OH$$

lipophilic   hydrophilic

Surface-active agents have been added to solutions of germicides to help penetrate wound and crevices in the skin by reducing the surface tension and to facilitate contact with bacteria by wetting their surfaces. When the solution is used by scrubbing with a swab, the detergent effect of the surface-active agent assists in removing dirt and bacteria.

Preservatives

Surface-active agents, particularly of the cationic type, may also function as germicides and preservatives. Cationic agents which are germicidal usually contain a quaternary nitrogen atom to which are attached two or three groups of low molecular weight and one long hydrocarbon chain of six to eighteen carbon atoms. These compounds are readily soluble in water and usually have no irritant or toxic effect on the tissues in the dilutions employed.

Surface-active germicides are stable in aqueous solution and may be used in normal saline solution or in alcohol–acetone–water mixtures. They have greater germicidal effect in neutral or alkaline solution than in acid solution,

thus differing from phenols, benzoates, and mercurials which increase in power as the pH decreases.

Cationic preservatives are compatible with certain vasoconstrictors such as epinephrine and ephedrine and also with procaine and many other local anesthetics. They are compatible with dyes containing quaternary nitrogen atoms, e.g., acriflavine and proflavine, but are incompatible with most of the germicidal dyes. The germicidal effect of cationic agents is greatly reduced or destroyed by anionic agents such as soap. Surface-active germicides are not effective orally or parenterally but are useful for local application in solution or in a suitable base such as pectin paste.

Oral Vehicles

See, e.g., *Raspberry Syrup,* page 595.

Injection Vehicles

Frequently used vehicles for the administration of drugs by injection are sterile preparations of

(1) water,
(2) water with various salts,
(3) water with dextrose,
(4) water with proteins,
(5) water with various buffers, and
(6) combinations of all of them in addition to various preservatives.

Incompatibilities of the vehicles themselves are usually unimportant. However, the vehicles are commonly used as a means of administering several drugs by intravenous infusion. To be certain of the compatibility of any one drug added to a certain vehicle a study should be made and an accounting preserved for future use. In most instances, the absence of an immediate physical incompatibility is taken as an indication of an acceptable preparation although it is recognized that both non-visible chemical and therapeutic incompatibilities may have occurred. Tabulations of extensive studies are available.[15] These demonstrate the importance of an informed knowledge of the effects of adding drugs to vehicles for intravenous use. More than 10,000 tests by Abbott personnel[16] have been reported. Many other studies available are based on a particular emphasis, such as pH effects, multiple additives, and a specific drug such as penicillin or steroids. There are an infinite number of possible combinations. The user must make studies of his particular needs or search out the results of other studies from reports such as those cited previously.

When reconstituting parenterals, the product insert should be consulted and the proper (recommended) vehicle used. The pharmacist should not misconstrue this information and use a vehicle that is similar but not the same; for example, interchanging bacteriostatic water for injection with sterile water for injection. In the former, the antimicrobial preservative present (such as benzyl alcohol or methylparaben and propylparaben) may have an effect on the solubility and stability of the drug. If bacteriostatic water for injection containing benzyl alcohol is used to solubilize Chloromycetin-Intramuscular, the material thickens slowly and makes it difficult to remove the antibiotic from the vial unless used within 2 hours. Another form of this drug, Chloromycetin succinate, is compatible with solvents containing benzyl alcohol and may be used either intramuscularly or intravenously.

Drugs such as thiopental sodium, atropine sulfate, phenobarbital sodium, sulfadiazine sodium, and sulfathiazole sodium are incompatible with bacteriostatic water for injection containing the parabens. Erythromycin glucceptate must be reconstituted with preservative-free sterile water for injection. If sodium chloride injection and bacteriostatic sodium chloride injection are used, again, the compatibility of the drug with the solvent must be recognized. The reconstitution of erythromycin lactobionate with sodium chloride injection (instead of sterile water for injection) will cause gel formations.

A further concern for injection vehicle incompatibilities is related to the stability of drugs after reconstitution. A rather comprehensive summary of the stability of reconstituted solutions of commonly used drugs has been prepared and published.[17] Hazards include the possibilities of using improper diluents, nonaseptic techniques, improper labeling, and improper storage. A careful inspection of the insert and labeling of commercially available injectable drugs provides good indications for proper use and stability.

Specific Compounding and Dispensing Information

The following section contains compounding and dispensing information for more than 1400 widely prescribed drugs and drug products. The data are arranged alphabetically by nonproprietary name and/or tradename. The information was compiled from a variety of sources.

ABDEC Drops [*P-D*]—Multivitamin. *Known compatibilities* and *incompatibilities:* mixtures not recommended by manufacturer.

Acacia USP [gum arabic]—Pharmaceutic aid. Aqueous solutions of acacia are slightly acid in reaction. Acacia is precipitated from its aqueous solutions by alcoholic preparations; this precipitation may be avoided by adding the alcoholic liquid, drop by drop with agitation, provided the final concentration of alcohol does not exceed about 35%. Mucilage of acacia is gelatinized by solutions of ferric chloride or ferric sulfate, unless the solutions are well diluted; aluminum chloride gives similar results. Concentrated solutions of sodium borate gelatinize mucilage of acacia but not if the alkalinity of the borax solution has been reduced by addition of glycerin or an acid. Lead subacetate solution produces a gelatinous precipitate in solutions of acacia. Due to the presence of an oxidizing enzyme in solutions of acacia, a blue color is obtained on mixing with fresh tincture of guaiac; the enzyme is inactivated in a short time at 100°C; hence, the blue color will not appear if the acacia has been subjected to heat. Because of the oxidizing enzyme, acacia gives a coloration with other substances such as Adrenalin, phenol, thymol, resorcinol, physostigmine, tannin, etc. The oxidizing enzymes of acacia oxidize morphine, as well as other alkaloids and glucosides, even in pill masses containing as little as 2% of water. These enzymes are also reported to cause thinning of emulsions. Acacia is decomposed by strong acids. When boiled with nitric acid, acacia is oxidized to mucic, saccharic, and oxalic acids.

Acenocoumarol NF [Sintrom (*Geigy*); $C_{19}H_{15}NO_6$]—Anticoagulant. Off-white powder. Practically insoluble in water, alcohol, and ether; slightly soluble in chloroform.

Acetaminophen USP [(*Various Mfrs.*)]—Analgesic; antipyretic. White, odorless, crystalline powder with a slightly bitter taste; pH (sat soln) 5.3–6.5; melts 168–172°. 1 g in about 10,000 ml cold water, 20 ml boiling water, 10 ml alcohol, and 15 ml NaOH TS. The hydrolysis in various hydrochloric acid solutions and buffered solutions has been studied and the hydrolysis found to be both hydrogen and hydroxyl ion catalyzed. The energy of activation for the hydrolysis (17.5 kcal/mole) appears to be in good agreement with that reported for similar compounds.

Dispensing Information: Consult physician for use in children under 3 years of age or for periods longer than 10 days. Generally, keep medication away from young children since large overdoses have resulted in massive hepatic necrosis and death. (Unlike aspirin, acetaminophen is not anti-inflammatory.)

Acetarsone [Stovarsol]—Antiprotozoal. White, odorless powder which is stable at ordinary temperatures. It is only slightly soluble in water but readily soluble in solutions of alkali hydroxides or carbonates. It is administered orally in the treatment of amebic dysentery and is used as a dusting powder in certain types of vaginitis.

Acetazolamide USP [Diamox (*Lederle*)]—Carbonic anhydrase inhibitor. White to faintly yellowish white, crystalline, odorless powder. Very slightly soluble in water; sparingly soluble in nearly boiling water; slightly soluble in alcohol.

Dispensing Information: May cause tingling sensation on initial therapy; consult physician if rapid shallow breathing occurs. Contraindicated in low Na^+ or K^+ levels and in pregnancy. Increased frequency of urination may occur. Notify physician if sore throat, fever, unusual bleeding, bruising, or skin rash occur. Drowsiness may occur which may impair the ability to drive or perform other tasks requiring alertness.

Acetest Reagent Tablets [*Ames*]—Diagnostic agent, ketone determination (*in vitro* use only). Contains nitroprusside sodium.

Dispensing Information: Patients should be familiar with the test procedure and should be provided with a color chart.

Acetic Acid USP [pK$_a$ 4.76]—Pharmaceutic aid; caustic; rubefacient. It is a weak acid. pH (1% aqueous solution) about 3. It causes effervescence with carbonates and bicarbonates. It neutralizes metallic hydroxides (e.g., NaOH, KOH), some of the oxides (e.g., PbO and HgO) and phosphates (e.g., Na_2HPO_4). Acetates of the metals act as buffers toward strong acids, forming acetic acid and a salt of the strong acid. All of the acetates are quite water-soluble except sparingly soluble silver or mercurous acetate, which sometimes separate out of prescriptions if the concentrations of the ions present exceed the solubility product. The acetates of aluminum, bismuth, iron, and tin will hydrolyze in water liberating some insoluble basic salt and free hydrogen ions. The chief incompatibilities of the alkali acetates (sodium acetate or potassium acetate) result from the hydroxyl ions liberated on hydrolysis: $CH_3COONa + HOH \rightarrow Na^+ + OH^- + CH_3COOH$. This alkalinity is made use of in solubilizing theophylline and theobromine for injection. It may explain the precipitation of quinine acetate (unless the solution is acid) from prescriptions containing acetates and soluble quinine salts. Ferric salts give a deep red color with the acetate ion, possibly due to basic ferric acetate. This hydrolyzes further if the solution is heated, forming a precipitate of ferric hydroxide. The coloration with ferric salts does not appear at lower pH values.

Acetohexamide USP [Dymelor (*Lilly*); $C_{15}H_{20}N_2O_4S$]—Hypoglycemic. White, crystalline powder; practically odorless; melts 184–189°. 1 g in about 10,000 ml cold water, 230 ml alcohol, and 210 ml chloroform; soluble in dilute solutions of alkali hydroxides.

Dispensing Information: Do not skip doses or exceed labeled dose. Consult physician if yellowing of eyes or skin occurs. See also *Hypoglycemic Agents (Oral)*.

Acetone NF [2-propanone; dimethyl ketone]—Pharmaceutic aid. Acetone is a useful pharmaceutical solvent miscible with water, alcohol, chloroform, ether, and most volatile and fixed oils. pH (1% aqueous solution) about 7.5. It is used as a solvent and drying agent in several official topical solutions in 2 to 50% concentrations, e.g., merbromin solution (2%), surgical merbromin solution (2%), carbolfuchsin solution (5%), nitromersol tincture (50%), and thimerosal solution (10%). *Caution:* Acetone is inflammable. Excessive inhalation may cause headache, bronchial irritation, and other symptoms leading to narcosis. Repeated topical use may produce dryness of skin.

Acetophenazine Maleate NF [Tindal (*Schering*); $C_{23}H_{29}N_3O_2S\cdot 2C_4H_4O_4$]—Tranquilizer. Fine, yellow powder; odorless; bitter taste; melts at 165° with decomposition; light-sensitive; reasonably stable in dry air. 1 g dissolves in about 10 ml water, 250 ml alcohol, 2800 ml chloroform, and 6000 ml ether.

Acetosulfone Sodium [Promacetin (*P-D*); $C_{14}H_{14}N_3NaO_5S_2$]—Antibacterial (leprostatic). White, crystalline powder; sparingly soluble in water; insoluble in alcohol.

Acetylcholine Chloride [Miochol (*SMP*); $C_7H_{16}ClNO_2$]—Miotic. Hygroscopic, crystalline powder. Very soluble in cold water and alcohol; decomposed by hot water or alkalies.

Acetylcysteine NF [Mucomyst (*Mead-Johnson*); $C_5H_9NO_3S$]—Mucolytic agent. White, crystalline powder; slight odor. 1 g dissolves in about 5 ml water and 4 ml alcohol; practically insoluble in chloroform and ether.

Dispensing Information: Patients need to be familiar with the equipment and method of preparation for administration of this agent by aerosolization. If worsening of bronchospasm occurs after use, notify physician.

Acetyldigitoxin [digitoxin monoacetate; Acylanid (*Sandoz*); $C_{43}H_{66}O_{14}$]—Cardiotonic. White, microcrystalline powder; odorless; melts 217–221°; hygroscopic; 1 g dissolves in about 6100 ml water, 62.5 ml alcohol, and 12 ml chloroform; insoluble in ether.

Acriflavine—Topical antiseptic. Acriflavine base (neutral acriflavine) has a deep orange color. It is incompletely soluble in alcohol. pH (1% aq. soln.) about 3.5. Acriflavine hydrochloride is a brick-red powder that is soluble in water or alcohol, giving distinctly acid solutions (pH, *circa* 1.5). It is incompatible with solutions of phenol, chlorine, silver nitrate, or mercuric salts. Solutions of acriflavine hydrochloride (1: 1000) in normal saline solution remain clear and free from sediment for 1 day if kept in the dark. Solutions of acriflavine and acriflavine hydrochloride may be boiled or autoclaved without decomposition. The solutions are sensitive to light and should be stored in amber-colored bottles. Solutions more than a week old should be discarded.

Acriflavine Hydrochloride—See under *Acriflavine.*

Acrisorcin NF [Akrinol (*Schering*); $C_{12}H_{18}O_2 \cdot C_{13}H_{10}N_2$]—Topical antifungal. Yellow powder; odorless; melts with decomposition about 190°. 1 g dissolves in about 1000 ml water, 18 ml alcohol, and 320 ml chloroform.

Actidil Syrup [*B-W*] Antihistaminic. Contains triprolidine HCl (1.25 mg/5 ml), glycerin (8%), alcohol (5%), sodium benzoate, methylparaben. pH 6. *Known incompatibilities:* Elixir Nembutal, elixir terpin hydrate.

Actifed Preparations [*B-W*]—Nasal decongestant. Tablets contain triprolidine HCl 2.5 mg (syrup 0.25 mg/ml), pseudoephedrine HCl 60 mg (syrup 6 mg/ml).

Dispensing Information: Use with caution in hypertension. May cause either drowsiness or stimulation and nervousness; patients should be so advised. Do not drive or operate machinery.

Actifed C Expectorant [*B-W*]—Expectorant liquid. Contains (per ml) triprolidine HCl 0.4 mg, pseudoephedrine HCl 6 mg, codeine phosphate 2 mg, guaifenesin 20 mg.

Dispensing Information: See *Actifed Preparations* and *Codeine.*

ADC Drops [*P-D*]—Multivitamin. *Known compatibilities* and *incompatibilities:* mixtures not recommended by manufacturer.

Adrenal Cortex Extract [*Various Mfrs.*]—Agent for Addison's disease and adrenal insufficiency of other types. It is a mixture of the endocrine principles derived from the cortex of adrenal glands of healthy domestic animals used for food by man. Adrenal cortex extract is a water-soluble extract obtained following extraction of the adrenal glands with fat solvents. Each cc is obtained from not less than 40 g of gland and contains not less than 50 dog units.

The activity of the extract is relatively stable, especially if maintained at refrigerator temperature. Alcohol (10%) is used as a preservative (pH approx 4.7). Adrenal cortex extract is reported to be compatible with thiamin HCl, vitamin B complex, potassium chloride, desoxycorticosterone acetate; it is compatible at 50 ml/liter in dextrose 5%-water, dextrose 5%-saline, Levugen 10%-Water, Levugen 10%-Saline, Levugen 10%-Electrolytes. Amigen 5%-Levugen 10%, Amigen 5%-Dextrose 5%.

Afrin [*Schering*]—Nasal decongestant. Contains (per ml): oxymetazoline HCl 0.5 mg, glycine 3.8 mg, sorbitol 40 mg, phenylmercuric acetate 0.02 mg, benzalkonium chloride 0.2 mg. pH 4–6.5. See also *Sympathomimetic Agents (Nasal).*

Agar USP—Pharmaceutic aid. Aqueous solutions of agar may be prepared by the use of boiling water. Agar is a negatively charged colloid; it is precipitated by tannic acid and also by alcohol in concentrations over 50%.

Albamycin Mix-O-Vial [*Upjohn*]—Injectable novobiocin. Contains (per 5 ml): Albamycin sodium 500 mg, *N,N*-dimethylacetamide (10%), benzyl alcohol (0.9%), nicotinamide (175 mg). pH about 8.3. *Known incompatibilities:* ingredients lowering pH below about 6.5 may liberate novobiocin acid.

Albamycin Syrup [*Upjohn*]—Oral antibiotic. Contains Albamycin Calcium (125 mg/5 ml novobiocin), methylparaben (0.075%), propylparaben (0.025%), rose pink color, cherry custard flavored syrup base. pH 6.9 (approx). *Known incompatibilities:* Ambodryl Elixir (1:1), Chloromycetin Palmitate Suspension (1:1 and 2:1), Pyribenzamine Citrate Elixir (1:1).

Albumin, Normal Human Serum, USP [(*Hyland*); Albumisol (*MSD*); Albuspan (*P-D*); Proserum (*Dow*)]—Blood volume supporter. Moderately viscous, clear, brownish fluid; substantially odorless. May develop a slight granular or flaky deposit during storage. Preserve at temperature directed on the label. The expiration date varies between not later than 3 years and not later than 10 years after date of manufacture depending on the storage temperature, the kind of outer container, and whether the air space of the latter has or has not been evacuated or filled with an inert gas. *Compatibilities:* dextrose 5% in water, whole blood, plasma, normal saline, sodium lactate solution. *Known incompatibilities:* protein hydrolysate.

Albumin, Normal Human Serum (Salt Poor) [Albuminar (*Armour*); Albutein (*Abbott*); Buminate N.H.S.A. (*Hyland*); Pro-Bumin (*Lederle*)]—Blood volume supporter.

Dispensing Information—see *Albumin, Normal Human Serum.*

Alcohol USP [ethyl alcohol, ethanol]— Topical anti-infective; pharmaceutic aid (solvent). Clear, colorless, mobile, volatile liquid with a characteristic odor and produces a burning sensation on the tongue; readily volatilized even at low temperatures and boils about 78°C; flammable. Miscible with water, ether, and chloroform. Gums, albumin, and some inorganic salts are insoluble in alcohol and tend to be precipitated when alcohol is added to aqueous solutions containing them. Alcohol is incompatible with chlorine and with other oxidizing agents such as chromates and permanganates in acid solution.

40

R	Potassium Iodide	1.125 g	
	Tr. Belladonna	1.125 ml	
	Essence of Pepsin	45	ml
	Syrup Sarsaparilla Comp.		
	q.s.	120	ml

Potassium iodide causes precipitation of some of the pepsin and a part of the extractive matter in the tincture. Dilution of the tincture with liquids of low alcohol content also induces some precipitation. If sufficient alcohol is added to dissolve the precipitate from the tincture, there will be a precipitation of sugar, potassium iodide, and pepsin. Hence, it seems best to make no changes in the vehicle other than the addition of a few grams of acacia to facilitate uniform dispersion of the precipitate.

Dispensing Information: For external use; apply topically as a 70% solution. Label: flammable.

Alginic Acid NF [pK_a 3.42]—Pharmaceutic aid (tablet binder and emulsifying agent). White to yellowish white, fibrous powder; odorless; tasteless; pH (3 in 100 aqueous dispersion) 1.5–3.5. Very slightly soluble in water; soluble in alkaline solutions.

Alidase (*Searle* brand of hyaluronidase)—Enzyme. Contains hyaluronidase in dry form (150 USP Units/ampul).

Allopurinol USP [Zyloprim (*B-W*); $C_5H_4N_4O$]—Xanthine oxidase inhibitor. White to off-white powder with only a slight odor. Very slightly soluble in water and alcohol; soluble in solutions of fixed alkali hydroxides. *Known compatibilities* (sodium salt): appears to be soluble in dextrose 5% in water. *Known incompatibilities* (sodium salt): 6-mercaptopurine sodium, prednisolone sodium succinate, acidic materials.

Dispensing Information: Notify physician if skin rash occurs; it can be severe at times.

Aloin—Laxative. A mixture of crystalline pentosides from various aloes. It is a light yellow powder, soluble in water and alcohol. It is decomposed and rendered inert by alkalies. Aloin gives color changes with some compounds, e.g., red with alkalies or ethyl nitrite spirit and a greenish-black with ferric chloride.

Alphaprodine Hydrochloride NF [Nisentil Hydrochloride (*Roche*); $C_{16}H_{23}NO_2 \cdot HCl$]—Narcotic analgesic. White, crystalline, bitter powder with a fishy odor; pH (1% aq. soln.) 4.5–5.2; stable to air, light, and heat. 1 g in about 1 ml water; freely soluble in alcohol; insoluble in ether.

Alum NF [purified alum]—Local astringent. Alum is composed of aluminum ammonium sulfate or aluminum potassium sulfate. Large, colorless crystals, crystalline fragments, or white powder; odorless, and has a sweetish, strongly astringent taste; solutions are acid to litmus. 1 g dissolves in 1–10 ml water, less than 1 ml boiling water, 10,000 ml alcohol, 1–10 ml glycerin, but slowly. *Known incompatibilities:* protein precipitants, carbonates, soluble organic salts, alkalies, and borax.

Alumina and Magnesia Oral Suspension USP [Aludrox (*Wyeth*)]—Antacid. Contains aluminum hydroxide, hydrated aluminum oxide, magnesium hydroxide, flavors, and antimicrobial agents. pH 7.3–7.9. Avoid freezing. *Known incompatibilities:* electrolytes, acids, fixed alkalies.

Alumina and Magnesia Tablets USP [Aludrox (*Wyeth*)]—Antacid. Occurs as tablets which may be chewed or swallowed. Contains aluminum hydroxide and magnesium hydroxide. *Known incompatibilities:* absorbs other drugs.

Aluminum Acetate Solution USP [Burow's solution]—Astringent. Clear, colorless liquid having a faint odor of acetic acid, and a sweetish, astringent taste; specific gravity about 1.02; pH: 3.6–4.4. *Known incompatibilities:* alkalies, carbonates, borax.

Aluminum Chloride NF[AlCl₃·6H₂O]—Local astringent. White or yellowish white, deliquescent, crystalline powder; nearly odorless, and has a sweet, very astringent taste; solutions are acid to litmus. 1 g dissolves in less than 1 ml water, 1–10 ml alcohol, and 10–30 ml glycerin. *Known incompatibilities:* alkalies, carbonates, borax, and many soluble organic salts.

Aluminum Hydroxide Gel USP [Amphogel (*Wyeth*)]—Antacid. Contains aluminum hydroxide, flavors, and antimicrobial agents. White, viscous suspension, from which small amounts of clear liquid may separate on standing; avoid freezing; pH 5.5–8. *Known incompatibilities:* acids, electrolytes, fixed alkalies, absorbs other drugs.

Aluminum Hydroxide Gel, Dried, USP—Antacid. Contains aluminum hydroxide, with varying amounts of basic aluminum carbonate and bicarbonate. White, odorless, tasteless, amorphous powder. Insoluble in water and alcohol; 1 part in 10–30 parts dilute mineral acids and solutions of fixed alkali hydroxides. *Known incompatibilities:* acids, electrolytes, fixed alkalies, absorbs other drugs.

Aluminum Hydroxide Gel, Dried, Tablets USP—Antacid. Occurs as tablets which may be chewed or swallowed. *Known incompatibilities:* adsorbs other drugs.

Aluminum Monostearate USP—Pharmaceutic aid; suspending agent for penicillin preparations. Contains aluminum monostearate and aluminum monopalmitate. Fine, white to yellowish white, bulky powder with a faint, characteristic odor. Insoluble in water, alcohol, and ether. *Known incompatibilities:* acids, alkalies, adsorbs other drugs.

Aluminum Nicotinate [Nicalex (*Merrell-National*)]—Peripheral vasodilator. White, amorphous powder; odorless; slight acidulous taste. Insoluble in water and alcohol.

Aluminum Subacetate Solution USP—Astringent. Contains aluminum sulfate, precipitated calcium carbonate, and acetic acid. Clear, colorless, or faintly yellow liquid, having an odor of acetic acid and an acid reaction to litmus; gradually becomes turbid on standing, through separation of a more basic salt; pH 3.8–4.6. *Known incompatibilities:* fixed alkalies, acids.

Aluminum Sulfate USP[Al₂(SO₄)₃·xH₂O]—Pharmaceutic aid for *Aluminum Subacetate Solution.* White crystalline powder, shining plates, or crystalline fragments; stable in air; odorless and has a sweet taste, becoming mildly astringent. 1 g in 1–10 ml of water; insoluble in alcohol. *Known incompatibilities:* alkalies, carbonates, borax, and many soluble organic salts.

Alurate Elixir (*Roche* brand of aprobarbital)—Barbiturate. Contains Alurate (40 mg/5 ml). *Known incompatibilities:* low alcoholic solutions, potassium iodide, strontium bromide (precipitates red color in Elixir Alurate Red).

Alurate Elixir Verdum—see *Alurate Elixir.*

Amantadine Hydrochloride NF [Symmetrel (*Endo*); $C_{10}H_{17}N \cdot HCl$]— Antiviral (prophylactic). Whitish, crystalline powder; bitter taste; pH (1 in 5 soln) 3.0–5.5. Freely soluble in water; soluble in alcohol and chloroform.

Dispensing Information: Parkinsonism patients first receiving this drug may experience such rapid clinical benefit that they should be cautioned not to resume their past activities too rapidly.

Ambenonium Chloride NF [Mytelase (*Winthrop*); $C_{28}H_{42}Cl_4N_4O_2$ and the tetrahydrate]—Cholinergic. White powder; odorless; melts about 200°. 1 g dissolves in 5 ml water and 20 ml alcohol; insoluble in chloroform and ether.

Americaine Aerosol [*Arnar-Stone* brand of benzocaine]—Local anesthetic. Contains 20% dissolved benzocaine and 0.5% 8-hydroxyquinoline in a base of polyethylene glycol 400 dilaurate; propellants P-11 and P-12. Nonaqueous, but base is water-dispersible.

Americaine Ointment [*Arnar-Stone*]—Contains 20% dissolved benzocaine and 0.1% benzethonium chloride in a base of PEG 300 and 4000. Nonaqueous, but base is water-soluble. Manufacturer does not recommend mixing with any other ointment, but it can be cut with additional PEG.

Americaine Otic [*Arnar-Stone*]— Contains 20% dissolved benzocaine and 0.1% benzethonium chloride in a base of PEG 300 and 1% glycerin. Nonaqueous, but base is water-soluble. Do not mix with other aural preparations.

Amesec Enseals [*Lilly*]—Antiasthmatic. Contains aminophylline, ephedrine HCl, amobarbital. Enteric tablet must be administered in intact form; cannot be crushed for ingestion as this destroys enteric coating.

Aminoacetic Acid USP [glycocoll glycine; pK_a 9.78, pK_b 11.65]—Irrigating solution. White crystalline nutrient compound; 1 g dissolves in 4 ml water

and 1254 ml alcohol. It should not be confused with the poisonous photographic developer "Glycin." pH (1% aq soln) about 5.7.

The darkening of solutions of aminoacetic acid in mixtures of water and low isoalcoholic elixir is ascribed to hydrolysis of the sucrose present in the elixir with formation of glucose and levulose. The glucose darkens in alkaline solution and levulose darkens in neutral or acid solutions. To mask the color change the solutions may be colored with compound cudbear tincture or some other suitable coloring agent. Discoloration may be prevented by omitting sugars entirely. Glycine is said to give a deep wine color with ferric chloride. This disappears with an excess of hydrochloric acid and reappears on adding an excess of ammonia. It also causes a color change with phenol or sodium hypochlorite (blue color).

Aminobenzoic Acid USP [*p*-aminobenzoic acid; pK_a 4.65 and 4.80]—Topical protectant (sun screen). White, or slightly yellow, crystalline powder which darkens on exposure to light. 1 g dissolves in 170 ml water and 8 ml alcohol; freely soluble in alkaline solutions; sparingly soluble in acid solutions. pH (0.5% aq soln) about 3.5. It is incompatible with ferric salts and oxidizing agents.

Sodium para-aminobenzoate is freely soluble in water, yielding an alkaline solution; it is slightly soluble in alcohol. *Caution:* Sodium para-aminobenzoate should not be administered with sulfonamides as it inhibits the antibacterial effect of these drugs; it is not antagonistic to penicillin.

Aminocaproic Acid NF [Amicar (*Lederle*)]—Antifibrinolytic; hemostatic. *Known compatibilities* (injection): dextrose 5% in water, Ringer's injection, normal saline, sterile water for injection. *Known incompatibilities* (injection): none.

Aminohippurate Sodium [*MSD*; $C_9H_9N_2NaO_3$]—Diagnostic aid (renal function determination). See also *Aminohippuric Acid.*

Aminohippuric Acid USP [*p*-aminohippuric acid; PAH; PAHA]—Diagnostic aid (renal function determination). pK$_a$ 3.64 1 g dissolves in 45 ml water, 50 ml alcohol, and 5 ml diluted hydrochloric acid; freely soluble in solutions of alkali hydroxides or carbonates with some decomposition. It is chiefly used as the water-soluble sodium salt which is alkaline hence must be buffered to pH 7 with citric acid before injection.

Aminophylline USP [theophylline ethylenediamine compound (2:1); (*Various Mfrs.*)]—Bronchodilator and smooth muscle relaxant. White or slightly yellowish granules or powder having a slight ammoniacal odor and bitter taste. It gradually loses ethylenediamine and adsorbs CO_2 with the liberation of free theophylline; alkaline to litmus. 1 g in 25 ml water to give a clear solution (in 5 ml, it crystallizes on standing but redissolves when a small amount of ethylenediamine is added); insoluble in alcohol and ether. Aminophylline is prone to liberate ethylenediamine, especially when prescribed in solutions or suppositories. Sorensen's phosphate buffer is said to prevent decomposition.

Dispensing Information: May cause nervousness or insomnia; use with caution in epilepsy, peptic ulcer, and renal failure; may be taken after meals to lessen gastric distress. See also *Smooth Muscle Relaxants (Xanthine Type)*.

Aminophylline Injection USP—Aqueous 2.5% injection; pH 6–9. Not for rectal use. Store in a cool place. *Known incompatibilities* (aminophylline injection): alkaline-labile drugs (e.g., epinephrine, Isuprel, levophed, penicillin G potassium), strong acid solutions; theophylline crystals tend to form if solution pH drops below 8.

Dispensing Information: See *Aminophylline*.

Aminosalicylic Acid [*p*-aminosalicylic acid; (*Various Mfrs.*); pK$_a$ 3.25] — Antibacterial (tuberculostatic). 1 g dissolves in 500 ml water or 21 ml alcohol. pH (0.1% aq soln) about 3.5. The aqueous solution decomposes to *m*-aminophenol with liberation of carbon dioxide.

Amitriptyline Hydrochloride USP [Elavil HCl (*MSD*); C$_{20}$H$_{23}$N·HCl] — Antidepressant. Whitish, crystalline powder or small crystals; odorless or almost so; melts about 197°; pH (1 in 100 soln) 5–6. Freely soluble in water, alcohol, and chloroform; insoluble in ether.

Dispensing Information: Consult physician if fever, eye pain, sore throat, ulcers in the mouth, or easy bleeding or bruising occur. There is often a time lag of up to 2 weeks before full therapeutic response is achieved. Patients taking guanethidine concurrently may lose guanethidine's antihypertensive effect. See also *Antidepressants (Tricyclic)*.

Ammonia Solution, Strong, NF [stronger ammonia water; spirit of Hartshorn]—Pharmaceutic aid; solvent; source of ammonia. 27–30% (*w/w*) NH$_3$. Clear, colorless liquid having an exceedingly pungent, characteristic odor; specific gravity about 0.90. *Known incompatibilities:* tartaric acid, fixed alkalies.

Ammonia Spirit, Aromatic, NF—Respiratory stimulant. Contains ammonium carbonate, strong ammonia solution, and flavors. Nearly colorless liquid when recently prepared, but gradually acquires a yellow color on standing; it has the taste of ammonia, an aromatic and pungent odor, and is affected by light; specific gravity about 0.90. *Known incompatibilities:* acids, fixed alkalies.

Ammonium Carbonate NF [mixt. of ammonium bicarbonate and ammonium carbonate]—Pharmaceutic aid (source of ammonia). Usually a white powder having a strong odor of ammonia, without empyreuma, and a sharp, ammoniacal taste; solutions are alkaline to litmus; on exposure to air, it loses ammonia and CO_2, becoming opaque, and is finally converted into friable porous lumps or a white powder of ammonium bicarbonate. 1 part in 1–10 parts water; decomposed by hot water. *Known incompatibilities:* fixed alkalies, acids.

Ammonium Chloride NF[NH$_4$Cl] —Acidifier; diuretic. Colorless crystals or white, fine or coarse, crystalline powder; cool, saline taste; somewhat hygroscopic; pH (1 in 20 solution) 4.5–6. 1 g dissolves in 1–10 ml water and glycerin (even more soluble in boiling water), 30–100 ml alcohol. *Known incompatibilities:* (ammonium chloride injection): alkalies and their carbonates, chlortetracycline HCl, codeine phosphate, dimenhydrinate, Furadantin, Gantrisin, iodine, Leritine, Levo-Dromoran, methadone HCl, Panwarfin, sulfadiazine sodium, tartaric acid.

Ammonium Salicylate—See under *Salicylic Acid.*

Ammonium Valerate, Acid—See under *Valeric Acid.*

Ammonium Valerianate—See under *Valeric Acid.*

Amobarbital NF [Amytal (*Lilly*); C$_{11}$H$_{18}$N$_2$O$_3$]—Hypnotic. White, crystalline powder, odorless and with a bitter taste; pH (sat soln) about 5.6; melts 156–161°; pK$_a$ 7.94. Soluble 1 g in 1300 ml water, 5 ml alcohol, 17 ml chloroform. *Known incompatibilities:* The addition of water to alcoholic solutions tends to precipitate the amobarbital. See also *Sedatives and Hypnotics.*

Amobarbital Sodium USP [Amytal Sodium (*Lilly*); C$_{11}$H$_{17}$N$_2$NaO$_3$]—Hypnotic. White, friable granular powder; odorless, has a bitter taste, and is hygroscopic; solutions decompose on standing, the decomposition being accelerated by heat; pH (5% aq soln) 9.6–10.4. Very soluble in water; soluble in alcohol; practically insoluble in chloroform and ether.

Known incompatibilities (amobarbital sodium for injection): codeine phosphate, Demerol, dimenhydrinate HCl, diphenhydramine HCl, insulin, Keflin, Leritine, Levo-Dromoran, Levophed, methadone HCl, methylphenidate HCl, morphine sulfate, penicillin G potassium, phytonadione, procaine HCl, Solu-Cortef, tetracycline HCl.

Dispensing Information: See *Sedatives and Hypnotics.*

Amodiaquine Hydrochloride USP [Camoquin Hydrochloride (*P-D*); C$_{20}$H$_{22}$ClN$_3$O·2HCl·2H$_2$O or anhydrous]—Antimalarial. Yellow, crystalline powder; odorless; bitter taste. 1 g dissolves in about 25 ml water and 78 ml alcohol; insoluble in chloroform and ether.

Amoxicillin [Amoxil (*Beecham-Massengill*); Larocin (*Roche*); C$_{16}$H$_{19}$N$_3$O$_5$S·3H$_2$O or anhydrous]— Antibacterial. White or slightly off-white highly hygroscopic powder; free-flowing with an ammoniacal odor; pH (0.2% solution in CO$_2$-free water at room temperature) 3.5–5.5; pK$_a$ 2.8. Soluble 1 g in about 370 ml water, about 2000 ml alcohol. See also *Penicillins.*

Amphetamine [Benzedrine (*SK&F*); C$_9$H$_{13}$N]—CNS stimulant. A colorless, slowly volatile liquid which is slightly soluble in water and soluble in alcohol, yielding alkaline solutions. It readily absorbs carbon dioxide from the air.

Amphetamines—*Dispensing Information:* May cause nervousness and anxiety. Patients should not exceed the recommended dose. Palpitations and fast heart rate should be brought to the attention of the physician.

Amphotericin B USP [Fungizone (*Squibb*); C$_{47}$H$_{73}$NO$_{17}$]—Antifungal. Heat-labile and light-sensitive insoluble polyene (heptaene). Both the dry powder and its solutions should be stored in the refrigerator and protected against exposure to light. Unused solutions should be discarded after 24 hours.

Known incompatibilities (amphotericin B for injection): Achromycin, Benadryl, calcium chloride, calcium gluconate, carbenicillin, chlorpromazine HCl, chlortetracycline HCl, Furadantin, kanamycin sulfate, metaraminol bitartrate, normal saline, penicillin G potassium, Terramycin.

Ampicillin USP [Omnipen (*Wyeth*); Penbritin (*Ayerst*); C$_{16}$H$_{19}$N$_3$O$_4$S]— Antibacterial. White, crystalline powder; practically odorless. Slightly soluble in water; insoluble in chloroform.

Dispensing Information: Take on an

empty stomach, 1 hour before or 2 hours after meals. Take as directed until all medication is consumed. Discontinue use and contact physician immediately if rash (10% of population) occurs. Diarrhea occurs in a large number of patients and usually subsides a day or two after therapy is discontinued. Patients allergic to penicillin will be allergic to ampicillin. See also *Penicillins*.

Ampicillin Sodium [Omnipen N (*Wyeth*); Polycillin-N (*Bristol*); SK-Ampicillin (*SK&F*); $C_{16}H_{18}N_3NaO_4S$]—Antibacterial. Whitish, crystalline powder; odorless or almost so; hygroscopic. Very soluble in water, isotonic sodium chloride solution, and dextrose solutions.

Known compatibilities: normal saline for 24 hours only at room temperature and refrigerated in concentrations less than 3 g/100 ml. *Known incompatibilities:* (ampicillin sodium for injection): Should not be mixed with other drugs as these may change the pH, thus affecting stability or compatibility of the injection.

Dispensing Information: See *Ampicillin* and *Penicillins*.

Ampicillin Trihydrate [Amcill (*P-D*); Pensyn (*Upjohn*); Polycillin (*Bristol*); (*Various Other Mfrs.*)]—Antibacterial. White, practically odorless, crystalline powder. Soluble in water and methanol; insoluble in benzene, carbon tetrachloride, and chloroform.

Amylene Hydrate NF [tertiary amyl alcohol]—Pharmaceutic aid (solvent). Liquid having a camphoraceous odor and a burning taste. Soluble in 8 parts water; miscible with alcohol and glycerin.

Amyl Nitrite NF [isoamylnitrite]—Vasodilator. Very slightly soluble in water but miscible with alcohol, chloroform, or ether. It is incompatible with alcohol (alcohol interchange); alkalies, alkaline carbonates (hydrolysis); iodides and bromides (liberates halogen); antipyrine and sodium salicylate (color changes). Ethyl nitrite and spirit of ethyl nitrite show similar incompatibilities.

Amytal Elixir [*Lilly*]—pH 8–9; 34% alcohol; hydroalcoholic-propylene glycol solvent system; 165 mg saccharin sodium/100 ml; $Na^+ < 1$ mg/5 ml; $K^+ < 1$ mg/5 ml. *Known incompatibilities:* May form a precipitate when mixed with a solution with a low pH.

Amytal Sodium Ampoules [*Lilly*]—pH (1:20 soln) 9.6–10.4. *Known incompatibilities:* when combined with acid solutions (e.g., codeine, morphine, lactated Ringer's solution, bacteriostatic water for injection, etc.), barbituric acid will precipitate; this precipitation is gradual, but will occur.

Anethole USP [*p*-methoxypropenyl-benzene]—Pharmaceutic aid (flavor); carminative; perfume. A relatively inert aromatic ether. It is insoluble in water but miscible with organic solvents.

Anileridine NF [Leritine (*MSD*); $C_{22}H_{28}N_2O_2$]—Narcotic analgesic. White to yellowish white, crystalline powder; practically odorless; slight, bitter taste; darkens in air and light; melts (2 polymorphic forms) about 80° and about 89°. Very slightly soluble in water; 1 g dissolves in 2 ml alcohol and 1 ml chloroform.

Anileridine Hydrochloride NF [Leritine Hydrochloride (*MSD*); $C_{22}H_{28}N_2O_2\cdot2HCl$]—Narcotic analgesic. White, crystalline powder; odorless; stable in air; melts about 270° with decomposition; pH (1 in 20 soln) 2.5–3. Freely soluble in water; sparingly soluble in alcohol.

Anileridine Phosphate [Leritine Phosphate (*MSD*); $C_{22}H_{28}N_2O_2\cdot H_3PO_4$]—Narcotic analgesic (parenteral). See also *Anileridine Hydrochloride*.

Anisotropine Methylbromide [Valpin (*Endo*); $C_{16}H_{29}NO_2\cdot CH_3Br$]—Anticholinergic. White, glistening powder or plates; extremely bitter taste. Soluble in water; sparingly soluble in alcohol; insoluble in ether.

Dispensing Information: With phenobarbital, do not drive or operate heavy equipment upon initiation of therapy. Consult physician if skin rash occurs.

Antacids—*Dispensing Information:* Patients should be told whether the agent being used is more likely to produce diarrhea or constipation.

Antacids (Aluminum-Containing)—*Dispensing Information:* These agents produce constipation; in combination preparations with magnesium salts the propensity to produce constipation may be balanced or overriden by the magnesium salt that produces diarrhea.

Antacids (Magnesium-Containing)—*Dispensing Information:* These antacids are used in a preponderance of antacid mixtures; the magnesium ion has a tendency to cause diarrhea.

Antazoline Hydrochloride [$C_{17}H_{19}N_3$·HCl]—Antihistaminic. White, crystalline powder; odorless; bitter taste; produces temporary numbness of tongue; melts 237–241°; pH (1% soln) 6.3. 1 g dissolves in about 40 ml water and 25 ml alcohol; practically insoluble in chloroform and ether.

Antazoline Phosphate NF —Antihistamine. White, crystalline powder; soluble in water. A 2% solution in water is slightly acidic (pH about 4.5).

Anthelmintics—*Dispensing Information:* Explain personal hygiene to avoid reinfestation.

Anthralin USP [1,8-dihydroxyanthranol; cignolin; dithranol]—Topical anti-eczematic. Yellowish crystalline powder. It is practically insoluble in water and slightly soluble in alcohol. It is soluble in alkalies but alkaline solutions turn red in the presence of air.

Antibiotics (Oral)—*Dispensing Information:* In order for an infection to clear, it is very important to take the antibiotic for the entire number of days for which it has been prescribed. The patient *should not stop* taking it even if he begins to feel better before the regimen is completed. A calendar may be provided to assist the patient in remembering when to take the medication. Most antibiotics should be taken with water on an empty stomach so that large amounts will enter the blood-stream; it is best taken *every* 6 hours (4 doses in 24 hours) $\frac{1}{2}$ hour before meals and at bedtime or it may be taken at least 2 hours after each meal and at bedtime. Notify the physician at once if any type of skin rash or itching occurs while taking an antibiotic. Occasionally, anorexia, nausea, or diarrhea can result from an antibiotic and this should be brought to the physician's attention.

Anticholinergic Agents—*Dispensing Information:* The patient should be advised that dry mouth, difficulty in urination, blurred vision, constipation, paralysis of accommodation, and sensitivity to light due to mydriasis may occur.

Antidepressants (Tricyclic)—*Dispensing Information:* The patient may experience extreme drowsiness when beginning therapy; this effect may diminish in 2 weeks. Other depressants including alcohol should be avoided or taken cautiously. Anticholinergic side effects may be seen in certain patients.

Antihistamines—*Dispensing Information:* Patients should be warned that drowsiness (sometimes profound depending on the agent) can occur. Extreme caution is essential when operating an automobile or machinery. Dry mouth and blurred vision can also sometimes occur. Individual patients differ markedly in their susceptibility to these side effects. Children occasionally respond to some antihistamines with symptoms of excitation, restlessness, and insomnia. Medication should be kept out of reach of children since large overdoses have resulted in death, especially in children.

Anti-inflammatory Agents—*Dispensing Information:* These agents may cause stomach upset and should be taken with meals, a buffer, or milk to reduce this effect. Advise the physician if sore throat, fever, other evidence of infection, any bleeding tendency, or any change in stool color occurs.

Antimony Potassium Tartrate USP [tartar emetic; $C_8H_4K_2Sb_2O_{12}$·$3H_2O$ or anhydrous]—Antischistosomal. Colorless, transparent crystals or white powder; odorless; efflorescent (crystals) in air; solutions acid to litmus. 1 g dissolves in about 12 ml water, 15 ml glycerin, and 3 ml boiling water; insoluble in alcohol.

Antineoplastic Agents (Bone Marrow-Suppressant)—*Dispensing Information:* Routine blood counts are indicated. Patients should be advised to bring to their physician's attention symptoms of infection (fever, sore throat, etc. due to leukopenia) and symptoms of bleeding (easy bruising, stool color change, etc. due to thrombocytopenia).

Antipsychotic Agents (Phenothiazine Type)—*Dispensing Information:* Patients should be cautioned about drowsiness which occurs early in therapy. Cholestatic jaundice may occur generally in the first months of therapy. Yellowing of the skin or sclera should be brought to the attention of the physician. Agranulocytosis may occur early in therapy; the patient should be told to be aware of the appearance of a sore throat or fever and report these symptoms to the physician. Anticholinergic effects are likely to be experienced (see *Atropine*). Any abnormal movement disorder should be reported to the physician. Hyperpigmentation and ocular side effects may occur in patients receiving high-dose long-term therapy.

Antipyrine [phenazone; analgesine; $C_{11}H_{12}N_2O$]—Antipyrine is a largely obsolete analgesic-antipyretic. 1 g dissolves in less than 1 ml of water, yielding a neutral solution, and 1 ml of alcohol. Antipyrine has a slightly bitter taste.

Aqueous solutions of antipyrine form precipitates with alkalies, mercuric salts, tannic acid, iodine, iodides, lead subacetate, and some other alkaloidal precipitants. With ethyl nitrite spirit a green color develops due to formation of isonitrosoantipyrine which has been found to be comparatively nontoxic; the appearance of the green color is retarded by $NaHCO_3$. Antipyrine gives a red color with ferric chloride. A liquid or soft mass is formed when antipyrine is triturated with a number of substances, e.g., sodium salicylate, chloral hydrate, or phenol. Antipyrine and calomel should not be dispensed together because in presence of moisture the mixture darkens, and the calomel is partially converted into metallic mercury and poisonous mercury bichloride; this change is hastened by $NaHCO_3$. Antipyrine is incompatible with methenamine, a physiologically inactive product being formed. On addition of antipyrine to concentrated solutions of salts of the alkali metals, e.g., potassium citrate, sodium acetate, and ammonium carbonate, there is a separation of an immiscible liquid which dissolves when the mixture is diluted with water.

Antithyroid Agents—*Dispensing Information:* These agents may cause rash. Advise the physician of any unusual bleeding or symptoms of infection.

Antivert Tablets [*Roerig*]—Contain meclizine 12.5 mg.

Dispensing Information: See *Antihistamines.*

Apomorphine [$C_{17}H_{17}O_2N$; pK_a = 8.92, pK_b = 7.0]—Apomorphine is usually used as the hydrochloride, qv.

Apomorphine Hydrochloride [$C_{17}H_{17}NO_2 \cdot HCl \cdot \frac{1}{2}H_2O$]—Emetic. 1 g dissolves in about 50 ml of water and 50 ml of alcohol. A 0.3% aqueous solution has a pH of 4.8. The salt and its solutions turn green on exposure to light and air and must then be rejected. Decomposition is a function both of pH and atmospheric (or dissolved) oxygen. The decomposition product appears devoid of nitrogen and is possibly an 8-substituted phenanthrene-3,4-dione which has no emetic properties. Apomorphine hydrochloride is decomposed by oxidizing agents, producing a green color with iodine and a dark purple with nitric acid.

Arginine Hydrochloride [Argivine (*Gray*); R-Gene (*Cutter*); $C_6H_{14}N_4O_2 \cdot HCl$]—Ammonia detoxicant. Crystalline plates or prisms. Soluble in water; slightly soluble in hot alcohol.

Ascorbic Acid USP [vitamin C; Cecon (*Abbott*); Cevalin (*Lilly*); Ce-Vi-

Sol (*M-J*); $C_6H_8O_6$; pK_{a1} 4.1; pK_{a2} 11.6]—Antiscorbutic vitamin. 1 g dissolves in about 3 ml water, 40 ml alcohol. It is insoluble in ether, chloroform, benzene, petroleum ether, oils, fats, and fat solvents. It is stable to air when dry.

Ascorbic acid is a strong monobasic acid which liberates carbon dioxide from carbonates and bicarbonates and forms well-defined salts with calcium, magnesium, potassium, and sodium. The most reactive portion of the molecule is the α-keto-diol system which is responsible for the high acidity of the compound and for the reducing properties. Like all α-keto-ene-diols, ascorbic acid is a powerful reducing agent in acid and neutral solutions. It reacts with iodine and other halogens and reduces Fehling's solution and ammoniacal silver nitrate without heating. The lactone portion of the molecule is remarkably resistant to hydrolysis and the principal decomposition is oxidation.

The first oxidation product of ascorbic acid is dehydroascorbic acid. This reaction is reversible and dehydroascorbic acid is reduced back to ascorbic acid by hydrogen sulfide or hydrogen iodide. L-Dehydroascorbic acid possesses the full biological activity of L-ascorbic acid (some of the naturally-occurring vitamin exists in the oxidized form). Further oxidation leads to oxalic acid and L-threonic acid with loss of activity. The latter decomposition is accelerated first by air then by alkali so neutral solutions of sodium ascorbate often retain their potency for a long time in the absence of air. The pH rate profile of the disappearance of ascorbic acid solutions under anaerobic conditions at 96°C has been determined and a small maximum at pH 4.1 can be rationalized as due to a salt-acid complex. In impure preparations and in many natural products the vitamin oxidizes on exposure to air and light. Aqueous solutions have an acid reaction, i.e., pH = 3 (5 mg/ml); pH = 2 (50 mg/ml).

Aqueous solutions of ascorbic acid are rapidly inactivated by atmospheric oxidation, particularly at high temperatures. The deterioration is hastened by light, alkali, oxidizing agents, and some metals, particularly iron and copper. Acids, reducing agents, and potassium iodide retard decomposition. In absence of oxygen, ascorbic acid is fairly stable to heat. Concentrated solutions are more stable than dilute solutions.

Data on the stability of ascorbic acid in water, syrup, 90% glycerin, propylene glycol, corn syrup, sorbitol, and 3% methocel vehicles have been recorded. The addition of gums to increase viscosity appeared to accelerate loss of the vitamin, however, the syrups and polyhydroxy liquids were significantly more stable than water. Stability of ascorbic acid also increased with increasing concentrations of sodium chloride. This is possibly associated with a lower concentration of dissolved oxygen in the vehicle. It has been found that the higher the content of ethylene glycol, 1,2-propylene glycol or 1,3-butylene glycol, the better the stability, while glycerol was not as effective. The auto-oxidation of ascorbic acid is accelerated in the presence of a Sorensen phosphate buffer. This is attributed to the formation of complexes by trace metal impurities.

The effect of various metal sulfates on the stability of ascorbic acid tablets indicates copper sulfate is most destructive, followed in order by cobalt, manganese, zinc, and iron. Other data show the order to be: copper, zinc, tin, iron, and aluminum. It has been found that biotin retards the copper catalysis best at pH 6, rutin at pH 7–8, and hesperidin at pH 6–8. An alkaline solution of ascorbic acid acquires a dark violet color when allowed to stand with ferrous sulfate.

Ascorbic acid causes darkening of tablet granulations prepared with the aid of liquids; in such cases it is necessary to use the precompression method or to add the ascorbic acid to a previously prepared granulation. It was found that sodium metabisulfite and thiourea had little or no effect.

For parenteral therapy ascorbic acid may be administered intravenously dissolved in an appropriate quantity of sterile distilled water or sterile normal saline. The acidity of such solutions renders them unsuitable for subcutaneous or intramuscular administration. On studying the effects of pH adjustment on 10% ascorbic acid injections autoclaved 1 hour at 120°C, decomposition was greatest at pH 4–6. Neutralized solutions for subcutaneous or intramuscular administration may be prepared by dissolving 0.1 g of ascorbic acid in 2 ml of sterile, pyrogen-free distilled water and adding 3 ml of a 0.1 M solution of Na_3PO_4. The latter may be prepared by dissolving 3.8 g of Na_3PO_4·$12H_2O$ in sufficient sterile, pyrogen-free water to make 100 ml. The phosphate solution may be sterilized by boiling. Solutions of ascorbic acid prepared in this manner have a pH of about 6.8 and are approximately isotonic. Because of the deterioration of ascorbic acid, the solutions should be prepared immediately before administration.

Vitamin C tablets may be administered to very young infants by dissolving the tablets in one or two teaspoonfuls of water and adding this solution to the milk. The whole tablets should not be added to milk because the acidity of ascorbic acid has a curdling effect.

Dispensing Information: Large quantities (over several grams/day) that produce urinary acidification can affect the excretion of several drugs. Patient medication history should be known where a history of ascorbic acid ingestion is known. pH paper may be a useful guide to assure the urine is adequately acidified when this is the therapeutic goal.

Ascorbyl Palmitate NF [$C_{22}H_{38}O_7$]— Pharmaceutic aid (antioxidant). White to yellowish powder; characteristic odor; melts 107–117°. Insoluble in water, chloroform, and ether; 1 g dissolves in 125 ml alcohol.

Aspirin USP [acetylsalicylic acid; salicylic acid acetate; $C_9H_8O_4$; $pK_a \simeq$ 3.62]—Analgesic; antipyretic; antirheumatic. White crystals. 1 g dissolves in 300 ml water, 5 ml alcohol, 17 ml chloroform, and 10–15 ml ether. Aspirin is the most widely used analgesic-antipyretic. A saturated solution of aspirin has a pH value of about 2.5 and is reported to be most stable in the neighborhood of this value. In the presence of moisture or in aqueous or hydroalcoholic solutions, this aromatic acid which is also an ester gradually hydrolyzes into acetic and salicylic acids. The hydrolysis is hastened by heat and by acids and alkalies. The rate is essentially independent of the concentration and nature of the additive at a given pH value. The solubility of aspirin may be increased by the addition of alcohol, but the aspirin is more stable if left undissolved and suspended with the aid of gums, or sorbitol solution. It has been reported that bentonite and kaolin are unsatisfactory as suspending agents (since they are too alkaline). Sodium alginate is also unsatisfactory due to liberation of sticky alginic acid. The stability of aspirin has been studied in absolute alcohol and the solutions found stable for at least 2 years at 37°C; however as little as 1% water gave up to 4% hydrolysis in this time.

It has been reported that the hydrolysis of aspirin suspensions is zero-order; e.g., *The British Pharmaceutical Codex* mixture of acetylsalicylic acid hydrolyzes only 1–4% after 1 week and only 3–5% after 2 weeks at room temperature. This formula contains 3.43% aspirin suspended in chloroform water, using 2.29% compound powder of tragacanth. Acetates and citrates of the alkali metals increase the solubility of aspirin but do not prevent the hydrolysis; at room temperature about ½ of the aspirin is hydrolyzed after 1 week. After testing the effect of various buffers and solubilizers on the stability of aspirin in solution (e.g., sodium acetate, sodium acetate and acetic acid, potassium citrate, potassium citrate and citric acid, sodium phosphate, and ammonium chloride), it was reported the most stable solution formula to be a solution containing 4.4% aspirin solubilized by 8.8% potassium citrate. Even this formula hydrolyzed 25% in 1 week at room temperature. Aspirin then is apparently one drug where it may be better to prepare a suspension with a "Shake Well" label than a clear solution.

The preparation of a powder mixture to which water can be added at the time of dispensing has been recommended. This formula, which hydrolyzed only 6.6% 1 month after reconstitution (hence, appears satisfactory), contains: aspirin (6.0 g), aromatic raspberry imitation flavor (1.0 g), hydroxyethylcellulose (1 g), *d*-sorbitol (crystalline), Citric Acid USP (0.1 g), Methylparaben USP (0.12 g), and Propylparaben USP (0.02 g). This formula makes 100 ml of finished suspension when shaken with 56 ml of deionized water.

Aspirin gives a violet color with ferric salts after some hydrolysis has occurred to set the salicylate ion free.

Salts of aspirin are hydrolyzed, and the resulting solutions have the incompatibilities of acetate and salicylate ions. These are not very stable even in the solid form, and soluble calcium acetylsalicylate is achieved in the BP with a combination of aspirin (0.324 g), calcium carbonate (0.097 g), and citric acid (0.032 g) dissolved in water before use.

Aspirin gives a sticky mass on trituration with some compounds, e.g., antipyrine, hexamethyleneamine, potassium acetate, sodium phosphate, acetanilid, aminopyrine, and phenol or phenyl salicylate.

It has been reported that aspirin can be buffered with certain antacids to produce mixtures that are stable for a year. The antacids recommended were aluminum dihydroxyaminoacetate or calcium gluconate since these liberated only 0.65 to 0.80% free salicylic acid in one year at 25 or 37°C. The antacids tested with the amounts of free salicylic acid present 2, 4, and 52 weeks after mixing are as follows: aluminum hydroxide dried gel (0.22, 0.53, 3.9%); calcium carbonate (0.18, 0.20, 4.4%); calcium gluconate (0.16, 0.15, 0.8%); calcium lactate pentahydrate (0.09, 0.09, 71.0%); aluminum dihydroxyglycinate (0.05, 0.08, 0.65%); magnesium carbonate (0.22, 0.57, 11.0%); magnesium hydroxide (1.2, 1.2, 19.5%); magnesium oxide (0.4, 1.4, 18.0%); magnesium trisilicate (0.22, 3.9, 100%); sodium bicarbonate (0.22, 3.8, 100%); and sodium phosphate dibasic anhydrous (0.2, 0.36, 100%).

Dispensing Information: Use with extreme caution with anticoagulant therapy and with sulfonylureas. Aspirin may cause GI upset. Discontinue use if rectal bleeding occurs or if severe heartburn develops. To help decrease gastric side effects it is prudent to take aspirin with a large quantity of water. (There is evidence to support the contention that aspirin in solution causes less gastrointestinal blood loss than aspirin tablets.) Buffered preparations probably do not decrease the amount of gastrointestinal blood loss in aspirin recipients. Patients receiving high doses of aspirin should be aware of tinnitus (ringing in the ears, head noises) as a symptom of toxicity; patients with a history of hearing loss will not experience this side effect. Keep aspirin away from children; aspirin remains the leading poisonous substance ingested by children. Patients receiving high-dose therapy may need serum level assessments to monitor therapy. Advise physician of any change in stool color.

Atropine [*dl*-tropine tropate pK_b 4.35]—Atropine is a crystalline solid anticholinergic and mydriatic; 1 g dissolves in 460 ml of water, 2 ml of alcohol, or 27 ml of glycerin.

Considering the solubility of the alkaloid and its small dosage, it follows that it is not as likely to be precipitated by alkalies as are the alkaloids of higher doses; the presence of alcohol or glycerin would further lessen the chances of precipitation. Atropine is incompatible with alkaloidal precipitants. In the presence of alkalies it is hydrolyzed to tropine and tropic acid, particularly if heated. The free base is useful in oily vehicles, ointment bases, and other nonaqueous preparations. See also *Anticholinergic Agents.*

Atropine Methylbromide—A synthetic quaternary derivative of the atropine alkaloids. Atropine methylbromide has been reported to turn gray when mixed with cerium oxalate or yellow when mixed with ascorbic acid or potassium bitartrate. Slight to no color changes or eutectic mixtures are observed with other drugs.

Atropine Methylnitrate—See *Atropine Methylbromide*.

Atropine Sulfate USP [$(C_{17}H_{23}NO_3)_2 \cdot H_2SO_4 \cdot H_2O$]—1 g of atropine sulfate dissolves in 0.5 ml of water, 2.5 ml of glycerin, or 5 ml of alcohol. In aqueous solution the free alkaloid is alkaline (pH approximately 9.5 for the saturated solution), and a 1% solution of the sulfate has a pH of 5.4. Atropine sulfate is efflorescent in dry air and must be protected from light to avoid decomposition. It has been reported that 95% decomposition occurs within three hours on exposure to ultraviolet light. Atropine solutions decompose least if slightly acid (pH 4 to 5). Atropine or its salts should ordinarily not be dispensed in alkaline mixtures that are to be kept for more than a few days.

Atropine Sulfate Ophthalmic Solution USP—*Dispensing Information:* Patients may experience long-lived blurred vision due to atropine's persistent mydriatic/cycloplegic effect.

Aurothioglucose USP [Solganol (*Schering*); $C_6H_{11}AuO_5S$]—Antirheumatic. Yellow powder; nearly odorless; stable in air; pH (1 in 100 soln) about 6.3; aqueous solutions unstable on long standing. Freely soluble in water; practically insoluble in alcohol, chloroform, and ether.

AVC Cream [*Merrell-National*]—Contains aminacrine HCl 0.2%, sulfanilamide 15%, allantoin 2%, with lactose in a water-miscible base. See also *Vaginal Creams*.

AVC Suppositories [*Merrel-National*]—Contains aminacrine HCl 14 mg, sulfanilamide 1.05 g, allantoin 140 mg, with lactose buffered to an acid pH.

Aventyl Hydrochloride [*Lilly*]—Antidepressant. Nortriptyline Hydro-chloride. *Liquid* (10 mg base/5 ml): pH 3–3.5; alcohol 4%; solvent, purified water; sweetener, approx 3 g sorbitol solution/5 ml; $Na^+ < 1$ mg/5 ml; $K^+ < 1$ mg/5 ml.

Azapetine Phosphate [Ilidar (*Roche*); $C_{17}H_{17}N \cdot H_3PO_4$]—Antiadrenergic. White crystalline powder; odorless; melts 210–213°. 1 g dissolves in about 25 ml water and 500 ml absolute alcohol; practically insoluble in chloroform and ether.

Azathioprine USP [Imuran (*B-W*); $C_9H_7N_7O_2S$]—Antineoplastic. Yellow powder; odorless; slightly bitter taste; nonhygroscopic; light-sensitive; decomposes about 245°. Practically insoluble in water; very slightly soluble in alcohol and chloroform.

Azo-Gantanol Tablets [*Roche*]—Urinary anti-infective. Contain sulfmethoxazole 500 mg, phenazopyridine HCl 100 mg.

Dispensing Information: See *Phenazopyridine Hydrochloride*.

Azo-Gantrisin Tablets [*Roche*]—Urinary anti-infective. Contain sulfisoxazole 500 mg, phenazopyridine HCl 50 mg.

Dispensing Information: See *Phenazopyridine Hydrochloride*.

Bacitracin USP [*Various Mfrs.*]—Antibacterial. Bacitracin is the name given to a family of sulfur-containing basic polypeptides formed by *Bacillus subtilis* and *Bacillus licheniformis*. The exact structural formula has not been established; however, the main peptide, Bacitracin A, has two acidic groups and three basic groups. The molecular weight is about 1470. Bacitracin is a white to pale buff hygroscopic powder and is odorless or has a slight odor.

Bacitracin is most effective in treating penicillin-resistant and other Gram-positive organisms. Although used intramuscularly at doses of 60,000–80,000 units per day, it is subject to possible renal irritation. Accordingly it is chiefly used topically. It is believed to act on bacteria by inhibiting synthesis of the cell wall.

Bacitracin is soluble in water (800

mg/ml), ethanol, and methanol. It has a bitter taste. It is slightly soluble in acetone and insoluble in ether or petroleum ether. It is usually neutral (pH range 5.5–7.5).

Bacitracin powder is relatively thermostable. Samples containing less than 1% water have been stored at 5° to 37°C for 15 months without loss of potency. It is generally accepted that bacitracin is unstable in water dispersions. However, properly buffered aqueous dispersions of bacitracin can be kept for months at refrigerator temperatures. It is rapidly inactivated in aqueous solutions below pH 4 and above pH 9. The most suitable pH range appears to be about pH 4 to 5, although solutions adjusted to a pH between 5 to 7 lose only about 10% of their potency in 2 to 3 months at 4°C. The latter solutions deteriorate within 2 to 3 days at room temperature, however.

It has been noted that prolonged exposure of bacitracin solutions to light results in pronounced inactivation.

Stable ointments can be formulated in the anhydrous grease type of base containing petrolatum, lanolin, mineral oil, peanut oil, etc. Bacitracin is not very stable in Carbowaxes or the glycol type of ointment base. The instability of bacitracin in a base composed of Carbowax 4000, 45 parts, and propylene glycol, 55 parts, was reported to be such that 50% of the potency was lost in one week at room temperature, while the potency was retained for two months in the refrigerator. While the glycols might have some effect upon the stability of the antibiotic, one should consider the fact that the glycols are hygroscopic, and more or less water can be incorporated with different lots. Some polyethylene glycols might also contain aldehydes or peroxides.

Bacitracin has been reported to be unstable in aqueous ointment bases unless buffered and refrigerated as noted with previously mentioned aqueous preparations. Bacitracin has been shown to be rapidly inactivated in bases containing water, macrogols, propylene glycol, glycerin, cetylpyridium chloride, benzalkonium chloride, ichthammol, phenol, and tannic acid; and slowly inactivated in bases containing stearyl alcohol, cholesterol, polyoxyethylene derivatives, and sodium lauryl sulfate.

Nose drops of the dry powder type for reconstitution with water are stable in the dry state for long periods of time. When reconstituted, these nasal solutions are stable for one week under refrigeration. In this type of product one can use *dl*-desoxyephedrine HCl, ephedrine sulfate, amphetamine, phenylephrine HCl, lactose, and various antihistamines such as Bristamin. These nasal solutions should be isotonic with a pH of 5.5 to 6.5.

Bacitracin is precipitated by heavy metal salts. This precipitation is accompanied by inactivation if the metals are low in the electromotive series, but those high in this series such as zinc do not produce inactivation. Tannic, trichloroacetic, benzoic, furoic, and salicylic acids precipitate bacitracin, the first two producing complete inactivation. High concentrations of sodium chloride and acetone will also precipitate bacitracin from aqueous solution. One can use sterile water, isotonic saline, or 2% procaine HCl as topical solvents, however.

Bacitracin is reported to be absorbed on charcoal, aluminum oxide, and Lloyd's reagent. It is not inactivated by proteolytic enzymes such as pepsin or trypsin but is inactivated by hydrogen peroxide. It is said to be partially inactivated by BAL or sodium thiosulfate.

Bacitracin   Zinc—Antibacterial. This is a salt of bacitracin precipitated at pH 5 to 9 by adding a water-soluble zinc salt to aqueous bacitracin. It is only slightly soluble in water (0.5%) but is very soluble in aqueous vehicles at pH 4. It is soluble in ethanol (0.2%) and methanol but is insoluble in benzene, petroleum ether, ether, and chloroform.

Bacitracin zinc is reported to have a much less bitter taste than bacitracin; i.e., 1/5 to 1/7 that of bacitracin. It has also been reported that bacitracin zinc is markedly more stable than bacitracin, both as a powder and in formulated troches, ointments, and tablets.

Bactrim Tablets [*Roche*]—Urinary anti-infective. Contain trimethoprim 80 mg, sulfamethoxazole 400 mg.

Dispensing Information: See *Trimethoprim* and *Sulfamethoxazole.*

Barbital [diethylbarbituric acid; barbitone; Veronal; diethylmalonylurea; pK_a 7.91]—Sedative; hypnotic. Barbital is unstable in the presence of hydroxyl ions and will undergo hydrolytic cleavage to form therapeutically inactive products in alkaline solutions. Barbital (1 g) dissolves in 130 ml of water (pH $\cong$ 5.1) or 15 ml of alcohol; it forms water-soluble salts with alkalies. Barbital and calomel are incompatible; the mixture becomes dark.

Barbital Sodium [soluble barbital; soluble barbitone]—Sedative; hypnotic. Soluble barbital is derived from barbital by replacing the hydrogen of one of the NH groups with sodium. Barbital sodium is freely soluble in water but only slightly soluble in alcohol. The addition of acids to solutions of barbital sodium precipitates the insoluble barbital. This precipitation is also brought about by acid salts, and preparations which are only weakly acidic. Solutions of soluble barbital are unstable; hydrolysis soon occurs with precipitation of barbital and the formation of diethylacetylurea and other decomposition products. Such hydrolysis has occurred up to 50% in only a few months at room temperature; hence, aqueous solutions should be freshly prepared.

Solutions of barbital sodium are alkaline in reaction; a 2% solution has a pH of 9.4. Hence, barbital sodium will precipitate alkaloids from aqueous solutions of alkaloidal salts; with ammonium salts, ammonia is liberated, and the barbiturate base is precipitated.

Barbital sodium also should not be dispensed with chloral hydrate since the alkalinity decomposes the latter to chloroform and sodium formate with liberation of barbital free acid.

Barium Hydroxide Lime USP—Carbon dioxide absorbant. White or grayish granules; may have a color if an indicator has been added.

Barium Sulfate USP [Barosperse (*Mallinckrodt*); $BaSO_4$]—Diagnostic aid (radiopaque medium). Fine, white, odorless, tasteless, bulky powder, free from grittiness. Practically insoluble in water, organic solvents, and solutions of acids and alkalies.

Basic Fuchsin [a mixture of pararosaniline and rosaniline hydrochlorides; basic magenta]—This is a dark green or bronzelike, crystalline powder that is soluble in water and alcohol. It is used in preparing carbol-fuchsin solution (Castellani's paint).

Bellergal Tablets [*Dorsey*]—Sedative with antispasmodic. Contains Bellafoline 0.1 mg, ergotamine tartrate 0.3 mg, phenobarbital 20 mg.

Dispensing Information: May cause drowsiness, dry mouth, blurred vision, and flushing. Gum or candied mints may relieve dry mouth. See individual ingredient listings for other warnings.

Benadryl Elixir [*P-D*]—Antihistaminic. *Known ingredients* (per 4 ml); Benadryl HCl (10 mg), alcohol (14%); pH 7.2. *Known incompatibilities:* none listed.

Bendectin Tablets [*Merrell-National*]—Antiemetic. Contains dicyclomine HCl 10 mg, doxylamine succinate 10 mg, pyridoxine HCl 10 mg.

Dispensing Information: Do not drive or operate heavy machinery.

Bendroflumethiazide NF [Naturetin (*Squibb*); $C_{15}H_{14}F_3N_3O_4S_2$]—Diuretic; antihypertensive.

White, crystalline powder; odorless or slight floral odor; melts about 220°. Practically insoluble in water; 1 g dissolves in about 23 ml alcohol and 200 ml ether.

Benoxinate Hydrochloride NF [Dorsacaine (*Dorsey*); $C_{17}H_{28}N_2O_3 \cdot HCl$]—Topical anesthetic. White crystals or crystalline powder; odorless; salty taste; produces numbness of the tongue; melts about 155°. Very soluble in water and chloroform; soluble in alcohol; insoluble in ether.

Benylin Cough Syrup [*P-D*]—Expectorant cough mixture. Contains (per 30 ml) diphenhydramine HCl 12.5 mg, alcohol 5%, chloroform 4%. Has a tendency to darken and develop a slight haze with age; pH 5; light-sensitive; protect from freezing; specific gravity 1.291–1.322. *Known incompatibilities:* none listed.

Benzaldehyde USP [artificial essential almond oil; C_7H_6O]—Pharmaceutic aid (flavor). Colorless, strongly refractive liquid; odor resembling bitter almond oil; burning, aromatic taste; light-sensitive; boils about 180°; solidifies about −56.5°; specific gravity 1.041–1.046; refractive index 1.544–1.546 at 20°. 1 volume dissolves in about 350 volumes water; miscible with alcohol, chloroform, and ether.

Benzalkonium Chloride USP [Zephiran Chloride (*Winthrop*); alkylbenzylammonium chloride]—Topical anti-infective. This is a mixture of alkyldimethylbenzylammonium chlorides of the general formula $[C_6H_5CH_2N-(CH_3)_2R]Cl$, in which R represents a mixture of the alkyls from C_8H_{17} to $C_{18}H_{37}$. Benzalkonium chloride is a white or yellowish white, amorphous powder or gelatinous pieces. It has an aromatic odor and a very bitter taste. It is very soluble in alcohol and in water. Its solutions in water are alkaline and foam strongly when shaken. It is hygroscopic and is affected by air and light. The aqueous solutions give an oily precipitate with acids, a white precipitate with mercury salts, and a gelatinous precipitate with soaps.

Dispensing Information: Readily inactivated when in contact with organic matter. Readily contaminated with Gram-negative organisms (i.e., *Pseudomonas*).

Benzene Hexachloride, Gamma, USP [Kwell (*R&C*); $C_6H_6Cl_6$]—Pediculicide; scabicide. White, crystalline powder with a slight musty odor. 1 g in >10,000 ml water, 3.5 ml chloroform, 40 ml ether, and 20 ml dehydrated alcohol.

Dispensing Information: Detailed instructions for use of cream, lotion, and shampoo are supplied by the manufacturer. Patients should be totally familiar with the administration directions on the package. Notify physician if skin rash occurs and discontinue use. Irritating to eyes and mucous membranes. Explain method of application and hygienic measures to minimize reinfestation. Label: Poison. For external use.

Benzestrol NF [*Various Mfrs.;* $C_{20}H_{26}O_2$]—Estrogen. Benzestrol is an odorless, white, crystalline powder. It is soluble in alcohol and practically insoluble in water.

Benzethonium Chloride NF [Phemerol (*P-D*); $C_{27}H_{42}ClNO_2$]—Topical anti-infective. Phemerol chloride is an odorless, white powder which is freely soluble in water and alcohol; aqueous solutions have a pH of 5 to 6. It is hygroscopic and is affected by air and light. Solutions of phemerol chloride are incompatible with soap and iodides.

Benzocaine NF [anesthesin; ethyl aminobenzoate; $C_9H_{11}NO_2$]—Topical anesthetic. White, crystalline powder that is stable in air. 1 g dissolves in about 2500 ml of water (solubility is greatly increased by HCl). The hydrochloride salt cannot be used as it is too irritating. 1 g dissolves in 5 ml of alcohol or in 30 to 50 ml of fixed oils. An acid solution is incompatible with oxidizing agents and gives a precipitate with iodine. It forms colored mixtures with bismuth subnitrate and a sticky mass with resorcinol. It is used in local powders (up to 20%), sun creams (2%), ointments (5–10%), and suppositories and troches.

A number of workers have reported the complexation of benzocaine with xanthines and derivatives. These usually are effective in decreasing the hydrolytic breakdown of the drug. Studies of polyvinylpyrrolidone and derivatives, dimethylacetamide, polyethylene glycols, urea, and derivatives have indicated some delay in hydrolysis. The effect of surfactants suggests that the reduction in rate of hydrolysis varied with the type and concentration of surfactant. Anionic and cationic surfactants appeared to stabilize the drug while a quaternary salt had the opposite effect.

Benzoic Acid USP [$C_7H_6O_2$; pK_a 4.16]—Benzoic acid, useful as a preservative and antiseptic, is only slightly soluble in water (0.34%) and, hence, is precipitated when an alcoholic solution is diluted with water or when an aqueous solution of a benzoate is acidified. It is soluble in chloroform, ether, volatile and fixed oils and alcohol (1:2.3). It is solubilized in water by alkalies such as sodium hydroxide and by borax, trisodium citrate, or other alkaline materials, but it loses its preservative effectiveness in neutral or alkaline preparations. The pH of a saturated solution is about 2.8–3.1. Soluble benzoates give precipitates with solutions of Pb, Ba, Mn, Ag, and Hg salts and with neutral solutions of ferric salts. Benzoic acid is used as a preservative in cherry syrup and raspberry syrup; hence, these syrups are incompatible with salts of silver, mercury, lead, and quinine.

Benzoin USP [Sumatra benzoin; Siam benzoin]—Topical protectant. Balsamic resin obtained from *Styrax benzoin* or from *Styrax tonkinensis,* or other species of the Section *Anthostyrax* of the genus *Styrax*. Alcoholic solution is acid to litmus; becomes milky on addition of water.

Benzonatate NF [Tessalon (*Ciba*); $C_{30}H_{53}NO_{11}$]—Antitussive. A mixture of the *p*-butylaminobenzoate esters of the monomethyl ethers from a mixture of polyethylene glycols. Pale-yellow, clear, viscous liquid; faint, characteristic odor; bitter taste; produces numbness of the tongue. Miscible with water in all proportions; freely soluble in alcohol and chloroform.

Benzoyl Peroxide [Benoxyl (*Steifel*); Oxy-5 (*USV*); Persadox (*Texas Pharmacal*); $C_{14}H_{10}O_4$]—Keratolytic. Benzoyl peroxide is practically insoluble in water but is slightly soluble in olive oil. Its use as an antiseptic depends on its oxidizing power; it is incompatible with reducing agents.

Benzoyl Peroxide, Hydrous, USP [Epi-Clear (*Squibb*); Oxy-5 (*USV*);

Persadox (*Texas Pharmacal*); $C_{14}H_{10}O_4$]—Keratolytic. Contains 65–75% of benzoyl peroxide and about 30% water (to reduce flammability and shock-sensitivity). White, granular powder; characteristic odor. Sparingly soluble in water and alcohol; soluble in chloroform and ether.

Benzoylpas Calcium NF [Therapas (*Barnes-Hind*); $C_{28}H_{20}CaN_2O_8 \cdot 5H_2O$ or anhydrous]—Antitubercular. White or cream-colored, crystalline powder; odorless; tasteless at first but develops a characteristic, slightly bitter taste and a saccharin-like sweet aftertaste. 1 g dissolves in about 700 ml water; very slightly soluble in alcohol; practically insoluble in chloroform and ether.

Benzphetamine Hydrochloride [Didrex (*Upjohn*); $C_{17}H_{21}N \cdot HCl$]—Anorexiant. White to off-white, crystalline powder; odorless. 1 g in 1.5 ml water, 1.5 ml alcohol, 1.5 ml chloroform, and 1200 ml ether.

Benzquinamide Hydrochloride [Emete-con (*Roerig*); $C_{22}H_{32}N_2O_5 \cdot HCl$; pK_a 5.9]—Antiemetic. White or pale-yellow, crystalline powder; melts 222–230°; light-sensitive; stable in solution pH 2–4. One g dissolves in about 12.5 ml water and 43 ml alcohol.

Benzthiazide NF [Aquatag (*Tutag*); Exna (*Robins*); $C_{15}H_{14}ClN_3O_4S_3$]—Diuretic; antihypertensive. Fine, white, crystalline powder; characteristic odor and taste; stable in light and air; melts about 242°. Practically insoluble in water and chloroform; 1 g dissolves in about 260 ml alcohol and 2900 ml ether.

Benztropine Mesylate USP [Cogentin (*MSD*); $C_{21}H_{25}NO \cdot CH_4O_3S$]—Anticholinergic; antiparkinson agent. White, slightly hygroscopic, crystalline powder. 1 g in 1 ml water and 1–10 ml alcohol; very slightly soluble in ether.

Dispensing Information: Drowsiness may occur which may impair ability to drive or perform other tasks requiring alertness. Notify physician if eye pain occurs. Additive anticholinergic toxicity can occur when taken with phenothiazines.

Benzyl Alcohol NF [phenylcarbinol;

C_7H_8O]—Benzyl alcohol, sometimes used as a solvent or preservative, is soluble in about 25 volumes of water; it is miscible with alcohol. Aqueous solutions may be sterilized by boiling without danger of decomposition. *Caution:* Injection of 3% or higher solutions may produce edema and local inflammation.

Benzyl Benzoate USP [$C_{14}H_{12}O_2$]—Benzyl benzoate is an oily scabicide liquid which is practically insoluble in water but soluble in alcohol and oils. It is neutral and easily saponified with potassium hydroxide. *Caution:* Irritating to eyes. Allergic reactions have also been reported. Slight irritation of skin is common. Chiefly used as a lotion, i.e., Benylate Lotion, Vanzoate Lotion, Zylate Emulsion.

Bephenium Hydroxynaphthoate USP [Alcopara (*B-W*); $C_{28}H_{29}NO_4$]—Anthelmintic. Yellow powder; odorless; somewhat bitter taste; melts 168–173°. Practically insoluble in water; soluble in hot alcohol; 1 g dissolves in about 50 ml cold alcohol.

Berocca C [*Roche*]—Multivitamin injection. *Known ingredients:* thiamine HCl (10 mg/2 ml), riboflavin-5′-phosphate sodium (10 mg/2 ml), niacinamide (80 mg/2 ml), *d*-panthenol (20 mg/2 ml), *d*-biotin (0.2 mg/2 ml), ascorbic acid (100 mg/2 ml). *Known incompatibilities:* Ferro-Arsen (*Breon*), calcium levulinate (*Nion*), Solu-Cortef (*Upjohn*).

Berocca C-500 [*Roche*]—*Known ingredients:* (Same as Berocca C except 2-ml ampul supplied contains 400 mg additional ascorbic acid. *Known incompatibilities:* none listed.

Betamethasone   NF   [Celestone (*Schering-White*); $C_{22}H_{29}FO_5$]—Hormone (glucocorticoid). White to practically white, crystalline powder; odorless. 1 g in 5300 ml water, 65 ml alcohol, and 325 ml chloroform. See also *Corticosteroids (Systemic)*.

Betamethasone   Acetate   NF [$C_{24}H_{31}FO_6$]—Glucocorticoid. White powder; odorless; sinters and resolidifies about 165° (remelts with decomposition 200–220°). 1 g dissolves in about

2000 ml water, 9 ml alcohol, and 16 ml chloroform.

Betamethasone Sodium Phosphate NF [$C_{22}H_{28}FNa_2O_8P$]—Glucocorticoid. White powder; odorless; hygroscopic. 1 g dissolves in about 2 ml water and 470 ml alcohol; insoluble in chloroform and ether.

Betamethasone Valerate NF [Valisone (*Schering-White*); $C_{27}H_{37}FO_6$]—Hormone (glucocorticoid). White to practically white powder; odorless. 1 g in 10,000 ml water, 16 ml alcohol, <10 ml chloroform, and 400 ml ether. See also *Corticosteroids (Topical)*.

Betapen VK [*Bristol*]—Antibacterial. Penicillin V potassium. *Oral Solution (125 mg/5 ml):* pH 5–7; buffer, sodium citrate anhydrous; sweetener, 86.9% sugar; contains (per 5 ml) Na⁺ 0.464 mEq; K⁺ 0.407 mEq. *Oral Solution (250 mg/5 ml):* same as above, excepting (per 5 ml) sugar 82.2%; Na⁺ 0.539 mEq; K⁺ 0.816 mEq.

Betazole Hydrochloride USP [Histalog (*Lilly*); $C_5H_9N_3$·2HCl]—Diagnostic aid (gastric secretion indicator). White, crystalline powder; nearly odorless; softens about 215° (finally melts not higher than 240°); pH (1 in 20 soln) about 1.5. Soluble in water; practically insoluble in chloroform.

Bethanechol Chloride NF [Myocholine (*Glenwood*); Urecholine Chloride (*MSD*); $C_7H_{17}ClN_2O_2$]—Cholinergic. This carbamate and quaternary compound is a colorless or white crystalline powder that is stable in air. It is freely soluble in water and freely soluble in alcohol. A 1% aqueous solution has a pH of about 5.5.

Bili - Labstix   [*Ames*] — Reagent strips for urinalysis: pH, protein, glucose, ketones, bilirubin, and blood in urine.

Dispensing Information: Protection against exposure to light, heat, and moisture is mandatory to guard against altered reagent activity. The patient should be advised of the recommended procedures for handling and use.

Biperiden NF [Akineton (*Knoll*);

$C_{21}H_{29}NO$]—Anticholinergic. White, crystalline powder; practically odorless; nonhygroscopic; melts 112–116°. Practically insoluble in water; freely soluble in chloroform; sparingly soluble in alcohol.

Biperiden Hydrochloride NF [Akineton Hydrochloride (*Knoll*); $C_{21}H_{29}NO \cdot HCl$]—Anticholinergic. White, crystalline powder; practically odorless; slightly bitter taste; nonhygroscopic; melts about 275° with decomposition. Slightly soluble in water, alcohol, chloroform and ether.

Biphetamine Capsules [*Pennwalt*]—Appetite control. Contains equal amounts of *d*-amphetamine resin and *dl*-amphetamine resin.

Dispensing Information: Contraindicated in diabetes, hypertension, and coronary disease. Do not take a dose later than 5 p.m.; may cause nervousness, dryness of mouth, and insomnia. See also *Amphetamines.*

Bisacodyl USP [Dulcolax (*B-I*); $C_{22}H_{19}NO_4$]—Cathartic. This phenolic diacetate ester is a white to off-white, crystalline powder. 1 g in >10,000 ml water, 210 ml alcohol, 2.5 ml chloroform, and 275 ml ether.

Dispensing Information: Store in cool, dry place. Prolonged use may result in dependence. Tablets are enteric-coated; should not be chewed or taken with alkalies (i.e., milk or antacid). Irritant cathartics should not be taken when abdominal pain, nausea, or vomiting is present.

Bismuth, Milk of, NF—Astringent; antacid. Thick, white, opaque suspension which separates on standing; odorless; almost tasteless. Miscible with water and alcohol. Prepared from bismuth subnitrate, nitric acid, ammonium carbonate, and strong ammonia solution. *Known incompatibilities:* salicylates, alkaline preparations.

Bismuth Salicylate—See under *Salicylic Acid.*

Bismuth Subnitrate NF [$Bi_5O-(OH)_9(NO_3)_4$] — Pharmaceutic aid. White, slightly hygroscopic powder. Practically insoluble in water and alcohol; readily dissolved by hydrochloric acid or nitric acid. *Known incompatibilities:* carbonates, salicylates, reducing agents, iodides, gallic acid, tannic acid; aqueous suspensions yield nitric acid.

Bone Marrow Suppressants (Nonantineoplastic)—*Dispensing Information:* When a drug is known to suppress bone marrow activity, routine blood counts are indicated. Patients should be advised to bring to their physician's attention symptoms of infection (fever, sore throat, etc. due to leukopenia) and symptoms of bleeding (easy bruising, stool color change, etc. due to thrombocytopenia).

Boric Acid NF [H_3BO_3]—Pharmaceutic aid. Colorless scales, crystals, or white powder; somewhat unctuous to the touch; stable in air. Soluble in water and alcohol (1 g in 10–30 ml); glycerin, boiling water, and boiling alcohol (1 g in 1–10 ml). *Known incompatibilities:* alkalies, alkaloids, heavy metals.

Bromelains [Ananase-100 (*Rorer*)]—Anti-inflammatory. A concentrate of proteolytic enzymes derived from the pineapple plant, *Ananas sativus.* Buff-colored, amorphous powder. Partially soluble in water; insoluble in alcohol.

Bromisovalum [Bromural (*Knoll*); $C_6H_{11}BrN_2O_2$] — Central depressant. Soluble in alcohol and very slightly soluble in water. It is soluble in a 1 in 10 aqueous solution of sodium hydroxide from which it is precipitated by acids. In aqueous suspensions, alkalies induce slow decomposition.

Bromodiphenhydramine Hydrochloride NF [Ambodryl Hydrochloride (*P-D*); $C_{17}H_{20}BrNO \cdot HCl$]—Antihistaminic. White, crystalline powder; no more than a faint odor; very bitter taste; solutions unstable in direct sunlight; melts 148–152°. 1 g dissolves in about 1 ml water and 2 ml alcohol; insoluble in ether.

Bromophenol Blue [$C_{19}H_{10}Br_4O_5S$; pK_a 4.0]—*In vitro* diagnostic aid (urine content). Elongated, hexagonal prisms; decomposes about 279°; 1 g dissolves in about 250 ml water (more soluble in alcohol).

Brompheniramine Maleate NF [Dimetane (*Robins*); $C_{16}H_{19}BrN_2 \cdot C_4H_4O_4$]—Antihistaminic. White, crystalline powder; odorless; melts 130–135°; pH (1% aq soln) 4–5. One g dissolves in 5 ml water, 15 ml alcohol, and 15 ml chloroform; slightly soluble in ether and benzene. See also *Antihistamines.*

Brondecon Preparations [*W-C*]— Expectorant; bronchodilator. *Tablets:* Contain oxtriphylline 200 mg, glyceryl guaiacolate 100 mg. *Elixir:* Contains (per 15 ml): oxtriphylline 300 mg, glyceryl guaiacolate 150 mg.

Busulfan USP [Myleran (*B-W*); $C_6H_{14}O_6S_2$]—Antineoplastic. See *Antineoplastic Agents* (*Bone Marrow-Suppressant*).

Butabarbital Sodium NF [Butisol Sodium (*McNeil*); $C_{10}H_{15}N_2NaO_3$]— Sedative. White, bitter powder. 1 g dissolves in 2 ml water, 7 ml alcohol, and 7000 ml chloroform. See also *Sedatives and Hypnotics.*

Butacaine Sulfate NF [Butyn Sulfate (*Abbott*); $(C_{18}H_{30}N_2O_2)_2 \cdot H_2SO_4$]— Topical anesthetic. On addition of alkali hydroxides or carbonates to aqueous solutions, the free base separates as a colorless oily liquid; with soluble bicarbonates the precipitate is a crystalline carbonate of butyn. Incompatible with alkaloidal precipitants and silver-protein preparations. It also has the incompatibilities of sulfates. Chlorides react in presence of water to form nearly insoluble butacaine chloride; bromides are similarly incompatible. Solutions are stable; they are not decomposed by boiling. A 2% solution has a pH of 6.

Butamben NF [butyl aminobenzoate; Butesin (*Abbott*); $C_{11}H_{15}NO_2$]— Topical anesthetic. Almost insoluble in water or liquid petrolatum but is soluble in alcohol, dilute acids, or fatty oils. Being an ester, butamben is slowly hydrolyzed by boiling water. It is usually used as the picrate.

Butamben Picrate [Butesin Picrate (*Abbott*)]—Minor-burn therapy. 1 g dissolves in 2000 ml of water or about 100 ml of fatty oils; it is readily soluble in alcohol.

Metaphen in Oil (1:4000) has a mineral oil base in which the butamben will not dissolve. A clear solution can be obtained by using Metaphen in Oil "A," which contains peanut oil.

Butaperazine Maleate [Repoise Maleate (*Robins*); $C_{24}H_{31}N_3OS \cdot 2C_4H_4O_4$]—Tranquilizer. Bright-yellow powder; odorless; moderately bitter taste; degrades before it melts. 1 g dissolves in about 400 ml water; sparingly soluble in alcohol; insoluble in chloroform and ether.

Butibel Elixir [*McNeil*]—Antispasmodic with sedative. Contains (per 5 ml) butabarbital sodium 15 mg belladonna extract 15 mg. pH 5.5; alcohol 7%; hydroalcoholic vehicle; sugar and artificial sweetener; $Na^+/5$ ml, <5 mg; hypertonic; may be mixed with dilute hydroalcoholic substances of approx. the same pH for short-term use; do not use if precipitation is observed.

Butisol Sodium Elixir [*McNeil*]— Sedative. Contains (per 5 ml) butabarbital sodium 30 mg. pH 9.4; alcohol 7%; hydroalcoholic vehicle; artificial sweetener; $Na^+/5$ ml, <5 mg; hypertonic. May be mixed with dilute hydroalcoholic substances of approx. the same pH for short-term use; do not use if precipitation is observed.

Butyl Aminobenzoate—see *Butamben.*

Butylated Hydroxyanisole NF [Tenox BHA (*Eastman*); $C_{11}H_{16}O_2$]— Pharmaceutic aid (antioxidant). White, waxy solid; faint, characteristic odor. Insoluble in water; 1 g dissolves in 4 ml alcohol, 2 ml chloroform, and 1.2 ml ether.

Butylated Hydroxytoluene NF [Butylated Hydroxytoluene Crystalline (*Diamond-Shamrock*); Tenox BHT (*Eastman*); $C_{15}H_{24}O$]—Pharmaceutic aid (antioxidant). White crystals; tasteless; mild odor; melts 70°; boils 265°. Insoluble in water; 1 g dissolves in about 4 ml alcohol; freely soluble in chloroform and ether.

Butylparaben USP $[C_{11}H_{14}O_3]$—Pharmaceutic aid (antifungal agent). Small, colorless crystals or white powder; melts 68–72°. Very slightly soluble in water; freely soluble in alcohol and ether.

Cafergot Preparations [*Sandoz*]—Migraine therapy. *Tablets:* Contain ergotamine tartrate 1 mg, caffeine 100 mg. *Suppositories:* Contain ergotamine tartrate 2 mg, caffeine 100 mg.

Dispensing Information: May cause numbing and tingling of fingers and toes. Consult physician if chest pain develops or heart beat changes. See individual ingredients for other warnings. See also *Oxytocic Agents.*

Caffeine USP [1,3,7-trimethylxanthine; $C_8H_{10}N_4O_2$; $pK_a \simeq 13$, pK_b 14.15]—Diuretic and central nervous system stimulant; 1 g dissolves in 50 ml of water or 75 ml of alcohol; the aqueous solution is neutral. Caffeine is precipitated by tannic acid but is solubilized by an excess. With HCl and iodine it forms a red brown precipitate which is soluble in NaOH solution. *Citrated caffeine* is a mixture of caffeine and citric acid containing approximately 50% caffeine. Citrated caffeine dissolves in about 4 parts of warm water, but, if this solution is diluted with an equal volume of water, some of the caffeine gradually separates; the caffeine redissolves if more water is added. An aqueous solution of citrated caffeine is acid in reaction; a 4% solution has a pH of 2.3. As indicated by the solubility data, the presence of citric acid increases the solubility of caffeine. However, in presence of buffer salts, i.e., salts of weak acids, the acidity of the citric acid may be reduced sufficiently to bring about a considerable reduction in the solubility of caffeine.

Caffeine, Citrated—See under *Caffeine.*

Caffeine and Sodium Benzoate [1:1 mixture]—This stimulant is soluble in water; a 4% solution has a pH of 7.4.

Caladryl [*P-D*]—Antipruritic; antihistaminic. *Known ingredients:* Benadryl HCl (1%), calamine, camphor, glyc-

erin. *Known compatibilities and incompatibilities:* mixtures not recommended by manufacturer.

Calamine USP [prepared calamine]—Topical protectant. Contains iron oxide and zinc oxide. Pink, fine powder; odorless; practically tasteless. Insoluble in water; practically completely soluble in mineral acids. *Known incompatibilities:* reducing agents, alkalies, borax, alkali phosphates, tannic acid, acetates, salicylates, antipyrine.

Calcidrine Syrup [*Abbott*]—Antitussive. Contains (per 5 ml) codeine 8.4 mg, ephedrine 4.2 mg, calcium iodide anhydrous 152 mg. pH 4–5; alcohol 6% (*v/v*); glucose 1.55 g; sucrose 2.45 g; Na$^+$ none; K$^+$ none.

Calcitonin [*Armour*; $C_{159}H_{232}$-$N_{46}O_{45}S_3$]—Hypocalcemic. Light-yellow, hygroscopic powder; odorless. 1 g dissolves in about 700 ml water and 300 ml alcohol.

Dispensing Information: Patients should be familiar with injection instructions and technique of preparation of the solution.

Calcium Aminosalicylate NF [Pasara Calcium (*Dorsey*); $C_{14}H_{12}CaN_2O_6 \cdot 3H_2O$ or anhydrous]—Antibacterial (tuberculostatic). 1 g dissolves in about 7 ml of water and slightly soluble in alcohol. It is somewhat hygroscopic, and its aqueous solutions decompose slowly and darken in color. "Under no circumstances should a solution be used if it is darker than that of a freshly prepared solution"—NF. Solutions should be prepared within 24 hours of administration.

Calcium Carbonate, Precipitated, USP [$CaCO_3$]—Pharmaceutic aid (for antacid oral suspension dosage form). Fine, white, microcrystalline powder; odorless and tasteless. Practically insoluble in water (its solubility is increased by the presence of any ammonium salt or of CO_2; alkali hydroxide reduces its solubility); insoluble in alcohol; dissolves with effervescence in dilute acetic, hydrochloric, or nitric acids. *Known incompatibilities:* acids, alkalies.

Calcium Chloride USP [$CaCl_2 \cdot$

$2H_2O$]—Calcium replenisher. White, hard fragments or granules; odorless; deliquescent. Soluble in water, alcohol, and boiling alcohol (1 g in 1–10 ml); boiling water (1 part in <1 part). *Known incompatibilities:* phosphates, sulfates, hydroxides, carbonates, bicarbonates, borates, oxalates, arsenates.

Calcium Folate—See under *Folic Acid.*

Calcium Gluceptate [calcium glucoheptonate; (*Lilly*); $C_{14}H_{26}CaO_{16}$]—Nutrient. Crystals; hygroscopic; somewhat acrid taste; decomposes 200°. Soluble in water. *Known incompatibilities* (calcium gluceptate injection): cephalothin sodium, magnesium sulfate, oxytetracycline HCl, prednisolone sodium phosphate, tetracycline HCl. See also *Calcium Lactate.*

Calcium Gluconate USP [calcinol; *Various Mfrs.;* $C_{12}H_{22}CaO_{14}$]—Calcium replenisher. White, crystalline granules or powder; odorless; tasteless; it is neutral to litmus. 1 g dissolves slowly in about 30 ml water and 5 ml boiling water; more soluble in the presence of chlorides, citrates, or glycerophosphates of the alkali metals; insoluble in alcohol. The USP allows calcium gluconate solutions for injection to be stabilized by addition of a small proportion of calcium *d*-saccharate and addition of sodium hydroxide to give a pH not exceeding 8.2. *Known incompatibilities* (calcium gluconate injection): Achromycin, Albamycin, amphotericin B, Keflin, magnesium sulfate, Phenergan, Terramycin. See also *Calcium Lactate.*

Calcium Hydroxide USP [$Ca(OH)_2$]—Astringent. White powder; alkaline, slightly bitter taste. Soluble in water (1 g in 100–1000 ml), glycerin, and syrup (1 g in 10–30 ml), boiling water (1 g in 1000–10,000 ml); insoluble in alcohol. *Known incompatibilities:* acids.

Calcium Lactate USP [$C_6H_{10}CaO_6$·xH_2O or anhydrous]—Calcium replenisher. White powder or granules; nearly odorless; somewhat efflorescent; becomes anhydrous at 120°; aqueous solutions can develop mold. 1 g dissolves in about 20 ml water; practically insoluble in alcohol. *Known incompatibilities:* borates, carbonates, citrates, oxalates, phosphates, sulfates, tartrates.

Calcium Levulinate USP [*Various Mfrs.;* $C_{10}H_{14}CaO_6$·$2H_2O$ or anhydrous]—Calcemic. White, crystalline or amorphous powder; faint, burnt-sugar odor; bitter, salty taste. Freely soluble in water; slightly soluble in alcohol; insoluble in chloroform and ether. *Known incompatibilities:* see *Calcium Lactate.*

Calcium Pantothenate USP [dextro calcium pantothenate; Pantholin (*Lilly*); $C_{18}H_{32}CaN_2O_{10}$]—Enzyme cofactor vitamin. White, odorless powder which is slightly hygroscopic but reasonably stable to light and air. It is freely soluble in water, soluble in glycerin, and slightly soluble in alcohol. Aqueous solutions are neutral or slightly alkaline. Calcium pantothenate solutions are most stable in a pH range of 5.5–7; hydrolysis occurs at an increasing rate as the pH moves away from this range on either the acid or alkaline side. The pantothenate ion hydrolyzes to β-alanine and $d(+)$-α,γ-dihydroxy-β,β-dimethylbutyric acid, which then forms a lactone. Nicotinamide has a stabilizing effect on calcium pantothenate at pH 7–9, but not at pH 4–5. The stability of some other vitamins, i.e., thiamine, pyridoxine, and ascorbic acid, is poor at the pH of optimal stability of calcium pantothenate. *Known incompatibilities:* see *Calcium Lactate.*

Calcium Phosphate, Dibasic, NF [$CaHPO_4$]—Calcium supplement; pharmaceutic aid (tablet base). White, powder; odorless; tasteless; stable in air. 1 g dissolves in >10,000 ml water, 10–30 ml diluted hydrochloric acid and nitric acid; insoluble in alcohol.

Calcium Phosphate, Tribasic, NF [mixture of calcium phosphates; $Ca_5(OH)(PO_4)_3$]—Calcium supplement. White powder; odorless and tasteless; stable in air. Dissolves readily in dilute hydrochloric and nitric acids; insoluble in alcohol; practically insoluble in water.

Calcium Preparations—*Dispensing*

Information: Patients should be advised as to whether tablets are to be chewed or swallowed whole.

Calcium Stearate NF—Pharmaceutic aid (tablet lubricant). Compound of calcium with a mixture of solid organic acids obtained from fats and consists chiefly of variable proportions of stearic and palmitic acids; contains equivalent of 9–10.5% CaO. Fine, white, bulky powder; slight, characteristic odor; unctuous; free from grittiness. Insoluble in water, alcohol, and ether. *Known incompatibilities:* see *Calcium Lactate.*

Calcium Sulfate NF [CaSO₄]— Pharmaceutic aid (tablet diluent). Fine, white to slightly yellow-white powder; odorless. Dissolves in dilute hydrochloric acid; 1 g dissolves in 100–1000 ml water.

Calusterone [Methosarb (*Upjohn*); $C_{21}H_{32}O_2$]—Antineoplastic. White to off-white, crystalline powder; odorless; tasteless; melts 128–134°; degrades about 210°. Insoluble in water; freely soluble in alcohol.

Camphor USP [$C_{10}H_{16}O$]—Convulsant, counterirritant, local anesthetic and analeptic terpene ketone. It liquefies or forms a soft mass when triturated with some compounds, e.g., resorcinol, betanaphthol, thymol, urethane, phenol, chloral hydrate, butylchloral hydrate, menthol, and salol. 1 g of camphor dissolves in about 800 ml of water and in 1 ml of alcohol; hence, it is precipitated when alcoholic solutions are diluted with water. Camphor is precipitated from camphor water when soluble salts are added in sufficient quantity.

Candicidin NF [Vanobid (*Merrell-National*)]—Local antifungal. Yellow to brown powder; store in refrigerator. Sparingly soluble in water; very slightly soluble in alcohol.

Dispensing Information: See *Vaginal Creams.*

Capreomycin Sulfate, Sterile, USP [Capastat Sulfate (*Lilly*)]—Antibacterial (tuberculostatic). A polypeptide antibiotic produced by *Streptomyces capreolus.* White, amorphous powder; essentially odorless; solutions darken on standing (no loss in potency or increase in toxicity); affected by heat and moisture. Freely soluble in water; practically insoluble in most organic solvents.

Caprylic Acid [$C_8H_{16}O_2$; pK_a 4.90]—Colorless, oily liquid with an unpleasant odor used in preparing pharmaceutical salts and esters. It is very slightly soluble in water and soluble in alcohol. *Sodium caprylate* is freely soluble in water and sparingly soluble in alcohol. *Zinc caprylate* is practically insoluble in water or alcohol. This solubility profile also fits the longer chain fatty acids.

Caramel USP [burnt sugar coloring] —Pharmaceutic aid (color). Thick, dark-brown liquid; characteristic odor of burnt sugar; pleasant, bitter taste. Miscible with water in all proportions; immiscible with chloroform and ether.

Carbachol USP [Carcholin (*MSD*); carbamylcholine chloride; $C_6H_{15}ClN_2O_2$]— Cholinergic (ophthalmic). Crystalline, hygroscopic carbamate and quaternary compound; 1 g dissolves in 1 ml of water, yielding a neutral solution. 1 g is soluble in 50 ml of alcohol.

Carbamazepine USP [Tegretol (*Ciba-Geigy*); $C_{15}H_{12}N_2O$]—Analgesic; anticonvulsant. Practically insoluble in water; soluble in alcohol.

Dispensing Information: Discontinue use and consult physician if fever, sore throat, ulcers in mouth, easy bruising, or purple spots under the skin occur. Drowsiness may occur which may impair ability to drive or perform other tasks requiring alertness. See also *Bone Marrow Suppressants (Nonantineoplastic).*

Carbarsone NF [(*Lilly*); C_7H_9-AsN_2O_4]—This amebacide and trichomonicide is only slightly soluble in water or alcohol, yielding acid solutions. It is soluble in alkaline solutions.

Carbenicillin Disodium USP [Geopen (*Roerig*); $C_{17}H_{16}N_2Na_2O_6S$]—Antibacterial. White to off-white, crystalline powder. Freely soluble in water; soluble in alcohol; practically insoluble in chloroform and ether. See also *Penicillins.*

Known incompatibilities (carbenicillin disodium for injection): amphotericin B, gentamicin sulfate, multiple B vitamins with C, oxytetracycline HCl, tetracycline HCl.

Carbenicillin Indanyl Sodium [Geocillin (*Roerig*); $C_{26}H_{25}N_2NaO_6S$]—Antibacterial. White powder; hygroscopic; odorless; bitter taste. Soluble in water; insoluble in chloroform and ether. See also *Penicillins*.

Carbethyl Salicylate [Sal Ethyl Carbonate (*P-D*)]—Nonaddictive analgesic ester which is insoluble in water and in the acid secretions of the stomach but is broken down by the alkaline intestinal secretions. It is incompatible with any material having an alkaline pH.

Carbinoxamine Maleate NF [Clistin Maleate (*McNeil*); $C_{16}H_{19}ClN_2O \cdot C_4H_4O_4$]—Antihistaminic. White, crystalline powder. It is very soluble in water and freely soluble in alcohol. A 1% aqueous solution is slightly acidic (pH range, 4.6–5.1).

Carbomer NF [carboxypolymethylene]—Pharmaceutic aid (suspending agent). Polymer of acrylic acid, crosslinked with a polyfunctional agent. White, fluffy powder; slight, characteristic odor; hygroscopic; pH (1 in 100 dispersion) about 3. When neutralized with alkali hydroxides or amines, dissolves in water, alcohol, and glycerin.

Carbon Tetrachloride NF [tetrachloromethane; CCl_4]—Pharmaceutic aid (solvent); anthelmintic (hookworm). Clear, colorless liquid; boils about 77°. Dissolves in about 2000 volumes water; miscible with alcohol, chloroform, and ether.

Carboxymethylcellulose Sodium USP [Carbose D; Carboxymethocel S; C.M.C. Cellulose Gum (*Hercules*)]—Pharmaceutic aid (suspending agent; tablet excipient; viscosity-increasing agent). The Tablets (NF) are used as a cathartic. Sodium salt of a polycarboxymethyl ether of cellulose. White powder (hygroscopic) or granules; pH (1 in 100 aq susp) 6.5–8.5. Easily dispersed in water to form colloidal suspensions; insoluble in alcohol and ether.

Carbrital Elixir [*P-D*]—Hypnotic; sedative. Contains (per 30 ml) carbromal 0.4 g, pentobarbital sodium 0.12 g, several inert ingredients. Clear, dark orange-reddish liquid with sweet taste and flavor and odor of anise; alcohol 17–19%; stable for up to 60 months under normal room storage conditions; not affected by normal high or low temperature changes.

Known incompatibilities: the use of the Elixir in compounding with other agents is not recommended. It exhibits the same basic incompatibilities as that of phenobarbital, usually resulting in the precipitation of pentobarbital. It reacts with acids, acid salts including many alkaloidal salts, and many of the common vehicles which have an acid reaction. All elixirs and syrups of thiamine HCl liberate pentobarbital from the sodium compound and subsequent solution or precipitation of this substance depends on the alcohol concentration of the product. Even if precipitation does not occur, the combination is incompatible due to the neutralizing effect of the sodium compound on the acidity of the liquid with resultant destruction of the thiamine. Pentobarbital sodium liberates ammonia from ammonium salts and decomposes chloral hydrate with the formation of chloroform; with alkaloidal salts, pentobarbital and the free alkaloids are produced and may be precipitated.

Dispensing Information: Do not drive or operate heavy machinery. Do not take with alcohol.

Carisoprodol [Rela (*Schering*); Soma (*Wallace*); $C_{12}H_{24}N_2O_4$]—Skeletal muscle relaxant. Crystals; melts 92–93°. Very slightly soluble in water; soluble in most common organic solvents; insoluble in vegetable oils.

Dispensing Information: Do not drive or operate heavy equipment. May be potentiated by other CNS depressants and alcohol. May cause tremor, headache, nausea, or vomiting.

Carnauba Wax—Pharmaceutic aid (tablet polishing agent). From the leaves of *Copernicia cerifera*. Light-brownish powder; moderately coarse; bland odor; no rancidity; sp gr about 0.99; melts about 83°. Insoluble in water; soluble in warm chloroform; slightly soluble in boiling alcohol.

Castor Oil USP—Cathartic. Fixed oil from the seed of *Ricinus communis.* Pale, yellowish, transparent, viscid liquid; faint, mild odor; bland followed by slightly acrid, usually nauseating taste; sp gr about 0.955. Soluble in alcohol; miscible with chloroform and ether.

Cathartics and Laxatives—*Dispensing Information:* Patients should be made aware of the dangers of excessive laxative use or "laxative abuse."

Cefazolin Sodium [Ancef (*SK&F*); Kefzol (*Lilly*); $C_{14}H_{13}N_8NaO_4S$]—Antibacterial. *Known incompatibilities:* Amytal Sodium, calcium gluceptate, calcium gluconate, chlortetracycline HCl, colistimethate sodium injection, garamycin, kanamycin, Ilotycin Gluceptate I.V., oxytetracycline HCl, pentobarbital sodium, polymyxin B sulfate, tetracycline HCl.

Celestone Preparations [*Schering*]—Anti-inflammatory. *Soluspan Injection:* contains (per ml): betamethasone sodium phosphate 6 mg. pH 6.8–7.2; monobasic and dibasic sodium phosphate buffer. *Syrup* (per 5 ml): contains betamethasone 0.6 mg. pH 3–4; sweetener, sugar.

Cellulose Acetate Phthalate USP—Pharmaceutic aid (tablet-coating agent). Reaction product of phthalic anhydride and a partial ester of cellulose. White powder; may have slight odor of acetic acid. Insoluble in water and alcohol; soluble in acetone.

Cellulose, Microcrystalline, NF—Pharmaceutic aid (tablet base). Purified, partially depolymerized cellulose prepared by treating alpha cellulose with mineral acids. Fine, white, crystalline powder; odorless. Insoluble in water and most organic solvents; slightly soluble in NaOH (1 in 20) solution.

Cellulose, Oxidized, USP [absorbable cellulose; cellulosic acid; absorbable cotton; Oxycel (*P-D*)]—Local hemostatic. Sterile gauze or cotton chemical-ly oxidized to make it both hemostatic and absorbable. Slightly off-white gauze or lint; acid taste; slight, charred odor. Insoluble in water and acids; soluble in dilute alkalies.

Cellulose, Powdered, NF [$(C_6H_{10}O_5)_n$]—Pharmaceutic aid (tablet diluent; adsorbent; suspending agent). Purified, mechanically disintegrated cellulose prepared by processing alpha-cellulose. White substance existing in various grades; pH (supernatant liquid of 10 g/90 ml aq susp after 1 hour) 5–7.5. Insoluble in water, dilute acids, and nearly all organic solvents; slightly soluble in NaOH (1 in 20) solution.

Cephalexin Monohydrate USP [Keflex (*Lilly*); $C_{16}H_{17}N_3O_4S\cdot H_2O$]—Antibacterial. White to off-white, crystalline powder. Slightly soluble in water; practically insoluble in alcohol, chloroform, and ether.

Dispensing Information: See *Cephalosporins* (*Oral*).

Cephaloglycin NF [Kafocin (*Lilly*); $C_{18}H_{19}N_3O_6S$]—Antibacterial. Whitish, crystalline powder. Slightly soluble in water; practically insoluble in most organic solvents.

Dispensing Information: Should only be used to treat urinary tract infections. See *Cephalosporins* (*Oral*).

Cephaloridine NF [Loridine (*Lilly*); $C_{19}H_{17}N_3O_4S_2$]—Antibacterial. White to off-white, crystalline powder. 1 g dissolves in 5 ml water, 1000 ml alcohol, and 10,000 ml chloroform and ether.

Known incompatibilities (cephaloridine for injection): Amobarbital, chlortetracycline HCl, colistimethate sodium, Ilotycin Gluceptate, pentobarbital sodium, tetracycline HCl.

Dispensing Information: See *Cephalosporins* (*Oral*).

Cephalosporins (**Oral**)—*Dispensing Information:* Patients allergic to penicillin may be allergic to cephalosporins. It is estimated that 0.1–10% of patients allergic to penicillin G are cross-sensitive. Give false positive to Clinitest Reagent Tablets. See *Penicillins.*

Cephalothin Sodium USP [Keflin

(*Lilly*); $C_{16}H_{15}N_2NaO_6S_2$]—Antibacterial. White to off-white, crystalline powder; practically odorless. Freely soluble in water, saline, and dextrose solutions; insoluble in most organic solvents. *Known incompatibilities:* colistimethate sodium injection, Ilotycin Gluceptate (10 mg/ml or above), polymyxin B sulfate, tetracycline HCl, kanamycin, calcium gluceptate, calcium gluconate, chlortetracycline HCl, oxytetracycline HCl, Amytal Sodium, pentobarbital sodium, protamine sulfate. Stable in the dry state; upon reconstitution it should be refrigerated. It may be injected intramuscularly or intravenously but is not absorbed following oral administration.

Known incompatibilities (cephalothin sodium for injection): Achromycin HCl, Amytal, Aureomycin, calcium gluceptate, calcium gluconate, Compazine, colistimethate sodium, Coly-Mycin-M, Dilantin, erythromycin gluceptate, Kantrex, penicillin G sodium, pentobarbital sodium, phenobarbital sodium, polymyxin B sulfate, Terramycin HCl, tetracycline HCl, thiopental, Thorazine.

Cephapirin Sodium [Cefadyl (*Bristol*); $C_{17}H_{16}N_3NaO_6S$; pK_{a1} 2.15; pK_{a2} 5.44]—Antibacterial. White, crystalline powder; odorless. 1 g dissolves in 1.7 ml water; insoluble in chloroform.

Cetyl Alcohol NF [$C_{16}H_{34}O$]—Pharmaceutic aid (emulsifying and stiffening agent). White solid useful in creams, lotions, etc. It is insoluble in water but soluble in oils and organic solvents; stable in the presence of acids, alkalies, light, and air.

Cetylpyridinium Chloride NF [Cepacol (*Merrell-National*); $C_{21}H_{38}$-ClN·H_2O] — Topical anti-infective. White powder; slight characteristic odor. 1 g dissolves in 4.5 ml water, 2.5 ml alcohol, and 4.5 ml chloroform. A 1% solution is nearly neutral to indicators (pH range 6–7) but instruments with glass electrodes give variable pH's.

Dispensing Information: Mouth washes are of no value in the prevention or treatment of "colds."

Cherry Juice NF—Pharmaceutic aid (flavor). Liquid expressed from the fresh, ripe fruit of *Prunus cerasus.* Clear, red liquid; aromatic, characteristic odor; sour taste; affected by light. Acidic material may cause precipitation of those substances insoluble at low pH.

Cherry Syrup NF—Pharmaceutic aid (flavored vehicle). Prepared from cherry juice. The coloring matter is a cyanidin derivative which is practically decolorized on addition of alkalies. The syrup is decolorized by even feebly alkaline substances such as methenamine, aminopyrine, potassium citrate, sodium phosphate, and sodium borate. Since the syrup is acid in reaction, it causes effervescence with carbonates. Thus, sodium bicarbonate, dissolved in cherry syrup, causes precipitation; the color of the syrup changes to a dirty gray and the mixture effervesces for hours. Cherry syrup contains benzoic acid and, thus, has the incompatibilities of benzoates, such as the formation of precipitates with salts of silver, lead, mercury, and quinine.

Chloral Betaine NF [Beta-Chlor (*Mead-Johnson*)]—Sedative. Adduct formed from chloral hydrate and betaine. White, crystalline powder; faint odor characteristic of chloral hydrate; slightly bitter taste; darkens slightly on long exposure to light; slightly hygroscopic; melts (with decomposition) about 124°. 1 g dissolves in 1 ml water and 4 ml alcohol; insoluble in chloroform and ether.

Chloral Hydrate USP [Felsules (*Fellows*); Noctec (*Squibb*); $C_2H_3Cl_3O_2$]—Hypnotic. Colorless, transparent, or white crystals; slightly bitter, caustic taste; aromatic, penetrating, and slightly acrid odor; melts about 55°; slowly volatilizes when exposed to air. 1 g dissolves in 0.25 ml water, 1.3 ml alcohol, 2 ml chloroform, and 1.5 ml ether. It slowly decomposes in aqueous solution with the formation of hydrochloric acid; in alkaline solutions (e.g., borax, sodium phosphate, alkali hydroxides, and carbonates) it decomposes into chloroform and formic acid, the latter being neutralized by the alkali. Aqueous solutions of chloral hydrate and its butyl derivative, owing to the acidity which develops, are incompatible with phenobarbital sodium and other soluble barbiturates, the insoluble barbituric acids being precipitated on standing. They are also incompatible with aqueous solutions of soluble iodides and may release free iodine on standing.

A liquid or soft enteric mass is formed when chloral hydrate or butyl chloral hydrate is triturated with a number of compounds, e.g., camphor, menthol, monobromated camphor, quinine sulfate, theobromine and sodium salicylate, urea, urethane, acetophenetidin, and salol. The softening effect of chloral hydrate on gelatin makes encapsulation difficult unless diluted with suitable excipient, e.g., $MgCO_3$.

In hydroalcoholic solutions of some salts (e.g., potassium bromide) chloral hydrate is converted into chloral alcoholate, which separates as an oily liquid unless the concentration of alcohol is sufficiently high. The oily layer consists of chloral alcoholate, chloral, alcohol, and a small quantity of dissolved salt. The oily layer rises to the top or settles to the bottom, according to the concentration of the solution. When the concentration of alcohol is about 10% or less, either the reaction does not take place or not enough chloral and chloral alcoholate are formed to be thrown out of solution. With a vehicle containing 50% or more alcohol, the chloral alcoholate may remain in solution. The saline ingredients such as potassium, ammonium, or calcium bromide have the effect of salting out the substances composing the oily layer. The omission of the salt prevents the layering. Sugar affects the salting-out process, making a smaller amount of salt necessary to cause separation. There is some evidence that chloral alcoholate is slightly less hypnotic and less toxic than chloral hydrate. Even so, the separation of the alcoholate as an oily layer is objectionable since an excessive quantity is more likely to be taken at one dose.

Dispensing Information: Drowsiness may occur; alcohol will exaggerate the depressant effect. May have a variable effect on prothrombin times in patients receiving warfarin-type anticoagulants.

Chlorambucil USP [Leukeran (*B-W*); $C_{14}H_{19}Cl_2NO_2$]—Antineoplastic. Off-white, slightly granular powder; melts about 67°. Very slightly soluble in water; soluble in dilute alkali. *Caution: Great care should be taken to prevent inhaling particles and exposing the skin to them.*

Dispensing Information: See *Antineoplastic Agents (Bone Marrow-Suppressant).*

Chloramine-T [*Various Mfrs.;* $C_7H_7ClNNaO_2S$]—Antibacterial; deodorant. Soluble in 7 parts of water; the aqueous solution is alkaline (pH 7–8). It is soluble in alcohol, but the solution decomposes on standing. It is insoluble in oils and fats and is incompatible with them. Chloramine slowly decomposes in air, liberating chlorine, and thus has the incompatibilities of chlorine. It slowly tarnishes most metals and is incompatible with acids and organic substances. Chloramine gives color changes with dihydric phenols, e.g., a yellow-green color with resorcinol. It is incompatible with hydrogen peroxide.

Chloramphenicol USP [Chloromycetin (*P-D*); $C_{11}H_{12}Cl_2N_2O_5$]—Antibacterial; antirickettsial. Colorless, elongated plates or fine needles. It is soluble in water (about 2.5 mg/ml) and in propylene glycol (150 mg/ml). It is very soluble in methanol, ethanol, and acetone. It is insoluble in benzene, petroleum ether, or vegetable oils. Saturated solutions are acidic to nearly neutral (pH range 4.5–7.5). Chloramphenicol is most effective against Salmonella, typhoid, proteus, rickettsias, large viruses, grampositive and Gram-negative organisms, and staphylococci. It is used orally in 1–3 g/day dosage; intramuscularly and intravenously at 2–4 g/day. *Caution:* It may depress bone marrow. It apparently acts by blocking protein synthesis.

Chloramphenicol is thermostable but alkali-labile. The degradation is acid-base catalyzed with the rate independent of the ionic strength of the medium. Degradation in aqueous solution below pH 7 occurs through hydrolytic cleavage of the amide group. Below pH 2, specific hydrogen-ion catalysis plays a major role. Decomposition is catalyzed by monohydrogen phosphate, mono- and dihydrogen citrate ions and by undissociated acetic acid. At room temperature, aqueous solutions are stable at pH 2 to 9 for at least 25 hours. Neutral and acid solutions are stable on heating, e.g., aqueous solutions are still active after boiling for 5 hours. Chloramphenicol has been found to be most stable in borate buffer at a pH of 6 by dissolving the drug in borate buffer at 95–98°C and heating at 100°C for 30 min rather than autoclaving. Alkaline solutions are rapidly inactivated. Aqueous solutions and solvent solutions also darken on exposure to light. The color changes are associated with a loss in potency but are apparently not directly related. It has been noted that the yellow color of chloramphenicol in propylene glycol becomes more intense with time, but the loss in antibacterial activity is not directly related to the increase in color intensity. It is recommended that such solutions should not be used after 1 year. Also, it has been found that lotions and creams in which the chloramphenicol is dissolved in propylene glycol before incorporation are much more active than ointments containing only dispersed chloramphenicol. Storage of from 5–9 months apparently did not decrease the clinical effectiveness of the ointments. Only a 10% loss in potency has been noted after 9–12 months in chloramphenicol ointments or suppositories containing up to 2% water. It has been reported that chloramphenicol is reasonably stable in carbowax and petrolatum-lanolin-beeswax type ointments.

Chloramphenicol also appears satisfactory in cocoa butter suppositories and in eye drops in which 0.2% chloramphenicol is dissolved in 0.5% boric acid solution.

The chlorine is nonionic; thus, chloramphenicol is compatible with chloride precipitants. Chloramphenicol is not hydrolyzed by papain, trypsin, chymotrypsin, or pepsin. It is hydrolyzed by some bacterial enzymes.

Dispensing Information: Complete the entire prescribed course; discard the remaining quantity, if any. Discontinue use and consult physician immediately if sore throat, fever, mouth ulcers, easy bruising, or purple spots under the skin develop; also, notify physician if these signs develop within several months after use.

Chloramphenicol Palmitate USP [Chloromycetin Palmitate (*P-D*); $C_{27}H_{42}Cl_2N_2O_6$]—Slightly soluble in water (0.1%) and benzene. It is soluble in ethanol, isopropanol, and ether. It is insoluble in petroleum ether.

Dispensing Information: See *Chloramphenicol.*

Chloramphenicol Sodium Succinate USP [Chloromycetin Sodium Succinate (*P-D*); $C_{15}H_{15}Cl_2N_2NaO_8$]—Light-yellow powder. 1 g dissolves in less than 1 ml of water and alcohol.

Known compatibilities: In a concentration of 1 mg/ml it is stable for 24 hours in the following intravenous solutions—5% dextrose in water, 5% sodium chloride injection, 5% lactated ringer's injection, 10% dextrose in water, lactated ringer's injection, Normosol-M in D-5-W, Normosol-R, ringer's injection, sodium chloride injection. *Known incompatibilities:* when reconstituted with water for injection (10 mg/ml), it has been reported to be physically incompatible with solutions containing polymyxin B sulfate (200 μg/ml) or tetracycline HCl (1.5 μg/ml); however, it is compatible 1 mg/ml for 24 hours with tetracycline HCl (500 μg/ml); in a concentration of 1 mg/ml, it is incompatible with sulfadiazine sodium (2.5 mg/ml).

Dispensing Information: See *Chloramphenicol.*

Chlorcyclizine Hydrochloride NF [$C_{18}H_{21}ClN_2 \cdot HCl$]—Antihistaminic. White, crystalline powder. It is freely soluble in water and soluble in alcohol.

A 1% aqueous solution is slightly acidic (pH range, 5–5.5).

Chlordantoin [comp. of Sporostacin (*Ortho*); $C_{11}H_{17}Cl_3N_2O_2S$]—Topical antifungal. White, crystalline powder. Practically insoluble in water; soluble in alcohol.

Chlordiazepoxide NF [Libritabs (*Roche*); $C_{16}H_{14}ClN_3O$]—Tranquilizer (minor). Yellow, crystalline powder; practically odorless; sensitive to sunlight. 1 g dissolves in >10,000 ml water, 50 ml alcohol, 134 ml ether, and 6250 ml chloroform.

Dispensing Information: Interacts with alcohol and CNS depressants. Do not drive or operate heavy equipment. Do not drink alcohol. See also *Tranquilizers (Chlordiazepoxide Type)*.

Chlordiazepoxide Hydrochloride USP [Librium (*Roche*); $C_{16}H_{14}ClN_3O\cdot HCl$]—Tranquilizer (minor). White or practically white crystalline powder; odorless; affected by sunlight. Soluble in water and alcohol.

Known incompatibilities (chlordiazepoxide for injection): ascorbic acid, heparin sodium, pentobarbital, phenytoin, promethazine HCl, secobarbital sodium.

Dispensing Information: Drowsiness may occur which may impair ability to drive or perform other tasks requiring alertness. May enhance response to alcohol and other CNS depressants. Notify physician if sore throat, fever, or unusual bleeding or bruising occurs.

Chlormezanone [Trancopal (*Winthrop*); $C_{11}H_{12}ClNO_3S$]—Tranquilizer. Crystals; melt about 117°. 1 g dissolves in about 400 ml water and 100 ml alcohol.

Chlorobutanol USP [Chloretone (*P-D*), acetonechloroform, tertiary trichlorobutyl alcohol; $C_4H_7Cl_3O$ or the hemihydrate]—Pharmaceutic aid (antimicrobial agent); dental analgesic. Chlorobutanol is commonly used in two forms: i.e., anhydrous and hydrated with up to one-half molecule of water. The anhydrous form is used as a preservative in oil solutions and must be stored carefully so as to avoid moisture.

Cloudiness due to water droplets will be observed if the hydrate is used with oils. The drug is volatile and, hence, cannot be dried by heat. The use of a desiccator is recommended.

The hydrate form is more readily soluble in water (1:125) and is frequently used as a preservative in aqueous solutions at 0.5% concentrations. It is soluble in alcohol (1:1), glycerin (1:10), and all oils and organic solvents.

Aqueous solutions become more acid on autoclaving due to the liberation of hydrochloric acid, e.g.,

$$
\underset{\underset{CCl_3}{|}}{\overset{\overset{CH_3}{|}}{CH_3-C-OH}} + H_2O \longrightarrow \underset{\underset{HOCCl_2}{|}}{\overset{\overset{CH_3}{|}}{CH_3-C-OH}} +
$$

other decomposition products + HCl

This reaction may also occur in aqueous solutions on prolonged storage.

Chlorobutanol is rather volatile and, hence, is not suitable for dispensing in powders. It is readily decomposed by weak acids or alkalies. It has been reported that 0.5% chlorobutanol in 0.2 M acetate buffers is stable at pH 5, 6, and 7 but unstable at pH's above 7 based on decomposition rate studies. A liquid or soft mass is formed on trituration with some compounds, e.g., menthol, phenol, and antipyrine. Concentrations of chlorobutanol above 0.5% are salted out by normal saline solution.

Chloroform NF [$CHCl_3$]—Pharmaceutic aid (solvent). Soluble in 210 volumes of water and is miscible with alcohol and oils. On exposure to light and air, chloroform is gradually decomposed into phosgene and HCl. It usually contains 0.75% ethanol as a stabilizer. Chloroform is occasionally prescribed as a carminative vehicle in the form of chloroform water, chloroform spirit, or emulsion of chloroform. *Caution:* Large oral or inhalation overdoses may cause narcosis and death from respiratory and myocardial depression.

Chloroguanide Hydrochloride [proguanil HCl; Paludrine (*Ayerst*); $C_{11}H_{16}ClN_5\cdot HCl$] — Antimalarial (against *P. falciparum*). White, crystalline powder; pH (sat aq soln) 5.8–6.3; melts about 243°. 1 g dissolves in about 75 ml water and 30 ml alcohol; insoluble in chloroform and ether.

Chloromycetin Palmitate Suspension [*P-D*]—Antibiotic. *Known ingredients:* Chloromycetin Palmitate (125 mg chloromycetin equivalent/4 ml). *Known compatibilities and incompatibilities:* mixtures not recommended by manufacturer.

Chloromycetin Sodium Succinate Steri-Vial [*P-D*]—Antibacterial; antirickettsial. When reconstituted as directed—pH 6.4–7; stable for 30 days at room temperature; Na$^+$ 2.7 mEq. *Known compatibilities and incompatibilities: see Chloramphenicol Sodium Succinate.*

Dispensing Information: See Chloramphenicol.

Chlorophenothane NF [$C_{14}H_9Cl_5$]—Pediculicide. Colorless or white crystals or white, crystalline powder; odorless or slight, aromatic odor; bitter taste; slowly discolored in light; congeals not lower than 89°. Insoluble in water; 1 g dissolves in about 50 ml alcohol (greater the purity, lower the solubility), 3.5 ml chloroform, and 4 ml ether.

Chloroprocaine Hydrochloride NF [Nesacaine HCl (*Pennwalt*); $C_{13}H_{19}ClN_2O_2 \cdot HCl$]—Local anesthetic. White, crystalline powder; odorless; solutions acid to litmus; produces numbness of the tongue; melts about 174°. 1 g dissolves in about 20 ml water and 100 ml alcohol; very slightly soluble in chloroform; practically insoluble in ether. Similar in structure and pharmacological activity to *Procaine Hydrochloride*.

Chloroquine USP [Aralen (*Winthrop*); $C_{18}H_{26}ClN_3$]—Antiamebic; antimalarial. Whitish, crystalline powder; odorless; bitter taste; melts about 90°. Very slightly soluble in water; soluble in chloroform and ether.

Dispensing Information: Contraindicated in pregnancy, alcoholism, or previous history of blood dyscrasia. Do not coadminister with gold salts, phenylbu-

tazone, or hepatotoxic drugs. *Keep out of reach of children.* Consult physician immediately if any changes in vision or hearing are detected or if sore throat, fever, easy bruising, or purple spots beneath the skin occur. Periodic eye examinations should routinely be undertaken. Note: Short-term administration does not result in ocular toxicity. When administered for connective tissue diseases, visual acuity and ophthalmoscopic assessment is mandatory. Diarrhea may occur.

Chloroquine Phosphate USP [Aralen Phosphate (*Winthrop*); $C_{18}H_{26}ClN_3 \cdot 2H_3PO_4$] — Bitter antimalarial powder which is almost insoluble in alcohol but freely soluble in water; a 1% solution has a pH of about 4.5 and darkens on exposure to light. It is less soluble at pH 7 or above and is stable to heat at pH 4 to 6.5.

Chlorothiazide USP [Diuril (*MSD*); $C_7H_6ClN_3O_4S_2$]—Diuretic; antihypertensive. White or practically white, crystalline powder; odorless; melts about 355°. Very slightly soluble in water; practically insoluble in chloroform and ether.

Dispensing Information: Notify physician if loss of appetite, nausea, lethargy, muscle weakness, or other signs of electrolyte imbalance occur. Drug will cause increased urination. Potassium sources (such as orange or tomato juice, bananas, citrus fruits, melons) usually may be included in the diet to prevent electrolyte imbalance. See also *Diuretics (Chlorothiazide Type).*

Chlorothiazide Sodium for Injection NF [Diuril Lyovac (*MSD*); $C_7H_5ClN_3NaO_4S_2$]—Diuretic; antihypertensive. *Known incompatibilities* (chlorothiazide sodium for injection): very pH-sensitive (below pH 7.4 precipitation occurs).

Chlorotrianisene NF [Tace (*Merrell-National*); $C_{23}H_{21}ClO_3$]—Estrogen. Small, white crystals or crystalline powder; odorless; stable in air; pH (aq sat soln) 5–7. Very slightly soluble in water; slightly soluble in alcohol; freely soluble in chloroform.

Chlorphenesin Carbamate [Maolate (*Upjohn*); $C_{10}H_{12}ClNO_4$]—Skeletal muscle relaxant. White, crystalline powder; melts about 90°. Practically insoluble in cold water; readily soluble in alcohol.

Chlorpheniramine Maleate USP [Chlor-Trimeton (*Schering*); Teldrin (*SK&F*); $C_{16}H_{19}ClN_2 \cdot C_4H_4O_4$]—Antihistaminic. White, crystalline powder; odorless; pH (aq soln) 4–5. 1 g dissolves in 4 ml water, 10 ml alcohol, and 10 ml chloroform; slightly soluble in ether. *Known incompatibilities* (chlorpheniramine maleate injection): alkaline materials, calcium chloride, kanamycin sulfate, Levophed, Nembutal.

Dispensing Information: Drowsiness may occur which may impair ability to drive or perform other tasks requiring alertness. Avoid alcohol.

Chlorphenoxamine Hydrochloride NF [Phenoxene (*Dow*); $C_{18}H_{22}ClNO \cdot HCl$]—Anticholinergic. White, crystalline powder; melts about 133°. Very soluble in water, alcohol, and chloroform; very slightly soluble in ether.

Chlorphentermine Hydrochloride [Pre-Sate (*W-C*); $C_{10}H_{14}ClN \cdot HCl$]—Anorexic. White powder; odorless; bitter taste; melts about 233°. Freely soluble in water and alcohol; sparingly soluble in chloroform; practically insoluble in ether.

Chlorpromazine USP [Thorazine (*SK&F*)]—Tranquilizer. See *Chlorpromazine Hydrochloride.*

Chlorpromazine Hydrochloride USP [Thorazine Hydrochloride (*SK&F*); $C_{17}H_{19}ClN_2S \cdot HCl$]—Tranquilizer (major). White or slightly creamy white, crystalline powder; odorless; darkens on prolonged exposure to light. 1 g dissolves in less than 1 ml water, 1.5 ml alcohol, and 1.5 ml chloroform. *Known incompatibilities* (chlorpromazine HCl injection): aminophyllin, amphotericin B, benzylpenicillin, chloramphenicol, chlorothiazide, cloxacillin sodium, cyanocobalamin, dexamethasone, dimenhydrinate, ethamivan, herapin sodium, kanamycin, Keflin, methicillin sodium, Nembutal, par-

aldehyde, penicillin G potassium, Pentothal, phenobarbital sodium, secobarbital sodium, sodium bicarbonate, sulfadiazine sodium, vitamin B complex with C.

Dispensing Information: Drowsiness may occur which may impair ability to drive or perform other tasks requiring alertness. Consult physician if yellowing of skin or eyes occur. See also *Antipsychotic Agents (Phenothiazine Type).*

Chlorpropamide USP [Diabenese (*Pfizer*); $C_{10}H_{13}ClN_2O_3S$]—Hypoglycemic. White, crystalline powder; slight odor. Practically insoluble in water; soluble in alcohol; sparingly soluble in chloroform.

Dispensing Information: Consult physician immediately if yellowing of skin or eyes or a skin rash develop. Potentiation of hypoglycemic effects occur with sulfonamides, phenylbutazone, oxyphenbutazone, probenecid, coumarins, and MAO inhibitors. See also *Hypoglycemic Agents (Oral).*

Chlorprothixene NF [Taractan (*Roche*); $C_{18}H_{18}ClNS$]—Tranquilizer. Yellow, crystalline powder; slight amine-like odor; unstable in light and air; melts about 99°. Practically insoluble in water; 1 g dissolves in about 9 ml alcohol, 2 ml chloroform, and 4 ml ether.

Chlortetracycline Hydrochloride NF [Aureomycin Hydrochloride (*Lederle*); $C_{22}H_{23}ClN_2O_8 \cdot HCl$]—Antibacterial; antiprotozoal. Bitter, odorless, yellow, crystalline powder. It is sparingly soluble in water (14 mg/ml) and slightly soluble in alcohol. A 0.5% aqueous solution is acidic (pH range, 2.3–3.3). It is stable in air but may be affected by light.

Chlortetracycline is thermolabile in strong acids and bases. It has been noted that dry chlortetracycline, oxytetracycline, and tetracycline are relatively stable; however, when ascorbic acid is present, decomposition occurs and is marked at high humidities. It has also shown similar inactivation by riboflavin. The mechanism seemed to be photochemical oxidation and is prevented by antioxidants.

The stability of chlortetracycline at different pH values was studied and it was found that it was completely dehydrated in 60 hours at pH 1 to anhydroaureomycin, with its bacteriostatic activity lowered to about $\frac{1}{20}$ that of chlortetracycline. In alkaline solutions above pH 7 the antibiotic was rearranged to isoaureomycin, which has no color or bacteriostatic activity. The half-lives (i.e., loss of 50% activity) at 20°C were reported to be as follows: 72 hours at pH 7.4, 29 hours at pH 8, 10 hours at pH 8.6, and 6 hours at pH 9.2. These half-lives are greatly shortened at 30°C and 40°C (e.g., at pH 8 the half-life at 30°C is 6 hours and at 40°C is 2 hours. Chlortetracycline is fairly stable at pH 2.5. The base is amphoteric and will form salts with acids (e.g., chlortetracycline HCl) and bases (e.g., chlortetracycline calcium, magnesium, barium, strontium, etc.). The base is only slightly soluble in water (0.05%) and may precipitate out of solution above pH 5. It is freely soluble in dioxane, Carbitol, and various Cellosolves, and is slightly soluble in the lower alcohols, acetone, ethyl acetate, and benzene. It is insoluble in ether and petroleum ether. Chlortetracycline is mostly used as the hydrochloride, which is extremely bitter and nauseating in taste. The hydrochloride is soluble to the extent of about 1% in normal saline. The pH of such solutions is about 2.5 to 2.9. Solutions of the hydrochloride are stable for considerable periods of time, if acidified and stored under refrigeration. Chlortetracycline is stable in air, but light slightly affects the potency. A 0.5% solution of chlortetracycline in normal saline at a pH of 7.5 to 7.8 is inactivated in 24 hours at room temperature. Solutions should be freshly prepared and should be refrigerated.

A commercially available (*Lederle*) powder mixture useful in ophthalmic work contains 25 mg of Aureomycin HCl, 62.5 mg of sodium chloride, 25 mg of sodium borate, and 5 ml of sterile distilled water. This is essentially a solution of the borate, which is less stable than the hydrochloride. This solution can be refrigerated for no longer than two days. The addition of 0.25% methylcellulose to this ophthalmic solution is said to give a less irritating product.

It is doubtful that sodium carboxymethylcellulose could be substituted for the methylcellulose since it has been found that an insoluble chlortetracycline - carboxymethylcellulose compound is formed when aqueous solutions of chlortetracycline HCl and carboxymethylcellulose are mixed. Nitrates should also be avoided since it has been reported that insoluble Aureomycin nitrate may crystallize from mixtures of Aureomycin HCl and common nitrates, e.g., sodium, potassium, ammonium, barium, calcium, lead, magnesium, bismuth, cadmium, chromium, manganese, and strontium. Precipitates did not form with the nitrates of aluminum, cerium, cobalt, copper, iron, mercury(ic), nickel, zinc, or zirconium. It has also been reported that Aureomycin HCl gives water-soluble red, violet, and deep green iron complexes with ferric nitrate, as would be expected from the phenolic groups present in the molecule.

Aureomycin for intravenous use is buffered with sodium glycinate and is reconstituted with saline or glucose solution.

Chlortetracycline was quite stable in distilled water on standing at low temperature, but it lost antibiotic activity in a short time in tap water containing 1–4 ppm of chlorine. Water containing 5 ppm of chlorine destroyed the biological activity completely in one hour at room temperature. When the tap water was acidified with citric acid to approximately pH 5, chlortetracycline was as stable as in distilled water. In water made faintly alkaline by adding NaOH, chlortetracycline was stable for a few days, but the activity decreased gradually on standing. Tap water, boiled and cooled, showed a smaller effect on the antibiotic activity of chlortetracycline than did the unboiled water, but the biological activity was also decreased gradually. Chlorine was most detrimental, pH was secondary.

Chlorthalidone USP [Hygroton (*USV*); $C_{14}H_{11}ClN_2O_4S$]—Diuretic. White to yellowish white, crystalline powder. Practically insoluble in water, ether, and chloroform; slightly soluble in alcohol.

Dispensing Information: Take with orange juice. Consult physician if abdominal pain, nausea, vomiting, muscle weakness, cramps, or loss of appetite occur (sign of low K$^+$). See also *Diuretics (Chlorothiazide Type).*

Chlor - Trimeton Expectorant [*Schering*]—Contains (per 5 ml) chlorpheniramine maleate 2 mg, phenylephrine HCl 10 mg, ammonium chloride 100 mg, sodium citrate 50 mg, glyceryl guaiacolate 50 mg, chloroform 12.5 mg. pH 5.5–6.5; sweetener, sugar; solvent, water.

Chlor-Trimeton Expectorant with Codeine [*Schering*]—Contains (per 5 ml) same as *Chlor-Trimeton Expectorant* plus codeine 10 mg. Sweetener, sugar; solvent, water.

Chlor-Trimeton Syrup [*Schering*]— Contains (per 5 ml) chlorpheniramine maleate 2 mg. pH 4.4–5.6; alcohol 7%; sweetener, sugar; solvent, water.

Chlorzoxazone [Paraflex (*McNeil*); $C_7H_4ClNO_2$; pK$_a$ 8.3]—Skeletal muscle relaxant. Whitish, glistening, crystalline powder; odorless; melts about 191°. Very slightly soluble in water; moderately soluble in acetone and methanol.

Cholecalciferol USP [vitamin D; activated 7-dehydrocholesterol; $C_{27}H_{44}O$]—Antirachitic vitamin. White crystals; odorless; affected by air and light; melts about 86°. Insoluble in water; soluble in alcohol and chloroform.

Choledyl Elixir [*W-C*]—Theophylline therapy. Contains (per 5 ml) oxtriphylline 100 mg; alcohol 20%.

Dispensing Information: See *Smooth Muscle Relaxants (Xanthine Type).*

Cholesterol USP [cholesterin; $C_{27}H_{46}O$]—Pharmaceutic aid (emulsifying agent); ingredient of *Hydrophilic*

Petrolatum. Whitish, pearly leaflets or granules; almost odorless; usually sensitive to prolonged exposure to light or elevated temperatures; melts about 148.5°. Insoluble in water; 1 g dissolves in about 100 ml alcohol (slowly); soluble in chloroform, ether, and vegetable oils.

Cholestyramine Resin USP [Cuemid (*MSD*); Questran (*Mead-Johnson*)]— Ion-exchange resin (bile salts). White, fine powder; pH (1 in 100) 4–5. Slightly soluble in water and alcohol; insoluble in chloroform and ether.

Dispensing Information: Patients should be familiar with dose preparation and administration instructions. Since there is a potential to bind other drugs taken concurrently, cholestyramine is best administered at the greatest interval possible from other medications. Constipation routinely occurs.

Choline [$C_5H_{15}NO_2$]—Colorless, viscous liquid, very soluble in water and alcohol. It is the basic constituent of lecithin. It is very alkaline and absorbs carbon dioxide from the air. It readily forms stable salts, e.g., bicarbonate, borate, bitartrate, chloride, choline dihydrogen citrate, gluconate, salicylate, and tricholine citrate. Many of these salts are quite hygroscopic. They are mainly used as lipotropic agents.

Chymoral-100 Tablets [*Armour*]— Anti-inflammatory enzymes. Contain trypsin 100,000 u, chymotrypsin 100,000 u.

Dispensing Information: Take 1 hour before meals. Discontinue use and consult physician if hematuria, skin rash, or itching develop.

Chymotrypsin USP [Avazyme (*Wampole*); Chymar (*Armour*)—Proteolytic enzyme. Crystallized from an extract of the pancreas of the ox, *Bos taurus.* Whitish, crystalline or amorphous powder; odorless. An amount equivalent to 100,000 USP Units is soluble in 10 ml water and 10 ml saline TS.

Cinchophen [$C_{16}H_{11}O_2$]—Antipyretic and analgesic amine almost insoluble in water but forms soluble salts with hydroxides of the alkali metals. It is soluble in alcohol (1:120).

Citric Acid USP [$C_6H_8O_7$; pK_{a1} 3.08, pK_{a2} 4.74, pK_{a3} 5.40]—Weak acid used as a pharmaceutic aid (buffer, salt former, and complexing agent) and an acidulant. The pH of a 1% solution is about 2.6. Citric acid is soluble in water (1:0.5) and alcohol (1:2). Citric acid gives a greenish color with ferric chloride; effervesces with alkali and alkaline earth carbonates and bicarbonates and releases H_2S from soluble sulfides; incompatible with potassium tartrate and acetates. The following citrates are soluble in water: sodium citrate (1:1.5), potassium citrate (1:1), ferric ammonium citrate (very soluble), green ferric ammonium citrate (very soluble), magnesium citrate dibasic (1:5), soluble manganese citrate (manganese sodium citrate, 1:4), lithium citrate (1:1.5). These are insoluble or only slightly soluble in alcohol. The normal citrates of many of the other metals are insoluble, although the acid citrates are generally soluble. Calcium and strontium citrate will frequently separate out of mixtures containing these ions. This may be due partially to formation of high molecular weight polymer-like compounds, where the divalent calcium or strontium ions link a number of citric acids together.

$$CH_2COO\!-\!Ca\!-\!R$$
$$|$$
$$HO\!-\!C\!-\!COOH$$
$$|$$
$$CH_2\!-\!COO$$
$$\qquad\qquad\diagdown Ca$$
$$CH_2\!-\!COO\diagup$$
$$|$$
$$HO\!-\!C\!-\!COOH$$
$$|$$
$$CH_2COO\!-\!Ca\!-\!R$$

The citrates of sodium and potassium are neutral to slightly alkaline and may precipitate alkaloidal citrates or free alkaloids from solutions of alkaloidal salts (e.g., potassium citrate will precipitate quinine citrate from solutions of quinine bisulfate; it also precipitates the alkaloids of opium, nux vomica, and belladonna).

Potassium citrate is very soluble in water (1:1) and almost insoluble in alcohol; in hydroalcoholic solutions it tends to dissolve in the water and salt out the alcohol as a separate layer. Thus, if camphorated opium tincture is saturated with potassium citrate, the alcoholic and aqueous portions separate into two layers, the lower being a saturated aqueous solution of potassium citrate and the water soluble constituents of the tincture, the upper consisting of alcohol and the substances soluble in it. On standing, a precipitate appears between the two layers; this contains, among other things, the alkaloids of the tincture. Tinctures of belladonna, cinchona, nux vomica, etc., behave similarly.

Disodium hydrogen citrate is frequently prescribed as Liquid Citralka (*P-D*). This is a palatable, clear, light yellow solution. Although the marketed solution is slightly acid (ph 4.5 to 5), it is a systemic alkalizer (the citrate radical is oxidized, and there is an increase in the alkali reserve due to liberation of sodium ions). Among the drugs which may be prescribed with Liquid Citralka are: codeine sulfate, ferric ammonium citrate, potassium bromide, sodium bromide, hydriodic acid syrup, elixir IQ and S, Elixir Crysto-Vibex, Cosanyl, and Citronin. Because of insolubility or precipitation, the following drugs should not be dispensed in a mixture with Liquid Citralka, although they may be administered separately: acetylsalicylic acid, sodium barbital, phenobarbital elixir, sodium phenobarbital, calcium bromide, strontium bromide, sulfapyridine, sulfanilamide, sodium sulfanilamide, and preparations containing white pine or wild cherry.

Sodium citrate is a neutral to slightly alkaline salt that is soluble in water (1: 1.5) and insoluble in alcohol, which gives the same compatibilities as potassium citrate (*qv*). *Caution:* Repeated large doses may produce systemic alkalosis.

Cleocin Pediatric [*Upjohn*]—Clindamycin palmitate hydrochloride for oral solution. Na^+ 0.025 mg/5 ml; K^+ 0.05 mg/5 ml.

Clindamycin Hydrochloride USP [Cleocin (*Upjohn*); $C_{18}H_{33}ClN_2O_5S\cdot$ HCl]—Antibacterial. White or practically white, crystalline powder; odorless or has a faint mercaptan-like odor; stable in air and light; solutions are acidic and dextrorotatory. Freely soluble in water; soluble in alcohol.

Dispensing Information: Diarrhea, at times severe with blood and mucus, can occur. Patients experiencing significant diarrhea should report the symptoms to their physician. Supportive therapy for the diarrhea is indicated; no specific antiperistaltic agents should be used. Patients should be encouraged to take the entire quantity prescribed as is the case with any antibacterial medication.

Clindamycin Palmitate Hydrochloride NF [Cleocin Pediatric (*Upjohn*); $C_{34}H_{63}ClN_2O_6S\cdot$HCl]—Antibacterial. White to off-white amorphous powder; characteristic odor and taste. 1 g dissolves in about 10 ml water (pH 6), 3 mg/ml water (pH 7.4), 4 ml anhydrous alcohol, and 4 ml chloroform.

Clindamycin Phosphate NF [Cleocin Phosphate (*Upjohn*); $C_{18}H_{34}$-ClN_2O_8PS]—Antibacterial. White to off-white, crystalline powder; odorless or nearly so; hygroscopic; degrades to free clindamycin in temperatures of 50°; melts about 175°. 1 g dissolves in about 2.5 ml water; practically insoluble in alcohol, chloroform, and ether. *Known incompatibilities* (clindamycin phosphate injection): B complex vitamins.

Clinitest Reagent Tablets [*Ames*]— Quantitative determination of reducing sugars in urine.

Dispensing Information: Patient should understand use. See also *Reagent Tablets or Strips.*

Clofibrate USP [Atromid-S (*Ayerst*); $C_{12}H_{15}ClO_3$]—Anticholesterolemic. Colorless to pale-yellow liquid; characteristic odor. Insoluble in water; soluble in alcohol and chloroform.

Dispensing Information: Interacts with oral anticoagulants; the dose of the anticoagulant must be reduced by $\frac{1}{2}$–$\frac{1}{3}$. Consult physician if nausea, vomiting,

headache, or skin irritation (itching or rash) occur.

Clomiphene Citrate USP [Clomid (*Merrell-National*); $C_{26}H_{28}ClNO\cdot$ $C_6H_8O_7$]—Gonad-stimulating principle (ovulation-inducing agent). White to pale-yellow powder; essentially odorless. Slightly soluble in water and chloroform; sparingly soluble in alcohol; insoluble in ether.

Dispensing Information: Notify physician if visual disturbance occurs. Dizziness, lightheadedness, or visual disturbance may occur which may impair ability to drive or perform other tasks requiring alertness.

Clonidine Hydrochloride [Catapres (*B-I*); $C_9H_9Cl_2N_3\cdot$HCl; pK_a 8.2]—Antihypertensive. White, crystalline powder; odorless; bitter taste. 1 g dissolves in about 13 ml water, about 25 ml alcohol, and about 5000 ml chloroform.

Dispensing Information: Drowsiness can occur when therapy is initiated. Patients should be warned not to discontinue therapy without their physician's knowledge; abrupt discontinuation has led to severe rebound increases in blood pressure.

Clorazepate Dipotassium [Tranxene (*Abbott*); $C_{16}H_{11}ClK_2N_2O_4$]—Tranquilizer (minor). Light-yellow, crystalline powder; slight burning taste. Very soluble in water; very slightly soluble in alcohol; insoluble in chloroform and ether.

Dispensing Information: See *Tranquilizers (Chlordiazepoxide Type).*

Cloxacillin Sodium USP [Tegopen (*Bristol*); $C_{19}H_{17}ClN_3NaO_5S\cdot H_2O$]— Antibacterial. White, crystalline powder; odorless. Freely soluble in water; soluble in alcohol; slightly soluble in chloroform.

Dispensing Information: Notify physician if skin rash occurs. See also *Penicillins.*

Cobalamin Concentrate NF [*Various Mfrs.*]—Source of vitamin B_{12} (cyanocobalamin). Dried, partially purified product from the growth of selected *Streptomyces* cultures or other cobalamin-producing microorganisms. Pink to brown granules or fine powder.

Cocaine NF [methylbenzoylecgonine; $C_{17}H_{21}NO_4$; pK_b 5.59]—Cocaine alkaloid is a local anesthetic sometimes used as a narcotic. It is a crystalline solid of which 1 g dissolves in about 600 ml of water, 7 ml of alcohol, 80 to 100 ml of liquid petrolatum, or 12 ml of olive oil. The aqueous solution is alkaline and slowly decomposes on standing into benzoic acid, methyl alcohol, and ecgonine, the hydrolysis being promoted by heat, strong acids, and alkalies. The alkaloid is most stable in slightly acid solutions.

Cocaine hydrochloride (1 g) dissolves in 0.5 ml of water or 3.5 ml of alcohol; a 2% solution has a pH of 4.6. Cocaine reduces salts of mercury and silver and is incompatible with iodine.

Cocaine Hydrochloride—See under *Cocaine.*

Cocoa Butter USP [cacao butter; theobroma oil]—Pharmaceutic aid (suppository base). A fat from the roasted seed of *Theobroma cacao.* Yellowish white solid; faint, agreeable odor; bland, chocolate-like taste (if obtained by pressing) or bland taste (if by extraction); sp gr about 0.861; usually brittle below 25°. Slightly soluble in alcohol; freely soluble in chloroform and ether.

Codeine NF [methylmorphine; $C_{18}H_{21}NO_3$; pK_b 6.05]—Codeine and its salts are narcotic-analgesic; antitussive. Codeine alkaloid (1 g) dissolves in 120 ml of water or 2 ml of alcohol. Because of its appreciable solubility in water, the free alkaloid is not precipitated from dilute solutions of its salts on addition of alkalies. A saturated aqueous solution of the free alkaloid has a pH of 9.8; the alkalinity is sufficiently great to liberate ammonia from ammonium salts and to precipitate the oxide or hydroxide of numerous metals from solutions of their salts. *Codeine sulfate* (1 g) dissolves in 30 ml of water (pH 5.0) or 1280 ml of alcohol. *Codeine phosphate* (1 g) dissolves in 2.5 ml of water or 325 ml of alcohol. The pH is about 4.5.

Iodides form insoluble codeine iodide with codeine salts if the concentration of alkaloid is about 1% and the concentration of KI is about 3 to 5% or the concentration of HI is 2.5 to 3%. Lower concentrations give clear solutions if the ingredients are mixed as dilute solutions. The addition of 10 to 20% alcohol prevents or delays the formation of a precipitate in the more concentrated solutions.

Tannins present in Cheracol, wild cherry syrup, and raspberry syrup may also form insoluble codeine tannate.

Among the codeine derivatives are dihydrocodeinone bitartrate; dihydrohydroxycodeinone hydrochloride; dihydrocodeine bitartrate, etc.

Dispensing Information: May cause drowsiness, produce tolerance, be habit forming, or cause constipation.

Codeine Phosphate USP—See under *Codeine.*

Codeine Sulfate NF—See under *Codeine.*

Colchicine USP [$C_{22}H_{25}NO_6$; *Various Mfrs.;* pK_b 12.35]—Gout suppressant. Alkaloid (1 g) dissolves in 25 ml of water; freely soluble in alcohol. The aqueous solution is almost neutral (pH 0.5% solution = 5.9); the alkaloid, being an amide, has weakly basic properties and does not form stable salts. The alkaloid and its solutions are yellow and darken on exposure to light. Colchicine is decomposed by strong acids and alkalies and is precipitated by the usual alkaloidal precipitants. It has been reported that there is no significant hydrolysis of colchicine in solutions having a neutral or slightly alkaline pH (pH 8.1) during storage for 2 months.

Dispensing Information: Begin dosage immediately upon the first sign of a gout attack. Consult the physician if nausea, vomiting, or diarrhea are persistent.

Colistimethate Sodium USP [Coly-Mycin M (*W-C*); $C_{58}H_{105}N_{16}Na_5O_{28}S_5$]—Antibacterial. White to slightly yellow, fine powder; odorless. Freely soluble in water; insoluble in ether. Its solubility behavior is similar to that of colistin sulfate, but it hydrolyzes gradually in solutions above pH 9 with precipitation of colistin base. It has also shown no significant loss in potency during 4 weeks storage at room temperature in citrate buffered aqueous solutions (30 mg base/5 ml) at pH 4, 5, 6, and 7, or in dry formulations such as those given above for 18 months at room temperature. *Known incompatibilities* (colistimethate sodium for injection): cephalothin sodium, erythromycin lactobionate, hydrocortisone sodium succinate, kanamycin sulfate.

Colistin—Colistin is an antibiotic substance produced by *Bacillus polymyxa* var. *colistinus.* It is closely related to the polymyxins since it is a cyclic polypeptide composed of 10 amino acid fragments as follows: six of L-α-γ-diaminobutyric acid, one of 6-methyloctanoic acid, two of L-threonine, and one each of L-leucine and D-leucine.

Its spectrum is chiefly Gram-negative (*Pseudomonas, Escherichia, Klebsiella, Aerobacter, Salmonella, Shigella,* and *Hemophilus*). It does not appear very active against *Proteus* species or Grampositive organisms. It is bactericidal, probably acting through its cationic surfactant effect on cell membranes. Two forms of colistin are available for therapeutic use: colistin sulfate used by oral administration and colistimethate sodium, used by intramuscular injection.

Colistin Sulfate USP [Coly-Mycin S (*W* - *C*)] — Antibacterial (intestinal). White crystalline compound which is very soluble in water and glycerin. It is somewhat soluble in 70% alcohol and in propylene glycol. The base precipitates from aqueous solutions at pH 7.5 and above. These aqueous solutions are practically odorless and tasteless, and in citrate buffers (30 mg base/5 ml) were stable for 4 weeks at room temperature at pH 4, 5, 6, and 7. It is very stable in the dry state and formulated mixtures containing such ingredients as sodium chloride, thimerosal, sorbitol, sugar, nonfat milk solids, guar gum, phosphate buffers, dibucaine hydrochloride, cocoa powder, flavors, and parabens have shown insignificant loss-

es after 12–18 months at room temperature.

Collodion USP—Topical protectant. *Preparation:* Add 250 ml alcohol and 750 ml ether to 40 g pyroxylin contained in a suitable container, and stopper the container well. Shake the mixture occasionally until the pyroxylin is dissolved. *Caution: Highly flammable.* Clear, or slightly opalescent, viscous liquid; colorless or slightly yellowish; odor of ether. Also available with camphor and castor oil added as *Flexible Collodion USP.*

Combid Spansules [*SK&F*]—Anticholinergic and antiemetic/tranquilizer. Contain isopropamide iodide 5 mg, prochlorperazine maleate 10 mg.

Dispensing Information: Drowsiness may occur which may impair ability to drive or perform other tasks requiring alertness. Do not take with sedatives.

Compazine Preparations [*SK&F*]—Antiemetic; tranquilizer. Prochlorperazine. *Concentrate* (as the edisylate): pH 4–5; aqueous solvent; sweetener, sugar; Na$^+$ 6.5 mg/5 ml. *Syrup* (as the edisylate): pH 4.1–5.1; aqueous solvent; sweetener, sugar; Na$^+$ 1 mg/5 ml.

Contraceptives (Oral) [birth control pills]—*Dispensing Information:* Oral contraceptives are the most effective of all contraceptive methods if the patient follows the directions for their use and is careful not to skip doses or take them irregularly. The patient is best protected if they take the tablet at about the same time every day (with the evening meal or at bedtime are the most acceptable times). The oral contraceptives are powerful and effective drugs which can cause some side effects. The patient is urged to follow their doctor's instructions and to familiarize themself with the information about these contraceptives as follows:

1. Call your doctor immediately and stop taking the tablets if you experience any of the following: severe leg or chest pains, cough up blood, have difficulty in breathing, sudden severe headache or vomiting, dizziness or fainting, disturbance of vision or speech, weakness or numbness of any arm or leg.

2. A few women experience unpleasant side effects similar to complaints women have in the early stages of pregnancy (nausea or vomiting, spotting or bleeding between menstrual periods, some gain or loss in weight, slight enlargement or tenderness of the breasts, darkening of patches of skin on the face or elsewhere). These symptoms generally last only a few days, rarely more than a few months.

3. If you forget to take one or more tablets refer to the patient instructions provided with your medication or the following suggestions: (a) If one tablet is missed, take it as soon as remembered, or take two tablets the next day. (b) If two consecutive tablets are missed, take two tablets daily for the next two days, then resume the regular schedule. (c) If you forget your tablets on three consecutive days, stop taking your pill and start a new packet seven days after the last tablet was taken. When three consecutive tablets are missed you should use alternative means of contraception until the start of the next menstrual period.

Co-Pyronil Suspension [*Lilly*]— Antiallergic therapy. Contains (per 5 ml) pyrrobutamine phosphate 7.5 mg, methapyrilene HCl 12.5 mg, cyclopentamine HCl 6.25 mg. pH 7–7.5; solvent, purified water; buffer, sodium citrate; sweetener, saccharin sodium 5 mg/5 ml and sucrose 2.5 g/5 ml; Na$^+$ approx 10 mg/5 ml; K$^+$ <1 mg/5 ml. *Known incompatibilities:* Mixing with other products is not recommended; such mixing will upset balance of suspension system and will result in possible dosing error.

Dispensing Information: Use with caution in elderly males, and in hypertensive, diabetic, and cardiac patients. Do not drive or operate heavy equipment on initiation of therapy.

Corn Oil USP [maize oil]—Pharmaceutic aid (solvent). Fixed oil from the embryo *Zea mays.* Clear, light-yellow, oily liquid; faint, characteristic odor and taste; sp gr about 0.917. Slightly soluble in alcohol; miscible with chloroform and ether.

Corticosteroids (Ophthalmic)— *Dispensing Information:* Explain administration technique and hazard of not discontinuing therapy when advised to do so (may cause glaucoma). Label: for the eye.

Corticosteroids (Systemic)—*Dispensing Information:* Where long-term

high-dose therapy is being conducted, consider providing the patient with identification indicating the use of a corticosteroid. Instruct long-term users not to discontinue therapy without physician's advice. Advise physician if excessive weight gain (due to fluid retention), muscle weakness, tiredness, or any change in stool appearance occur.

Corticosteroids (Topical)—*Dispensing Information:* Should be used sparingly for the period of time directed by the physician. Repeated or overuse can result in a number of dermatologic side effects. Patients should be advised that "a little goes a long way."

Cortisone Acetate USP [Cortogen Acetate (*Schering*), Cortone Acetate (*MSD*); C$_{23}$H$_{30}$O$_6$]—Glucocorticoid. White, crystalline powder. It is practically insoluble in water (0.03 mg/ml), and slightly soluble in alcohol (1.6 mg/ml), glycerin (0.5 mg/ml), and propylene glycol (0.4 mg/ml). It does not hydrolyze readily in neutral or weakly acidic vehicles but is rapidly decomposed by alkaline and strong acids (see *Hydrocortisone*).

Cottonseed Oil USP—Pharmaceutic aid (solvent). Fixed oil from the seed of *Gossypium hirsutum* or other species of *Gossypium.* Pale yellow, oily liquid; odorless or nearly so; bland taste; solid fat particles may separate below 10°; solidifies 0° to −5°; sp gr about 0.918. Slightly soluble in alcohol; miscible with chloroform and ether.

Co-Tylenol Liquid Cold Formula [*McNeil*]—Decongestant; analgesic. pH 5; alcohol 7%; hydroalcoholic vehicle; artificial sweetener present; Na$^+$ <5 mg/dosage unit; K$^+$ none; hypertonic. May be mixed with dilute hydroalcoholic substances of approx the same pH for short-term use; do not use if precipitation is observed.

Cough Preparations—See *Expectorants and Cough Preparations.*

Cromolyn Sodium USP [Aarane (*Syntex*); Intal (*Fisons*); C$_{23}$H$_{14}$Na$_2$O$_{11}$]— Bronchodilator. White powder; odorless; hygroscopic; melts 261°. 1 g dissolves in 20 ml water; insoluble in alcohol and organic solvents.

Dispensing Information: Patients should be familiar with the operation and maintenance of the unique inhalation device. Patients should understand that the capsules are not to be taken orally and that the partially filled capsules represent no error; rather, they are partially filled by intent. Patients should understand that cromolyn will not abort an acute asthmatic attack. Increased wheezing (or other asthmatic symptoms) following cromolyn's use should be reported to the physician.

Crotamiton [Eurax (*Geigy*); $C_{13}H_{17}NO$]—Scabicide. Light yellow, oily liquid; faint, fishy odor. Slightly soluble in water; very soluble in alcohol.

Cryptennamine Acetates [Unitensin Aqueous (*Mallinckrodt*)]—Antihypertensive. Acetates of a mixture of alkaloids from *Veratrum viride*. Whitish, amorphous powder; odorless; melts over a wide range. Very soluble in water and alcohol.

Cryptennamine Tannates [Unitensin (*Mallinckrodt*)]—Antihypertensive. Tannates of a mixture of alkaloids from *Veratrum viride*. Tan, amorphous powder; odorless; melts over a wide range. Very slightly soluble in water; soluble in alcohol.

Crystodigin Tablets [*Lilly*]—Cardiotonic. Digitoxin.

Dispensing Information: Due to the importance of accurate dosing, the manufacturer does not recommend mixing with any other product.

Cupric Sulfate NF [copper sulfate; bluestone; blue vitriol; blue copperas; $CuSO_4 \cdot 5H_2O$ or anhydrous]—Antidote to phosphorus. Deep blue crystals or blue, crystalline granules or powder; nauseous, metallic taste; effloresces slowly in dry air; solution acid to litmus. 1 g dissolves in about 3 ml water, 500 ml alcohol, 3 ml glycerin (very slowly), and 0.5 ml boiling water. *Known incompatibilities:* alkali hydroxides, ammonium hydroxide, alkali carbonates, phosphates, borax, tannic acid, soluble iodides, lead, barium, strontium, calcium.

Cyanocobalamin USP [vitamin B_{12}; (*Various Mfrs.*); $C_{63}H_{90}CoN_{14}O_{14}P$]—Hematopoietic vitamin.

In addition to being a polyacidic base with six weakly basic amide groups, cyanocobalamin is a coordination compound of cobalt, with a cyano group attached to the cobalt. This cyano group is replaceable by other groups, e.g., in vitamin B_{12b} the cyano group is replaced by a hydroxo group and in vitamin B_{12c} the cyano group is replaced by nitroso. Similarly the cyano group may also be replaced by acetate, chloride, nitrate, and other anions to form other B_{12} analogs. Cyanocobalamin is soluble in alcohol but sparingly soluble in water, e.g., 1 g dissolves in about 80 ml water. It is insoluble in acetone, chloroform, and ether. Aqueous solutions are neutral. The most stable range has been found as pH 4 to 7 at normal temperatures. Solutions in the pH range 4.5–5 can be autoclaved for 20 min at 120°C.

Cyanocobalamin occurs as hygroscopic, dark-red crystals. When exposed to air, it may absorb about 12% water. It is inactivated by acids and alkalies. Exposure to sunlight or even traces of reducing substances such as reducing sugars, sodium bisulfite, ferrous salts, some flavors, decomposition products of thiamine, etc., have been reported as destructive.

Ascorbic acid causes rapid decomposition of vitamin B_{12} in solution, i.e., 1.5% loss per day at pH 2.5–3.0 and 100% loss in 1 hour at pH 7 (room temperature). Saccharated iron oxide or soluble iron salts at 17–1700 $\mu g/ml$ have successfully been employed as preservatives.

The successful use of 70% sorbitol either alone or in mixture with glycerin as a vehicle for oral products containing ascorbic acid, cyanocobalamin, and ferrous gluconate has been noted and also these vehicles have been found satisfactory for B_{12} alone.

Riboflavin may absorb light and cause rapid and complete photo-oxidation of cyanocobalamin. Niacinamide accelerates this photolysis while the antioxidants thiourea and ethylhydrocaffeate inhibit it.

Cyclandelate [Cyclospasmol (*Ives*); $C_{17}H_2O_3$]—Antispasmodic. Crystals; melts 50–53°. Insoluble in water; soluble in lipids and their solvents.

Cyclizine NF [Marezine (*B-W*); $C_{18}H_{22}N_2$]—Antinauseant. Whitish, crystalline powder; practically odorless; melts about 106°; pH (sat soln) about 8. Slightly soluble in water; soluble in alcohol and chloroform.

Cyclizine Hydrochloride USP [Marezine HCl (*B-W*); $C_{18}H_{22}N_2 \cdot$ HCl]—Antinauseant. White, crystalline powder or small, colorless crystals; odorless or nearly so; bitter taste; melts (indistinctly and with decomposition) about 285°; pH (potentiometric) about 5. One g dissolves in about 115 ml water, 115 ml alcohol, and 75 ml chloroform; insoluble in ether.

Cyclomethycaine Sulfate NF [Surfacaine (*Lilly*); $C_{22}H_{33}NO_3 \cdot H_2SO_4$]— Topical anesthetic. 1 g dissolves in about 100 ml of water, yielding a faintly acid solution which is soluble and retains its potency after boiling.

Cyclopentamine Hydrochloride NF [Clopane (*Lilly*); $C_9H_{19}N \cdot HCl$]— Adrenergic (vasoconstrictor). White, crystalline powder; mild, characteristic odor; bitter taste; melts (within 2° range) 111–117°; pH about 6. One g dissolves in about 1 ml water, 2 ml alcohol, and 1 ml chloroform; slightly soluble in ether.

Cyclopentolate Hydrochloride USP [Cyclogyl (*Schieffelin*); $C_{17}H_{25}NO_3 \cdot HCl$]—Adrenergic (ophthalmic). White, crystalline powder; characteristic odor on standing; solution acid to litmus; melts about 139°; pH (1 in 100) about 5.2. Very soluble in water; freely soluble in alcohol; insoluble in ether.

Cyclophosphamide USP [Cytoxan (*Mead-Johnson*); $C_7H_{15}Cl_2N_2O_2P \cdot H_2O$]—Antineoplastic. White, crystalline powder; liquefies on loss of water of crystallization; pH (3.33% aq soln) 3.6–4.7. Soluble in water and alcohol. *Caution:* Great care should be taken to pre-

vent inhaling particles and exposing the skin to it.

Dispensing Information: Keep from heat. This drug should be taken only under strict medical supervision. Notify physician if fever, sore throat, pain on urination, or unusual bleeding or bruising occurs. Reversible hair loss may occur beginning after 3 weeks of therapy. Preferably taken on an empty stomach, but may be taken with meals if gastric upset is severe. Maintain high fluid intake since this is an effective means of inhibiting the development of hemorrhagic cystitis which occurs with cyclophosphamide. Blood in the urine must be brought to the attention of the physician. See also *Antineoplastic Agents* (*Bone Marrow-Suppressant*).

Cycloserine USP [Seromycin (*Lilly*); $C_3H_6N_2O_2$; pK_a 4.4, 7.4]—Antibacterial (tuberculostatic). An antibiotic obtained from *Streptomyces orchidaceus* or *Streptomyces garyphalus*.

It resembles streptomycin in antibacterial activity and is most effective in INH-resistant tubercle bacilli. It is commonly given orally at 1 g/day. It may produce central nervous system irritation, principally convulsions, at higher dosage. It apparently acts by competing with D-alanine as a cell wall precursor.

Cycloserine is a white crystalline, amphoteric material, soluble in water (100 mg/ml) and partially soluble in glycols and isopropanol. It is insoluble in hexane, benzene, chloroform, ether, petroleum ether, methanol, ethanol, acetone, or dioxane. It is stable in aqueous solution for at least 1 week at 4°C. It is inactivated slowly at 37°C at pH 6.8. It is very unstable in acid or neutral solutions but stable in alkaline solutions.

Cyclothiazide NF [Anhydron (*Lilly*); $C_{14}H_{16}ClN_3O_4S_2$]—Diuretic; antihypertensive. Whitish powder; practically odorless; melts (within 4° range) 217–225°. Practically insoluble in water, chloroform, and ether; freely soluble in acetone and methanol; 1 g dissolves in about 70 ml alcohol.

Cycrimine Hydrochloride NF

[Pagitane (*Lilly*); $C_{19}H_{29}NO \cdot HCl$]—Anticholinergic. White solid; odorless; bitter taste; melts with decomposition about 241°; pH about 5.5. One g dissolves in about 175 ml water, 35 ml chloroform, and 50 ml alcohol.

Cyproheptadine Hydrochloride NF [Periactin Hydrochloride (*MSD*); $C_{21}H_{21}N \cdot HCl \cdot 1\frac{1}{2}H_2O$ or anhydrous]—Antihistaminic; antipruritic. White to slightly yellow, crystalline powder; slightly bitter taste; odorless or practically so; melts about 162° (sesquihydrate) or 250° (anhydrous). 1 g dissolves in about 275 ml water, 16 ml chloroform, 35 ml alcohol; practically insoluble in ether.

Dispensing Information: Contraindicated in glaucoma and urinary retention. Do not drive or operate heavy machinery. Avoid alcohol. See also *Antihistamines.*

Cytarabine USP [Cytosar (*Upjohn*); $C_9H_{13}N_3O_5$]—Antineoplastic; antiviral. Whitish, crystalline powder; odorless; nonhygroscopic; melts about 216°. 1 g dissolves in about 5 ml water, 500 ml alcohol, and 1000 ml chloroform.

Dactinomycin USP [Lyovac Cosmegen (*MSD*); $C_{62}H_{86}N_{12}O_{16}$]—Antineoplastic. Bright red, crystalline powder; light-sensitive (also protect from excess heat and moisture); melts about 246.5° with decomposition. 1 g dissolves in about 25 ml water (at 10°), 1000 ml water (at 37°), 8 ml alcohol, and 1666 ml ether.

Danthron NF [Dorbane (*Riker*); $C_{14}H_8O_4$]—Cathartic. Orange, crystalline powder; sublimes about 75°; melts 190–197°. Practically insoluble in water; very slightly soluble in alcohol; slightly soluble in ether; sparingly soluble in chloroform.

Dispensing Information: Prolonged use may cause brownish mucosal staining and drug dependence. Urine may appear pink.

Dantrolene Sodium [Dantrium (*Eaton*); $C_{14}H_9N_4NaO_5 \cdot x H_2O$ or anhydrous; pK_a (free acid) about 7.5]—Skeletal muscle relaxant. Deep-orange, fine powder; odorless; melts (with decomposition) 225–230°.

Dispensing Information: Main side effect is weakness, which may be profound; drowsiness may occur. These effects may diminish after the initial weeks of therapy. Advise physician if hepatitis-like symptoms occur.

Dapsone USP [sulfoxone sodium; DDS; Diasone Sodium (*Abbott*); $C_{12}H_{12}N_2O_2S$]—Antibacterial (leprostatic); dermatitis herpetiformis suppressant. Water-soluble and remains so if kept in evacuated ampuls but is slowly oxidized and becomes insoluble if exposed to air. The addition of 10% of sodium bicarbonate stabilizes the product in air for some time in the solid state or in solution. Acids cause precipitation of dapsone from its alkaline solutions.

Darvon-N Suspension (M-135) [*Lilly*]—Analgesic. pH 4–5.5; alcohol 0.1%; aqueous solvent; contains (per 5 ml) sweetener, approx 2.5 g sucrose; Na^+ approx 10 mg; K^+ <1 mg. *Known incompatibilities:* Manufacturer does not recommend mixing with other products as such mixing will upset the balance of the suspension system and will result in possible dosing error.

Deanol Acetamidobenzoate [Deaner (*Riker*); $C_{14}H_{11}NO \cdot C_9H_9NO_3$]—Antidepressant. White, crystalline powder; melts 159–163°. 1 g dissolves in about 2 ml water and 25 ml alcohol; slightly soluble in ether and chloroform.

Decamethonium Bromide [Syncurine (*B-W*); $C_{16}H_{38}Br_2N_2$]—Skeletal muscle relaxant. This diquaternary compound occurs as crystals which decompose 255–267°; aqueous solutions are stable and may be autoclaved. Freely soluble in water and alcohol; very slightly soluble in chloroform; insoluble in ether. It is compatible with thiopental sodium. Decamethonium iodide is similarly used. The pH of a 1% aqueous solution is about 6.6, while that of a 0.1% solution is about 6.1.

Decamethonium Iodide—See under *Decamethonium Bromide.*

Deconamine Elixir [*Cooper*]—Antihistaminic and decongestant. Contains (per 5 ml) chlorpheniramine maleate 2 mg, d-pseudoephedrine HCl 30 mg. pH 5.2–6.2; alcohol 15%; solvent system, water/alcohol/sorbitol; sweeteners: sucrose, sorbitol, saccharin sodium; Na^+ 0.74 mEq/100 ml.

Deferoxamine Mesylate [Desferal Mesylate (*Ciba*); $C_{25}H_{48}N_6O_8 \cdot CH_4O_3S$]—Chelating agent (iron). White crystals. Freely soluble in water.

Dehydrocholic Acid NF [Cholan-DH (*Pennwalt*); Decholin (*Dome*); $C_{24}H_{34}O_5$]—Choleretic. White, fluffy powder; odorless; bitter taste; melts (within 3° range) 231–242° (for parenteral use, 237–242°); the higher the melting temperature, the greater the purity. Practically insoluble in water; slightly soluble in ether; 1 g dissolves in about 100 ml alcohol and 35 ml chloroform.

Demazin Syrup [*Schering-White*]—Antihistaminic. Contains (per 5 ml) chlorpheniramine maleate 1 mg, phenylephrine HCl 2.5 mg. pH 4.5–6; alcohol 7.5%; sweetener, sugar; solvent, water.

Demecarium Bromide NF [Humorsol (*MSD*); $C_{32}H_{52}Br_2N_4O_4$]—Cholinergic (ophthalmic). Whitish, crystalline powder; slightly hygroscopic; melts with decomposition about 165°; aqueous solution neutral. Freely soluble in water and alcohol; soluble in ether.

Demeclocycline NF [demethylchlortetracycline; Declomycin (*Lederle*) $C_{21}H_{21}ClN_2O_8 \cdot 1\frac{1}{2}H_2O$; p$K_a'$ = 4.45 (50% dimethylformamide - water)] — Antibacterial. Slightly soluble in water (45 mg per ml). This broad-spectrum antibiotic produced by a mutant strain of *Streptomyces aureofaciens* is closely related to earlier tetracyclines. The absence of the methyl group at position 6 on the ring gives the molecule greater stability to acid and alkali and to elevated storage temperatures. This antibiotic is said to have about the same spectrum as the other tetracyclines, however it is slightly more active against a greater proportion of the strains. See *Demeclocycline Hydrochloride.*

Demeclocycline Hydrochloride [demethylchlortetracycline hydrochloride; Declomycin Hydrochloride (*Lederle*); $C_{21}H_{21}ClN_2O_8 \cdot HCl$]—Antibacterial. Yellow, crystalline powder; odorless; bitter taste; pH (1% soln) about 2.5. Sparingly soluble in water.

Dispensing Information: Do not expose to intense sunlight as this may cause a severe sunburn-like reaction. May cause nausea and vomiting or skin rash. See also *Tetracyclines.*

Denatonium Benzoate NF [$C_{28}H_{34}N_2O_3$]—Pharmaceutic aid (alcohol denaturant; flavor). White, crystalline powder; odorless; intensely bitter taste; melts about 168°. 1 g dissolves in about 20 ml water, 2.4 ml alcohol, 2.9 ml chloroform, and 5000 ml ether.

Deprol Tablets [*Wallace*]—Antidepressant. Contain meprobamate 400 mg, benactyzine HCl 1 mg.

Dispensing Information: Do not drive or operate heavy machinery on starting therapy. Avoid alcohol.

Dermatologic Preparations—*Dispensing Information:* Administration advice is essential.

Deserpidine [Harmonyl (*Abbott*); 11-desmethoxyreserpine; $C_{32}H_{38}N_2O_8$]—This is an ester alkaloid isolated from *Rauwolfia canescens.* *Side effects:* Qualitatively similar to those of reserpine with less incidence and severity.

Desipramine Hydrochloride NF [Norpramin (*Lakeside*); $C_{18}H_{22}N_2 \cdot HCl$]—Antidepressant. White to off-white, crystalline powder. 1 g dissolves in 12 ml water, 14 ml alcohol, 3.5 ml chloroform, and >10,000 ml ether.

Dispensing Information: See *Antidepressants* (*Tricyclic*).

Deslanoside NF [Cedilanid D (*Sandoz*); $C_{47}H_{74}O_{19}$]—Cardiotonic. Colorless or white crystals or white, crystalline powder; odorless; hygroscopic; melts (indistinctly) about 220°. Very slightly soluble in water; 1 g dissolves in about 300 ml alcohol; very slightly soluble in chloroform.

Desonide [Tridesilon (*Dome*); $C_{24}H_{32}O_6$]—Anti-inflammatory. Whitish, fine, crystalline powder. Practically insoluble in water.

Desoxycorticosterone Acetate USP [Cortate (*Schering*), D.O.C.A. (*Organon*), Percorten (*Ciba*); $C_{23}H_{32}O_4$]—Adrenocortical steroid (salt-regulating). White, crystalline powder. It is practically insoluble in water and sparingly soluble in alcohol. It is stable in air but is sensitive to light.

Desoxycorticosterone Pivalate NF [Percorten Trimethylacetate (*Ciba*); $C_{26}H_{38}O_4$]—Whitish, crystalline powder; odorless; melts about 203°. Practically insoluble in water; slightly soluble in alcohol and ether.

Dexamethasone USP [Decadron (*MSD*); Hexadrol (*Organon*); $C_{22}H_{29}FO_5$]—Adrenocortical steroid (anti-inflammatory). White to practically white, crystalline powder; odorless; stable in air; melts about 250° with some decomposition. Practically insoluble in water; sparingly soluble in alcohol; slightly soluble in chloroform; very slightly soluble in ether.
Dispensing Information: See *Corticosteroids (Systemic).*

Dexamethasone Sodium Phosphate USP [Decadron Turbinaire (*MSD*); $C_{22}H_{28}FNa_2O_8P$]—Adrenocortical steroid (anti-inflammatory). White or slightly yellow, crystalline powder; odorless or slight odor of alcohol; extremely hygroscopic; pH (1% soln) 7.5–10.5. One g dissolves in 2 ml water; slightly soluble in alcohol; insoluble in chloroform and ether. *Known incompatibilities* (dexamethasone sodium phosphate injection): Compazine, Vancocin.

Dexamyl Preparations [*SK&F*]—Contain (per tablet or 5 ml elixir) dextroamphetamine sulfate 5 mg, amobarbital 30 mg.
Dispensing Information: Interacts with MAO inhibitors. Do not exceed labeled dosage. *Spansules:* Take dose in early morning. *Elixir* and *Tablets:* Take last dose before 6 p.m.

Dexbrompheniramine Maleate NF [Disomer (*Schering*); $C_{16}H_{19}BrN_2 \cdot C_4H_4O_4$]—Antihistaminic. White, crystalline powder; odorless; melts about 108°; pH (1 in 100 soln) about 5. One g dissolves in about 1.2 ml water, 2.5 ml alcohol, 2 ml chloroform, and 3000 ml ether.

Dexchlorpheniramine Maleate NF [Polaramine (*Schering*); $C_{16}H_{19}ClN_2 \cdot C_4H_4O_4$]—Antihistaminic. White, crystalline powder; odorless. 1 g dissolves in 1.1 ml water, 2 ml alcohol, 1.7 ml chloroform, and 2500 ml ether.

Dexpanthenol [Ilopan (*Warren-Teed*); Motilyn (*Abbott*); Cozyme (*Travenol*); $C_9H_{19}NO_4$]—Cholinergic. Viscous liquid; somewhat hygroscopic; slightly bitter taste. Freely soluble in water and alcohol; slightly soluble in ether.

Dextran 40 [Gentran 40 (*Travenol*); LMD (*Abbott*); Rheomacrodex (*Pharmacia*); $(C_6H_{10}O_5)_n$]—Blood flow adjuvant; plasma volume extender. White, amorphous powder; odorless; tasteless; 10% solution in D5W darkens slightly over long storage as with other dextrose-containing solutions (darkening accelerated by increased ambient temperatures). Freely soluble in water; insoluble in alcohol and ether.

Dextran 75 [Gentran 75 (*Travenol*); Macrodex (*Pharmacia*); $(C_6H_{10}O_5)_n$]—Plasma volume extender. Fine, white, amorphous powder; odorless; tasteless; very hygroscopic. Freely soluble in hot water; insoluble in alcohol and ether.

Dextrin [British gum; starch gum; $(C_6H_{10}O_5)_n$]—Pharmaceutic aid (excipient; emulsifier). White or yellow, amorphous powder (yellow has a characteristic odor). Soluble in 3 parts boiling water (forms gummy solution); less soluble in cold water.

Dextroamphetamine Phosphate NF [*Various Mfrs.;* $C_9H_{13}N \cdot H_3PO_4$]—Central stimulant. White, crystalline powder; odorless; bitter taste; pH (1 in 20 soln) 4–5. One g dissolves in 20 ml water; slightly soluble in alcohol; practically insoluble in chloroform and ether.
Dispensing Information: Take last dose 6 hours before bedtime (12 hours for sustained-action preparations). May cause dry mouth, nervousness, sweating, diarrhea, headache, and increased blood pressure. See also *Amphetamines.*

Dextromethorphan Hydrobromide NF [Dormethan (*Dorsey*); Romilar Hydrobromide (*Roche*); $C_{18}H_{25}NO·HBr·H_2O$ or anhydrous]—Antitussive. Synthetic, nonnarcotic drug; said to have the same antitussive action as codeine without sharing its drawbacks. It resembles the narcotics in incompatibilities.

Dextrose USP [D-glucose, corn sugar; $C_6H_{12}O_6·H_2O$ or anhydrous]—Fluid and nutrient replenisher. Dextrose is official in the form of the monohydrate. 1 g dissolves in 1 ml of water or 60 ml of alcohol. Alkaline solutions of dextrose darken on standing, but this color change does not occur in neutral or acid solutions. Dextrose is a reducing agent, especially in alkaline solution. Iodine and similar oxidizing agents convert it into gluconic acid. Aqueous solutions of dextrose dissolve calcium hydroxide, forming glucosates of calcium. Concentrated dextrose syrups crystallize in the cold; this difficulty may be overcome by reducing the concentration of dextrose and adding 0.1% of benzoic acid or sodium benzoate as a preservative.

At a given temperature, the rate of decomposition of glucose in solution varies inversely with its concentration, the decomposition reaction of glucose is subject to general acid-base catalysis, and, therefore, solutions containing combinations of glucose with inorganic ions might be expected to decompose upon autoclaving to a greater extent than solutions containing glucose alone.

Dextrose 5% in Lactated Ringer's Injection [*Cutter*]—Fluid and nutrient replenisher. pH 4.9; solvent, water for injection; buffer, lactic acid; Na^+ 130 mEq/liter; K^+ 4 mEq/liter; osmolarity, 524 mOs/liter.

Dextrothyroxine Sodium NF [Choloxin (*Flint*); $C_{15}H_{10}I_4NNaO_4·xH_2O$ or anhydrous]—Anticholesteremic. Light yellow to buff-colored powder; odorless; tasteless; may assume slight pink color in light; pH (sat soln) about 8.9. One g dissolves in about 700 ml water and 300 ml alcohol; insoluble in chloroform and ether.

Diatrizoate Meglumine USP [Hypaque Meglumine (*Winthrop*); $C_7H_{17}NO_5·C_{11}H_9I_3N_2O_4$]—Diagnostic aid (radiopaque medium). White powder; odorless. Freely soluble in water.

Diatrizoate Sodium USP [Hypaque Sodium (*Winthrop*); Renografin (*Squibb*); $C_{11}H_8I_3N_2NaO_4$]—Diagnostic aid (radiographic medium). White powder; odorless. Soluble in water; slightly soluble in alcohol; practically insoluble in ether.

Diatrizoic Acid USP [$C_{11}H_9I_3N_2O_4$ or dihydrate]—Pharmaceutic aid. White powder; odorless. Very slightly soluble in water and alcohol.

Diazepam USP [Valium (*Roche*); $C_{16}H_{13}ClN_2O$]—Tranquilizer (minor). Off-white to yellow, crystalline powder; practically odorless; melts 131–135°. 1 g dissolves in about 400 ml water, 17 ml alcohol, 2 ml chloroform, and 40 ml ether. *Known incompatibilities* (diazepam injection): D5W (precipitate), normal saline (precipitate).

Dispensing Information: Interacts (potentiation) with phenothiazines, narcotics, barbiturates, and other antidepressants. See also *Tranquilizers (Chlordiazepoxide Type).*

Diazoxide [Hyperstat (*Schering*); $C_8H_7ClN_2O_2S$]—Antihypertensive. Whitish crystals or crystalline powder; odorless; melts about 330°. Insoluble in water; soluble in dilute alkali solutions. *Known incompatibilities* (diazoxide injection): do not dilute; should not be mixed in an IV infusion.

Dibucaine NF [$C_{20}H_{29}N_3O_2$]—Local anesthetic. Whitish powder; slight, characteristic odor; somewhat hygroscopic; darkens in light; melts about 63.5°. Slightly soluble in water; soluble in ether.

Dibucaine Hydrochloride NF [Nupercaine (*Ciba*); $C_{20}H_{29}N_3O_2·HCl$]—Local anesthetic. White, crystalline, hygroscopic powder. 1 g dissolves in about 2 ml water; freely soluble in alcohol and chloroform. Aqueous solutions may be sterilized by heat without decomposition. Even the slightest alkalinity is sufficient to precipitate the free base from solutions of the hydrochloride. Aqueous solutions (5%) of dibucaine have a pH of 4.7 as determined electrolytically, although with litmus there is an unexplained indefinite color change, which gives an erroneous indication of faint alkalinity. Dibucaine is incompatible with oxidizing agents and salts of heavy metals but is compatible with tannin and with high dilutions of mercuric chloride and mercuric oxycyanide.

Dichlorodifluoromethane   NF [CCl_2F_2]—Pharmaceutic aid (aerosol propellant No. 12). Clear, colorless gas; faint, ethereal odor; vapor pressure (25°) about 4883 mm Hg.

Dichlorotetrafluoroethane   NF [$C_2Cl_2F_4$]—Pharmaceutic aid (aerosol propellant No. 114 and 114a). Clear, colorless gas; faint, ethereal odor; vapor pressure (25°) about 1620 mm Hg.

Dichlorphenamide USP [Daranide (*MSD*);   Oratrol   (*Alcon*); C_6H_6-$Cl_2N_2O_4S_2$]—Carbonic anhydrase inhibitor. Whitish, crystalline powder; not more than slight, characteristic odor; melts about 237.5°. Very slightly soluble in water; soluble in alcohol; slightly soluble in ether.

Dicloxacillin Sodium USP [Dynapen (*Bristol*); Pathocil (*Wyeth*); Veracillin (*Ayerst*); $C_{19}H_{16}Cl_2N_3NaO_5S\cdot H_2O$ or anhydrous; pK_a 2.67]—Antibacterial. Whitish, crystalline powder; faint, characteristic odor; melts about 223° with decomposition. Freely soluble in water; soluble in alcohol.

Dicumarol USP [biscumarol; bishydroxycoumarin; dicoumarol; (*Various Mfrs.*); $C_{19}H_{12}O_6$]—Anticoagulant. Whitish,   crystalline   powder;   faint, pleasant odor; slightly bitter taste; melts about 290°. Practically insoluble in water, alcohol, and ether; slightly soluble in chloroform.

Dicyclomine Hydrochloride USP [Bentyl Hydrochloride (*Merrell-National*); $C_{19}H_{35}NO_2\cdot HCl$]—Anticholinergic. Fine, white, crystalline powder; practically odorless; very bitter taste; pH (1% soln) 5–5.5. One g dissolves in

13 ml water, 5 ml alcohol, 2 ml chloroform, and 770 ml ether.

Dispensing Information: See *Anticholinergic Agents.*

Didrex Tablets [*Upjohn* brand of benzphetamine   hydrochloride]—Contain (per tablet): *25 mg tablet:* Na$^+$ 0.03 mg, K$^+$ 0.01 mg, calories <1; *50 mg tablet:* Na$^+$ 0.02 mg, K$^+$ 0.01 mg, calories 1.

Dienestrol NF [Synestrol (*Schering*); $C_{18}H_{18}O_2$]—Estrogen. Consists of colorless or white or practically white, needle-like crystals or is a white or practically white, crystalline powder. It is odorless. It is soluble in alcohol and practically insoluble in water. It is sensitive to light.

Diethylcarbamazine Citrate USP [Hetrazan   (*Lederle*); $C_{10}H_{21}N_3O\cdot$ $C_6H_8O_7$]—Anthelmintic. White, crystalline powder; odorless or slight odor; slightly hygroscopic; melts about 138°. Very soluble in water; sparingly soluble in alcohol; practically insoluble in chloroform and ether.

Diethylpropion Hydrochloride NF [Tenuate Hydrochloride (*Merrell-National*); Tepanil Hydrochloride (*Riker*); $C_{13}H_{19}NO\cdot HCl$]—Anorexic. White to off-white,   fine,   crystalline   powder; slight, characteristic odor; melts about 175° with decomposition. 1 g dissolves in 0.5 ml water, 3 ml alcohol, and 3 ml chloroform.

Dispensing Information: See *Amphetamines.*

Diethylstilbestrol USP [stilbestrol; *Various   Mfrs.*; $C_{18}H_{20}O_2$]—Estrogen. White,   crystalline   powder;   odorless; melts 169–175°. Practically insoluble in water; soluble in alcohol, chloroform, and ether.

Dispensing Information: May cause menstrual spotting, breast tenderness, headache, and rash.

Diethylstilbestrol   Dipropionate NF [$C_{24}H_{28}O_4$]—Estrogen. Odorless, tasteless, white, crystalline powder. It is soluble in hot alcohol and very slightly soluble in water. A suspension of 0.1 g of diethylstilbestrol dipropionate in 10 ml of diluted alcohol is neutral to litmus paper (pH range, 4.5–8).

Diethyltoluamide NF [$C_{12}H_{17}NO$]—Arthropod repellant. Colorless liquid; faint, pleasant odor; sp gr about 0.999; boils about 111° at 1 mm Hg. Practically insoluble in water and glycerin; miscible with alcohol, chloroform, and ether.

Digitalis NF [digitalis leaf; foxglove; Digifortis (*P-D*); Digitora (*Upjohn*)]—Cardiotonic. Dried leaf of *Digitalis purpurea*. When digitalis is prescribed *Powdered Digitalis NF* is to be dispensed.
Dispensing Information: See *Digitalis and Related Preparations.*

Digitalis, Powdered, NF [prepared digitalis]—Cardiotonic. Digitalis dried at a temperature not exceeding 60°, reduced to a fine or a very fine powder, and adjusted, if necessary, to conform to the official potency.
Dispensing Information: See *Digitalis and Related Preparations.*

Digitalis and Related Preparations—*Dispensing Information:* The importance of precise compliance with the patient's medication regimen cannot be emphasized enough since there is a narrow therapeutic index. Advise physician if slow heart rate or palpitations occur. Patients receiving digitalis and diuretics should be given potassium supplements or instructed in daily consumption of potassium-containing foods. Advise physician if nausea, vomiting, mood or mental changes, or visual changes (especially in color perception) occur since these may be early signs of digitalis toxicity.

Digitoxin USP [Crystodigin (*Lilly*); $C_{41}H_{64}O_{13}$]—Cardiotonic. White or pale-buff, microcrystalline powder; odorless. Practically insoluble in water; 1 g dissolves in 150 ml alcohol and 40 ml chloroform; very slightly soluble in ether. *Known incompatibilities* (digitoxin injection): should not be added directly to IV infusions.
Dispensing Information: See *Digitalis and Related Preparations.*

Digoxin USP—[Lanoxin (*B-W*); $C_{41}H_{64}O_{14}$]—Clear to white crystals or white, crystalline powder; odorless.

Practically insoluble in water and ether; slightly soluble in alcohol (diluted) and chloroform. *Caution: Handle with exceptional care; extremely poisonous. Known incompatibilities* (digoxin injection): should not be added to IV infusions.
Dispensing Information: See *Digitalis and Related Preparations.*

Dihydroergotamine Mesylate NF [D.H.E. 45 (*Sandoz*); $C_{33}H_{37}N_5O_5 \cdot CH_4O_3S$]—Vasoconstrictor (specific in migraine). White, yellowish, or faintly red powder; pH (1 in 1000 soln) about 5.5. One g dissolves in about 125 ml water, 90 ml alcohol, 175 ml chloroform, and 2600 ml ether.

Dihydrostreptomycin Sulfate [$(C_{21}H_{41}N_2O_{12})_2 \cdot 3H_2SO_4$; pK_a 7.75]—Antibacterial. This is a white powder that is hygroscopic but stable toward air and light. Dihydrostreptomycin sulfate is very slightly soluble in alcohol and freely soluble in water. It is insoluble in benzene, petroleum ether, chloroform, and ether. A 20% solution is slightly acidic to nearly neutral (pH range, 4.5–7). It is stable in neutral and alkaline solution. Its compatibilities and incompatibilities are discussed under *Streptomycin.*

Dihydrotachysterol USP [Hytakerol (*Winthrop*); $C_{28}H_{46}O$]—Blood calcium regulating steroid prepared in noncrystalline form as an oil solution, which is standardized biologically and adjusted to a potency equivalent to 1.25 mg of the crystalline material per ml.

Dihydroxyaluminum Aminoacetate NF [Alglyn (*Brayten*); Alzinox (*Patch*); Robalate (*Robins*); C_2H_6-$AlNO_4 \cdot xH_2O$]— A basic antacid salt which is insoluble in water and alcohol. The pH of a saturated aqueous solution is about 7.4.

Dihydroxyaluminum Sodium Carbonate NF [Rolaids (*Am. Chicle*); $CH_2AlNaO_5 \cdot xH_2O$ or anhydrous]—Antacid. Fine, white powder; odorless; tasteless; slightly hygroscopic at room temperature; dehydrates and loses CO_2 above 100°. Practically insoluble in organic solvents; dissolves in dilute mineral acids.

Diiodohydroxyquin USP [(*Panray*);Yodoxin (*Glenwood*);$C_9H_5I_2NO$]—Antitrichomonal and amebicide extremely insoluble in water, dilute acids, or alkalies and only slightly soluble in common organic solvents.

Dimacol Liquid [*Robins*]—Cough and cold therapy. Contains (per 5 ml) pseudoephedrine HCl 30 mg, pheniramine maleate 7.5 mg, dextromethorphan HBr 15 mg, glyceryl guaiacolate 100 mg. pH 2–3; alcohol 4.75%; solvent, aqueous; sweeteners: sugar, saccharin sodium; K^+ <0.01 mg/5 ml; Na^+ 3.9 mg/5 ml.

Dimenhydrinate USP [Dramamine (*Searle*); $C_{17}H_{21}NO \cdot C_7H_7ClN_4O_2$]—Antinauseant. White, crystalline powder; odorless; melts 102–107°. Slightly soluble in water; freely soluble in alcohol and chloroform; sparingly soluble in ether. *Known incompatibilities* (dimenhydrinate injection): aminophylline, ammonium chloride, amobarbital sodium, chlorpromazine HCl, Compazine, heparin, hydrocortisone sodium succinate, hydroxyzine HCl, Luminal, Nembutal, Pentothal, Phenergan, protein hydrolysates, Sparine, streptomycin, trifluoperazine HCl, tetracycline.

Dispensing Information: Drowsiness may occur which may impair ability to drive or perform other tasks requiring alertness; avoid alcohol as it may enhance the drowsiness. See also *Antihistamines.*

Dimercaprol USP [British Anti-Lewisite; BAL in Oil (*HW&D*); $C_3H_8OS_2$]—Antidote to arsenic, gold, and mercury poisoning. Colorless liquid; mercaptan-like odor; sp gr about 1.243; boils about 67° (0.2 mm Hg). 1 g dissolves in about 20 ml water; soluble in alcohol.

Dimetane Preparations [*Robins*]—*Elixir:* Antihistaminic. Contains (per 5 ml) brompheniramine maleate 2 mg. pH 2.5–3.5; alcohol 3%; aqueous solvent system; sugar; saccharin sodium; K^+/5 ml, <0.01 mg, Na^+/5 ml, 2.1 mg. *Expectorant:* Antihistaminic; antitussive. Contains (per 5 ml): brompheniramine maleate 2 mg, glyceryl guaiacolate 100 mg, phenylephrine HCl 5 mg, phenyl-propanolamine HCl 5 mg. pH 2.3–3; alcohol 3.5%; aqueous solvent system; sugar; saccharin sodium; K^+/5 ml, <0.05 mg; Na^+/5 ml, 1.94 mg. *Expectorant-DC:* Antihistaminic; antitussive. Contains (per 5 ml) same as the Expectorant plus codeine phosphate 10 mg. pH 2.3–3; alcohol 3.5%; aqueous solvent system; sugar; saccharin sodium; K^+/5 ml, <0.01 mg; Na^+/5 ml, 1.8 mg.

Dimethicone [$(C_2H_6OSi)_n$]—Protectant. Water-white liquid; viscous; oil-like. Immiscible with water and alcohol; miscible with chloroform and ether.

Dimethindene Maleate NF [Forhistal Maleate (*Ciba*); Triten (*Marion*); $C_{20}H_{24}N_2 \cdot C_4H_4O_4$]—Antihistaminic. Colorless crystalline powder soluble in water (about 1.8%). Due to the presence of the tertiary hydrogen, dimethindene maleate is prone to oxidative degradation which may be catalyzed by free radical-inducing agents. It is most stable in the acid range (i.e., greater than 12 months at 6° or 25°C or 12 weeks at 40° and 50°C).

Dimethisoquin Hydrochloride NF [Quotane (*SK&F*); $C_{17}H_{24}N_2O \cdot HCl$]—Topical anesthetic. Whitish, crystalline powder; odorless; melts about 146°; pH (1 in 100 soln) about 4.5. One g dissolves in about 8 ml water, 3 ml alcohol, and 2 ml chloroform; very slightly soluble in ether.

Dimethisterone NF [$C_{23}H_{32}O_2 \cdot H_2O$ or anhydrous]—Progestin. White, crystalline powder; odorless; tasteless; melts (with decomposition) about 110°. Practically insoluble in water; 1 g dissolves in about 3 ml alcohol and 0.7 ml chloroform.

Dimethyl Tubocurarine Iodide NF [Metubine Iodide (*Lilly*); $C_{40}H_{48}I_2N_2O_6$]—This diquaternary polyether is a white or pale yellow, odorless, crystalline powder that is slightly soluble in water and very slightly soluble in alcohol. It is compatible with intravenous barbiturates (e.g., thiopental sodium) in the concentrations normally used in anesthesia but may accelerate formation of insoluble acid barbiturate on storage.

Cloudy or precipitated solutions should not be used.

Dioctyl Calcium Sulfosuccinate NF [Doxidan (*Hoescht*); Surfak (*Hoescht*); $C_{40}H_{74}CaO_{14}S_2$]—Wetting agent; nonlaxative fecal matter softener. White, gelatinous solid; characteristic odor of octyl alcohol. Slightly soluble in water; freely soluble in alcohol and glycerin.

Dispensing Information: See *Dioctyl Sodium Sulfosuccinate.*

Dioctyl Sodium Sulfosuccinate USP [Colace (*Mead-Johnson*); Dio-Medicone (*Medicone*); Doxinate (*Hoescht*); $C_{20}H_{37}NaO_7S$]—Cathartic. White, wax-like, plastic solid; characteristic odor suggestive of octyl alcohol. 1 g dissolves slowly in 70 ml water.

Dispensing Information: May take 2–3 days before it is effective. Take liquid in ½ glass of milk or fruit juice or for infants in infant's formula (to mask bitter taste). Do not take concurrently with mineral oil. Do not take when abdominal pain, nausea, or vomiting occur.

Dioxybenzone USP [Cyasorb UV 24 (*Lederle*); $C_{14}H_{12}O_4$]—Ultraviolet screen. Off-white to yellow powder; congeals not lower than 68°. Practically insoluble in water; freely soluble in alcohol.

Dioxyline Phosphate [Paveril Phosphate (*Lilly*); $(C_{22}H_{25}NO_4)_2\cdot3H_3PO_4$]—Vasodilator. Whitish crystals or white, crystalline powder; practically odorless; slight bitter taste; melts about 199°; may slightly discolor in light; nonhygroscopic (may absorb water in high humidity). 1 g dissolves in about 25 ml water and 320 ml alcohol.

Diperodon NF [Diothane (*Merrell*); $C_{22}H_{27}N_3O_4\cdot H_2O$ or anhydrous]—Anesthetic. Whitish powder; characteristic odor. Insoluble in water.

Diperodon Hydrochloride [Diothane Hydrochloride (*Merrell*); $C_{22}H_{27}N_3O_4\cdot HCl$]—Anesthetic. Since this is a salt of a weak base and a strong acid, it is partially hydrolyzed in solution. When the solutions are aged in hard glass, the acidity gradually increases, but in bottles of soft glass there is a progressive decrease in acidity with attendant precipitation of diperodon base. On heating or prolonged aging of diothane solutions, some of the free base decomposes with liberation of aniline. Diperodon hydrochloride solutions may be sterilized by gentle boiling in nonalkaline containers without affecting the anesthetic activity. Cotton or gauze should not be used to stopper the flask during sterilization since condensate from such stoppers causes precipitation. Adjustment of the pH to 4.8 by the addition of HCl stabilizes the solution, provided it is stored in bottles of resistant glass. If solutions are to be stored for more than a few days, they should be stabilized by the addition of one drop of diluted hydrochloric acid to each 500 ml of solution. Solutions which have become colored or cloudy should not be used. Alkalies precipitate diperodon base from aqueous solutions. 1 g dissolves in about 100 ml water; soluble in alcohol; insoluble in ether.

Diphemanil Methylsulfate NF [Prantal Methylsulfate (*Schering*); $C_{21}H_{27}NO_4S$]—Anticholinergic. White, somewhat hygroscopic quaternary compound that is sparingly soluble in water and alcohol. A 1% aqueous solution has a pH value of about 4–6. It is stable to heat and light.

Diphenadione NF [Dipaxin (*Upjohn*); $C_{23}H_{16}O_3$]—Anticoagulant. Yellow crystals or yellow, crystalline powder; odorless; melts about 147°. Insoluble in water; 1 g dissolves in <100 ml alcohol and <100 ml chloroform; soluble in ether.

Diphenhydramine Hydrochloride USP [Benadryl Hydrochloride (*P-D*); $C_{17}H_{21}NO\cdot HCl$] — Antihistaminic. White, crystalline powder; odorless; slowly darkens on exposure to light. Its solutions in water are nearly neutral (pH, about 7); 1 g dissolves in 1 ml water, 2 ml alcohol or chloroform. Its elixir is incompatible with aspirin, quinine sulfate, and sulfathiazole, which are insoluble in the elixir. Its elixir and most antihistamines are incompatible with alkaline substances as these tend to liberate the free base which gradually collects as an oily material on the surface of the liquid. Citrated caffeine may be dissolved in a small portion of the elixir by heating to 60°C and this solution may be mixed with the remainder of the elixir, or the citrated caffeine may be dissolved in water and the solution mixed with the elixir.

41

℞	Potassium Iodide		5 g
	Ephedrine Sulfate		0.12 g
	Elixir of Benadryl HCl	q.s.	30 ml

In this combination long, needle-like crystals develop on standing, sometimes almost immediately. This difficulty can be avoided by reducing the potassium iodide content about ½.

Dispensing Information: Drowsiness may occur which may impair ability to drive or perform other tasks requiring alertness. Avoid alcohol. This antihistamine is extremely sedating, so much so that it is used occasionally as a hypnotic. See also *Antihistamines.*

Diphenidol [Vontrol (*SK&F*); $C_{21}H_{27}NO$]—Antiemetic. White, crystalline powder; odorless; slightly bitter taste; melts about 105°. Insoluble in water; freely soluble in chloroform and ether; sparingly soluble in alcohol.

Diphenidol Hydrochloride [Vontrol HCl (*SK&F*); $C_{21}H_{27}NO \cdot HCl$]—Antiemetic. White, crystalline powder; melts about 104°. 1 g dissolves in about 1.25 ml water and 5 ml alcohol.

Diphenoxylate Hydrochloride USP [ingred. of Lomotil (*Searle*); $C_{30}H_{32}N_2O_2 \cdot HCl$]—Antiperistaltic. White, crystalline powder; odorless; melts about 223°; pH (sat soln) about 3.3. Slightly soluble in water; sparingly soluble in alcohol; freely soluble in chloroform; practically insoluble in ether.

Diphenylhydantoin—See *Phenytoin.*

Diphenylpyraline Hydrochloride [Diafen (*Riker*); Hispril (*SK&F*); $C_{19}H_{23}NO \cdot HCl$]—Antihistaminic. Crystals; melts about 206°. Soluble in water and alcohol; insoluble in ether.

Dipyridamole [Persantine (*B-I*); $C_{24}H_{40}N_8O_4$; pK_{a1} about 6.3; pK_{a2} about 0.8]—Coronary vasodilator. Yellow, crystalline powder. Very slightly soluble in water; freely soluble in alcohol.

Disodium Hydrogen Citrate—See under *Citric Acid.*

Disulfiram NF [Alcophobin (*Consolidated*); Antabuse (*Ayerst*); $C_{10}H_{20}N_2S_4$]—Alcohol deterrent. Whitish, crystalline powder; odorless; melts about 70°. Very slightly soluble in water; soluble in alcohol and chloroform.

Dispensing Information: Avoid alcohol rigorously. Instruct patient as to unusual sources of alcohol that could precipitate reaction, i.e., cooking wine, aftershave lotion. Do not drive or operate heavy equipment during initial therapy. Advise physician if skin rash occurs.

Diuretics (Chlorothiazide Type)—*Dispensing Information:* Patients may be given information as follows if these agents are being used as antihypertensives:

This medication is called a diuretic and is designed to help the body lose excess fluid. Diuretics work by acting on the kidneys to cause the excretion of more than the usual amount of urine. This loss of fluid will help decrease your blood pressure.

The excess urine that is lost carries a chemical called potassium along with it. To avoid excess potassium loss you should take your diuretic with one or more of the following fruits or juices that are high in potassium content:

Juices	Fruit
Apricot juice	Apricots
Grapefruit juice	Bananas
Orange juice (fresh)	Fruit cocktail
Pineapple juice	Oranges
Prune juice	Peaches (dried)
Tomato juice	Prunes

Diuretics (Ethacrynic Acid Type)—*Dispensing Information:* Patients should be aware of the symptoms of hypokalemia. Drug should not be given late in the day since diuresis occurring during the night may be troublesome. Anorexia may occur.

Donnagel [*Robins*]—Antidiarrheal. Contains (per 30 ml) hyoscyamine sulfate 0.1037 mg, atropine sulfate 0.0194 mg, hyoscine HBr 0.0065 mg, sodium benzoate 60 mg, kaolin 6 g, pectin 142.8 mg. pH 4–5.5; alcohol 3.8%; aqueous solvent; sweeteners: sugar, saccharin sodium; Na^+ 5.2 mg/5 ml; $K^.$ <0.01 mg/5 ml.

Donnatal Elixir [*Robins*]—Sedative; antispasmodic. Contains (per 5 ml) hyoscyamine sulfate 0.1037 mg, atropine sulfate 0.0194 mg, hyoscine HBr 0.0065 mg, phenobarbital 16.2 mg. pH 4–5.5; alcohol 23%; sweeteners: sugar, saccharin sodium; Na^+ 0.56 mg/5 ml; K^+ <0.05 mg/5 ml.

Dispensing Information: May cause dry mouth and/or blurring of vision. Consider *Phenobarbital* warnings.

Donnagel-PG [*Robins*]—Antidiarrheal. Contains (per 30 ml) *Donnagel* formula plus opium 24 mg. pH 4–5.5; alcohol 5%; aqueous solvent; sweeteners: sugar, saccharin sodium; Na^+ 5.79 mg/5 ml; K^+ 0.24 mg/5 ml.

Dopamine Hydrochloride [Intropin (*Arnar-Stone*); $C_8H_{11}NO_2 \cdot HCl$]—Adrenergic. White powder; odorless; bitter tasting; extremely unstable in alkaline media; light- and oxygen-sensitive; melts (with decomposition) about 244°. 1 g dissolves in about 4 ml water and 100 ml alcohol; practically insoluble in chloroform and ether.

Doxapram Hydrochloride NF [Dopram (*Robins*); $C_{24}H_{30}N_2O_2 \cdot HCl \cdot H_2O$ or anhydrous]—Antihistaminic. Whitish, crystalline powder; odorless; melts about 220°. 1 g dissolves in about 50 ml water; soluble in chloroform; sparingly soluble in alcohol; practically insoluble in ether.

Doxepin Hydrochloride [Adapin (*Pennwalt*);   Sinequan   (*Pfizer*); $C_{19}H_{21}NO \cdot HCl$]—Antidepressant.

Dispensing Information: Interacts with guanethidine and MAO inhibitors. Do not drive or operate heavy machinery on initial therapy. Avoid alcohol. See also *Antidepressants* (*Tricyclic*); doxepin is least likely to interfere with guanethidine's antihypertensive effect.

Doxycycline USP [Vibramycin (*Pfizer*); $C_{22}H_{24}N_2O_8 \cdot H_2O$]—Antibac-

terial. Yellow, crystalline powder. Very slightly soluble in water; sparingly soluble in alcohol; practically insoluble in chloroform and ether.

Dispensing Information: May discolor developing teeth in young children. Avoid exposure to direct sunlight. See also *Tetracyclines;* unlike the tetracyclines, the patient need *not* be cautioned about taking doxycycline with meals or milk.

Doxycycline Hyclate USP [Doxychel Hyclate (*Rachelle*); Doxy II (*USV*); Vibramycin Hyclate (*Pfizer*); $(C_{22}H_{24}N_2O_8 \cdot HCl)_2 \cdot C_2H_6O \cdot H_2O$]—Antibacterial. Yellow, crystalline powder. Soluble in water; slightly soluble in alcohol; practically insoluble in chloroform and ether.

Doxylamine Succinate NF [Decapryn Succinate (*Merrell*); $C_{17}H_{22}N_2O \cdot C_4H_6O_4$]—Antihistaminic. White or creamy white powder. It is freely soluble in water and in alcohol. A 1% aqueous solution is slightly acidic (pH range, 4.9–5.1).

Dramamine Liquid [*Searle* brand of   dimenhydrinate] — Antinauseant. *Known ingredients:* Dramamine (12.5 mg/4 ml), alcohol (5%), glycerin, methylparaben. pH 7. *Known compatibilities:* none listed. *Known incompatibilities:* iodides, acidic or alkaline substances.

Dromostanolone Propionate NF [Drolban (*Lilly*); $C_{23}H_{36}O_3$]—Whitish, crystalline powder; odorless or faint odor; melts (2° range) 127–133°. Practically insoluble in water; 1 g dissolves in about 30 ml alcohol, 2 ml chloroform, and 20 ml ether.

Droperidol NF [Inapsine, comp. of Innovar (*McNeil*); $C_{22}H_{22}FN_3O_2$; pK_a 7.6]—Tranquilizer. Pale yellow to yellowish orange liquid; viscous; characteristic odor; light-sensitive. Insoluble in water; 1 g dissolves in about 140 ml alcohol, 4 ml chloroform, and 500 ml ether.

Dyazide Capsules [*SK&F*]—Diuretic. Contain triamterene 50 mg, hydrochlorothiazide 25 mg.

Dispensing   Information: Consult

physician if sore throat or signs of cold develop. Take after meals to prevent nausea and vomiting. (Do not advise patient to take with orange juice; this is a *potassium-sparing* diuretic.)

Dyclonine Hydrochloride NF [Dyclone (*Dow*); $C_{18}H_{27}NO_2 \cdot HCl$]—Topical anesthetic. White crystals or white, crystalline powder; may have slight odor; produces numbing of tongue; melts about 175°; pH (1 in 100) 4–7. One g dissolves in about 50 ml water; soluble in alcohol and chloroform.

Dydrogesterone NF [Duphaston (*Philips-Roxane*); Gynorest (*Mead-Johnson*); $C_{21}H_{28}O_2$]—Progestin. Whitish, crystalline powder; melts about 169°. Practically insoluble in water; sparingly soluble in alcohol.

Dyphylline [Neothylline (*Lemmon*); Lufyllin (*Mallinckrodt*); $C_{10}H_{14}N_4O_4$]—Smooth muscle relaxant. White, amorphous solid similar in activity to *Aminophylline*. It is soluble in alcohol and freely soluble in water. A 1% solution in water is nearly neutral (pH 6.5–7).

Ear Drops—See *Eye, Ear, Nose, and Throat Preparations.*

Echothiophate Iodide USP [Phospholine Iodide (*Ayerst*); $C_9H_{23}INO_3PS$]—Cholinergic (ophthalmic).

Dispensing Information: To avoid systemic toxicity, patients should be instructed in the proper administration technique which includes digital compression of the nasal-lacrimal duct during and for a minute after ocular administration of the ophthalmic solution.

Edetate Calcium Disodium USP [Calcium Disodium Versenate (*Riker*); $C_{10}H_{12}CaN_2Na_2O_8 \cdot xH_2O$ or anhydrous]—Chelating agent (lead). White, crystalline granules or white, crystalline powder; odorless; slightly hygroscopic; faint, saline taste. Freely soluble in water. *Known incompatibilities* (edetate calcium disodium injection): chelates with cations of any metals.

Edetate Disodium USP [Disotate (*Fellows*); Endrate Disodium (*Abbott*); $C_{10}H_{14}N_2Na_2O_8 \cdot 2H_2O$ or anhydrous]—Chelating agent (calcium). White, crystalline powder. Freely soluble in water.

Edetic Acid NF [$C_{10}H_{16}N_2O_8$]—Pharmaceutic aid (metal complexing agent). White, crystalline powder; melts above 220° (with decomposition). Very slightly soluble in water.

Edrophonium Chloride USP [Tensilon Chloride (*Roche*); $C_{10}H_{16}ClNO$]—Antidote to curare principles. White crystalline powder which is very soluble in water and freely soluble in alcohol. A 1% solution is acidic (pH 4–5).

Efudex Cream [*Roche*]—Solar keratoses therapy. Fluorouracil. This cream, like most creams, is shear-dependent. The possibility exists that, in mixing this cream with other materials (powders and/or other semisolids), the mixing action (trituration) would result in a loss of viscosity of this cream causing it to become more fluid.

Elixophyllin [*Cooper*]—Theophylline 80 mg/15 ml. pH 3–4; alcohol 20%; solvent, water/alcohol/glycerin; sweetener: saccharin sodium, glycerin; Na^+ 0.49 mEq/100 ml.

Emetine [$C_{29}H_{40}N_2O_4$; pK_{b1} 5.77, pK_{b2} 6.64]—Emetine alkaloid is a useful amebicide soluble in alcohol and sparingly soluble in water. *Emetine hydrochloride* is readily soluble in water and in alcohol; a 2% aqueous solution is very slightly acid. Emetine gives precipitates with the usual alkaloidal precipitants. *Caution:* In weighing and handling emetine hydrochloride, special precautions must be taken (including wearing of goggles and rubber gloves) since the drug is irritating to the skin and very irritating to the eye; in one case a manufacturing pharmacist lost the sight of one eye after making tablet triturates of emetine hydrochloride. This drug is intended for intramuscular injection. It should never be injected intravenously.

Emetine Hydrochloride USP [$C_{29}H_{40}N_2O_4 \cdot 2HCl$]—Antiamebic. See under *Emetine.*

Emetrol [*Rorer*]—Antinauseant. Levulose, dextrose, and *o*-phosphoric acid solution.

Dispensing Information: Do not dilute or ingest other liquids for at least 15 min after dosage.

Ephedrine NF [$C_{10}H_{15}NO$]—Adrenergic (bronchodilator). Ephedrine alkaloid is a vasoconstrictor and adrenergic agent. It is a strong base that is soluble in water and alcohol. It is also soluble in liquid petrolatum, but the solutions are turbid if the ephedrine is not dry. Anhydrous ephedrine is about 2½ times as soluble in liquid petrolatum as the hemihydrate, which contains about 5% of water of hydration. Aqueous solutions of ephedrine are strongly alkaline, but solutions of its salts are neutral. Ephedrine alkaloid is volatilized by heat. Solutions of ephedrine in liquid petrolatum on exposure to light and air decompose and acquire an odor similar to that of garlic. Development of a foreign odor in ephedrine alkaloid is retarded by storage in a cold place. The *hydrochloride* is soluble in 3 ml of water or 14 parts of alcohol. The *sulfate* is soluble in 1.3 ml water and 90 ml alcohol. Many of the common alkaloidal precipitants do not form precipitates with ephedrine. *Ephedrine sulfate* is compatible with colloidal silver preparations. Ephedrine alkaloid in aqueous solution reduces silver salts to metallic silver, but salts of ephedrine do not have this reducing effect. *Ephedrine hydrochloride* is incompatible with colloidal silver preparations containing ionizable silver, forming insoluble silver chloride. Ephedrine and ephedrine sulfate appear to be stable in solution with colloidal silver chloride.

Known incompatibilities (ephedrine sulfate injection): hydrocortisone sodium succinate, pentobarbital sodium, phenobarbital sodium, secobarbital sodium, thiopental sodium.

Dispensing Information: Patients should report fast heart rate or palpitations to the physician. Nervousness, tremulousness, or anxiety may occur.

Ephedrine Hydrochloride NF—See under *Ephedrine.*

Ephedrine Sulfate USP—See under *Ephedrine.*

Epinephrine USP [Adrenalin (*P-D*); (*Various Mfrs.*); $C_9H_{13}NO_3$]—Adrenergic. Very slightly soluble in water or alcohol, but it combines with acids to form salts which are soluble in water (e.g., epinephrine hydrochloride and epinephrine bitartrate [Adrenatrate (*Crookes-Barnes*), Epitrate (*Ayerst*), Suprarenin Bitartrate (*Winthrop*)]. See under *Phenolic Compounds*, page 435.

It is insoluble in oils. An aqueous solution of the base is slightly alkaline. Solutions of epinephrine hydrochloride do not form precipitates on addition of alkaloidal precipitants such as tannic acid or potassium mercuric iodide. Weak alkalies precipitate epinephrine from solutions of its salts. Epinephrine is incompatible with iron and its ferrous and ferric salts, cupric and chromic ions, and traces of copper. It has been found that epinephrine solutions stored in certain kinds of yellow glass deteriorated rapidly because of the absorption of iron from the glass. Chelating agents such as disodium hydrogen edetate have been recommended to prevent metallic catalysis.

Under the influence of light and air, solutions of epinephrine salts and related compounds are oxidized, turning pink, red, and then brown and becoming physiologically inert; the change is hastened by oxidizing agents such as iodine, potassium permanganate, hydrogen peroxide, and salts of easily reduced metals. The first stage in the oxidation is probably the formation of the corresponding *o*-quinone which undergoes further changes with the formation of an indol derivative and other compounds. Oxidation is retarded by inorganic reducing agents such as 0.1% of sodium metabisulfite and by traces of mineral acids but is more rapid in alkaline solutions. It has been reported that 0.1% sodium metabisulfite may even accelerate oxidation in neutral solutions. The use of 1% fumaric acid at a pH of 3–3.5 is superior to solutions made with metabisulfite or hydrochloric acid. On the other hand, solutions of adrenaline tartrate or hydrochloride at a pH of 3.4 to 4 are stable for several years especially with 0.1% sodium metabisulfite added. Solutions of epinephrine also lose potency due to racemization; the official levorotatory form is between 15 and 20 times as active as the dextrorotatory form. Racemization follows the first-order law and is hastened by light and alkalies and is retarded by acids. The initial use of the racemic mixture with compensation for the less active dextrorotatory form has been recommended; also, filling the vial or ampoule as near capacity as is feasible has been suggested to limit the volume of air contacting the solution.

The use of a nitrogen atmosphere and storage at low temperature has also been recommended.

Solutions of epinephrine hydrochloride are incompatible with preparations of Butyn such as Butyn Metaphen ophthalmic ointment; the nearly insoluble Butyn chloride is precipitated, thus reducing the anesthetic effect. Formaldehyde destroys the activity of epinephrine. Quinine and epinephrine are therapeutically antagonistic; epinephrine accelerates cardiac action and exerts a hypertensive effect on the arterial pressure, while quinine reduces cardiac action and has a hypotensive effect on the arterial pressure.

Epinephrine Bitartrate USP—See under *Epinephrine.*

Epinephrine Hydrochloride—See under *Epinephrine.*

Epinephryl Borate Ophthalmic Solution NF [Epinal (*Alcon*); Eppy (*Barnes-Hind*); $C_9H_{12}BNO_4$]—Adrenergic.

Equagesic Tablets [*Wyeth*]—Analgesic and tranquilizer. Contain meprobamate 150 mg, ethoheptazine citrate 75 mg, aspirin 250 mg.

Dispensing Information: Drowsiness may occur which may impair ability to drive or perform other tasks requiring alertness. Avoid alcohol. Excessive or prolonged use may lead to dependence and/or habituation.

Ergocalciferol USP [calciferol; vitamin D$_2$; $C_{28}H_{44}O$]—Antirachitic vitamin. Insoluble in water and soluble in the usual organic solvents. Acetone (1 ml) dissolves 0.0695 g at 7°C. It is slightly soluble in vegetable oils. Commercial solutions are made usually with propylene glycol or sesame oil. Calciferol is particularly liable to oxidation and should also be protected from light.

Toxicity: 100,000 to 150,000 IU/day over a long period of time causes anorexia, thirst, lassitude, urinary frequency, nausea, vomiting, diarrhea, and abdominal discomfort. Hypercalcemia, renal impairment, and lithiasis may also occur.

Ergonovine Maleate NF [Ergotrate Maleate (*Lilly*); $C_{19}H_{23}N_3O_2\cdot C_4H_4O_4$; pK$_b$ (base) 6.8]—Oxytocic. White to grayish white or faintly yellow, microcrystalline powder; odorless; darkens with age and on exposure to light. 1 g dissolves in 36 ml water, 120 ml alcohol; insoluble in chloroform and ether.

Known incompatibilities (ergonovine maleate injection): should not be mixed with IV infusions.

Dispensing Information: Consult physician if severe sustained cramping occurs.

Ergotrate Maleate Ampoules [*Lilly*]—Oxytocic. pH 2.7–3.5; hypotonic.

Ergotamine Tartrate USP [Gynergen (*Sandoz*); $(C_{33}H_{35}N_5O_5)_2\cdot C_4H_6O_6$]—Oxytoxic frequently used as a specific for migraine headache. 1 g dissolves in 500 ml of water or alcohol.

Dispensing Information: See *Oxytocic Agents.*

Eriodictyon NF [yerba santa]—Pharmaceutic aid (flavor). Dried leaf of *Eriodictyon californicum.*

Erythrityl Tetranitrate, Diluted, NF [Cardilate (*B-W*); tetranitrol; $C_4H_6N_4O_{12}$]—It is soluble in alcohol or ether, but is insoluble in water. It is a crystalline mass which explodes on percussion. For this reason it is marketed in diluted form mixed with lactose. It is usually dispensed in tablet form.

Dispensing Information: Concurrent headaches may be relieved with aspirin.

Erythrocin Ethylsuccinate [*Abbott*]—Erythromycin ethylsuccinate.

Antibacterial. *Drops:* pH 7–9; sweeteners, 1.55 g sucrose/5 ml; Na^+ 29 mg/5 ml. *Granules:* Same data as for *Drops.*

Erythromycin USP [*Various Mfrs.;* $C_{37}H_{67}NO_{13}$; pK_a 8.6]—This is an antibacterial substance produced by the growth of *Streptomyces erythreus* Waksman.

Erythromycin is active against many penicillin-resistant Gram-positive organisms (staphylococci, streptococci, pneumococci, etc.); with some activity against Gram-negative bacteria, rickettsia, and protozoa. Resistance may develop to erythromycin; and cross resistance is to be expected with carbomycin, oleandomycin, triacetyloleandomycin, staphylomycin, and streptogramin. Erythromycin mechanism of action may be related to that of chloramphenicol and may involve an interaction with one or several categories of RNA that mediate protein biosynthesis.

It is soluble in alcohol and slightly soluble in water (1 g in 1000 ml). It is very soluble in acetone, ether, and chloroform. A saturated solution is alkaline (pH range, 8–10.5).

Erythromycin is a very bitter-tasting base which readily forms organic or inorganic salts. Structurally, it consists of a large lactone ring linked glycosidically to a dimethylamino sugar (desosamine) and to another sugar (cladinose). It is similar in this respect to oleandomycin and carbomycin. Erythromycin is stable at pH 6 to 8 with optimum stability at pH 7. It is rapidly destroyed at a pH below 4. Accordingly, erythromycin tablets are sometimes enteric coated to protect the drug from destruction by the gastric juice. Aqueous solution of erythromycin salts are stable for about 7 days at room temperature and for several weeks at 4°C. The hydrochloride and other salts are very soluble in water and lower alcohols.

Erythromycin esters prepared by esterifying one or more of the hydroxyl groups of the molecule have been prepared by various workers. Some of these esters are practically insoluble in water, e.g., erythromycin ethylcarbonate.

The antibacterial activity of erythromycin in various suppository bases has been studied and it was found that the base employed influences the effectiveness and stability of the incorporated antibiotic.

Also, the effect of various drugs on the antibacterial activity of erythromycin in ointments was investigated and it was determined that the activity of erythromycin is enhanced for a period up to 1 week by ammoniated mercury, benzoic acid, and salicylic acid; is mildly enhanced by mercurous chloride; is not affected by mercuric chloride, yellow mercuric oxide, and zinc oxide; and is destroyed by boric acid, benzocaine, phenol, and red mercuric oxide. Erythromycin ointments containing 5 to 10% yellow or white wax in white petrolatum rapidly lost erythromycin potency. Similar ointments prepared from white petrolatum and incorporating 1 to 4% water, 1 to 10% liquid petrolatum, 1 to 10% glycerin, 1 to 50% wool fat; or 1 to 100% yellow petrolatum showed no appreciable change over a period of 6 months.

Dispensing Information: Tablets should be taken on an empty stomach. Full course of therapy should be completed.

Erythromycin Estolate NF [Ilosone (*Dista*); $C_{40}H_{71}NO_{14} \cdot C_{12}H_{26}O_4S$]—Antibacterial. White, crystalline powder; odorless or practically so; practically tasteless. 1 g dissolves in 10,000 ml water, 20 ml alcohol, 10 ml chloroform. This ester salt has advantages over the base and simple esters in that it is acid-stable and capable of producing therapeutic blood levels without requiring fasting. It is more palatable in suspension than the propionate.

Ilosone for oral suspension is prepared by adding water to a granulated base and such suspensions are then stable for at least 2 weeks at room temperature. Acidic liquids or salts can be added without serious loss of antibiotic activity (e.g., Cosanyl, Co-Pyronil Suspension, Suspension Chlormycetin Palmitate, Compazine Syrup, Neotrizine

Suspension, Fluid Cortef, Elixir Tylenol, Triaminic Syrup, methadone hydrochloride, promethazine hydrochloride, codeine phosphate). Here the salts should be dissolved in the water before making the suspension. Equal volumes of the liquids listed are apparently acceptable. Robitussin, Robitussin AC, and Histadyl EC give stable suspensions but when combined with equal parts of Ilosone for oral suspension, the estolate ester floats on the surface of the liquid and care must be taken not to take all of the antibiotic in the first dose. All combinations require a "Shake Well" label. Refrigeration is desirable. The admixture of alkaline liquids or those of high alcoholic content should be avoided because these hasten hydrolysis.

Dispensing Information: Discontinue use if skin becomes yellow, or if eyeballs become yellow, skin rash occurs, or itching develops.

Erythromycin Ethylcarbonate [Ilotycin Ethyl Carbonate (*Lilly*); $C_{40}H_{71}NO_{15}$]—Antibacterial. Freely soluble in alcohol and practically insoluble in water.

Erythromycin Ethylsuccinate USP [Pediamycin (*Ross*); $C_{43}H_{75}NO_{16}$]—Antibacterial. White or slightly yellow, crystalline powder; odorless or practically so; almost tasteless. Very slightly soluble in water; freely soluble in alcohol and chloroform.

Erythromycin Gluceptate, Sterile, USP [Ilotycin Glucoheptonate (*Lilly*)]; $C_{37}H_{67}NO_{13}\cdot C_7H_{14}O_8$]—Antibacterial. Freely soluble in alcohol and in water. It is nearly neutral (pH range, 6–7.5) in a 2% solution.

Erythromycin Lactobionate for Injection USP [Erythrocin Lactobionate (*Abbott*); $C_{37}H_{67}NO_{13}\cdot C_{12}H_{22}O_{12}$]—Antibacterial. Freely soluble in alcohol and in water and nearly neutral (pH range 6–7.5) in a 2% solution. *Known incompatibilities* (erythromycin lactobionate for injection): chloramphenicol sodium succinate, Coly-Mycin M, heparin sodium, Keflin, tetracycline HCl.

Erythromycin Stearate USP [Bristamycin (*Bristol*); $C_{37}H_{67}NO_{13}\cdot C_{18}H_{36}O_2$]—Antibacterial. White or slightly yellow crystals or powder; practically odorless; slightly bitter taste. Practically insoluble in water; soluble in alcohol, chloroform, and ether.

Erythrosine Sodium USP [Trace (*Lorvic*); $C_{20}H_6I_4Na_2O_5$ or anhydrous]—Dental disclosing agent. Reddish powder; odorless. Soluble in water (dissolves to a bluish red solution that shows no fluorescence in ordinary light); sparingly soluble in alcohol.

Eskatrol spansules [*SK&F*]—Obesity therapy. Contain dextroamphetamine sulfate 15 mg; prochlorperazine maleate 7.5 mg.

Dispensing Information: Contraindicated in hyperthyroidism, diabetes, anxiety, pregnancy, and lactating mothers. Take last dose of the day before 6 p.m. Consult physician if yellowing of the eyes or skin, skin rash, severe sudden headaches, sore throat, fever, easy bruising, or ulcers of the mouth occur.

Estradiol NF [dihydrotheelin; (*Merrell-National*); Progynon (*Schering*); $C_{18}H_{24}O_2$]—Estrogen. White or slightly yellow, small crystals or is a crystalline powder. It is odorless. It is practically insoluble in water (0.015 mg/ml); 1 g dissolves in about 28 ml alcohol, 435 ml chloroform, and 50 ml ether. It is stable in air but is sensitive to light.

Estradiol Benzoate NF [Progynon Benzoate (*Schering*), beta-estradiol benzoate; $C_{25}H_{28}O_3$]—Estrogen. White or slightly off-white crystals or is a crystalline powder. It is odorless. It is almost insoluble in water and soluble in alcohol. It is stable in air but is sensitive to light.

Estradiol Cypionate USP [estradiol cyclopentylpropionate; Depo-Estradiol Cypionate (*Upjohn*); $C_{26}H_{36}O_3$]—Estrogen. White, odorless, crystalline solid. It is practically insoluble in water and sparingly soluble in alcohol.

Estradiol Dipropionate NF [Ovocylin Dipropionate (*Ciba*); $C_{24}H_{32}O_4$]—Estrogen. Small, white or slightly off-white crystals or is a crystalline powder. It is practically insoluble in water and soluble in alcohol. It is sensitive to light.

Estradiol Valerate USP [Delestrogen (*Squibb*); Duratrad (*Ascher*); $C_{23}H_{32}O_3$]—Estrogen. White, crystalline powder; usually odorless or faint, fatty odor; melts about 146°. Practically insoluble in water; soluble in castor oil.

Estrogens, Conjugated, USP [Amnestrogen (*Squibb*); Conestron (*Wyeth*); Menest (*Beecham-Massengill*); Premarin (*Ayerst*)]—Estrogen. Buff-colored, amorphous powder; odorless or slight, characteristic odor. This is an amorphous preparation containing the naturally occurring, water-soluble, conjugated forms of the mixed estrogens obtained from the urine of pregnant mares. Conjugated estrogenic substances may be prepared by either selective extraction or selective adsorption of concentrated urine from mares pregnant 5 months or longer. The principal estrogen present in conjugated estrogenic substances is sodium estrone sulfate. Varying small amounts of other equine estrogens and relatively large quantities of nonestrogenic material are also present in the mixture. The total estrogenic potency of the preparation is expressed in terms of an equivalent quantity of sodium estrone sulfate. *Known incompatibilities* (estrogenic substances, conjugated, injection): ascorbic acid, protein hydrolysate.

Dispensing Information: Take as directed.

Estrogens, Esterified, USP—Estrogen. Mixture of the sodium salts of the sulfate esters of estrogenic substances, principally estrone, excreted by pregnant mares. Whitish, amorphous powder; odorless or slight, characteristic odor.

Estrone NF [Menformin (*Organon*); Theelin (*P-D*); $C_{18}H_{22}O_2$]—Estrogen. Insoluble in water (0.03 mg/ml), slightly soluble in alcohol, vegetable oils, soluble in solutions of fixed alkali hydroxides.

Ethacrynate Sodium for Injection USP [Lyovac Sodium Edecrin (*MSD*); $C_{13}H_{11}Cl_2NaO_4$]—Diuretic. Prepared by the neutralization of ethacrynic acid with the aid of NaOH. Cryodesiccated powder. *Known incompatibilities* (ethacrynate sodium for injection): solutions or drugs with pH 5 or below, blood and its derivatives.

Ethacrynic Acid USP [Edecrin (*MSD*); $C_{13}H_{12}Cl_2O_4$]—Diuretic. Whitish, crystalline powder; odorless or almost so. Very slightly soluble in water; freely soluble in alcohol, chloroform, and ether.

Dispensing Information: Take with orange juice to prevent K^+ loss. Do not exceed prescribed dosage. (Nausea and vomiting may indicate low K^+.) See also *Diuretics (Ethacrynic Acid Type)*.

Ethambutol Hydrochloride USP [Myambutol (*Lederle*); $C_{10}H_{24}N_2O_2 \cdot 2HCl$]—Antibacterial (tuberculostatic). White, crystalline powder; essentially odorless; bitter taste; melts 198–202°. Freely soluble in water; slightly soluble in alcohol; insoluble in chloroform.

Dispensing Information: Patients should be encouraged to advise the physician of any visual symptoms including a drop in visual acuity or change in color vision. Routine ophthalmologic monitoring is suggested. Since therapy can require many months, compliance should be encouraged.

Ethamivan NF [Emivan (*USV*); $C_{12}H_{17}NO_3$]—Central and respiratory stimulant. Whitish, crystalline powder; faint, characteristic odor; melts about 95°. 1 g dissolves in about 100 ml water; very soluble in chloroform; freely soluble in alcohol; sparingly soluble in ether. *Known incompatibilities* (ethamivan injection): chlorpromazine HCl, hydralazine HCl, prochlorperazine mesylate, promazine HCl, promethazine HCl, protein hydrolysate, lactated Ringer's, Ringer's injection, invert sugar.

Ethchlorvynol NF [Placidyl (*Abbott*); C_7H_9ClO]—Sedative. Colorless to yellow liquid; characteristic pungent odor; darkens on exposure to light and air. Immiscible with water; miscible with most organic solvents.

Dispensing Information: See *Sedatives and Hypnotics*.

Ether USP [diethyl ether; $C_4H_{10}O$]—Anesthetic (inhalation). Although ether is usually considered immiscible with water, water will dissolve about 8% ether, and ether will dissolve about 1 to 1.5% of water. Ether is miscible with alcohol, chloroform, benzene, and petroleum ether.

Ethinamate NF [Valmid (*Dista*); $C_9H_{13}NO_2$]—Sedative. White powder; essentially odorless; melts about 96°; pH (sat soln) about 6.5. One g dissolves in about 400 ml water and 2.9 ml alcohol; freely soluble in chloroform and ether.

Ethinyl Estradiol USP [*Various Mfrs.;* $C_{20}H_{24}O_2$]—Estrogen. Fine, white, odorless, crystalline powder. It is soluble in alcohol and practically insoluble in water. It is sensitive to light.

Ethiodized Oil USP [Ethiodol (*Fougera*)]—Diagnostic aid (radiopaque medium). Iodine addition product of the ethyl ester of the fatty acid of poppyseed oil; contains about 37% organically combined iodine. Straw- to amber-colored liquid; oily; may have an odor. Insoluble in water; soluble in chloroform and ether.

Ethionamide USP [Trecator S.C. (*Ives*); $C_8H_{10}N_2S$]—Antibacterial (tuberculostatic). Yellow powder; faint to moderate sulfide-like odor; melts about 161°. Slightly soluble in water, chloroform, and ether; sparingly soluble in alcohol.

Ethopropazine Hydrochloride USP [Parsidol HCl (*W-C*); $C_{19}H_{24}N_2S\cdot HCl$]—Anticholinergic. Whitish, crystalline powder; odorless; melts (with decomposition) about 210°. 1 g dissolves in about 400 ml water, 35 ml alcohol, and 7 ml chloroform; insoluble in ether.

Ethosuximide USP [Zarontin (*P-D*); $C_7H_{11}NO_2$]—Anticonvulsant. Whitish, crystalline powder or waxy solid; characteristic odor; melts about 50°. Freely soluble in water and chloroform; very soluble in alcohol and ether.

Ethoxzolamide USP [Cardrase (*Upjohn*); Ethamide (*Allergan*); $C_9H_{10}N_2O_3S_2$]—Carbonic anhydrase inhibitor. Whitish, crystalline powder; odorless; melts about 192°. Practically

insoluble in water; slightly soluble in alcohol, chloroform, and ether.

Ethyl Acetate NF [acetic ether; $C_4H_8O_2$]—Pharmaceutic aid (flavor). Transparent, colorless liquid; fragrant, slightly acetous odor; acetous, burning taste; sp gr about 0.896; distils about 77°. 1 ml dissolves in about 10 ml water; miscible with alcohol, chloroform, and ether.

Ethyl Aminobenzoate—see *Benzocaine.*

Ethylcellulose NF—Pharmaceutic aid (tablet binder). An ethyl ether of cellulose containing ethoxy groups (about 46.5%); medium type viscosity grade, below 46.5%; standard type viscosity grade, above 46.5%. Free-flowing whitish powder; aqueous suspensions neutral to litmus. Medium type freely soluble in chloroform; standard type freely soluble in alcohol and chloroform; both types insoluble in water.

Ethyl Chloride NF [chloroethane; C_2H_5Cl]—Topical anesthetic. Gas above 12°; under 12° (or under sufficient pressure) a colorless, mobile liquid; very volatile; boils about 12°; sp gr about 0.921 (0°); characteristic odor; at ordinary room temperature it rapidly vaporizes, lowering the temperature; burns with a smoky greenish flame, forming hydrogen chloride. Slightly soluble in water; freely soluble in alcohol and ether.

Ethylenediamine USP [$C_2H_8N_2$]—Pharmaceutic aid (component of Aminophylline Injection USP). Clear, colorless, or slightly yellow liquid; ammonia-like odor; strong alkaline reaction; anhydrous boils about 116° and solidifies about 8°; volatile with steam; strong base, readily combining with acids to form salts with evolution of much heat. Miscible with water and alcohol. *Caution: Use care in handling because of caustic nature and irritating properties of vapor. Note:* Strongly alkaline and may readily absorb CO_2 from the air to form a nonvolatile carbonate; protect against undue exposure to air.

Ethylestrenol [Maxibolin (*Organon*); $C_{20}H_{32}O$]—Anabolic. Whitish, crystalline powder; odorless; tasteless; unstable in heat and light; melts about 76°. Practically insoluble in water; freely soluble in alcohol; soluble in chloroform.

Ethylnorepinephrine Hydrochloride [ethylnoradrenaline HCl; Bronkephrine (*Breon*); $C_{10}H_{15}NO_3 \cdot HCl$]—Bronchodilator. Crystalline solid; 3.32% aqueous solution iso-osmotic with serum. Soluble in water.

Ethyl Oleate NF [$C_{20}H_{38}O_2$]—Pharmaceutic aid (vehicle for certain IM preparations). Pale yellow liquid; oily; strong odor and taste; sp gr about 0.870; boils about 207°. Insoluble in water; miscible with alcohol and ether.

Ethylparaben USP [ethyl *p*-hydroxybenzoate; $C_9H_{10}O_3$]—Pharmaceutic aid (antifungal agent). Small, colorless crystals or white powder; melts about 116°. Slightly soluble in water and glycerin; freely soluble in alcohol and ether.

Ethyl Vanillin NF [$C_9H_{10}O_3$]—Pharmaceutic aid (flavor). Fine, whitish crystals; vanillin-like odor and taste; affected by light; solutions acid to litmus; melts about 77°. 1 g dissolves in about 100 ml water and 2 ml alcohol; freely soluble in chloroform and ether.

Ethynodiol Diacetate USP [$C_{24}H_{32}O_4$]—Progestin. White, crystalline powder; odorless; melts about 129°. Insoluble in water; very soluble in chloroform; freely soluble in ether; soluble in alcohol.

Eucalyptus Oil NF—Pharmaceutic aid (flavor). Volatile oil distilled with steam from the fresh leaf of *Eucalyptus globulus* or some other species of *Eucalyptus;* contains not less than 70% of eucalyptol. Colorless or pale yellow liquid; characteristic odor; pungent taste; sp gr about 0.915 (25°). Soluble in 5 volumes alcohol (70%).

Eucatropine Hydrochloride USP [$C_{17}H_{25}NO_3 \cdot HCl$]—Anticholinergic (ophthalmic). Freely soluble in water and alcohol. Aqueous solutions are neutral and are precipitated by alkaline substances and alkaloidal precipitants.

Eugenol USP [synthetic clove oil; $C_{10}H_{12}O_2$]—Dental analgesic. Colorless or pale yellow liquid; strong odor of clove; pungent taste; becomes darker and thicker in air; sp gr about 1.067; distils about 253°. Slightly soluble in water; miscible with alcohol, chloroform, and ether.

Evans Blue USP [$C_{34}H_{24}N_6Na_4O_{14}S_4$]—Diagnostic aid (blood volume determination). This is a green, bluish-green, or brown, hygroscopic powder that is very soluble in water, very slightly soluble in alcohol, and soluble in acids and alkalies. It is destroyed by strong oxidizing and reducing agents. It is precipitated from solution by strong solutions of neutral salts. It is stable and may be autoclaved at 15 psi for 30 min.

Expectorants and Cough Preparations—*Dispensing Information:* Patients should be encouraged to maintain a high fluid intake to insure hydration of secretions; this aids expectoration. Patients should be discouraged in their use of antitussive preparations for "loose" or productive coughs.

Eye, Ear, Nose, and Throat Preparations—*Dispensing Information:* Administration advice is essential as follows:

Eye Ointments—When instilling an eye ointment, lie down or sit with your head tilted back (see Fig. 1). Draw the lower eyelid down; then look up. Place the ointment about ½ in. along the inside margin of the lower eyelid. Do not touch the eye or the eyelid with the tip of the ointment tube. Close your eye; then with a tissue gently remove any excess ointment from the eyelid lashes.

Eye Drops—In administering eye drops, lie down or sit with your head tilted back with your chin up (see Fig. 2). After checking the tip of the dropper to see it is not chipped or cracked, you should draw the medication into the dropper. The dropper should be held with the tip end down. Open both eyes and look up; with one finger draw the lower eyelid down. With the dropper in the other hand, hold it as near as possible to the eyelid without touching it and

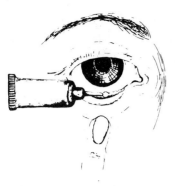

Fig. 1—Using eye ointments.

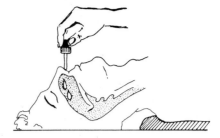

Fig. 3—Using nose drops.

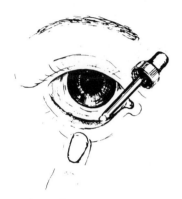

Fig. 2—Using eye drops.

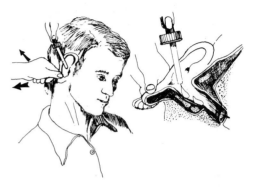

Fig. 4—Using ear drops.

drop the prescribed number of drops into the pocket made when the lower lid is pulled down. The solution should not fall on the sensitive cornea which will cause stinging. Do not touch the eye or the eyelid with the tip of the dropper. Close your eye; then with a tissue gently remove any excess solution from the eyelid and lashes. For some agents (e.g., *Echothiophate*), nasolacrimal duct compression should be employed.

Nose Drops—In administering nose drops, lie down or sit with your head tilted back (see Fig. 3). After checking the tip of the dropper to see it is not chipped or cracked, you should breathe through your mouth and place the prescribed number of drops into the nose. Do not touch the sides of the nasal openings with the dropper. Remain in this position for several minutes so the medication can spread through the nasal cavity.

Ear Drops—In administering ear drops, be sure to tilt your head horizontally raising the ear into which the medication will be administered (see Fig. 4). After checking the tip of the dropper to see it is not chipped or cracked, you should place the tip of the dropper just above the opening of the ear canal. Press gradually, counting each drop as it falls into the ear. The number of drops used must agree with your physician's instructions. After administration of the medication, pull your ear gently upward toward the top of your head, once or twice, to help straighten the ear canal and to help the flow of drops into the inner areas of the ear canal.

If medication has been prescribed for both ears, wait in this position for an extra minute, before tilting head to the other side, and then repeat the procedure.

Fenfluramine Hydrochloride [Pondimin (*Robins*); $C_{12}H_{16}F_3N \cdot HCl$]—Anorexic.

Dispensing Information: In contrast to the other anorexic agents, this drug will cause drowsiness or sedation.

Fennel Oil NF—Pharmaceutic aid (flavor). Volatile oil from dried ripe fruit of *Foeniculum vulgare.* Colorless or pale yellow liquid; characteristic odor; fennel-like taste; sp gr about 0.963; congeals not below 3°. 1 ml soluble in about 8 ml alcohol (80%) and 1 ml alcohol (90%).

Fentanyl Citrate USP [Sublimaze (*McNeil*); $C_{22}H_{28}N_2O\cdot C_6H_8O_7$]—Narcotic analgesic. White, crystalline powder or white, glistening crystals. Sparingly soluble in water; slightly soluble in chloroform.

Feosol Elixir [*SK&F*]—Iron supplement. Contains (per 5 ml) ferrous sulfate 220 mg. pH 2–3; alcohol 5%; aqueous solvent; Na^+ 0.5 mg/5 ml; sweeteners: saccharin sodium, sugar.

Ferric and Ferrous Salts—Iron supplements taken with meals will decrease the amount of iron available to the patient; however, taking these agents with meals is often mandatory to avoid the most profound side effects of all oral iron preparations (nausea and anorexia). To decrease nausea, it may be possible to take less iron at each dose (i.e., take smaller doses more frequently) such as in a liquid form. Sustained-action iron is of no value in preventing gastrointestinal upset compared to regular tablets of equivalent iron content. Stools may be colored black during administration.

Ferric Cacodylate [iron cacodylate; $C_6H_{18}As_3FeO_6$]—This hematinic is a yellow powder that is soluble in water (1:30) and very slightly soluble in alcohol.

Ferric Valerate—See under *Valeric Acid.*

Ferrous Fumarate USP [$C_4H_2FeO_4$]—Hematinic. Reddish powder; odorless. Slightly soluble in water; very slightly soluble in alcohol.

Ferrous Gluconate NF [*Various Mfrs.;* $C_{12}H_{22}FeO_{14}\cdot 2H_2O$]—Iron supplement. Yellowish gray or pale greenish yellow, fine powder or granules; slight odor of burned sugar; pH (5% aq soln) acid to litmus. 1 g dissolves in 5 ml water with slight heating; practically in-

soluble in alcohol. Oxidation of ferrous gluconate solutions may be retarded by use of a citric acid–sodium citrate buffer at pH 3.5–4.5. In making ampuls, it is desirable to prepare the solution in an atmosphere of nitrogen or CO_2 and to sterilize by filtration through a bacteria-removing filter.

Dispensing Information: See *Ferric and Ferrous Salts.*

Ferrous Salts—See *Ferric and Ferrous Salts.*

Ferrous Sulfate USP [copperas (contains no copper); green vitriol; Feosol (*SK&F*); Fer-In-Sol (*Mead-Johnson*); $FeSO_4\cdot 7H_2O$]—Hematinic. Pale, bluish green crystals or granules; odorless; saline, styptic taste; efflorescent in dry air; oxidizes readily in moist air to form brownish yellow basic ferric sulfate; pH (1 in 10 soln) about 3.7. One g dissolves in 1–10 ml water and <1 ml boiling water; insoluble in alcohol. *Known incompatibilities:* oxidizing agents, carbonates, arsenites, arsenates, oxalates, phosphates, alkalies.

Dispensing Information: Keep out of reach of children. Take after meals to prevent GI upset.

Ferrous Sulfate, Dried, USP [dried iron sulfate; $FeSO_4\cdot xH_2O$]—Pharmaceutic aid (ferrous sulfate tablets). Grayish white to buff powder. Dissolves very slowly in water; insoluble in alcohol. *Known incompatibilities:* See *Ferrous Sulfate.*

Fiorinal [*Sandoz*]—Analgesic sedative. *Tablets:* Contain butalbital 50 mg, aspirin 200 mg, phenacetin, 130 mg, caffeine 40 mg.

Dispensing Information: Drowsiness may occur which may impair ability to drive or perform other tasks requiring alertness. Prolonged use may be habit-forming.

Flavoxate Hydrochloride [Urispas (*SK&F*); $C_{24}H_{25}NO_4\cdot HCl$]—Smooth muscle relaxant. Off-white powder; odorless; extremely bitter taste; melts (with decomposition) about 232°. 1 g dissolves in about 6 ml water (at 80°) and 500 ml alcohol; insoluble in ether.

Floxuridine NF [FUDR (*Roche*);

$C_9H_{11}FN_2O_5$]—Antiviral. Whitish solid; odorless; melts about 151°. 1 g dissolves in about 2 ml water and 12 ml alcohol; insoluble in chloroform and ether.

Flucytosine USP [Ancobon (*Roche*); $C_4H_4FN_3O$]—Antifungal. Whitish, crystalline powder; odorless or slight odor; melts (with decomposition) about 295°. 1 g dissolves in about 83 ml water and 650 ml alcohol; practically insoluble in chloroform and ether.

Fludrocortisone Acetate USP [Florinef Acetate (*Squibb*); $C_{23}H_{31}FO_6$]—Anti-inflammatory. White, crystalline powder. It is very slightly soluble in water and sparingly soluble in alcohol.

Flumethasone Pivalate NF [Locorten (*Squibb*); $C_{27}H_{36}F_2O_6$]—Glucocorticoid. Whitish, crystalline powder. Insoluble in water; very slightly soluble in chloroform.

Fluocinolone Acetonide USP [Synalar (*Syntex*); $C_{24}H_{30}F_2O_6$]—Glucocorticoid. White or practically white, crystalline powder; odorless; stable in air; melts about 270°. 1 g dissolves in >1000 ml water, 45 ml alcohol, 25 ml chloroform, and 350 ml ether.

Dispensing Information: Contraindicated, as with all steroids, in fungal or viral lesions. Discontinue use and consult physician if signs of spreading infection occur at the site of use or if topical rash appears. See also *Corticosteroids* (*Systemic*).

Fluocinonide [fluocinolide; Lidex; Topsyn (*Syntex*); $C_{26}H_{32}F_2O_7$]—Glucocorticoid. Whitish, crystalline powder; odorless; melts (3° range) about 300° with decomposition. Insoluble in water; slightly soluble in chloroform.

Fluorescein Sodium USP [$C_{20}H_{10}Na_2O_5$]—Diagnostic aid (corneal trauma indicator). Orange-red powder; odorless; hygroscopic; aqueous solutions strongly fluorescent even in extreme dilution (acids cause fluorescence to disappear; reappears with alkalies). Freely soluble in water; sparingly soluble in alcohol.

Fluorometholone NF [Oxylone (*Upjohn*); $C_{22}H_{29}FO_4$]—Glucocorticoid. Whitish, crystalline powder; odor-

less; melts (with decomposition) about 280°. Practically insoluble in water and ether; 1 g dissolves in about 200 ml alcohol and 2200 ml chloroform.

Fluorouracil USP [*Roche;* $C_4H_3FN_2O_2$]—Antineoplastic. White to practically white, crystalline powder; practically odorless. Sparingly soluble in water; slightly soluble in alcohol; practically insoluble in chloroform and ether.

Dispensing Information: Severe GI toxicity could be expected in a large percentage of recipients. See also *Antineoplastic Agents* (*Bone Marrow-Suppressant*).

Fluoxymesterone USP [Halotestin (*Upjohn*); Ora-Testryl (*Squibb*); Ultandren (*Squibb*); $C_{20}H_{29}FO_3$]—Androgen. White solid; odorless; tasteless; melts (with decomposition) about 240°. Practically insoluble in water; soluble in alcohol; slightly soluble in chloroform.

Fluphenazine Decanoate [Prolixin Decanoate (*Squibb*); $C_{32}H_{44}F_3N_3O_2S$]—Tranquilizer. Yellowish liquid; viscous; characteristic odor; light-sensitive. Insoluble in water; soluble in alcohol and ether.

Fluphenazine Enanthate USP [Prolixin Enanthate (*Squibb*); $C_{29}H_{38}F_3N_3O_2S$]—Tranquilizer. Yellowish, clear to slightly turbid liquid; viscous; characteristic odor; *do not taste;* unstable in strong light. Insoluble in water; 1 g dissolves in <1 ml alcohol, <1 ml chloroform, and 2 ml ether.

Fluphenazine Hydrochloride USP [Prolixin HCl (*Squibb*); $C_{22}H_{26}F_3N_3OS\cdot2HCl$]—Tranquilizer. Whitish, crystalline powder; odorless; melts (5° range) above 225°. 1 g dissolves in about 2 ml water and 7 ml alcohol; slightly soluble in chloroform; practically insoluble in ether.

Flurandrenolide USP [Cordran (*Dista*); $C_{24}H_{33}FO_6$ — Glucocorticoid; adrenocortical steroid (topical anti-inflammatory). White to off-white, fluffy, crystalline powder; odorless. Practically insoluble in water; 1 g dissolves in 72 ml alcohol and 10 ml chloroform. *Known compatibilities* (Cordran topical preparations): ammoniated mercury 10%, bacitracin ointment, Peruvian balsam 10%, benzocaine 5%, boric acid 10%, Burow's solution 20%, camphor 0.3–3%, chrysarobin 0.1–2%, coal tar solution 10%, cold cream, Garamycin cream and ointment, hydrophilic ointment, ichthammol 10%, Ilotycin Crystalline Ointment, iodochlorhydroxyquin 3%, juniper tar 10%, lime water qs to make lotion, Lubriderm Cream, menthol 0.3–3%, Merthiolate Cream and Ointment, olive oil qs to make lotion, petrolatum (as desired), phenol 0.25–1%, resorcinol 5%, resorcinol monoacetate 6%, salicylic acid 10%, sulfur precipitated 10%, Surfacaine Cream/Jelly/Ointment, Surfacaine Compound Cream, Surfadil Cream and Lotion, tars (pine and crude coal) 5%, titanium dioxide 5%, undecylenic acid 5%, urea 40%, white ointment, zinc oxide 20%, zinc oxide paste, zinc undecylenate 5%.

Dispensing Information: Do not apply to "fever blisters" or "cold sores." For external use, only a very thin layer is necessary on the skin.

Flurazepam Hydrochloride NF [Dalmane (*Roche*); $C_{21}H_{23}ClFN_3 \cdot 2HCl$]—Hypnotic. Whitish, crystalline powder; slight odor or odorless; moderately hygroscopic; melts (with decomposition) about 212°. 1 g dissolves in about 2 ml water; freely soluble in alcohol; slightly soluble in chloroform.

Flurothyl NF [Indoklon (*Ohio Med.*); $C_4H_4F_6O$]—Central stimulant. Clear, colorless liquid; volatile; mild odor; boils about 64°. 1 g dissolves in about 500 ml water; miscible with alcohol and ether.

Fluroxene NF [Fluoromar (*Ohio Med.*); $C_4H_5F_3O$]—Anesthetic (inhalation). Clear, colorless liquid; volatile; mild odor; boils about 43°. 1 g dissolves in about 220 ml water; miscible with alcohol and ether.

Folic Acid USP [pteroylglutamic acid, PGA; Folvite (*Lederle*); $C_{19}H_{19}N_7O_6$]—Hematopoietic vitamin. Yellowish powder which is insoluble in water and alcohol but soluble in dilute acids and alkalies. It is partially or completely inactivated by heat, sunlight, oxidation, reduction, acids, and alkalies. Sulfadiazine inactivates folic acid. On addition of calcium salts, elixirs containing sodium folate give a precipitate of calcium folate.

In alcoholic solution folic acid is incompatible with chloral hydrate, ferrous sulfate, sulfonamides, mucilage of acacia, acidic vitamin preparations, and cherry and raspberry syrups.

At pH 3–4, folic acid is insoluble hence forms suspensions stable in the presence of all the B vitamins. Solutions are much less stable and considerable decomposition takes place in solutions containing riboflavin and thiamine. It has been found that the rapid decomposition of folic acid which occurs in the presence of riboflavin and light can be minimized by adjustment of the pH to 6.5, exclusion of air and light, and addition of antioxidants. It has been discovered that aminoacetic acid sometimes used as a solvent for folic acid causes decomposition within a few weeks. Solutions containing propylene glycol have also been reported as rather unstable.

At pH 6 folic acid and cyanocobalamin solutions will precipitate. It has been found that nicotinamide will maintain clarity and stabilize such solutions containing 5 mg/ml of folic acid.

Injectable solutions are prepared by dissolving folic acid in normal sodium bicarbonate solution (which should be sterilized by filtration) or by preparing solutions of the sodium or methylglucamine salt.

Forhistal Maleate Syrup [*Ciba*]—Antihistaminic. A clear, pink unflavored syrup containing per 5 ml: dimethindene maleate (1 mg), sodium benzoate (0.2%), Versene Fe-3 (0.01%), FD&C Red No. 4, sodium phosphate monobasic (qs ad pH 5), and commercially available liquid sugar (89.6%). *Known incompatibilities (per 5 ml):* Alcohol 95% USP (excess of 40%, precipitation); ascorbic acid (200 mg, color bleached); amobarbital (15 mg, incomplete solution); pentobarbital (15 mg, incomplete solution); phenobarbital sodium (15 mg, precipitation); secobarbital sodium (15 mg, precipitation); ferric pyrophosphate (250 mg, possible chemical reaction occurs); ferrous sulfate (300 mg, possible chemical reaction occurs).

Formaldehyde Solution USP [formol, formalin, CH_2O]—Disinfectant. Official formaldehyde solution is an aqueous disinfectant solution containing at least 37% formaldehyde plus methanol to inhibit formation of paraformaldehyde polymer. It is miscible with water and alcohol.

Formaldehyde and other simple aldehydes are incompatible with tannins iron preparations, gelatin, bisulfites, salts of copper, iron, and silver.

Formic Acid [HCOOH; pK_a 3.77]— Sometimes used as a caustic, counterirritant, or astringent, it is the strongest aliphatic acid. It possesses both carboxyl (COOH) and aldehyde (CHO) groups, and, hence, acts both as an acid and an aldehyde. Formic acid and formates are accordingly strong reducing agents, e.g., they reduce mercury bichloride to the insoluble mercurous chloride and silver ions to free silver. With ferric salts, formates give a red color which changes to yellow on addition of mineral acids. Formic acid is soluble in water and alcohol. Most metallic formates are soluble in water.

Fructose NF [$C_6H_{12}O_6$]—Fluid and nutrient replenisher. A sugar usually obtained by the inversion of aqueous solutions of sucrose and subsequent separation of fructose from glucose. Colorless crystals or white, crystalline or granular powder; odorless; sweet taste. Freely soluble in water; 1 g dissolves in about 15 ml alcohol.

Furacin Preparations [*Eaton*]— Topical Antibacterial. Nitrofurazone. *Soluble Dressing* (0.2%): yellow, opaque, water-miscible ointment; characteristic glycol odor; PEG base; pH 4–7. *Solution* (0.2% w/w): light-yellow, clear, somewhat viscous liquid; faint, characteristic glycol odor; aqueous glycol vehicle; pH 4.5–7. *Topical Cream*

(0.2% w/w): water-miscible base; pH 5–7.

Furadantin Oral Suspension [*Eaton*]—Antibacterial (urinary). Nitrofurantoin (25 mg/5 ml). Opaque, yellow, liquid suspension; pH 4.5–6.5; buffer, citrate; sweetener, saccharin; Na^+ 7 mg/5 ml.

Furazolidone [Furoxone (*Eaton*); $C_8H_7N_3O_5$]—Topical anti-infective; topical antiprotosoal (Trichomonas).

Dispensing Information: Contraindicated in hypertension, diabetes. May impart a brown color to urine. Avoid alcohol while taking or for 4 days after cessation of therapy.

Furosemide USP [Lasix (*Hoescht*); $C_{12}H_{11}ClN_2O_5S$]—Diuretic. White to slightly yellow, crystalline powder. Practically insoluble in water; sparingly soluble in alcohol; slightly soluble in ether; very slightly soluble in chloroform. *Known incompatibilities:* (furosemide injection): solutions are pH-dependent (therefore, recommended that no other additive be mixed), acidic solutions.

Dispensing Information: Take with orange juice. Do not exceed labeled dosage. Consult physician if weakness, dizziness, leg cramp, nausea and vomiting, or mental confusion occur. Report any changes in hearing. See also *Diuretics (Ethacrynic Acid Type)*.

Furoxone Liquid [*Eaton*]—Furazolidone (50 mg/15 ml): Yellow, aqueous suspension; pH 7.5; sweetener, saccharin sodium; Na^+ 1.2 mg/15 ml.

Fusidate Sodium [Fucidin (*Leo*); $C_{31}H_{47}NaO_6$]—Antibacterial. Steroid antibiotic from the fermentation broth of *Fusidium coccineum*. White powder; less stable in alkaline than in neutral or acid media. Freely soluble in water.

Gallamine Triethiodide USP [Flaxedil (*Lederle*); $C_{30}H_{60}I_3N_3O_3$]—Skeletal muscle relaxant. Hygroscopic powder freely soluble in water and soluble in alcohol. A 2% solution in water has a pH of about 5.8.

Gallic Acid [3,4,5-trihydroxybenzoic acid; $C_7H_6O_5$; pK_a 4.42]—Gallic acid is an astringent slightly soluble in water

(1:87) and is soluble in alcohol (1:6) and glycerin (1:10). The pH of a 1% solution is about 2.9. An aqueous solution of gallic acid decomposes in the presence of air, the solution turning dark; this change is hastened by alkalies, hydroxides, and carbonates plus oxidizing agents such as chlorates or permanganates. Gallates of the alkali metals are soluble, but gallates of the other metals are only sparingly soluble; with ferric salts a bluish-black solution or precipitate is formed. Ethyl nitrite spirit effervesces and gives a red color with gallic acid.

Gantanol Pediatric Suspension [*Roche*]—Antibacterial. pH 4.8–5; buffer, citric acid/sodium citrate; sweetener, sucrose 50%/sorbitol 10%/saccharin 0.3%; Na^+ 319.7 mg%; solvent, distilled water. *Known compatibilities* (for immediate consumption with the following diluents): Coca-Cola, milk, dilute syrup. Also compatible with Benylin Cough Syrup, Elixir Benadryl, Tylenol Elixir, phenobarbital elixir, Butibel Elixir, and Lomotil Liquid. *Known incompatibilities:* orange juice, Butibel Gel Suspension.

Gantrisin Ampul [*Roche*]—Injectable sulfonamide. *Known ingredients:* Sulfisoxazole diethanolamine (2 g/5 ml). *Known incompatibilities:* none listed.

Gantrisin Ophthalmic Solution [*Roche*]—*Known Ingredients:* Sulfisoxazole diethanolamine (4%). *Known incompatibilities:* acid salts, Adrenalin, Argyrol, boric acid, Butyn Sulfate 2%, cocaine HCl 2%, ephedrine sulfate, homatropine HBr, homatropine methylbromide, Metycaine, Neo-Synephrine HCl ¼%, Nupercaine 0.2%, penicillin, pontocaine, Privine, pilocarpine HCl, silver nitrate.

Gantrisin Vaginal Cream [*Roche*]—*Known ingredients:* Sulfisoxazole (10%) vanishing cream base. pH 4.6. *Known incompatibilities:* none listed.

Gantrisin Acetyl Pediatric Suspension [*Roche*]—Antibacterial. Sulfisoxazole acetyl (0.5 g/5 ml). pH 5–5.5; alcohol 0.3075% *v/v;* buffer, citric acid/

sodium citrate; sucrose 62%; Na^+ 141 mg%; aqueous solvent. *Known incompatibilities:* none listed.

Gantrisin Acetyl Syrup [*Roche*]—Antibacterial. Sulfisoxazole acetyl. pH 4.7–4.9; alcohol 0.9% *v/v;* buffer, sodium citrate; sucrose 70%; Na^+ 82 mg%; aqueous solvent. *Known incompatibilities:* see *Gantrisin Acetyl Pediatric Suspension.*

Gantrisin Acetyl, Lipo [*Roche*]—Antibacterial. Sulfisoxazole acetyl in vegetable oil emulsion. pH 4.3–4.8; buffer, sodium hydroxide; sucrose 5.5%; Na^+ 14.4 mg%; aqueous solvent. *Known incompatibilities:* none listed.

Gelatin USP [white gelatin]—Pharmaceutic aid (suspending agent). Obtained from the partial hydrolysis of collagen from the skin, white connective tissue, and bones of animals. Occurs as Type A (from acid-treated precursor) or Type B (from alkali-treated precursor). Sheets, flakes, shreds, or coarse to fine powder; faintly yellow; characteristic odor; undergoes microbial decomposition when moist or in solution. Insoluble in cold water; soluble in hot water; insoluble in alcohol, chloroform, and ether.

Gelusil Liquid [*W-C*]—Antacid. Contains (per 5 ml) magnesium trisilicate 500 mg, aluminum hydroxide 250 mg. Has adsorbent, demulcent, and antifoaming properties. Alginates added to the liquid provide smoothness and palatability in Gelusil. Peppermint-flavored. *Known incompatibilities:* acids, electrolytes, fixed alkalies; absorbs drugs.

Dispensing Information: Contraindicated in impaired renal function. May inhibit absorption of anticoagulants, penicillins, phenylbutazone, sulfonamides, tetracyclines.

Gentamicin [gentamycin]—This is a basic broad-spectrum antibiotic produced by *Micromonospora purpurea* and related species. It is active against both Gram-positive and Gram-negative organisms. Gentamycin is a white amorphous powder. It is very soluble in water, soluble in dilute acid, moderately soluble in the lower alcohols, and insoluble in ether, benzene, and halogenated hydrocarbons. It is stable for 30 min at 100°C at pH 2–12.

Gentamicin Sulfate USP [Garamycin (*Schering*)]—Antibacterial. Sulfate of the antibiotic substances from *Micromonospora purpurea*. Potency at least 590 μg base/mg. Whitish powder; odorless; melts (with decomposition) 200–250°. Soluble in water; insoluble in alcohol. *Known incompatibilities* (gentamicin sulfate injection): Berocca C, cephalothin sodium, chloramphenicol sodium succinate, erythromycin ethylsuccinate, heparin sodium, nafcillin sodium, oxacillin sodium; should not be combined physically with other drugs but can be administered separately.

Gentian Violet USP [crystal violet; methyl violet; methylrosaniline chloride]—1 g dissolves in 30 to 40 ml of water, 15 ml of glycerin, and 10 ml of alcohol. Its solutions give a precipitate with tannic acid. Gentian violet stains may be removed from the hands by alcohol acidified with HCl.

Glucagon USP [*Lilly;* $C_{153}H_{225}N_{43}O_{49}S$]—Hyperglycemic. Polypeptide from the pancreas of domestic food mammals; increases blood glucose concentrations; used as the hydrochloride. Fine, whitish, crystalline powder; practically odorless and tasteless. Soluble in dilute acid and alkali solutions; insoluble in most organic solvents. *Known incompatibilities* (glucagon injection): admixtures with final pH 3–9.5.

Gluconic Acid [$C_6H_{12}O_7$]—Liquid acid useful as a salt former, which interconverts to delta gluconolactone. It is miscible with water but insoluble in alcohol. A 5% solution has pH of 2.7. It is present in several important salts; e.g., calcium gluconate, ferrous gluconate, and potassium gluconate.

Glutamic Acid [$C_5H_9NO_4$]—Anticonvulsant which apparently acts by assisting in the removal of blood ammonia. Soluble only about 0.86% in water; quite insoluble in alcohol.

Glutamic Acid Hydrochloride [Acidulin *Lilly*); $C_5H_9NO_4 \cdot HCl$]—HCl-releasing digestive. It is soluble in about 3 parts of water, yielding an acid solution; it is almost insoluble in alcohol. The pH of a 1% aqueous solution is about 2.2.

Glutethimide NF [Doriden (*USV*); $C_{13}H_{15}NO_2$]—Sedative. White, crystalline powder; saturated solution acid to litmus. Practically insoluble in water; soluble in alcohol; freely soluble in chloroform and ether.

Dispensing Information: Avoid alcohol (potentiation). Do not drive or operate heavy machinery. Keep out of reach of children; accidental ingestion of only a few tablets has led to severe intoxication. May antagonize the effects of anticoagulants.

Glycerin USP [glycerol, propanetriol, trihydroxypropane; $C_3H_8O_3$]—Pharmaceutic aid (humectant; solvent). Faintly hydroscopic and miscible with alcohol or water but insoluble in organic solvents and immiscible with fixed oils. Strong oxidizing agents such as potassium permanganate, nitric acid, or potassium chlorate may produce an explosion. It is more polar than the monohydric or dihydric alcohols and is accordingly a better solvent for many salts. It is chemically similar to the monohydric alcohols. Glycerin combines with boric acid or borates to form an acid stronger than boric acid. This mixture is incompatible with carbonates and other acid sensitive compounds:

$$\underset{\text{glycerin}}{C_3H_5(OH)_3} + H_3BO_3 + K_2CO_3 \rightarrow$$

$$C_3H_5BO_3 + CO_2\uparrow + 2K^+ + H_2O$$

With oxidizing agents it will form oxalic acid and carbon dioxide:

$$C_3H_5(OH)_3 \xrightarrow{(O)} HOOC\!-\!COOH +$$

$$CO_2\uparrow + 3H_2O$$

With phosphoric acid, glycerin forms glycerophosphoric acid ($pK_{a1} = 1.47$; $pK_{a2} = 6.19$):

$$C_3H_5(OH)_3 + H_3PO_3 \rightarrow$$

$$C_3H_5(OH)_2PO_4H_2 + H_2O$$

Glyceryl Guaiacolate—see *Guaifenesin NF*

Glyceryl Monostearate NF [monostearin]—Pharmaceutic aid (emulsifying agent). Glyceryl monostearate is a white, waxlike substance which is insoluble in water but may be emulsified in hot water with aid of soap or some other emulsifying agent. The NF grade is not self-emulsifying, but various commercial, self-emulsifying brands are available, containing different emulsifying agents and intended for a variety of purposes.

Glyceryl Triacetate [triacetin; $C_9H_{14}O_6$]—Solvent. Soluble in water and alcohol. It is hydrolyzed by alkalies.

Glycobiarsol NF [Milibis (*Winthrop*); $C_8H_9AsBiNO_6$]—Antiprotozoal. Yellowish, flesh-colored, amorphous powder that is very slightly soluble in water and alcohol.

Glycopyrrolate NF [Robinul (*Robins*); $C_{19}H_{28}BrNO_3$]—Anticholinergic. White, crystalline powder; odorless; bitter taste; melts (2° range) 193–198°. 1 g dissolves in about 4.2 ml water, 30 ml alcohol, and 260 ml chloroform; insoluble in ether.

Glycyrrhiza USP and Its Preparations—Glycyrrhizin, the sweet principle of glycyrrhiza, is a mixture of calcium and potassium salts of glycyrrhizic acid. It is incompatible with acids, which precipitate the free acid and take away the sweetness. Salts of heavy metals and of some of the alkaloids precipitate glycyrrhizin.

Gold Sodium Thiomalate USP [sodium aurothiomalate; Myochrysine (*MSD*); $C_4H_3AuNa_2O_4S\cdot H_2O$]—Antirheumatic. Fine, whitish powder; odorless; light-sensitive; pH (1 in 10 soln) about 6.2. Very soluble in water; insoluble in alcohol and ether. *Known incompatibilities* (gold sodium thiomalate injection): should not be mixed in IV infusions.

Gonadotropin, Chorionic, USP [*Various Mfrs.*] — Gonadotropin. Gonad-stimulating principle from the urine of pregnant women; potency at least 1500 USP Units/mg. Whitish, amorphous powder. Freely soluble in water.

Gramicidin   NF—Antibacterial. From the growth of *Bacillus brevis;* may be obtained from tyrothricin; potency at least 900 μg/mg. Whitish, crystalline powder; odorless; melts not below 229°. Insoluble in water; soluble in alcohol.

Griseofulvin USP [Fulvicin (*Schering*); Grifulvin (*McNeil*); Grisactin (*Ayerst*); $C_{17}H_{17}ClO_6$]—Antifungal. White to creamy white powder; odorless. Very slightly soluble in water; sparingly soluble in chloroform.

Dispensing Information Avoid exposure to intense sunlight. Consult physician if sore throat, fever, or other signs of infection occur, or if lesions of mouth, throat, or skin develop. May antagonize warfarin effects.

Guaifenesin NF [glyceryl guaiacolate; *Various Mfrs.;* $C_{10}H_{14}O_4$]—Expectorant. Whitish, crystalline powder; bitter taste; may have slight odor; melts (3° range) 78–82°. 1 g dissolves in 60–70 ml water; soluble in alcohol, chloroform, and glycerin.

Guanethidine Sulfate USP [Ismelin Sulfate (*Ciba*); $(C_{10}H_{22}N_4)_2\cdot H_2SO_4$]—Antihypertensive. White, crystalline powder; characteristic odor. Sparingly soluble in water; slightly soluble in alcohol; practically insoluble in chloroform.

Dispensing Information: Contraindicated in bronchial asthma, pheochromocytoma, peptic ulcer, and pregnancy. Patients should be told to exercise care in rapidly changing from a sitting or lying to a standing position since dizziness or faintness may occur; the problem can be avoided by rising slowly. Avoid strenuous exercise. Nasal stuffiness, tiredness, diarrhea, and nausea can be produced by this drug.

Guar Gum NF—Pharmaceutic aid (tablet binder; tablet disintegrant). Gum from the ground endosperms of *Cyamopsis tetragonolobus.* Whitish powder; nearly odorless. Dispersible in hot or cold water (forms colloidal solution).

Gutta Percha USP—Dental restoration agent. Lumps or blocks of variable size; externally brownish to grayish color; internally reddish color; slight odor and taste. Insoluble in water; about 90% soluble in chloroform.

Halazone NF [(*Abbott*); $C_7H_5Cl_2NO_4S$]—Disinfectant. White powder having the odor of chlorine. It is affected by light. It is slightly soluble in water and soluble in alkaline solutions.

Haldol [*McNeil*]—Tranquilizer (major). Haloperidol. *Concentrate:* Contains 2 mg/ml. pH 3.4; aqueous solvent; hypotonic.

Haloperidol USP [Haldol (*McNeil*); $C_{21}H_{23}ClFNO_2$]—Tranquilizer (major). Whitish, amorphous or microcrystalline powder; saturated solution is neutral to litmus; melts about 150°. Practically insoluble in water; soluble in chloroform; sparingly soluble in alcohol; slightly soluble in ether.

Dispensing Information: Do not drive or operate heavy machinery on initial therapy. Consult physician if mask-like facial expression or incoordination develop. See also *Antipsychotic Agents (Phenothiazine Type)*.

Halothane USP [Fluothane (*Ayerst*); $C_2HBrClF_3$]—General inhalation anesthetic. Mobile, heavy liquid; colorless; nonflammable; characteristic odor resembling chloroform; sweet taste producing a burning sensation. Slightly soluble in water; miscible with alcohol, chloroform, and ether.

Helium [He]—Diluent for gases. Gas; colorless; odorless; tasteless; noncombustible and does not support combustion.

Heparin Sodium USP [*Various Mfrs.*]—Anticoagulant. White or pale-colored, amorphous powder; odorless or nearly so; hygroscopic. pH (1% soln) 5–7.5. One g dissolves in 20 ml water. *Known incompatibilities* (heparin sodium injection): Albamycin, chlordiazepoxide, chlorpromazine HCl, codeine phosphate, Compazine, Demerol, Dramamine, erythromycin lactobionate, gentamicin sulfate, hyaluronidase, Ilotycin, Kantrex, Leritine, Levo-Dromoran, methadone HCl, penicillin G potassium, Phenergan, polymyxin B sulfate, Pronestyl, Solu-Cortef, streptomycin sulfate, Vancocin, viomycin sulfate, Vistaril.

Hetacillin Potassium [Versapen-K (*Bristol*); $C_{19}H_{22}KN_3O_4S$]—Antibacterial. Fine, whitish, crystalline powder; odorless or faint odor of penicillins; bitter taste; slightly hygroscopic; melts about 176°. Freely soluble in water; 1 g dissolves in about 70 ml absolute alcohol.

Hexachlorophene USP [*Various Mfrs.*; $C_{13}H_6Cl_6O_2$]—Topical anti-infective; detergent. Whitish, crystalline powder; odorless or slight phenolic odor; melts about 164°. Insoluble in water; freely soluble in alcohol and ether; soluble in chloroform.

Hexachlorophene Cleansing Preparations—*Dispensing Information:* Patients should be advised to thoroughly rinse all residual detergent from the skin to avoid absorption.

Hexafluorenium Bromide NF [Mylaxen (*Mallinckrodt*); $C_{36}H_{42}Br_2N_2$]—Skeletal muscle relaxant; succinylcholine synergist. White, crystalline powder; melts about 188°. Sparingly soluble in water; soluble in alcohol; insoluble in chloroform and ether.

Hexestrol [*Various Mfrs.*; $C_{18}H_{22}O_2$]—Estrogen. Odorless, white, crystalline powder. It is soluble in alcohol and practically insoluble in water. It is sensitive to light.

Hexocyclium Methylsulfate [Tral (*Abbott*); $C_{21}H_{36}N_2O_5S$]—Anticholinergic. Crystals; melts about 205°. 1 g dissolves in about 2 ml water; slightly soluble in chloroform; insoluble in ether.

Hexylcaine Hydrochloride NF [Cyclaine (*MSD*); $C_{16}H_{23}NO_2 \cdot HCl$]—Local anesthetic. White powder; bitter taste; slight odor; melts about 183°; pH (1 in 20 soln) about 5. One g dissolves in about 17 ml water; freely soluble in alcohol and chloroform; practically insoluble in ether.

Hexylresorcinol NF [*Various Mfrs.*; $C_{12}H_{18}O_2$]—Anthelmintic (intestinal roundworms and pinworms). Soluble in about 2000 parts of water and is readily soluble in alcohol, glycerin, and fixed oils. It is white but becomes brownish-pink on exposure to light and air. Hexylresorcinol solution (ST-37) is a 1:1000 solution of hexylresorcinol in a mixture of glycerin and water; it is odorless, stainless, and does not attack any of the heavy metals. It has been reported to be stable in tablet form; however, capsules containing an oil solution lost 37% in 6 months. (Note—The hexylresorcinol was held in the gelatin capsule enveloping the oil solution; thus, it would undoubtedly still be active.)

Histamine Phosphate USP [$C_5H_9N_3 \cdot 2H_3PO_4$]—Diagnostic aid (gastric secretion indicator). Colorless, long, prismatic crystals; odorless; light-sensitive; aqueous solution acid to litmus; melts about 140°. 1 g dissolves in about 4 ml water.

Homatropine [tropine mandelate; $C_{16}H_{21}NO_3$]—The incompatibilities of this anticholinergic and mydriatic are similar to those of *Atropine,* except that tannin does not cause precipitation in dilute aqueous solutions.

Homatropine Hydrobromide USP [$C_{16}H_{21}NO_3 \cdot HBr$]—Anticholinergic (ophthalmic). White crystals or a white, crystalline powder; melts 214–217°; affected by light; aqueous solution practically neutral or faintly acid. 1 g dissolves in 6 ml water, 40 ml alcohol, and 420 ml chloroform; insoluble in ether.

Homatropine Methylbromide NF [novatropine; Mesopin (*Endo*); $C_{17}H_{24}BrNO_3$]—Anticholinergic. White powder; odorless; slowly darkens on exposure to light; melts about 190°. Very soluble in water; freely soluble in alcohol; almost insoluble in ether. See also *Atropine Methylbromide.*

Hyaluronidase for Injection NF [Alidase (*Searle*); Hyazyme (*Abbott*); Wydase (*Wyeth*)]—This spreading agent is supplied in dry vials or as a specially stabilized solution. Hyaluronidase is compatible with most local anesthetics, procaine, and epinephrine. Dilute aqueous solutions stabilized with heavy metal complexing agents have been patented. The preferred stabilizing agent is 0.075 *M* glycine.

Hycanthone Mesylate [Etrenol Mesylate (*Winthrop*); $C_{20}H_{24}N_2O_2S \cdot CH_4O_3S$]—Antischistosomal.

Hycodan Syrup [*Endo*] Narcotic antitussive. Contains (per 5 ml) hydrocodone bitartrate 5 mg, homatropine methylbromide 1.5 mg.

Dispensing Information: Take with food or milk. May cause constipation or GI upset. Do not drive or operate heavy machinery.

Hydralazine Hydrochloride USP [Apresoline (*Ciba*); $C_8H_8N_4 \cdot HCl$]—Antihypertensive. White to off-white, crystalline powder; odorless; melts 270–280° with decomposition. 1 g dissolves in about 25 ml water and 500 ml alcohol; very slightly soluble in ether.

Known incompatibilities (hydralazine hydrochloride injection): aminophylline, Calcium Disodium Versenate, chlorothiazide, dextrose 10% in lactated Ringer's, ethamivan, fructose 10%, hydrocortisone sodium succinate, mephentermine sulfate, phenobarbital sodium.

Dispensing Information: The following will give the patient a better understanding of this medication:

1. This medication may occasionally cause headaches, palpitations, nausea, and flushing.

2. This medication should be taken at the same time every day and on an evenly spaced schedule, i.e., every 6 hours (if 4 times a day) or every 8 hours (if 3 times a day).

3. Notify your physician if fever, chest, muscle, or joint pains occur while taking this drug.

Hydrochloric Acid USP [HCl, 37%]—Pharmaceutic aid (acidifying agent). Fuming liquid; colorless; pungent odor; ceases to fume when diluted with 2 volumes of water; specific gravity about 1.18. *Known incompatibilities:* carbonates, sulfides, basic preparations.

Hydrochloric Acid, Diluted, USP [HCl 10%]—Pharmaceutic aid (acidifying agent). Liquid; colorless; odorless. *Known incompatibilities:* carbonates, sulfides, basic preparations.

Hydrochlorothiazide USP [Esidrix (*Ciba*); HydroDiuril (*MSD*); $C_7H_8ClN_3O_4S_2$]—Diuretic. White or practically white, crystalline powder; odorless; melts with decomposition about

268°. Slightly soluble in water; insoluble in chloroform and ether.

Dispensing Information: Take with orange juice (K⁺ depletion). Consult with physician if nausea, vomiting, or muscle weakness develop (sign of low K^+). See also *Diuretics (Chlorothiazide Type)*.

Hydrocodone Bitartrate NF [dihydrocodeinone bitartrate; Dicodid (*Knoll*); Hycodan (*Endo*); $C_{18}H_{21}NO_3 \cdot C_4H_6O_6 \cdot 2\frac{1}{2}H_2O$ or anhydrous]—Antitussive. White, odorless, crystalline narcotic. It is soluble in water and slightly soluble in alcohol. A 0.1 *M* solution in freshly boiled and cooled water is acidic (pH range, 3–4). It is affected by light. Alkalies precipitate the free base from solution.

Hydrocortamate Hydrochloride [Ulcort (*Ulmer*); $C_{27}H_{41}NO_6 \cdot HCl$]—Adrenocortical steroid. Crystals; decompose about 222°.

Hydrocortisone USP [Cort-Dome (*Dome*); Cortef (*Upjohn*); Cortril (*Pfizer*); Hydrocortone (*MSD*); $C_{21}H_{30}O_5$]—Glucocorticoid. White to practically white, crystalline powder; odorless; melts about 215°; slightly sensitive to light. 1 g dissolves in >1000 ml water or ether and 40 ml alcohol. Readily decomposed by alkalies and strong acids.

Dispensing Information: See *Corticosteroids (Systemic)*.

Hydrocortisone Acetate USP [*Various Mfrs.;* $C_{23}H_{32}O_6$]—Glucocorticoid. White to practically white, crystalline powder; odorless; melts about 220°. Insoluble in water; 1 g dissolves in 230 ml alcohol and 200 ml chloroform.

Hydrocortisone Cypionate NF [hydrocortisone cyclopentylpropionate; Cortef Fluid (*Upjohn*); $C_{29}H_{42}O_6$]—Glucocorticoid. White, tasteless solid. It is insoluble in water.

Hydrocortisone Sodium Phosphate USP [Hydrocortone Phosphate (*MSD*); $C_{21}H_{29}Na_2O_8P$]—Glucocorticoid. Whitish powder; odorless or almost so; bitter taste; very hygroscopic; pH (1% soln) about 8. One g dissolves in about 1.5 ml water; slightly soluble in alcohol; practically insoluble in chloroform and ether.

Hydrocortisone Sodium Succinate USP [Solu-Cortef (*Upjohn*); $C_{25}H_{33}NaO_8$]—Glucocorticoid. White or nearly white, amorphous solid; odorless; hygroscopic. Very soluble in water and alcohol; insoluble in chloroform.

Known incompatibilities (hydrocortisone sodium succinate for injection): Achromycin, Albamycin, Amytal, Aramine, chlortetracycline HCl, colistimethate sodium, Compazine, Dramamine, ephedrine sulfate, Folbesyn, heparin sodium, hydralazine HCl, Kantrex, pentobarbital sodium, Phenergan, phenobarbital sodium, protein hydrolysate, Sparine, Seconal, Terramycin, Vancocin.

Hydroflumethiazide NF [Diucardin (*Ayerst*); Saluron (*Bristol*); $C_8H_8F_3N_3O_4S_2$]—Antihypertensive; diuretic. Whitish, crystalline powder; odorless; pH (1 in 100 aq disp) 4.5–7.5; melts about 272°. 1 g dissolves in >5000 ml water and chloroform, 39 ml alcohol, and 2500 ml ether.

Hydrogen Peroxide Solution USP—Topical anti-infective. Contains about 3 g H_2O_2/100 ml. Colorless liquid; odorless or ozone-like odor; slightly acid to taste and litmus; froths in the mouth; deteriorates on standing; sp gr about 1.01. *Known incompatibilities:* oxidizing agents, reducing agents, rapid heating, metals, metallic salts, alkalies, light, agitation, heat, phenol.

Hydromorphone NF [Dilaudid (*Knoll*); $C_{17}H_{19}NO_3$]—Narcotic analgesic. Fine, whitish, crystalline powder; odorless; light-sensitive; melts about 265°. 1 g dissolves in about 3 ml water; freely soluble in alcohol; very soluble in chloroform.

Hydromorphone Hydrochloride NF [dihydromorphinone hydrochloride; Dilaudid (*Knoll*); $C_{17}H_{19}NO_3 \cdot HCl$;]—White narcotic-analgesic powder 1 g of which is soluble in about 3 ml of water and sparingly soluble in alcohol. The aqueous solution is neutral to litmus and can be sterilized with heat. Hydromorphone differs from morphine in that the secondary alcohol group has been oxidized to a ketone group, and a double bond has been saturated with hydrogen. Hydromorphone is marketed only in the form of the hydrochloride. Alkalies precipitate the free base, dihydromorphinone, which is soluble in excess of the alkali. In general, hydromorphone has the incompatibilities of alkaloids.

Hydroquinone USP [Eldopaque (*Elder*); $C_6H_6O_2$]—Depigmentor. Fine, white needles; darkens in air; melts about 173°. 1 g dissolves in about 17 ml water, 4 ml alcohol, 51 ml chloroform, and 17 ml ether.

Hydroxocobalamin NF [vitamin B_{12a}; *Various Mfrs.*; $C_{62}H_{89}CoN_{13}O_{15}P$]—Hematopoietic vitamin. Red crystals or crystalline powder; odorless or slight acetone odor; anhydrous form very hygroscopic; pH (2 in 100 soln) about 9. One g dissolves in about 50 ml water and 100 ml alcohol; practically insoluble in chloroform and ether.

Hydroxyamphetamine Hydrobromide NF [Paredrine (*SK&F*); $C_9H_{13}NO \cdot HBr$]—Adrenergic (ophthalmic). White, crystalline powder; solution slightly acid to litmus (pH about 5); melts about 190°. 1 g dissolves in about 1 ml water and 2.5 ml alcohol; slightly soluble in chloroform; practically insoluble in ether.

Hydroxychloroquine Sulfate USP [Plaquenil (*Winthrop*); $C_{18}H_{26}ClN_3O \cdot H_2SO_4$]—Lupus erythematosus suppressant. Whitish, crystalline powder; odorless; bitter taste; pH (aq soln) about 4.5; two forms (melt about 240° and 198°). Freely soluble in water; practically insoluble in alcohol, chloroform, and ether.

Hydroxyethyl Cellulose [Cellosize (*Union Carbide*); Natrosol (*Hercules*)]—Pharmaceutic aid (thickener; binder; stabilizer; suspending agent). White, free-flowing powder; odorless, tasteless; softens about 138°; browns about 207°; pH about 7. Dissolves readily in cold or hot water; insoluble in most organic solvents.

Hydroxyprogesterone Acetate [Prodox (*Upjohn*); $C_{23}H_{32}O_4$]—Progestin. A white, crystalline solid. Slightly

soluble in water; soluble in alcohol.

Hydroxyprogesterone Caproate USP [Delalutin (*Squibb*); $C_{27}H_{40}O_4$]—Progestin. Whitish, crystalline powder; odorless or slight odor; melts about 122°; light- and heat-sensitive. Insoluble in water; 1 g dissolves in about 20 ml ether.

Hydroxypropyl Cellulose [Klucel (*Hercules*)]—Pharmaceutic aid (binder; granulating agent; film-coater; thickener; suspending agent; stabilizer). Off-white powder; odorless; tasteless; softens at 130°; burns out completely 450–500° in N_2 or O_2; pH (aq soln) 5–8.5. Soluble in water below 40° (insoluble above 45°); soluble in many polar organic solvents.

Hydroxystilbamidine Isethionate USP [*Merrell-National*; $C_{16}H_{16}N_4O \cdot 2C_2H_6O_4S$]—Antileishmanial. Fine, yellow, crystalline powder; odorless; decomposes in light; pH (1 in 100 soln) about 4.3; melts about 280°. Soluble in water; slightly soluble in alcohol; insoluble in ether. *Known incompatibilities* (hydroxystilbamidine isethionate for injection): heparin sodium.

Hydroxyurea [Hydrea (*Squibb*); $CH_4N_2O_2$]—Antineoplastic. Whitish powder; odorless; essentially tasteless; light-, air-, and heat-sensitive; melts about 135°. Freely soluble in water and hot alcohol.

Hydroxyzine Hydrochloride NF [Atarax (*Roerig*); Vistaril HCl (*Pfizer*); $C_{21}H_{27}ClN_2O_2 \cdot 2HCl$]—Tranquilizer (minor). White powder; odorless; melts with decomposition 196–204°. 1 g dissolves in 1 ml water, 4.5 ml alcohol, 13 ml chloroform, and >1000 ml ether. *Side effects:* transient drowsiness may occur shortly after administration.

Dispensing Information: An extremely sedating antihistamine; caution with other CNS depressants. See also *Antihistamines.*

Hydroxyzine Pamoate NF [Vistaril (*Pfizer*); $C_{21}H_{27}ClN_2O_2 \cdot C_{23}H_{16}O_6$]—Tranquilizer (minor). Yellow powder; practically odorless. Practically insoluble in water, chloroform, and ether; 1 g dissolves in about 700 ml alcohol.

Hydryllin Compound [*Searle*]—Antihistaminic. *Known ingredients:* Dramamine (8 mg/4 ml), aminophylline (32 mg/4 ml), ammonium chloride (30 mg/4 ml), chloroform (8 mg/4 ml), sugar (2.8 g/4 ml), alcohol (5%), glycerin (5%), methylparaben, flavor, color. *Known incompatibilities:* citrates, iodides, and phenobarbital.

Hydryllin Elixir [*Searle*]—Antihistaminic. *Known ingredients:* Dramamine (12.5 mg/4 ml), aminophylline (50 mg/4 ml), propylene glycol. alcohol (19%), sugar, flavor, color. pH 8.5.. *Known incompatibilities:* iodides, citrates, acids, calcium and magnesium salts, some alkaloidal salts, phenobarbital.

Hyoscyamine NF [*l*-tropine tropate; levo form of atropine; $C_{17}H_{23}NO_3$; pK_b 11.72]—Hyoscyamine is a cholinergic similar to atropine in its solubilities and incompatibilities. 1 g dissolves in 281 parts of water (pH 9.5). It is freely soluble in alcohol.

The racemization of hyoscyamine in tablet formulations due to wet granulation, high temperatures, and presence of alkaline substances has been reported. *Hyoscyamine hydrobromide* is affected by light. It is freely soluble in water and alcohol (1:2.8). The aqueous solutions are neutral to litmus. Hyoscyamine sulfate [Donnazyme, Levsin Sulfate, and Levsinex] is deliquescent and affected by light. It is soluble in water (1:0.4) and alcohol (1:5). Its aqueous solutions are acid to litmus.

Hyoscyamine Hydrobromide NF —See under *Hyoscyamine.*

Hyoscyamine Sulfate NF—See under *Hyoscyamine.*

Hypaque Preparations [*Winthrop*]—Diagnostic aid (radiographic medium). *Hypaque Sodium 20%:* pH 7–8; alcohol 0.9–1%; solvent, benzyl alcohol/water; buffer, HI or NaOH; stabilizer, edetate calcium disodium. *Hypaque Sodium Oral Liquid:* pH 4.5–7.5; solvent, water; buffer, HCl; sugar 35.4%; preservatives, methylparaben/propylparaben/butylparaben. *Hypaque Sodium Oral Powder:* Dispersing agent, polysorbate 80.

Hypaque Sodium 25%: pH 6.5–7.7; solvent, water; buffer, Na_2CO_3 or HCl; stabilizer, edetate calcium disodium. *Hypaque Sodium 50%:* pH 6.5–7.7; solvent, water; buffer, Na_2CO_3 or HCl; stabilizer, edetate calcium disodium. *Hypaque Meglumine 30%:* pH 6.5–7; solvent, water; buffer, meglumine or HCl; stabilizer, edetate calcium disodium. *Hypaque Meglumine 60%:* pH 6.5–7.7; solvent, water; buffer, diatrizoic or *N*-methyl glucamine; stabilizer, edetate calcium disodium. *Hypaque-M 75%* and *90%* (sodium and meglumine diatrizoates): pH 6.5–7.7; solvent, water; buffer, HCl or NaOH; stabilizer, edetate calcium disodium.

Hypnotics—See *Sedatives and Hypnotics.*

Hypoglycemic Agents (Oral)—*Dispensing Information:* Patients should know symptoms of hypoglycemia and its corrective measures.

Hypophosphorous Acid NF [phosphinic acid; H_3PO_2]—Pharmaceutic aid (antioxidant). Colorless or slightly yellow liquid; odorless; solution acid to litmus even if highly diluted; sp gr about 1.13. Miscible with water and alcohol. *Known incompatibilities:* oxidizing agents, ferric compounds, salts of bismuth, mercury, and silver.

Ichthammol NF [Ichthyol (*Stiefel*)] —Topical anti-infective. The principal constituents of this local antibacterial and irritant are ammonium salts of sulfonic acids of hydrocarbons and sulfur compounds of hydrocarbons. Ichthammol is soluble in water, incompletely soluble in alcohol, and miscible with glycerin, oils, and fats. Aqueous solutions of ichthammol have a faintly acid reaction.

Ichthammol is incompatible with acids (which precipitate a dark, resinous mass) and with alkali hydroxides and carbonates (which decompose it with liberation of ammonia). Precipitates are formed with some salts, e.g., zinc sulfate, alum, ferric chloride, ferrous sulfate, lead acetate, copper sulfate, silver nitrate, calcium chloride, and mercuric chloride. Ichthammol precipitates alkaloids. Uniform distribution of ichthammol in ointments is best obtained in bases containing considerable wool fat.

Idoxuridine USP [IDU; Dendrid (*Alcon*); Herplex (*Allergan*); Stoxil (*SK&F*); $C_9H_{11}IN_2O_5$]—Antiviral (ophthalmic). White, crystalline powder; practically odorless; turns black 168–171°; pH (0.1% aq soln) about 6. Slightly soluble in water and alcohol; practically insoluble in chloroform and ether.

Dispensing Information: Do not use with other ophthalmic preparations except on advice of physician. Consult physician if irritation, pain, pruritus, edema, or inflammation of eye or lids occur.

Ilosone [*Dista*]—Erythromycin estolate. Manufacturer does not recommend mixing with other products; such mixing will upset the balance of the suspension system and will result in possible dosing error. *Dry 125:* pH 5–5.5; solvent, purified water; buffer, citrate; sweetener, approx 1.6 g sucrose/5 ml; Na$^+$ 11 mg/5 ml; K$^+$ <1 mg/5 ml. Reconstitute with water according to directions. Product is to be used within 14 days and stored in refrigerator. *Liquid 125:* pH 3.5–6.5; solvent, purified water; buffer, citric acid/sodium citrate; sweetener, approx 2 g sucrose/5 ml; Na$^+$ 12 mg/5 ml; K$^+$ <1 mg/5 ml. *Liquid 250:* Same as *Liquid 125*, except: sweetener, approx 1.7 g sucrose/5 ml. *Ready-Mixed Drops:* pH 3.5–6.5; solvent, purified water; buffer, citric acid/sodium citrate; sweetener, 360 mg sucrose/ml; Na$^+$ approx 12 mg/ml; K$^+$ <1 mg/ml.

Imipramine Hydrochloride USP [Presamine (*USV*); Tofranil (*Geigy*); $C_{19}H_{24}N_2 \cdot HCl$] — Antidepressant. White to off-white, crystalline powder; odorless; melts 170–174°. Freely soluble in water and alcohol; insoluble in ether.

Dispensing Information: The ability to drive or perform other tasks requiring alertness may be impaired. Avoid alcoholic beverages. Take no other medication without consent of physician. Notify physician if fever, sore throat, or unusual bleeding or bruising occurs. There is often a time lag of up to 2 weeks before full therapeutic response is achieved. See also *Antidepressants* (*Tricyclic*).

Inapsine Injection [*McNeil*]—Droperidol. pH 3.4; solvent, aqueous with lactic acid; hypotonic.

Indigotindisulfonate Sodium USP [soluble indigo blue; indigo carmine; $C_{16}H_8N_2Na_2O_8S_2$]—Blue powder or granules; coppery luster; light-sensitive. 1 g dissolves in about 100 ml water; slightly soluble in alcohol; practically insoluble in most organic solvents.

Indocyanine Green USP [Cardio-Green (*HW&D*); $C_{43}H_{47}N_2NaO_6S_2$]— Diagnostic aid (blood volume, cardiac output, and hepatic function determination). Green, brown, blue, or black powder; odorless or slight odor; unstable in solution; pH (1 in 200 soln) about 6. Soluble in water; practically insoluble in most organic solvents.

Indomethacin NF [Indocin (*MSD*); $C_{19}H_{16}ClNO_4$] — Nonsteroid anti-inflammatory. Pale yellow to yellow tan, crystalline powder; odorless (or with a slight odor); sensitive to light; polymorphic forms melt about 155° and 162° (mixture melts 155–162°). 1 g dissolves in >10,000 ml water, 50 ml alcohol, 30 ml chloroform, and 40 ml ether.

Dispensing Information: May be taken with meals or milk. Headache may occur; if so, advise physician. Unless directed otherwise, aspirin should not be taken concurrently.

Innovar Injection [*McNeil*]—Tranquilizer; analgesic. Contains (per ml) fentanyl citrate 0.05 mg, droperidol 2.5 mg. pH 3.5; solvent system, aqueous with lactic acid; hypotonic.

Inositol [meso-inositol, hexahydroxycyclohexane; $(CHOH)_6$]—This B-complex factor is a stable, white crystalline substance. It is soluble in water (14%), slightly soluble in alcohol, practically insoluble in ether and common organic solvents. It is neutral to litmus and has a sweet taste.

Insulin Preparations—*Dispensing Information:* Patients need to be familiar with injection technique (including site rotation); injection preparation (including mixing instructions); syringe and needle care; adverse reactions (including symptoms of hypoglycemia and corrective treatment); storage conditions; urine testing materials and methods; nature of the disease and what to expect from treatment.

Intropin Injection [*Arnar-Stone*]— Dopamine hydrochloride. Adrenergic. pH 3–4.5; solvent, water for injection; Na^+ approx 2.2 mg/ml; antioxidant, 1% sodium bisulfite. This product must be diluted in a sterile intravenous solution before use. *Known compatibilities:* compatible with and stable for 24 hours at 25°C in sodium chloride injection, dextrose (5%) injection, dextrose (5%) and sodium chloride (0.9%) injection, dextrose (5%) and sodium chloride (0.45%) injection, dextrose (5%) in lactated Ringer's solution, sodium lactate (⅙ M) injection, and lactated Ringer's injection.

Iocetamic Acid [Cholebrine (*Mallinckrodt*); $C_{12}H_{13}I_3N_2O_3$; pK_a (isomer A 4.25; B 4.10)]—Diagnostic aid (radiopaque medium). Whitish powder; odorless or faint acetic acid odor; light-sensitive; melts 190–222° (isomer A about 232°; B about 201°); insoluble in water; slightly soluble in alcohol and chloroform; very slightly soluble in ether.

Iodine USP [I]—Topical anti-infective. Heavy, grayish black plates or granules; metallic luster; characteristic odor. 1 g dissolves in 1000–10,000 ml water, 1–10 ml chloroform and ether, 10–30 ml alcohol, and 30–100 ml glycerin. *Known incompatibilities:* reducing agents, volatile oils, alkaloids, strong oxidizing agents.

Iodipamide USP [$C_{20}H_{14}I_6N_2O_6$]— Diagnostic aid (radiopaque medium). White, crystalline powder; nearly odorless. Very slightly soluble in water, chloroform, and ether; slightly soluble in alcohol.

Iodochlorhydroxyquin NF [Vioform (*Ciba*); C_9H_5ClINO]—Topical anti-infective. Practically insoluble in water or alcohol.

Dispensing Information: Topical— may stain clothes and skin yellow.

Iopanoic Acid USP [Telepaque (*Winthrop*); $C_{11}H_{12}I_3NO_2$]—Diagnostic aid (radiopaque medium). Cream-colored powder; tasteless or nearly so; faint, characteristic odor; affected by light; melts with decomposition 152–158°. Insoluble in water; soluble in alcohol, chloroform, and ether.

Dispensing Information: To have the gall bladder adequately visualized, patient should be fully aware of dosage instructions, including dietary instructions, before x-ray examination is performed.

Iophendylate USP [Pantopaque (*Lafayette*); $C_{19}H_{29}IO_2$]—Diagnostic aid (radiopaque medium). Colorless to pale yellow, viscous liquid; color darkens on long exposure to air; odorless or a faintly ethereal odor. Very slightly soluble in water; freely soluble in alcohol, chloroform, and ether.

Iothalamate Meglumine Injection USP [Conray (*Mallinckrodt*); $C_7H_{17}NO_5 \cdot C_{11}H_9I_3N_2O_4$]—Diagnostic aid (radiopaque medium). Clear, colorless to pale yellow, slightly viscous liquid.

Iothalamic Acid USP [$C_{11}H_9I_3N_2O_4$]— Diagnostic aid (radiopaque medium). White powder; odorless. Slightly soluble in water and alcohol.

Ipecac USP [ipecacuanha]—Expectorant; emetic; amebicide. Dried rhizome and roots of *Cephaelis acuminata*.

Ipodate Calcium USP [Oragrafin Calcium (*Squibb*); $C_{24}H_{24}CaI_6N_4O_4$]— Fine, whitish, crystalline powder; odorless; chalky, very bitter taste; light- and heat-sensitive; melts (with decomposition) about 300°. 1 g dissolves in about 1700 ml water and 2.6 ml chloroform; slightly soluble in alcohol.

Ipodate Sodium USP [Oragrafin Sodium ˙(*Squibb*); $C_{12}H_{12}I_3N_2NaO_2$]— Whitish, crystalline powder; odorless; light- and heat-sensitive; melts (with decomposition) about 303°. 1 g dissolves in <1 ml water and about 2 ml alcohol; very slightly soluble in chloroform.

Iron Salts—see *Ferric and Ferrous Salts.*

Isobucaine Hydrochloride NF [$C_{15}H_{23}NO_2 \cdot HCl$]—Local anesthetic. White, crystalline solid; odorless; melts about 183°. 1 g dissolves in about 1 ml water, 8 ml alcohol, 6 ml chloroform, and >100 ml ether.

Isocarboxazid NF [Marplan (*Roche*); $C_{12}H_{13}N_3O_2$]—Antidepressant. Whitish, crystalline powder; slight odor; melts about 106°. 1 g dissolves in about 2000 ml water, 83 ml alcohol, 2 ml chloroform, and 58 ml ether.

Isoflurophate USP [Floropryl (*MSD*); $C_6H_{14}FO_3P$]—Cholinergic (ophthalmic). Clear, colorless, or faintly yellow liquid; moisture-sensitive (decomposes and loses activity); sp gr about 1.05. Sparingly soluble in water; soluble in alcohol. *Caution: vapor extremely irritating to the eye and mucous membranes.*

Isometheptene Hydrochloride [Octin HCl (*Knoll*); $C_9H_{19}N \cdot HCl$]—Adrenergic. Crystals; extremely hygroscopic; melts about 68°. Soluble in water and alcohol.

Isometheptene Mucate [Octin Mucate (*Knoll*); $(C_9H_{19}N)_2 \cdot C_6H_{10}O_8$]—Adrenergic. White, crystalline powder; bitter taste. Freely soluble in water; 1 g dissolves in about 20 ml alcohol; practically insoluble in chloroform and ether.

Isoniazid USP [Niconyl (*P-D*); Nydrazid (*Squibb*); $C_6H_7N_3O$]—Antibacterial (tuberculostatic). 1 g dissolves in about 8 ml water and 50 ml alcohol; slightly soluble in chloroform and ether.

Dispensing Information: Patient card may contain the following information:

May occasionally cause nausea or vomiting. These symptoms usually occur when you are starting therapy and should clear up after a short period of time. You should notify your physician if you notice any fever, fatigue, tiredness, muscle aches or pains, or any other "flu-like" symptoms. In addition loss of appetite, darkening of the urine, and yellowing of the skin or eyes should also be brought to your doctor's attention. You should take your TB medication at the same time every day, preferably in the morning. This will help you to develop a continuous and regular treatment schedule. However, if you forget your morning dose, you can take it later in the day.

Isopropamide Iodide NF [Darbid (*SK&F*); $C_{23}H_{33}IN_2O$]—Anticholinergic. Whitish, crystalline powder; practically odorless; bitter taste; melts about 183°. 1 g dissolves in about 50 ml water, 10 ml alcohol, and 5 ml chloroform; very slightly soluble in ether.

Isopropyl Alcohol NF [2-propanol; C_3H_8O]—Pharmaceutic aid (solvent). Isopropyl alcohol is miscible in all proportions with water and alcohol. Because of its toxicity, isopropyl alcohol is not used internally but is considered safe for external use as there is little danger from inhalation of the vapors, owing to its moderate volatility. Ingestion of 10 ml or more (or excessive inhalation) has produced dizziness, depression, vomiting, coma, and death. Compared with alcohol, isopropyl alcohol has a lower surface tension and is a better fat solvent. Isopropyl alcohol is a good solvent for removing creosote from the skin to prevent burns, but its use as a solvent for inorganic salts is limited because it is easily salted out, forming two layers.

Isopropyl Myristate NF [$C_{17}H_{34}O_2$]—Pharmaceutic aid (emollient). Liquid; low viscosity; practically odorless; congeals about 5°; decomposes about 208°. Practically insoluble in water; soluble in alcohol and chloroform.

Isopropyl Rubbing Alcohol NF—Rubefacient. Contains about 70% isopropyl alcohol, by volume. Transparent, mobile liquid; volatile; slightly bitter taste; characteristic odor; sp gr about 0.877. Do not drink.

Isoproterenol Hydrochloride USP [Isuprel (*Winthrop*); (*Various Mfrs.*); $C_{11}H_{17}NO_3 \cdot HCl$]—Bronchodilator; adrenergic. White to practically white, crystalline powder; odorless; slightly bitter taste; gradually darkens in air and light; solutions become pink to brownish pink in air and almost so when rendered alkaline; pH (1% soln) about 5. One g dissolves in 3 ml water and 50 ml alcohol; insoluble in chloroform and ether. *Known incompatibili-*

ties (isoproterenol HCl injection): protein hydrolysate.

Dispensing Information: Advise physician if fast heart beat or palpitations occur.

Isoproterenol Sulfate NF [Norisodrine (*Abbott*); $(C_{11}H_{17}NO_3)_2 \cdot H_2SO_4 \cdot 2H_2O$]—Bronchodilator; adrenergic. White to practically white, crystalline powder; odorless; gradually darkens in air; pH (1% soln) about 5. Freely soluble in water; slightly soluble in alcohol; very slightly soluble in ether.

Dispensing Information: See *Isoproterenol Hydrochloride.*

Isopto-Carpine [*Alcon*]—Cholinergic (ophthalmic). Pilocarpine hydrochloride. *0.25%* (*and 0.5%*): pH 5; aqueous solvent; citrate buffer; Na^+ 0.1585% (0.1192%); isotonic. *1%:* same as above, excepting Na^+ 0.0636%.

Isopto - Cetamide Suspension [*Alcon*]—Antibacterial (ophthalmic). Contains sulfacetamide sodium 15%, methylcellulose 0.5%. pH 7.4; aqueous solvent; buffer, phosphate; Na^+ 0.1131%; hypertonic.

Isopto - Cetapred Suspension [*Alcon*]—Antibacterial (ophthalmic). Contains sulfacetamide sodium 10%, prednisolone 0.25%, methylcellulose 0.5%. pH 6.8; aqueous solvent; buffer, phosphate; Na^+ 0.0650%; hypertonic.

Isosorbide Dinitrate, Diluted, USP [Isordil (*Ives*); Sorbitrate (*Stuart*); Sorquad (*Tutag*); $C_6H_8N_2O_8$]—Antianginal therapy. Ivory-white powder; odorless. *Caution* (*pure material only*): *store in tight containers and prevent exposure to excessive heat; powerful explosive which can be exploded by percussion or excessive heat.* Very slightly soluble in water; freely soluble in chloroform; sparingly soluble in alcohol.

Dispensing Information: May cause flushing and headache. Avoid alcohol (potentiation).

Isoxsuprine Hydrochloride NF [Vasodilan (*Mead-Johnson*); $C_{18}H_{23}-NO_3 \cdot HCl$]—Vasodilator. White, crystalline powder; odorless; bitter taste; melts 201–208°; pH (1% soln) 4.5–6. One g dissolves in 500 ml water, 100 ml alcohol, and >10,000 ml chloroform and ether.

Dispensing Information: Consult physician if dizziness or palpitations occur.

Isuprel Solution (1:5000 injection) [*Winthrop*]—Bronchodilator; adrenergic. Isoproterenol HCl. pH 3.5–4.5; aqueous solvent; buffer, HCl; preservative, sodium bisulfite.

Kanamycin Sulfate USP [Kantrex Sulfate (*Bristol*)]—This antibiotic is produced by deep-tank fermentation of cultures of *Streptomyces kanamyceticus*. Kanamycin is active against many penicillin-resistant staphylococci coliform organisms, salmonella, shigella. It is given intramuscularly at 15 mg/kg of body weight/day but due to possible eighth nerve or renal damage it is usually given only in severe resistant infections. It may be used preoperatively by mouth at 1 g/day. It probably acts by increasing cytoplasmic membrane permeability.

Kanamycin is a water-soluble basic antibiotic. It is structurally similar to both neomycin and streptomycin, and it appears to have two amino sugars (hexosamines) glycosidically linked to the hydroxylated base, deoxystreptamin.

Kanamycin sulfate [$C_{18}H_{36}N_4O_{11} \cdot H_2SO_4 \cdot H_2O$] occurs as a white, odorless, crystalline powder that is freely soluble in water (360 mg/ml). It is insoluble in common alcohols and nonpolar solvents. It is stable over a pH range of 2 to 11, and aqueous solutions at pH 6 to 8 are stable to boiling for 30 min. Gradual darkening of the solution does not reflect a loss of potency. It is compatible with such local anesthetics as procaine hydrochloride and lidocaine hydrochloride. *Known incompatibilities* (kanamycin sulfate for injection): amphotericin B, chlorpromazine HCl, Coly-Mycin M, Compazine, Dilantin, Dimocillin, Furadantin, Keflin, Luminal, Panheparin, pentobarbital sodium, secobarbital sodium, Solu-Cortef, sulfadiazine sodium.

Dispensing Information: Used only as inpatient drug. Significant ototoxicity can occur without patient being able to discern symptoms. Sophisticated audiometric testing should be employed.

Kantrex Injections [*Bristol* brand of kanamycin]—Antibacterial. *Injection (0.5 g)*: pH 4.2–4.8; solvent, water for injection; buffer, sodium citrate 2.2% adjusted to pH 4.5 with H_2SO_4; Na^+ 0.6 mEq/2 ml; ionic strength, 1.511. *Injection (1 g)*: pH 4.2–4.8; solvent (see above); buffer (see above); Na^+ 0.8 mEq/3 ml; ionic strength, 1.23. *Injection (75 mg)*: pH 4.2–4.8; solvent (see above); buffer (see above); Na^+ 0.079 mEq/2 ml; ionic strength, 0.71.

These solutions contain methyl and propyl parabens, sodium bisulfite, and sodium citrate with a pH approximately 4.5. These solutions are stable for at least 3 years under normal storage conditions. Tests of the compatibility of this solution with 15 common intravenous solutions have shown that mixtures containing varying concentrations developed no physical changes and had less than 6.8% loss in potency after 8 hours at 25°C.

Kaolin NF [approx $H_2Al_2Si_2O_8 \cdot H_2O$]—Adsorbent. Soft, white or yellowish white powder or as lumps; earthy or clay-like taste; when moistened with water, assumes a darker color and develops a marked clay-like odor. Insoluble in water, cold dilute acids, and solutions of alkali hydroxides. *Known incompatibilities:* adsorbs other drugs.

Kay Ciel Elixir [*Cooper*]—Electrolyte replenisher (potassium and chloride). pH 4–6; alcohol 4%; solvent, water/alcohol/sorbitol; sweetener: saccharin sodium, sorbitol; Na^+ 0.26 mEq/100 ml; preservative, methylparaben/propylparaben.

Keflex Preparations [*Lilly* brand of cephalexin]—Antibacterial. *For Oral Suspension (M-201)*: pH 4–5; solvent, purified water; sweetener, approx 3 g sucrose/5 ml; Na^+ <1 mg/5 ml; K^+ <1 mg/5 ml. *For Oral Suspension (M-202)*: pH 4–5; solvent, purified water; sweetener, approx 3 g sucrose/5 ml; Na^+ <1 mg/5 ml; K^+ <1 mg/5 ml; *For Pediatric Drops (M-204)*: pH 4–5; solvent, purified water; sweetener, approx 670 mg sucrose/ml; Na^+ <1 mg/ml; K^+ <1 mg/ml. *Known incompatibilities:* Manufacturer does not recommend mixing these products with other products; such mixing will upset the balance of the suspension system and will result in possible dosing errors.

Keflin Preparations [*Lilly* brand of cephalothin sodium]—Antibacterial. *Ampoules No. 698:* pH 4.5–7 in 4 ml water for injection; Na^+ 2.4 mEq; hypotonic. *Ampoules No. 706:* pH 4.5–7 in 20 ml water for injection; Na^+ 4.8 mEq; hypotonic. *Ampoules No. 738:* pH 4.5–7 in 20 ml water for injection; Na^+ 9.6 mEq; hypotonic. *Ampoules No. 7001, Neutral:* pH 6–8.5 in 4 ml water for injection; buffer, sodium bicarbonate; Na^+ 2.8 mEq; hypotonic. *Ampoules No. 7002, Neutral:* pH 6–8.5 in 20 ml water for injection; buffer, sodium bicarbonate; Na^+ 5.5 mEq; hypotonic. *Ampoules No. 7004, Neutral:* pH 6–8.5 in 20 ml water for injection; buffer, sodium bicarbonate; Na^+ 11 mEq; hypotonic. *Known incompatibilities:* see *Cephalothin Sodium.*

Kefzol Preparations [*Lilly* brand of cefazolin sodium]—Antibacterial. *Ampoules No. 766:* pH 4–6 (10% solution in water for injection); Na^+ 0.5 mEq; K^+ none; hypertonic. *Ampoules No. 767:* pH 4–6; Na^+ 1 mEq; K^+ none; hypertonic. *Ampoules No. 768:* pH 4–6; Na^+ 2 mEq; K^+ none; hypertonic. *Known incompatibilities:* see *Cefazolin Sodium.*

Ketamine Hydrochloride NF [Ketaject (*Bristol*); Ketalar (*P-D*); $C_{13}H_{16}ClNO \cdot HCl$]—Anesthetic (inhalation). White, crystalline powder; characteristic odor; solution acid to litmus; melts (with decomposition) about 259°; solution precipitates free base at high pH. 1 g dissolves in about 5 ml water, 14 ml alcohol, 60 ml chloroform, and 60 ml absolute alcohol.

Keto-Diastix [*Ames*] Reagent strips; test for glucose and ketones in urine. Contain sodium nitroprusside.

Dispensing Information: Patient must be familiar with the procedures. See also *Reagent Tablets and Strips.*

K-Lyte Tablets [*Mead-Johnson*]—

Oral potassium supplement. Contain potassium bicarbonate 2.5 g, citric acid 2.1 g; K$^+$ 25 mEq. *Known incompatibilities:* acid solutions of tartrates.

Labstix [*Ames*]—Test for pH, protein, glucose, ketones, and blood in urine.

Dispensing Information: Advise patient of recommended procedures for handling and use. See also *Reagent Tablets or Strips.*

Lactic Acid USP [$C_3H_6O_3$; pK$_a$ 3.86]—Lactic acid, a useful acidifier, is miscible with water, alcohol, and ether. The pH of a 1% solution is about 2.5. It is incompatible with oxidizing agents and is reduced by concentrated hydriodic acid to propionic acid. Lactates are excellent solubilizing agents for many inorganic cations, probably due to chelate formation. Lactates of the alkali metals are very soluble in water and alcohol (e.g., sodium lactate injection), those of the other metals are less soluble in water (e.g., calcium lactate, 1:20; ferrous lactate, 1:40; silver lactate, 1:15; and strontium lactate, 1:3) and insoluble in alcohol. Most lactates are freely soluble in sodium citrate solution. Calcium lactate is slightly acid (pH 6–7).

Lactinex [*HW&D*]—To restore intestinal flora. Contains *Lactobacillus acidophilus* and *L. bulgaricus.*

Dispensing Information: Keep in refrigerator.

Lactose USP [milk sugar, saccharum lactis; $C_{12}H_{22}O_{11}H_2O$]—Pharmaceutic aid (tablet and capsule diluent). Lactose is soluble in 5 parts of water and is very slightly soluble in alcohol. Hydrolysis of lactose yields dextrose and galactose.

Lanolin USP [hydrous wool fat]—Pharmaceutic aid (W/O emulsion ointment base). Purified, fat-like substance from wool of sheep (*Ovis aries*). Yellowish ointment-like mass; slight odor; on heating, separates into oil and water layers. Insoluble in water; soluble in chloroform and ether with separation of its water.

Lasix Injection [*Hoechst*]—Diuretic. Furosemide. Contains Lasix in solution as the sodium salt of a carboxylic acid; pH 9. *Known compatibilities:* Although Lasix Injection should, in general, not be mixed with infusion solutions or other drugs, the following directions should be observed when such mixtures are believed to be necessary: Lasix Injection can usually be mixed with weakly alkaline and neutral solutions (pH 7 to 10). Examples of this type are physiological saline and Ringer's solution. Lasix Injection may generally also be mixed with weakly acid solutions provided they have a low buffer capacity. Lasix Injection should *not* be mixed with acid solutions, particularly those having a marked buffer capacity in the acid range, since free Lasix may precipitate. Examples of this type are solutions containing ascorbic acid, tetracycline, epinephrine, and norepinephrine. Lasix Injection should *not* be mixed with salts of organic bases. Examples of this type are solutions containing local anesthetics, alkaloids, antihistamines, hypnotics, demerol, and morphine.

Dispensing Information: See *Furosemide.*

Laxatives—see *Cathartics and Laxatives.*

Leucovorin Calcium USP [Calcium Folinate SF (*Lederle*); $C_{20}H_{21}CaN_7O_7 \cdot 5H_2O$ or anhydrous]—Antidote for folic acid antagonists. Insoluble in water.

Levallorphan Tartrate NF [Lorfan Tartrate (*Roche*); $C_{19}H_{25}NO \cdot C_4H_6O_6$]—Antagonist to narcotics. Whitish, crystalline powder; odorless; melts about 175°. 1 g dissolves in about 20 ml water and 60 ml alcohol; practically insoluble in ether; insoluble in chloroform.

Levarterenol Bitartrate USP [Levophed Bitartrate (*Winthrop*); $C_8H_{11}NO_3 \cdot C_4H_6O_6 \cdot H_2O$ or anhydrous]—Adrenergic (vasopressor). 1 g dissolves in about 2.5 ml water and 100 ml alcohol. It darkens slowly on exposure to air and light. The conditions for levarterenol stability are reported to be very similar to those for epinephrine and dilute solutions in distilled water, 5% dextrose, or plasma are more stable than solutions in saline or whole blood. The deleterious effects of copper have also been reported. *Caution:* Constant attention is required when administering this adrenergic drug since dangerously high blood pressure may result in sensitive patients. Levarterenol is contraindicated in cyclopropane anesthesia and heart disease. *Known incompatibilities* (levarterenol bitartrate for injection): Albamycin, Amytal, ascorbic acid, Chlor-Trimeton, Dilantin, Gantrisin, Luminal, Nembutal, normal saline, oxytocin, Pentothal, Seconal, sodium bicarbonate, sodium iodide, streptomycin sulfate, sulfadiazine sodium.

Levodopa USP [Larodopa (*Roche*); Levopa (*SK&F*); $C_9H_{11}NO_4$]—Anticholinergic. Whitish, crystalline powder; odorless; in moisture, rapidly oxidized by oxygen and darkens. Slightly soluble in water; insoluble in alcohol.

Dispensing Information: Patient should be familiar with the disease and treatment schedule. GI disturbances can result if the dosing schedule is not adhered to. Report fainting or dizziness, palpitations, or any abnormal bowel movements to the physician. Do not take multivitamins or vitamin-fortified foods without the physician's attention.

Levo-Dromoran Ampul [*Roche* brand of levorphanol tartrate]—Narcotic; analgesic. *Known ingredients:* levorphan tartrate (2 mg/ml). *Known compatibilities:* atropine sulfate, magnesium sulfate 50% solution (1:1 and 1:10), Phenergan HCl 25 mg/ml Vial Solution (compatible if ratio of Phenergan HCl to *l*-Dromoran is 25:2 or less), prostigmine methylsulfate ampul solution, scopolamine HBr. *Known incompatibilities:* Dramamine Ampul Solution (*Searle*) (50 mg/ml) (solution becomes opalescent).

Levonordefrin NF [$C_9H_{13}NO_3$]—Adrenergic (vasoconstrictor). Whitish, crystalline solid; odorless; melts about 210°. Practically insoluble in water; slightly soluble in alcohol, chloroform, and ether.

Levophed Bitartrate Injection (*Winthrop*)—Vasopressor. *Known ingredients:* Levarterenol bitartrate 0.1% (or 0.02%). *Known compatibilities:* Dextran 6%, dextrose 5% in water (or saline), Levugen 10% in water, Levugen 10% in saline, Levugen 10% in electrolytes.

Levopropoxyphene Napsylate NF [Novrad Napsylate (*Lilly*); $C_{22}H_{29}NO_2$·$C_{10}H_8O_3S$·H_2O or anhydrous]—Antitussive. White powder; essentially odorless; bitter taste; melts (4° range) 158–165°. Very slightly soluble in water; 1 g dissolves in about 17 ml alcohol and 2 ml chloroform.

Levorphanol Tartrate NF [Levo-Dromoran Tartrate (*Roche*); $C_{17}H_{23}$·NO·$C_4H_6O_6$·$2H_2O$ or anhydrous]—Narcotic analgesic. White, odorless, bitter, crystalline narcotic. It is slightly soluble in alcohol and sparingly soluble in water. A 1% solution in water is acidic (pH range, 3.4–4). Levorphanol tartrate is stable to light, air, heat, and moisture.

Levothyroxine Sodium USP [Letter (*Armour*); Synthroid (*Flint*); Titroid (*Century*); $C_{15}H_{10}I_4NNaO_4$·x H_2O or anhydrous]—Thyroid hormone. 1 g dissolves in 700 ml water and 300 ml alcohol; insoluble in chloroform and ether.

Dispensing Information: Consult physician if cramps, diarrhea, tremors, nervousness, vomiting, weight loss, or rapid heartbeat develop (all are signs of excess dosage and necessitate a lowering of dose).

Librax Capsules [*Roche*]—Antianxiety agent. Contain clidinium bromide 2.5 mg, chlordiazepoxide HCl 5 mg.

Dispensing Information: Interacts with MAO inhibitors, alcohol, phenothiazines. Drowsiness may occur which may impair ability to drive or perform other tasks requiring alertness. Librax may enhance response to alcohol and other CNS depressants. Consult physician immediately if sore throat, high fever, easy bruising, or purple spots beneath the skin develop.

Lidocaine USP [Xylocaine (*Astra*); $C_{14}H_{22}N_2O$; pK_a 7.86]—Topical anesthetic. Whitish, crystalline powder; characteristic odor; melts about 67°.

Practically insoluble in water; very soluble in alcohol and chloroform; freely soluble in ether; dissolves in oils.

Lidocaine Hydrochloride USP [Xylocaine Hydrochloride (*Astra*); $C_{14}H_{22}N_2O \cdot HCl \cdot H_2O$]—Local anesthetic. White, crystalline powder; odorless; slightly bitter taste; melts 74–79°. Very soluble in water and alcohol; soluble in chloroform; insoluble in ether. *Known incompatibilities* (lidocaine hydrochloride injection): certain acid-stable preparations (e.g., epinephrine, Isuprel, and Levophed) because of lidocaine's buffering action in IV admixtures.

Dispensing Information: Label: For topical use. Notify physician if skin rash or irritation occur.

Lime NF [calcium oxide; CaO]— Pharmaceutic aid. Hard, white or grayish white masses or granules or as a white or grayish white powder; odorless. 1 g dissolves in 100–1000 ml water; less soluble in boiling water. *Known incompatibilities:* hydroxides, citrates, carbonates, oxalates, tartrates, phosphates.

Lime Solution, Sulfurated, NF— Scabicide. Clear, orange liquid; slight odor of hydrogen sulfide; alkaline to litmus. Contains calcium oxide and sulfur. *Known incompatibilities:* acids, alkalies.

Lincocin Syrup [*Upjohn*]—Antibacterial. Lincomycin hydrochloride (250 mg/5 ml). Red-colored; raspberry-flavored; pH 4.5–5. *Known incompatibilities:* novobiocin, kanamycin.

Lincomycin [Lincocin (*Upjohn*)]— Lincomycin is a basic water-soluble antibiotic produced by *Streptomyces lincolnensis* var. *lincolnensis, et al.* It is active against Gram-positive cocci and Neisseriae, unaffected by penicillinase. It is relatively nontoxic and cross-resistance with currently available antibiotics has not been noted. It is useful by the oral, intramuscular, and intravenous route giving rapid peak serum levels; bioglogical half-life for all three routes of administration is 5.4 ± 1 hour.

Dispensing Information: See *Lincomycin Hydrochloride.*

Lincomycin Hydrochloride USP [Lincocin Hydrochloride (*Upjohn*); $C_{18}H_{34}N_2O_6S \cdot HCl \cdot H_2O$]—Antibacterial. White or practically white, crystalline powder; odorless or faint odor; stable in air and light; solutions are dextrorotatory and acid. Freely soluble in water; slightly soluble in acetone. *Known incompatibilities* (lincomycin HCl injection): Dilantin, penicillin G potassium, penicillin G sodium, sulfadiazine sodium.

Dispensing Information: Consult physician if serious diarrhea develops. Take 1 hour before or 2 hours after eating. Discontinue use and consult physician if blood or mucus appear in stools.

Liothyronine Sodium USP [Cytomel (*SK&F*); $C_{15}H_{11}I_3NNaO_4$]—Thyroid hormone. Light-tan, crystalline powder; odorless. Very slightly soluble in water; slightly soluble in alcohol; practically insoluble in most other organic solvents.

Dispensing Information: Advise physician if signs of overdose (sweating, diarrhea, headache, or heart palpitations) occur.

Lithium Carbonate USP [Eskalith (*SK&F*); Lithane (*Roerig*); Lithonate (*Rowell*); Li_2CO_3]—Antidepressant. White, granular powder; odorless. Sparingly soluble in water; very slightly soluble in alcohol.

Dispensing Information: If diarrhea, vomiting, drowsiness, or muscular weakness occur, advise physician. Do not change your normal salt or water intake without advising physician.

Lomotil Preparations [*Searle*]— Antidiarrheal. Contains (per tablet or 5 ml) atropine sulfate 0.025 mg, diphenoxylate HCl 2.5 mg.

Dispensing Information: Contraindicated in hepatic dysfunction. Potentiates barbiturates. Do not exceed labeled dosage. May cause drowsiness.

Loridine Ampoules [*Lilly* brand of cephaloridine]—Antibacterial. Reconstituted with specified amount of either water for injection, sodium chloride injection, or bacteriostatic sodium chloride injection; when reconstituted—pH

3.5–6; hypertonic; Na^+ depends on reconstitution medium.

Lututrin [Lutrexin (*HW&D*)]— Uterine relaxant. Polypeptide factor from the corpus luteum of sow ovaries. Soluble in water.

Lypressin [8-L-lysinevasopressin; Diapid (*Sandoz*); $C_{46}H_{65}N_{13}O_{12}S_2$]— Antidiuretic; vasodepressor.

Maalox [Rorer]—Antacid. Balanced combination of magnesium and aluminum hydroxides; supplied as oral suspension or tablets. *Known incompatibilities:* acids.

Dispensing Information: see *Gelusil Liquid.*

Mafenide Acetate USP [Sulfamylon (*Winthrop*); $C_7H_{10}N_2O_2S \cdot C_2H_4O_2$]— Antibacterial (topical). White, crystalline powder; melts 162–171°. Freely soluble in water.

Dispensing Information (cream): This is an inpatient medication. Label: For the skin. Note: A painful or burning sensation may follow application.

Magaldrate USP [Riopan (*Ayerst*); $Al_2H_{14}Mg_4O_{14} \cdot 2H_2O$]—Antacid. White, crystalline powder; odorless. Insoluble in water and alcohol.

Magnesia, Milk of, USP [$Mg(OH)_2$] —Antacid; cathartic. White, opaque, more or less viscous suspension from which varying proportions of water usually separate on standing; pH about 10. *Known incompatibilities:* acids.

Dispensing Information: See *Antacids (Magnesium-Containing).*

Magnesia and Alumina Oral Suspension USP—Antacid. Suspension containing magnesium hydroxide and variable amounts of aluminum oxide; pH 7.3–8.5. *Known incompatibilities:* acids.

Magnesia and Alumina Tablets USP—Antacid. Tablets which may be chewed or swallowed. Contain magnesium hydroxide and aluminum hydroxide. *Known incompatibilities:* acids, absorption of other drugs.

Magnesium Carbonate NF [magnesium carbonate, basic; $MgCO_3$]—Antacid. Light, white, friable masses or bulky, white powder; odorless; stable in air.

Practically insoluble in water (to which, however, it imparts a slightly alkaline reaction); insoluble in alcohol; dissolved by dilute acids with effervescence. *Known incompatibilities:* acids.

Magnesium Chloride USP [$MgCl_2 \cdot 6H_2O$]—Electrolyte replenisher; pharmaceutic aid (hemodialysis and peritoneal dialysis fluids). Colorless, flakes or crystals; odorless; deliquescent; loses water when heated to 100° and HCl when heated to 110°. *Known incompatibilities:* alkalies.

Magnesium Citrate Solution NF [$C_{12}H_{10}Mg_3O_{14}$]—Cathartic. Colorless to slightly yellow, clear, effervescent liquid; sweet, acidulous taste, lemon flavor. Contains magnesium carbonate, citric acid, potassium bicarbonate, and flavors. Store in cool place and in bottles containing not less than 200 ml.

Magnesium Hydroxide NF [$Mg(OH)_2$]—Antacid; cathartic. Bulky, white powder. Dissolves in dilute acids; practically insoluble in water and alcohol. *Known incompatibilities:* acids, sodium bicarbonate.

Magnesium Oxide USP [MgO]— Pharmaceutic aid (sorbent). Very bulky, white powder (light magnesium oxide) or relatively dense white powder (heavy magnesium oxide); 5 g of light magnesium oxide occupies a volume of approx 40–50 ml (heavy, 10–20 ml). Soluble in dilute acids (10–30 parts); 1 g dissolves in >10,000 ml water and alcohol.

Magnesium Phosphate NF [$Mg(PO_4)_2 \cdot 5H_2O)$]—Antacid. White powder; odorless; tasteless. Readily soluble in diluted mineral acids; almost insoluble in water.

Magnesium Stearate USP [approx $Mg(C_{18}H_{35}O_2)_2$] — Pharmaceutic aid (lubricant). Fine, white, bulky powder; faint, characteristic odor; unctuous, adheres readily to the skin, and free from grittiness. Insoluble in water, alcohol, and ether. *Known incompatibilities:* dilute acids.

Magnesium Sulfate USP [$MgSO_4 \cdot 7H_2O$]—Cathartic; anticonvulsant (injection); electrolyte replenisher. Small, colorless crystals; usually needle-like; cooling, saline, bitter taste; solutions neutral to litmus; effloresces in warm, dry air. 1 g dissolves in 1–10 ml water, 1–10 ml glycerin (slowly), <1 ml boiling water, and 30–100 ml alcohol. *Known incompatibilities:* alkalies, phosphates, carbonates, silicates.

Magnesium Trisilicate USP [$2MgO \cdot 3SiO_2 \cdot x\,H_2O$]—Pharmaceutic aid; antacid. Fine, white, powder; odorless; tasteless; free from grittiness. Insoluble in water and alcohol; readily decomposed by mineral acids. *Known incompatibilities:* acids, dyes, toxins; adsorbs alkaloids.

Mandelic Acid [$C_8H_8O_3$; pK_a 3.37]—The pH of a 1% solution of mandelic acid is approximately 2.4.

Mandelic acid (racemic mandelic acid) useful as a urinary antiseptic is a white, crystalline compound which is soluble in 6.3 parts of water and freely soluble in alcohol. On exposure to light it gradually decomposes and darkens. Aqueous solutions of mandelic acid are decomposed on boiling. *Ammonium mandelate* in crystalline form is hygroscopic and unstable; it is freely soluble in water and soluble in alcohol. *Sodium mandelate* is quite stable in the solid form, but its solutions should be protected from light; it is soluble in water and slightly soluble in alcohol. *Calcium mandelate* is slightly soluble in water and insoluble in alcohol.

Mannitol USP [Osmitrol (*Travenol*); $C_6H_{14}O_6$]—Diuretic. White, crystalline powder or free-flowing granules; odorless; sweet taste; melts 165–168°; pH (sat soln) 4.5–7. One g dissolves in 5.5 ml water; very slightly soluble in alcohol; practically insoluble in ether. *Known incompatibilities* (mannitol injection): strong acidic and basic solutions, blood, protein hydrolysate.

Maolate Tablets [*Upjohn* brand of chlorphenesin carbamate]—Skeletal muscle relaxant. Contains (per tablet) Na$^+$ 1.1 mg K$^+$ 0.17 mg; calories 2.

Marax Tablets [*Roerig*]—Bronchodilator. Contain hydroxyzine HCl 10 mg, ephedrine sulfate 25 mg, theophylline 130 mg.

Dispensing Information: Use with caution in elderly males. Interacts with CNS depressants. Do not drive or operate heavy machinery. Should be taken with food to prevent GI irritation.

Maxitrol Ophthalmic Suspension [*Alcon*]—Anti-inflammatory. Contains (per ml) dexamethasone 0.1%, neomycin sulfate 3.5 mg, polymyxin B sulfate 6000 u. pH 5.5; aqueous solvent; buffer, NaOH/HCl; Na$^+$ 0.3343%; isotonic.

Mecamylamine Hydrochloride NF [Inversine HCl (*MSD*); $C_{11}H_{21}N \cdot$ HCl]—Antihypertensive. White, crystalline powder; odorless or almost so; melts (with some decomposition) about 245°. Freely soluble in water and chloroform; 1 g dissolves in about 28 ml isopropyl alcohol; practically insoluble in ether.

Mechlorethamine Hydrochloride USP [nitrogen mustard; Mustargen HCl (*MSD*); $C_5H_{11}Cl_2N \cdot HCl$]—Antineoplastic. White, crystalline powder; hygroscopic; melts about 109°; pH (1 in 500 aq soln) about 4. *Caution: A vesicant; the powder or its solution is irritating to the respiratory tract.* Very soluble in water; soluble in alcohol. *Known incompatibilities* (mechlorethamine HCl for injection): should not be diluted and prepared as an IV infusion.

Meclizine Hydrochloride USP [Bonine (*Roerig*); $C_{25}H_{27}ClN_2 \cdot 2HCl \cdot H_2O$]—Antinauseant. White or slightly yellowish, crystalline powder; slight odor; tasteless; melts 217–224°. Practically insoluble in water and ether; freely soluble in chloroform; slightly soluble in alcohol.

Dispensing Information: Contraindicated in pregnancy. Use due precaution when engaging in activities where alertness is mandatory. See also *Antihistamines.*

Medroxyprogesterone Acetate USP [Depo-Provera, Provera (*Upjohn*); $C_{24}H_{34}O_4$]—Progestin. White to off-white, crystalline powder; odorless; stable in air. Insoluble in water; freely soluble in chloroform; sparingly soluble in alcohol; slightly soluble in ether.

Medrysone USP [HMS Liquifilm (*Allergan*); Medrocort (*Upjohn*); $C_{22}H_{32}O_3$]—Glucocorticoid. Whitish, crystalline powder; odorless or slight odor; melts (with decomposition) about 158°. Sparingly soluble in water; soluble in chloroform.

Mefenamic Acid [Ponstel (*P-D*); $C_{15}H_{15}NO_2$]—Anti-inflammatory. Whitish, crystalline powder; odorless; very little initial taste, but bitter aftertaste; darkens in light; melts about 230° (decarboxylates above melting point). Insoluble in water; 1 g dissolves in about 220 ml alcohol.

Megestrol Acetate [Megace (*Mead-Johnson*); $C_{24}H_{32}O_4$]—Antineoplastic. Whitish, crystalline powder; odorless; tasteless; melts (3° range) 213–219°. Insoluble in water; sparingly soluble in alcohol; slightly soluble in ether; very soluble in chloroform.

Meglumine USP [$C_7H_{17}NO_5$]—Pharmaceutic aid (preparing radiopaque media). White to faintly yellowish white crystals or powder; odorless; melts 128–132°. Freely soluble in water; sparingly soluble in alcohol.

Mellaril Preparations [*Sandoz*]—Tranquilizer. Thioridazine hydrochloride. *Concentrate (30 mg/ml)*: pH 4.1–5.3; alcohol 2.56–3.14%; aqueous solvent; sweetener, sorbitol. *Concentrate (100 mg/ml)*: pH 3.5–4.5; alcohol 3.7–4.7%; aqueous solvent; sweetener: sucrose, sorbitol.

Melphalan USP [Alkeran (*B-W*); $C_{13}H_{18}Cl_2N_2O_2$]—Antineoplastic. *Caution: Do not inhale.* Whitish powder; faint odor; light-, heat-, and moisture-sensitive; melts (with decomposition) about 180°. Practically insoluble in water, chloroform, and ether; slightly soluble in alcohol.

Menadiol Sodium Diphosphate NF [vitamin K_4; $C_{11}H_8Na_4O_8P_2$·$6H_2O$ or anhydrous]—Prothrombogenic vitamin. Insoluble in alcohol and very soluble in water. It occurs as a white to pink, hygroscopic powder. A 1% solution in water is slightly alkaline (pH range,

7.8–8.5). *Known incompatibilities* (menadiol sodium diphosphate injection): protein hydrolysate.

Menadione NF [vitamin K_3; $C_{11}H_8O_2$]—Prothrombogenic vitamin. This is a synthetic compound which possesses the activity of vitamin K. Menadione is a yellow, crystalline powder; it is stable in air when protected from light. This compound is very slightly soluble in water and soluble in about 60 parts of alcohol. It is soluble in fixed oils. It is incompatible with reducing agents, halogens, and alkalies.

Menadione Sodium Bisulfite NF [$C_{11}H_9NaO_5S$·$3H_2O$ or anhydrous]—Prothrombogenic vitamin. This may be prepared by the interaction of menadione and sodium bisulfite to form the addition product. This substance is a white, odorless, crystalline powder. It is soluble in about 2 parts of water and is slightly soluble in alcohol. It is less affected by light than menadione. *Known incompatibilities* (menadione sodium bisulfite injection): Dilantin, Sparine; should not be added to IV infusions.

Menthol USP [$C_{10}H_{20}O$]—This terpene alcohol useful as a skin coolant and counterirritant is only slightly soluble in water, but it is soluble in alcohol, fixed oils, volatile oils, and organic solvents.

The addition of water to alcoholic solutions of menthol causes separation of the menthol. Menthol forms a liquid or soft mass (eutectic mixture) when triturated with a number of substances, e.g., camphor, phenol, thymol, butyl chloral hydrate, chloral hydrate, betanaphthol, resorcinol, and *N*-methylacetanilide. It is also incompatible with pyrogallol, potassium permanganate, and chromic acid.

Mepenzolate Bromide NF [Cantil (*Lakeside*); $C_{21}H_{26}BrNO_3$]—Anticholinergic. Whitish powder; melts (with decomposition) about 230°. 1 g dissolves in about 110 ml water and 630 ml chloroform; practically insoluble in ether.

Meperidine Hydrochloride USP [Demerol Hydrochloride (*Winthrop*);

(*Various Other Mfrs.*); $C_{15}H_{21}NO_2 \cdot$ HCl]—Narcotic analgesic. Fine, white, crystalline powder; odorless; pH (5% soln) about 5; stable in air at ordinary temperatures; *Known incompatibilities:* addition of alkalies to aqueous solutions precipitates the free base.

Dispensing Information: Contraindicated in bronchial asthma, atrial flutter. May be habit-forming. Do not drive or operate heavy machinery. Reduce dose or discontinue use if tremors or incoordination occur. May cause nausea, vomiting, dizziness, sweating, flushing of face, dryness of mouth, antidiuretic effect.

Mephenesin [$C_{10}H_{14}O_3$]—Skeletal muscle relaxant. Freely soluble in alcohol, propylene glycol and chloroform but soluble in water only 1 part in 85. Aqueous solutions (pH *circa* 6) are stable and compatible with saline, glucose, barbiturates, and thiobarbiturates.

Mephentermine Sulfate NF [Wyamine Sulfate (*Wyeth*); $(C_{11}H_{17}N)_2 \cdot H_2SO_4$ or the dihydrate]— Adrenergic (vasopressor). White crystals or crystalline powder; odorless; pH (aq soln) about 6. One g dissolves in 20 ml water and about 150 ml alcohol; practically insoluble in chloroform. *Known incompatibilities* (mephentermine sulfate injection): epinephrine HCl, hydralazine HCl.

Mephenytoin NF [Mesantoin (*Sandoz*); $C_{12}H_{14}N_2O_2$]—Anticonvulsant. White, crystalline powder; melts about 137°; pH about 8. One g dissolves in about 1400 ml water, 15 ml alcohol, 3 ml chloroform, and 90 ml ether.

Mephobarbital NF [Mebaral (*Winthrop*); $C_{13}H_{14}N_2O_3$; pK_a 8.8]—Anticonvulsant; sedative. White, crystalline powder; odorless; bitter taste; sat soln acid to litmus; melts about 178°. 1 g dissolves in >1000 ml water, alcohol, and ether, and about 50 ml chloroform.

Mepivacaine Hydrochloride USP [Carbocaine HCl (*Winthrop*); $C_{15}H_{22}N_2O \cdot HCl$; pK_a 7.73]—Local anesthetic. White, crystalline solid; odorless; melts (with decomposition) about 258°. Freely soluble in water; very slightly soluble in chloroform; practically insoluble in ether.

Meprednisone NF [Betapar (*P-D*); $C_{22}H_{28}O_5$]—Glucocorticoid. Whitish powder; odorless; melts (with decomposition) about 200°. 1 g dissolves in about 3300 ml water, 10 ml chloroform, and 1700 ml ether; soluble in alcohol.

Meprobamate USP [Equanil (*Wyeth*), Miltown (*Wallace*); (*Various Other Mfrs.*); $C_9H_{18}N_2O_4$]—Tranquilizer (minor). White powder; characteristic odor; bitter taste; melts 103–107°; pH (aq soln) about 7; stable in dilute alkali and acid, thus stable in intestinal and gastric juice. *Side effects:* Although overall toxicity is low, it is capable of producing a variety of side effects and untoward reactions. Among the more common of these are hypersensitivity reactions in addition to dermal manifestations (urticaria and erythematous and maculopapular skin rashes), shaking chills and fever, acute nonthrombocytopenic purpura, etc.

Dispensing Information: Do not drive or operate heavy equipment on initial therapy. Contact physician if excessive drowsiness, staggering, or unusual disturbances occur. May enhance response to alcohol and other CNS depressants.

Meprylcaine Hydrochloride NF [$C_{14}H_{21}NO_2 \cdot HCl$]—Local anesthetic. White, crystalline solid; odorless; melts about 151°; pH (1 in 50 soln) about 5.7. 1 g dissolves in about 6 ml water, 5 ml alcohol, 3 ml chloroform, and 12 ml ether.

Meralluride NF [Mercuhydrin (*Lakeside*); $C_{16}H_{22}HgN_6O_7$] — Diuretic. Slightly soluble in water, yielding an acid solution; it is soluble in alkaline solutions.

Merbromin [Mercurochrome (*HW&D*); $C_{20}H_8Br_2HgNa_2O_6$]—Antibacterial. Freely soluble in water and practically insoluble in alcohol. The gel which sometimes forms in solutions containing more than 10% of merbromin may be prevented by the addition of 1% of sodium carbonate. The mercury atom is in an ortho position to a phenolic hydroxyl group and, hence is easily removed by acids. Merbromin is precipitated from aqueous solutions by acids and acid reacting salts and gives a precipitate with solutions of most alkaloidal salts and local anesthetics. It is incompatible with higher alcohols, reducing substances, heavy metal salts, and substances capable of liberating chlorine or other halogens. Merbromin is incompatible with all strengths of ethyl alcohol above 50%. Precipitation of mercurochrome is immediate from aqueous solutions more acid than pH 4.8. In solutions of pH 5.4 to 4.8, precipitation takes place slowly, the complete process requiring from 6 to 8 hours. Solutions should not be heated above 70°C since decomposition occurs at higher temperatures. Stains of mercurochrome may be removed by washing the affected area with a dilute solution of chlorinated soda.

Mercaptomerin Sodium USP [Thiomerin Sodium (*Wyeth*); $C_{16}H_{25}HgNNa_2O_6S$]—Diuretic. White powder or amorphous solid; hygroscopic; 1 in 50 soln neutral or slightly alkaline to litmus. Freely soluble in water; soluble in alcohol; slightly soluble in chloroform and ether.

Mercaptopurine USP [Purinethol (*B-W*); $C_5H_4N_4S\cdot H_2O$ or anhydrous]—Antineoplastic. Yellow, crystalline powder; odorless or almost so; melts (with decomposition) above 308°. Insoluble in water and ether; soluble in hot alcohol. *Known incompatibilities* (mercaptopurine sodium injection): allopurinol sodium, prednisolone sodium succinate.

Mercresin Tincture [*Upjohn*]— This product contains 1 part of mercarbolide and 1 part of pentacresol (mixture of five isomeric secondary-amyltricresols) in 1000 parts of solution, the solvent being a mixture of alcohol, water, and acetone. For the purpose of defining the area of application, the tincture contains a small proportion of a water-soluble, inert coloring material which is easily removed from the skin or linens by soap and water. A stainless

tincture containing no coloring material is also available.

Mercresin Tincture is compatible with both acids and alkalies. It does not react with sodium chloride of the body fluids and does not precipitate serum proteins. It is miscible with water in any proportion.

Merethoxylline Procaine [Dicurin Procaine (*Lilly*)]—Diuretic. Mixture of procaine merethoxylline and theophylline in a ratio of 1:1.4. Whitish powder; melts about 139°. Practically insoluble in water; soluble in alkaline solutions.

Mesoridazine Besylate NF [Serentil (*B-I*); $C_{21}H_{26}N_2OS_2\cdot C_6H_6O_3S$]— Tranquilizer. Whitish, crystalline powder; faint odor; melts (with decomposition) about 178°. 1 g dissolves in about 1 ml water, 11 ml alcohol, 3 ml chloroform, and 6300 ml ether.

Mestranol USP [$C_{21}H_{26}O_2$]—Estrogen. Whitish powder or small plates; odorless; melts (4° range) 146–154°. Insoluble in water; freely soluble in chloroform; sparingly soluble in ether; slightly soluble in alcohol.

Metaproterenol Sulfate [Alupent (*B-I*); Metaprex (*Dorsey*); $(C_{11}H_{17}NO_3)_2\cdot H_2SO_4$]—Bronchodilator. Whitish, crystalline powder; odorless; bitter taste; light-sensitive; oxidizes in air; melts about 206°. Freely soluble in water and alcohol.

Metaraminol Bitartrate USP [Aramine (*MSD*); $C_9H_{13}NO_2\cdot C_4H_6O_6$]— Adrenergic. White, crystalline powder; practically odorless; melts about 173°; pH about 3.3. Freely soluble in water; practically insoluble in chloroform and ether; 1 g dissolves in about 100 ml alcohol. *Known incompatibilities* (metaraminol bitartrate injection): amphotericin B, fibrinogen, hydrocortisone sodium succinate, methicillin sodium, morphine sulfate, nitrofurantoin sodium, penicillin G salts, phenytoin sodium, sulfadiazine sodium, thiopental sodium, warfarin sodium.

Metaxalone [Skelaxin (*Robins*); $C_{12}H_{15}NO_3$]—Skeletal muscle relaxant. White, crystalline powder; melts about

122°. Practically insoluble in water; soluble in alcohol.

Methacholine Bromide NF [Mecholyl Bromide (*MSD*); $C_8H_{18}BrNO_2$]—Cholinergic. This ester and quaternary compound is a white, crystalline, very hygroscopic powder that is readily soluble in water and alcohol. A 5% aqueous solution is slightly acidic (pH about 4.6).

Methacholine Chloride NF [Mecholyl Chloride (*MSD*); $C_8H_{18}ClNO_2$]—Cholinergic. Colorless or white crystalline ester and quaternary compound that is very soluble in water and freely soluble in alcohol. Its aqueous solutions are nearly neutral (pH *circa* 7). It is very deliquescent.

Methacycline Hydrochloride NF [Rondomycin Hydrochloride (*Wallace*); $C_{22}H_{22}N_2O_8 \cdot HCl$]—Antibacterial. Yellow to dark-yellow, crystalline powder; pH (1% soln) 2–3. One g dissolves in 100 ml water, 300 ml alcohol, and >1000 ml chloroform and ether.

Dispensing Information: See *Tetracyclines.*

Methadone Hydrochloride USP [amidone hydrochloride; Dolophine Hydrochloride (*Lilly*); $C_{21}H_{27}NO \cdot HCl$]—Narcotic analgesic. White, crystalline powder or colorless crystals. It is soluble in water and freely soluble in alcohol. Solutions in water are acidic (pH range, 3–6.5). Methadone is precipitated from solution by alkalies and alkaloidal reagents and is incompatible with wild cherry syrup. It has a bitter taste.

Methamphetamine Hydrochloride [Desoxyn Hydrochloride (*Abbott*); (*Various Other Mfrs.*); $C_{10}H_{15}N \cdot HCl$]—Central stimulant. 1 g dissolves in 2 ml of water or 3 ml of alcohol. An aqueous solution has a slightly acid reaction and gives a precipitate with iodine or mercury bichloride.

Dispensing Information: Interacts with MAO inhibitors. Sustained-action preparations, take dose in early morning; tablets, do not take dose after 6 p.m.

Methandrostenolone NF [Dianabol (*Ciba*); $C_{20}H_{28}O_2$]—Androgen. Whitish crystals or crystalline powder; odorless; melts about 165°. Insoluble in water; soluble in alcohol and chloroform; slightly soluble in ether.

Dispensing Information: Contraindicated in pregnancy. Potentiates oral anticoagulants and oxyphenbutazone. Avoid excess salt intake. Consult physician immediately if yellowing of eyes or skin occur.

Methantheline Bromide NF [Banthine Bromide (*Searle*); $C_{21}H_{26}BrNO_3$]—Anticholinergic. This quaternary compound is a white, microcrystalline powder that is very soluble in water and freely soluble in alcohol. Its aqueous solutions decompose on standing. It is very rapidly hydrolyzed in alkaline solution. A freshly prepared aqueous solution has a pH of 5–5.5

Methapyrilene Hydrochloride NF [Histadyl Hydrochloride (*Lilly*), $C_{14}H_{19}N_3S \cdot HCl$]—Antihistaminic. White, crystalline powder. It is very soluble in water and freely soluble in alcohol. A 5% solution in water is slightly acidic (pH range, 5–6).

Methaqualone NF [Quaalude (*Rorer*); (*Various Other Mfrs.*); $C_{16}H_{14}N_2O$; pK_a 2.54]—Hypnotic. White, crystalline powder; little or no odor; bitter taste; aq soln alkaline to litmus; melts about 115°. 1 g dissolves in about 3300 ml water, 8 ml alcohol, 2 ml chloroform, and 27 ml ether.

Methaqualone Hydrochloride NF [Parest (*P-D*); Somnafac (*Cooper*); $C_{16}H_{14}N_2O \cdot HCl$]—Hypnotic. White, crystalline powder; odorless; melts (with decomposition) about 250°. 1 g dissolves in about 64 ml water; sparingly soluble in alcohol; soluble in chloroform; very slightly soluble in ether.

Metharbital NF [Gemonil (*Abbott*); $C_9H_{14}N_2O_3$; pK_a 8.45]—Anticonvulsant. Whitish, crystalline powder; faint odor; pH (sat soln) about 6; melts about 153°. 1 g dissolves in about 830 ml water, 23 ml alcohol, and 40 ml ether.

Methazolamide USP [Neptazane (*Lederle*); $C_5H_8N_4O_3S_2$]—Carbonic anhydrase inhibitor. Whitish, crystalline powder; slight odor; melts about 213°.

Very slightly soluble in water and alcohol.

Methdilazine NF [Tacaryl (Mead-Johnson); $C_{18}H_{20}N_2S$; pK_a 7.45]—Antipruritic. Light-tan, crystalline powder; characteristic odor; sensitive to light and oxidizing agents; melts (2° range) 83–88°. Practically insoluble in water; 1 g dissolves in about 2 ml alcohol, 1 ml chloroform, and 8 ml ether.

Methdilazine Hydrochloride NF [Tacaryl HCl (Mead-Johnson); $C_{18}H_{20}N_2S \cdot HCl$]—Antipruritic. Light-tan, crystalline powder; slight odor; bitter anesthetic taste; solution unstable in light; melts about 187°. 1 g dissolves in about 2 ml water, 2 ml alcohol, and 6 ml chloroform; insoluble in ether.

Methenamine NF [Uritone (P-D); $C_6H_{12}N_4$]—Antibacterial (urinary). 1 g dissolves in about 1.5 ml of water or 12.5 ml of alcohol. It is alkaline in aqueous solution and, hence, has the incompatibilities of weak alkalies. A damp mass is formed when methenamine is triturated with acetylsalicylic acid. In the presence of acids methenamine is slowly converted into formaldehyde and ammonium salts of the acids.

Dispensing Information: Provide advice for making urine acid with food stuffs or ascorbic acid if indicated. Explain ways of testing for acid urine.

Methenamine Mandelate USP [Mandelamine (W-C); $C_6H_{12}N_4 \cdot C_8H_8O_3$]—Antibacterial (urinary). White, crystalline powder; practically odorless; sour taste; pH (solutions) about 4; melts about 127° with decomposition. 1 g dissolves in 1 ml water, 10 ml alcohol, 20 ml chloroform, and 350 ml ether.

Dispensing Information: May cause nausea and vomiting or rash. See *Methenamine.*

Methicillin Sodium USP [Staphcillin (Bristol); $C_{17}H_{19}N_2NaO_6S \cdot H_2O$]—Antibacterial. Fine, white, crystalline powder; odorless or slight odor. Freely soluble in water; slightly soluble in chloroform; insoluble in ether.

This is a semisynthetic penicillin, stable in dry form and soluble in water; Aqueous solutions are labile to heat and storage and gradually darken to a deep orange color and acquire an odor of hydrogen sulfide, hence should be used within 24 hours at room temperature or within 4 days if refrigerated. Frozen solutions may apparently be stored in a freezer several months without decomposition. This frozen solution thaws after several minutes at room temperature and is then ready for administration. Solutions should be neutral as it is extremely unstable in acid solution. Accordingly it is used by injection; principally in penicillin G-resistant, staphylococcic infections. Although resistant to penicillinase and demonstrating a low degree of serum protein binding, the possibility of serious toxicity has been noted. Label directions should be carefully followed. *Known incompatibilities* (methicillin sodium for injection): acidic solutions, anileridine HCl, Aramine, chlorpromazine HCl, chlortetracycline HCl, codeine phosphate, Compazine, Demerol, hydrocortisone sodium succinate, kanamycin sulfate, Levo-Dromoran, Lorfan, methadone, morphine sulfate, Phenergan, sodium bicarbonate, sulfadiazine sodium, Terramycin, tetracycline HCl, Vancocin.

Methimazole USP [Tapazole (Lilly); $C_4H_6N_2S$]—Thyroid inhibitor. White to buff, crystalline powder which has almost no taste and a very faint odor. It is freely soluble in water and in alcohol. A 2% aqueous solution is nearly neutral (pH range, 6.7–6.9). It is sensitive to light.

Dispensing Information: See *Antithyroid Agents.*

Methiodal Sodium NF [Skiodan (Winthrop); CH_2INaO_3S]—Diagnostic aid (radiopaque medium—urographic). White, crystalline powder; odorless; slight saline taste (sweetish aftertaste); decomposes in light and turns yellow; solution neutral to litmus. 1 g dissolves in about 1 ml water and 200 ml alcohol; practically insoluble in chloroform and ether.

Methionine NF [DL-methionine; Meonine (Ives); $C_5H_{11}NO_2S$; pK_a 9.21; pK_b 11.72]—Lipotropic. The pH of a

1% aqueous solution of this essential amino acid is about 5.6–6.1. Soluble in water (3.38%), soluble in dilute acids (forming acid salts, e.g., hydrochlorides), and dilute alkalies (forming, e.g., sodium salts). Very slightly soluble in alcohol. *Caution:* Never administer on an empty stomach as large doses may produce ketosis.

Methisazone [Marboran (*B-W*); $C_{10}H_{10}N_4OS$]—Antiviral. Crystals; melts about 245°.

Methixene Hydrochloride [Trest (*Dorsey*); $C_{20}H_{23}NS \cdot HCl$]—Smooth muscle relaxant. White, crystalline powder; practically odorless; bitter taste; darkens slowly in light; melts about 215°. Soluble in water, alcohol, and chloroform; practically insoluble in ether.

Methocarbamol NF [Robaxin (*Robins*); $C_{11}H_{15}NO_5$]—Skeletal muscle relaxant. White powder; odorless or with slight, characteristic odor; melts 93–97°. 1 g dissolves in 40 ml water; sparingly soluble in chloroform; freely soluble in alcohol.

Methohexital USP [Brevital (*Lilly*); $C_{14}H_{18}N_2O_3$]—General anesthetic (intravenous). Whitish, crystalline powder; odorless; melts (3° range) 92–96°. Very slightly soluble in water; slightly soluble in alcohol and chloroform. Also available as Methohexital Sodium for Injection USP.

Methotrexate USP [*Lederle;* $C_{20}H_{22}N_8O_5$]—Antineoplastic. Orange-brown, crystalline powder; pH (injection) 8.3–8.6. Practically insoluble in water, alcohol, chloroform, and ether. *Caution:* Great care should be taken to prevent inhaling particles of methotrexate and exposing the skin to it.

Methotrimeprazine NF [Levoprome (*Lederle*); $C_{19}H_{24}N_2OS$]—Analgesic. Fine, white, crystalline powder; practically odorless; light-sensitive; melts about 126°. 1 g dissolves in about 10 ml water, 10 ml alcohol, and 2 ml chloroform; freely soluble in ether.

Methoxamine Hydrochloride USP [Vasoxyl HCl (*B-W*); $C_{11}H_{17}NO_3 \cdot HCl$]—Adrenergic (vasopressor). Whitish, plate-like crystals or white, crystalline powder; odorless or slight odor; solution acid to litmus; pH about 5; melts about 216°. 1 g dissolves in about 2.5 ml water and 12 ml alcohol; almost insoluble in chloroform and ether.

Methoxsalen USP [Meloxine (*Upjohn*); Oxsoralen (*Elder*); $C_{12}H_8O_4$]—Aid to dermal pigmentation. Whitish, needle-like crystals; odorless; melts about 145°. Practically insoluble in cold water (sparingly soluble in boiling water); freely soluble in chloroform; soluble in boiling alcohol.

Methoxyflurane NF [Penthrane (*Abbott*); $C_3H_4Cl_2F_2O$]—General anesthetic by inhalation as required. Clear, practically colorless, mobile liquid; characteristic odor; boils about 105°. Miscible with acetone, alcohol, chloroform, ether, benzene, and fixed oils.

Methoxyphenamine Hydrochloride NF [Orthoxine HCl (*Upjohn*); $C_{11}H_{17}NO \cdot HCl$]—Adrenergic. White, crystalline powder; melts about 130°. Freely soluble in water, alcohol, and chloroform; slightly soluble in ether.

Methscopolamine Bromine NF [Pamine Bromide (*Upjohn*); $C_{18}H_{24}BrNO_4$]—Anticholinergic. This quaternary derivative of the ester alkaloid scopolamine is a white crystalline powder that is freely soluble in water and sparingly soluble in alcohol. A 0.1% aqueous solution is nearly neutral (pH about 6.5). Alkaline solutions hydrolyze this and related compounds, breaking the ester linkage.

It has been reported that Pamine solutions and compounded mixtures are usually stable for long periods of time below pH 6, are apparently stable enough for prescription use between pH 6 and 7, and should not be dispensed above pH 8 as they are very rapidly hydrolyzed. Simple, aqueous Pamine solutions were initially compatible with 30 potentially incompatible test solutions but later developed delayed incompatibilities with 10 of these. Only one of the 10 gave any physical evidence of incompatibility, i.e., sodium stearate. Nine of the ten were slightly to extensively hydrolyzed, e.g., mixtures with arsenates, arsenites, bicarbonates, glycerophosphates, laurylsulfates p-aminobenzoates, propionates, soluble parabens, and other alkaline materials, although no physical change had occurred in 1 to 2 weeks.

Similar results were obtained when a Pamine Syrup and Pamine and Phenobarbital Elixir were tested as dispensing vehicles for a number of likely ingredients. These Pamine liquids had no adverse effects on the stability or potency of penicillin, sulfonamides, or multivitamin products. They were also compatible with ammonium chloride, Cheracol, Citrocarbonate Syrup, Cryobeta, ephedrine hydrochloride, Hydrolose, Hydrolose Fortified, methamphetamine hydrochloride, Orthoxine Syrup, Orthoxicol, pyridoxine hydrochloride, sodium biphosphate, sodium bromide, Sugracillin, Sulfa-Sugracillin, Syrasulfas, thiamine hydrochloride, Vitikon, Zymalixir, and Zymasyrup. They were incompatible with aluminum hydroxide gel, Emulserol with Cascara, Malcogel, fluidextract of cascara sagrada aromatic, 20% sodium citrate, 20% potassium citrate, terpin hydrate and codeine elixir, and camphorated opium tincture, although physical changes were not always evident. Pamine Syrup and Pamine and Phenobarbital Elixir are stable for several years.

Methsuximide NF [Celontin (*P-D*); $C_{12}H_{13}NO_2$]—Anticonvulsant. Whitish, crystalline powder; odorless or slight odor; melts about 53°. 1 g dissolves in about 350 ml water, 3 ml alcohol, <1 ml chloroform, and 2 ml ether.

Methyclothiazide NF [Enduron (*Abbott*); $C_9H_{11}Cl_2N_3O_4S_2$]—Diuretic; antihypertensive. White or practically white, crystalline powder; odorless or slight odor. 1 g dissolves in >10,000 ml water and chloroform, 92.5 ml alcohol, and >2703 ml ether.

Dispensing Information: See *Diuretics (Chlorothiazide Type)*.

Methyl Alcohol NF [methanol; wood alcohol; CH_4O]—Pharmaceutic aid (solvent). Clear, colorless liquid; characteristic odor; flammable; sp gr not more than 0.790; distils (1° range) including 64.6°. Miscible with water, alcohol, ether, and most other organic solvents.

Methylbenzethonium Chloride NF [Diaparene Chloride (*Breon*); $C_{28}H_{44}ClNO_2 \cdot H_2O$ or anhydrous]—Topical anti-infective. White crystals; hygroscopic; very bitter taste; mild odor; solutions neutral or slightly alkaline to litmus. Effective in preventing ammonia dermatitis in children and incontinent adults.

Dispensing Information: Diapers and other articles to be rinsed should be soap-free to avoid inactivation of methylbenzethonium.

Methylcellulose USP [cellulose methyl ether; Cellothyl (*W-C*); Methocel (*Dow*); Syncelose (*Blue Line*)]—Pharmaceutic aid (suspending agent). Methylcellulose is a cellulose ether which is soluble in water, yielding clear, neutral, viscous solutions that are stable for a long period without the addition of a preservative. Solutions are prepared by mixing methylcellulose with about half of the required amount of water at 80° to 90°C allowing to stand for a few minutes, and then bringing to volume with cold water. Solutions can also be made at room temperature, provided the methylcellulose has been thoroughly triturated with other dry ingredients of a prescription.

The mucilages are compatible with alcohol, glycerin, alkalies, diluted acids, and soap but are coagulated by tannic acid and many salts. Methylcellulose is available in six viscosity types that are classified according to the viscosity in centipoises of a 2% aqueous solution at 20°C as follows: 15, 25, 100, 400, 1500, and 4000 cps. Methylcellulose is used as a dispersing, thickening, and emulsifying agent. The mucilages can be blended with aqueous dispersions of starch, glue, casein, and gums.

Methyldopa USP [Aldomet (*MSD*); $C_{10}H_{13}NO_4 \cdot 1\frac{1}{2}H_2O$] — Antihypertensive. White to yellowish white, fine powder which may contain friable lumps; odorless. Sparingly soluble in water; slightly soluble in alcohol; practically insoluble in ether.

Dispensing Information: Contraindicated in hepatic disease or dysfunction. May cause sedation during initial period of therapy.

A patient card may include the following:

This drug is used to lower your blood pressure and is often prescribed along with other blood pressure medications to increase the effectiveness of each. High blood pressure usually has few or no symptoms, yet if left untreated can result in complications that endanger health. You are urged to follow your doctor's treatment instructions.

1. This medication may cause dizziness or fainting when arising rapidly from a lying or sitting position. This problem *can be avoided* by getting up *slowly* from a lying or sitting position.

2. This medication may occasionally cause nasal stuffiness, tiredness, diarrhea and nausea. Drowsiness is common during the first weeks of therapy, but it usually diminishes over a period of 2 weeks. If this medication causes a feeling of tiredness or drowsiness please exercise care in driving a car or operating equipment.

Methyldopate Hydrochloride USP [Aldomet Ester HCl (*MSD*); $C_{12}H_{17}NO_4 \cdot HCl$]—Antihypertensive. Whitish, crystalline powder; odorless or nearly so; bitter taste; melts about 160°. Freely soluble in water and alcohol; slightly soluble in chloroform; practically insoluble in ether. *Known incompatibilities* (methyldopate HCl injection): amphotericin B, sulfadiazine sodium, tetracycline HCl.

Methylene Blue USP [methylthionine chloride; aniline violet; $C_{16}H_{18}ClN_3S \cdot 3H_2O$] — Antimethemoglobinemic; antidote to cyanide poisoning. Methylene blue is soluble in water and alcohol. Solutions of methylene blue are changed to a lighter shade of blue by acids and to a purplish shade by alkalies; sodium hydroxide added in excess produces a violet precipitate on standing. Reducing agents decolorize methylene blue. Methylene blue also gives a precipitate with mercuric salts, permanganates, and thiocyanates.

Methylergonovine Maleate NF [Methergine (*Sandoz*); $C_{20}H_{25}N_3O_2 \cdot C_4H_4O_4$]—Oxytocic. Whitish, micro-crystalline powder; odorless; bitter taste; light- and heat-sensitive; pH (1 in 5000 soln) about 4.8. One g dissolves in about 100 ml water, 175 ml alcohol, 1900 ml chloroform, and 8400 ml ether.

Methylhexamine [Forthane (*Lilly*); $C_7H_{17}N$]—Sympathomimetic. Colorless to pale-yellow liquid; ammonia-like odor. Very slightly soluble in water; freely soluble in alcohol, chloroform, and ether.

Methyl Isobutyl Ketone NF [$C_6H_{12}O$]—Pharmaceutic aid (alcohol denaturant). Colorless liquid; mobile; volatile; faint odor; distils about 115°. Slightly soluble in water; miscible with alcohol and ether.

Methylparaben USP [$C_8H_8O_3$—Pharmaceutic aid (antifungal agent). Methylparaben is a crystalline substance which is soluble in 400 parts of water, approximately 40 parts of warm oil, 70 parts of warm glycerin, or 2.5 parts of alcohol.

While the esters of *p*-hydroxybenzoic acid are very useful preserving agents, they have some undesirable properties. These esters are volatile and, therefore, should not be subjected to high temperatures during the compounding or manufacturing process. The methyl ester is only slightly soluble in water, and this solubility decreases further when certain substances such as salts are included in the formula.

Alcoholic solutions are sometimes used as a means of adding the esters. These solutions have the unfavorable habit of "creeping" up the walls of the flask. The alcohol evaporates, and the ester crystallizes and is hard to redissolve. The addition of Tween 80 to the alcoholic solution has been recommended.

However, it was found that a relatively high degree of interaction occurred between the Tween and the parabens, and that the binding is a function of the concentration of unbound paraben and the concentration of Tween 80. Analysis of the data indicated that the binding is a result of complex formation. Calculation of the quantity of methylparaben or propylparaben which must be added to a system containing a known concentration of Tween 80 in order to have the desired concentration of unbound preservative is possible from the data.

The bactericidal and preservative action of *p*-hydroxybenzoate esters may also be reduced by hydroxyethyltheophylline and methylcellulose. This appears to be due to the formation of complex compounds.

Methylphenidate Hydrochloride USP [Ritalin Hydrochloride (*Ciba*); $C_{14}H_{19}NO_2 \cdot HCl$]—Central stimulant. White, fine, crystalline powder; odorless; solutions are acid to litmus. Freely soluble in water; soluble in alcohol; slightly soluble in chloroform.

Dispensing Information: Occasionally patients experience nervousness, insomnia, anorexia, dizziness, palpitation, headache, and nausea. Significant changes in blood pressure and pulse rate may occur. See also *Amphetamines.*

Methylprednisolone NF [Medrol (*Upjohn*); $C_{22}H_{30}O_5$]—Glucocorticoid. White to practically white, crystalline powder; odorless; melts with some decomposition about 240°. 1 g dissolves in > 10,000 ml water, 100 ml alcohol, and 800 ml chloroform and ether.

Dispensing Information: See *Corticosteroids (Systemic).*

Methylprednisolone Acetate USP [Depo-Medrol, Medrol Acetate Veriderm (*Upjohn*); $C_{24}H_{32}O_6$]—Glucorticoid. White or practically white, crystalline powder; odorless; melts with decomposition about 215°; pH (sterile suspension) 3.5–7. One g dissolves in 1500 ml water and ether, 400 ml alcohol, and 250 ml chloroform.

Dispensing Information: See *Corticosteroids (Systemic).*

Methylprednisolone Sodium Succinate USP [Solu-Medrol (*Upjohn*); $C_{26}H_{33}NaO_8$]—Glucorticoid. White or nearly white, amorphous solid; odorless; hygroscopic. 1 g dissolves in 1.5 ml water, 12 ml alcohol, and >10,000 ml chloroform and ether. *Known incompatibilities* (methylprednisolone sodium succinate for injection): promethazine HCl.

Methylrosaniline Chloride—see *Gentian Violet.*

Methyl Salicylate USP [betula oil; gaultheria oil; wintergreen oil; $C_8H_8O_3$]—Pharmaceutic aid (flavor). Obtained from the leaves of *Gaultheria procumbens* or from the bark of *Betula lenta.* Colorless, yellowish or reddish liquid; characteristic odor and taste of wintergreen; boils (with some decomposition) about 221°. Slightly soluble in water; soluble in alcohol. *Known incompatibilities:* alkalies (decomposition).

Methyltestosterone USP [Metandren (*Ciba*); Neo-Hombreol M (*Organon*), Oreton (*Schering*); $C_{20}H_{30}O_2$]—Androgen. White or creamy-white crystals or is a crystalline powder. It is odorless. It is soluble in alcohol and practically insoluble in water. It is stable in air but is sensitive to light.

Methylthiouracil NF [antibason; $C_5H_6N_2OS$]—Thyroid inhibitor. White, odorless, crystalline powder. It is very slightly soluble in water and sparingly soluble in alcohol. It is sensitive to light.

Methyprylon NF [Noludar (*Roche*); $C_{10}H_{17}NO_2$]—Sedative. White or nearly white, crystalline powder; slight characteristic odor; melts 75–78.5°. 1 g dissolves in 11 ml water, 2 ml each of alcohol, chloroform, and ether.

Dispensing Information: Avoid alcohol. Do not drive or operate heavy machinery after ingestion. See also *Sedatives and Hypnotics.*

Methysergide Maleate USP [Sansert (*Sandoz*); $C_{21}H_{27}N_3O_2 \cdot C_4H_4O_4$]—Vasoconstrictor (specific in migraine). Whitish, crystalline powder; odorless or almost so; pH (1 in 500 soln in CO_2-free water) 3.7–4.7. Slightly soluble in water and alcohol; very slightly soluble in chloroform; practically insoluble in ether.

Dispensing Information: Contraindicated in pregnancy, most vascular conditions, phlebitis or cellulitis of lower limbs. Consult physician immediately if cold, numb, and painful hands or feet, leg spasms on walking, or any type of chest or girdle or flank pain is noted.

Metolazone [Zaroxolyn (*Pennwalt*); $C_{16}H_{16}ClN_3O_3S$; pK_a 9.72]—Diuretic; antihypertensive. Colorless, crystalline powder; odorless; tasteless; light-sensitive. Insoluble in water and alcohol.

Metronidazole USP [Flagyl (*Searle*); $C_6H_9N_3O_3$]—Antitrichomonal. White to pale yellow crystal or crystalline powder; odorless; stable in air; darkens in light. Sparingly soluble in water, alcohol, and chloroform; slightly soluble in ether.

Dispensing Information: Avoid alcohol. May darken urine. May cause nausea, vomiting, or headache, and may develop Monilia superinfection (furry tongue, glossitis, stomatitis).

Metyrapone USP [Metopirone (*Ciba*); $C_{14}H_{14}N_2O$]—Diagnostic aid (pituitary function determination). Fine, whitish, crystalline powder; characteristic odor; darkens in light. Soluble in chloroform; forms water-soluble salts with acids. Also available as Metyrapone Tartrate Injection NF.

Miconazole Nitrate [Mica Tin (*J&J*); Monistat (*Ortho*); $C_{18}H_{14}Cl_4N_2O \cdot HNO_3$]—Antifungal. White, microcrystalline powder. Very slightly soluble in water; slightly soluble in alcohol.

Mineral Oil USP [liquid paraffin; liquid petrolatum; heavy liquid petrolatum; white mineral oil]—Mixture of liquid hydrocarbons from petroleum. Colorless, transparent liquid; oily; odorless; and tasteless when cold (faint odor of petroleum when heated); sp gr 0.860–0.905. Insoluble in water and alcohol; miscible with most fixed oils excepting castor oil; soluble in volatile oils.

Minocycline Hydrochloride USP [Minocin (*Lederle*); Vectrin (*P-D*); $C_{23}H_{27}N_3O_7 \cdot HCl$]—Antibacterial. Yellow, crystalline powder. Soluble in water and solutions of alkali hydroxides and carbonates; slightly soluble in alcohol; practically insoluble in chloroform and ether.

Dispensing Information: Possible interference with absorption by divalent and trivalent cations. Discoloring of teeth of infants and children may occur. A photosensitivity reaction may occur in patients who are exposed to ultraviolet light or direct sunlight. CNS reactions (e.g., dizziness) are known to occur with this member of the tetracycline family. See also *Tetracyclines*.

Mithramycin USP [Mithracin (*Pfizer*); $C_{52}H_{76}O_{24}$]—Antineoplastic. Obtained from a suitable strain of *Streptomyces*. Yellow, crystalline powder; odorless; hygroscopic; birefringent; decomposes in light and heat; melts (with decomposition) about 182°. 1 g dissolves in <200 ml water and about 2000 ml alcohol.

Mitotane USP [Lysodren (*Calbiochem*); $C_{14}H_{10}Cl_4$]—Antineoplastic. White, crystalline powder; slight odor; tasteless; melts about 78°. Practically insoluble in water; soluble in alcohol and ether.

Molindone Hydrochloride [Moban (*Endo*); $C_{16}H_{24}N_2O_2 \cdot HCl$]—Sedative; tranquilizer. White, crystalline powder. Freely soluble in water and alcohol.

Monobenzone NF [Benoquin (*Elder*); $C_{13}H_{12}O_2$]—Depigmentor. White, crystalline powder; odorless; melts about 118°. Insoluble in water; 1 g dissolves in about 15 ml alcohol, 29 ml chloroform, and 14 ml ether.

Monoethanolamine NF [ethanolamine; C_2H_7NO]—Pharmaceutic aid (surfactant). Clear, colorless liquid; moderately viscous; ammoniacal odor; light-sensitive; sp gr about 1.015; distils about 170°. Miscible with water, alcohol, glycerin, and chloroform; immiscible with ether.

Monothioglycerol NF [$C_3H_8O_2S$]—Pharmaceutic aid (preservative). Colorless or yellow liquid; viscous; slight odor; hygroscopic; sp gr about 1.245; pH (1 in 10 soln) 3.5–7. Freely soluble in water; miscible with alcohol; insoluble in ether.

Morphine [$C_{17}H_{19}NO_3$; pK_a 9.85, pw_b 6.13]—Narcotic analgesic. 1 g of morphine alkaloid dissolves in 3340 ml of water or 210 ml of alcohol. The pH of a saturated solution is about 8.5. Morphine sulfate (1 g) dissolves in 16 ml of water or 570 ml of alcohol. Morphine hydrochloride is soluble in 17.5 ml of water or 52 ml alcohol. Aqueous solutions of the salts are very slightly acid; an 8% solution of the sulfate has a pH of 4.8. The morphine molecule has an alcoholic hydroxyl group.

$$(H\overset{|}{\underset{|}{C}}-OH),$$

a phenolic hydroxyl group,

$$(=\overset{|}{C}-OH)$$

an ether bridge,

$$(=\overset{|}{C}-O-\overset{|}{\underset{|}{C}}-)$$

an alicyclic unsaturated linkage (—CH=CH—), and a tertiary nitrogen (>N—CH$_3$). Various substitutions on these groups give rise to the many official morphine derivatives. The free alkaloid is precipitated from solutions of its salts when the pH is raised above 6 but redissolves in an excess of fixed alkali hydroxides such as sodium hydroxide or limewater. Morphine is oxidized by chlorates, permanganates, and other oxidizing agents. A number of workers have correlated the decomposition (darkening of solutions and formation of oxydimorphine) with the pH of the solution and the presence of atmospheric oxygen. The addition of 0.005–0.01% EDTA and adjustment of the solution to pH 3–3.5 or the addition of sodium bisulfite in 0.1 *M* phosphate buffer have been recommended. Morphine injection (2%) has been reported stable up to 10 years (pH 4.1 with sulfite). Adding 0.2% NaHSO$_3$ and filling under carbon dioxide has also been suggested. The solubility of morphine in alkalies and its susceptibility to oxidation are properties which may be correlated with the presence of phenolic groups in the molecule.

Morphine   Hydrochloride—See under *Morphine.*

Morphine Sulfate USP—See under *Morphine.*

Multistix   [*Ames*]—Dip-and-read test for pH, protein, glucose, ketones, bilirubin, blood, and urobilinogen in urine.

Dispensing Information: Patient should be made familiar with recommended procedures for handling Multistix. See also *Reagent Tablets or Strips.*

Nafcillin Sodium USP [Unipen (*Wyeth*);   C$_{21}$H$_{21}$N$_2$NaO$_5$S]—Antibacterial. White to yellowish white powder; not more than a slight, characteristic odor. Freely soluble in water and chloroform; soluble in alcohol. *Known incompatibilities* (nafcillin sodium for injection): vitamin B complex with C.

Dispensing Information: See *Penicillins.*

Naldecon Preparations [*Bristol*]—*Syrup:* Aqueous solution containing per 5 ml: Phenylephrine HCl (5 mg), phenylpropanolamine hydrochloride (20 mg), phenyltoloxamine dihydrogen citrate (7.5 mg), chlorpheniramine maleate (2.5 mg), in a red strawberry-raspberry flavored syrup having a pH of 4.5; sweetener, sugar 77.9%; Na$^+$ 0.03 mEq/5 ml. It is reported to be stable for at least 2 years at 25°C or 12 months at 37°C.

Pediatric: pH 4.5–5.5; solvent, purified water; sweetener, sugar 77.9%; Na$^+$ 0.03 mEq/5 ml; K$^+$ 0.006 mEq/5 ml. *Pediatric Drops:* pH 4–5; solvent, purified water; sweetener, sugar 77.9%; Na$^+$ 0.006 mEq/ml. *Known incompatibilities:* Butisol Sodium Elixir, Co-Pyronil, erythromycin ethyl succinate, Hydryllin Elixir, Nembutal Elixir, Kaopectate with Neomycin, paregoric tincture, Polymagma.

Dispensing Information: Drowsiness may occur which may impair ability to drive or perform other tasks requiring alertness. Take with food to avoid GI symptoms.

Nalidixic Acid NF [NegGram (*Winthrop*);   C$_{12}$H$_{12}$N$_2$O$_3$]—Antibacterial. White to slightly yellow, crystalline powder; odorless; melts 225–231°. 1 g dissolves in >1000 ml water and ether, 910 ml alcohol, and 29 ml chloroform.

Dispensing Information: Contraindicated in pregnancy, epilepsy. Drowsiness may occur. Visual disturbances with vertigo or dizziness should be brought to the attention of the physician. Avoid excessive exposure to direct sunlight.

Nalorphine Hydrochloride NF [Nalline Hydrochloride (*MSD*); $C_{19}H_{21}NO_3 \cdot HCl$]—Antidote for morphine, meperidine, and methadone. Nalorphine hydrochloride is soluble in water (1:8) (pH *circa* 5) and alcohol (1:35).

Naloxone Hydrochloride USP [Narcan (*Endo*); $C_{19}H_{21}NO_4 \cdot HCl \cdot H_2O$]—Antidote to narcotic overdose. White to slightly off-white powder; solution is acid to litmus. Soluble in water; slightly soluble in alcohol; practically insoluble in chloroform and ether.

Nandrolone Decanoate NF [Deca-Durabolin (*Organon*); $C_{28}H_{44}O_3$]—Androgen. Fine, whitish, crystalline powder; odorless or slight odor; melts about 35°. Practically insoluble in water; soluble in chloroform and alcohol.

Nandrolone Phenpropionate NF [Durabolin (*Organon*); $C_{27}H_{34}O_3$]—Androgen. Fine, whitish, crystalline powder; slight odor; melts about 97°. Practically insoluble in water; soluble in chloroform and ether; 1 g dissolves in about 2 ml alcohol.

Naphazoline Hydrochloride USP [Privine Hydrochloride (*Ciba*); $C_{14}H_{14}N_2 \cdot HCl$]—Adrenergic (vasoconstrictor). Nasal decongestant. White powder; bitter taste; pH (1% soln) 6.2; melts 255–260°. Freely soluble in water and alcohol; slightly soluble in chloroform.

Dispensing Information: Do not use in aluminum containers.

Nembutal Elixir [*Abbott*]—Sedative. Pentobarbital. pH 3.7–4; alcohol 18%; contains (per 5 ml) sweetener, sucrose 2.6 g; Na^+ 0.16 mg.

Neocinchophen [$C_{19}H_{17}NO_2$]—Analgesic. Whitish, crystalline powder; odorless; tasteless; light-sensitive; melts about 75°. Practically insoluble in water; soluble in hot alcohol; very soluble in chloroform and ether.

Neomycin Sulfate USP [*Various Mfrs.*]—Antibacterial. This is the sulfate of an antibacterial substance produced by the growth of *Streptomyces fradiae* Waksman.

Neomycin is effective against many topical bacterial infections. It is used orally for suppression of enteric organisms (up to 6–10 g/day). It is sometimes injected intramuscularly at 10–15 mg/kg body weight/day (not to exceed 10 days) for severe Gram-negative infections resistant to other antibiotics. It may produce eighth nerve and renal damage in some patients upon injection, but is remarkably free of topical and oral side effects.

Neomycin sulfate contains not less than 60% neomycin base. Neomycin is a very stable complex base which has been shown to consist almost entirely of two isomers, neomycin B and neomycin C. Both have the molecular formula $C_{23}H_{46}N_6O_{13}$. Neomycin C consists of the following fragments: neamine (neosamine C + 2-deoxy-D-streptamine) and neobiosamine C (D-ribose + neosamine C). Neomycin B is identical except that it is the epimer of Neomycin C. Neomycin sulfate occurs as a white to slightly yellow crystal or powder. It is odorless or practically odorless and is hygroscopic. The pH value of a solution containing 33 mg of neomycin sulfate in each milliliter is not less than 5.0 and not more than 7.5. Aqueous solutions of neomycin sulfate are stable for 2 years at room temperature but should be refrigerated to prevent color changes unless antioxidants and preservatives are present. Neomycin sulfate is highly soluble in water, e.g., 1 g dissolves in about 1 ml of water. It is soluble in propylene glycol and slightly soluble in methanol and ethanol (0.01%). It is insoluble in other organic solvents.

Neomycin is a base and can form salts with inorganic and organic acids. The dry powder is very stable, even at elevated temperatures for long periods of time. Aqueous solutions are quite stable over the pH range of 2 to 9 for long periods of time, even at elevated temperatures. The highest activity is in alkaline solutions.

Neomycin is stable in many types of ointment bases such as the water-miscible or Carbowax type, the grease type (with petrolatum, lanolin, and beeswax), and the oil-in-water or vanishing cream type. A water-miscible ointment of neomycin sulfate can be made with Carbowax 4000, Carbowax 1500, polysorbate 20, and propylene glycol. An oil-in-water vanishing cream type ointment or lotion can be made using glyceryl monostearate, polysorbate, propylene glycol, spermaceti, parabens, and water. A grease type of ointment can be made with petrolatum, lanolin, and mineral oil.

Neomycin has been reported to be incompatible with anionic substances. It was found to become firmly bound to bentonite, crack emulsions prepared with sodium lauryl sulfate, and precipitate some gums such as carboxymethylcellulose.

In nasal solutions neomycin is compatible and stable with *dl*-desoxyephedrine HCl, ephedrine sulfate, amphetamine, phenylephrine HCl, lactose, sodium chloride, and antihistamines such as Bristamin.

In oral solutions or suspensions neomycin is compatible with sweetening agents such as soluble and insoluble saccharin, sugar, hydrophilic colloids (pectin, polyvinylpyrrolidone) FD&C dyes, many flavoring oils, bismuth subcarbonate, kaolin, sodium benzoate, parabens, and various sulfonamides such as sulfadiazine, sulfathiazole, and sulfaguanidine.

Neosporin Ophthalmic Solution [*B-W*]—*Known ingredients:* polymyxin B sulfate (5000 u/ml), neomycin sulfate (2.5 mg/ml), gramicidin (0.025 mg/ml), alcohol (0.5%), propylene glycol (0.5%), thimerosal (0.001%), saline vehicle qs. pH 5.5–6. *Known incompatibilities:* Butyn, physostigmine salicylate, epinephrine HCl.*

---

* Discolors rapidly.

Neostigmine Bromide USP [Prostigmin Bromide (*Roche*); $C_{12}H_{19}BrN_2O_2$]—Cholinergic. 1 g dissolves in 1 ml of water and is soluble in alcohol. The crystals are much less hygroscopic than are those of the methylsulfate and thus may be used in tablets. Solutions are stable and may be sterilized by boiling.

Neostigmine Methylsulfate USP [Prostigmin Methylsulfate (*Roche*); $C_{13}H_{22}N_2O_6S$]—Cholinergic. White, crystalline, hydroscopic carbamate and quaternary compound. 1 g dissolves in 10 ml of water and is less soluble in alcohol. Solutions of the drug are stable and may be sterilized by boiling. Aqueous solutions are neutral to litmus. It is used by subcutaneous or intramuscular injection for the treatment of postoperative distention and diminished tone of intestinal and bladder musculature.

Neo-Synephrine [*Winthrop*]—IV Vasoconstrictor. *Known ingredients:* phenylephrine 0.2% (1%). *Known compatibilities:* Dextran 6%, dextrose 5% in water, dextrose 5% in saline, Levugen 10% in water (or saline).

Niacin NF [nicotinic acid; *Various Mfrs.*; $C_6H_5NO_2$]—Vitamin B-complex vitamin. White crystals or crystalline powder; odorless or slight odor; melts about 235°; pH (1% soln) about 3. One g dissolves in 60 ml water; freely soluble in boiling water and boiling alcohol; practically insoluble in ether. The sodium and potassium salts of niacin are very soluble in water; solutions are alkaline. *Known incompatibilities:* oxidizing agents; niacin readily attacks copper vessels with loss of stability.

Dispensing Information: Contraindicated in peptic ulcer, diabetes, impaired liver function. May cause flushing of skin; this will usually disappear with continued use. Toxicity noted by tingling sensation.

Niacinamide USP [nicotinamide; $C_6H_6N_2O$]—White crystals with a slightly bitter taste. 1 g dissolves in about 1 ml of water, 1.5 ml of alcohol, or 10 ml of glycerin. The pH of a 1% aqueous solution is approximately 6. Niacinamide is slightly hygroscopic but otherwise is stable in the dry form. In aqueous solutions it is quite stable in the absence of added acid or alkali, which cause hydrolysis.

Nialamide [Niamid (*Pfizer*); $C_{16}H_{18}N_4O_2$]—Antidepressant. White, crystalline powder; practically odorless; melts about 153°. 1 g dissolves in about 600 ml water; soluble in alcohol.

Dispensing Information: Patient may experience light-headedness upon arising rapidly. Avoid prolonged exposure to sunlight. Avoid cheese, wine, beer, or chocolate. Discontinue use and consult physician if fever, headache, blurred vision, GI upset, or severe abdominal pain occur. Avoid alcohol or other sedatives.

Niclosamide [Yomesan (*Bayer*); $C_{13}H_8Cl_2N_2O_4$]—Anthelmintic. Although not marketed in the US, the tablets may be obtained by licensed physicians from the Parasitic Disease Drug Service, Center for Disease Control, Atlanta, GA 30333.

Nisentil Solution [*Roche* brand of alphaprodine hydrochloride]—Narcotic; analgesic. *Known ingredients:* Nisentil Hydrochloride (40–60 mg/ml). *Known incompatibilities:* Nembutal, Synkayvite.

Nitric Acid NF [HNO_3]—Pharmaceutic aid (acidifying agent). Highly corrosive, fuming liquid; characteristic, highly irritating odor; stains animal tissues yellow; boils about 120°; specific gravity about 1.41. *Known incompatibilities:* Reducing agents, alkaloids, sulfuric acid and glycerin, charcoal, sulfur, sucrose.

Nitrofurantoin USP [Furadantin (*Eaton*); (*Various Other Mfrs.*); $C_8H_6N_4O_5$]—Antibacterial (urinary). Lemon-yellow crystals or fine powder; odorless; bitter aftertaste. Very slightly soluble in water and alcohol. *Caution:* Nitrofurantoin and its solutions are discolored by alkali and exposure to light, and are decomposed on contact with metals other than stainless steel and aluminum. *Known incompatibilities* (nitrofurantoin sodium for injection): ammonium chloride, Aramine, codeine phosphate, Demerol, insulin, levartere-

nol bitartrate, methylparaben, morphine sulfate, Phenergan, procaine HCl, Pontocaine, streptomycin sulfate, vitamin B complex with C.

Dispensing Information: Take with food or milk to prevent nausea. Consult physician if yellowing of eyes or skin occurs. May cause fever, chills, muscle pains.

Nitrofurazone NF [Furacin (*Eaton*); $C_6H_6N_4O_4$]—Local anti-infective. Lemon-yellow crystalline powder; odorless; darkens in light; melts with decomposition about 236°; pH (filtrate from 1% susp) 5–7.5.

Dispensing Information: Protect nonaffected areas from accidental application. Discontinue use and contact physician if rash, pruritus, or irritation occur.

Nitrogen USP [N_2]—Pharmaceutic aid (air displacement). Colorless gas; odorless; tasteless; nonflammable, does not support combustion; 1 liter at 0° and 760 mm Hg weighs about 1.251 g.

Nitroglycerin USP [glyceryl trinitrate; glonoin; *Various Mfrs.;* $C_3H_5N_3O_9$]—Vasodilator. Practically colorless liquid, odorless; sweet taste; hydrolyzed by alkalies. *Caution:* Nitroglycerin is a violent explosive; hence, if any spirit of glyceryl trinitrate is spilled, a solution of NaOH or KOH should be poured over it immediately to cause decomposition and avert an explosion. Nitroglycerin is commonly supplied to pharmaceutical manufacturers as a 10% trituration with lactose or chalk, or as a 10% solution in alcohol.

Dispensing Information: Label: Do not swallow. Explain sublingual administration and proper storage conditions. Explain that potent nitroglycerin will produce a burning sensation when placed under the tongue. Make certain a patient knows total number that can be taken per event or day before chest pain should be brought to the attention of the physician. Administration technique (i.e., stop, rest, or sit down) should be stressed.

Nitromersol NF [Metaphen (*Abbott*); $C_7H_5HgNO_3$]—Topical antiseptic very slightly soluble in water, alcohol, acetone, ether. Metaphen Solution 1:500 is an aqueous solution containing Metaphen (1:500) dissolved with the aid of sodium hydroxide, thus forming the sodium salt. Metaphen (1:2500) is an aqueous solution containing Metaphen which has been converted into the sodium salt by means of sodium bicarbonate and sodium carbonate. Tincture Metaphen is a solution of Metaphen (1:200) in a mixture of alcohol, water, and acetone. The tincture is tinted to produce an amber stain which temporarily outlines the area of application; the stain may be removed, when desired, with soap and water. Tincture Metaphen Untinted is also available. Metaphen is incompatible with chlorazene, hydrogen peroxide, sodium perborate, tannic acid, salts of copper, zinc, and silver, and with acids and acid reacting drugs such as alkaloidal salts and local anesthetics. Anesthesin is soluble in Tincture Metaphen up to 7.5 g in 100 ml, and this mixture is pharmaceutically stable.

Nitroprusside Sodium—See *Sodium Nitroprusside*.

Nitrous Oxide USP [nitrogen oxide; *Various Mfrs.*; N_2O]—General anesthetic (inhalation). Colorless gas; no appreciable odor or taste; 1 liter at 0° and 760 mm Hg weighs about 1.97 g. Preserve in cylinders. 1 volume dissolves in about 1.4 volumes water at 20° and 760 mm Hg; soluble in alcohol (1 in 1–10) and ether and oils (1 in 10–30). *Known incompatibilities:* oxidizing agents, reducing agents.

Norethindrone USP [Micronor (*Ortho*); Nor-QD (*Syntex*); Norlutin (*P-D*); $C_{20}H_{26}O_2$]—Progestin. Whitish, crystalline powder; odorless; melts about 205°. Practically insoluble in water; soluble in chloroform; sparingly soluble in alcohol; slightly soluble in ether.

Dispensing Information: See *Contraceptives (Oral)*.

Norethindrone Acetate USP [Norlutate (*P-D*); $C_{22}H_{28}O_3$]—Progestin. Available as 5-mg tablets used for progestational deficiencies and as a combination with estrogen—Norlestrin (*P-D*)—for use as an oral contraceptive; in combination, e.g., (Norlutate, 2.5 mg, and ethinylestradiol, 0.05 mg).

Norethynodrel NF [$C_{20}H_{26}O_2$]—Progestin. Whitish, crystalline powder; odorless; melts (3° range) about 179°. Very slightly soluble in water; freely soluble in chloroform; sparingly soluble in alcohol and ether.

Norgesic Tablets [*Riker*]—Analgesic. Contain orphenadrine citrate 25 mg, aspirin 225 mg, caffeine 30 mg, phenacetin 160 mg.

Dispensing Information: Consult physician immediately if severe headache or eye pain develop.

Norgestrel USP [Ovrette, comp. of Ovral (*Wyeth*); $C_{21}H_{28}O_2$]—Progestin. Whitish, crystalline powder; odorless; melts about 128°. Practically insoluble in water; soluble in alcohol.

Norinyl-1 + 50 (21-Day) Tablets [*Syntex*]—Oral contraceptive. Contain norethindrone acetate 1 mg, mestranol 0.05 mg.

Dispensing Information: See *Contraceptives (Oral)*.

Norlestrin-21 Tablets [*P-D*]—Oral Contraceptive. Contain norethindrone acetate 1 mg, ethinyl estradiol 0.05 mg.

Dispensing Information: See *Contraceptives (Oral)*.

Nortriptyline Hydrochloride NF [Aventyl Hydrochloride (*Lilly*); $C_{19}H_{21}N \cdot HCl$]—Antidepressant. White to off-white powder; slight characteristic odor. 1 g dissolves in 90 ml water, 30 ml alcohol, 20 ml chloroform; practically insoluble in ether.

Dispensing Information: May enhance response to alcohol and other CNS depressants. Drowsiness may occur which may impair ability to drive or perform other tasks requiring alertness. Avoid alcohol.

Nose Drops—See under *Eye, Ear, Nose, and Throat Preparations*.

Novobiocin [Albamycin (*Upjohn*), $C_{31}H_{36}N_2O_{11}$; pK$_{a1}$ 4.2, pK$_{a2}$ 9.1]—Novobiocin is a dibasic antibiotic derived from cultures of *Streptomyces niveus* or *Streptomyces spheroides*.

Novobiocin is active against many penicillin-resistant staphylococci and proteus strains. It is administered orally and intravenously at 1–2 g/day. Novobiocin occurs as pale yellow crystals having two crystalline forms. It is soluble in aqueous solution above pH 7.5 and usually begins to precipitate below this pH value. The acid form is soluble in acetone, ethyl acetate, amyl acetate, methanol, ethanol, and pyridine. Dry material of both crystal forms is stable at room temperature in the absence of light. Dilute aqueous solutions are stable between pH 2 to 6.5 at room temperature. The half-life is said to be 60 days at pH 7 to 10. The sodium salt is moderately water-soluble (approx 1.5%) but not very stable in solution; hence, it is usually supplied as a dry powder reconstituted before use in parenteral preparations or for oral solutions. Ready-mixed oral liquid preparations are usually prepared with the less soluble, but more stable, calcium salt (pH 6.6).

Monosodium novobiocin solid is reasonably stable for 2 years at 20–37°C, but increases in temperature and pH and the presence of nickel, lead, and zinc at certain pH values adversely affect the antibacterial activity. Ultraviolet radiation, sulfate, phosphate, and metabisulfite decrease potency.

At pH 10 or above novobiocin is converted in about 30% yield to an isomeric product called iso-novobiocin. This change is accompanied by the loss of about one-third of the original activity.

It has been reported that sodium novobiocin combines with all of the common basic antibiotics to form water insoluble salts of novobiocin. The molar proportions found for the combinations of novobiocin with basic antibiotics were: streptomycin 3:1 (i.e., novobiocin-3; streptomycin-1); neomycin, 6:1, spiramycin, 1:1; viomycin, 1:2; erythromycin, 1:1; and eulicin, 1:2. The solubility in water found for these combinations were: novobiocin-streptomycin, 0.8 mg/ml; novobiocin-neomycin, 0.5 mg/ml; novobiocin-spiramycin, 0.4 mg/ml;

novobiocin-viomycin, 1.1 mg/ml; novobiocin-erythromycin, 0.3 mg/ml; and novobiocin-eulicin, less than 1 mg/ml. Antibiotics having neutral, acidic, or amphoteric properties did not form insoluble salts with novobiocin. These included bacitracin, penicillin, synnematin, cycloserine, tetracyline, carbomycin, tyrothricin, and candicidin.

Novobiocin Calcium [Albamycin Calcium (*Upjohn*); $C_{62}H_{70}CaN_4O_{22} \cdot 2H_2O$ or anhydrous]—Antibacterial. Whitish, crystalline powder; odorless or nearly so; pH (sat soln) about 7.5. One g dissolves in about 250 ml water, 30 ml alcohol, 1100 ml chloroform, and 450 ml ether.

Novobiocin Sodium [Albamycin (*Upjohn*); $C_{31}H_{35}N_2NaO_{11}$]—Antibacterial. Whitish, crystalline powder; odorless or nearly so; hygroscopic; pH about 7.5. Very soluble in water; freely soluble in alcohol and glycerin. *Known incompatibilities* (novobiocin sodium injection): solutions pH below 6, dextrose-containing solutions, chloramphenicol sodium succinate. See also under *Novobiocin*.

Novocain [*Winthrop* brand of procaine]—Local anesthetic. *Known compatibilities* (1 g/liter): dextrose 5% in water or saline, Levugen 10% in water, Levugen 10% in saline, Levugen 10% in electrolytes, Amigen 5%-Levugen 10%, Amigen 5%-dextrose 5%, Sodium R-Lactate $\frac{1}{6}$ M, Ringer's lactate.

Nupercainal [*Ciba* brand of dibucaine]—Local anesthetic ointment, cream, ophthalmic ointment, or suppositories. *Known ingredients:* dibucaine. *Known incompatibilities:* resorcin (darkens on exposure to air; catalyzed by alkalies).

Nupercaine [*Ciba* brand of dibucaine hydrochloride]—Local anesthetic in ampuls 2% topical solution, tablets for preparation of topical solutions, or spinal anesthetic solution. *Known ingredients:* dibucaine hydrochloride. *Known incompatibilities* (of nupercaine): alkaline solution, Merthiolate Solution and Tincture, soap solutions;

(of 2% topical solution): aqueous iodine solution, iodine tincture 2%.

Nylidrin Hydrochloride NF [Arlidin Hydrochloride (*USV*); $C_{19}H_{25}NO_2 \cdot HCl$]—Peripheral vasodilator. White, crystalline powder; odorless; practically tasteless; pH (1% soln) 4.5–6.5. One g dissolves in 65 ml water, 40 ml alcohol; very slightly soluble in chloroform and ether.

Dispensing Information: Contraindicated in angina, thyrotoxicosis, myocardial infarction. Consult physician if dizziness or palpitation occur.

Nystatin USP [*Various Mfrs.*; $C_{47}H_{75}NO_{17}$ (nystatin A)]—Nystatin is an antifungal substance (mixture) which is isolated from cultures of *Streptomyces nursei* Brown, *et al.* It is active against *Candida albicans* and other fungi and yeasts. Since it is not absorbed it is administered topically or given as oral suspensions, tablets, capsules, etc., to control the growth of susceptible organisms in the intestine. Nystatin inhibits uptake of phosphate by the sensitive fungi.

The stability of dry powder, tablets, and pills of nystatin has been investigated. Tablets and pills were more stable than the powder. Pills were reported more stable when tetracycline was present. The chemical identity of nystatin has not been fully determined.

Nystatin is a yellow powder which does not form salts. It is unstable to heat, light, moisture, and air. Its solubility depends to a considerable degree on its purity, and its rate of solution depends on its particle size but it is quite insoluble in water and most organic solvents, while it is quite soluble in aqueous alcohols. It is precipitated by sodium chloride. It is unstable at pH 2–9 in aqueous or hydroalcoholic solutions. The pH value of a saturated solution is about 6.2. A suspension may be prepared which is stable for 7 days at room temperature or 10 days under refrigeration. It has been prepared in stable ointment, powder, and tablet forms.

Dispensing Information: May cause diarrhea or GI distress in large doses.

Patient should retain in mouth as long as possible and then swallow.

Octoxynol NF [$C_{34}H_{62}O_{11}$]—Pharmaceutic aid (surfactant). Clear, pale yellow liquid; viscous; faint odor; bitter taste; sp gr about 1.063; pH (1 in 20 aq soln) about 8. Miscible with water and alcohol.

Oleic Acid USP [consists chiefly of $CH_3(CH_2)_7CH{=}CH(CH_2)_7COOH$]—Pharmaceutic aid (solvent). Oleic acid is a rarely used salt-former almost insoluble in water but is soluble in alcohol. The pH of a saturated aqueous solution is about 4.4. The oleates of the alkali metals (soaps) are soluble, but the oleates of the other metals (e.g., Zn, Cu, Pb, and Bi) are insoluble. Metallic and alkaloidal oleates are generally soluble in fats and are sometimes used in ointments, e.g., mercury oleate, which is insoluble in water, slightly soluble in alcohol, and soluble in fixed oils. Oleic acid decolorizes iodine, which adds at the double bond.

Other unsaturated acids and their derivatives used in pharmacy include sodium morrhuate solution (a mixture of cod liver oil sodium salts), sodium ricinoleate (a castor oil soap, pH 8.2–8.5) and sodium psylliate injection (a mixture of sodium soaps from plantago seed oil, pH 8.5–9).

Oleovitamin A and D NF—Source of vitamins A and D. Solution of these two vitamins in fish liver oil or in an edible vegetable oil. Yellow to red liquid (clear at temperatures above 65°); oily; may crystallize on cooling; nearly odorless or fish-like odor; does not have rancid odor or taste; air- and light-sensitive. Insoluble in water and glycerin; very soluble in chloroform and ether; soluble in alcohol (dehydrated) and vegetable oils.

Oleyl Alcohol NF [$C_{18}H_{36}O$]—Pharmaceutic aid (emulsifying agent; emollient). Mixture of saturated and unsaturated high molecular weight fatty alcohols (chiefly oleyl alcohol). Clear liquid; oily; faint odor; bland taste. Insoluble in water; soluble in alcohol and ether.

Opium USP—Narcotic analgesic exudate from unripe capsules of *Papaver somniferum* or *Papaver album;* contains not less than 9.5% of anhydrous morphine. Pale, olive masses (internally, reddish brown); coarse surface; plastic when fresh (becomes hard in storage); characteristic odor; very bitter taste. Also available as Powdered Opium USP. Sale and use of opium, its derivatives and related synthetic compounds, subject to Controlled Substances Act.

Ornacol Liquid [*SK&F*]—Cough and cold therapy. Contains (per 5 ml): dextromethorphan HBr 15 mg, phenylpropanolamine HCl 12.5 mg. pH 3.8–4.5; alcohol 8%; Na^+ 19 mg/5 ml; sweeteners: saccharin sodium, sorbitol.

Ornade Spansules [*SK&F*]—Cough and cold therapy. Contain chlorpheniramine maleate 8 mg, phenylpropanolamine HCl 50 mg, isopropamide iodide 2.5 mg.

Dispensing Information: Contraindicated in peptic ulcer, hypertension, hyperthyroidism, coronary artery disease, pregnancy. Drowsiness may occur which may impair ability or drive to perform other tasks requiring alertness. May cause nervousness, insomnia, and dry mouth.

Orphenadrine Citrate NF [Norflex (*Riker*); $C_{18}H_{23}NO \cdot C_6H_8O_7$]—Skeletal muscle relaxant. White, crystalline powder; practically odorless; bitter taste; pH (injection) 5–6. One g dissolves in 45 ml water, 63 ml alcohol, and >10,000 ml chloroform.

Orphenadrine Hydrochloride [Disipal (*Riker*); $C_{18}H_{23}NO \cdot HCl$]— Skeletal muscle relaxant. Crystalline powder; melts about 156°; pH (aq soln) about 5.5. Soluble in water, alcohol, and chloroform; insoluble in ether.

Ortho-Novum Tablets [*Ortho*]— Oral contraceptive. Contain varying strengths of norethindrone, mestranol.

Dispensing Information: See *Contraceptives (Oral)*.

Orthotolidine [*Ames*; $C_{14}H_{16}N_2$]— *In vitro* diagnostic aid (blood or hemoglobin). Whitish, crystalline powder; melts about 130°. Slightly soluble in water; soluble in alcohol, chloroform, and ether.

Otobiotic Otic Solution [*Schering-White*]—Antibacterial. Contains (per ml) neomycin sulfate 5 mg, sodium propionate 50 mg, sodium metabisulfite 0.1%, qs glycerin, isopropanol, and water. pH (undiluted) 4–7; aqueous solvent.

Ouabain USP [$C_{29}H_{44}O_{12} \cdot 8H_2O$ or anhydrous]—Cardiotonic. *Caution: Extremely poisonous.* Glycoside from the seeds of *Strophanthus gratus* and the wood of *Acokanthera Schimperi*. White crystals or crystalline powder; odorless; light-sensitive; solution neutral to litmus; melts (indistinctly with decomposition) about 190°. 1 g dissolves in about 75 ml water (slowly) and 100 ml alcohol (more soluble in hot water and hot alcohol).

Oxacillin Sodium USP [Prostaphlin (*Bristol*); $C_{19}H_{18}N_3NaO_5S \cdot H_2O$]—Antibacterial. Fine, white, crystalline powder; odorless or slight odor; Freely soluble in water; slightly soluble in absolute alcohol and chloroform; insoluble in ether. Highly resistant to gastric acidity, thus is used orally. It is reported to be stable for about 24 hours at room temperature in aqueous solution buffered with sodium citrate. Its stability, absorption, and serum levels resemble penicillin V; however, it binds more strongly to serum than other penicillins. *Known incompatibilities* (oxacillin sodium for injection): oxytetracycline HCl, tetracycline HCl.

Dispensing Information: Discontinue use if skin rash, itching, chills, or edema occur. See also *Penicillins*.

Oxalic Acid [$C_2H_2O_4 \cdot 2H_2O$; pK_{a1} 1.23, pK_{a2} 4.19]—Oxalic acid is incompatible with oxidizing agents. It forms insoluble compounds with most other metallic ions except those of the alkali group. Cerium oxalate is a mixture of insoluble rare earth oxalates, chiefly $Ce_2(C_2O_4)_3$. The acid salts of oxalic acid and the alkali metals are less soluble than the normal salts. Oxalates of the heavy metals are insoluble in water, but many of them dissolve in solutions of alkali oxalates with formation of complex salts.

Oxandrolone NF [Anavar (*Searle*); $C_{19}H_{30}O_3$]—Androgen. White, crystalline powder; odorless; darkens in light; melts about 225°. 1 g dissolves in about 5200 ml water, 57 ml alcohol, <5 ml chloroform, and 860 ml ether.

Oxazepam NF [Serax (*Wyeth*); $C_{15}H_{11}ClN_2O_2$]—Sedative. Creamy white to pale-yellow powder; practically odorless; pH (2% susp) 4.8–7. One g dissolves in >10,000 ml water, 220 ml alcohol, and 270 ml chloroform.

Dispensing Information: See *Sedatives and Hypnotics.*

Oxtriphylline NF [choline theophyllinate; Choledyl (*W-C*); $C_{12}H_{21}N_5O_3$]— Bronchodilator. White, crystalline solid similar in activity to aminophylline. It is very soluble in water. A 1% aqueous solution is alkaline (pH around 10).

Dispensing Information: See *Smooth Muscle Relaxants* (*Xanthine Type*).

Oxybenzone USP [Cyasorb UV 9 (*Lederle*); $C_{14}H_{12}O_3$]—Ultraviolet screen. Whitish powder. Practically insoluble in water; freely soluble in alcohol.

Oxymetazoline Hydrochloride USP [Afrin (*Schering*); $C_{16}H_{24}N_2O$·HCl]—Adrenergic (vasoconstrictor). Fine, whitish, crystalline powder; odorless; melts (with decomposition) about 300°. 1 g dissolves in about 7 ml water, 4 ml alcohol, and 862 ml chloroform; practically insoluble in ether.

Oxymetholone NF [Anadrol (*Syntex*); $C_{21}H_{32}O_3$]—Androgen. Whitish crystals or crystalline powder; odorless; can exist as either of two tautomers or mixture of both; melts about 176°. Practically insoluble in water; 1 g dissolves in about 40 ml alcohol, 5 ml chloroform, and 82 ml ether.

Oxymorphone Hydrochloride NF [Numorphan (*Endo*); $C_{17}H_{19}NO_4$·HCl]—Narcotic analgesic. White crystals or whitish powder; odorless; darkens in light; aqueous solution acid to litmus; pH about 5. One g dissolves in about 4 ml water, 100 ml alcohol, and >1000 ml chloroform and ether.

Oxyphenbutazone NF [Tandearil (*Geigy*); $C_{19}H_{20}N_2O_3$·H_2O]—Antiarthritic; anti-inflammatory (nonsteroid). White to yellowish white, crystalline powder; odorless; melts (over a wide range) 85–100°. 1 g dissolves in >10,000 ml water, 1.5 ml alcohol, 4 ml chloroform, and 15 ml ether.

Oxyphencyclimine Hydrochloride NF [Daricon (*Beecham-Massengill*); Vio-Thene (*Rowell*); $C_{20}H_{28}N_2O_3$·HCl]—Anticholinergic. White, crystalline powder; odorless; bitter taste; melts (with decomposition) about 232°. 1 g dissolves in about 100 ml water, 75 ml alcohol, 500 ml chloroform, and >1000 ml ether.

Oxytetracycline NF [Terramycin (*Pfizer*); (*Various Other Mfrs.*); $C_{22}H_{24}N_2O_9$·$2H_2O$; pK_a = 3.49, 7.55, 9.24]—Amphoteric broad-spectrum antibiotic obtained from *Streptomyces rimosus*. It is a yellow, odorless, crystalline powder with a very bitter taste. It is stable in air for prolonged periods, but exposure to strong sunlight causes it to darken. It deteriorates in solutions below pH 2 and is rapidly destroyed by alkaline hydroxide solutions. It is stable in aqueous solution at pH 2 to 5 at 25°C. Its saturated solution in water has a pH value of about 6.5. One g dissolves in about 2000 ml of water and in about 100 ml of alcohol. It readily dissolves in dilute hydrochloric acid. It is soluble in propylene glycol, acids, and alkalies and insoluble in ether.

Oxytetracycline is amphoteric and will readily form acid and alkali salts (e.g., HCl salts and sodium salts). The chemical properties of Terramycin closely resemble those of tetracycline (*qv*) since it is oxytetracycline, e.g., it has a high affinity for divalent cations of heavy metals such as calcium, magnesium, and barium.

Oxytetracycline dihydrate forms soluble complexes in water with sodium salicylate, sodium *p*-aminobenzoate, sodium *p*-hydroxybenzoate, sodium saccharin, and caffeine.

Terramycin has been found to be compatible with petrolatum, sodium borate, sodium chloride, and sugar. Aluminum hydroxide gel should not be used with Terramycin. Milk should not be used in the oral administration of Terramycin.

Dispensing Information: See *Oxytetracycline Hydrochloride.*

Oxytetracycline Calcium NF [Calcium Terramycin (*Pfizer*); $C_{44}H_{46}$-CaN_4O_{18}]—Antibacterial. Yellowish, crystalline powder; odorless; tasteless; discolors in light; sensitive to air oxidation; pH (1 in 40 susp) about 7. One g dissolves in >1000 ml of water, alcohol, chloroform, and ether.

Dispensing Information: See *Oxytetracycline Hydrochloride.*

Oxytetracycline Hydrochloride USP [Terramycin Hydrochloride (*Pfizer*); (*Various Other Mfrs.*); $C_{22}H_{24}N_2O_9$·HCl]—Antibacterial. Yellow, crystalline powder. It is odorless, has a bitter taste, and is hygroscopic. On exposure to strong sunlight or to temperatures above 90°C in moist air it will darken, but with no appreciable loss in potency. It decomposes below pH 2 and is rapidly destroyed by alkali hydroxide solutions. The pH of a 1% aqueous solution is about 2.5. One g dissolves in 2 ml of water, but the solution soon becomes cloudy or turbid due to liberation of oxytetracycline base. 1 g dissolves in 35 ml of alcohol and in 45 ml of methanol. It is less soluble in dehydrated alcohol and is insoluble in ether or chloroform.

In the dry state the base and hydrochloride show no loss in activity after very prolonged storage at 25°C. The hydrochloride shows a loss of 5% activity after 4 months at 56°C. No loss in activity occurred after 4 days at 100°C.

An aqueous solution of the hydrochloride at a pH of 1 to 2.5 retains its potency for at least 30 days at 25°C. At pH 7 this solution shows a 50% loss in activity after 7 days and a greater loss in activity when the pH is above 7. Aqueous solutions in the pH range of 3 to 9 have been found to be satisfactory in stability for at least 1 month at 5°C. The acid salts of Terramycin slowly hydrolyze in solution and deposit Terramycin base.

Terramycin HCl powder for intrave-

nous use is buffered with sodium glycinate. The powder for intramuscular use is combined with procaine HCl and magnesium chloride. *Known incompatibilities* (oxytetracycline HCl for injection): can precipitate the free acids of barbituric acid and sulfanilamide derivatives, acid-labile additives (e.g., erythromycin, penicillin, oxacillin, methicillin, and nafcillin).

Dispensing Information: Do not take with milk or antacid. Take 1 hour before meals or 2 hours after meals. Discontinue use and consult physician if rash occurs. Avoid intense sunlight.

Oxytocic Agents—*Dispensing Information:* Patients should be cautioned as to the maximum dose allowable per period of time.

Oxytocin Injection USP [Pitocin (*P-D*)]—Oxytocic hormone. Synthetic or natural oxytocic principle in sterile water for injection; pH 2.5–4.5. *Known incompatibilities* (oxytocin injection): levarterenol bitartrate, Panwarfin, protein hydrolysate.

Paladac [*P-D*] — Multivitamin. *Known compatibilities and incompatibilities:* mixtures not recommended by manufacturer.

Pancreatin NF [viokase; Panteric (*P-D*)]—Pancreatin is an enzyme substance containing principally pancreatic amylase, trypsin, and lipase. It is slowly and incompletely soluble in water and is insoluble in alcohol. Its digestive power is greatest in neutral or faintly alkaline solutions. The activity of pancreatin is adversely affected by mineral acids, excessive alkalinity, heat, alcohol, and salts of heavy metals.

Pancuronium Bromide [Pavulon (*Organon*); $C_{35}H_{60}Br_2N_2O_4$]—Skeletal muscle relaxant. Fine, white powder; odorless; hygroscopic; heat-sensitive; melts 215°. More than 1 g dissolves in 100 ml water; soluble in alcohol and chloroform.

Panmycin Syrup [*Upjohn*]—Oral Antibiotic. *Known ingredients:* tetracycline (equivalent to 125 mg/5 ml), methylparaben (0.075%), propylparaben (0.025%), sodium metabisulfite (0.1%), aqueous vehicle qs pH 4.6 (approx.).

Known incompatibilities: none listed. Very acid ingredients i.e., *circa* pH 2 may solubilize the tetracycline. Such mixtures will usually be satisfactory if stored in a refrigerator and if no more than a 1-week supply is dispensed.

Pantopon [*Roche* brand of alkaloids of opium]—Narcotic. *Known ingredients:* Pantopon (bulk powder). *Known incompatibilities:* none listed.

Pantothenic Acid [$C_9H_{17}NO_5$]— Yellow viscous oil not used as such in pharmacy. It is water-soluble, thermostable, but destroyed by alkali. Its more stable calcium salt is widely used in pharmaceuticals (see *Calcium Pantothenate*).

Papain [Papase (*W-C*)]—This proteolytic enzyme is used orally and bucally for edema and inflammatory conditions. Papain causes precipitation in quince seed mucilage, decoction of chondrus, and solutions of karaya gum and sodium alginate. It appears to be compatible with acacia, tragacanth, and gelatin. Papain is partially soluble in water and almost insoluble in alcohol. A stable topical composition comprising aqueous papain solutions stabilized with urea and boron has been patented. Papain is available in commercial products with official malt extract.

Papaverine [$C_{20}H_{21}NO_4$; pK_b 8.07]—Papaverine is a white crystalline vasodilator. It is a narcotic almost insoluble in water and soluble in 45 ml of alcohol. The solubility is decreased by the presence of certain salts, including sodium chloride, sodium bromide, and potassium bromide.

The presence of decomposition products was observed immediately after sterilization unless injections were prepared with inert gas or antioxidant.

Papaverine Hydrochloride NF [*Various Mfrs.*; $C_{20}H_{21}NO_4 \cdot HCl$]— Smooth muscle relaxant. White, crystalline powder; odorless; slightly bitter taste; melts with decomposition about 220°; pH (2% soln) 3–4.5. One g dissolves in 30 ml water and 120 ml alcohol. Aqueous solutions of the hydrochloride are acid in reaction and will act to neutralize sodium barbiturates, sodium sulfonamides, etc.

Parachlorophenol USP [C_6H_5ClO; pK_a 9.38]—Topical antibacterial (dental). Sparingly soluble in water and liquid petrolatum but very soluble in alcohol, glycerin, caustic alkali solutions, and fixed oils. It resembles phenol in many of its properties, e.g., it burns the skin, forms a liquid when triturated with camphor, and gives a violet-blue color with ferric chloride.

Paraffin NF—Pharmaceutic aid (stiffening agent). Mixture of solid hydrocarbons from petroleum. Colorless or white mass; more or less translucent; crystalline structure; slightly greasy; odorless; tasteless; congeals 47–65°. Insoluble in water and alcohol; freely soluble in chloroform and ether.

Paraldehyde USP [paracetaldyde; $C_6H_{12}O_3$]—Hypnotic. Colorless liquid sedative with a disagreeable taste, is soluble in about 8 parts of water and is readily soluble in alcohol. It should be kept in well-closed and filled single-dose ampoules, or capsules protected from light and heat; preferably in a refrigerator. On standing in light and air, it oxidizes to dangerous glacial acetic acid. Flavoring vehicles which have an acid reaction promote deterioration of paraldehyde. Strong alkalies convert paraldehyde into aldehyde resins. Paraldehyde liberates iodine and reacts with chlorine to form substitution products. It is incompatible with oxidizing agents. Hydrocyanic acid promotes the depolymerization of paraldehyde and forms addition compounds with the acetaldehyde which is set free.

Paramethadione USP [Paradione (*Abbott*); $C_7H_{11}NO_3$]—Anticonvulsant. Clear, colorless liquid; may have aromatic odor; pH (1 in 40 soln) about 6. Sparingly soluble in water; freely soluble in alcohol, chloroform, and ether.

Paramethasone Acetate NF [Haldrone (*Lilly*); $C_{24}H_{31}FO_6$]—Glucocorticoid. Whitish, crystalline powder; odorless; light-sensitive; melts (with decomposition) about 240°. Insoluble in water; very soluble in alcohol; soluble in ether; 1 g dissolves in about 50 ml chloroform.

Paregoric USP [camphorated opium tincture]—Antiperistaltic. Contains about 40 mg anhydrous morphine/100 ml; contains also anise oil, benzoic acid, camphor, diluted alcohol, and glycerin. See USP for preparation. Alcohol about 45%.

Pargyline Hydrochloride NF [Eutonyl (*Abbott*); $C_{11}H_{13}N \cdot HCl$; pK_a 6.9]—Antihypertensive. Fine, whitish, crystalline powder; slight odor; sublimes at high temperatures (slowly); melts about 160°. 1 g dissolves in about 1 ml water, 5 ml alcohol, and 7 ml chloroform.

Paromomycin Sulfate NF [Humatin (*P-D*); $C_{23}H_{45}N_5O_{14} \cdot x\,H_2SO_4$]—Antiamebic. Sulfate of an antibiotic substance(s) from *Streptomyces rimosus* var. *paromomycinus* or by other means. Potency equivalent to at least 675 μg base/mg. Whitish powder; amorphous; odorless or nearly so; slightly bitter taste; stable but very hygroscopic in air; stable but may darken in heat. 1 g dissolves in <1 ml water; insoluble in alcohol, chloroform, and ether.

Peanut Oil USP [arachis oil]—Pharmaceutic aid (solvent). Refined fixed oil from seed kernels of varieties of *Arachis hypogaea*. Colorless or pale yellow liquid; oily; nutty odor; bland taste; sp gr about 0.916. Very slightly soluble in alcohol; miscible with chloroform and ether.

Pectin NF—Protectant. The cellular tissues of citrus fruits, apples, and many other fruits contain pectin, which is the mucilaginous carbohydrate that makes possible the preparation of jellies from fruit juices. A jelly is formed when a warm, dilute solution of pectin containing a very small proportion of acid is allowed to cool.

Pectin is soluble in about 20 parts of water, yielding a viscous, opalescent colloidal solution which is slightly acid in reaction. When pectin is mixed with water, it is likely to form clumps which retard the process of solution. Clumping may be diminished by adding the pectin to the water slowly, with agitation, or by first moistening the pectin with alcohol, glycerin, or syrup. Pectin is insoluble in alcohol.

Pectin is considered to be made up of chain molecules, consisting largely of polygalacturonic acids which are partially in the form of methyl esters. Hence, the incompatibilities of pectin are essentially those of an organic acid of high molecular weight.

Certain ions with large positive charges precipitate the negatively charged colloidal particles of pectin from solution. Thus, solutions of pectin yield precipitates with various metallic ions, e.g., lead, copper, aluminum, iron, nickel, and calcium. Pectin forms soluble salts with ammonia and the alkali metals.

Pectin contains a trace of iron which gives a black color with tannic acid and a purple color with salicylic acid.

In making jellies or pharmaceutical pastes, excessive boiling must be avoided because pectin hydrolyzes, particularly in presence of acids or alkalies, and the resulting solution does not set to a jelly on cooling.

Pediamycin Preparations [*Ross*]—Erythromycin ethylsuccinate. Antibacterial. *Drops:* pH 7–9; sweetener, 1.55 g sucrose/5 ml; Na^+ 29 mg/5 ml. *Liquid:* Same data as for *Drops*, except: sweetener, 3.6 g sucrose/5 ml. *400:* pH 6.5–8.5; sweetener, 3.5 g sucrose/5 ml; Na^+ 135 mg/5 ml. *Suspension:* Same data as for *400*.

Penicillamine USP [Cuprimine (*MSD*); $C_5H_{11}NO_2S$]—Chelating agent. Fine, whitish, crystalline powder; slight odor; slightly bitter taste; melts (with decomposition) about 200°. Freely soluble in water; slightly soluble in alcohol; insoluble in chloroform and ether.

Penicillinase [Neutrapen (*Riker*)]—Enzyme for treatment of penicillin reactions. White, mixed crystals; odorless. Soluble in water.

Penicillin G Benzathine USP [Bicillin (*Wyeth*) $C_{16}H_{20}N_2 \cdot 2C_{16}H_{18}$-$N_2O_4S \cdot 4H_2O$ or anhydrous]—Antibacterial. White, crystalline salt with no odor, and it is virtually tasteless. The dry powder is quite stable for long periods of time even at temperatures of 37° and 56°C.

Aqueous suspensions for parenteral or oral use are also stable for long periods of time at 37°C. The aqueous suspension given by the intramuscular route gives detectable low blood levels for 7 to 10 days. Orally, this salt gives blood levels of about 30% of the magnitude of sodium or potassium penicillin G. Benzathine penicillin is slightly soluble in alcohol (1.5%), benzene, chloroform, ether, and petroleum ether (0.03%). A saturated solution is slightly acidic to nearly neutral (USP pH range, 5.0–7.5).

Dispensing Information: Take on an empty stomach. See also *Penicillins.*

Penicillin G Potassium USP [benzyl penicillin potassium; *Various Mfrs.,* $C_{16}H_{17}KN_2O_4S$]—Antibacterial. Slightly soluble in alcohol (1%) but is inactivated by this solvent and is very soluble in water. The USP specifies a pH range of 5.0–7.5.

Both sodium and potassium penicillin G are chemical compounds with a definite chemical structure. These are crystalline compounds with little odor and a very bitter taste. They are hygroscopic, very soluble in water, and are relatively insoluble in most organic solvents. Penicillin is thermolabile with maximal stability in the dry state and minimal stability in solution. It is decomposed by prolonged exposure to temperatures of 100°C. However, in the crystalline state it will stand heating at this temperature for at least four days. The presence of moisture accelerates decomposition. It is not affected by air or light. If the moisture content is less than 0.5 to 1%, the dry salt will be stable for at least three years at room temperature and for many months at elevated temperatures of 37–56°C.

Sodium and potassium penicillin G are unstable in aqueous solution. They deteriorate very rapidly at room temperature but can be kept for several days under refrigeration. Stability is greatly affected by pH, temperature, concentration, and the presence of other substances. The optimum pH range for aqueous solutions is 6.0 to 6.5. The deterioration is more rapid on the alkaline side than it is on the acid side. Hence, buffer substances such as sodium citrate and some sodium and potassium phosphates help to lessen the decomposition in aqueous solution. Buffered solutions are stable for one to two weeks at room temperature and two to three weeks under refrigeration. Aqueous solutions are also stabilized to some degree by the addition of methenamine and ethylenediamine tetraacetate. Aqueous solutions are rapidly inactivated by acids, alkalies, alcohols, glycerin, glycols, traces of heavy metals (such as copper, lead, mercury, and zinc), cysteine, hydrogen peroxide, zinc peroxide, certain aldehydes, phenols, rubbers, tannins, oxidizing agents, and certain enzymes (such as clarase and penicillinase).

Gastric juice, because of its acidity, rapidly destroys penicillin sodium, but saliva, bile, and enteric juices do not cause inactivation. For intravenous or intramuscular injection, penicillin sodium may be dissolved in sterile, pyrogen-free distilled water, normal saline solution, or 5% dextrose solution.

Penicillin ointments may be made by triturating penicillin with petrolatum, taking precautions against moisture. Suppositories may be made by triturating penicillin with melted cocoa butter and pouring into molds.

Penicillin is compatible for a few days with many antiseptic solutions, providing the pH is controlled and no heavy metal ions are present, e.g., Al^{3+} or Fe^{3+}. These may precipitate insoluble penicillinates which retain their activity when taken orally.

Penicillin is compatible with alkaloidal salts of atropine and epinephrine, benemid, dehydrocholates, eucalyptol, heparin, methyl salicylate, organic arsenicals, silicone fluids, sulfamylon, and thymol. The pH must be controlled since some of these are quite acid and would destroy penicillin unless buffered.

An isotonic solution with a 0.56°C feeezing point depression contains 77,000 units per ml.

Penicillin G Procaine USP [*Various Mfrs.;* $C_{16}H_{18}N_2O_4S \cdot C_{13}H_{20}N_2O_2 \cdot H_2O$ or anhydrous]—Antibacterial. White, crystalline compound with very little odor and a somewhat bitter taste. In the dry state it is quite stable for at least 3 years at room temperature and many months at 37° and 56°C. It cannot be heated in the dry state much above 60°C without decomposition. In this respect, sodium and potassium penicillin are more stable than procaine. However, procaine penicillin is much more stable in aqueous suspension, in which it is stable for 2 years under refrigeration. Procaine penicillin is slightly soluble in 2-propanol (0.65%), soluble in ethanol (0.68%) and chloroform, and insoluble in benzene and petroleum ether. The solubility of procaine penicillin in water can be decreased to about 1.5 mg per ml by the use of 2% of procaine HCl. This increases the stability of the aqueous procaine penicillin suspension and enables it to be kept at room temperature for 1 year without significant loss in activity. Citrate and phosphate buffers slightly decrease the solubility and help the stability to some extent. The pH of a 1% suspension is about 5.7 (USP range 5.0–7.5).

It has been found that the sodium salt of sulfamethoxypyridazine exerts a protective action on penicillin degradation in aqueous solutions above pH 7.

Penicillin G Sodium NF [$C_{16}H_{17}N_2NaO_4S$]—Antibacterial. Moderately soluble in alcohol (1%) but is inactivated by this solvent. It is very soluble in water. It is insoluble in acetone, benzene, chloroform, ether, and petroleum ether. The USP specifies a pH range of .5.0–7.5. For compatibility data, see *Penicillin G Potassium. Known incom-*

patibilities (penicillin G sodium injection): Achromycin, Aramine, Compazine, Dilantin, Keflin, Pentothal, Phenergan, Sparine, Vancocin, Vistaril.

Penicillins—The patient may be given a card containing the following information:

Your doctor has prescribed an antibiotic drug for you.

In order that your infection clears it is very important that you take this medication for the entire —— days for which it is prescribed. *Do not stop taking it even if you begin to feel better before the* —— days are completed. A calendar on the other side of this card has been completed to assist you in remembering when to take this medication.

The medication should be taken with water on an empty stomach so that large amounts will enter your bloodstream. This drug is best taken *every 6 hours* throughout the 24-hour day unless the physician has expressly prescribed another frequency.

Call your doctor if you notice any type of skin rash or itching while taking this medication. Occasionally, stomach upset or diarrhea can result from this drug and should be brought to the attention of your physician.

Penicillin V USP [phenoxymethyl penicillin; Compocillin-V (*Abbott*); Pen-Vee (*Wyeth*); V-Cillin (*Lilly*); $C_{16}H_{18}N_2O_5S$]—Antibacterial. An antibiotic (produced by fermentation) that contains a phenoxymethyl group instead of the benzyl group present in penicillin G.

Penicillin V is very slightly soluble in water (0.09%), benzene, and petroleum ether. It is soluble in acetone, alcohol, and chloroform.

Penicillin V Benzathine NF [penicillin benzathine phenoxymethyl; Pen-Vee (Suspension) (*Wyeth*); ($C_{16}H_{18}N_2O_5S)_2 \cdot C_{16}H_{20}N_2$] — Antibacterial. Whitish, crystalline powder; characteristic odor; tasteless; pH (sat aq susp) 4–6.5. One g dissolves in about 3200 ml water, 42 ml chloroform, 330 ml alcohol, and 910 ml ether.

Penicillin V Hydrabamine NF [hydrabamine phenoxymethyl penicillin; Compocillin-V Hydrabamine (*Abbott*); ($C_{16}H_{18}N_2O_5S)_2 \cdot C_{42}H_{64}N_2$] — Antibacterial. Insoluble in water (0.005%), slightly soluble in ethanol (0.58%), benzene, and petroleum ether, and soluble in chloroform.

Penicillin V Potassium USP [potassium phenoxymethyl penicillin; *Various Mfrs.;* $C_{16}H_{17}KN_2O_5S$]—Antibacterial. This compound resembles penicillin G potassium in most properties.

Dispensing Information: Discontinue use if skin rash, itching, chills, fever, edema, or exhaustion occur.

Pentaerythritol Tetranitrate [Pentritrol (*Armour*); Peritrate (*W-C*); Vasitol (*Rowell*); $C_5H_8N_4O_{12}$]—Vasodilator. White to ivory colored powder; faint, mild odor.

Dispensing Information: Use with caution in glaucoma and with nitrates. Take exactly as prescribed. Discontinue use if rash appears. Arise slowly if dizziness occurs.

Pentapiperium   Methylsulfate [pentapiperide methylsulfate; Quilene (*W-C*); $C_{20}H_{33}NO_6S$]—Anticholinergic. White, crystalline powder; odorless; bitter taste; melts (2° range) 140–148°. Soluble (80% *w/v*) in water; 1 g dissolves in about 7100 ml absolute alcohol.

Pentazocine NF [Talwin (*Winthrop*); $C_{19}H_{27}NO$]—Analgesic. Whitish powder; melts about 153°. Practically insoluble in water; freely soluble in chloroform; soluble in alcohol and ether.

Dispensing Information: Drowsiness may occur which may impair ability to drive or perform other tasks requiring alertness. This drug has the properties of a narcotic antagonist. Use only as directed. Advise physician of any nervous system complaint.

Pentazocine   Hydrochloride   NF [Talwin HCl (*Winthrop*); $C_{19}H_{27}NO\cdot$ HCl]—Analgesic. White, crystalline powder; polymorphic forms melt about 254° and 218°. 1 g dissolves in about 30 ml water, 7 ml alcohol, and 3 ml ether; insoluble in chloroform.

Pentazocine Lactate Injection NF [Talwin Injection (*Winthrop*)]—Analgesic. Usually occurs as a sterile solution of pentazocine prepared with the aid of lactic acid and water for injection; pH 4–5. *Known incompatibilities* (pentazocine lactate injection): aminophylline, amobarbital sodium, pentobarbital sodium, phenobarbital sodium, secobarbital sodium, sodium bicarbonate.

Dispensing Information: See *Pentazocine.*

Pentobarbital NF [Nembutal (*Abbott*); (*Various   Other   Mfrs.*); $C_{11}H_{18}N_2O_3$]—Sedative. White to practically white, fine powder; practically odorless; melts 127–131°. One g dissolves in >2000 ml water, 4.5 ml alcohol, 4 ml chloroform, and 10 ml ether.

When mixed with solutions of ammonium salts, pentobarbital (pH 8–10) liberates ammonia and gives a precipitate of 2-ethyl-2-(1-methylbutyl)barbituric acid. It forms a sticky mass with acetylsalicylic acid, chloral hydrate, and ephedrine salts. Mixtures of pentobarbital with bismuth subgallate or bismuth subcarbonate are stable for 10–20 days, after which a foreign odor develops. In the presence of moisture, a mixture of pentobarbital and calomel turns gray. In powders or dry filled capsules there is no change in mixtures of pentobarbital with acetophenetidin, acetanilid, antipyrine, aminopyrine, bismuth subnitrate, calomel, sodium bromide, sodium salicylate, or salicylic acid.

Pentobarbital is incompatible with certain liquid preparations. In lactated pepsin elixir it precipitates and changes color. It is compatible for a short time with pepsin essence, but precipitates in 3–5 days. A mixture of pentobarbital with milk of bismuth turns yellow and develops a foreign odor. When it is dissolved in compound white pine syrup, pentobarbital does not change for 10–20 days but thereafter shows a precipitate.

Dispensing Information: See *Sedatives and Hypnotics.*

Pentobarbital Sodium USP [Nembutal Sodium (*Abbott*); Pental (*Mallinckrodt*);   Napental   (*Massengill*); $C_{11}H_{17}N_2NaO_3$]—Hypnotic. White, crystalline granules or white powder; odorless or slight, characteristic odor; slightly bitter taste; pH (10% soln) 9.8–11; pH (10% parenteral soln) 10–10.5.

Very soluble in water; freely soluble in alcohol; practically insoluble in ether. Aqueous solutions decompose when boiled or on standing.

Dispensing Information: See Sedatives and Hypnotics.

Pentobarbital Sodium Injection— This is usually supplied as a dry powder for reconstitution or as a propylene glycol solution (usually with 2% benzyl alcohol or a local anesthetic). The injection pH must fall in the pH range 9–10.5.

The compatibility of Nembutal Sodium Solution (50 mg/ml) with a number of parenteral solutions has been studied. Incompatibilities reported were: Benadryl HCl (at approx 5 mg/ml), Compazine Ethylenedisulfonate (1 mg), Demerol HCl (10 mg), Dramamine (5 mg), Phenergan HCl (10 mg), Thorazine HCl (5 mg). These probably involved liberation of the amine free base by the alkalinity of the Nembutal Sodium. Compatible mixtures were reported for the Nembutal Sodium Solution (50 mg/ml) containing: Aminophylline Injection (50 mg/ml approx), Coramine (50 mg), Desoxyn HCl (1.5 mg), ephedrine sulfate (5 mg), Hyazyme (15 units), Megimide (20 mg), Metrazole (30 mg), morphine sulfate (1.62 mg), Norisodrine Sulfate (1:500,000), Pentothal Sodium (100 mg), Polybrene (10 mg), procaine HCl (10 mg), Prostigmin Methylsulfate (0.05 mg), Quelicin Chloride (3 mg), scopolamine HBr (0.013 mg), sodium bicarbonate (0.375 g), sodium iodide (100 mg), Solu-Cortef (25 mg), Tral (1 mg), tubocurarine chloride (0.225 mg).

Pentolinium Tartrate NF [Ansolysen Tartrate (*Wyeth*); $C_{23}H_{42}N_2O_{12}$]— Antihypertensive. This diquaternary compound is a white to light cream colored crystalline powder that is very soluble in water and slightly soluble in alcohol. A 1% solution in water has a pH of about 3–4. It is stable to autoclaving.

Pentylenetetrazol [Metrazol (*Knoll*); $C_6H_{10}N_4$]—Central stimulant. White, crystalline powder which is an analeptic and antidote to the barbiturates. It is very soluble in alcohol and water. Its solutions are neutral, stable to light, and may be sterilized by heat. Pentylenetetrazol is extremely stable and, hence, does not have very many incompatibilities. Heavy metal salts such as mercuric chloride give crystalline precipitates.

Pepsin—Proteolytic enzyme. Pepsin is freely soluble in water, yielding opalescent solutions; it is almost insoluble in alcohol. The activity of most enzymes in solution is destroyed by alkalies and by heating above 70°C; dry pepsin is not inactivated by heating to 100°C. Aqueous solutions of pepsin are slightly acid in reaction. Pepsin solutions yield precipitates with tannic acid, gallic acid, and salts of many of the heavy metals. Agitation of pepsin solutions lowers or destroys the activity. Pepsin solutions show no marked deterioration if less than 30% of alcohol or 50% of glycerin is present. Solutions of pepsin retain their activity longer in the presence of 20% of glycerin. Preparations of pepsin having a pH of 4.5–5.5 retain their proteolytic activity longer than if the pH is 2.5. Thus, preparations of pepsin containing the proper concentration of HCl for optimum proteolytic effect should not be kept for long periods of time. It has been reported that pepsin solutions containing hydrochloric acid should be prepared by adding the pepsin after the acid has been fully diluted. The use of glass filters has been suggested since both cotton or paper filters adsorb pepsin.

Liquids containing pepsin are frequently used as vehicles for prescription use. Common pepsin fluids (with the pepsin concentration indicated in parentheses) are: pepsin elixir (3.5% pepsin), compound pepsin elixir (3.5%), saccharated pepsin (10%), pepsin and rennin elixir (4.5%). Other products (which may contain rennin in addition to pepsin) are essence of pepsin, Enzymol, Gastron, Neo-Gastricine, Pepsencia, and Pepsin Cordial. A combination of pepsin with lactic acid is Peptalac. Combinations of pepsin with other enzymes are Diastanol, Liquenzyme, Liquor Diastos and Pava-Pepsin. Others are Alphaden, Caltase, and Pan-peptic Elixir.

Percodan Tablets [*Endo*]—Narcotic; analgesic. Contain dihydrocodeinone HCl 4.5 mg, dihydrocodeinone terephthalate 0.38 mg, aspirin 224 mg, phenacetin 160 mg, caffeine 32 mg.

Dispensing Information: May enhance response to alcohol or other CNS depressants. Drowsiness may occur which may impair ability to drive or perform other tasks requiring alertness. Do not exceed labeled dosage. May be taken with meals or milk to prevent GI effects.

Perphenazine NF [Trilafon (*Schering*); $C_{21}H_{26}ClN_3OS$]—Tranquilizer. *Side effects:* Infrequent blurred vision, dryness of the mouth, constipation, and skin rash. Nausea and vomiting, urinary frequency, or polyphagia are uncommon. With high dosages, a Parkinson-like syndrome may develop.

Petrolatum NF [petroleum jelly]—Pharmaceutic aid (ointment base). Purified mixture of semisolid hydrocarbons from petroleum. Yellowish, unctuous mass; transparent in thin layers; odorless and tasteless or almost so; sp gr 0.815–0.880; melts 38–60°. Insoluble in water; almost insoluble in cold or hot alcohol; freely soluble in chloroform; solvent in ether.

Petrolatum, Hydrophilic, USP—Pharmaceutic aid (absorbent ointment base); topical protectant. Preparation: Melt stearyl alcohol (30 g), white wax (80 g), and white petrolatum (860 g) together on a steam bath, then add cholesterol (30 g), and stir until it completely dissolves. Remove from the bath, and stir until the mixture congeals.

Phenacaine Hydrochloride NF [holocaine hydrochloride; $C_{18}H_{22}N_2O_2 \cdot HCl$]—Topical anesthetic (ophthalmic). Phenacaine is precipitated by alkaline substances and alkaloidal precipitants. Phenacaine hydrochloride (1 g) is soluble in 50 ml of water and is freely soluble in alcohol. The aqueous solution is almost neutral. Solutions should be prepared in receptacles of porcelain or alkali-free glass since the alkali derived from soft glass causes precipitation.

Phenacemide NF [Phenurone (*Abbott*); $C_9H_{10}N_2O_2$]—Anticonvulsant. Fine, whitish, crystalline powder; odorless or almost so; melts about 213°. Practically insoluble in water; slightly soluble in alcohol; very slightly soluble in chloroform and ether.

Phenacetin [acetophenetidin; acetphenetidin; *p*-ethoxyacetanilid; $C_{10}H_{13}NO_2$]—Analgesic. 1 g dissolves in 1300 ml water or 15 ml alcohol. With oxidizing agents, phenacetin gives a pink to red color, while with spirit of ethyl nitrite it gives a yellow color which gradually deepens to a red-brown. Phenacetin yields a pasty mass on trituration with some substances, e.g., chloral hydrate, phenol, and pyrocatechin. It is decomposed by strong acids or alkalies and forms a compound with iodine.

Phenaglycodol [Ultran (*Lilly*); $C_{11}H_{15}ClO_2$]—Tranquilizer. Practically insoluble in water. *Side effects:* Occasional drowsiness.

Phenaphen Tablets (or Capsules) [*Robins*]—Analgesic. Contain phenacetin 194 mg, aspirin 162 mg, phenobarbital 16.2 mg. Also available with codeine: 16.2 mg, 32.4 mg, and 65 mg.

Dispensing Information: May cause GI upset, nausea, vomiting, and constipation. Drowsiness may occur which may impair ability to drive or perform other tasks requiring alertness. (See warnings of individual ingredients also.)

Phenaphthazine [Nitrazine paper (*Squibb*); $C_{18}H_8N_4Na_2O_{11}S_2$]—*In vitro* diagnostic aid (urine pH).

Phenazopyridine Hydrochloride NF [Pyridium (*W-C*); $C_{11}H_{11}N_5 \cdot HCl$]—Analgesic (urinary tract). Light or dark-red to dark-violet, crystalline powder; odorless or slight odor; melts with decomposition about 235°. One g dissolves in <10 ml water, 59 ml alcohol, 331 ml chloroform, >5000 ml ether, 300 ml cold water, 20 ml boiling water, and 100 ml glycerin.

Dispensing Information: Produces a reddish-orange discoloration of urine.

Phencyclidine Hydrochloride [Sernylan (*P-D*); $C_{17}H_{25}N \cdot HCl$]—Anesthetic. Whitish, crystalline powder or granules; odorless; slightly bitter taste; melts about 225°. Freely soluble in water, alcohol, and chloroform.

Phenelzine Sulfate NF [Nardil (*W-C*); $C_8H_{12}N_2 \cdot H_2SO_4$]—Antidepressant. Whitish powder; characteristic odor; subject to oxidation; heat- and light-sensitive; melts about 166°. 1 g dissolves in about 7 ml water; practically insoluble in alcohol, chloroform, and ether.

Phenethicillin Potassium NF [Maxipen (*Roerig*); Syncillin (*Bristol*); $C_{17}H_{19}KN_2O_5S$]—Antibacterial. This water-soluble penicillin, closely related to penicillin V, is acid-stable and exceedingly well-absorbed but binds somewhat to serum protein. The rate of degradation in aqueous solution follows the general pattern of penicillin G, although the rates were slower. The pH of maximum stability is 6.5. Combinations of phenethicillin with 77 common liquid prescription preparations have been studied and most had no effect on stability for 3 days at 4°C. Those which had the greatest effect were products which changed the pH outside the range for maximum stability.

Phenetsal [Phenosal; Salophen; $C_{15}H_{13}NO_4$]—Analgesic; antipyretic. Crystalline powder; solution neutral to litmus; melts about 187°. Practically insoluble in water (more soluble in warm water); soluble in alcohol and ether. *Known incompatibilities:* alkalies (an alkaline solution) which dissolve it with decomposition (forms blue color when boiled).

Phenformin Hydrochloride USP [DBI (*Geigy*); Meltrol (*USV*); $C_{10}H_{15}N_5 \cdot HCl$]—Hypoglycemic. White or practically white, crystalline powder; odorless; bitter taste; pH (2.5% soln) 6–7. Freely soluble in water; soluble in alcohol; practically insoluble in chloroform and ether.

Dispensing Information: May cause gastric upset; if vomiting occurs, advise physician. Avoid alcohol. Do not skip or exceed labeled dosage. See also *Acetohexamide.*

Phenindamine Tartrate NF [Thephorin (*Roche*); $C_{19}H_{19}N \cdot C_4H_6O_6$]— This antihistaminic, anticholinergic agent is soluble about 2.5% in water, sparingly soluble in propylene glycol, and insoluble in ethanol and glycerin.

Phenindione NF [Danilone (*Schieffelin*); Hedulin (*Merrell-National*); $C_{15}H_{10}O_2$]—Anticoagulant. Whitish crystals or crystalline powder; practically odorless; melts about 149°. Very slightly soluble in water; slightly soluble in alcohol and ether; freely soluble in chloroform.

Pheniramine Maleate [Trimeton Maleate (*Schering*); $C_{16}H_{20}N_2 \cdot C_4H_4O_4$]— Antihistaminic. White solid. It is very soluble in water and in alcohol. A 1% aqueous solution is slightly acidic (pH range, 4.5–5.5).

Phenmetrazine Hydrochloride NF [Preludin (*B-I*); $C_{11}H_{15}NO \cdot HCl$]—Anorexic. Whitish, crystalline powder; melts (3° range) 172–182°; pH (1 in 40 soln) 4.5–5.5. Very soluble in water; freely soluble in alcohol and chloroform.

Dispensing Information: May cause dry mouth and insomnia. Last dose should be taken 6 hours before bedtime (12 hours for Preludin Endurets).

Phenobarbital USP [Luminal (*Winthrop*); $C_{12}H_{12}N_2O_3$; pK_a 7.41]—Anticonvulsant; hypnotic; sedative. Slightly soluble in water (1:1000), soluble in alcohol (1:8), and soluble in alkaline hydroxides and carbonates. A number of studies have been made of the solubility of phenobarbital in mixtures of water and alcohol, water–alcohol–glycerin, water–alcohol–propylene glycol, and water–alcohol–propylene glycol-sorbitol. It has been found necessary to go to fairly high concentrations of alcohol before the solubility of free phenobarbital increases significantly. Thus, 35% alcohol at pH 7, or 10% alcohol at pH 8, is required to solubilize 30 mg in about 5 ml.

Caution (especially in pediatric prescriptions): Alcohol may potentiate the depressant action of barbiturates and produce toxic effects.

42

R̶   Tincture Belladonna   8 ml
     Phenobarbital   1.5 g
     Elixir Lactated Pepsin   q.s.   120 ml

The alcohol strength is too low to dissolve the phenobarbital. A clear solution can be obtained by replacing 12 ml of the elixir with alcohol.

Dispensing Information: Discontinue use and consult physician if skin rash occurs. See also *Sedatives and Hypnotics.*

Phenobarbital Sodium USP [Luminal Sodium (*Winthrop*), soluble phenobarbital, soluble phenobarbitone, sodium gardenal; $C_{12}H_{11}N_2NaO_3$]—Anticonvulsant; hypnotic. Very soluble in water; soluble in alcohol; practically insoluble in chloroform and ether. A 10% solution of phenobarbital sodium (Luminal Sodium) has a pH of about 9.7 and undergoes about 1% decomposition in 3 weeks at room temperature. The reaction kinetics of phenobarbital sodium have been studied and found to be first order. On addition of acids to a solution of phenobarbital sodium, precipitation of phenobarbital acid occurs when the pH is lowered to 8.8. Hydroalcoholic solutions of phenobarbital sodium are more stable to heat than aqueous solutions; after heating at 115°C for 30 min, a 10% solution of phenobarbital sodium containing 46% of alcohol showed a 1.5% deterioration, as compared with 9% deterioration in an aqueous solution. Solutions of phenobarbital sodium containing a high proportion of propylene glycol are considerably more stable than aqueous solutions but may acquire a light amber color upon heating.

Similar stabilization of hexobarbital has been attributed to the decrease of dielectric constant of the medium. Along this line, a stable 10% phenobarbital injection which contains 20% glycerol, 20% urethane, and piperazine equimolar to the phenobarbital has been described.

Known incompatibilities (phenobarbital sodium injection): Achromycin, acidic solutions, Benadryl, calcium chloride, codeine phosphate, codeine sulfate, Compazine, Demerol, Dilantin, ephedrine sulfate, hydralazine HCl, Ilotycin, insulin, Keflin, Leritine, Levo-Dromoran, Levophed, magnesium sulfate, methadone HCl, methylphenidate HCl, methylparaben, morphine sulfate, papaverine, para-aminobenzoic acid, penicillin G potassium, Phenergan, phytonadione, procaine HCl, propylparaben, Pyribenzamine, sodium bicarbonate, Solu-Cortef, Sparine, streptomycin sulfate, succinylcholine chloride, Terramycin, thiamine, Thorazine, Vancocin, Vistaril.

Phenol USP [carbolic acid; C_6H_5OH; pK_a 9.94]—Phenol is a useful germicide and preservative soluble 1 g in 15 ml of water or about 70 ml of liquid petrolatum and is very soluble in alcohol and glycerin. It forms a liquid or soft mass when triturated with compounds such as camphor, menthol, thymol, acetanilid, chloral hydrate, acetophenetidin, monobromated camphor, naphthalene, naphthol, pyrogallol, resorcinol, salol, terpin hydrate, sodium phosphate, or other eutectic formers. Phenol decolorizes dilute solutions of iodine, forming HI and iodophenol; stronger solutions of iodine react with phenol to form the insoluble 2,4,6-triiodophenol. On exposure to light and air, phenol turns red or brown, the color being influenced by metallic impurities; oxidizing agents hasten the color change. Phenol coagulates albumin and burns the skin (alcohol is used as an external antidote). Aqueous solutions stronger than 2% should not be applied to the surface of the body. *Note:* The corrosive effect on the tissues is lost when phenol is mixed with twice its weight of camphor, forming a liquid containing addition compounds of camphor and phenol. The addition of water to camphorated phenol precipitates camphor and liberates phenol, yielding a corrosive mixture.

Phenolphthalein NF [$C_{20}H_{14}O_4$]—Cathartic. Almost insoluble in water but soluble in solutions of alkali hydroxides; 1 g dissolves in 15 ml of alcohol. Phenolphthalein gives a red color with alkaline solutions.

Phenolsulfonphthalein NF [phenol red; $C_{19}H_{14}O_5S$]—Diagnostic aid (renal function determinations). Reddish, crystalline powder. 1 g dissolves in about 1300 ml water and 350 ml alcohol; practically insoluble in chloroform and ether.

Phenoxybenzamine Hydrochloride NF [Dibenzyline HCl (*SK&F*); $C_{18}H_{22}ClNO\cdot HCl$] — Antiadrenergic. White, crystalline powder; odorless; melts about 138°. 1 g dissolves in about 25 ml water, 6 ml alcohol, 3 ml chloroform, and >1000 ml ether.

Phenprocoumon NF [Liquamar (*Organon*); $C_{18}H_{16}O_3$]—Anticoagulant. Fine, white, crystalline powder; odorless or slight odor; melts about 179°. Practically insoluble in water; soluble in chloroform and alkali hydroxides.

Phensuximide NF [Milontin (*P-D*); $C_{11}H_{11}NO_2$]—Anticonvulsant. Whitish, crystalline powder; odorless or slight odor; melts about 71°. 1 g dissolves in about 210 ml water, 11 ml alcohol, <1 ml chloroform, and 19 ml ether.

Phentermine [Ionamin (*Pennwalt*); $C_{10}H_{15}N$]—Anorexic. Colorless, mobile liquid; oily; characteristic odor; boils about 200°. Slightly soluble in water; soluble in alcohol, chloroform, and ether.

Phentolamine Hydrochloride NF [Regitine Hydrochloride (*Ciba*); $C_{17}H_{19}N_3O\cdot HCl$]—Antiadrenergic. Whitish, crystalline powder; odorless; solution acid to litmus (pH about 5) (foams on shaking); melts about 240°. 1 g dissolves in about 50 ml water and 120 ml alcohol; very slightly soluble in chloroform and ether.

Phentolamine Mesylate USP [Regitine Methanesulfonate (*Ciba*); $C_{17}H_{19}N_3O\cdot CH_4O_3S$]—Antiadrenergic. White, crystalline powder; odorless; solution acid to litmus (pH about 5) and slowly deteriorates; melts about 177°. 1 g dissolves in about 1 ml water, 4 ml alcohol, and 700 ml chloroform.

Phenylbutazone USP [Azolid (*USV*); Butazolidin (*Geigy*); $C_{19}H_{20}N_2O_2$]—Antirheumatic. White to off-white, crystalline powder; odorless; melts 104–107°. Very slightly soluble in water; freely soluble in ether; soluble in alcohol.

Dispensing Information: See *Anti-inflammatory Agents.*

Phenylephrine Hydrochloride USP [Neo-Synephrine Hydrochloride (*Winthrop*); $C_9H_{13}NO_2\cdot HCl$]—Adrenergic. Adrenergic and vasoconstrictor compound readily soluble in water or alcohol. Its aqueous solutions are slightly acid; the addition of alkalies causes precipitation of phenylephrine base. Phenylephrine is related chemically to ephedrine and epinephrine but is more stable than epinephrine. Solutions of phenylephrine hydrochloride can be sterilized (by boiling) without decomposition. The solution should not be allowed to come in contact with metals; when used as a spray, it should be placed in glass bottles with connections made of glass or hard rubber.

It has been noted that 0.1% edetate sodium prevents the discoloration of phenylephrine solutions stored in amber bottles while sodium metabisulfite does not. Trace quantities of manganese and iron are believed to accelerate the discoloration.

Phenylethyl Alcohol NF [$C_8H_{10}O$]—Pharmaceutic aid (antimicrobial agent). This rose perfume is sometimes used as a preservative in 0.5% concentrations. It is soluble in water (2%), very soluble in alcohol, glycerin, oils, propylene glycol, and slightly soluble in mineral oil.

Phenylmercuric Acetate NF [$C_8H_8HgO_2$]—Pharmaceutic aid (antimicrobial agent). Whitish, crystalline powder or small, white prisms or leaflets; odorless; melts about 151°. 1 g dissolves in about 180 ml water, 225 ml alcohol, 7 ml chloroform, and 200 ml ether.

Phenylmercuric Nitrate NF—This substance is an antiseptic and preservative mixture of $C_6H_5HgNO_3$ and C_6H_5HgOH. 1 g dissolves in 1200 ml of water, 800 ml of alcohol, or 200 ml of glycerin. A 0.1% aqueous solution has a pH of 3.7. The phenylmercuric ion is more stable in acid solutions than in alkaline solutions. Aqueous solutions of phenylmercuric nitrate are incompatible with halides and soaps, both of which cause precipitation.

Phenylpropanolamine Hydrochloride NF [Propadrine HCl (*MSD*); $C_9H_{13}NO \cdot HCl$]—Adrenergic (vasoconstrictor). It is a synthetic analog of ephedrine. The hydrochloride is readily soluble in water. Aqueous solutions appear to be stable over long periods of time. The 1% solution, as marketed by the manufacturers, contains 0.5% chlorobutanol as a preservative.

Dispensing Information: Caution in hypertension, cardiac disease, hyperthyroidism, or persons taking MAO inhibitors.

Phenytoin USP [diphenylhydantoin; Dilantin (*P-D*); $C_{15}H_{12}N_2O_2$]—Anticonvulsant. White powder; odorless; melts about 295°. Practically insoluble in water; soluble in hot alcohol; slightly soluble in cold alcohol, chloroform, and ether.

Dispensing Information: Potentiates coumarins, potentiates griseofulvin, and potentiated by phenylbutazone. Good dental hygiene is required due to gingival hyperplasia. Drowsiness may occur which may impair ability to drive or perform other tasks requiring alertness. Take with meals to prevent GI upset. Patients should be familiar with symptoms of toxicity (i.e., ataxia). Enforce compliance with exact instructions and describe close range between efficacy and toxicity.

Phenytoin Sodium USP [diphenylhydantoin sodium; Dilantin Sodium (*P-D*); (*Various Other Mfrs.*); $C_{15}H_{11}N_2NaO_2$]—Anticonvulsant. White, hygroscopic powder; on exposure to air it gradually absorbs carbon dioxide, which liberates diphenylhydantoin. It is freely soluble in water and soluble in alcohol. Due to hydrolysis, aqueous solutions are alkaline and contain a shiny, silky precipitate of diphenylhydantoin,

which dissolves completely when the alkalinity is increased to pH 11.7. *Known incompatibilities* (phenytoin sodium for injection): should not be mixed with any drugs or added to any IV infusions; very pH-dependent.

Phosphoric Acid NF [H_3PO_4]—Pharmaceutic aid (solvent). Colorless liquid; syrupy consistency; odorless; sp gr about 1.71. Miscible with water and alcohol, evolving heat.

Phthalylsulfathiazole NF [Sulfathalidine (*MSD*); $C_{17}H_{13}N_3O_5S_2$; pK_a 3]—Antibacterial (intestinal). Slightly soluble in alcohol, very slightly soluble in ether, practically insoluble in chloroform and water, and readily soluble in sodium or potassium hydroxide solution, ammonia water, and concentrated hydrochloric acid. A 10% solution of the sodium salt has a pH of approximately 8.5.

Physostigmine USP [eserine; $C_{15}H_{21}N_3O_2$; pK_{b1} 6.12, pK_{b2} 12.24]—Physostigmine is a cholinergic (ophthalmic) ester alkaloid slightly soluble in water and readily soluble in alcohol. The free alkaloid absorbs moisture from the air and changes to a red mass, especially on exposure to heat, light, air, or traces of metals. This red color also develops in aqueous solutions of the salts of physostigmine; boric acid and carbonic acid retard the change, but alkalies hasten decomposition.

Physostigmine in solution first hydrolyzes to methyl carbonic acid and eserinol (a phenol), which is readily oxidized to the red-colored compound, rubreserine. In the absence of an antioxidant, the color change may be taken as an index of activity. In the presence of an antioxidant (e.g., sulfite) no color change takes place; however, the ester may still be inactive. Accordingly, only about a week's supply should be prepared at a time, and the solution should be sterilized by filtration so as to avoid heat. The pH of optimum stability was found to be 4–5.5 and it was recommended that sodium metabisulfite be used as an antioxidant and benzalkonium chloride as the best preservative.

It has been reported that the buffer components of eserine eye drops affect the hydrolysis rate constants. Aliphatic dibasic acids and aromatic carboxylic and monohydroxycarboxylic acids are effective stabilizers.

Physostigmine Salicylate USP [Isopto-Eserine (*Alcon*); $C_{15}H_{21}N_3O_2 \cdot C_7H_6O_3$]—Cholinergic (ophthalmic). 1 g dissolves in 75 ml of water or 16 ml of alcohol; the aqueous solution is neutral or only faintly acid (the pH of a 0.5% aqueous solution is about 5.8). A solution of physostigmine salicylate, adjusted to pH 6.2 by a phosphate buffer and containing sodium formaldehydesulfoxylate as a preservative in a concentration of 1:5000, has been kept for 6 months without developing a pink color; this solution is nonirritating to the conjunctiva. Solutions which remain colorless for weeks may be prepared by dissolving physostigmine salicylate in an almost saturated solution of benzoic acid. The latter solution is made by dissolving 1 g of benzoic acid in 290 ml of distilled water, previously warmed to 70°C, and cooling it to room temperature. The container should be rinsed with a 1% solution of HCl and then with distilled water, in order to neutralize the alkalinity of the glass.

Physostigmine Sulfate USP [$(C_{15}H_{21}N_3O_2)_2 \cdot H_2SO_4$] — Cholinergic (ophthalmic). White, microcrystalline powder; odorless; deliquescent in moist air; acquires red tint in light, air, and heat or with contact with traces of metals. 1 g dissolves in about 4 ml water, <1 ml alcohol, and 1200 ml ether. *Known incompatibilities:* see *Physostigmine Salicylate.*

Phytonadione USP [vitamin K_1; Mephyton (*MSD*); $C_{31}H_{46}O_2$]—Prothrombogenic vitamin. This is a viscous liquid that is insoluble in water, sparingly soluble in methanol, and soluble in ethanol, acetone, benzene, petroleum ether, hexane, dioxane, chloroform, ether, other fat solvents, and vegetable oils.

Phytonadione is stable to air and moisture but decomposes in sunlight. It is unaffected by dilute acids but is destroyed by solutions of alkali hydroxides and by reducing agents. Keep well closed and protected from light.

A solution of 1 part phytonadione and 20 parts alcohol is neutral to litmus (pH range, 4.5–8).

Pilocarpine [$C_{11}H_{16}N_2O_2$; pK_{b1} 7.15, pK_{b2} 12.57]—Pilocarpine is a cholinergic liquid alkaloid which is easily soluble in water. Aqueous solutions of the alkaloid or its salts are precipitated by the general alkaloidal reagents, except that alkalies do not cause precipitation because of the solubility of the free alkaloid in water. Oxidizing agents convert the alkaloid into homopilopic and pilopic acids.

Dispensing Information: Explain nature of chronic disease (glaucoma) and necessity for continuous treatment.

Pilocarpine Hydrochloride USP [Isopto-Carpine (*Alcon*); $C_{11}H_{16}N_2O_2 \cdot HCl$]—Cholinergic (ophthalmic). Colorless, translucent crystals; odorless; faintly bitter; hygroscopic; affected by light; solution is acid to litmus. 1 g dissolves in 0.3 ml water, 3 ml alcohol, and 360 ml chloroform.

Dispensing Information: See *Pilocarpine.*

Pilocarpine Nitrate USP [P.V. Carpine (*Allergan*); $C_{11}H_{16}N_2O_2 \cdot HNO_3$]—Cholinergic (ophthalmic). White, shiny crystals; light-sensitive; solution acid to litmus; melts about 173°. 1 g dissolves in about 4 ml water and 75 ml alcohol; insoluble in chloroform and ether. *Known incompatibilities:* see *Pilocarpine Hydrochloride.*

Piminodine Esylate NF [Alvodine Ethanesulfonate (*Winthrop*); $C_{23}H_{30}N_2O_2 \cdot C_2H_6O_3S$]—Narcotic analgesic. Colorless, crystalline solid; slightly bitter taste; pH (1 in 125 soln) about 4.8; discolors in strong light; melts about 131°. 1 g dissolves in >1000 ml water and ether, 6 ml alcohol, and 2 ml chloroform.

Pipenzolate Bromide [Piptal (*Lakeside*); $C_{22}H_{28}BrNO_3$]—Anticholinergic. Whitish powder; melts (with decomposition) about 179°. 1 g dissolves in about 2 ml water, 10 ml anhydrous alcohol, and 5 ml chloroform.

Piperacetazine NF [Quide (*Dow*); $C_{24}H_{30}N_2O_2S$]—Tranquilizer. Yellow powder; granular; melts about 104°. Practically insoluble in water; soluble in alcohol; freely soluble in chloroform.

Piperazine USP [diethylenediamine; $C_4H_{10}N_2$]—Anthelmintic (intestinal pinworms and roundworms). Whitish lumps or flakes; ammoniacal odor; boils about 145°; melts about 111°. Soluble in water and alcohol; insoluble in ether. *Known incompatibilities:* salts of heavy metals, salts of alkaloids, acetanilid, phenacetin, nitrates.

Piperazine Citrate USP [Antepar Citrate (*B-W*); $(C_4H_{10}N_2)_3 \cdot 2C_6H_8O_7 \cdot xH_2O$ or anhydrous]—Anthelmintic (intestinal pinworms and roundworms).

Dispensing Information: Interacts with chlorpromazine. Take exactly as directed. Do not skip doses.

Piperazine Estrone Sulfate NF [Ogen (*Abbott*); $C_{18}H_{22}O_5S \cdot C_4H_{10}N_2$] —Estrogen. Fine, white to creamy white, odorless, crystalline powder. It is slightly soluble in water and alcohol.

Piperazine Phosphate NF [Anthalazine (*Bowman*); Pinrou (*Century*); $C_4H_{10}N_2 \cdot H_3PO_4 \cdot H_2O$ or anhydrous]— Anthelmintic (intestinal pinworms or roundworms). White, crystalline powder; may have slight odor; pH (1 in 100 soln) about 6.2. Sparingly soluble in water and alcohol.

Piperidolate Hydrochloride NF [Dactil (*Lakeside*); $C_{21}H_{25}NO_2 \cdot HCl$]— Anticholinergic. Whitish powder; melts about 196°. 1 g dissolves in about 18 ml water, 53 ml alcohol, and 4 ml chloroform.

Piperocaine Hydrochloride [Metycaine Hydrochloride (*Lilly*); $C_{16}H_{23}$- $NO_2 \cdot HCl$]—Local anesthetic. Easily soluble in water and alcohol but insoluble in fixed oils. Solutions of piperocaine hydrochloride are stable and retain their potency after sterilization by boiling. Aqueous solutions are faintly acid in reaction; on addition of alkali hydroxides or carbonates, the free base separates as an oily liquid.

Pipobroman NF [Vercyte (*Abbott*); $C_{10}H_{16}Br_2N_2O_2$]—Antineoplastic.] Whitish, crystalline powder; slight, sharp, fruity odor; slight, bitter taste; melts about 103°. 1 g dissolves in about 230 ml water, 35 ml alcohol, 5 ml chloroform, and 530 ml ether.

Podophyllum Resin USP [podophyllin]—Caustic. Powdered mixture of resins from podophyllum. Amorphous powder; light brown to greenish yellow (turns darker at temperatures above 25° and in light); slight, faintly bitter taste; alcohol solution acid to litmus. Soluble in alcohol (slight opalescence); partially soluble in chloroform and ether; insoluble in water. *Caution: highly irritating to the eye and mucous membranes.*

Polacrilin Potassium [Amberlite IRP-88 (*Rohm & Haas*)]—Pharmaceutic aid (tablet disintegrant). Potassium salt of a methacrylic acid polymer with divinylbenzene. Dry, free-flowing powder; buff-colored; odorless; tasteless. Insoluble in water.

Polaramine Preparations [*Schering*]—*Expectorant:* Antihistaminic and antitussive. Contains (per 5 ml) dexchlorpheniramine maleate 2 mg, *d*-isoephedrine sulfate 20 mg, glyceryl guaiacolate 100 mg. pH 5.1–5.7; alcohol 7.2%; sweetener, sugar; solvent, water. *Syrup:* Antihistaminic. Contains (per 5 ml) dexchlorpheniramine maleate 2 mg. pH 5.5–6.5; alcohol 6%; sweetener, sugar; solvent, water.

Poldine Methylsulfate NF [Nacton (*McNeil*); $C_{22}H_{29}NO_7S$]—Anticholinergic. Whitish, crystalline powder; odorless; melts about 136°. 1 g dissolves in about 1 ml water, 20 ml alcohol, and 1000 ml chloroform; practically insoluble in ether.

Poloxalkol [Magcyl (*Elder*); Polykol (*Upjohn*)]—Cathartic. Polymer of ethylene oxide and polypropylene glycol. White granules or flakes; slightly soapy taste; faint, bitter aftertaste. Freely soluble in water, alcohol, and chloroform; sparingly soluble in ether.

Polycarbophil NF [comp. of Sorboquel (*Schering*)]—Cathartic. Polyacrylic acid cross-linked with divinyl glycol. Whitish granules; slight, characteristic odor. Swells in water (insoluble); insoluble in most organic solvents.

Polycillin Preparations [*Bristol*]— Antibacterial. Ampicillin trihydrate. *Oral Suspension 125 mg/5 ml:* pH 5–7.5; sugar 74.7%; Na$^+$ 0.174 mEq. *Oral Suspension 250 mg/5 ml:* pH 5–7.5; sugar 69.5%; Na$^+$ 0.174 mEq. *Oral Suspension 500 mg/5 ml:* pH 5–7.5; sugar 59%; Na$^+$ 0.165 mEq. *Pediatric Drops:* pH 5–7.5; sugar 59%; Na$^+$ 0.033 mEq.

Polyestradiol Phosphate [Estradurin (*Ayerst*); approx $(C_{18}H_{23}PO_4)_n$]— Antineoplastic; estrogen. White, crystalline powder. Slightly soluble in water.

Polyethylene Glycols [Carbowaxes (*Carbide & Carbon*)]—Pharmaceutic aids (vehicle). The polyglycols are water-soluble vehicle components which are also soluble in many organic solvents including aromatic hydrocarbons but are only slightly soluble in aliphatic hydrocarbons. They are physically incompatible with petrolatum ointments.

Polymyxin B Sulfate USP [Aerosporin Sulfate (B-W)]—Antibacterial. Polymyxin B sulfate is derived from various stains of the spore-forming soil bacterium, *Bacillus polymyxa* (*Bacillus aerosporus* Greer). Chemically, the polymyxins are basic polypeptides with 5 basic amino groups. Polymyxin B contains leucine, threonine, phenylalanine, α,γ-diaminobutyric acid, and a fatty acid of empirical formula, $C_9H_{18}O_2$, and has a molecular weight of about 1000.

The polymyxins are bactericidal against Gram-negative bacteria (e.g., *Pseudomonas*) and resistance is moderate and slow to develop. These antibiotics apparently act through their cationic surface action (rupture of cell membranes). They are not absorbed orally and are rapidly excreted in the urine after injection. They should probably be limited to use in infections resistant to other antibiotics due to their potential renal damaging effects, and bizarre neurological effects (ataxia, paresthe-

sias, etc.) after injection. These difficulties are not observed with topical or intrathecal use.

It has been reported that calcium, magnesium, manganese, and ferrous ions inhibit the action of polymyxin.

Polymyxin B sulfate is a white to buff powder. It is slightly soluble in alcohol (0.0114%) and freely soluble in water. Its solutions in water are slightly acidic to nearly neutral (pH range, 5–7.5). It is insoluble in benzene, chloroform, ether, and petroleum ether. There is some solubility in glycerin and propylene glycol. The dry powder is stable indefinitely and is quite heat stable. Aqueous solutions are rather stable and can be kept for many months at room temperature, and longer under refrigeration. Moderate changes in pH do not greatly influence the potency. A pH of 3 to 5 favors maximum stability. Alkaline solutions are considerably less stable especially since the free base may be liberated which is only slightly soluble in water and almost insoluble in alcohol. The activity of aqueous solutions is partly destroyed by boiling for more than 10 min. Activity is rapidly lost in strong acids or alkalies. Polymyxin is stable in petrolatum, lanolin, carbowaxes, and polyethylene glycol diesters.

Polyoxyl Stearates [Polyoxyl 40 Stearate USP; Polyoxyethylene 50 Stearate NF; Myrjs (*Atlas*)]—Pharmaceutic aid (surfactant). Mixture of the monostearate and distearate esters of mixed polyoxyethylene diols and corresponding free glycols. *40 USP:* Whitish, waxy solid; odorless or faint odor; congeals about 42°. Soluble in water, alcohol, and ether. *50 NF:* Soft, cream-colored, waxy solid; faint odor; melts about 45°. Soluble in water.

Polysorbates [Polysorbate USP; Monitans (*Ives*); Sorlates (*Abbott*); Tweens (*Atlas*)]—Pharmaceutic aid (surfactant). Fatty acid esters of sorbital and its anhydrides copolymerized with a varying number of moles of ethylene oxide. *80 USP:* Lemon- to amber-colored liquid; oily; faint odor; warm, somewhat bitter taste; sp gr about 1.08;

pH (1 in 20 aq soln) about 7. Very soluble in water (produces odorless and nearly colorless solution); soluble in alcohol.

Polythiazide NF [Renese (*Pfizer*); $C_{11}H_{13}ClF_3N_3O_4S_3$]—Diuretic; antihypertensive. White, crystalline powder; characteristic odor. 1 g dissolves in >1000 ml water, 150 ml alcohol, 175 ml chloroform, and >1000 ml ether.

Dispensing Information: See *Diuretics (Chlorothiazide Type).*

Polyvinyl Alcohol USP [$(C_2H_4O)_n$]— Pharmaceutic aid (vehicle). Vinyl alcohol polymer. Whitish powder or granules; odorless. Freely soluble in water.

Pontocaine HCl Solution 0.5% [*Winthrop*]—Eye Drop. *Known ingredients:* Tetracaine HCl (0.5%), sodium chloride (0.75%), chlorobutanol (0.4%). *Known compatibilities:* Suprarenin (1: 1000).

Pontocaine HCl Solution 2% [*Winthrop*]—Surface anesthetic. *Known ingredients:* Tetracaine HCl (2%), methylene blue, chlorobutanol (0.4%). *Known compatibilities:* Suprarenin 1: 1000.

Potash, Sulfurated, NF [K_2S_x]— Pharmaceutic aid (source of sulfide). Contains potassium polysulfides and potassium thiosulfates. Irregular, liver-brown pieces when freshly made, changing to a greenish yellow; odor of hydrogen sulfide; bitter, acrid, and alkaline taste; decomposes on exposure to air; 1 in 10 solution is light-brown and alkaline to litmus. 1 g dissolves in 10 ml water leaving a slight residue; alcohol dissolves only the sulfides. Containers from which it is to be taken for immediate use in compounding prescriptions contain not more than 120 g. *Known incompatibilities:* acids (hydrogen sulfide being liberated), forms insoluble zinc sulfide and various polysulfides with zinc sulfate.

Potassium Acetate USP [$C_2H_3KO_2$]— Electrolyte replenisher. Colorless, monoclinic crystals or white, crystalline powder; saline and slightly alkaline taste; odorless or faint, acetous odor; deliquesces in moist air; pH (1 in 20

soln) 7.5–8.5. One g dissolves in <1 ml water and 10 ml alcohol.

Potassium Aminosalicylate NF [$C_7H_6KNO_3$]—Antibacterial (tuberculostatic). Whitish, crystalline powder; almost odorless; saline taste; solution decomposes slowly and darkens on standing. Freely soluble in water; sparingly soluble in alcohol; very slightly soluble in chloroform and ether. *Caution: Prepare solutions within 24 hours of administration. Under no circumstances use a solution if its color is darker than the freshly prepared solution.*

Potassium Bicarbonate NF [$KHCO_3$]—Pharmaceutic aid. Colorless, transparent, monoclinic prisms or white, granular powder; odorless; stable in air; solutions are neutral or alkaline to phenolphthalein TS. 1 g dissolves in 10 ml water and >10,000 ml alcohol. *Known incompatibilities:* acids (with liberation of gas).

Potassium Chloride USP [Kay Ciel (*Cooper*); KCl]—Electrolyte replenisher (potassium and chloride). Colorless, elongated, cubical or prismatic crystals or granular powder; odorless; saline taste; stable in air; solution is neutral to litmus. 1 g dissolves in 2.8 ml water and 2 ml boiling water; insoluble in alcohol. *Known incompatibilities* (potassium chloride injection): amphotericin B.

Potassium Citrate NF [$C_6H_5K_3O_7 \cdot H_2O$]—Alkalizer. Transparent crystals or white, granular powder; odorless; cooling, saline taste; deliquescent in moist air. 1 g dissolves in 1 ml water and >10,000 ml alcohol. See also under *Citric Acid.*

Potassium Gluconate NF [Kaon (*Warren-Teed*); $C_6H_{11}KO_7$]—Electrolyte replenisher. White to yellowish white, crystalline powder or granules; odorless; slightly bitter taste; solution is slightly alkaline to litmus. 1 g dissolves in 3 ml water; practically insoluble in dehydrated alcohol, chloroform, and ether.

Potassium Hydroxide USP [KOH]— Pharmaceutic aid (alkalizing agent). White or nearly white, fused masses, small pellets, flakes, sticks, or other forms; hard and brittle; shows a crystalline fracture; in air it rapidly absorbs carbon dioxide and moisture and deliquesces; melts about 360° (380° when anhydrous); produces much heat on solution. 1 g freely soluble in water, alcohol, and glycerin; 1 g in <1 ml boiling alcohol. *Caution:* Exercise great care in handling as it rapidly destroys tissues. *Known incompatibilities:* acids.

Potassium Iodide USP [KI]—Antifungal; expectorant; source of iodine. Crystals; colorless; odorless; characteristic salty taste; hygroscopic; affected by light; solution is neutral or alkaline to litmus. 1 g dissolves in 0.7 ml water, 0.5 ml boiling water, 22 ml alcohol, and 2 ml glycerin. *Known incompatibilities:* acids, precipitates alkaloids.

Potassium Iodide Solution—Antifungal; expectorant; source of iodine. Clear, colorless liquid; odorless; characteristic, strongly salty taste; pH neutral or alkaline to litmus; specific gravity about 1.7. *Known incompatibilities:* reducing agents, acids.

Potassium Metaphosphate NF [KPO_3]—Pharmaceutic aid (buffering agent). White powder; odorless. Insoluble in water; 1 g dissolves in 10–30 ml dilute solutions of sodium salts.

Potassium Permanganate USP [$KMnO_4$]—Topical anti-infective. Dark-purple crystals, almost opaque by transmitted light and of a blue metallic luster by reflected light; its color is sometimes modified by a dark, bronze-like appearance; stable in air. 1 g dissolves in 10–30 ml water and 1–10 ml boiling water. *Known incompatibilities:* reducing agents, sulfides, sulfites, hypophosphites, chlorides, bromides, iodides, arsenites, ferrous salts, most organic substances.

Potassium Phosphate, Monobasic, NF [KH_2PO_4]—Pharmaceutic aid (buffering agent). Colorless crystals or white, granular or crystalline powder; odorless; stable in air; pH (1 in 100 soln) about 4.5. One g dissolves in 1–10 ml water; insoluble in alcohol. *Known incompatibilities* (potassium phosphate

injection): calcium chloride, calcium gluconate.

Potassium Replacement Preparations—*Dispensing Information:* Explain different ways of improving taste of oral liquid supplements (i.e., addition to tomato juice, full dilution, or serving over ice). Explain method of preparation of oral powder dosage forms. Patients who are taking digitalis should be made aware of the hazard of not taking potassium.

Potassium Sodium Tartrate NF [Rochelle Salt; $C_4H_4KNaO_6 \cdot 4H_2O$ or anhydrous]—Cathartic. Colorless crystals or white, crystalline powder; cooling saline taste; effloresces slightly in warm, dry air (crystals often coated with white powder); aqueous solution alkaline to litmus. 1 g dissolves in about 1 ml water; practically insoluble in alcohol. *Known incompatibilities:* acids, calcium salts, magnesium salts, tartrates.

Potassium Sorbate NF [$C_6H_7KO_2$]—Pharmaceutic aid (antimicrobial agent). White crystals or powder; characteristic odor; melts (with decomposition) about 270°. 1 g dissolves in about 5 ml water, 35 ml alcohol, and >1000 ml chloroform and ether.

Povidone-Iodine USP [Betadine (*P-F*): Isodine (*Blair*); complex of iodine with povidone]—Local anti-infective. Yellowish brown, amorphous powder; slight characteristic odor; aqueous solution acid to litmus. Soluble in water and alcohol; practically insoluble in chloroform and ether.

Dispensing Information: Discontinue use if skin rash occurs. Easily removed from skin and most fabrics.

Pralidoxime Chloride USP [Protopam Chloride (*Ayerst*); $C_7H_9ClN_2O$]—Cholinesterase reactivator. Whitish, crystalline powder; odorless; melts (with decomposition) about 220°. Freely soluble in water; slightly soluble in anhydrous alcohol.

Pramoxine Hydrochloride NF [Tronothane (*Abbott*); $C_{17}H_{27}NO_3 \cdot$ HCl]—Topical anesthetic. Whitish, crystalline powder; numbing taste; may have slight odor; pH (1 in 100 soln) about 4.5; melts about 172°. Freely soluble in water and alcohol; 1 g dissolves in about 35 ml chloroform; very slightly soluble in ether.

Prednisolone USP [*Various Mfrs.;* $C_{21}H_{28}O_5$]—Glucocorticoid. White to practically white, crystalline powder; odorless; melts about 235° with slight decomposition. Very slightly soluble in water; sparingly soluble in alcohol; slightly soluble in chloroform.

Dispensing Information: See *Corticosteroids (Systemic).*

Prednisolone Acetate USP [Meticortelone (*Schering*); Nisolone (*Ascher*); Sterane (*Pfizer*); $C_{23}H_{30}O_6$]—Glucocorticoid. Whitish, crystalline powder; odorless; melts (with some decomposition) about 235°. Practically insoluble in water; slightly soluble in chloroform; 1 g dissolves in about 120 ml alcohol and 150 ml chloroform.

Prednisolone Sodium Phosphate USP [Hydeltrasol (*MSD*); $C_{21}H_{27}Na_2O_8P$]—Glucocorticoid. The white, slightly hygroscopic powder is stable at room temperature. It is soluble in water, methanol, ethanol. The pH of a 1% aqueous solution is 7.5–8.5. *Known incompatibilities* (prednisolone sodium phosphate injection): calcium gluconate glucoheptonate, polymyxin B sulfate.

Dispensing Information: See *Corticosteroids (Systemic).*

Prednisolone Sodium Succinate USP [Meticortelone (*Schering*); $C_{25}H_{31}NaO_8$]—Glucocorticoid. Soluble form suitable for parenteral injection. *Known incompatibilities* (prednisolone sodium succinate for injection): allopurinol sodium, mercaptopurine sodium.

Prednisolone Succinate USP [$C_{25}H_{32}O_8$]—Glucocorticoid. Used to prepare *Prednisolone Sodium Succinate.* Fine, creamy white powder with friable lumps; practically odorless; melts (with decomposition) about 205°. 1 g dissolves in about 4200 ml water, 6 ml alcohol, 1100 ml chloroform, and 250 ml ether.

Prednisolone Tebutate USP [prednisolone *tert*-butylacetate; Hydeltra T.B.A. (*MSD*); $C_{27}H_{38}O_6$ or monohydrate]—Glucocorticoid. Whitish powder; odorless or not more than moderate odor; practically tasteless; hygroscopic (absorbs moisture equilibrating at monohydrate); melts about 245°. Very slightly soluble in water; freely soluble in chloroform; sparingly soluble in alcohol.

Prednisone USP [*Various Mfrs.;* $C_{21}H_{26}O_5$]—Glucocorticoid. White to practically white, crystalline powder; odorless; melts about 225° with slight decomposition. Very slightly soluble in water; slightly soluble in alcohol and chloroform.

Dispensing Information: Do not exceed directed dosage. Consult physician if signs of infection (sore throat, cold, etc.), blood in stools, or vomiting of coffee-ground-colored material (ulcerogenic) develop. See also *Corticosteroids (Systemic).*

Prilocaine Hydrochloride NF [Citanest HCl (*Astra*); $C_{13}H_{20}N_2O \cdot HCl$; p$K_a$ 7.89]—Local anesthetic. White, crystalline powder; odorless; initial acid, followed by bitter taste; melts about 167°. 1 g dissolves in about 4 ml water, 5 ml alcohol, and 175 ml chloroform.

Primaquine Phosphate USP [*Winthrop;* $C_{15}H_{21}N_3O \cdot 2H_3PO_4$]—Antimalarial. Orange-red, crystalline powder; odorless; bitter taste; solution acid to litmus; melts about 200°. 1 g dissolves in about 15 ml water; insoluble in chloroform and ether.

Primidone USP [Mysoline (*Ayerst*); $C_{12}H_{14}N_2O_2$]—Anticonvulsant. White, crystalline powder; odorless; slightly bitter; melts 279–284°. Very slightly soluble in water and most organic solvents; slightly soluble in alcohol.

Dispensing Information: Do not drive or operate heavy machinery during first few weeks of therapy.

Probenecid USP [Benemid (*MSD*); $C_{13}H_{19}NO_4S$]—Uricosuric. Whitish, fine, crystalline powder; practically odorless; melts about 199°. Practically insoluble in water; soluble in alcohol, chloroform, and ether.

Dispensing Information: Contraindicated in previous history of blood dyscrasias. Interactions: antagonized by salicylates; increases penicillin and sulfonamide plasma levels; potentiates sulfonylureas; causes false positive Benedict's test. Mild nausea may occur at onset of therapy. Do not take aspirin-containing products without consulting physician. Discontinue use and consult physician if dermatitis, dizziness, or flushing occur.

Procainamide Hydrochloride USP [Pronestyl (*Squibb*); $C_{13}H_{21}N_3O \cdot HCl$] —Cardiac depressant (anti-arrhythmic). Whitish, crystalline powder; odorless; pH (1 in 10 soln) 5–6.5; melts about 167°. Very soluble in water; soluble in alcohol; slightly soluble in chloroform; very slightly soluble in ether. *Known incompatibilities* (procainamide HCl injection): phenytoin sodium.

Dispensing Information: The patient may be given a card containing the following information:

It is important that you take this medication as specified on the package label. If you unexpectedly run out of medication before your next doctor's appointment, call your doctor and inform him of this. As with all medications, *procainamide* can cause some side effects. Nausea, vomiting or diarrhea, may occur with this drug. If these symptoms are particularly troublesome or persist for several days notify your physician. Skin rash, fever, chills, sore throat, joint and muscle pains may rarely result from taking procainamide. If you develop any of these symptoms they should be brought to the attention of your physician without delay.

Procaine Hydrochloride USP [Novocain (*Winthrop*); (*Various Other Mfrs.*); $C_{13}H_{20}N_2O_2 \cdot HCl$]—Local anesthetic. Precipitated by the hydroxides and carbonates of the alkali metals and by alkaloidal precipitants such as iodine, picric acid, and tannic acid. It is also incompatible with mercurous chloride, mercuric chloride, iodides, dichromates, permanganates, and silver salts. Procaine hydrochloride is a white, crystalline powder and is stable in air. It is soluble in water (1:1) and alcohol (1:30). When reacted with an equivalent of sodium carbonate, soluble procaine carbonate is formed. This soon breaks down to insoluble procaine base, i.e.,

$$2 \text{ Procaine HCl} + Na_2CO_3 \rightarrow$$
$$(\text{Procaine})_2 \, H_2CO_3 \rightarrow$$
$$\text{Procaine} \downarrow + CO_2 + H_2O$$

Excess sodium carbonate immediately precipitates the free base.

Sodium bicarbonate even in excess forms a solution of procaine bicarbonate which is stable for several days before forming procaine, carbon dioxide, and water.

A decrease in anesthetic activity in mixtures of glucose and procaine has been noted. This is apparently due to formation of procaine *N*-glucoside. This reaction is exothermic so refrigerator storage of the procaine solution is not advised.

Procaine hydrochloride, being the salt of a weak base and a strong acid, undergoes hydrolysis to a slight extent in aqueous solution at ordinary temperature to yield a slightly acid solution, a 2% solution having a pH of 5.8. Procaine HCl solutions are stable for long periods at pH 4.5. The extent of hydrolysis is increased during sterilization of the solution by heat. Alkaline solutions of procaine cannot be stored for any considerable length of time or sterilized by heating, owing to the decomposition which ensues

The yellow degradation product of procaine which appears in bisulfite solutions at pH 2 is reported to be the sulfonic acid derivative which may be prevented from forming by using the proper amount of bisulfite at pH above 4. Potassium metabisulfite has no inhibiting influence on the hydrolytic cleavage of procaine but prevents the oxidative discoloration of para-aminobenzoic acid. Acetone-bisulfite and bisulfite-metabisulfite are very effective in stabilizing procaine-epinephrine solutions. Sodium sulfite is less effective while ascorbic acid is entirely unsuitable.

Procarbazine Hydrochloride USP [Matulane (*Roche*); $C_{12}H_{19}N_3O \cdot HCl$; pK_a (room temp) 6.8]—Antineoplastic. Whitish, crystalline powder; slight odor; bitter taste; solution acid to litmus; slowly oxidized in air; melts (with decomposition) about 223°. 1 g dissolves in about 7 ml water, 100 ml alcohol, and 1000 ml chloroform and ether.

Prochlorperazine USP [Compazine (*SK&F*); $C_{20}H_{24}ClN_3S$]—Tranquilizer; antiemetic. *Side effects:* Contraindicated in coma and marked central nervous system depression of drug origin. Mild side effects include somnolence, dizziness, moderate hypotension, tachycardia, blurred vision, dryness of mouth, and spasms of the voluntary muscles of the neck region.

Dispensing Information: See *Antipsychotic Agents (Phenothiazine Type)*.

Prochlorperazine Edisylate USP [Compazine Ethanedisulfonate (*SK&F*); $C_{20}H_{24}ClN_3S \cdot C_2H_6O_6S_2$]— Antiemetic; tranquilizer. Whitish, crystalline powder; odorless; solution acid to litmus. 1 g dissolves in about 2 ml water and 1500 ml alcohol; insoluble in chloroform and ether. *Known incompatibilities* (prochlorperazine edisylate injection): aminophylline, amobarbital sodium, chloramphenicol sodium succinate, chlorothiazide sodium, cyanocobalamin, erythromycin glucceptate, heparin sodium, hydrocortisone sodium succinate, kanamycin sulfate, levallorphan, meralluride, methicillin sodium, oxytetracycline HCl, paraldehyde, penicillin G potassium, penicillin G sodium, pentobarbital sodium, pentylenetetrazol, phenobarbital sodium, phenytoin sodium, sulfisoxazole, tetracycline HCl, thiopental sodium, vancomycin HCl.

Prochlorperazine Maleate USP [Compazine Dimaleate (*SK&F*); $C_{20}H_{24}ClN_3S \cdot 2C_4H_4O_4$]—Antiemetic; tranquilizer. Whitish, crystalline powder; practically odorless; saturated solution acid to litmus. Practically insoluble in water; 1 g dissolves in about 1200 ml alcohol; slightly soluble in warm chloroform.

Procyclidine Hydrochloride NF [Kemadrin (*B-W*); $C_{19}H_{29}NO \cdot HCl$]— Anticholinergic. White, crystalline powder; moderate odor; melts about 226°. 1 g dissolves in about 33 ml water and 15 ml alcohol; more soluble in chloroform; very slightly soluble in ether.

Progesterone USP [Proluton (*Schering*); $C_{21}H_{30}O_2$]—Progestin. White, crystalline, odorless powder. It is practically insoluble in water (0.01 mg/ml) and soluble in alcohol. It is stable in air but is sensitive to light.

Promazine Hydrochloride NF [Sparine (*Wyeth*); $C_{17}H_{20}N_2S \cdot HCl$]— Tranquilizer (major). White to slightly yellow, crystalline powder; practically odorless; oxidizes upon prolonged exposure to air and acquires a blue or pink color. 1 g dissolves in 3 ml water; freely soluble in chloroform. *Side effects:* Drowsiness, dizziness, and postural hypotension may occur. It potentiates barbiturates. Transient leukopenia, agranulocytosis, and convulsive seizures have been observed.

Known incompatibilities (promazine hydrochloride injection): aminophylline, chloramphenicol sodium succinate, chlorothiazide sodium, chlortetracycline HCl, dimenhydrinate, ethamivan, heparin sodium, fibrinolysin, hydrocortisone sodium succinate, menadione sodium bisulfite, penicillin G potassium, penicillin G sodium, pentobarbital sodium, phenobarbital sodium, phenytoin sodium, phytonadione, protein hydrolysate, sodium bicarbonate, sulfisoxazole, thiopental sodium, vitamin B complex with C, warfarin sodium.

Promethazine Hydrochloride USP [Phenergan (*Wyeth*); Remsed (*Endo*); $C_{17}H_{20}N_2S \cdot HCl$] —Antihistaminic. Whitish, crystalline powder; practically odorless; slowly oxidized (particularly when moistened) in air turning blue; pH (1 in 20 soln) about 4.7; melts (3° range) about 220°. 1 g dissolves in about 0.6 ml water, 9 ml alcohol, and 2 ml chloroform; practically insoluble in ether. *Known incompatibilities* (promethazine HCl injection): aminophylline, calcium gluconate, chlordiazepoxide HCl, codeine sulfate, ethamivan, hydrocortisone sodium succinate, methylprednisolone, penicillin G salts, phenobarbital sodium, phenytoin sodium, sulfisoxazole, vitamin B complex with C.

Promethestrol Dipropionate [Meprane Dipropionate (*R&C*)]—Estrogen.

White, odorless, crystalline powder. It is slightly soluble in alcohol and practically insoluble in water. Solutions of promethestrol dipropionate in 90% alcohol are neutral to litmus (pH range, 4.5–8).

Propantheline Bromide USP [Pro-Banthine (*Searle*); $C_{23}H_{30}BrNO_3$]—Anticholinergic. Whitish crystals; odorless; bitter taste; melts (with decomposition) 156–162°. Very soluble in water, alcohol, and chloroform; practically insoluble in ether.

Dispensing Information: See *Anticholinergic Agents.*

Proparacaine Hydrochloride USP [Ophthaline (*Squibb*); Ophthetic (*Allergan*); $C_{16}H_{26}N_2O_3 \cdot HCl$]—Topical anesthetic (ophthalmic). Whitish, crystalline powder; odorless; discolors on heating or in air; solution discolors and becomes dark in air (some loss of potency); solution neutral to litmus; melts (2° range) about 182°. 1 g dissolves in about 30 ml water and warm alcohol; insoluble in ether. *Known incompatibilities:* alkalies (liberate free base).

Propiomazine Hydrochloride NF [Largon HCl (*Wyeth*); $C_{20}H_{24}N_2OS \cdot HCl$]—Sedative. Yellow powder; practically odorless; slowly oxidized when moistened or in aqueous solution in air and light; melts about 203°. 1 g dissolves in <1 ml water, 6 ml alcohol, and 2 ml chloroform; practically insoluble in ether.

Propionic Acid [methyl acetic acid; $C_3H_6O_2$; pK_a 4.88]—Propionic acid, useful as a topical fungicide, is a weaker acid than acetic acid, which it resembles in chemical properties. It is miscible with water and soluble in alcohol, ether, and chloroform. The pH of a 1% aqueous solution is about 3. Its salts are soluble in water; however, the acid can be salted out of water by calcium chloride and other salts. Sodium propionate is soluble in water (1:1) and alcohol (1:24). It is most effective as a fungicide at pH 5.5 in combination with propionic acid.

Propoxycaine Hydrochloride NF [Blockain (*Breon*); $C_{16}H_{26}N_2O_3 \cdot HCl$; pK_a 8.6]—Local anesthetic. White, crystalline solid; odorless; discolors in light and air; melts about 148°; pH (1 in 50 soln) about 5.4. One g dissolves in about 2 ml water, 10 ml alcohol, and 80 ml ether; insoluble in chloroform.

Propoxyphene   Hydrochloride USP [Darvon *Lilly*); SK-65 (*SK&F*); $C_{22}H_{29}NO_2 \cdot HCl$]—Analgesic.   White, crystalline powder; odorless; bitter taste; melts (3° range) 163.5–168.5°. Freely soluble in water; soluble in alcohol and chloroform; practically insoluble in ether.

Dispensing Information: Drowsiness, dizziness, and other nervous system effects can occur and should be brought to the attention of the physician.

Propoxyphene Napsylate NF [Darvon-N (*Lilly*); $C_{22}H_{29}NO_2 \cdot C_{10}H_8O_3S \cdot H_2O$ or anhydrous]—Analgesic. White, crystalline powder; essentially odorless; bitter taste; melts (4° range) 158–165°. 1 g dissolves in about 10,000 ml water, 15 ml alcohol, and 10 ml chloroform.

Propranolol Hydrochloride USP [Inderal (*Ayerst*); $C_{16}H_{21}NO_2 \cdot HCl$]—Cardiac depressant (antiarrhythmic). Whitish, crystalline powder; odorless; bitter taste; melts about 161°. Soluble in water and alcohol; slightly soluble in chloroform; practically insoluble in ether.

Dispensing Information: Do not abruptly stop therapy without consulting the physician. The patient may be given the following information with the medication.

The following will give you a better understanding of this medication: This medication may occasionally cause nausea, diarrhea and fatigue. This medication should be taken on an empty stomach, at the same time every day and on an evenly spaced schedule, i.e., every 6 hours (if 4 times a day). *If prescribed for high blood pressure, the pharmacist may advise patient as follows:* One of the mechanisms by which this drug works to lower your blood pressure is to slow down the rate at which your heart beats; notify your physician if your pulse is less than 50 beats/min.

Propylene Glycol USP [$C_3H_8O_2$]—Pharmaceutic aid (humectant; solvent). Propylene glycol is a viscous, hygroscopic solvent which has a lower specific gravity and viscosity than glycerin and a rather acrid taste. It is considered practically nontoxic, although many of the glycols are poisonous. Propylene glycol is miscible with water, chloroform, and acetone but not with fixed oils. It inhibits mold growth and fermentation. The pink color which frequently develops in preparations containing propylene glycol may be caused by impurities in the propylene glycol.

Propylene Glycol Monostearate NF—Pharmaceutic aid (emulsifying agent). Mixture of the propylene glycol mono- and diesters of stearic and palmitic acids. White solid, beads, or flakes; wax-like; slight odor and taste; congeals not lower than 45°. Insoluble in water (may be dispersed in hot water with small amount of soap or other surface-active agent); dissolves in alcohol and ether.

Propylhexedrine NF [Benzedrex (*SK&F*); $C_{10}H_{21}N$]—Adrenergic (vasoconstrictor). Clear, colorless liquid; characteristic odor; solution alkaline to litmus; volatilizes slowly at room temperature; sp gr about 0.850; boils about 205°. 1 g dissolves in >500 ml water, 0.5 ml alcohol and chloroform, and 0.1 ml ether.

Propyliodone USP [Dionosil (*Glaxco*); $C_{10}H_{11}I_2NO_3$]—Diagnostic aid (radiopaque medium). Whitish, crystalline powder; odorless or faint odor; melts about 188°. Practically insoluble in water; soluble in alcohol and ether.

Propylparaben USP [$C_{10}H_{12}O_3$]—Pharmaceutic aid (antifungal agent). Soluble in 2000 parts of water; it is soluble in alcohol (see *Methylparaben*).

Propylthiouracil USP [*Various Mfrs.;* $C_7H_{10}N_2OS$]—Thyroid inhibitor. White, crystalline powder; starch-like in appearance and to touch; bitter taste; melts about 219°. 1 g dissolves in about 900 ml water and 60 ml alcohol; slightly soluble in chloroform and ether.

Prostigmin Methylsulfate Ampul [*Roche*]—*Known ingredient:* neostigmine (1:2000). *Known compatibilities:* ascorbic acid, atropine, Berocca C, Demerol, Dromoran or Levo-Dromoran, morphine sulfate, Nisentil, Pantopon,

Synkavite Ampul, thiamine HCl. *Known incompatibilities:* none listed.

Protamine Sulfate USP—Antidote to heparin. Mixture of simple protein principles from the sperm or testes of suitable species of fish having the property of neutralizing heparin. Fine, whitish, crystalline powder; amorphous; hygroscopic. Sparingly soluble in water.

Protriptyline Hydrochloride NF [Vivactil HCl (*MSD*); $C_{19}H_{21}N \cdot HCl$]—Antidepressant. Whitish powder; odorless or slight odor; bitter taste; melts about 168°. 1 g dissolves in about 2 ml water, 4 ml alcohol, and 2.3 ml chloroform; practically insoluble in ether.

Pseudoephedrine Hydrochloride NF [Sudafed (*B-W*); $C_{10}H_{15}NO \cdot HCl$]—Adrenergic. Fine, white to off-white powder or crystals; faint, characteristic odor; solution is neutral to litmus; melts 181–186°. One g dissolves in 0.5 ml water, 3.6 ml alcohol, 90 ml chloroform, and 7000 ml ether.

Dispensing Information: Do not exceed recommended dosage. Do not use if hypertensive, diabetic, coronary patient, or thyroid patient except on the advice of the physician. Reduce dosage if nervousness, restlessness, or sleeplessness occur.

Pyrantel Pamoate [Antiminth (*Roerig*); $C_{11}H_{14}N_2S \cdot C_{23}H_{16}O_6$]—Anthelmintic. Yellowish powder; odorless; tasteless; decomposes slowly in light; melts (with decomposition) about 254°. Insoluble in water; very slightly soluble in alcohol.

Pyrazinamide USP [aldinamide; *MSD; Lederle;* $C_5H_5N_3O$]—Antibacterial (tuberculostatic). Whitish, crystalline powder; odorless or almost so; aqueous solution neutral to litmus; melts about 189°. 1 g dissolves in 67 ml water, 135 ml chloroform, and 1000 ml ether; slightly soluble in alcohol.

Pyribenzamine Ointment (and Cream) [*Ciba*]—*Known ingredients:* Pyribenzamine Hydrochloride 2% in a petrolatum base (or water-washable vehicle). *Known incompatibilities:* None of the commonly used ointments or creams that have been tested have been found incompatible.

Pyribenzamine Elixir [*Ciba*]— *Known ingredients:* Pyribenzamine Hydrochloride, alcohol, green dye, cinnamon flavor. *Known incompatibilities:* aminophylline (after 1 month), Amytal Sodium, Elkosin Suspension, iodides, pentobarbital sodium, phenobarbital sodium, Propadrine Elixir, sodium salicylate (slightly cloudy).

Pyribenzamine Expectorant with Ephedrine [*Ciba*] (with or without codeine)—*Known ingredients:* Pyribenzamine Citrate (30 mg/4 ml), ephedrine sulfate (10 mg/4 ml), ammonium chloride (80 mg/4 ml), codeine phosphate (4 or 8 mg/ml). *Known compatibilities and incompatibilities:* same as *Pyribenzamine Elixir.*

Pyridostigmine Bromide USP [Mestinon (*Roche*); $C_9H_{13}BrN_2O_2$]— Cholinergic. Whitish, crystalline powder; agreeable odor; hygroscopic; melts about 153°. Freely soluble in water, alcohol, and chloroform; practically insoluble in ether.

Pyridoxine Hydrochloride USP [vitamin B_6 hydrochloride; Hexabetalin (*Lilly*); $C_8H_{11}NO_3HCl$]—Enzyme cofactor vitamin. White, crystalline powder of which 1 g is soluble in about 5 ml of water or 100 ml of alcohol. A 1% aqueous solution has a pH of 3. In the solid form it is stable in air but slowly destroyed by light. Aqueous solutions are stable to heat and acid, but the stability decreases as the pH is raised. Solutions having a pH not greater than 5 may be autoclaved at 120°C for 20 min without significant deterioration.

Pyridoxine is amphoteric but is stronger as a base than as an acid and is generally used as the hydrochloride. Due to the phenolic group, it has some of the incompatibilities of phenols.

Pyrilamine Maleate NF [*Various Mfrs.;* $C_{17}H_{23}N_3O \cdot C_4H_4O_4$]—Antihistaminic. White crystalline powder. It is very soluble in water and freely soluble in alcohol. A 5% aqueous solution is slightly acidic (pH range, 4.5–5.5).

Pyrimethamine USP [Daraprim (*B-W*); $C_{12}H_{13}ClN_4$]—Antimalarial. White, crystalline powder; odorless; melts about 240°. Practically insoluble in water; 1 g dissolves in about 200 ml alcohol and 125 ml chloroform.

Pyroxylin USP [soluble guncotton]— Pharmaceutic aid for *Collodion.* From the action of a mixture of nitric and sulfuric acids on cotton; consists chiefly of cellulose tetranitrate. Light yellow mass of filaments (resembles raw cotton); decomposes in well-closed containers in light. Insoluble in water; dissolves slowly in 25 parts of a mixture of ether (3 vols) and alcohol (1 vol). *Caution: very flammable (burns very rapidly with luminous flame).*

Pyrrobutamine Phosphate NF [Pyronil (*Lilly*); $C_{20}H_{22}ClN \cdot 2H_3PO_4$]— Antihistaminic. Whitish, crystalline powder; may have a faint odor; melts about 129°. Soluble in water (1 g dissolves in about 10 ml warm water); 1 g dissolves in about 20 ml alcohol; practically insoluble in chloroform and ether.

Pyrrocaine Hydrochloride NF [Endocaine HCl (*Endo*); $C_{14}H_{20}N_2O \cdot HCl$]—Local anesthetic. White, crystalline powder; odorless; melts about 202°. 1 g dissolves in about 2 ml water, 12 ml alcohol, and 8 ml chloroform; soluble in ether.

Pyrvinium Pamoate USP [Povan (*P-D*); $C_{75}H_{70}N_6O_6$]—Anthelmintic (intestinal pinworms). Bright, orangy to almost black, crystalline powder. Practically insoluble in water and ether; slightly soluble in chloroform; very slightly soluble in alcohol.

Quinacrine Hydrochloride USP [Atabrine HCl (*Winthrop*); mepacrine hydrochloride; $C_{23}H_{30}ClN_3O \cdot 2HCl$]— Anthelmintic (intestinal tapeworms). 1 g of this amine is soluble in 35 ml of water and is soluble in alcohol; a 1% aqueous solution has a pH of about 4.5. In aqueous solution, quinacrine hydrochloride gradually hydrolyzes, forming a precipitate of 2-methoxy-6-chloroacridine. *Caution:* Quinacrine hydrochloride sometimes causes yellowing of the skin, urine, and eyes and other toxic reactions. *Known incompatibilities* (quinacrine HCl for injection): alkali metals, nitrates, oxidizing agents.

Quinethazone NF [Hydromox (*Lederle*); $C_{10}H_{12}ClN_3O_3S$]—Diuretic. Whitish, crystalline powder; odorless; bitter taste; discolors in strong light and alkaline materials; melts about 251°. Very slightly soluble in water; 1 g dissolves in about 500 ml alcohol.

Quinidine [$C_{20}H_{24}N_2O_2$; pK_{b1} 5.46, pK_{b2} 10.0]—Cardiac depressant. It is a stereoisomer of quinine and has similar incompatibilities. 1 g dissolves in about 2000 ml cold (800 ml boiling) water.

Dispensing Information: See *Quinidine Preparations.*

Quinidine Gluconate USP [Quinaglute (*Cooper*); $C_{20}H_{24}N_2O_2 \cdot C_6H_{12}O_7$]— Cardiac depressant (antiarrhythmic). The gluconate of an alkaloid from various species of *Cinchona* and hybrids, or from *Remijia pedunculata*. White powder; odorless; bitter taste. 1 g dissolves in about 9 ml water and 60 ml alcohol. *Known incompatibilities* (quinidine gluconate injection): alkaline solutions, iodides.

Quinidine Polygalacturonate — More water-soluble salt than *Quinidine Sulfate, qv.*

Quinidine Preparations—*Dispensing Information:* Patient may be given the following information concerning these medications. It is important that you take this medication as specified on the package label. If you unexpectedly run out of medication before your next doctor's appointment, call your doctor and inform him of this. As with all medications, *quinidine* can cause some side effects. Nausea, vomiting or diarrhea, may occur with this drug. If these symptoms are particularly troublesome or persist for several days notify your physician. Skin rash, ringing in the ears, and blurred vision also may occur. These symptoms should be brought to the attention of your physician without delay.

Quinidine Sulfate USP [*Various Mfrs.;* $(C_{20}H_{24}N_2O_2)_2 \cdot H_2SO_4 \cdot 2H_2O$]— Cardiac depressant (antiarrhythmic).

Fine, needle-like, white crystals or fine, white powder; odorless; very bitter taste; darkens in light; solution is neutral or slightly alkaline to litmus. Slightly soluble in water; soluble in alcohol and chloroform; insoluble in ether.

Dispensing Information: See *Quinidine Preparations.*

Quinine [pK_{b1} 6.0; pK_{b2} 9.89]—Quinine alkaloid is a white powder; 1 g dissolves in 1560 ml of water or 1 ml of alcohol. The alcoholic solution is alkaline as is the saturated aqueous solution (pH 8.8). Quinine has 2 nitrogen atoms which can form salts (pK_{b1} = 5.97; pK_{b2} = 9.9). This gives rise to diacid and monoacid salts. The diacid ("acid" or "bi" salts) may be quite acid, e.g., quinine bisulfate (pH *circa* 3.5) and quinine dihydrochloride (pH *circa* 2.6). The monoacid salts ("neutral salts") involve only the tertiary nitrogen in the quinuclidine nucleus and are approximately neutral, e.g., quinine sulfate (pH 6.2, saturated solution), quinine hydrochloride (pH *circa* 6), and quinine phosphate (pH slightly acid). The acid salts such as the bisulfate and dihydrochloride are soluble in water and alcohol, and the solutions are strongly acid. The hydrochloride, hydrobromide, and sulfate (in aqueous solution) are neutral or only slightly alkaline. The hydrochloride (1 g) dissolves in 16 ml of water or 1 ml of alcohol, the hydrobromide in 40 ml of water or 1 ml of alcohol, and the sulfate in 810 ml of water or 120 ml of alcohol. The phosphate and salicylate are only sparingly soluble in water.

In solutions of quinine salts there is a precipitate on addition of acetates, citrates, benzoates, and salicylates, except in acid solution, but bromides and iodides ordinarily do not cause precipitation. When quinine sulfate (in aqueous solution) is treated with acetic acid, citric acid, or hypophosphorous acid, and an excess of the corresponding potassium salt, quinine is precipitated in each case as a normal salt, e.g., quinine acetate, rather than as a complex compound. Alkalies and the general alkaloidal precipitants cause precipitation in solutions of quinine salts. In mixtures of organic acids and quinine there is a gradual darkening and formation of the toxic quinotoxine, which results from the opening of one of the piperidine rings in the quinine molecule. However, powders containing quinine and acetylsalicylic acid are considered perfectly safe to dispense and use unless they are kept for such a long time that darkening and decomposition occur, in which case they should be discarded.

Dispensing Information: Potentiates coumarins. Consult physician if tinnitus, dizziness, or other audio problems develop, or if skin rash occurs.

Quinine and Urea Hydrochloride [(*P-D*);$C_{20}H_{24}N_2O_2$·HCl+$CO(NH_2)_2$]— This sclerotic complex is soluble 1 g in 1 ml of water or 3 ml of alcohol. Its aqueous solutions are strongly acid (pH of 5% aqueous solution is about 3.1) and decompose on addition of alkali hydroxides with precipitation of quinine.

Quinine Salts—See under *Quinine.*

Quinine Sulfate USP [*Various Mfrs.;* $(C_{20}H_{24}N_2O_2)_2$·H_2SO_4·$2H_2O$]— Antimalarial. White, fine, needle-like crystals; usually lusterless; making a light and readily compressible mass; odorless; persistent, very bitter taste; darkens in light; saturated solution neutral or alkaline to litmus. Slightly soluble in water, alcohol, chloroform, and ether.

Dispensing Information: See under *Quinine.*

Raspberry Syrup—Raspberry syrup has the same incompatibilities as cherry syrup.

The pH values of a number of manufactured liquids often used as oral vehicles are given in *Husa's Pharmaceutical Dispensing,* 6th ed, Mack Publ. Co., Easton PA, 767–775, 1966.

Rauwolfia Serpentina NF [Raudixin (*Squibb*); (*Various Other Mfrs.*)]— Antihypertensive. This is the powdered whole root of *Rauwolfia serpentina* (Benth). The chief alkaloid is reserpine. This is a light brown, amorphous pow-

der. It is very slightly soluble in water and sparingly soluble in alcohol. *Side effects:* Commonly, nasal stuffiness, weight gain, diarrhea, dryness of mouth, insomnia, nervousness, chronic fatigue, agitated or paranoid depression, and nightmares. Peptic ulcers and skin eruptions occur rarely.

Dispensing Information: See under *Reserpine.*

Reagent Tablets or Strips—*Dispensing Information:* Make certain patient knows how to perform the test. Patient also needs color comparator insert. Patient should know when to report findings to the physician.

Regitine Injectable Solution [*Ciba* brand, phentolamine methanesulfonate]—Adrenergic blocking agent. *Known ingredients:* Regitine (5 mg/ml), water. *Known compatibilities:* Levophed Bitartrate Solution. *Known incompatibilities:* none listed.

Regroton Tablets [*USV*]—Contain chlorthalidone 50 mg, reserpine 0.25 mg.

Dispensing Information: Contraindicated in pregnancy; warnings in diabetes. and hyperuricemia. Consult physician immediately if yellowing of eyes or skin, sore throat, fever, easy bruising, purple spots beneath skin, or epigastric pain occur. Take with a glass of orange juice.

Rescinnamine [Moderil (*Pfizer*); $C_{35}H_{42}N_2O_9$]—Antihypertensive. From *Rauwolfia vomitoria,* other species of *Rauwolfia,* or produced synthetically. Whitish, crystalline powder; odorless; darkens slowly in light (more rapidly in solution); melts about 226°. Practically insoluble in water; 1 g dissolves in about 500 ml alcohol and 8 ml chloroform.

Reserpine USP [Serpasil (*Ciba*); (*Various Other Mfrs.*); $C_{33}H_{40}N_2O_9$]— Antihypertensive. This is a pure, crystalline alkaloid obtained from *Rauwolfia serpentina* (Benth).

It is a white to light yellow, crystalline material that is very slightly soluble in water (1:10,000) and in alcohol (1:1800). A saturated aqueous solution has a pH of about 4.5–6. Reserpine is reported easily isomerized and decomposed by air, light, and heat. Ultraviolet light changes the reserpine acid portion of the molecule to lumireserpine.

Investigators have reported that reserpine can be heated to 120°C at pH 2 for 2 hours without hydrolysis. At pH 8.5, 30% is hydrolyzed after 20 min heating in an autoclave. In an acid medium the amount of trimethoxybenzoic acid represents the degree of hydrolysis, whereas in an alkaline medium the amount of reserpic acid expresses the percentage that is hydrolyzed. Trimethoxybenzoic acid is decomposed in alkaline media.

Reserpine injection solutions can be autoclaved and stored for 6 months at pH 3 if they contain 25% Carbowax 400, 10% ethanol, and 1% citric acid.

Reserpine can be made soluble with a minimum of acid in the presence of metrazol, urethan, and succinonitrile. Solutions are stable during 20 min of sterilization.

Mixtures of rauwolfia alkaloids with sodium salicylate or with sodium salicylate and theobromine become discolored, wet, and liquid even in winter in less than a week. Rauwolfia alkaloids with other alkaloids such as quinine HCl or with ephedrine HCl become wet within 4–5 days after storing. Mixtures of rauwolfia alkaloids with pyrazolone derivatives, sulfamides, digestive enzyme preparations, or with theophylline derivatives also become wet or discolored and are not suited for storage, especially in summer.

Side effects: May include nasal stuffiness, weight gain, diarrhea, dryness of mouth, and insomnia; also nervousness, fatigue, agitated or paranoid depression, and nightmares. Peptic ulcers and skin eruptions occur rarely.

Dispensing Information: Consult physician if GI disturbances or any change in mood occur.

Reserpoid Elixir [*Upjohn*]—Reserpine 0.25 mg/ml in alcoholic vehicle. Reserpoid Elixir may be diluted with water or syrup and certain other fluid preparations provided the pH is maintained below pH 6. At pH 6.8–10 reserpine precipitates and crystals develop rapidly.

Resorcinol USP [resorcin; $C_6H_6O_2$; pK_a 9.44; pH 5.2]—Resorcinol is an antiseptic which dissolves 1 g in 1 ml of alcohol or water and is freely soluble in ether and glycerin. Aqueous solutions of resorcin darken on exposure to light and air and then become pink, red, and finally brown, the change being hastened by moisture, copper, alkalies, and oxidizing agents. The color change may be retarded by use of 0.5 to 1% ascorbic acid. The discoloration of resorcinol eye drops is catalyzed by copper, and the solution can be stabilized by the use of 0.05% sodium metabisulfite and double distilled water. It has been recommended that 0.01% thiourea, 0.005% oxyquinoline sulfate, or 0.005% disodium ethylenediamine tetraacetate with citrate buffer for this purpose. Resorcinol in hair preparations tends to discolor gray or white hair. Resorcinol gives a violet color with ferric salts; it is not precipitated by lead acetate. Resorcinol is a reducing agent; it reduces ammoniated mercury to metallic mercury, even in ointments. It also reduces bismuth compounds. With strong iodine solutions, resorcinol forms the insoluble 2,4,6-triiodoresorcinol.

Resorcinol Monoacetate NF [Euresol (*Knoll*); $C_8H_8O_3$]—Antiseborrheic; keratolytic. Yellowish liquid; viscous; faint odor; burning taste; sp gr about 1.205; boils (with decomposition) about 283°; saturated aqueous solution acid to litmus. Sparingly soluble in water; dissolves in alcohol and most organic solvents; soluble in fixed bases but solutions of such are not stable.

Riboflavin USP [vitamin B_2; lactoflavin, vitamin G; $C_{17}H_{20}N_4O_6$; pK_a 10.2, pK_b 1.7]—Enzyme co-factor vitamin. Riboflavin is an orange-yellow powder; it has a slight odor and a bitter taste. It is soluble 1 g in about 10,000 ml of water (from 3000 to 15,000 ml depending on the crystal structure) or 25,000 ml of alcohol. It is slightly more soluble in NaCl solutions and very soluble in alkaline solutions. The solubility of riboflavin in water is increased by *N*-methylacetamide, L-tyrosine amide, tryptophan, sodium acetyl tryptophan, urea, urethane, veratryl alcohol, benzyl alcohol, gallic acid, sodium 3-hydroxy-2-naphthoate or by liver extract, propylene glycol, or nicotinamide. The pH of a saturated aqueous solution of riboflavin is approximately 6.

Many of these solubilizers have been covered by patents, e.g., fusing riboflavin with urea, urethane, or niacinamide will give products which yield aqueous solutions up to 6% riboflavin.

Crystalline riboflavin is stable under ordinary conditions of storage. Solutions of riboflavin are sensitive to light and alkali, but decomposition is greatly retarded if the solutions are buffered in the acid range. At room temperature solutions buffered at pH 6 and 5 showed 3.1 and 1.2% decomposition, respectively, in 1 month. A solution of pH 5 showed a rate of decomposition of 0.25%/hour at 100°C in the dark. For intravenous use, sterile solutions of riboflavin in normal saline solution may be prepared. By heating to the boiling point, a concentration of 1 mg/ml can be attained; the solutions should be used within a few hours after preparation.

Rifamide [*Dow;* $C_{43}H_{58}N_2O_{13}$]— Antibacterial. Yellowish, crystalline powder; begins to soften at 140°; melts completely (with decomposition) about 170°.

Rifampin USP [Rifadin (*Dow*); Rimactane (*Ciba*); $C_{43}H_{58}N_4O_{12}$]—Antibacterial (tuberculostatic). Red-brown, crystalline powder. Very slightly soluble in water; freely soluble in chloroform.

Dispensing Information: Patient may be given a card containing the following information.

This medication may color your urine, stools, saliva, sweat or tears a red-orange. *Don't be alarmed.* This effect occurs in almost every patient who takes this medication. Nausea, vomiting, heartburn, gas and diarrhea may occasionally occur while taking this medication. These symptoms usually occur when you are starting therapy and should clear up after a short period of time.

You should take your TB medication at the same time every day, preferably in the morning. This will help you to develop a continuous and regular treatment schedule. However, if you forget your morning dose, you can take it later in the day. If you would like to have a sample of the rifampin capsule you are taking, the pharmacist will attach one to this card.

Ringer's Injection USP—Fluid and electrolyte replenisher. Sodium chloride, potassium chloride, and calcium chloride in water. Colorless, sterile, aqueous solution; pH 5–7.5. Ringer's Injection contains no antimicrobial agents. *Known incompatibilities:* immiscible with oil preparations.

Ringer's Injection, Lactated, USP —Systemic alkalizer; fluid and electrolyte replenisher. Sodium chloride, potassium chloride, calcium chloride, and sodium lactate in water. Colorless, sterile, aqueous solution; pH 6–7.5. Lactated Ringer's Injection contains no antimicrobial agents. *Known incompatibilities:* immiscible with oil preparations.

Ringer's Solution NF—Irrigation solution. *Do not use Ringer's Solution for parenteral administration.* Sodium chloride, potassium chloride, and calcium chloride in purified water. Sterile solution; pH 5–7.5. *Known incompatibilities:* immiscible with oil preparations.

Robaxisal Tablets [*Robins*]—Muscle relaxant; analgesic. Contain methocarbromal 400 mg, aspirin 325 mg.

Dispensing Information: Contraindicated in pregnancy. Interacts with oral anticoagulants. Do not drive or operate heavy machinery.

Robicillin-VK Preparations [*Robins*]—Antibacterial. Penicillin V potassium. *For Oral Solution 125 mg:* pH 7–7.5; solvent, purified water; sweeteners: sugar, saccharin sodium; contains (per 5 ml) K^+ 16 mg; Na^+ 13 mg. *For Oral Solution 250 mg:* See above, excepting (per 5 ml) K^+ 31 mg; Na^+ 15 mg.

Robitussin-DM Syrup [*Robins*]— Antitussive; expectorant. Contains (per 5 ml) glyceryl guaiacolate 100 mg, dextromethorphan HBr 15 mg. pH 2–3; alcohol 1.4%; aqueous solvent; sweeteners: sugar, saccharin sodium; Na^+ 6.12 mg/5 ml; K^+ 0.003 mg/5 ml.

Rolitetracycline NF [Syntetrin (*Bristol*); $C_{27}H_{33}N_3O_8$]—Antibacterial. Potency not less than 900 μg/mg. Light yellow, crystalline powder; characteristic odor; decomposes about 163°. 1 g dissolves in about 1 ml water and 200 ml alcohol; very slightly soluble in ether.

Rolitetracycline Nitrate [Tetriv, Tetrim (*Bristol*); $C_{27}H_{33}N_3O_8 \cdot HNO_3 \cdot 1\frac{1}{2}H_2O$ or anhydrous]—Antibacterial.

Rondec-DM Drops [*Ross*]—Cough mixture. Contains (per ml) sweeteners: sucrose 0.5 g, glucose 0.3 g, saccharin sodium 3 mg; Na^+ 1 mg. pH 4–4.5; alcohol <0.6% *v/v*.

Rondec-DM Syrup [*Ross*]—Cough mixture. Contains (per 5 ml) carbinoxamine maleate 2.5 mg, pseudoephedrine HCl 60 mg, dextromethorphan HBr 15 mg, glyceryl guaiacolate 100 mg, chloroform 3.5 mg; sweeteners: sucrose 2.5 g, glucose 1.5 g, saccharin sodium 0.5 mg; Na^+ 15 mg. pH 4–4.5; alcohol <0.6% *v/v*.

Rotoxamine Tartrate NF [Twiston R.A. (*McNeil*); $C_{16}H_{19}ClN_2O \cdot C_4H_6O_6$]—Antihistaminic. Whitish, crystalline powder; odorless; melts about 140°. 1 g dissolves in about 10 ml water, 100 ml alcohol, and >10,000 ml chloroform and ether.

Rynatan Pediatric Suspension [*Mallinckrodt*]—Cold, sinusitis, allergic rhinitis therapy. Contains (per 5 ml) phenylephrine tannate 5 mg, chlorpheniramine tannate 2 mg, pyrilamine tannate 12.5 mg; sugar 1 g; saccharin sodium 0.6 mg; Na^+ 0.06 mg. pH 4–5; solvent, glycerin/water.

Known incompatibilities: contains tannates; incompatible with iron-containing preparations.

Rynatuss Pediatric Suspension [*Mallinckrodt*]—Antitussive. Contains (per 5 ml) carbetapentane tannate 30 mg, chlorpheniramine tannate 4 mg, ephedrine tannate 5 mg, phenylephrine tannate 5 mg; sugar 1 g; saccharin sodium 0.75 mg; Na^+ 0.07 mg. pH 4–5; solvent, glycerin/water.

Known incompatibilities: contains tannates; incompatible with iron-containing preparations.

Saccharin USP [benzosulfimide; gluside; $C_7H_5NO_3S$; pK_a 1.60]—Pharmaceutic aid (flavor). Saccharin is soluble in 290 parts of water or 31 parts of alcohol; its solutions are acid in reaction. Saccharin is soluble in alkaline solutions.

Saccharin Calcium NF [$C_{14}H_8Ca$-$N_2O_6S_2 \cdot 3\frac{1}{2}H_2O$ or anhydrous]—Nonnutritive sweetener. White crystals or crystalline powder; odorless or faint odor; intensely sweet taste (even in dilute solutions). 1 g dissolves in about 3 ml water and 5 ml alcohol.

Saccharin Sodium NF [sodium benzosulfimide, soluble saccharin, soluble gluside; $C_7H_4NNaO_3S \cdot 2H_2O$]—Nonnutritive sweetener. Saccharin sodium is soluble 1 g in 1.5 ml of water or 50 ml of alcohol; its solutions are neutral or very slightly alkaline. It has been reported to be compatible with ephedrine sulfate, thiamine HCl, phenobarbital sodium, and potassium iodide, but incompatible with ascorbic aid, quinine HCl, aspirin, sulfanilamide, and sodium biphosphate.

Salicylanilide [Salinidol (*Doak*); $C_{13}H_{11}NO_2$]—Salicylanilide is a topical antifungal agent amide slightly soluble in water and freely soluble in alcohol. *Caution:* Do not confuse with salicylamide, an oral analgesic (see *Amides,* page 444).

Salicylazosulfapyridine— See *Sulfasalazine.*

Salicylic Acid USP [$C_7H_6O_3$; pK_a 2.97]—Keratolytic. The pH of a saturated solution is about 2.6. Salicylic acid useful as an antiseptic and keratolytic agent is soluble 1 g in 460 ml of water or 3 ml of alcohol and, hence, is precipitated when aqueous solutions of salicylates are acidified. The solubility curves for salicylic acid in alcohol–water mixtures (0–90% alcohol) demonstrate the solubility is little affected from 0–10% alcohol; 40% alcohol is recommended for 1% salicylic acid and 50% alcohol for any higher concentration normally used. *Sodium salicylate* widely used as an analgesic is soluble in water (1:0.9), in alcohol (1:9.2), and in glycerin (1:4). It is incompatible with ferric salts, lead acetate, silver nitrate, and limewater (forming insoluble metal salicylates) or with mineral acids (forming insoluble free salicylic acid). The pH of a 1% solution is about 5–6. The powder becomes pinkish on exposure to light. *Ammonium salicylate* is soluble in water (1:1) and alcohol (1:3). It may lose NH_3 on exposure to air and also discolors on exposure to light. It is incompatible with alkalies (NH_3 formation) and acids (salicylic acid formation). The pH of a 1% solution is slightly acid. *Bismuth salicylate* is practically insoluble in water and alcohol and is soluble in fixed oils. It is stable in air but unstable to light.

Aqueous solutions of salicylates darken on standing, the change being more rapid in alkaline solutions. The nature of the change is not definitely known, but it seems to involve oxidation; the darkening may be due to the formation of benzoquinone or its polymers. The darkening is accelerated by light, microorganisms, oxidizing agents, and traces of copper and iron. The color change has also been ascribed to traces of phenol in the sodium salicylate. The darkening can be retarded to some extent by using chemically pure materials and recently boiled water; it is also an advantage to protect the solution from light and air. Various stabilizers have been recommended to delay the darkening, including 0.1% of sodium bisulfite, sodium sulfite, sodium thiosulfate or sodium hypophosphite, or 0.5% of sodium citrate. The color change is believed to be harmless, and the patient may be advised to ignore it. It would be good practice for the physician to prescribe a colored vehicle such as glycyrrhiza syrup, compounded sarsaparilla syrup, or cinnamon syrup to mask the color change.

Scopolamine [hyoscine, scopine tropate; $C_{17}H_{21}NO_4$]—Scopolamine, in the form of the free alkaloid, is liquid which is slightly soluble in water but very soluble in alcohol.

Scopolamine Hydrobromide USP [hyoscine hydrobromide; $C_{17}H_{21}NO_4 \cdot$ $HBr \cdot 3H_2O$ or anhydrous]—Anticholinergic. Soluble 1 g in 1.5 ml of water or 20 ml of alcohol; the aqueous solution is neutral or only slightly acid (pH 0.05 *M* solution—*circa* 5.85). Due to the appreciable solubility of the free alkaloid, the addition of alkalies to dilute aqueous solutions of the salts does not cause precipitation.

"Scopolamine Stable" is an aqueous solution of scopolamine hydrobromide stabilized by the presence of 10% of mannitol.

Secobarbital USP [Seconal (*Lilly*); $C_{12}H_{18}N_2O_3$]—This short-acting sedative and hypnotic is more water-soluble than amobarbital thus Seconal Elixir (12% alcohol) is compatible with items found compatible with Amytal Elixir but the taste may be more bitter. The following items have been found compatible with Seconal Elixir (30 ml): ammonium bromide (1 g), sodium bromide (1 g), potassium bromide (1 g), lithium bromide (1 g), codeine sulfate (65 mg) potassium thiocyanate (0.5 g), ephedrine sulfate syrup (30 ml), phenobarbital elixir (30 ml), Ephedrol with Codeine (30 ml), Sedatussin (30 ml), terpin hydrate and codeine elixir (30 ml—may precipitate terpin hydrate if chilled). White Pine Compound Syrup (*Lilly*) was reported not acceptable (precipitate) and three bromides elixir produced a gradual color fading with seconal elixir.

Dispensing Information: See *Sedatives and Hypnotics*.

Secobarbital Sodium USP [Seconal Sodium (*Lilly*); $C_{12}H_{17}N_2NaO_3$]—Hypnotic, sedative. White powder; odorless; bitter taste; hygroscopic; solutions decompose on standing with heat accelerating the decomposition; pH (5% soln) 9.7–10.5. Very soluble in water; soluble in alcohol; practically insoluble in ether. *Known incompatibilities* (secobarbital sodium injection): anileridine HCl, chlordiazepoxide, chlorpromazine HCl, codeine phosphate, ephedrine sulfate, erythromycin gluceptate, hydrocortisone sodium succinate, insulin, levarterenol bitartrate, meperidine HCl, methadone HCl, methylphenidate HCl, penicillin G potassium, phenytoin sodium, phytonadione, procaine HCl, prochlorperazine, promethazine HCl, streptomycin sulfate, tetracycline HCl, vancomycin HCl.

Dispensing Information: See *Sedatives and Hypnotics.*

Seconal Sodium [*Lilly*]—Hypnotic; sedative. Secobarbital sodium. *Ampoules (No. 616):* pH 9.5–10.5; solvent, polyethylene glycol 50%; Na$^+$ 0.19 mEq/ml. *Hyporets (No. 27):* pH 9.4–9.6; solvent, polyethylene glycol 50%; Na$^+$ 0.38 mEq/2 ml. *Known incompatibilities:* Seconal Sodium combined with acid solutions (i.e., codeine, morphine, lactated Ringer's solution, and bacteriostatic water for injection) results in barbituric acid precipitation; this precipitation is gradual, but will occur.

Secretin [Secretin-Boots (*Warren-Teed*)]—Diagnostic aid (pancreatic disorders). Hormone from porcine duodenal mucosa.

Sedatives and Hypnotics—*Dispensing Information:* Drug dependence can occur insidiously in patients who chronically use hypnotics. "Hangover" or unwanted drowsiness can be experienced the morning after a nighttime dose with all hypnotics. Numerous drug interaction potentials exist in patients taking barbiturates, glutethimide, and chloral hydrate. Alcohol ingestion will produce additive hypnotic effects. Patients should be cautioned about the lingering CNS-depressant effects and should not ingest other CNS depressants concurrently with hypnotics. Recommended doses must not be exceeded. Advise physician if skin rash occurs.

Selenium Sulfide USP [Selsun (*Abbott*); SeS$_2$]—Antiseborrheic. Bright-orange powder; faint odor; pH (Selsun Suspension) 2.9–3.5. Practically insoluble in water and alcohol; 1 g dissolves in 161 ml chloroform and 1667 ml ether.

Senna NF [Glycennid (*Sandoz*)]—Cathartic. Dried leaflet of *Cassia acuti-folia* (Alexandria Senna) or *Cassia angustifolia* (Tinnevelly Senna).

Sennosides A and B NF [Senokot (*P-F*)]—Cathartic. Brownish powder; pH (1 in 10 aq soln) about 6.8. One g dissolves in about 35 ml water, 2100 ml alcohol, 3700 ml chloroform, and 6100 ml ether.

Serpasil Elixir [*Ciba* brand of reserpine]—Tranquilizer. *Known ingredients:* reserpine (0.2 or 1.0 mg/4 ml), alcohol, water. *Known incompatibilities: drugs incompatible with 1 mg/4 ml elixir include* belladonna tincture, Ephedrol with Codeine Expectorant, Hydryllin Syrup, lactated pepsin elixir, Propadrine Elixir, terpin hydrate with codeine elixir, Thephorin Expectorant with Codeine and Papaverine, Thorazine Syrup; *drugs incompatible with 0.2 mg/4 ml elixir include* Propadrine Elixir.

Serpasil Injectable Solution [*Ciba*]—*Known ingredients:* reserpine (2.5 mg/ml). *Known compatibilities:* 5% dextrose solution. *Known incompatibilities:* Apresoline Injectable Solution, normal saline solution, procaine HCl, vitamin B complex injection.

Siliceous Earth, Purified, USP [diatomaceous earth; purified infusorial earth; purified kieselguhr]—Filtering medium. Very fine, whitish powder; amorphous; gritty; absorbs about 4 times its weight without becoming liquid. Insoluble in water, acids, or dilute solutions of alkali hydroxides.

Silicon Dioxide, Colloidal, NF—Pharmaceutic aid (suspending agent; tablet base). Submicroscopic fumed silica. Light, white powder; nongritty; extremely fine particle size. Insoluble in water and acids (excepting HF); dissolves in hot solutions of alkali hydroxides.

Silver Nitrate USP [argenti nitras; AgNO$_3$]—Topical anti-infective. Colorless or white crystals; discolors in light (in the presence of organic matter) (reduction to metallic silver); sp gr about 4.3; melts about 212°; 1 in 10 aqueous solution neutral to litmus. 1 g dissolves in about 0.4 ml water, 0.1 ml alcohol, and 30 ml chloroform; slightly soluble in ether. *Known incompatibilities:* reducing agents, in neutral or alkaline solutions (borax, bromides, carbonates, chlorides, hydroxides, iodides, etc.), potassium permanganate, tannic acid, soluble citrates and sulfates, ammonia water.

Silver Nitrate, Toughened, USP [argenti nitras induratus; caustic stick or pencil; lunar caustic; silver nitrate pencils; $AgNO_3$]—Caustic. Contains some AgCl. White, crystalline masses (generally molded as pencils or cones); breaks with fibrous fracture; darkens in light; solution neutral to litmus. Soluble in water to the extent of its nitrate content (always a residue of AgCl); partially soluble in alcohol; slightly soluble in ether.

Simethicone NF [Mylicon(*Stuart*)]— Antiflatulent; pharmaceutic release agent. Translucent, gray, viscous liquid. Insoluble in water and alcohol; 1 g dissolves in 10 ml chloroform and ether.

Smooth Muscle Relaxants (Xanthine Type)—*Dispensing Information:* Patients with cardiovascular disease should report fast heart rate or palpitations to their physician. Orally, aminophylline is best taken on an empty stomach as uncoated tablets (nausea and vomiting produced by aminophylline may be related to serum levels and not simply an effect of the stomach mucosa); rectal administration may cause proctitis.

Soda Lime USP—Soda lime is a mixture of calcium hydroxide and sodium or potassium hydroxide or both; may contain an indicator that is inert toward anesthetic gases (i.e., ether, cyclopropane, and nitrous oxide) and that changes color when the soda lime no longer can absorb CO_2. White or grayish white granules; may have a color if an indicator has been added.

Sodium Acetate USP [$C_2H_3NaO_2 \cdot 3H_2O$]—Pharmaceutic aid (in solutions for hemodialysis and peritoneal dialysis). Colorless, transparent crystals or white, granular, crystalline powder or white flakes; odorless or faint acetous

odor; slightly bitter, saline taste; efflorescent in warm, dry air; pH (1 in 20 soln in CO_2-free water) 7.5–9.2. One g dissolves in <1 ml water and 10–30 ml alcohol.

Sodium Alginate NF—Sodium alginate is soluble 1 g in 20 ml of water. It is insoluble in acid solutions (pH less than 4) and hydroalcoholic solutions containing more than 30% (by weight) of alcohol. A 5% solution sets to an immobile gel; more dilute solutions have the viscosity of mucilages. Solutions are prepared by suspending sodium alginate in glycerin and adding water, with continuous stirring. Metallic ions, other than those of the alkali metals, ammonium, iron, and magnesium, thicken the mucilage due to formation of insoluble alginates of the metals. A preservative must be added to the mucilage to prevent fermentation.

Sodium Aminosalicylate USP [*Various Mfrs.;* $C_7H_6NNaO_3 \cdot 2H_2O$ or anhydrous]—Antibacterial (tuberculostatic). Whitish, crystalline powder; practically odorless; sweet, saline taste; aqueous solution decomposes slowly and darkens; pH (1 in 50 aq soln) 6.5–8.5. One g dissolves in about 2 ml water; sparingly soluble in alcohol; very slightly soluble in chloroform and ether.

Sodium Ascorbate USP [Cenolate (*Abbott*); $C_6H_7NaO_6$]—Pharmaceutic aid. This is prepared from ascorbic acid with the aid of sodium hydroxide, sodium carbonate, or sodium bicarbonate. The USP requires that the potency of ascorbic acid be expressed in terms of ascorbic acid on labels of its preparations.

Sodium Benzoate USP [$C_7H_5NaO_2$] —Pharmaceutic aid (antifungal agent). 1 g in 1.8 ml water and 75 ml alcohol. Incompatible with acids (liberating benzoic acid) and ferric salts (forming insoluble basic ferric benzoate).

Sodium Bicarbonate USP [$NaHCO_3$]—Systemic alkalizer; antacid; electrolyte replenisher. White, crystalline powder; stable in dry air; slowly decomposes in moist air; solutions, when freshly prepared with cold water without shaking, alkaline to litmus; alkalinity increases as solutions stand, are agitated, or are heated. 1 g dissolves in 12 ml water and >10,000 ml alcohol. *Known incompatibilities:* (sodium bicarbonate injection): acids, anileridine HCl, calcium chloride, calcium gluconate, chlorpromazine HCl, codeine phosphate, corticotropin, dihydromorphinone HCl, insulin, Levophed, magnesium sulfate, meperidine HCl methadone HCl, methicillin sodium, morphine sulfate, penicillin G potassium, pentobarbital sodium, Pentothal, phenobarbital sodium, procaine HCl, protein hydrolysate, Ringer's injection, lactated Ringer's, streptomycin sulfate, sodium lactate ($\frac{1}{6}$ *M*), Sparine, Terramycin, tetracycline HCl, vancomycin HCl, vitamin B complex with C.

Sodium Biphosphate USP [$NaH_2PO_4 \cdot H_2O$]—Anticoagulant for storage of whole blood; cathartic. Colorless crystals or white, crystalline powder; odorless; slightly deliquescent; solution is acid to litmus; solutions effervesce with sodium carbonate. 1 g dissolves in 1–10 ml water and >10,000 ml alcohol.

Sodium Bisulfite USP [Na_2SO_3]—Pharmaceutic aid (antioxidant). White or yellowish white crystals or granular powder; odor of sulfur dioxide; unstable in air. 1 g dissolves in 4 ml water and 100–1000 ml alcohol. *Known incompatibilities:* oxidizing agents, heavy metal salts.

Sodium Borate USP [borax; $Na_2B_4O_7 \cdot 10H_2O$]—Pharmaceutic aid (alkalizing agent). Colorless, transparent crystals or white, crystalline powder; odorless; solutions are alkaline to phenolphthalein TS; as it effloresces in warm, dry air, the crystals are often coated with white powder. 1 g dissolves in 16 ml water, 1 ml boiling water, and 1 ml glycerin; insoluble in alcohol. *Known incompatibilities:* Precipitates alkaloids and solutions of metals other than alkali metals, forms moist mass when triturated with alum, zinc sulfate, tartaric acid or benzoic acid, alkalinity is reduced by the addition of glycerin or mannitol.

Sodium Caprylate—See *Caprylic Acid.*

Sodium Carbonate USP [Na_2CO_3]—Pharmaceutic aid (alkalizing agent). Colorless crystals or white, crystalline powder or granules; stable in air under ordinary conditions; when exposed to dry air above 50°, hydrous salt effloresces and, at 100°, becomes anhydrous. 1 g dissolves in 3 ml water; more soluble in boiling water. *Known incompatibilities:* acids.

Sodium Chloride USP [NaCl]—Pharmaceutic aid (tonicity agent). Colorless, cubic crystals or white, crystalline powder; saline taste. 1 g dissolves in 2.8 ml water (slightly more so in boiling water), 10 ml glycerin, and 100–1000 ml alcohol.

Sodium Chloride Injection USP [normal saline; *Various Mfrs.*]—Sterile, isotonic solution of sodium chloride 0.9% in water for injection. Contains no antimicrobial agents; pH 4.5–7. *Known incompatibilities* (sodium chloride injection): amphotericin B.

Sodium Chloride Injection, Bacteriostatic, USP—Pharmaceutic aid (sterile isotonic vehicle). Clear, colorless solution; odorless or odor of bacteriostatic substances. *Known incompatibilities:* immiscible with oil preparations; characteristic incompatibilities of the bacteriostatic agent must be considered.

Sodium Citrate USP—See *Under Citric Acid.*

Sodium Fluoride USP [NaF]—Dental caries prophylactic. White powder; odorless. 1 g dissolves in 25 ml water; insoluble in alcohol. *Known incompatibilities:* acids; tooth mottling may occur with excess.

Dispensing Information: Before use of solutions, make certain that the local water supply is not fluoridated.

Sodium Folate [Folvite Sodium (*Lederle*); $C_{19}H_{18}N_7NaO_6$]—Water-soluble hematopoietic vitamin. A 1.5% solution in water is alkaline (pH range, 8.5–11). See also under *Folic Acid.*

Sodium Formaldehyde Sulfoxylate NF [$CH_3NaO_3S \cdot 2H_2O$ or anhydrous]— Antidote to mercury; antioxidant (in parenteral preparations). White crystals or hard masses; odor of garlic; pH (1 in 50 soln) about 10.1. One g dissolves in about 4 ml water, 510 ml alcohol, 175 ml chloroform, and 180 ml ether.

Sodium Hydroxide USP [NaOH]— Pharmaceutic aid (alkalizing agent). White or nearly white, fused masses, small pellets, flakes, sticks, or other forms; hard and brittle; shows a crystalline fracture; rapidly absorbs CO_2 and moisture in air; produces much heat on solution. 1 g dissolves in 1 ml water; freely soluble in alcohol. *Caution:* Exercise great care in handling as it rapidly destroys tissues. *Known incompatibilities:* acids.

Sodium Hypochlorite Solution NF [NaClO]—Disinfectant. Clear, pale greenish yellow liquid; odor of chlorine; affected by light. *Caution: not suitable for application to wounds. Known incompatibilities:* acids, oxidizing agents, reducing agents.

Sodium Hypochlorite Solution, Diluted, NF—Local anti-infective. Colorless or light-yellow liquid; odor suggesting chlorine; specific gravity not more than 1.025. *Known incompatibilities:* oxidizing agents, reducing agents.

Sodium Iodide USP [NaI]—Pharmaceutic aid (iodine tincture). Colorless crystals or white, crystalline powder; odorless; deliquescent in moist air; develops a brown tint on decomposition. 1 g dissolves in 0.6 ml water, 2 ml alcohol and 1 ml glycerin.

Known incompatibilities (sodium iodide injection): acids, alkaloids, codeine phosphate, Demerol, Leritine, Levo-Dromoran, Levophed, metallic ions, methadone HCl, morphine sulfate, procaine HCl, protein hydrolysate.

Sodium Lauryl Sulfate USP [Gardinol W A (*Procter & Gamble*), Duponol C (*Du Pont*), a mixture of sodium alkyl sulfates composed chiefly of sodium lauryl sulfate $CH_3(CH_2)_{10}CH_2$— SO_3—Na]—Pharmaceutic aid (surfactant). It is compatible with dilute acids, alkalies, soaps, and calcium and magnesium ions. It is incompatible with many cationic materials.

Sodium Metabisulfite NF [$Na_2S_2O_5$]— Pharmaceutic aid (antioxidant). White crystals or white to yellowish, crystalline powder; odor of sulfur dioxide. 1 g dissolves in 1–10 ml water and glycerin and 100–1000 ml alcohol. *Known incompatibilities:* oxidizing agents, heavy metal salts.

Sodium Nitrite USP [$NaNO_2$]— Antidote to cyanide poisoning. White to slightly yellow, granular powder or white or nearly white, opaque, fused masses or sticks; mild, saline taste; deliquescent in air; solution is alkaline to litmus. 1 g dissolves in 1.5 ml water and 30–100 ml alcohol. *Known incompatibilities:* reducing agents, oxidizing agents, alkaloids, antipyrine, acetanilid, acetophenetidin, phenolic compounds, tannic acid.

Sodium Nitroprusside [sodium nitroferricyanide; Nipride (*Roche*); Na_2-$Fe(CN)_5NO \cdot 2H_2O$ or anhydrous]—Antihypertensive. See *Keto-Diastix.*

Sodium Para-Aminobenzoate—See under *Aminobenzoic Acid.*

Sodium Phosphate USP [$Na_2HPO_4 \cdot 7H_2O$]—Cathartic. Colorless or white, granular salt; effloresces in warm, dry air; solutions are alkaline to phenolphthalein TS (0.1 M soln, pH about 9.5). 1 g dissolves in 1–10 ml water and 1000–10,000 ml alcohol.

Sodium Phosphate, Dried, NF [$Na_2HPO_4 \cdot x H_2O$]—Cathartic. White powder; readily absorbs moisture. 1 g dissolves in 8 ml water and >10,000 ml alcohol.

Sodium Phosphate and Biphosphate Enema USP [$Na_2HPO_4 \cdot 7H_2O$ and $NaH_2PO_4 \cdot H_2O$]—Cathartic. pH 5–5.8; specific gravity 1.121–1.128.

Sodium Phosphate and Biphosphate Oral Solution USP—Cathartic. pH 4.4–5.2.

Sodium Phosphate, Effervescent, NF—Cathartic. Contains dry mixture of granular salts: dried sodium phosphate, sodium bicarbonate, tartaric acid, and citric acid.

Sodium Phosphate Solution NF—Cathartic. Contains sodium phosphate, citric acid monohydrate, and glycerin. Clear, colorless liquid; thick, syrupy consistency; practically odorless; cooling, salty taste; acid to litmus; specific gravity about 1.39.

Sodium Polystyrene Sulfonate USP [Kayexalate (*Winthrop*)]—Ion-exchange resin (potassium). Fine, golden-brown powder; odorless; tasteless. Insoluble in water.

Dispensing Information: If not fully prepared for the patient, mixing instructions should be provided. Advise physician if constipation occurs or, if taken with sorbitol, excessive diarrhea develops. Importance of appropriate compliance should be stressed.

Sodium Propionate NF [$C_3H_5NaO_2 \cdot xH_2O$ or anhydrous]—Topical antifungal. Colorless, transparent crystals or granular, crystalline powder; deliquescent (in moist air); odorless or faint odor. 1 g dissolves in about 1 ml water and 24 ml alcohol. See also under *Propionic Acid.*

Sodium Salicylate NF [$C_7H_5NaO_3$]—Analgesic. Powder or scales; amorphous or microcrystalline; colorless or faint pink; odorless or faint odor; sweet, saline taste; light-sensitive; aqueous solution neutral or acid to litmus. 1 g dissolves in about 1 ml water, 10 ml alcohol, and 4 ml glycerin. *Known incompatibilities:* oxidizing agents (e.g., alkalies, iron), ferric salts (also bismuth, lead, mercury), mineral acids, soluble quinine salts. See also under *Salicylic Acid.*

Sodium Stearate USP [$C_{18}H_{35}NaO_2$]—Pharmaceutic aid (emulsifying and stiffening agent). Consists chiefly of sodium stearate and palmitate. Fine, white powder; soapy touch; may have slight odor; light-sensitive; solution alkaline to phenolphthalein TS. Slowly soluble in cold water and alcohol; readily soluble in hot water and alcohol. See also under *Stearic Acid.*

Sodium Succinate—See under *Succinic Acid.*

Sodium Sulfate USP [Glauber's Salt; $Na_2SO_4 \cdot 10H_2O$ or anhydrous]—Cathartic; antihypercalcemic (injection). Large, colorless, transparent crystals or granular powder; odorless; effloresces rapidly in air; liquefies in its water of hydration at about 33°; loses water of hydration at 100°; solution neutral to litmus. 1 g dissolves in about 2 ml water; soluble in glycerin; insoluble in alcohol.

Sodium Tetradecyl Sulfate [Sotradecol Sodium (*Elkins-Sinn*); $C_{14}H_{29}NaO_4S$]—Wetting agent; sclerosing agent. White, waxy solid; odorless. Soluble in water, alcohol, and ether.

Sodium Thiosulfate USP [$Na_2S_2O_3 \cdot 5H_2O$]—Antidote to cyanide poisoning. Large, colorless crystals or coarse, crystalline powder; deliquescent in moist air; effloresces in dry air at temperatures above 33°; solution is neutral or faintly alkaline to litmus. 1 g dissolves in <1 ml water; insoluble in alcohol. *Known incompatibilities:* acids, oxidizing agents, reducing agents; silver, lead, and bismuth salts.

Solu-B Sterile [*Upjohn*]—Injectable vitamin B complex. *Known ingredients* (per 5 ml after reconstitution): thiamine HCl (10 mg), riboflavin (10 mg), pyridoxine HCl (5 mg), calcium pantothenate (50 mg), nicotinamide (250 mg), cyanocobalamin (B_{12}, 25 µg). pH 5.5 (approx). *Known incompatibilities:* none listed.

Solu-B Sterile Mix-O-Vial [*Upjohn*]—*Known ingredients:* same as *Solu-B Sterile* except 2-ml volume. The water in the upper compartment is preserved with parabens. *Known compatibilities and incompatibilities:* see *Solu-B Sterile.*

Solu-B with Ascorbic Acid [*Upjohn*] *Known ingredients:* Same as *Solu-B Sterile* with a vial of aqueous ascorbic acid (500 mg/5 ml) supplied as diluent. pH 6 (approx). *Known compatibilities and incompatibilities:* See *Solu-B Sterile.*

Sorbic Acid NF [$C_6H_8O_2$]—Pharmaceutic aid (antimicrobial agent). White, crystalline powder; free-flowing; characteristic odor; melts about 133°. 1 g dissolves in about 1000 ml water, 10 ml alcohol, 15 ml chloroform, and 30 ml ether.

Sorbitan Esters [Spans (*Atlas*)]— Pharmaceutic aid (surfactant). *Monolaurate:* Amber liquid; oily. Dispersible in distilled water and hard water, 200 ppm (insoluble in hard water, 20,000 ppm); soluble in alcohol. *Monooleate:* Amber liquid. Dispersible in water; slightly soluble in ether. *Monopalmitate:* Tan, granular solid; waxy. Dispersible in distilled water and hard water, 200 ppm (insoluble in cold distilled water and hard water, 20,000 ppm). *Monostearate:* Cream to tan beads. Insoluble in water and alcohol. *Trioleate:* Amber liquid; oily. Insoluble in water; soluble in alcohol. *Tristearate:* Tan beads; waxy. Insoluble in water.

Sorbitol USP [Sorbo (*Atlas*), D-sorbitol, $C_6H_{14}O_6$]—Sorbitol is a pharmaceutical necessity (substitute for glycerin, sucrose, etc.). It is about $\frac{1}{2}$ as sweet as sugar but only 30% appears as glucose in the blood. It is soluble up to 83% in water and is available commercially as a 70% solution. It is soluble in hot ethanol, isopropanol, butanol, etc., but sparingly soluble in cold alcohol. It is resistant to attack by dilute acids, alkalies, or mild oxidizing agents. The pH is neutral (*circa* 7). A combination of 0.12% methylparaben and 0.02% propylparaben as preservatives for aqueous sorbitol solutions has been recommended and 0.15% sorbic acid was also effective but gave occasional failures. A poorly protected metal container can be the source of metal contamination giving inconsistent vitamin stability (i.e., ascorbic acid).

Sparteine [Tocosamine (*Trent*) $C_{15}H_{26}N_2$; pK$_{b1}$ 2.24, pK$_{b2}$ 9.46]—This drug is sometimes injected for uterine inertia. The pH of a 0.01 *M* solution is about 11.6. One gram dissolves in 325 ml of water. *Sparteine sulfate* ($C_{15}H_{26}N_2$·H_2SO_4·$5H_2O$) is soluble 1 g in 1.1 ml of water or 3 ml of alcohol. Alkalies do not precipitate the alkaloid from dilute solutions of its salts since the free liquid alkaloid is slightly soluble in water. The sulfate is hydroscopic.

The stability of sparteine and its salts in solution has been reported and it was found that the drug degrades in response to light and auto-oxidation.

Sparteine Sulfate—See under *Sparteine.*

Spectinomycin Hydrochloride, Sterile, USP [Trobicin (*Upjohn*); $C_{14}H_{24}N_2O_7$·$2HCl$·$5H_2O$ or anhydrous] —Antibacterial. White, crystalline powder; odorless; slightly bitter taste. 1 g dissolves in about 7 ml water; practically insoluble in alcohol, chloroform, and ether.

Spermaceti USP—Pharmaceutic aid (stiffening agent for consistency and texture in ointments). Waxy substance from the head of the sperm whale, *Physeter macrocephalus.* White, slightly unctuous mass; somewhat translucent; crystalline fracture; pearly luster; faint odor; bland taste; free from rancidity; sp gr about 0.94; melts about 46°. Insoluble in water; practically insoluble in cold alcohol (soluble in boiling alcohol); soluble in chloroform and ether.

Spermaceti, Synthetic, NF—Pharmaceutic aid (stiffening agent). Mixture primarily of esters of saturated fatty alcohols and fatty acids. Description and solubility similar to *Spermaceti.*

Spironolactone USP [Aldactone (*Searle*); $C_{24}H_{32}O_4S$]—Diuretic. Light, cream-colored to light-tan, crystalline powder; faint to mild mercaptan-like odor; stable in air. Practically insoluble in water; freely soluble in chloroform; soluble in alcohol; slightly soluble in fixed oils.

Dispensing Information: It should be ascertained if patient is receiving other potassium supplements; if so, this perhaps should be brought to the attention of the physician. Consult physician if drowsiness, dryness of mouth, erythematous or maculopapular eruption, hirsutism, irregular menses, or deepening of female voice occur. (Do not advise taking with orange juice, bananas, or other fruits as this is a potassium-sparing diuretic).

Stannous Fluoride USP [tin difluoride; fluoristan; SnF_2]—Dental caries prophylactic. White, crystalline powder; bitter, salty taste; melts about 213°. Freely soluble in water; practically insoluble in alcohol, chloroform, and ether.

Stanozolol NF [Winstrol (*Winthrop*); $C_{21}H_{32}N_2O$]—Androgen. Nearly colorless, crystalline powder; odorless or almost so; two forms: needles (melt about 155°), prisms (melt about 235°). Insoluble in water; 1 g dissolves in about 41 ml alcohol, 74 ml chloroform, and 375 ml ether.

Starch USP—Dusting powder; pharmaceutic aid (tablet disintegrant). Starch is insoluble in alcohol or cold water. Partial hydrolysis of starch forms dextrins and maltose; complete hydrolysis yields glucose. Free iodine gives a blue color with starch.

Starch Glycerite NF [starch glycerin]—Pharmaceutic aid (emollient). *Preparation:* Rub starch (100 g) and benzoic acid (2 g) with purified water (200 ml) in a porcelain dish until a smooth mixture is produced, then add glycerin (700 ml), and mix well. Heat the mixture on a sand bath to a temperature between 140° and 144°, with constant but gentle stirring until a translucent, jelly-like mass results, and then strain through muslin. *Note:* Should be freshly prepared.

Starch, Pregelatinized, USP—Pharmaceutic aid (tablet excipient). Starch that has been chemically or mechanically processed to rupture all or part of the granules in the presence of water and subsequently dried. Moderately coarse to fine, whitish powder; odorless; slight, characteristic taste. Slightly soluble to soluble in cold water; insoluble in alcohol.

Stearic Acid USP [a mixture of $CH_3(CH_2)_{14}COOH$ and $CH_3(CH_2)_{16}$-COOH; $pK_a = 5.75$ @ 35°C]—Pharmaceutic aid. Stearic acid useful in lotions, creams, etc., is almost insoluble in water but is soluble 1 g in about 20 ml of alcohol. The pH of a saturated solution is about 7–7.2. Stearates of the alkali metals are slowly soluble in water and alco-

hol (e.g., sodium stearate). Stearates of the other metals are insoluble in water and alcohol but soluble in fixed oils, especially when heated (e.g., aluminum stearate, magnesium stearate, and zinc stearate). These have been used to make water-repellent gels useful as repository vehicles for injectable penicillin.

Stearyl Alcohol USP—Pharmaceutic aid. This fatty alcohol ointment base constituent is insoluble in water, soluble in alcohol and ether.

Stelazine Concentrate [*SK&F*]—Tranquilizer (major). Trifluoperazine hydrochloride. pH 2–3.2; aqueous solvent; Na^+ 3 mg/5 ml; sweetener: saccharin sodium, sugar.

Stibophen NF [Fuadin (*Winthrop*) $C_{12}H_4Na_5O_{16}S_4Sb\cdot7H_2O$ or anhydrous]—Antischistosomal. Discolored by light. It is freely soluble in water and almost insoluble in alcohol. The aqueous solutions are alkaline. It is discolored by iron due to its phenolic character and the presence of sulfonic groups.

Storax USP [styrax; sweet gum]—Pharmaceutic aid (Compound Benzoin Tincture USP); expectorant. Balsam from the trunk of *Liquidambar orientalis* (Levant Storax) or *Liquidambar styraciflua* (American Storax). *Levant Storax:* semiliquid, grayish, sticky, opaque mass; deposits heavy, dark brown layer on standing. *American Storax:* semisolid, sometimes solid, mass; softened by gentle warming. Storax is transparent in thin layers; characteristic odor and taste; denser than water. Insoluble in water; soluble (usually incompletely) in equal weight of warm alcohol; soluble in ether, some residue usually remaining.

Streptomycin and Dihydrostreptomycin—Streptomycin is an antibiotic obtained from *Streptomyces griseus*. It contains two basic guanidino groups, a basic *N*-methylamino group and a free aldehyde group. The catalytic reduction of the latter to a hydroxyl group produces dihydrostreptomycin.

These antibiotics are most effective against Gram-negative rods, tuberculosis, etc., however, many strains formerly sensitive are now resistant. Accordingly, many medical authorities feel these drugs should be used only for infections shown to be sensitive by laboratory tests. They may produce vertigo, tinnitus or deafness, contact dermatitis or allergic reactions, under certain conditions of use (check insert). They are believed to act by causing formation of a faulty cellular membrane (inhibition of protein synthesis).

Streptomycin and dihydrostreptomycin are bases, and they form salts with anions. The salts are hygroscopic, very soluble in water and insoluble in most organic solvents. The dry powder is very stable for long periods of time, even at elevated temperatures. Some discoloration may occur, but this does not appear to interfere with potency. Aqueous solutions are quite stable at a pH of 3–7 for long periods of time, even at elevated temperatures. Strong acids or strong bases decompose them very rapidly and it has been noted that pH 6–8 is the optimal range for stability. They are inactivated by hydroxylamine HCl, and activity is diminished by potassium permanganate, hydrogen peroxide, potassium iodide, and potassium chloride. They are compatible with chlorocresol, formaldehyde, phenol, and phenylmercuric nitrate.

The inactivation of streptomycin sulfate in aqueous solution by Co, Mn, Cu, Ni, Hg, Cd, Ag, and Pb ions at various temperatures has been noted. Inactivation by these ions increased with temperature.

Isotonic solutions with a 0.56°C freezing point depression can be made using a 3.25% solution of the streptomycin-calcium chloride complex, a 2% solution of streptomycin HCl, or an 8% solution of streptomycin sulfate.

Aqueous nasal solutions (1000 or 3000 units/ml) can be made with additives such as amphetamine, antihistamines, chlorbutanol, *dl*-desoxyephedrine HCl, some dyes (e.g., FDC Yellow #5), ephedrine sulfate, lactose, the parabens, phenylephrine HCl, and sodium citrate.

These solutions are stable for long periods of time, even at 37°C.

Ear products can be made using glycerin or propylene glycol or a polyethylene glycol as the solvent. Various additives such as antihistamines, phenol, sodium citrate, sulfanilamide, urea, and urethane can be used. These solutions are stable for long periods of time, even at 37°C.

Isotonic ophthalmic solutions can be made using sodium or potassium chlorides and sodium or potassium phosphates.

In oral products streptomycin and dihydrostreptomycin are compatible with other antibiotics such as neomycin and bacitracin, calcium carbonate, various flavors and dyes, kaolin, lactose, pectin, saccharin, starch, Sucaryl, sugar, sulfaguanidine, sulfasuxidine and sulfathalidine. These tablets, solutions, and suspensions are stable for long periods of time, even at summer temperatures. Effervescent soluble tablets which are stable for long periods of time can be made with citric acid, sodium benzoate, and sodium bicarbonate.

Suppositories can be made with a cocoa butter base or with a water-soluble, Carbowax type base. These are stable for long periods of time.

Streptomycin and dihydrostreptomycin are very stable in polyethylene glycol type bases, in petrolatum bases and in a grease type base containing beeswax, lanolin, and petrolatum. They are also quite stable in an oil-in-water vanishing cream type base. One such ointment can be made with beeswax, nonionic emulsifiers, petrolatum, propylene glycol, stearic acid, and water. Various antihistamines and/or various sulfa drugs can also be incorporated in this type of ointment.

Aqueous solutions for intramuscular use are quite stable for long periods of time, even at elevated summer temperatures. At times these solutions develop color, but it apparently does not affect potency. Most of this color formation can be eliminated by the addition of substances such as sodium bisulfite or sodium formaldehyde sulfoxylate. A preservative such as phenol or the parabens is usually used, and about 2 to 3% of sodium citrate is also used in these solutions.

Streptomycin Sulfate USP [Strycin Sulfate (*Squibb*); $(C_{21}H_{39}N_7O_{12})_2$·$3H_2SO_4$]—Antibacterial (tuberculostatic). Streptomycin sulfate is a white or practically white, hygroscopic powder. It is stable toward air and light. It is very soluble in water (75%). It is very slightly soluble in alcohol (0.03%) and insoluble in benzene, chloroform, petroleum ether, and ether. The pH of a 20% aqueous is between 4.5 and 7.

It has been reported the color development in a streptomycin sulfate solution with procaine HCl is due to the reaction between the carbonyl group of streptomycin and the para amino group of procaine.

Sublimaze Injection [*McNeil*]— Fentanyl. Narcotic analgesic. pH 5.8; aqueous solvent; Na^+, trace; hypotonic.

Succinic Acid [$C_4H_6O_4$; pK_{a1} 4.19, pK_{a2} 5.48]—Succinic acid is soluble in water (1:13) and alcohol (1:18.5). The pH of a 1% solution is about 2.7. The sodium salt is soluble in water (1:5) but insoluble in alcohol. Succinic acid is sometimes used in manufacturing pharmacy since one carboxyl group can be reacted with an insoluble alcohol (e.g., hydrocortisone), while the other is converted to a sodium salt. The resulting compound (e.g., hydrocortisone sodium succinate) is usually very water-soluble.

Succinylcholine Chloride USP [Anectine Chloride (*B-W*); Quelicin Chloride (*Abbott*); Sucostrin Chloride (*Squibb*); Sux-Cert (*Travenol*); $C_{14}H_{30}Cl_2N_2O_4$]—Skeletal muscle relaxant. This diester and diquaternary compound is a white powder which is very soluble in water, slightly soluble in alcohol, and sensitive to light. A 2% aqueous solution is acid (pH 3–4.5). The injection of succinylcholine chloride has been reported to undergo a 20% hydrolysis after a year's storage at room temperature. *Known incompatibilities* (succinylcholine chloride injection): alkaline solutions, barbiturates (short-acting).

Succinylsulfathiazole [Sulfasuxidine (*MSD*); $C_{13}H_{13}N_3O_5S_2$·H_2O or anhydrous; pK_a 4.5]—Antibacterial (intestinal). It is very slightly soluble in water (1:4800) and is sparingly soluble in alcohol. It is stable in air but darkens slowly on exposure to light. It is readily soluble in sodium bicarbonate solution. A saturated solution in water is slightly acidic. A 10% aqueous solution of the sodium salt has a pH of approximately 9.

Dispensing Information: Contraindicated in renal or hepatic impairment, pregnancy, and lactation. Avoid prolonged exposure to sunlight. Discontinue use and contact physician immediately if sore throat, fever, or large red inflamed areas on body occur.

Succinylsulfathiazole   Sodium— See under *Succinylsulfathiazole*.

Sucrose USP [saccharum, sugar; $C_{12}H_{22}O_{11}$]—Pharmaceutic aid (flavor). Sucrose is soluble in 0.5 part of water or 170 parts of alcohol. Aqueous solutions of sucrose dissolve calcium hydroxide, forming sucrates of calcium. Sucrose likewise increases the solubility of various other medical agents and essential oils.

Sucrose is a disaccharide which is hydrolyzed by acids or enzymes into dextrose and levulose. The darkening of neutral or acid syrups is due to formation of levulose, which polymerizes to form dark colored compounds. In alkaline preparations the dextrose causes darkening.

Sucrose Octaacetate NF [$C_{28}H_{38}O_{19}$]— Pharmaceutic aid (alcohol denaturant). White powder; practically odorless; intensely bitter taste; hygroscopic; melts not below 78°. 1 g dissolves in about 1100 ml water and 11 ml alcohol; very soluble in chloroform; soluble in ether.

Sudafed Syrup [*B-W* brand of pseudoephedrine hydrochloride]—Nasal decongestant. *Known ingredients:* pseudoephedrine HCl (30 mg/5 ml), glycerin

(10%), sodium benzoate, methylparaben. pH 2.5–3. *Known incompatibilities:* Sudafed Syrup should not be combined in prescription but may be given separately with: Elixir Nembutal, elixir terpin hydrate, sodium salicylate.

Sulfacetamide [$C_8H_{10}N_2O_3S$; pK_a 5.38]—Antibacterial. Sulfacetamide is soluble 1 g in 150 ml water at 20°C, in 15 ml alcohol, and in 7 ml acetone. It is insoluble in ether. An aqueous solution is acid to litmus. It forms a very soluble sodium salt. Solutions in water are stable only when they are adjusted to be neutral or slightly alkaline (pH range, 7–9). Solutions in water are sensitive to light.

Sulfacetamide Sodium USP [Bleph (*Allergan*): Sulamyd Sodium (*Schering*); Sulf-30 (SMP); $C_8H_9N_2NaO_3S \cdot H_2O$]—Antibacterial. This is soluble 1 g in 1.5 ml water, and sparingly soluble in alcohol and in acetone. The pH of 10% (*w/v*) aqueous solution is 9; the pH of 30% aqueous solution is 7.4 (glass electrode). Ampuled solutions can be autoclaved with steam at 115°C for 30 min.

It has been reported that sulfacetamide sodium solutions discolor on exposure to air and light. Edetate sodium alone, sodium thiosulfate, or ascorbic acid did not retard discoloration. Metabisulfite alone retards discoloration until the bisulfite is oxidized, then the solutions discolor even more rapidly. Edetate sodium 0.1% and sodium metabisulfite 0.1% proved the most effective combination. All solutions were adjusted to pH 8–9.9.

Sulfacetamide, Sulfadiazine, and Sulfamerazine Suspension and Tablets [*Various Mfrs.*]—See separate drugs.

Sulfadiazine USP [Coco-Diazine (*Lilly*); $C_{10}H_{10}N_4O_2S$; pK_a 6.37]—Antibacterial. Sulfadiazine is sparingly soluble in water (13 mg/100 ml at pH 5.5) and sparingly soluble in alcohol and acetone. 1 g dissolves in about 620 ml of human serum at 37°C. It is freely soluble in dilute mineral acids and in solutions of potassium and sodium hydroxides and in ammonia water. A saturated solution in water is nearly neutral (pH, about 7) and is stable in air but slowly darkens on exposure to light.

Sulfadiazine Silver [Silvadene (*Marion*); $C_{10}H_9AgN_4O_2S$]—Antimicrobial (topical treatment of burns).

Sulfadiazine Sodium USP [soluble sulfadiazine; $C_{10}H_9N_4NaO_2S$]—Antibacterial. 1 g dissolves in about 2 ml of water. It is only slightly soluble in alcohol. Its solutions are alkaline to phenolphthalein (pH 9–11). Intravenous solutions are best prepared aseptically, sterile sulfadiazine sodium being dissolved in freshly boiled sterile distilled water under the atmosphere of nitrogen; the solutions should not be heated. A 4.5% solution has a pH of about 9.9

Solutions of sulfadiazine sodium undergo color changes and precipitation on prolonged storage. The nature of the degradation is concluded to be one of oxidation. The degradation products do not interfere with the therapeutic efficacy of the sulfadiazine but do make the product appear pharmaceutically objectionable.

In a study undertaken to disclose the nature of the coloration and precipitation, it was found that the infrared and ultraviolet spectra of the precipitate from a sulfadiazine sodium solution differed little from the spectra of pure sulfadiazine. The spectrophotometric evidence indicated that the precipitate is composed of at least 99% sulfadiazine.

The colored fraction of an aged sulfadiazine sodium solution was isolated, using a Soxhlet extractor. The product finally isolated was a yellow-colored oil, the infrared spectrum of which indicated that it consisted of intermediate oxidation products that were postulated to be sulfanilic type compounds which undergo further oxidation to colored compounds with a quinoid structure.

The analytical procedures demonstrated that degradation of the sulfadiazine sodium in ampuls stored at 60°C for 100 days was less than 2% in all quantitative procedures employed.

Sulfaethidole NF [Sul-Spansion,

Sul-Spantab (*SK&F*); $C_{10}H_{12}N_4O_2S_2$]—Antibacterial. Whitish, crystalline powder; practically odorless; melts about 188°. 1 g dissolves in >3000 ml water, 75 ml alcohol, 1300 ml chloroform, and 1700 ml ether.

Sulfamerazine USP [$C_{11}H_{12}N_4O_2S$; pK_a 7.06]—Antibacterial. The solubility in water of pH 5.5 is 35 mg/100 ml at 37°C; it is soluble in water of pH 7.5 (170 mg/100 ml at 37°C). It is readily soluble in dilute mineral acids and in solutions of potassium, ammonium, and sodium hydroxides. It is slightly soluble in alcohol and very slightly soluble in ether and in chloroform. It forms a soluble sodium salt. A saturated solution is nearly neutral (pH, about 7). It is stable in air but slowly darkens on exposure to light.

Sulfamerazine Sodium [soluble sulfamerazine; $C_{11}H_{11}N_4NaO_2S$]—Antibacterial. The sodium salt is hygroscopic. On prolonged exposure to humid air, it absorbs carbon dioxide with the liberation of sulfamerazine and becomes incompletely soluble in water. Its solutions are alkaline to phenolphthalein (pH, 10 or more). 1 g dissolves in 3.6 ml of water. It is slightly soluble in alcohol and insoluble in ether and chloroform.

Sulfamethazine USP [$C_{12}H_{14}N_4O_2S$; pK_a 7.37]—Antibacterial. It is slightly soluble in alcohol and very slightly soluble in water. Solubility in water at 29°C = 150 mg/100 ml; at 37°C = 192 mg/100 ml at pH 7. The solubility increases rapidly with an increase in pH, and the alkaline sodium salt is very soluble in water. A saturated solution in water is nearly neutral (pH, about 7). It may darken on exposure to light.

Sulfamethazine Sodium—See under *Sulfamethazine*.

Sulfamethizole NF [Thiosulfil (*Ayerst*); $C_9H_{10}N_4O_2S_2$]—Antibacterial. White powder or crystals; slightly bitter taste; almost odorless; no odor of hydrogen sulfide. 1 g dissolves in 2990 ml water, 38 ml alcohol, 1888 ml chloroform, and 1936 ml ether.

Sulfamethoxazole NF [Gantanol (*Roche*); $C_{10}H_{11}N_3O_3S$]—Antibacterial.

White powder or crystals; slight bitter taste; practically odorless. 1 g dissolves in 3400 ml water, 50 ml alcohol, and 1000 ml chloroform and ether.

Sulfamethoxypyridazine [Kynex (*Lederle*); Midicel (*P-D*); $C_{11}H_{12}N_4O_3S$; pK_a 7.17]—This sulfonamide is soluble in water at 37°C 1.1 mg/ml at pH 5; 1.2 mg/ml at pH 6; 1.46 mg/ml at pH 6.5.

Sulfamethoxypyridazine Acetyl [Kynex Acetyl (*Lederle*); Midicel Acetyl (*P-D*); $C_{13}H_{14}N_4O_4S$]—Antibacterial. Fine, whitish powder; essentially odorless and tasteless; melts about 186°. 1 g dissolves in about 5000 ml water and 500 ml alcohol.

Sulfanilamide [$C_6H_8N_2O_2S$; pK_a 10.43]—Antibacterial. This drug is soluble 1 g in about 125 ml of water or 37 ml of alcohol; it is soluble in glycerin. Aqueous solutions of sulfanilamide are neutral to litmus (pH of 0.5% solution 5.8–6.1). Sulfanilamide is readily oxidized in solution with the development of a yellow color. Because of this decomposition, sulfanilamide should not be marketed in aqueous solutions. Numerous fatalities resulted from the use of an elixir of sulfanilamide containing diethylene glycol as a solvent. The use of stearic acid as a lubricant in sulfanilamide tablets is not advisable as it apparently promotes photochemical decomposition of the drug.

Sulfapyridine USP [$C_{11}H_{11}N_3O_2S$; pK_a 8.43]—Antibacterial. Sulfapyridine is closely related to sulfanilamide, a hydrogen of the amido group being replaced by the pyridyl group. Sulfapyridine is a white, crystalline powder which is soluble 1 g in about 3500 ml of water or 440 ml of alcohol. It is freely soluble in dilute mineral acids and in aqueous solutions of potassium and sodium hydroxides and is more soluble in warm sugar solutions than in water alone. The aqueous solution of this compound is neutral.

Sulfapyridine Sodium [soluble sulfapyridine; $C_{11}H_{10}N_3O_2SNa \cdot H_2O$, the calcium salt was marketed at one time under the name "Orsulon"]—Antibacterial. Sulfapyridine sodium is soluble 1 g in 1.5 ml of water or 10 ml of alcohol. A 5% solution of sulfapyridine sodium has a pH of 10 to 11. Solutions for intravenous use should not be sterilized by heat because of the instability of the drug.

Sulfasalazine NF [salicylazosulfapyridine; Azulfidine (*Pharmacia*); $C_{18}H_{14}N_4O_5S$]—Antibacterial. Bright yellowish, fine powder; odorless; melts (with decomposition) about 255°. Practically insoluble in water, chloroform, and ether; very slightly soluble in alcohol.

Dispensing Information: Contraindicated in pregnancy. May impart an orange-yellow color to the urine. Take doses evenly spaced and take after meals. Consult physician immediately if skin rash, sore throat, high fever, easy bruising, or purple spots beneath skin appear. See also *Sulfonamides.*

Sulfathiazole [$C_9H_9N_3O_2S_2$]—Antibacterial. Whitish crystals, granules, or powder; melts about 202°. 1 g dissolves in about 1700 ml water and 200 ml alcohol. Now only of historical interest; cannot be recommended for therapeutic use because of the likelihood of hypersensitivity.

Sulfathiazole Sodium [$C_9H_8N_3O_2S_2Na \cdot 1\frac{1}{2} H_2O$ or anhydrous]—Antibacterial. Sulfathiazole sodium is soluble 1 g in 2.5 ml of water or 15 ml of alcohol; the solutions are alkaline. Aqueous solutions have a pH of about 10 and are stable for only a short time; the addition of even weakly acidic substances precipitates the sulfathiazole. Solutions of sulfathiazole sodium develop a precipitate on standing in air due to absorption of carbon dioxide, which liberates the sparingly soluble sulfathiazole. Hence, it is advisable to prepare the solution from distilled water which has been boiled and cooled, and to store the product in small, tightly stoppered bottles. The solution darkens on exposure to light. Parenteral solutions should not be boiled or autoclaved; the solutions should be prepared aseptically and used promptly.

Sulfinpyrazone USP [Anturane (*Geigy*); $C_{23}H_{20}N_2O_3S$]—Uricosuric. Whitish powder; melts about 132°. Practically insoluble in water; soluble in alcohol.

Sulfisoxazole USP [Gantrisin (*Roche*); $C_{11}H_{13}N_3O_3S$; $pK_a \simeq 4.79$]—Antibacterial. Sulfisoxazole is a white to slightly yellowish, odorless, slightly bitter, crystalline powder. It is soluble in alcohol and very slightly soluble in water. Sulfisoxazole is completely soluble, even in neutral or slightly acid body fluids. It is affected by light. The pH of a 10% aqueous solution of the sodium salt is about 9.

Dispensing Information: Potentiates oral anticoagulants and sulfonylureas. Take with large glass of water. Discontinue use if rash, nausea, vomiting, diarrhea, or eye infections occur.

Sulfisoxazole Acetyl USP [Gantrisin Acetyl, (*Roche*); $C_{13}H_{15}N_3O_4S$]—antibacterial. Acetylsulfisoxazole is a white to slightly off-white, crystalline solid, with a slight characteristic odor. It is very soluble in alcohol and practically insoluble in water.

Sulfisoxazole Diolamine NF [Gantrisin Diolamine (*Roche*); $C_{11}H_{13}N_3O_3S \cdot C_4H_{11}O_2$]—Antibacterial. Sulfisoxazole diethanolamine is made by adding enough diethanolamine to a solution of sulfisoxazole to bring the pH to about 7.5. This salt is more soluble at the physiologic pH range (6–7.8) than sulfisoxazole itself. *Known incompatibilities* (sulfisoxazole diolamine injection); acidic solutions, ammonium chloride, codeine phosphate, Demerol, hydroxyzine HCl, insulin, Kantrex, Leridine, levallorphan tartrate, levarterenol bitartrate, methadone HCl, morphine sulfate, oxytetracycline HCl, Phenergan, phenytoin, procaine HCl, prochlorperazine maleate, Sparine, streptomycin sulfate, tetracycline HCl, thiopental sodium, Vancocin, vitamin B complex with C.

Sulfisoxazole Sodium—See under *Sulfisoxazole.*

Sulfobromophthalein Sodium USP [Bromsulphalein (*HW&D*); $C_{20}H_8Br_4Na_2O_{10}S_2$]—Diagnostic aid (hepatic function determination). White, crystalline powder; odorless; bitter taste; hygroscopic. Soluble in water; insoluble in alcohol.

Sulfonamides—*Dispensing Information:* Patients should advise their physician of any dermatologic symptoms coming to their attention during therapy with sulfonamides. Patients allergic to thiazide diuretics and/or sulfonylurea oral hypoglycemic agents may be allergic to sulfonamides. Fever developing during therapy should be brought to the attention of the physician, as well as joint pains, sore throat, or easy bruising. High fluid intake during therapy should be encouraged. Ascorbic acid should not be taken so as to avoid a lowered urinary pH that facilitates the development of sulfonamide crystalluria that can occur with the more insoluble sulfonamides. Blacks who are deficient in glucose-6-phosphate dehydrogenase should receive sulfonamides only if other non-sulfonamide antibacterials cannot be used. Numerous drug interaction potentials exist in patients taking sulfonamides.

Sulfosalicylic Acid [$C_7H_6O_6S \cdot 2H_2O$ or anhydrous]—*In vitro* diagnostic aid (protein).

Sulfoxone Sodium NF [Diasone Sodium (*Abbott*); $C_{14}H_{14}N_2Na_2O_6S_3$; p$K_{a1}$ 11.51; pK_{a2} 12.70]—Antibacterial (leprostatic). Mixture (about 77% sulfoxone sodium plus buffers and inert ingredients). Whitish powder; characteristic odor. 1 g dissolves in about 14 ml water, >1000 ml alcohol and chloroform, and >2000 ml ether.

Sulfur Dioxide USP [SO_2]—Pharmaceutic aid (antioxidant). Colorless, nonflammable gas; strong, suffocating odor characteristic of burning sulfur. At 20° and standard pressure, approx 36 volumes dissolve in 1 volume water and approx 114 volumes dissolve in 1 volume alcohol; soluble also in chloroform and ether. *Known incompatibilities:* oxidizing agents.

Sulfur Ointment USP—Scabicide. Contains precipitated sulfur, mineral oil, and white ointment. *Known incompatibilities:* oxidizing agents, fixed alkalies.

Sulfur, Precipitated, USP [S]—Scabicide. Very fine, pale-yellow, amorphous or microcrystalline powder; no odor or taste. 1 g dissolves in >10,000 ml water, <1 ml carbon disulfide, 100 ml olive oil, and 1000–10,000 ml alcohol. *Known incompatibilities:* oxidizing agents, fixed alkalies.

Sulfur, Sublimed, NF [S]—Parasiticide; scabicide. Fine, yellow, crystalline powder; faint odor and taste. Practically insoluble in water and nearly so in alcohol; 1 g dissolves in 30–100 ml olive oil. *Known incompatibilities:* oxidizing agents, fixed alkalies.

Sulisobenzone [Spectra-Sorb UV 284 (*Am. Cyanamid*); Sungard (*Miles*); Uval (*Dome*); Uvinul MS-40 (*GAF*); $C_{14}H_{12}O_6S$]—Ultraviolet screen. Light-tan powder; odorless; characteristic taste; melts about 145°. 1 g dissolves in about 4 ml water and 3.3 ml alcohol.

Sutilains NF [Travase (*Flint*)]—Proteolytic enzymes derived from *Bacillus subtilis*. Potency at least 2,500,000 NF Casein Units of proteolytic activity/g. Cream-colored powder; odorless; irritating to oral membranes (do not taste); decomposes in heat; hygroscopic. 1 g dissolves in about 100 ml water; insoluble in alcohol and most other organic solvents.

Sympathomimetic Agents (Inhalation Aerosols)—*Dispensing Information:* Patients should be familiar with their inhalation equipment and directions for use. Advise physician if rapid heart beat, palpitations, anxiety, nervousness, or tremulousness occur. Overuse may lead to increased frequency of asthmatic attacks.

Sympathomimetic Agents (Nasal)—*Dispensing Information:* Overuse can lead to diminished effect and/or potentially a rebound or worsening nasal stuffiness after excessive use.

Synkayvite Ampuls [*Roche* brand of menadiol sodium diphosphate]—*Known ingredients:* Synkayvite (2, 5, 10, 37.5 mg/ml). *Known compatibilities:* atropine sulfate, Bejectal, Berocca

C, Berocca C-500, dextrose solution, fructose solution, Mercuhydrin, normal saline, Prostigmin Methylsulfate Ampul Solution, procaine penicillin aqueous for injection, Terramycin Intravenous, vitamin C ampul solution. *Known incompatibilities:* Nisentil.

Talbutal NF [Lotusate (*Winthrop*); $C_{11}H_{16}N_2O_3$]—Hypnotic; sedative. White, crystalline powder; may have slight odor; melts about 108° (polymorphic form about 111°). 1 g dissolves in about 500 ml water, 1 ml alcohol, 2 ml chloroform, and 40 ml ether.

Talwin Solution [*Winthrop*]—Analgesic. Pentazocine. *Injection, 30 mg/ml:* pH 4–5; aqueous solvent; buffer, NaOH; preservatives, acetone sodium bisulfite/methylparaben.

Tannates—See under *Tannic Acid.*

Tannic Acid [tannin, gallotannic acid]—Tannic acid used as an astringent, styptic, and alkaloidal antidote is a complex mixture obtained from nutgalls and consists largely of compounds in which the hydroxyl groups of glucose are esterified by gallic and digallic acids. Tannic acid is very soluble in water (1:0.35), alcohol, and warm glycerin (1:1). The pH of a 1% solution is about 2.9. *Caution:* Tannic acid is unstable in aqueous solution and hydrolyzes to gallic acid which decomposes and darkens in air. Consequently, tannic acid solutions should be freshly prepared and labeled "Store in a Refrigerator." Liver damage may result from application of tannic acid over large denuded areas or from combinations with barium sulfate.

Deterioration of solutions of tannic acid is retarded by glycerin, alcohol, or 0.1% of sodium bisulfite. Alkalies precipitate tannin from solution; the precipitate is soluble in excess, and the solution darkens on standing. Practically all alkaloids are precipitated as tannates from aqueous solution, but not from alcohol. Antipyrine and some glycosides, gums, and neutral principles are likewise precipitated by tannic acid. Gelatin, albumin, starch, and salts of many of the heavy metals form precipitates with tannic acid. Most ferric salts give a blue-black color or precipitate with tannic acid. Ferrous salts in concentrated solution form a white precipitate with tannin. This precipitate becomes blue as soon as some ferric iron is formed by exposure to air. The coloration with ferric salts is diminished or prevented by addition of sufficient phosphoric acid to form ferric phosphate. Tannic acid solutions reduce oxidizing agents, e.g., iodine, permanganates, and chlorates; if tannic acid is triturated dry with oxidizing agents, explosions are likely to occur. Tannic acid will frequently reduce ammoniated mercury to metallic mercury even in a grease base ointment. Ethyl nitrite spirit, when mixed with tannin, turns red and liberates oxides of nitrogen.

Preparations of gambir, krameria, kino, rubus, wild cherry, nux vomica, and other tannin-containing drugs have the same incompatibilities as tannin.

In some proprietary specialties, incompatibilities of tannin-bearing drugs are avoided by using preparations which have been detannated by special processes such as precipitation of the tannin with gelatin. Cinchona alkaloids elixir does not contain tannin as would be the case with an elixir made from the crude drug.

Tartaric Acid NF [$C_4H_6O_6$; pK_{a1} 2.96, pK_{a2} 4.16]—Pharmaceutic aid (buffering agent). Tartaric acid is a weak acid useful as a pharmaceutic. It is soluble in water (1:0.75), ethanol (1:3), and glycerin. *Caution:* Large doses sometimes used as a laxative may produce renal damage or acidosis. The pH of a 1% solution is about 2.2. The normal tartrates of the alkali metals are water-soluble, e.g., sodium tartrate (1:3), potassium and sodium tartrate (1:0.9), potassium tartrate (1:0.5), and ammonium tartrate (1:17). These compounds are useful as buffers, salt formers, solubilizers, and complexing agents. Potassium bitartrate is only slightly soluble in cold water (1:162); hence, it may be precipitated when solutions of tartaric acid are treated with solutions containing the potassium ion or when a Rochelle Salt (potassium sodium tartrate) solution is acidified. Other tartrates are less soluble, and calcium, barium, strontium, lead, silver, or copper tartrate may separate from mixtures of these ions unless excess tartrate is present to form complexes. Soluble complexes or chelates may form in slightly alkaline solutions through replacement of the hydrogen of the hydroxyl group: e.g., bismuth potassium tartrate ($K(BiO)C_4H_4O$) and antimony potassium tartrate ($K(SbO)C_4H_4O_6$). Strong oxidizing agents convert tartaric acid into oxalic acid.

Tartrates—See under *Tartaric Acid.*

Tedral Tablets [*W-C*]—Asthma therapy. Contain theophylline 130 mg, ephedrine HCl 24 mg, phenobarbital 8 mg.

Dispensing Information: Do not drive or operate heavy machinery upon initial therapy. May take with food if GI distress occurs. Discontinue use and consult physician if rash develops. Do not exceed two tablets in any 4-hour period.

Tegopen Oral Solution [*Bristol*]—Cloxacillin sodium 125 mg/5 ml. pH 5–7.5; buffer, sodium citrate anhydrous; sweetener, sugar 90.4%; Na^+ 1.43 mEq/5 ml.

Terbutaline Sulfate [Bricanyl Sulfate (*Astra*); $(C_{12}H_{19}NO_3)_2 \cdot H_2SO_4$; pK_{a1} 8.8; pK_{a2} 10.1; pK_{a3} 11.2]—Bronchodilator. Whitish, crystalline powder; odorless or faint odor; slightly bitter taste; light-sensitive. 1 g dissolves in about 2 ml water and 250 ml alcohol.

Terpin Hydrate NF [$C_{10}H_{20}O_2 \cdot H_2O$]—Expectorant. Colorless, lustrous crystals or white powder; slight odor; effloresces in dry air; 1% hot solution in water is neutral to litmus. 1 g dissolves in 200 ml water, 13 ml alcohol, 140 ml chloroform, 140 ml ether, 35 ml boiling water, and 3 ml boiling alcohol.

Terramycin Hydrochloride Crystalline Intravenous [*Pfizer*]—Intravenous antibiotic. *Known ingredients:* Terramycin HCl (250 mg/vial). *Known compatibilities:* dextrose 5% in water, dextrose 5% in saline, Levugen 10% in water, Levugen 10% in saline, Levugen 10% in electrolytes, Amigen 5%-Levugen 10%, Amigen 5%-dextrose 5%.

Testolactone NF [Teslac (*Squibb*); $C_{19}H_{24}O_3$]—Antineoplastic. Whitish, crystalline powder; practically odorless; melts about 218°. Slightly soluble in water; soluble in alcohol and chloroform; insoluble in ether.

Testosterone NF [*Various Mfrs.;* $C_{19}H_{28}O_2$]—Androgen. Testosterone consists of white or slightly creamy white crystals or is a crystalline powder. It is odorless. It is freely soluble in alcohol and practically insoluble in water (0.02 mg/ml). It is stable in air and to light.

Dispensing Information: May cause masculinization of female and gynecomastia in males. Take exactly as directed.

Testosterone Cypionate USP [testosterone cyclopentylpropionate; *Various Mfrs.;* $C_{27}H_{40}O_3$]—Androgen. Off-white, odorless, tasteless, crystalline powder. It is freely soluble in alcohol and slightly soluble in water.

Testosterone Enanthate USP [Delatestryl (*Squibb*); $C_{26}H_{40}O_3$]—Androgen. Whitish, crystalline powder; odorless or faint, characteristic odor; melts about 36°. Insoluble in water; 1 g dissolves in about 0.5 ml ether; soluble in vegetable oils.

Testosterone Propionate USP [*Various Mfrs.;* $C_{22}H_{32}O_3$]—Androgen. This is insoluble in water, freely soluble in alcohol and ether, and soluble in vegetable oils.

Tetracaine NF [$C_{15}H_{24}N_2O_2$]–Topical anesthetic. Whitish, waxy solid; melts about 43°. 1 g dissolves in >1000 ml water, 2 ml chloroform and ether, and 5 ml alcohol.

Tetracaine Hydrochloride USP [Pontocaine Hydrochloride (*Winthrop*); $C_{15}H_{24}N_2O_2 \cdot HCl$]—Local anesthetic. Tetracaine hydrochloride is a white, crystalline powder which is very soluble in water and soluble in alcohol.

A 2% solution of the drug has a pH of 5.4; the addition of alkali hydroxides or carbonates precipitates the free base as an oily liquid. Solutions of tetracaine hydrochloride are stable indefinitely and are unaffected by boiling. Tetracaine and related local anesthetics form unstable complexes with copper ions.

Pontocaine eye ointment contains 0.5% of pontocaine base incorporated in pure petrolatum. This ointment is incompatible with salts of mercury and silver but may be used in conjunction with zinc sulfate, boric acid, resorcin, eserine sulfate, atropine, pilocarpine, and epinephrine.

Tetrachloroethylene USP [carbon dichloride, perchloroethylene, tetrachloroethene; ethylene tetrachloride; C_2Cl_4]—Anthelmintic (hookworms and some trematodes). Tetrachloroethylene is a colorless liquid with an ethereal odor. 1 g is soluble in 1 ml of alcohol or about 10,000 ml of water, and is miscible with oils. This drug is usually given in soft capsules. Broken capsules or liquid which has been exposed to air should not be administered due to possible formation of toxic phosgene. Oils, fats, and alcohol should be avoided as they promote undesirable absorption of the drug, which is used as an anthelmintic. A dose of magnesium sulfate is usually given 1 or 2 hours after the tetrachloroethylene has been administered.

Tetracycline USP [*Various Mfrs.;* $C_{22}H_{24}N_2O_8$; pK_a 8.3, 9.2]—Antibacterial; antiamebic; antirickettsial. Tetracycline differs from chlortetracycline (Aureomycin) by a chlorine atom and from oxytetracycline (Terramycin) by an OH group. Tetracycline can be obtained chemically by the dechlorination of Aureomycin and by fermentation using *Streptomycetes Sp.*

Tetracycline is reported to be more stable and less toxic than Aureomycin and Terramycin.

Tetracycline is amphoteric with two acidic groups and one basic group and forms salts with acids and bases. Tetracycline base is hydrated (up to $6H_2O$) or anhydrous.

Tetracycline is a yellow, odorless powder. It is stable in air but darkens on exposure to strong sunlight. Its potency is affected in solutions below pH 2, e.g., it shows no loss at pH 1 after 2 days but a 40% loss in 8 days at room temperature. It is rapidly destroyed by alkali hydroxide solutions, e.g., it shows a 50% loss in 12 hours at pH 8.85. However, there have been patented stable tetracycline solutions for oral use buffered to pH 9.5 to 11 with calcium hydroxide and inorganic phosphates other than orthophosphates. True solutions were not obtained when citrate, tartrate, sulfate, chloride, etc., were present. In pH 4 buffer it undergoes a 40% loss in 3 weeks. It is reported to be stable as a suspension at pH 7.

1 g of tetracycline dissolves in about 2500 ml of water and in about 50 ml of alcohol. It readily dissolves in dilute hydrochloric acid and alkali hydroxide solutions. It is practically insoluble in chloroform and ether.

The pH of a saturated solution of tetracycline is between 3 and 7.

In capsules, tetracycline is compatible with ascorbic acid, calcium carbonate, monobasic calcium phosphate, kaolin, lactose, magnesium stearate, potassium dihydrogen phosphate, sodium bisulfite, stearic acid, sugar, and talc.

In tablets, tetracycline is compatible with acacia, dibasic calcium phosphate, monobasic calcium phosphate, carnauba wax, lactose, magnesium stearate, sodium citrate, starch, talc, and white wax.

In oral powders to be reconstituted with water, tetracycline is compatible with acacia, carboxymethylcellulose, cocoa, methylcellulose, soluble saccharin, insoluble saccharin, sugar, vanillin, various flavors, and dyes.

Tetracycline, oxytetracycline, and chlortetracycline have been reported to be inactivated under certain conditions by vitamin mixtures containing riboflavin. The inactivation reaction is said to be a photochemical oxidation of the tetracycline molecule in which riboflavin plays the part of a sensitizer. Inactivation does not take place in the dark or in the presence of nitrogen and a reducing agent, i.e., sodium metabisulfite.

Dispensing Information: See *Tetracyclines.*

Tetracycline Hydrochloride USP [*Various Mfrs.;* $C_{22}H_{24}N_2O_8 \cdot HCl$]— Category: See *Tetracycline.* Tetracycline HCl is a yellow, odorless, crystalline powder. It is moderately hygroscopic. It is stable in air but darkens on exposure to strong sunlight. Its potency is affected in solutions with a pH below 2 and is slowly destroyed by alkali hydroxide solutions (see *Tetracycline*). A 1% aqueous solution has a pH value of about 2.5.

1 g of tetracycline HCl dissolves in 10 ml of water and in about 100 ml of alcohol, the aqueous solution becoming turbid after some time because of hydrolysis. It is soluble in solutions of alkali hydroxides and carbonates and is practically insoluble in chloroform and in ether.

Known incompatibilities: Although the mechanism of incompatibility has not been precisely determined, tetracycline hydrochloride has been reported to be physically or chemically incompatible with solutions containing aminophylline, amobarbital sodium, amphotericin B, ampicillin sodium, calcium chloride, calcium gluconate, carbenicillin disodium, cephalothin sodium, chloramphenicol sodium succinate, chlorothiazide sodium, chlorpromazine hydrochloride, cloxacillin sodium, colistimethate sodium, corticotropin, diphenylhydantoin sodium, epinephrine hydrochloride, erythromycin gluceptate, erythromycin lactobionate, heparin sodium, hydrocortisone phosphate, hydrocortisone sodium succinate, hyaluronidase, levarterenol bitartrate, methicillin sodium, methyldopa hydrochloride, nafcillin sodium, nitrofurantoin sodium, novobiocin sodium, oxacillin sodium, potassium penicillin G, sodium penicillin G, pentobarbital sodium, phenobarbital sodium, polymyxin B sulfate, prochlorperazine edisylate, riboflavin, secobarbital sodium, sodium bicarbonate, streptomycin sulfate, sulfadiazine sodium, sulfisoxazole diolamine, thiopental sodium, warfarin sodium, and vitamin B complex with C. There are conflicting reports of incompatibilities of tetracycline with Ringer's injection, lactated Ringer's injection, and protein hydrolysate injection.

Tetracycline Phosphate Complex NF [Sumycin (*Squibb*); Tetrex (*Bristol*)]—Antibacterial. Yellow, crystalline powder; odorless; pH (sat soln) 2.5–2.6. Sparingly soluble in water; slightly soluble in methanol; very slightly soluble in acetone.

Tetracyclines—*Dispensing Information:* Tetracyclines generally should be administered on an empty stomach. Milk, food, antacids (containing calcium, magnesium, and aluminum salts), iron salts, and sodium bicarbonate should not be taken for at least 1 hour after tetracycline administration. Occasionally, tetracyclines will be prescribed with meals or milk to those patients who develop serious gastric disturbances to these agents. Superinfection with *Candida albicans* can develop during therapy. Female patients should report vaginal irritation or itching to the physician. Anorexia, nausea and vomiting, and rash are side effects patients frequently develop. Phototoxicity can occur; in summer months patients should be made aware that an exaggerated sunburn response can occur if exposure to the sun is prolonged or intense. Tetracyclines should not be given in pregnancy. Patients should be cautioned against prolonged storage of tetracyclines. Medication remaining after a completed course of therapy should be discarded appropriately. Tetracyclines should not be given to children 8 years old or younger because of the possibility of permanent staining or discoloration of the teeth.

Tetrahydrozoline Hydrochloride USP [Tyzine (*Pfizer*); Visine (*Leeming*); $C_{13}H_{16}N_2 \cdot HCl$]—Adrenergic (vasoconstrictor). White solid; odorless;

melts about 256°. 1 g dissolves in about 4 ml water, 8 ml alcohol, and >1000 ml chloroform and ether.

Tetranitrol—See *Erithrityl Tetranitrate, Diluted.*

Tetrex Syrup [*Bristol*]—Antibacterial. Tetracycline phosphate complex 125 mg/5 ml. pH 4–4.5; solvent, purified water; buffer, phosphoric acid (reagent grade) or potassium hydroxide solution 18.75%; sugar 65.37%; Na^+ 0.35 mEq/5 ml.

Theobromine [3,7-dimethylxanthine; $C_7H_8N_4O_2$; pK_a 10.05, pK_a 13.89]—Theobromine is a diuretic soluble 1 g in 1800 ml of water or 2400 ml of alcohol. It has a bitter taste.

Theobromine Calcium Salicylate [Theocalcin (*Knoll*)]—Diuretic; smooth muscle relaxant. Theobromine calcium and calcium salicylate in approx. equimolecular proportions (about 48% theobromine). White powder; odorless; saline taste. Slightly soluble in water; insoluble in alcohol.

Theobromine Sodium Acetate—Diuretic; smooth muscle relaxant. Theobromine sodium and sodium acetate in approx. equimolecular proportions (about 60% theobromine). White, crystalline powder; bitter taste; moderately hygroscopic; powder or its solution absorbs CO_2 in air, liberating theobromine. 1 g dissolves in about 2 ml water; slightly soluble in alcohol.

Theobromine Sodium Salicylate—Diuretic; smooth muscle relaxant. Theobromine sodium and sodium salicylate in approx. equimolecular proportions (at least 46.5% theobromine and 35% salicylic acid). Whitish powder; odorless or slight odor; sweetish, salty, somewhat alkaline taste; absorbs CO_2 in air becoming incompletely soluble in water; solution (1 in 20) alkaline to litmus. 1 g dissolves in about 1 ml water; slightly soluble in alcohol.

Theophylline USP [1,3-dimethylxanthine; Elixophyllin (*Cooper*); Optiphyllin (*Fougera*); $C_7H_8N_4O_2 \cdot H_2O$ or anhydrous]—Smooth muscle relaxant (bronchioles). White, crystalline powder; odorless; bitter taste; label to indi-

cate whether anhydrous or hydrous. There are reported incompatibilities of soluble theophylline derivatives when mixed with citric acid, tartaric acid, ascorbic acid, caffeine and sodium benzoate, ephedrine hydrochloride, pyribenzamine, etc. These acidic drugs will release the free xanthine from its complexes. Neutral compounds such as lactose, reserpine, aminopyrine, caffeine, etc., were compatible. The compatibilities of theophylline and its mixtures are similar to those of the other purine bases. Theophylline base is stable in air but produces a yellow discoloration on prolonged exposure to light; aqueous solutions are stable with mild acids or alkalies but are decomposed by strong acids or bases.

Dispensing Information: See *Smooth Muscle Relaxants (Xanthine Type).*

Theophylline Meglumine—Smooth muscle relaxant. Equimolecular mixture of theophylline and *N*-methylglucamine. More soluble than *Theophylline Sodium Acetate.*

Theophylline Olamine NF [(*Fleet*); Theamin (*Lilly*); $C_7H_8N_4O_2 \cdot C_2H_7NO$; pK_a 9.1]—Smooth muscle relaxant. Coarse, whitish, crystalline powder; not more than slight odor. 1 g dissolves in about 20 ml water.

Theophylline Sodium Acetate—Smooth muscle relaxant. Theophylline sodium and sodium acetate in approx. equimolecular proportions (about 60% theophylline). White, crystalline powder; odorless; bitter, salty taste; absorbs CO_2 in air, liberating theophylline; solution alkaline to phenolphthalein TS. 1 g dissolves in about 25 ml water; insoluble in alcohol, chloroform, and ether.

Theophylline Sodium Glycinate NF [Synophylate (*Central*)]—Smooth muscle relaxant. Theophylline sodium and aminoacetic acid in approx. equimolecular proportions with an additional mole of aminoacetic acid as buffer (about 50% theophylline). White, crystalline powder; slight ammoniacal odor; bitter taste; pH (sat soln) about 9. One g dissolves in about 6 ml water; very slightly soluble in alcohol; practically insoluble in chloroform.

Thiabendazole USP [Mintezol (*MSD*); Thibenzole (*Merck*); $C_{10}H_7N_3S$]—Anthelmintic. Whitish powder; odorless or almost so; tasteless; melts about 300°. Practically insoluble in water; very slightly soluble in ether; 1 g dissolves in about 150 ml alcohol and 300 ml chloroform.

Thiamine Hydrochloride USP [Betalin S (*Lilly*), vitamin B_1 hydrochloride; aneurine hydrochloride; $C_{12}H_{17}ClN_4OS \cdot HCl$]—Enzyme co-factor vitamin. Thiamine occurs in nature as the free compound, as salts, as protein complexes and as the ester with pyrophosphoric acid (cocarboxylase).

Thiamine hydrochloride deliquesces under high humidity. Despite its variable moisture content (up to 5%) crystalline thiamine hydrochloride is stable as a solid at room temperature and at elevated temperatures even in contact with air. 1 g dissolves in about 1 ml water, 18 ml glycerin, 100 ml 95% alcohol, and 315 ml absolute alcohol; it is more soluble in methanol and practically insoluble in ether, benzene, hexane, chloroform, and oils. The pH of a 1% *w/v* solution in water is 3.13; the pH of a 0.1% *w/v* solution in water is 3.58. The kinetics of thiamine hydrolysis has been studied and the pH profile of thiamine hydrolysis suggests at least four separate reactions.

Being a compound of the pyrimidinethiazole type, thiamine hydrochloride has many of the properties and incompatibilities of the alkaloids. In aqueous solution it forms a white precipitate with mercuric chloride, a red-brown precipitate with iodine, and also yields precipitates with picric acid and potassium mercuric iodide. Tannic acid precipitates thiamine hydrochloride; hence, wines used as vehicles should be completely detannated. It has been reported that thiamine hydrochloride gives precipitates with iodides, carbonates, bicarbonates, acetates, ferric ammonium citrate, ferric sulfate, sodium phosphate, sodium borate, Fowler's solution, and phenobarbital sodium. It also has the incompatibilities of chlorides.

Thiamine hydrochloride is incompatible with alkalies and alkaline salts, including magnesium carbonate, sodium citrate, ammonium citrate, and alkaloidal bases; such alkaline substances produce the unstable thiamine base. Thiamine hydrochloride is incompatible with iron, cobalt, and copper salts. It has been shown that the latter two metals are less likely to cause decomposition in the presence of phosphate and gluconate buffers.

In the solid form thiamine hydrochloride is not oxidized or destroyed by exposure to air or light. Even heating at 100°C for 24 hours in contact with air causes no loss in potency of the dry crystals. Thiamine hydrochloride in aqueous solution is stable at pH 2.5 to 4.5 at low temperatures (4°C) and fairly stable at room temperature. The vitamin potency is lowered by heat, especially if solution is alkaline. The vitamin effect is destroyed by heating at 115° to 120°C for 1 or 2 hours, but heating at 100°C for a short time causes little destruction. A relatively large proportion of the vitamin is destroyed or lost in cooking. Solutions of crystalline thiamine hydrochloride for parenteral injection may be sterilized by heating for 1 hour at 100°C or 20 min at 120°C without appreciable loss in potency if the pH is 3.5; solutions so sterilized remain stable for more than 4 months.

An intravenous solution of thiamine hydrochloride with a pH of 3.5 may be prepared by dissolving the crystals in freshly distilled water in the proportion of 5 mg/ml. When only 1 or 2 ml are used for intravenous injection, it is not considered necessary to neutralize the solution as would be done when larger amounts are injected. A solution with a pH of 6.2 (for intramuscular injection) may be prepared by dissolving 0.1 g of thiamine hydrochloride crystals in 1 ml of sterile distilled water and adding 1.5 ml of a 0.1 *M* solution of tribasic sodium phosphate of reagent grade; sufficient distilled water may be added to make 10 ml or any other desired volume. Both the intravenous and intramuscular solutions are filtered and ·placed in ampuls, which are then sealed and sterilized in live steam at 120°C for 20 min. There is some evidence that about 10% of the potency may be lost during sterilization of the buffered solution. To cover this loss, a 10% excess of thiamine hydrochloride may be used in preparing the solution. Thiamine hydrochloride is readily adsorbed by fuller's earth or charcoal.

Hydrogen peroxide, potassium permanganate, and other oxidizing agents convert thiamine hydrochloride into thiochrome, $C_{12}H_{14}N_4OS$. Small amounts of thiochrome are formed when alcoholic solutions of thiamine hydrochloride stand at room temperature for several months. Very little thiochrome is formed in aqueous solutions at pH 2, but it is produced more rapidly the nearer the pH is to 7.

Thiamine hydrochloride is decomposed by reducing agents such as formaldehyde, tannins, sulfur dioxide, sulfites, starch containing sulfites, etc.

Thiamine has been reported to interact with other vitamins (i.e., pantothenic acid, cyanocobalamin, and riboflavin).

The problem with thiamine-pantothenic acid combinations is largely a pH problem. Adjustment of pH to about 4 to insure thiamine stability results in rapid decomposition of pantothenate. The use of pantothenyl alcohol (*qv*) has largely eliminated this problem, at least for dispensing purposes.

Incompatibilities of thiamine hydrochloride with cyanocobalamin have been found by some workers but not by others. This has apparently been resolved as differences due to the concentrations of drugs present, the effects of heat and the presence of thiamine decomposition products (i.e., thiazole compounds which may function as reducing agents for cyanocobalamin). The use of ferric chloride as a stabilizer at

pH 4–4.5 to avoid this problem has been proposed. Special processing techniques have been reported (i.e., with a critical drug ratio, a critical pH, and avoiding heat) which may also help here. These procedures worked if the thiamine-cyanocobalamin ratio did not exceed 120 to 1 but at 5000 to 1 or 10,000 to 1 proved inoperative. One method which assures maximum stabilization involves lyophilization.

An incompatibility between thiamine and riboflavin has been noted in aqueous vitamin B complex solutions which manifests itself as trace precipitation of thiochrome or chloroflavin. The precipitation of thiochrome is brought about by the oxidative action of riboflavin on thiamine. The greater the riboflavin concentration or the greater the air or oxygen present, the faster the reaction. On the other hand, the reducing action of thiamine or its decomposition products on riboflavin results in the appearance of chloroflavin. This occurs more readily as the ratio between thiamine and riboflavin concentrations increases. This incompatibility has been reported to be entirely eliminated by the addition of ascorbic acid.

Thiamine hydrochloride is chemically compatible with acids and acid salts, including acid reacting salts of alkaloids and iron. In acid media it is compatible with benzoic acid, salicylic acid, and their derivatives. Thiamine hydrochloride is compatible with sucrose, dextrose, lactose, alcohol, glycerin, and gelatin (free from sulfites).

Numerous proprietary specialties contain thiamine hydrochloride in an elixir or wine base, e.g., Elixir Betalin S, Vinothiam, Lixa-Beta, Elixir Bewon, Thialixir, and Elixir Betaxin. Examples of similar preparations, containing thiamine hydrochloride and other vitamins of the B complex are Elixir B-G-Phos, Elixir Betalin Complex, and Elixir Beta-Concemin.

Thialixir contains vitamin B_1 in a base containing 22% of alcohol by volume. Being acid in reaction (pH about 3.5), it is incompatible with carbonates and alkalies. However, it has a wide range of compatibility, due in large measure to the fact that it contains no wine. Thialixir is pharmaceutically compatible with a considerable variety of drugs, including iodides, ammonium chloride, and such salts as bromides, acetates, and citrates. It is also compatible with numerous alkaloidal salts, barbiturates, tinctures, and fluidextracts.

Elixir Betalin S and Elixir Betalin Complex are compatible with bromides, potassium iodide, sodium citrate, sodium salicylate, pepsin, chloral hydrate, atropine sulfate, diluted hydrochloric acid, ferric ammonium citrate, and aminoacetic acid elixir. These elixirs should not be used as vehicles for alkalies, and they are also incompatible with tinctures of nux vomica and belladonna and other tinctures of high alcoholic content.

Thiamine Mononitrate USP [aneurine mononitrate; $C_{12}H_{17}N_5O_4S$; pK_a 4.8]—Enzyme co-factor vitamin. The solubility in water is 2.7 g/100 ml at 25°C and approximately 30 g/100 ml at 100°C.

In the dry form the vitamin is stable, and heating at 100°C for 24 hours does not diminish its potency. In aqueous solution it can be sterilized at 110°C, but if the pH of the solution is above 5.5, it is destroyed rapidly. It is practically nonhygroscopic. 1 g of thiamine mononitrate is equal to 343,000 International Units. It is more stable than the hydrochloride and is especially recommended for enrichment of flour mixes and the preparation of multivitamin capsules and tablets.

The pH of 2% aqueous solution is 6.5 to 7.1. Solutions of pH 4 show greater stability than neutral solutions and can be prepared in concentrations as high as 18.5 g/100 ml at room temperature. For preparing solutions of pH 4 approximately 2.6 ml of 1 N HCl is required for each gram of thiamine mononitrate when no other acidic or basic substances are present.

Thiethylperazine Malate NF [Torecan(*Sandoz*);$C_{22}H_{29}N_3S_2 \cdot 2C_4H_6O_5$]—

Antiemetic. Whitish, crystalline powder; slight odor; pH (fresh 1 in 100 soln) about 3.3. One g dissolves in about 40 ml water, 90 ml alcohol, 525 ml chloroform, and 3400 ml ether. This water-soluble salt is used to prepare the infection; see also *Thiethylperazine Maleate*.

Thiethylperazine Maleate NF [Torecan(*Sandoz*);$C_{22}H_{29}N_3S_2 \cdot 2C_4H_4O_4$]—Fine, yellowish, crystalline powder; odorless or slight odor; bitter taste; melts (with decomposition) about 183°. 1 g dissolves in about 1700 ml water and 530 ml alcohol; insoluble in chloroform and ether. This salt is used to prepare suppositories and tablets; see also *Thiethylperazine Malate*.

Thimerosal NF [Merthiolate (*Lilly*); $C_9H_9HgNaO_2S$]—Topical anti-infective. Merthiolate is an antiseptic and preservative soluble 1 g in about 1 ml of water or about 12 ml of alcohol. A 1% aqueous solution has a pH of 6.7.

Thioguanine USP [*B-W;* $C_5H_5N_5S$ or the hemihydrate]—Antineoplastic. Pale yellow, crystalline powder; odorless or almost so. Insoluble in water and chloroform; 1 g dissolves in about 7700 ml alcohol.

Thiopental Sodium USP [Pentothal Sodium (*Abbott*); $C_{11}H_{17}N_2NaO_2S$]—Anesthetic (intravenous). Thiopental sodium is a hygroscopic powder which is soluble in water and alcohol. The aqueous solution is alkaline and decomposes on standing; if the solution is boiled, a precipitate is formed.

Thiopropazate   Hydrochloride [Dartal   Hydrochloride   (*Searle*); $C_{23}H_{28}ClN_3O_2S \cdot 2HCl$]—Tranquilizer. *Side effects:* May show an extrapyramidal activity of pseudoparkinsonism on high dosage.

Thioridazine [Mellaril (*Sandoz*); $C_{21}H_{26}N_2S_2$]—Tranquilizer. Crystalline powder; melts about 73°.

Thioridazine Hydrochloride USP [Mellaril   Hydrochloride   (*Sandoz*); $C_{21}H_{26}N_2S_2 \cdot HCl$]—Tranquilizer. Whitish, granular powder; faint odor; very bitter taste; pH (1 in 10 soln) 3.5–4.5; melts about 162°. 1 g dissolves in about

9 ml water, 10 ml alcohol, and 2 ml chloroform; insoluble in ether.

Dispensing Information: See *Antipsychotic Agents (Phenothiazine Type).*

Thiotepa NF [Thio-Tepa (*Lederle*); $C_6H_{12}N_3PS$]—Antineoplastic. Fine, white, crystalline flakes; faint odor; melts about 54°. 1 g dissolves in about 13 ml water, 2 ml chloroform, 4 ml ether, and 8 ml alcohol. *Caution: Extremely poisonous.*

Thiothixene NF [Navane (*Roerig*); $C_{23}H_{29}N_3O_2S_2$]—Tranquilizer. Whitish, crystalline powder; practically odorless; very bitter taste; light-sensitive; melts about 149°. Practically insoluble in water; very soluble in chloroform; slightly soluble in alcohol.

Thiothixene Hydrochloride NF [Navane HCl (*Roerig*); $C_{23}H_{29}N_3O_2S_2\cdot2HCl\cdot2H_2O$ or anhydrous]—Tranquilizer. Whitish, crystalline powder; slight odor; light-sensitive. Soluble in water; slightly soluble in chloroform; practically insoluble in ether.

Thonzylamine Hydrochloride [$C_{16}H_{22}N_4O\cdot HCl$] — Antihistaminic. White, crystalline powder; faint odor; solution acid to litmus (pH about 5.5); melts about 174°. 1 g dissolves in about 1 ml water, 4 ml chloroform, and 6 ml alcohol; practically insoluble in ether.

Thorazine Concentrate [*SK&F* brand of chlorpromazine]—*30 mg/ml:* pH 3.2–4.2; Na$^+$ 0.43 mg/ml; sweetener, saccharin sodium. *100 mg/ml:* pH 2.4–3.4; Na$^+$ 1.2 mg/ml; sweetener, saccharin sodium.

Thorazine Syrup [*SK&F*]—*10 mg/5 ml:* pH 3.5–5.5; aqueous solvent; Na$^+$ 0.4 mg/5 ml; sweetener, sugar.

Throat Preparations—See under *Eye, Ear, Nose, and Throat Preparations.*

Thromboplastin [thrombokinase]—Diagnostic aid (prothrombin estimation). Powder or liquid suspension with thrombokinase activity from brain and/or lung tissue of freshly killed rabbits. *Dry form:* buff powder. *Liquid form:* opalescent or turbid suspension; solid matter may deposit on standing. May have characteristic odor; may contain antibacterial agent.

Thymol USP [$C_{10}H_{14}O$]—Thymol is a vermifuge and antiseptic soluble in water 1:1000. The solubility is increased by alkalies which form salts—the resulting solutions darken on standing. Thymol liquefies or forms a soft mass on trituration with menthol, camphor, monobromated camphor, acetanilid, antipyrine, caffeine, aminopyrine, methenamine salts of quinine, and some other substances, but not with phenacetin. Thymol is soluble 1:1 in alcohol and is soluble in vegetable and volatile oils. It was used in the formerly official antiseptic solution, alkaline aromatic solution (0.05%), and compound zinc sulfate powder (0.1%).

Thyroglobulin NF [Proloid (*W-C*)]—Thyroid supplement. Cream-colored to tan-colored, free-flowing powder; slight, characteristic odor. Insoluble in water, HCl, chloroform, and carbon tetrachloride.

Thyroid USP—Thyroid hormone. *Dispensing Information:* Patients should be aware of symptoms of hypo- and hyperthyroidism. Frequent checkups are a must for new patients. Remind them that they must make all return visits on time. Do not exceed daily dose or miss a dose.

Titanium Dioxide USP [TiO_2]—Topical protectant. White, infusible powder; amorphous; odorless; tasteless; sp gr about 4; 1 in 10 aqueous suspension neutral to litmus. Insoluble in water.

Tocamphyl [Gallogen (*Beecham-Massengill*); Syncuma (*Philips-Roxane*); $C_{23}H_{37}NO_6$]—Choleretic. Pale yellowish mass; unctuous; faint, aromatic odor; bitter taste. Slowly soluble in water (becomes turbid when diluted); soluble in alcohol, chloroform, and ether.

Tolazamide USP [Tolinase (*Upjohn*)]—Oral hypoglycemic. Whitish, crystalline powder; odorless or almost so; melts (with decomposition) about 165°. Very slightly soluble in water;

freely soluble in chloroform; slightly soluble in alcohol.

Dispensing Information: See *Hypoglycemic Agents* (*Oral*).

Tolazoline Hydrochloride NF [*Various Mfrs.;* $C_{10}H_{12}N_2 \cdot HCl$]—Antiadrenergic. Whitish, crystalline powder; solution slightly acid to litmus; melts about 174°. Freely soluble in water and alcohol.

Tolbutamide USP [Orinase (*Upjohn*)]—Oral hypoglycemic. Whitish, crystalline powder; slightly bitter; practically odorless; melts about 129°. Practically insoluble in water; soluble in alcohol and chloroform.

Dispensing Information: Do not take OTC medication without first consulting physician. Advise physician immediately if skin rash, yellowing of eyes, sore throat, fever, or other untoward symptoms appear. See also *Hypoglycemic Agents* (*Oral*).

Tolbutamide Sodium USP [Orinase Diagnostic (*Upjohn*); $C_{12}H_{17}N_2NaO_3S$]—Diagnostic aid (diabetes). Whitish, crystalline powder; practically odorless; slightly bitter taste; pH (1 in 20 soln) 8.5–9.8. Freely soluble in water; soluble in alcohol and chloroform; very slightly soluble in ether. See also *Reagent Tablets or Strips.*

Tolnaftate USP [Tinactin (*Schering-White*); $C_{19}H_{17}NOS$]—Antifungal. Whitish, fine powder; slight odor; melts about 111°. Practically insoluble in water; freely soluble in chloroform; slightly soluble in alcohol.

Dispensing Information: Discontinue use if sensitization, irritation, or worsening of skin condition occur.

Tolu Balsam USP—Pharmaceutic aid (flavored vehicle). Balsam from *Myroxylon balsamum.* Brownish, plastic solid; transparent in thin layers; vanilla-like odor; mild, aromatic taste. Practically insoluble in water; soluble (sometimes with residue or turbidity) in alcohol, chloroform, and ether.

Tolu Balsam Syrup NF—Pharmaceutic aid. Tolu contains vanillin which oxidizes and darkens in the presence of alkalies. Thus, a solution of ammonium

carbonate in tolu balsam syrup became colored and ultimately turned black.

Tragacanth USP—Pharmaceutic aid (suspending agent). Tragacanth contains a small proportion of water-soluble gum and a large proportion of bassorin, which is insoluble but absorbs water and swells, forming an adhesive paste.

Tragacanth is decomposed by alkalies and precipitated by alcohol in concentrations greater than 35%. The stability and viscosity of tragacanth is greatly affected by pH. Tragacanth, being a negatively charged colloid, is precipitated by bismuth subnitrate while bismuth subcarbonate does not cause this incompatibility.

Tragacanth can inactivate some cationic preservatives.

Tranquilizers (Chlordiazepoxide Type)—*Dispensing Information:* Drowsiness can occur. Concurrent administration of depressants (including alcohol) will lead to exaggerated effects.

Tranylcypromine Sulfate NF [Parnate (*SK&F*); $(C_9H_{11}N)_2 \cdot H_2SO_4$]—Antidepressant. White, crystalline powder; odorless or faint odor. Soluble in water; very slightly soluble in alcohol and ether; practically insoluble in chloroform.

Dispensing Information: Consult physician if headache or other unusual symptoms develop. Do not eat cheese or drink beer or wine (these will cause a hypertensive crisis with tranylcypromine). Do not take OTC preparations for cold, hay fever, or weight reduction (these will cause an exaggeration of pressor effects).

Tretinoin USP [retinoic acid; Aberel (*McNeil*); Retin-A (*J&J*); $C_{20}H_{28}O_2$]—Keratolytic. Yellowish, crystalline powder. Insoluble in water; slightly soluble in alcohol and chloroform.

Dispensing Information: Patients should be aware of the severe inflammation that this agent can produce. Caution is required with application to avoid mucous membranes.

Triamcinolone Acetonide USP [Aristocort Acetonide, Aristoderm (*Led-*

erle); Kenalog (*Squibb*); $C_{24}H_{31}FO_6$]—Glucocorticoid. Triamcinolone acetonide is insoluble in water, sparingly soluble in methanol, acetone, ethyl acetate.

Triamcinolone Diacetate NF [AristocortDiacetate(*Lederle*);$C_{25}H_{31}FO_8$]—Glucocorticoid. Fine, whitish crystals; not more than slight odor and slight, bitter taste; hydrate melts about 151°; anhydrous form melts about 177°. Practically insoluble in water; 1 g dissolves in about 13 ml alcohol and 80 ml chloroform; slightly soluble in ether.

Triamcinolone Hexacetonide USP [Aristospan (*Lederle*); $C_{30}H_{41}FO_7$]—Glucocorticoid. Whitish, crystalline powder; odorless; tasteless or slight, bitter taste; decomposes about 295°. Practically insoluble in water; 1 g dissolves in about 20 ml chloroform.

Triaminic Expectorant [*Dorsey*]—Decongestant; expectorant; antihistaminic. Contains (per 5 ml) pyrilamine maleate 6.25 mg, pheniramine maleate 6.25 mg, phenylpropanolamine HCl 12.5 mg, glyceryl guaiacolate 100 mg; sweetener: sucrose 3.6 g, saccharin 2.5 mg, saccharin sodium 3.75 mg; Na^+ 0.4 mg. pH 3.2–4.2; alcohol 5%; aqueous solvent.

Dispensing Information: Use with caution in hypertension, diabetes, heart disease, thyrotoxicosis. Do not drive or operate dangerous equipment.

Triaminic Oral Infant Drops [*Dorsey*]—Decongestant; antihistaminic. Contains (per ml) pyrilamine maleate 10 mg, pheniramine maleate 10 mg, phenylpropanolamine HCl 20 mg. pH 4–5; aqueous solvent; sweetener (per 5 ml): sucrose 1.45 g, saccharin sodium 8 mg; Na^+ 0.9 mg/5 ml.

Dispensing Information: See *Triaminic Expectorant.*

Triaminic Syrup [*Dorsey*]—Decongestant; antihistaminic. Contains (per 5 ml) pyrilamine maleate 6.25 mg, pheniramine maleate 6.25 mg, phenylpropanolamine HCl 12.5 mg; sweetener, sucrose 3.6 g. pH 3.5–4.5; aqueous solvent.

Dispensing Information: See *Triaminic Expectorant.*

Triamterene USP [Dyrenium (*SK&F*); $C_{12}H_{11}N_7$]—Diuretic. Yellow, crystalline powder; odorless. Practically insoluble in water, chloroform, and ether; very slightly soluble in alcohol.

Dispensing Information: Potassium supplements should be avoided.

Trichlormethiazide NF [Metahydrin (*Lakeside*); Naqua (*Schering*); $C_8H_8Cl_3N_3O_4S_2$]—Diuretic; antihypertensive. White, crystalline powder; odorless or slight odor; light-sensitive; melts (with decomposition) about 274°. 1 g dissolves in about 1100 ml water, 48 ml alcohol, 1400 ml ether, and 5000 ml chloroform.

Trichloroacetic Acid USP [$C_2HCl_3O_2$; $pK_a \simeq 0.65$]—Trichloroacetic acid is a strong caustic acid, pH 1.2 (0.1 *M*). It is highly reactive because it is soluble and because it is highly dissociated. It is soluble in water (1:0.1), alcohol, and most organic solvents. It forms a precipitate with albuminous substances and must be handled with care since it is very corrosive to the skin. *Caution:* When used topically as a caustic, use on small areas only. When sufficient penetration has occurred, neutralize area with sodium carbonate solution. On heating with strong alkalies it will decompose into chloroform and alkali carbonate.

Trichloroethylene NF [Trilene (*Ayerst*); Trimar (*Ohio Med.*); C_2HCl_3]—Analgesic (inhalation). Liquid which is miscible with alcohol but practically insoluble in water. It is gradually decomposed by light in presence of moisture. It is used by inhalation and must be dispensed in the original sealed ampuls.

Trichloromonofluoromethane NF [CCl_3F]—Pharmaceutic aid (aerosol propellant). Clear, colorless gas; faint odor; vapor preure (at 25°) about 796 mm Hg; boils about 24°. Practically insoluble in water; soluble in alcohol and ether.

Triclofos Sodium [Triclos (*Lakeside*); $C_2H_3Cl_3NaO_4P$]—Hypnotic; sedative. Whitish powder; odorless; saline taste; hygroscopic; heat-sensitive above room temperature. 1 g dissolves in about 2 ml water and 250 ml alcohol; practically insoluble in ether.

Tridihexethyl Chloride NF [Pathilon (*Lederle*); $C_{21}H_{36}ClNO$]—Anticholinergic. White, crystalline powder; odorless; melts about 199°. 1 g dissolves in about 3 ml water, 2 ml chloroform, and 3 ml alcohol; practically insoluble in ether.

Triethanolamine USP [$C_6H_{15}NO_3$]—Pharmaceutic aid (alkalizing agent). Strongly basic, viscous, hydroscopic liquid having a slight ammoniacal odor. It is miscible in all proportions with water and alcohol. Triethanolamine reacts with free fatty acids to form soaps, which tend to discolor on aging.

Triethylenemelamine NF [TEM; Triethylene Melamine (*Lederle*); $C_9H_{12}N_6$]—Antineoplastic. White, crystalline powder; odorless or slight odor; melts to a clear liquid about 160°, then polymerizes vigorously. 1 g dissolves in about 3 ml water, 4 ml chloroform, and 13 ml alcohol. *Caution: Triethylene - melamine is very poisonous.*

Trifluoperazine   Hydrochloride NF [Stelazine Hydrochloride (*SK&F*); $C_{21}H_{24}F_3N_3S\cdot2HCl$]—Tranquilizer (major). White to pale-yellow, crystalline powder; practically odorless; bitter taste; melts about 242° with decomposition; pH (5%) 1.7–2.6. One g dissolves in 3.5 ml water, 11 ml alcohol, and 100 ml chloroform.

Dispensing Information: May enhance response to alcohol or other CNS depressants. Drowsiness may occur which may impair ability to drive or perform other tasks requiring alertness. Discontinue use and consult physician if yellowing of eyes or skin occurs.

Triflupromazine   NF [Vesprin (*Squibb*); $C_{18}H_{19}F_3N_2S$]—Tranquilizer. Light amber liquid; viscous; oily; crystallizes on standing into large, irregular crystals. Practically insoluble in water.

Triflupromazine   Hydrochloride NF [Vesprin Hydrochloride (*Squibb*); $C_{18}H_{19}F_3N_2S\cdot HCl$]—Tranquilizer. Whitish, crystalline powder; slight odor; melts about 174°. Soluble in water and alcohol; insoluble in ether. *Side effects:*

Rarely observed skin eruptions, photosensitivity, and hyperthermia.

Trihexyphenidyl   Hydrochloride USP [Artane (*Lederle*); Pipanol (*Winthrop*); Tremin (*Schering*); $C_{20}H_{31}NO\cdot HCl$]—Anticholinergic. Whitish, crystalline powder; no more than very faint odor; melts (with slight decomposition) about 250°. Slightly soluble in water; soluble in alcohol and chloroform.

Dispensing Information: May cause constipation, urinary retention, drowsiness, or headache. Take before meals to prevent dry mouth; chewing gum or mint candy may also alleviate dry mouth.

Trimeprazine Tartrate USP [Temaril (*SK&F*); $(C_{18}H_{22}N_2S)\cdot C_4H_6O_6$]—Antipruritic. Whitish, crystalline powder; odorless. Freely soluble in water and chloroform; soluble in alcohol; very slightly soluble in ether.

Dispensing Information: See *Antipsychotic   Agents   (Phenothiazine Type).*

Trimethadione USP [Tridione (*Abbott*); $C_6H_9NO_3$]—Anticonvulsant. White, crystalline granules; slight odor; melts about 46°. 1 g dissolves in about 13 ml water and 2 ml alcohol; freely soluble in chloroform and ether.

Trimethaphan   Camsylate   USP [Arfonad (*Roche*); $C_{32}H_{40}N_2O_5S_2$]—Antihypertensive. White crystals or white, crystalline powder; odorless or almost so; 1 in 10 solution clear and practically colorless; melts (with decomposition) about 233°. 1 g dissolves in about 5 ml water and 2 ml alcohol; freely soluble in chloroform; insoluble in ether. *Known incompatibilities* (trimethaphan camsylate injection): alkaline solutions, bromides, iodides; infusion should not be used as vehicle for other drugs.

Trimethobenzamide   Hydrochloride NF [Tigan (*Beecham-Massengill*); $C_{21}H_{28}N_2O_5\cdot HCl$]—Antiemetic. White, crystalline powder; slight phenolic odor. 1 g dissolves in 2 ml water, 59 ml alcohol, and 67 ml chloroform; insoluble in ether.

Dispensing Information: Contraindicated in patients allergic to local anesthetics; use with caution with phenothiazines, barbiturates, or belladonna preparations. Drowsiness may occur which may impair ability to drive or perform other tasks requiring alertness. Discontinue use if yellowing of eyes or skin occurs and advise physician.

Trimethoprim [comp. of Bactrim (*Roche*); comp. of Septra (*B-W*); $C_{14}H_{18}N_4O_3$; pK_a about 6.6]—Antibacterial. Whitish crystals or crystalline powder; odorless; bitter taste; melts about 199°; pH (1% aq susp) about 8.2. Very slightly soluble in water; 1 g dissolves in about 53 ml chloroform and 285 ml anhydrous alcohol.

Trioxsalen USP [Trisoralen (*Elder*); $C_{14}H_{12}O_3$]—Pigmentation agent (photosensitizer). Whitish, crystalline solid; odorless; tasteless; melts about 230°. Practically insoluble in water; 1 g dissolves in about 84 ml chloroform and 1150 ml alcohol. *Caution: Avoid contact with the skin.*

Tripelennamine Citrate USP [Pyribenzamine Citrate (*Ciba*); $C_{16}H_{21}N_3 \cdot C_6H_8O_7$]—Antihistaminic. Tripelennamine citrate is a white, crystalline powder. It is very soluble in water and freely soluble in alcohol. A 1% aqueous solution is slightly acidic (pH, about 4.3).

Dispensing Information: May potentiate MAO inhibitors, other antihistamines, hypnotics, sedatives; antagonizes guanethidine. Drowsiness may occur which may impair ability to drive or perform other tasks requiring alertness. Discontinue use and advise physician if fever, sore throat, easy bruising, or purple spots beneath the skin occur. Avoid alcohol.

Tripelennamine Hydrochloride USP [Pyribenzamine Hydrochloride (*Ciba*); $C_{16}H_{21}N_3 \cdot HCl$]—Antihistaminic. Tripelennamine hydrochloride is a white, crystalline powder which darkens slowly on exposure to light. It is very soluble in water and freely soluble in alcohol. Its solutions in water are nearly neutral (pH, about 7).

Triprolidine Hydrochloride NF [Actidil)*B-W*); $C_{19}H_{22}N_2 \cdot HCl \cdot H_2O$]—

This antihistaminic is moderately soluble in water, ethanol, and methanol.

Troleandomycin [triacetyloleandomycin; Cyclamycin (*Wyeth*); TAO (*Roerig*); $C_{41}H_{67}NO_{15}$]—Antibacterial. White, crystalline powder; odorless; pH (1% soln in diluted alcohol) 7.5–9. One g dissolves in about 1000 ml water and ether and 10 ml alcohol.

Dispensing Information: Discontinue use and consult physician if yellowing of eyes or skin occurs.

Trolnitrate Phosphate [Metamine (*Pfizer*); $C_6H_{12}N_4O_9 \cdot 2H_3PO_4$]—Vasodilator. Colorless, crystalline powder; in moist air hydrolytic decomposition occurs; explosions are possible when handling the undiluted material; melts (with decomposition) about 102°. Dissociates in water (liberating phosphoric acid and trinitrotriethanolamine); soluble in alcohol; insoluble in chloroform and ether.

Tromethamine NF [Tham-E (*Abbott*); $C_4H_{11}NO_3$]—Alkalizer. White, crystalline powder; slight odor; faint, sweet, soapy taste; melts about 170°. 1 g dissolves in about 2 ml water and 46 ml alcohol; practically insoluble in chloroform.

Tropicamide USP [Mydriacyl (*Alcon*); $C_{17}H_{20}N_2O_2$]—Anticholinergic (ophthalmic). Fine, whitish, crystalline powder; odorless or slight odor; bitter taste; melts about 98°. 1 g dissolves in about 500 ml water and 3 ml chloroform; freely soluble in alcohol.

Trypsin Crystallized NF [Tryptar (*Armour*)]—Proteolytic enzyme. Extracted from beef pancreas and crystalized. It is a yellow or yellowish-gray crystalline powder that is soluble in water, saline, and vegetable oils; it is insoluble in alcohol or glycerin. It is stable indefinitely at room temperature in the dry state but in solution it loses activity. It has been found that polyethylene glycol ointment containing calcium chloride as a stabilizer retains 80% of its trypsin activity after 6 months. Stable trypsin solutions stabilized by 0.5–20% amino acids, 0.3–5% calcium salts at pH 5.5 have been patented. Polyethylene glycol of molecular weight 100–800 at 20–40% is a desirable additive as are preservatives such as thimerosal, methylparaben, or propylparaben.

Tuaminoheptane NF [2-aminoheptane; Tuamine (*Lilly*); $C_7H_{17}N$]— Vasoconstrictor and adrenergic drug chiefly used in inhaler form. It is a colorless to pale yellow liquid, sparingly soluble in water and freely soluble in alcohol. A 1% aqueous solution is alkaline (pH about 11.5). *Caution:* Excessive use of sympathomimetic inhalers may produce tachycardia and hypertension headache.

Tuaminoheptane Sulfate NF [Tuamine Sulfate (*Lilly*) $(C_7H_{17}N)_2 \cdot H_2SO_4$]—Adrenergic. White, crystalline powder which is freely soluble in water and readily soluble in alcohol. The aqueous solution is neutral to litmus (pH of 1% solution = 5.4) but may corrode the metal parts of atomizers. Tuamine Sulfate may be used with other drugs commonly used for intranasal therapy, with the possible exception of silver nitrate or drugs which liberate the insoluble free base.

Tubocurarine Chloride USP [*d*-tubocurarine chloride (*Various Mfrs.*); $C_{37}H_{41}ClN_2O_6 \cdot HCl \cdot 5H_2O$ or anhydrous]— Skeletal muscle relaxant. This diquaternary polyether is a white or yellowish-white to gray or light tan crystalline powder. It is soluble in water and sparingly soluble in alcohol. The pH of tubocurarine chloride injection is about 3 to 5. The compatibility of tubocurarine solutions with injectable barbiturates appears to be dependent on the tertiary alkaloids present as impurities in the tubocurarine, the stabilizers and buffers present, and the age of the barbiturate solution. Mixtures containing cloudiness or precipitate should not be used.

Tuinal Pulvules [Lilly]—Sedative; hypnotic. Contain equal amounts of secobarbital sodium and amobarbital sodium (45 mg, 90 mg, and 180 mg).

Dispensing Information: Do not exceed labeled dosage. Avoid alcohol. Do not drive or operate heavy machinery.

Tussagesic Suspension [*Dorsey*]—

Cold therapy. Contains (per 5 ml) phenylpropanolamine HCl 12.5 mg, pheniramine maleate 6.25 mg, pyrilamine maleate 6.25 mg, dextromethorphan HBr 15 mg, terpin hydrate 90 mg, acetaminophen 120 mg; sweetener: sucrose 3.6 g, saccharin sodium 16.18 mg; Na^+ 1.8 mg; pH 4.5–6; alcohol, trace; aqueous solvent.

Tuss-Ornade Liquid [*SK&F*]— Cough/cold therapy. Contains (per 5 ml) caramiphen edisylate 5 mg, chlorpheniramine maleate 2 mg, phenylpropanolamine HCl 15 mg, isopropamide 0.75 mg; Na^+ 11 mg; pH 3.8–4.8; alcohol 7.5%; aqueous solvent; sweetener: saccharin sodium, sorbitol.

Tylenol Drops [*McNeil* brand of acetaminophen]—Analgesic; antipyretic. pH 4.1; alcohol 7%; hydroalcoholic vehicle; sweetener essentially absent; Na^+ <5 mg/dosage unit; K^+ none; hypertonic. May be mixed with dilute hydroalcoholic substances of approx the same pH for short-term use; do not use if precipitation is observed.

Tylenol Elixir [*McNeil* brand of acetaminophen]—Analgesic; antipyretic. pH 5; alcohol 7%; hydroalcoholic vehicle. Artificial sweetener present; Na^+ <5 mg/dosage unit; K^+ none; hypertonic. May be mixed with dilute hydroalcoholic substances of approx the same pH for short-term use; do not use if precipitation is observed.

Tyloxapol NF [Enuclene (*Alcon*); Superinone (*Winthrop*)]—Detergent. Amber liquid; viscous; may have slight turbidity; slight odor; sp gr about 1.072; aqueous solution grows molds in air; chemically stable during sterilization and in the presence of acids, bases, and salts; oxidized by metals; pH (5% aq soln) 4–7. Freely soluble in water (slowly); soluble in chloroform and many organic solvents.

Tyropanoate Sodium [Bilopaque Sodium (*Winthrop*); $C_{15}H_{17}I_3NNaO_3$]— Whitish powder; odorless; bitter taste; hygroscopic; decomposes on heating. Soluble in water and alcohol; very slightly soluble in ether.

Tyzine Nasal Solution [*Pfizer*

brand of tetrahydrozoline hydrochloride]—*Known ingredients:* tetrahydrozoline HCl (0.1%), citrate buffer, yellow dye, thimerosal. pH 5.5. *Known incompatibilities:* oxytetracycline HCl (5 mg/ml, residue after 3 days), chlortetracycline HCl (5 mg/ml, residue after 3 days), tyrothricin (0.2 mg/ml), cetyldimethylbenzyl ammonium chloride ($\frac{1}{50.000}$—precipitate forms slowly), cetylpyridinium chloride ($\frac{1}{50.000}$—precipitate forms slowly), benzalkonium chloride ($\frac{1}{50.000}$—precipitate forms slowly), butacaine sulfate (1%—residue after few hours), tetracaine HCl (2%—crystals formed after 2 weeks), silver nitrate (0.5%), mild silver protein (10–20%—residue formed after 1 month), strong silver protein (1%—not soluble).

Undecylenic Acid USP [Desenex Solution (*WTS*); $C_{11}H_{20}O_2$]—Yellow antifungal liquid which is almost insoluble in water but is soluble in alcohol and oils. The pH of a saturated solution in water is about 4.2. Undecylenic acid may be liberated from solutions of the sodium salt on addition of acids. Zinc undecylenate is practically insoluble in water and alcohol.

Uracil Mustard NF [*Upjohn;* $C_8H_{11}Cl_2N_3O_2$]—Antineoplastic. Whitish, crystalline powder; odorless; melts (with decomposition) about 200°. 1 g dissolves in >1000 ml water and chloroform and 150 ml alcohol.

Urea USP [carbamide; Ureaphil (*Abbott*); Urevert (*Travenol*); CH_4N_2O]—Diuretic. 1 g dissolves in 1.5 ml of water or 10 ml of alcohol. The solutions are neutral.

Uticillin VK Preparations [*Upjohn*]—Antibacterial. Penicillin V potassium. *For Oral Solution (125 mg/5 ml):* Contains (per 5 ml) Na^+ 22 mg; K^+ 17 mg. *For Oral Solution (250 mg/5 ml):* Contains (per 5 ml) Na^+ 24 mg; K^+ 31 mg.

Vaginal Creams—*Dispensing Information:* Vaginal creams should not be administered, if possible, when the patient is pregnant; there is the danger of membrane perforation with the hard, plastic applicator. Instead, comparable vaginal tablets, inserts, or suppositories should be used and inserted with the fingers. Patients should be encouraged to complete the entire prescribed course. Applicator care should be stressed.

Valeric Acid [$C_5H_{10}O_2$; pK_a 4.78]—Valeric acid forms soluble salts with the alkali metals, but some of the heavy metal valerates such as the ferric salt are insoluble. All have an objectional odor that is characteristic of the anion. These compounds may be useful as placebos. Acid ammonium valerate (ammonium valerinate) is soluble in water (1:0.3) and alcohol (1:0.6). This compound of 1 mole of ammonium valerate and 2 moles of valeric acid will separate the free acid when the saturated solution is diluted with 5 volumes of water. Valeric acid (C_5) is, thus, the upper limit for water solubility (about 1:30).

Vancomycin Hydrochloride USP [Vancocin (*Lilly*)]—Antibacterial. Vancomycin is an amphoteric antibiotic obtained from *Streptomyces orientalis*. It is active against Gram-positive organisms and spirochetes (bactericidal). It has an isoelectric point of 5 and a molecular weight of 3200–3500. Vancomycin hydrochloride is a white solid that is very soluble in water (200 mg/ml). The pH value is about 5.8. It is moderately soluble in aqueous methanol and insoluble in higher alcohols, acetone, or ether. Low concentrations of urea increase the solubility in neutral, aqueous solutions.

Vancomycin is precipitated from aqueous solution by heavy metals; and ammonium sulfate and sodium chloride precipitate it from acid solutions. It apparently has carboxylic, amino, and phenolic groups. It is stable in aqueous solution in the pH range 2.5–9.

Vanilla NF [vanilla bean]—Pharmaceutic aid (flavor). Fruit of *Vanilla planifolia* (Mexican or Bourbon Vanilla) or *Vanilla tahitensis* (Tahiti Vanilla). *Note: Do not use if it has become brittle.*

Vanillin USP [$C_8H_8O_3$]—Pharmaceutic aid (flavor). Fine, whitish crystals (usually needle-like); vanilla-like odor and taste; light-sensitive; solution acid to litmus; melts about 82°. 1 g dissolves in about 100 ml water (20 ml at 80°) and 20 ml glycerin; freely soluble in alcohol, chloroform, and ether. *Known incompatibilities:* glycerin (forming alcohol-insoluble compound), alkalies, oxidized in air.

Vasocidin Ophthalmic [*Cooper*]— Ocular anti-inflammatory; decongestant. Contains prednisolone sodium phosphate 0.25%, sulfacetamide sodium 10%, phenylephrine HCl 0.125%. pH 6.8–7.2; aqueous solvent; hypertonic; preservative, methylparaben/propylparaben.

Vasocon Ophthalmic [*Cooper*]— Ocular decongestant. Contains naphazoline HCl 0.1%; pH 5.5–6; aqueous solvent; buffers, sodium carbonate/boric acid; isotonic; preservative, phenylmercuric acetate 0.002%.

Vasocon-A Ophthalmic [*Cooper*]— Decongestant; antihistaminic. Contains naphazoline HCl 0.05%, antazoline phosphate 0.5%; pH 5.5–6; aqueous solvent; buffers, sodium carbonate/boric acid; isotonic; preservative, phenylmercuric acetate 0.002%.

V-Cillin Drops (M-130) [*Lilly*]— Antibacterial. Penicillin V. pH 2.3–2.8; solvent, purified water; buffer, citrate; contains (approx per 0.6 ml) sweeteners: 200 mg sucrose, 4 mg saccharin; Na$^+$ 2 mg; K$^+$ <1 mg. *Known incompatibilities:* Manufacturer does not recommend mixing this product with other products; such mixing will upset the balance of the suspension system and will result in possible dosing error.

V-Cillin Preparations, Other [*Lilly*]—Antibacterial. Penicillin V potassium. *For Oral Solution (M-126):* pH 5–6; solvent, purified water; buffer, citrate; contains (approx per 5 ml) sweeteners: 3 g sucrose, 5 mg saccharin; Na$^+$ 15 mg; K$^+$ 15 mg. *For Oral Solution (M-142):* pH 5.2–5.8; solvent, purified water; buffer, citrate; contains (approx per 5 ml) sweeteners: 3.5 g sucrose, 3.5 mg saccharin sodium; Na$^+$ 30 mg; K$^+$ 35 mg. *Known incompatibilities:* Manufacturer does not recommend

mixing this product with other products as such mixing will upset the balance of the suspension system and will result in possible dosing error.

Versapen Preparations [*Bristol*]— Antibacterial. *Oral Suspension (112.5 mg/5 ml):* pH 2.3–2.8; buffer, citric acid anhydrous; sugar 88.7%; Na$^+$ 0.03 mEq. *Oral Suspension (225 mg/5 ml):* pH 2.3–2.8; buffer, citric acid anhydrous; sugar 65.2%; Na$^+$ 0.02 mEq. *Oral Suspension (112.5 mg/ml):* pH 2.3–2.8; buffer, citric acid anhydrous; sugar 69.6%; Na$^+$ 0.006 mEq.

Dispensing Information: See *Penicillins.*

Vinblastine Sulfate USP [Velban (*Lilly*); $C_{46}H_{58}N_4O_9 \cdot H_2SO_4$]—Antineoplastic. Whitish, crystalline powder; amorphous; odorless; hygroscopic. Freely soluble in water.

Vincristine Sulfate USP [Oncovin (*Lilly*); $C_{46}H_{56}N_4O_{10} \cdot H_2SO_4$]—Antineoplastic. Whitish, crystalline powder; amorphous; odorless; hygroscopic. Freely soluble in water.

Vinyl Ether NF [Vinethene (*MSD*); divinyl oxide; divinyl ether; C_4H_6O]— Vinyl ether is an anesthetic slightly soluble in water, miscible with alcohol, oils, and other organic solvents.

Vioform (or Vioform-Hydrocortisone) Lotion [*Ciba*]—*Known ingredients:* Vioform. *Known compatibilities:* benzocaine, liquor carbonis detergens 5%, phenol 1%. *Known incompatibilities:* none listed.

Vioform-Hydrocortisone Cream [*Ciba*]—Anti-inflammatory. *Known ingredients:* Vioform (3%), hydrocortisone (1%), in a water-washable base. *Known compatibilities:* menthol, phenol, Pyribenzamine Cream. *Known incompatibilities:* none listed.

Vioform Ointment (and Cream) [*Ciba*]—Topical antiseptic. *Known ingredients:* Vioform (3% in petrolatum or washable cream base). *Known compatibilities:* camphor, cortisone, 1% hydrocortisone ointment, Lassar's paste (yellow color), menthol, phenol, Pyribenzamine Ointment and Cream, resorcin, salicylic acid, sulfur, zinc oxide (yellow color). *Known incompatibilities:* ammoniated mercury ointment, calomel ointment. 10% inactivation by bacitracin.

Viomycin Sulfate USP [Viomycin (*P-D*); Viocin Sulfate (*Pfizer*); $C_{25}H_{43}N_{13}O_{10} \cdot x H_2SO_4$]—Antibacterial (tuberculostatic). Viomycin is the salt of an antibiotic substance or substances produced by the growth of *Streptomyces puniceus* on suitable culture media.

Viomycin is a strongly basic polypeptide. Viomycin loses its activity at high temperatures. The half-life at 100°C is about 12 hours.

Viomycin sulfate is very soluble in water and very slightly soluble in alcohol. It is moderately hygroscopic. It is insoluble in most organic solvents.

Viomycin is very stable in acid and less stable in alkaline solution. A 1% solution is acidic to nearly neutral (pH range, 4.5–7).

Visine Eye Drops [*Pfizer* brand of tetrahydrozoline hydrochloride]— *Known ingredients:* tetrahydrozoline HCl (0.05%), borate buffer, thimerosal. pH 6.2–6.3.

Known incompatibilities: oxytetracycline hydrochloride (5 mg/ml—residue after 3 days), chlortetracycline hydrochloride (5 mg/ml—residue after 3 days), silver nitrate (0.5%—precipitate formed), strong silver protein (1%—not readily dispersible, precipitate formed), Butyn Sulfate (2%—residue formed after 2 days).

Vitamin A [retinol; antixerophthalmic vitamin; $C_{20}H_{29}OH$; an unsaturated alcohol which crystallizes in yellowish prisms]—Vitamin A contains a series of five conjugated double bonds, four of which are in the side chain. Addition reactions can therefore occur with bisulfite and certain solvents. Numerous *cis-trans* isomers with differing vitamin potency are also possible. The conversion of all *trans* to certain *cis* structures may reduce activity 65–70% without affecting the chemical assay significantly.

Vitamin A is insoluble in water but soluble in fats and oils. Vitamin A is oxidized by air, and readily undergoes autoxidation and polymerization in the presence of peroxides and catalysts. Preparations containing vitamin A should thus be processed with careful precautions against oxidation. In the absence of air vitamin A is not affected by moderate heat.

Much of the vitamin A used in manufacturing pharmaceuticals is prepared by synthesis. Esters such as the acetate and palmitate are the preferred form due to greater stability. Vitamin A is found in the liver oils of salt-water fish partly in the form of the free alcohol but predominantly in esterified form. Another form, vitamin A_2, $C_{20}H_{27}OH$, predominates in the liver oils of freshwater fish. Certain fruits and vegetables contain substances such as carotene and cryptoxanthin which are converted into vitamin A in the body.

In cod liver oil emulsions vitamin D is very resistant to decomposition, but vitamin A is unstable. Preparation of the emulsion in an atmosphere of carbon dioxide protects the vitamin A from the oxygen of the air, but the emulsifying agent used should not contain oxidases, and the essential oil used for flavoring must be free from peroxides. When oils showing a great tendency to absorb oxygen (such as lemon and clove oils) are used they should always be freshly distilled. The oxidizing enzymes in acacia mucilage may be destroyed by heating at 100°C for a few minutes.

Certain trace metals seem to promote oxidation of vitamin A and it has been reported that copper and iron decreased the stability of vitamin A in dispersions made with Tween 20 and 80. Chelating agents had very little effect on iron and copper, however the presence of antioxidants increased vitamin stability and a mixture of NDGA and ascorbyl palmitate was found most effective. In a study of vitamin A in natural fish oils it was also found that iron and copper were most deleterious of the metal ions added but found *N,N'*-diphenyl-*p*-phenylene diamine was the best antioxidant. The latter compound has been patented as a stabilizer of vitamin A under conditions of high heat and humidity. Antioxidant combinations have been recommended as vitamin A stabilizers. The use of malt extract as a filler and antioxidant for vitamin A preparations and tocopherol and 2,6-di-tertiary-butyl-4-methylphenol as vitamin A stabilizers has been patented. It was also discovered that gelatin-coated vitamin A showed the best stability in feed supplements. A stable aqueous suspension of vitamin A as an aliphatic ester of synthetic vitamin A has also been patented.

Data on the relative stability of vitamin A in aqueous and oily media at 28°, 45°, and 85°C show the destruction of vitamin A in aqueous dispersions is more pronounced than in oily solvents. Tocopherol and lecithin stabilized vitamin A in oily media but had no significant effect in aqueous media; ascorbic acid was the best protectant in the latter. Vitamin A alcohol was apparently more stable than the palmitate in aqueous dispersions but less stable in oil. The stability of vitamin A at pH 3 was markedly lower than at pH 8; tocopherol at pH 3 had no significant antioxidant property.

It has been found that oxidation seems to be the principal degradation mechanism in hydrocarbon solvents, however oxidation and elimination reactions took place in hydroxylated solvents. Fatty acids showed a stabilizing effect in both vehicles. It has been noted that in addition to oxidation, vitamin A isomerizes from an all *trans*-form into a mixture containing two *cis*-isomers of much lower potency. This occurs in multivitamin drops.

The destruction of vitamin A by mineral acids results in the formation of anhydrovitamin A, a hydrocarbon practically devoid of biological activity.

The stability of vitamin A alcohol and palmitate in aqueous dispersions containing polysorbate 80 were compared and vitamin A alcohol appeared quite stable in suspensions at room temperature in contrast to the palmitate. Changes observed were oxidations and dehydration.

A one-phase, water-miscible, transparent solution of vitamin A palmitate in polysorbate 80:glycerol:water vehicle has been reported.

An investigation of the stability of vitamin A in oral liquid formulations containing thiamine hydrochloride determined that the optimum pH for vitamin A stability in the four vehicles used was pH 6 while that for thiamine hydrochloride was pH 4. Vitamin A combined with thiamine hydrochloride was unstable in two of the vehicles.

Dispensing Information: Patients should be warned of the hazard of self-medication with large doses.

Vitamin A Acetate—See under *Vitamin A.*

Vitamin A Palmitate—See under *Vitamin A.*

Vitamin D [antirachitic vitamin, sunshine vitamin]—Vitamin D is necessary for the proper utilization of calcium and phosphorus. Fish liver oils are the richest natural sources of this vitamin.

Vitamin D exists in several forms. Ultraviolet irradiation of ergosterol, a constituent of yeast, produces vitamin D_2 (calciferol), which is identical with one of the natural forms of vitamin D. Vitamin D_3 is a form contained in most fish liver oils. Vitamin D_3 is an activation product of 7-dehydrocholesterol. Other sterols are also precursors of vitamin D, the properties of vitamin D being exhibited by at least ten different sterol derivatives. Vitamin D is formed by the effect of sunlight on sterols which naturally occur in the skin. Activation of sterols by ultraviolet light consists in changing these compounds into isomers possessing antiarchitic properties by shifting the position of a double bond in the molecule.

Vitamin D is insoluble in water but soluble in oils, fats, and alcohol. It is relatively stable to heat and oxidation, but prolonged exposure to light may cause some deterioration. Vitamins D_2 and D_3 in pure form are white, odorless crystals.

Solutions of vitamin D in fixed oils are not miscible with milk. Drisdol, which is a brand of vitamin D_2, is available in the form of a solution in propylene glycol; this preparation readily dissolves in milk.

Dispensing Information: Patients should be warned of the hazard of self-medication with large doses.

Vitamin E NF [α-tocopherol; antisterility vitamin; $C_{29}H_{50}O_2$]—Alpha-tocopherol is an odorless, yellowish, viscous, oily liquid with an insipid taste. It is practically insoluble in water but is soluble in fats. It is stable toward heat and alkali. It is liable to oxidation and because of this is sometimes used as a nontoxic antioxidant in oils. It undergoes slow oxidation in the air and is incompatible with ferric salts, silver nitrate, and other oxidizing agents. Contact with lead or iron should be avoided.

In its natural sources vitamin E is apparently associated with certain protective substances or antioxidants which tend to stabilize it. Wheat germ oil is rich in antioxidants and, hence, is a good medium for this vitamin. Wheat germ oil, if sealed *in vacuo* in glass, appears to keep its vitamin E content unimpaired for several years at room temperature. Lard and other fats which are low in protective substances are poor vehicles for the vitamin and may even cause its destruction. The development of rancidity in the oil vehicle destroys vitamin E.

Warfarin   Potassium   NF [$C_{19}H_{15}KO_4$]—Anticoagulant. White, crystalline powder; odorless; slightly bitter taste; light-sensitive (discoloration). 1 g dissolves in about 1.5 ml water and 1.9 ml alcohol; very slightly soluble in chloroform and ether.

Warfarin Sodium USP [Coumadin Sodium (*Endo*); Panwarfin (*Abbott*); $C_{19}H_{15}NaO_4$]—Anticoagulant. White, amorphous or crystalline powder; odorless; slight bitter taste; discolors in light; pH (1 in 100 soln) 7.2–8.3. Very soluble in water; freely soluble in alcohol; very slightly soluble in chloroform and ether. *Known incompatibilities* (warfarin sodium for injection): ammonium chloride, cyanocobalamin, dextrose, epinephrine HCl, metaraminol

bitartrate, oxytocin, promazine HCl, tetracycline HCl, vitamin B complex with C.

Dispensing Information: Patients may be given a card containing the following information:

Warfarin has been prescribed for you. This drug is called an anticoagulant. That means it prevents blood clots from forming in your veins. The amount of drug that you take is determined by the rate at which your blood normally clots or coagulates. The "prothrombin time" is the blood test that measures this rate. You will be having this test performed according to your doctor's instructions. If you take this drug exactly as requested by your physician the possibility of complications during therapy is greatly reduced. You are urged to follow your doctor's treatment instructions and to familiarize yourself with the instructions and precautions about this medication. NOTE: The purse or wallet card pictured below may be obtained at the pharmacy.

> **IN CASE OF EMERGENCY**
> **THE BEARER IS BEING TREATED WITH COUMADIN* (crystalline warfarin sodium),** an anticoagulant, which slows down the clotting of the blood.
> In case of bleeding, injury or illness, call the physician whose name appears on the reverse side of this card.
> **Bearer** ....
> **Address** ....

The following instructions and precautions should be observed while taking warfarin or coumadin:

1. Avoid aspirin or aspirin-containing products such as Anacin, Bufferin, Alka-Seltzer, Excedrin, etc. Use Tylenol or Nebs for pain or fever.

2. If you are taking any other medication be certain to let your doctor know. This includes such common drugs as vitamins, cold preparations or any other non-prescription or prescription drugs. Do not start or stop taking drugs without consulting your doctor. If you are in need of a cold, cough, headache or pain remedy contact your doctor for advice or inform your pharmacist that you are taking coumadin and ask him to recommend a preparation that will not interfere with your anticoagulant.

3. Avoid injury to gums by using a medium or soft toothbrush.

4. Avoid food fads, crash diets, and other changes in eating habits.

5. Never increase, decrease or change your dosage schedule without specific instructions from your physician.

6. Whenever you visit any other physician (or dentist) be certain to inform him that you are taking coumadin.

7. Avoid situations, whether at work or play, that may result in injury to yourself, that is cuts, bruises, etc.

8. Harsh laxatives such as Dulcolax, Citrate of Magnesia, Cascara Sagrada or Ex-Lax should be avoided. Mild laxatives such as Milk of Magnesia, Colace or Mineral Oil should be used if needed.

9. If you are pregnant, or think you have become pregnant while taking this medication your doctor should be told.

10. Inform your doctor if any of the following happen:
   a. excessive bleeding after cuts, as during shaving—particularly any bleeding that does not stop by itself with reasonable promptness
   b. excessive menstrual bleeding
   c. the sudden appearance of "black & blue" spots on the skin
   d. the appearance of red or dark-brown urine
   e. the appearance of red or black stools

Water USP [H_2O]—Pharmaceutic aid (solvent). Clear, colorless liquid; odorless. *Known incompatibilities:* immiscible with oil preparations, hydrolyzes salts which may form precipitates.

Water for Injection USP—Pharmaceutic aid (solvent). Clear, colorless liquid, odorless. *Known incompatibilities:* see *Water.*

Water for Injection, Bacteriostatic, USP—Pharmaceutical aid (sterile vehicle). Contains water and an antimicrobial substance such as benzyl alcohol, chlorobutanol, phenol, parabens, phenylmercuric nitrate or thimerosal. Clear, colorless liquid; odorless; or odor of the antimicrobial substance. *Known incompatibilities:* see *Water;* also, characteristic incompatibilities of the bacteriostatic agent must be considered.

Water for Injection, Sterile, USP—Pharmaceutic aid (solvent). Clear, colorless liquid; odorless. *Known incompatibilities:* see *Water.*

Water for Irrigation, Sterile, USP—Irrigating solution; pharmaceutic aid (solvent). Clear, colorless liquid; odorless. *Known incompatibilities:* see *Water.*

Water, Purified, USP—Pharmaceutic aid (solvent). Clear, colorless liquid; odorless; pH 5–7. *Known incompatibilities:* see *Water.*

Wax, White, USP [white beeswax; bleached wax]—Pharmaceutic aid (stiffening agent). Bleached and purified yellow wax from the honeycomb of the bee, *Apis mellifera.* Yellowish white, somewhat translucent solid; faint odor; nearly tasteless; no rancidity; sp gr about 0.95; melts about 63°. Insoluble in water; sparingly soluble in cold alcohol; completely soluble in chloroform and ether.

Wax, Yellow, NF [beeswax; yellow beeswax]—Pharmaceutic aid (stiffening agent). Purified wax from the honeycomb of the bee, *Apis mellifera.* Yellowish solid; honey-like odor; faint taste; somewhat brittle when cold; has a dull, granular, noncrystalline fracture when broken; pliable in heat of the hand; sp gr about 0.95; melts about 63°. Insoluble in water; sparingly soluble in cold alcohol; completely soluble in chloroform and ether.

White Lotion NF—Local astringent; local protectant. Contains zinc sulfate and sulfurated potash. White suspension. *Known incompatibilities:* acids.

Wild Cherry Syrup—Pharmaceutic aid (flavored vehicle). The pH of wild cherry syrup is 4.1; hence, it is incompatible with carbonates and bicarbonates which produce with it a very slow but definite effervescence. The addition of acids such as diluted hydrochloric acid causes precipitation on standing. Wild cherry syrup has all the incompatibilities of tannic acid.

Xanthan Gum NF [Keltrol (*Kelco*)]—Pharmaceutic aid (to thicken, suspend, emulsify, and stabilize aqueous systems). High molecular weight polysaccharide gum from fermentation of a carbohydrate with *Xanthomonas campestris.* Whitish powder; slight odor; tasteless; aqueous solution neutral to litmus; chars about 240°. Soluble in hot or cold water; 1 g dissolves in about 3 ml alcohol.

Xylometazoline Hydrochloride NF [Otrivin (*Ciba*); $C_{16}H_{24}N_2 \cdot HCl$]—Adrenergic (vasoconstrictor). White to off-white, crystalline powder; odorless; melts with decomposition above 300°; pH (5%) 5.5–6.6. One g dissolves in 35 ml water; freely soluble in alcohol; sparingly soluble in chloroform; practically insoluble in ether.

Zinc Acetate USP [$C_4H_6O_4Zn \cdot$

2H₂O]—Pharmaceutic aid (zinc-euge-nol cement). White crystals or granules; slight, acetous odor; astringent taste; slightly effervescent; pH 6–8. One g dis-solves in 1–10 ml water and boiling al-cohol and 100–1000 ml alcohol. *Known incompatibilities:* alkalies, carbonates, phosphates, fatty acids.

Zinc Caprylate—See *Caprylic Acid.*

Zinc Chloride USP [ZnCl₂]—Dentin desensitizer. White or practically white, crystalline powder or crystalline gran-ules; may also be in porcelain-like mass-es or molded into cylinders; very deli-quescent; solution (1 in 10) acid to lit-mus. 1 g dissolves in 0.5 ml water, 1.5 ml alcohol, and 2 ml glycerin; solution in water or alcohol is usually slightly tur-bid; turbidity disappears when a small quantity of HCl is added. *Known in-compatibilities:* alkalies, carbonates, phosphates, fatty acids.

Zinc Gelatin USP—Topical protect-ant. Smooth jelly containing zinc oxide and gelatin. *Known incompatibilities:* acids, alkalies.

Zinc Oxide USP [ZnO]—Astringent; topical protectant; topical protectant (dental). Very fine, white or yellowish white powder; odorless; amorphous; free from gritty particles; gradually absorbs CO₂ from air. Insoluble in water and al-cohol; 1 g dissolves in 10–30 ml dilute acids. *Known incompatibilities:* acids, alkalies.

Zinc Stearate USP—Dusting pow-der. Compound of zinc with a mixture of solid organic acids from fats consist-ing chiefly of variable proportions of zinc stearate and palmitate; contains about 13% ZnO. Fine, white, bulky pow-der; faint odor; no grittiness; neutral to moistened litmus. Insoluble in water, alcohol, and ether.

Zinc Sulfate USP [ZnSO₄·7H₂O]—Astringent. Colorless, transparent prisms, small needles, or granular, crys-talline powder; odorless; efflorescent in dry air; solutions acid to litmus. 1 g dis-solves in 0.6 ml water and 2.5 ml glycer-in; insoluble in alcohol. *Known incom-patibilities:* alkalies, carbonates, phos-phates, fatty acids.

Zinc Undecylenate USP [C₂₂H₃₈O₄Zn]—Topical antifungal. Fine, white powder. Practically insolu-ble in water and alcohol. See also under *Undecylenic Acid.*

Zymalixir [*Upjohn*]—Hematinic vi-tamin. *Known ingredients* (per 5 ml): ferrous gluconate (130 mg), liver con-centrate (65 mg), thiamine HCl (1 mg), riboflavin (1 mg), nicotinamide (8 mg), pyridoxine HCl (0.5 mg), folic acid (1 mg), vitamin B₁₂ activity (2 μg), alcohol (1.5%). pH 3.6 (approx).

Zymasyrup [*Upjohn*]—Multivitam-in. *Known ingredients* (per 5 ml): vita-min A (5000 u), vitamin D₃ (1000 u), thiamine HCl (1 mg), riboflavin (1 mg), pyridoxine HCl (0.5 mg), *d*-pantothenyl alcohol (3 mg), nicotinamide (10 mg), ascorbic acid (60 mg), folic acid (0.25 mg), cyanocobalamin (3 μg), alcohol (2%), in an orange-colored, fruit-fla-vored emulsion. pH 3.1 (approx).

References

1. Drug Interactions That Can Affect Your Patients. *Patient Care,* Miller & Find Publ. Co., Stamford, CT, Nov., 1967.
2. Block LH, Lamy PP: *JAPhA NS9:*202, 1969.
3. Smith WE: *Am J Hosp Pharm 24:*228, 1967.
4. Modell W: *GP 20:*129, 1959.
5. Anon: *The Sciences 4:*17, 1964.
6. Honigfeld G: *Dis Nervous Syst 25:*145, 225, 1964.
7. Fellner CH: Cited by Ref. 5.
8. *The Rx Legend—An FDA Manual for Pharmacists,* USDHEW, FDA Leaflet #12, rev April 1962.
9. Hodgman CD: *Handbook of Chemistry and Physics,* Chemical Rubber Publ. Co., Cleveland, OH, 1964.
10. Braude EA, Nachod FC: *Determination of Organic Structures by Physical Methods,* Aca-demic, New York, 14, 1955.
11. Glasstone S: *Textbook of Physical Chemis-try,* 2nd ed, Van Nostrand, Princeton, NJ, 729, 1946.
12. Miller OH: *JAPhA Prac Ed 13:*657, 1952.
13. Buchi J, Schlumpf R: *Pharm Acta Helv 18:* 673, 1943.
14. Kline W: *The Chemistry of Steroids,* Neth-nen & Co., Ltd., London, 1957.
15. Fowler TJ: *Am J Hosp Pharm 24:* 450, 1967.
16. Parker EA: *Ibid:* 434, 1967.
17. Latiolais CJ, *et al: Ibid 24:* 667, 1967; *25:* 209, 1968.

Bibliography

Absorption and Distribution of Drugs (Saunders L), Williams & Wilkins, Baltimore, 1974.

Accepted Dental Therapeutics, American Dental Assoc., Chicago, IL (annual).

AMA Drug Evaluations, 2nd ed, Publ. Sci. Group, Inc., Acton, MA, 1973.

American Drug Index (Wilson CO, Jones TE, eds), Lippincott, Philadelphia (annual).

American Druggist Blue Book, Hearst Corp., New York (annual, incl. suppl.).

American Hospital Formulary Service, Am. Soc. Hosp. Pharm., Washington, DC (loose-leaf, bimonthly updates).

Current Contents, Inst. Sci. Inform., Philadelphia (weekly).

Dispensing of Medication (Dale JK; Martin EW, ed), 7th ed, Mack Publ. Co., Easton, PA, 113–176, 1971. *Ibid* (Dale JK, Booth RE; Martin EW, ed), 177–384.

Drug-Induced Diseases, Vol 4 (Meyler L), Am. Elsevier, New York, 1973.

Drug Interactions (Hansten PD), 2nd ed, Lea & Febiger, Philadelphia, 1973.

Drugs in Current Use and New Drugs (Modell W), Springer, New York (annual).

Drugs of Choice (Modell W), 1974–75, Mosby, St. Louis, 1974.

Drug Topics Red Book, Medical Economics, Oradell, NJ (annual, incl. suppl.).

Evaluations of Drug Interactions—1973, APhA, Washington, DC, 1973; also *Supplement—1974* and *Supplement—1975.*

Facts and Comparisons (Kastrup EK, ed), Facts and Comparisons, Inc., St. Louis (loose-leaf, monthly updates).

FDA, Reports of Suspected Adverse Reactions, FDA, Washington, DC.

Guide to Parenteral Admixtures, Cutter Labs., St. Louis.

Handbook of Chemistry and Physics (Weast RC, Selby SM), 52nd ed., Chem. Rubber Co., 1971.

Handbook of Drug Interactions, 2nd ed (Hartshorn EA), Drug. Intel. Publ., Cincinnati, 1973.

Handbook of Non-Prescription Drugs (Griffenhagen GB, Hawkins LL, eds), APhA, Washington, DC (annual).

Handbook of Poisoning (Dreisbach R), Lange Med. Publ., Los Altos, CA (freq. rev.).

Hazards of Medication (Martin EW, ed), Lippincott, Philadelphia, 1971.

Manual of Medical Therapeutics (Rosenfeld MG, ed), 20th ed, Little-Brown, Boston, 1973.

Martindale: The Extra Pharmacopeia (Blacow NW, Wade E, eds), The Pharmaceutical Press, London, 1972.

Merck Index, 8th ed, Merck & Co., Inc., Rahway, NJ, 1968.

Merck Manual of Diagnosis and Therapy (Holvey DN, ed), 12th ed, Merck Sharp & Dohme Res. Labs., 1972.

Modern Drug Encyclopedia and Therapeutic Index, 13th ed, Dun-Donnelley, New York, 1975.

The National Formulary, 14th ed, Mack Publ. Co., Easton, PA, 1975.

Parenteral Drug Information Guide (Trissel LA, Grimes CR, Gallelli JF), Am. Soc. Hosp. Pharm., Washington, DC, 1974.

Pediatric Dosage Handbook (Shirkey HC), APhA, Washington, DC, 1975.

Pediatric Therapy (Shirkey HC), 4th ed, Mosby, St. Louis, 1972.

The Pharmacological Basis of Therapeutics (Goodman LS, Gilman A), 5th ed, Macmillan, New York, 1975.

pharmIndex, Skyline Publ., Inc., Portland, OR (loose-leaf, monthly updates).

Physical Pharmacy (Martin AN, et al) 2nd ed, Lea & Febiger, Philadelphia, 1969.

Physicians' Desk Reference, Medical Economics Co., Oradell, NJ (annual).

Remington's Pharmaceutical Sciences, 15th ed, Mack Publ. Co., Easton, PA, 1975.

The Stability and Stability Testing of Pharmaceuticals (annotated bibliography), 1939–1963, Pharm. Mfrs. Assoc., Washington, DC, 1964.

USAN and the USP Dictionary of Drug Names, USP Conv., Inc., Rockville, MD, 1975.

The United States Dispensatory (Osol A, Pratt R, eds), 27th ed, Lippincott, Philadelphia, 1973.

The United States Pharmacopeia, 19th rev., Mack Publ. Co., Easton, PA, 1975.

Index

A

Aarane, 508
Abbreviations, medication order, 3
ABDEC drops, 468
Aberel, 622
Absorbable cellulose, 495
  cotton, 495
Absorption and elimination
  kinetics, parenteral
    products, 59
  dermatological preparations, 77
  drug, patient factors, 50
  drugs, effect of food, 52
    modification, 52
  effect of particle size, 72
  elimination kinetics, 57
  gastrointestinal, 41
  mathematical relationships, 55–60
  methods of prolonging, 71
  models, 55–58
  of drugs, effect of pH, 42
  ophthalmic drugs, 230
  percutaneous, 77
  rectal products, 79
  theory, 44
Acacia, 468
  emulsifying agent, 194
  suspending agent, 204
Acenocoumarol, 469
Acetaminophen, 210, 469
  antipyretic effect, 210
  suppositories, 79
Acetarsone, 469
Acetazolamide, 469
Acetest reagent tablets, 469
Acetic acid, 469
  ether, 527
Acetohexamide, 470
Acetone, 470
Acetophenazine maleate, 470
Acetophenetidin, 578
Acetosulfone sodium, 470
Acetylcholine chloride, 470
Acetylcysteine, 470
Acetyldigitoxin, 470
N-acetylparaminophenol, 210
Acetylsalicylic acid, 481
Acids, Brønsted-Lowry theory, 184
  categories, 399
  incompatibilities, 399
  oxidizing, incompatibilities, 400
  reducing, incompatibilities, 403
  strong, incompatibilities, 399
  weak, incompatibilities, 400
Acidulin, 535
Acriflavine, 470
  hydrochloride, 471
Acrisorcin, 471
Actidil, 625
  syrup, 471
Actifed preparations, 471
Activated 7-dehydrocholesterol, 503
Active transport, 44
Acylanid, 470
Adapin, 520
ADC drops, 471
Adrenal cortex extract, 471

Adrenalin, 522
Adrenatrate, 522
Adsorption, 72
Adverse drug reactions, 385–389
  reactions, classification, 387
  reactions, genetic factors, 386
  reactions, selected, 359
Aerosol(s), 296
  actuators, 307, 309, 310
  advantages, 296
  aspirator (Venturi), 316
  bag-in-can, 316
  co-dispensing, 316
  compressed gas systems, 300
  containers, 304
    aluminum, 305
    glass, 305
    plastic, 306
    protective caps, 310
    stainless steel, 305
    tin-plate, 304
    valves, 306–309
  definition, 297
  dermatological, 150
  dermatologic, products, 315
  dispensing, 317
  emulsions, 300
  external use, 218
  gas systems, liquefied, 298
  groups, 297
  history, 297
  inhalation, products, 309
    therapy, 313
  internal use, 311
  metering valves, 308
  nasal therapy, 314
  oral therapy, 314
  pharmaceutical applications, 311
  powder, 117
  pressure, 298
  principle, 298
  propellants, 301
    compressed gas, 302, 303
    fluorocarbon, 301, 302
    hydrocarbon, 302, 303
    requirements, 301
    toxicity, 302, 303
  respiratory medication, 311
  special systems, 316
  suspensions, 300
  three-phase systems, 299
  topical therapy, 315
  two-phase, system, 298
  vaginal therapy, 314
Aerosporin sulfate, 585
Afrin, 471, 570
Agar, 471
Agents, anticholinergic, 478
  anti-inflammatory, 478
  antineoplastic, 479
  antipsychotic, 479
  antithyroid, 479
  emulsifying, 193
  suspending, 203–205
Air suspension coating, 143
Akineton, 488
  hydrochloride, 489
Akrinol, 471
Albamycin, 566, 567
  calcium, 567
  Mix-O-Vial, 471
  syrup, 471

Albumin, normal human serum, 471
  human serum (salt poor), 472
Albuminar, 472
Albumisol, 471
Albuspan, 471
Albutein, 472
Alcohol, 472
Alcohols, incompatibilities, 434, 435
Alcopara, 488
Alcophobin, 519
Aldactone, 605
Aldehydes, incompatibilities, 437, 438
Aldinamide, 592
Aldomet, 558
  ester hydrochloride, 559
Alginic acid, 472
Alglyn, 516
Alidase, 472, 538
Alkaloids, incompatibilities, 445, 448
Alkeran, 552
Allergic reactions, 388
Allopurinol, 472
Aloin, 472
Alpha-Keri, 151
Alphaprodine hydrochloride, 472
Aludrox, 473
Alum, 472
Alumina and magnesia oral
  suspension, 473
  magnesia tablets, 473
Aluminum acetate solution, 473
  chloride, 473
  hydroxide gel, 473
  gel, dried, 473
  monostearate, 473
  nicotinate, 473
  salts, incompatibilities, 395
  stearate, thickener, 204
  subacetate solution, 473
  sulfate, 473
Alupent, 554
Alurate elixir, 473
Alvodine ethanesulfonate, 583
Alzinox, 516
Amantadine hydrochloride, 474
Ambenonium chloride, 474
Amberlite IRP-88, 584
Ambodryl hydrochloride, 489
Amcill, 477
Americaine preparations, 474
Amesec enseals, 474
Amicar, 474
Amides, incompatibilities, 444, 445
Amidone hydrochloride, 555
Amines, incompatibilities, 442, 443
Aminoacetic acid, 474
Aminobenzoic acid, 474
Aminocaproic acid, 474
Aminohippurate sodium, 474
Aminohippuric acid, 475
Aminophylline, 475
  injection, 475
Aminosalicylic acid, 475
Amitriptyline hydrochloride, 475
Ammoniacal silver nitrate
  solution, 219
Ammonia solution, strong, 475

P